Derby Hospitals NHS Foundation
Trust
Library and Knowledge Service

KU-537-484
B08797

WITHDRAWN

This b   e for retu   on

Epilepsy in children

Epilepsy in children

Second Edition

Edited by

The late
SHEILA J WALLACE
Paediatric Neurologist, Department of Child Health
University Hospital of Wales, Cardiff, UK

and

KEVIN FARRELL
Professor, Division of Pediatric Neurology
University of British Columbia, and
Director, Epilepsy Service
British Columbia's Children's Hospital, Vancouver,
British Columbia, Canada

ARNOLD

A member of the Hodder Headline Group
LONDON

First published in Great Britain in 2004 by Arnold, a member of the
Hodder Headline Group,
338 Euston Road, London NW1 3BH

http://www.arnoldpublishers.com

Distributed in the United States of America by
Oxford University Press Inc.,
198 Madison Avenue, New York, NY 10016
Oxford is a registered trademark of Oxford University Press

© 2004 Arnold

All rights reserved. No part of this publication may be reproduced or
transmitted in any form or by any means, electronically or mechanically,
including photocopying, recording or any information storage or retrieval
system, without either prior permission in writing from the publisher or a
licence permitting restricted copying. In the United Kingdom such licences
are issued by the Copyright Licensing Agency: 90 Tottenham Court Road,
London W1T 4LP.

Whilst the advice and information in this book are believed to be true and
accurate at the date of going to press, neither the author[s] nor the publisher
can accept any legal responsibility or liability for any errors or omissions
that may be made. In particular (but without limiting the generality of the
preceding disclaimer) every effort has been made to check drug dosages;
however it is still possible that errors have been missed. Furthermore,
dosage schedules are constantly being revised and new side-effects
recognized. For these reasons the reader is strongly urged to consult the
drug companies' printed instructions before administering any of the drugs
recommended in this book.

British Library Cataloguing in Publication Data
A catalogue record for this book is available from the British Library

Library of Congress Cataloging-in-Publication Data
A catalog record for this book is available from the Library of Congress

ISBN 0 340 80814 4

1 2 3 4 5 6 7 8 9 10

Commissioning Editor: Joanna Koster
Development Editor: Sarah Burrows
Project Editor: Zelah Pengilley
Production Controller: Deborah Smith
Cover Design: Lee-May Lim
Index: Indexing Specialists (UK) Ltd

Typeset in 10/12 Minion by Charon Tec Pvt. Ltd, Chennai, India
Printed and bound in the UK by Butler & Tanner Ltd

What do you think about this book? Or any other Arnold title?
Please send your comments to **feedback.arnold@hodder.co.uk**

To the memory of Sheila Wallace
and to my wife, Kate,
and my children, Seonaid, Alastair and Nicholas,
for their love and inspiration.

Contents

Contributors

Jean Aicardi MD FRCP
Professor, Service de Pédiatrie,
Hôpital Robert Debré, Paris, France

Joan K Austin DNS RN FAAN
Distinguished Professor, Department of Environments for Health,
Indiana University School of Nursing, Indianapolis, USA

Frank MC Besag
Professor and Consultant Neuropsychiatrist,
University of Luton, and Specialist Medical Department,
Learning Disability Service, Twinwoods Health
Resource Centre, Bedfordshire and Luton Community
NHS Trust, Bedfordshire, UK

Paulo Rogério M de Bittencourt MD PhD
Clinical Director, Unidade de Neurologia Clínica,
Curitiba, Brazil

Blaise FD Bourgeois MD
Professor of Neurology, Harvard Medical School, and
Director, Division of Epilepsy and Clinical Neurophysiology,
Children's Hospital, Boston, USA

Harry T Chugani MD
Professor of Pediatrics, Neurology and Radiology, Wayne State
University School of Medicine, and Chief, Division of Pediatric
Neurology and Co-Director, Positron Emission Tomography
Center, Children's Hospital of Michigan, Detroit, Michigan, USA

Mary B Connolly MB MRCP(I) MRCP(UK) FRCP(C)
Head of Epilepsy Surgery Program and Clinical Associate Professor,
Division of Neurology, Department of Paediatrics,
British Columbia's Children's Hospital, Vancouver, BC, Canada

Paolo Curatolo
Professor of Pediatric Neurology and Chief, Division of Pediatric
Neurology, Department of Neurosciences, Tor Vergata University
of Rome, Italy

JoAnne Dahl PhD
Associate Professor, Department of Education and
Psychology, University of Gävle, Sweden

Sharon Davies MB BS MRCPsych
Specialist Registrar in Child and Adolescent Psychiatry,
Great Ormond Street Hospital for Children, London, UK

Thierry Deonna
Professor, Unité de Neuropédiatrie, Centre Hospitalier
Universitaire Vaudois, Lausanne, Switzerland

Charlotte Dravet
Centre Saint-Paul – Hôpital Henri Gastaut, Marseille, France

Olivier Dulac
Professor, Service de Pédiatrie Neurologique,
Hôpital Saint Vincent-de Paul, Paris, France

David W Dunn MD
Associate Professor, Departments of Psychiatry and Neurology,
Indiana University School of Medicine, Indianapolis, USA

Kevin Farrell MB FRCP(E) FRCP(C)
Professor, Division of Pediatric Neurology,
University of British Columbia, and Director,
Epilepsy Service, British Columbia's Children's Hospital,
Vancouver, British Columbia, Canada

Natalio Fejerman
Department of Neurology, Hospital de Pediatria,
Prof. Juan P Garrahan Hospital, Buenos Aires, Argentina

Colin D Ferrie MD FRCPCH
Department of Paediatric Neurology, The General Infirmary at
Leeds, UK

Andrew Fisher PhD
Pharmacology and Therapeutics Unit, Department of Clinical
and Experimental Epilepsy, Institute of Neurology, London, UK

Lars Forsgren MD PhD
Professor of Neurology, Department of Neurology,
Umeå University Hospital, Sweden

Elena Gardella
Department of Neurological Sciences, University of Bologna,
Bellaria Hospital, Bologna, Italy

R Mark Gardiner MD FRCPCH FMedSci
Professor, Department of Paediatrics and Child Health,
Royal Free and University College Medical School University
College London, The Rayne Institute, London, UK

Richard A Grünewald MA DPhil FRCP
Consultant Neurologist and Honorary Senior Clinical Lecturer,
Sheffield Teaching Hospitals NHS Trust and University of Sheffield,
Royal Hallamshire Hospital, Sheffield, UK

Renzo Guerrini
Professor of Child Neurology and Psychiatry, University of Pisa,
DUNPI–IRCCS Stella Maris, Calambrone, Pisa, Italy

The late Olaf Henriksen
Formerly of Statens Senter for Epilepsi, Sandvika, Norway

Isobel Heyman MB BS PhD MRCPsych
Consultant Child and Adolescent Neuropsychiatrist and
Honorary Senior Lecturer, Maudsley Hospital/Institute of
Psychiatry, and Great Ormond Street Hospital for Children,
London, UK

Sara Hudson LPN CCRC
Executive Director, Pediatric Epilepsy Research Center,
Children's Mercy Hospital, Kansas City, Missouri, USA

John GR Jefferys FMED SCI
Professor of Neuroscience and Head of Neurophysiology,
University of Birmingham Medical School, Birmingham, UK

Csaba Juhász MD PhD
Assistant Professor, Department of Pediatrics, Division of
Pediatric Neurology, Wayne State University School of
Medicine, and Positron Emission Tomography Center,
Children's Hospital of Michigan, Detroit, Michigan, USA

Dorothée GA Kasteleijn–Nolst Trenité MD PhD MPH
Medical Center Alkmaar, The Netherlands

Rüdiger Köhling
Professor, Experimental Neurophysiology, Department of
Epileptology, University of Bonn, Germany

Eric H Kossoff MD
The Johns Hopkins Medical Institutions, Baltimore,
Maryland, USA

Michael Koutroumanidis MD
Consultant and Honorary Senior Lecturer,
GKT School of Medicine, Department of Clinical Neurophysiology
and Epilepsies, Guy's and St. Thomas' NHS Trust,
St. Thomas' Hospital, London, UK

Ruben I Kuzniecky MD
Professor of Neurology, New York University
Epilepsy Center, Department of Neurology, New York University,
New York, USA

John H Livingston
Department of Paediatric Neurology, Leeds General Hospital, UK

Alain Malafosse
Professor, Hôpitaux Universitaires de Genève, Instituts
Universitaires de Psychiatrie, Chêne-Bourg, Switzerland

Roberto Michelucci MD
Department of Neurosciences, University of Bologna,
Bellaria Hospital, Bologna, Italy

Hajime Miyata MD PhD
Section of Neuropathology, Department of Pathology and
Laboratory Medicine, UCLA Medical Center, Los Angeles,
CA, USA and Department of Neuropathology, Institute of
Neurological Sciences, Faculty of Medicine, Tottori University,
Yonago, Tottori, Japan

Eli M Mizrahi MD
Head, Peter Kellaway Section of Neurophysiology,
Professor of Neurology and Pediatrics, Director,
Baylor Comprehensive Epilepsy Center, Baylor College
of Medicine, and Chief, Neurophysiology Services,
The Methodist Hospital and Texas Children's Hospital,
Houston, Texas

Jerome V Murphy MD
Principle Investigator Pediatric Epilepsy Research Center
Children's Mercy Hospital Kansas City MO USA

Shunsuke Ohtahara MD PhD
Professor emeritus, Department of Child Neurology,
Okayama University Medical School,
Shikatacho, Okayama, Japan

Yoko Ohtsuka MD PhD
Department of Child Neurology
Okayama University Medical School,
Shikatacho, Okayama, Japan

CP Panayiotopoulos MD PhD FRCP
Department of Clinical Neurophysiology and Epilepsies,
St Thomas' Hospital, London, UK

Lucio Parmeggiani MD PhD
DUNPI – IRCCS Stella Maris, Calambrone, Pisa, Italy

Philip N Patsalos FRCPath PhD
Professor of Clinical Pharmacology,
Pharmacology and Therapeutics Unit,
Department of Clinical and Experimental Epilepsy,
Institute of Neurology, London, UK

Daniela T Pilz FRCP MD
Consultant in Medical Genetics, Institute for Medical Genetics,
University Hospital of Wales, Cardiff, UK

Charles E Polkey MD FRCS
Emeritus Professor of Neurosurgery, Division of Clinical
Neurosciences, Kings College Hospital, London, UK

Bwee Tien Poll-The MD PhD
Professor in Child Neurology, Academic Medical Center,
University of Amsterdam, The Netherlands

Jean-Paul Rathgeb
Service de Pédiatrie Neurologique,
Hôpital Saint Vincent-de Paul, Paris, France

David Ravine FRACP MRCPath MD
Professor of Medical Genetics, University of Western Australia,
Perth, Western Australia

Anna Lecticia Ribeiro Pinto MD PhD
Pediatric Neurologist, Clinica Neurológica de Joinville,
Brazil

Raili Riikonen
Professor of Child Neurology, University of Kuopio,
Head, Department of Child Neurology,
Central Hospital of Kuopio University,
Kuopio, Finland

Robert Robinson BA(Hons) MBBS MRCP
Department of Paediatrics and Child Health, Royal Free and
University College Medical School, University College London,
The Rayne Institute, London, UK

Guido Rubboli
Department of Neurological Sciences, University of Bologna,
Bellaria Hospital, Bologna, Italy

Anne de Saint-Martin
Service de Pédiatrie, CHU Hautepierre, Strasbourg, France

Matti Sillanpää MD PhD
Professor of Child Neurology, Departments of
Child Neurology and Public Health, Turku University,
Turku, Finland

John Stephenson
Professor in Paediatric Neurology, Fraser of Allander
Neurosciences Unit, Royal Hospital for Sick Children,
Glasgow, UK

Carlo Alberto Tassinari
Professor, Department of Neurological Sciences,
University of Bologna, Bellaria Hospital, Bologna,
Italy

Eileen PG Vining MD
Associate Professor of Neurology and Pediatrics, Johns Hopkins
University School of Medicine, Baltimore, MD, USA

Harry V Vinters MD
Departments of Pathology and Laboratory Medicine
(Neuropathology and Neurology), and Brain Research Institute,
Mental Retardation Research Center and
Neuropsychiatric Institute, UCLA Medical Center
Los Angeles, CA, USA

The late Sheila J Wallace
Formerly Paediatric Neurologist, Department of Child Health,
University Hospital of Wales, Cardiff, UK

Katherine Wambera
Division of Neurology, British Columbia's Children's Hospital,
Vancouver, British Columbia, Canada

Kazuyoshi Watanabe MD PhD
Department of Paediatrics, Nagoya University Graduate School
of Medicine, Showa-ku, Nagoya, Japan

William P Whitehouse
Senior Lecturer in Paediatric Neurology, The University of
Nottingham and Queen's Medical Centre, University Hospital,
Nottingham, UK

Peter KH Wong MD FRCPC
Division of Pediatric Neurology, Department of Pediatrics,
University of British Columbia, and
Department of Clinical Neurophysiology,
British Columbia's Children's Hospital,
Vancouver, British Columbia, Canada

Yasuko Yamatogi MD PhD
Faculty of Health and Welfare Science,
Okayama Prefectural University,
Soja, Okayama, Japan

Sameer Zuberi
Consultant Paediatric Neurologist, Fraser of Allander
Neurosciences Unit, Royal Hospital for Sick Children,
Yorkhill, Glasgow, UK

Foreword

At one time epilepsy was epilepsy, and the field of epilepsy was dominated by adult epileptologists who seemed to believe that children were only small adults, that adult epilepsy was identical to epilepsy in children of all ages and sizes. They appeared to think that the underlying pathology, pathogenesis, and treatment of children with epilepsy were similar, only the dosing of medications was different. Sheila Wallace was one of the pioneers in pediatric epilepsy, and played a prominent role in beginning to change the perceptions of adult epileptologists, helping them to recognize that epilepsy in children was different.

A limp may have many varied causes: from a nail in a shoe, a bad knee or hip, to a stroke or cerebral palsy. The differential diagnosis of a limp and its pathogenesis and treatment will vary with the age of the patient and the course of the condition. However, all the patients hobble. Just so, seizures are a manifestation of a dysfunction within the nervous system, but their manifestations, etiology, pathogenesis, and management will often differ by age, even within childhood, and will often be different from those of seizures in adults. Children are not small adults, and epilepsy in children is different than epilepsy in adults.

This second edition of *Epilepsy in Children* is testimony to those differences. A perusal of the table of contents reveals the breadth and depth to which the editors have gone to cover this increasingly extensive field. The authors of chapters not only cover, in depth, the myriad aspects and multiple types of epilepsy in children, but also further cover the many aspects by which children and their families are affected by epilepsy. Authors come from around the world, and represent many of the best, brightest, and most forward thinking in this field. The editors have chosen well.

As my mother would have said, "If only Sheila could have lived to see it – she would have been justly proud." Kevin Farrell, as the co-editor, should be proud as well, of having completed the editing of a book that will add to the growing field of epilepsy in children.

John M. Freeman, MD
October 2003

Preface

This second edition of *Epilepsy in Children* reflects not only Sheila Wallace's vision of the problem of epilepsy in this age group but also her ability to translate the science of epilepsy into a practical clinical approach. There have been many major advances in both the basic and clinical science of epilepsy since this work was first published, and the purpose of this edition is to demonstrate the relevance of these discoveries to the practical management of epilepsy in this age group. This book is written therefore for those who are involved in the management of children with epilepsy.

Seizures are a symptom and many diseases manifest with this problem. In addition, the management of patients with epilepsy often involves a wide variety of fields including pediatrics, neurology, neurophysiology, nursing, pharmacology, neuroradiology, genetics, neurosurgery, neuropathology, psychiatry, psychology, social work and education. Consequently, the contributors come from a wide variety of different disciplines. On behalf of Sheila, I must thank all of these authorities for helping to make this edition relevant to those who care for children with epilepsy.

During the writing of this book, Sheila developed a brain tumor that made it increasingly difficult for her to edit. Her approach to this illness and her ability to retain her spirit despite her problems reflected the outstanding nature of Sheila's character and contributed greatly to the completion of this edition. I had the good fortune to work with Sheila on her last major work and was supported by her warmth, experience and strength of character. We were helped considerably by Joanna Koster, Sarah Burrows, Zelah Pengilley of Arnold Publishing and the proof reader, Rose James. I need also to thank Leila Laakso, Julie Baron, Pam Sekhon and Francesca Zanotto at British Columbia's Children's Hospital, who kept the ship afloat; Drs Mary Connolly, Olivia O'Mahony, Peter Wong, Kati Wambera and Alan Hill, who helped me complete the work; and Pnina Granirer for her artistic work. Finally, my greatest thanks must be to my wife, Kate, and my children, Seonaid, Alastair and Nic, who make it all worthwhile.

Kevin Farrell

Sheila Wallace – an appreciation

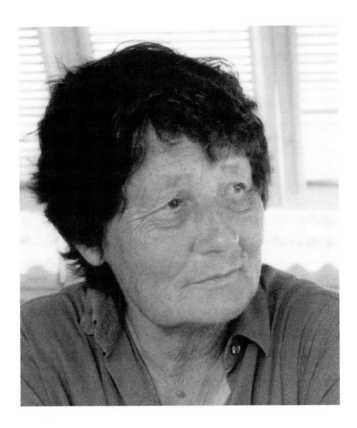

This is not an obituary for Sheila but rather an appreciation, a dedication, indeed an attempt at a celebration of the remarkable individual who began the venture that is this book, not knowing that it was to become her memorial.

Sheila's early life and education were in England. She went to the sort of school that instils a certain language and accent of authority, her voice precise, concise, well-modulated and even pukka. I first met her when we were both junior doctors doing paediatrics in the fertile intellectual breeding ground of East Anglia, a flat part of England very different from her later haunts in hilly Wales and mountainous Scotland. Ever since she was amused to boast that she had been senior to me in rank although younger than I by several months. Later she said that being tough-minded and competitive was necessary for a woman in medicine in those days. Humour was certainly an integral part of her make-up throughout her life, and many readers will remember her hearty laugh and almost conspiratorial guffaw.

Then she took off northwards to Edinburgh where in paediatric neurology Tom Ingram was king. He it was who suggested that she immerse herself in the study of febrile seizures. This led to her book *The Child with Febrile Seizures*, published in 1988, and to a lifetime studying the phenomenology and treatment of epileptic seizures that culminated in the present volume.

It is important to recognize that Sheila was not merely an epileptologist in an ivory tower but was a fully qualified wide-ranging child neurologist. She was fortunate in having been able to join the Department of Neurology at Great Ormond Street Hospital for Sick Children under Drs John Wilson and Edward Brett and to become the Consultant Paediatric Neurologist at the University Hospital of Wales in Cardiff. In a busy career in the British National Health Service – predominantly single-handed – she found time to contribute to the literature on the varied problems of paediatric neurology that came her clinical way: genetic, metabolic, infectious or whatever.

I have mentioned and illustrated Sheila's lifelong and often irrepressible sense of humour, but three other facets of her character are worthy of note. These were common sense, the ability to communicate, and innate skills in the organization of space and time. Kevin Farrell tells me that the attribute of common sense was very apparent to him as a co-editor. She was down to earth, with a no-nonsense style and the ability to give political correctness the lack of respect it deserves. There is a web site devoted to common sense that includes a discussion of its localization within the brain. No-one will be surprised to hear that the answer is not clear: I can only imagine Sheila's reaction to the question!

Sheila was a master – or mistress – of communication. To many worldwide she was known not only for her spoken presentations and lectures, given with great clarity and effect, particularly on the epilepsies of childhood and their medical management, but also for her quiet but clear and penetrating questions given at the microphone in a serious rather deep voice with inflections of humour and accompanied by a quizzically-raised eyebrow. To leaders in the field of child neurology and epilepsy she was known for her work in committees and boards. She was elected more than once to the boards of both the International Child Neurology Association and the European Paediatric Neurology Association. She was chairman of the Professional Group of the Epilepsy Task Force (UK), member of the Scientific Advisory Committee of the Epilepsy Research Foundation, and member of the teaching faculty for the Master of Science degree in Epileptology at King's College, London. She served on the editorial boards of *Developmental Medicine and Child Neurology* and the *European Journal of Paediatric Neurology*. That she was able to persuade so many to collaborate with her (and the number of contributors to this book is now over 60 from 14 countries) is a tribute to her pre-eminent communication skills.

Turning now from her left to her right hemisphere, Sheila was also gifted with immense skills in space and in time. At international meetings it was she who arrived by the most adventurous route, and afterwards backpacked into byways off the path of the official post-conference tours. She was indeed an inveterate traveller. She managed 49 countries, and only regretted not making the half-century. My most relaxed memory of her is of a long lunch in the open air under a plane tree – in truth, the identity of the tree was in dispute, despite Sheila's botanical expertise (she had made a beautiful garden in the grounds of her personally restored 500 year old home in Wales where she came first with her late husband) – by some water in Strasbourg, en route to a board meeting of the European Paediatric Society in Baden-Baden. We ate a fish called sander and drank wine from Alsace. When Sheila got home she sent me a post card to confirm that sander = pike-perch.

It was fun to write chapters for Sheila's most important book. When I queried the title of our chapter in the second edition she replied:

Good! I told Kevin you would want to write about anoxic-epileptic seizures, and I give you permission to do so. As

for the title: I do not like 'nonepilepsy' it sounds too gimmicky and I should remind you, this is a serious book! We can sort out something which we agree on later, but call it differential diagnosis for now.

But when we were late another email arrived:

I hope it really is nearly done, and that you are able to send it to Kevin before I die of the glioblastoma which has recently raised its ugly head in the mid/posterior part of my corpus callosum! A little bit of neuroanatomical knowledge is undoubtedly helpful in directing one to the relatively intact verbal skills that I still retain! Please finish it soon. I hope you are reasonably well at the moment, and I salute our years of comradeship. I have always enjoyed your company.

Sheila.

What do you do then? I telephoned and spoke with her for at least an hour or maybe two. She had lost her sense of space and time because the tumour had invaded her right parietal lobe. She wanted to stay in her old house and beautiful garden, but could not and soon had to be moved to hospital. I told her nurse that she was world class, and wrote to Sheila that her voice was in the heads of thousands throughout the world. To be destroyed by a glioblastoma in one's own brain must have been an extraordinary hardship for her, but her reaction was typical of the robust bravery that had characterized her life for decades before. When I asked her if she was still going to the International Child Neurology Association meeting in Beijing in October 2002, Sheila replied that no, she would have no more deadlines, no more deadlines – just one. Her sense of humour, now black humour, had not deserted her.

Kevin wrote to me that in her final illness:

she demonstrated a wonderful ability to enjoy the moment and to live life to the fullest. In many ways, I think that she had many of the qualities of a good highland lady, which may stem from the fact that she had the good luck to train in Scotland.

Be that as it may, she is not easily pigeonholed: she was truly her own person. I fancy she might smile to think that through this new edition of her book she will now easily attain and exceed the 50 countries into which she strove to communicate about epilepsy and about children.

John B.P. Stephenson

Abbreviations

ABPEC	atypical benign partial epilepsy of childhood	CA	conceptional age
ACTH	adrenocorticotropic hormone	CAE	childhood absence epilepsy
ADHD	attention deficit/hyperactivity disorder	CAG	cytosine-adenine-guanosine
ADJME	autosomal dominant juvenile myoclonic epilepsy	CBC	complete blood count
		CBCL	Child Behavior Checklist
ADNFLE	autosomal dominant nocturnal frontal lobe epilepsy	CBPS	congenital bilateral perisylvian syndrome
		CD	cortical dysplasia
ADPEAF	autosomal dominant partial epilepsy with auditory features	CMV	cytomegalovirus
		CNS	central nervous system
AEA	acquired epileptic aphasia	CPS	complex partial seizures
AED	antiepileptic drug	CPSE	complex partial status epilepticus
AES	anoxic-epileptic seizure	CRF	cortisol releasing factor
AGAT	arginine:glycine amidinotransferase	CRH	corticotrophin
AHS	Ammon's horn sclerosis	CSF	cerebrospinal fluid
AMPA	α-amino-3-hydroxy-5-methyl-4-isoxazolepropionic acid	CSWS	continuous spike-waves during slow wave sleep
AMT	α-[^{11}C]-methyl-L-tryptophan	CVST	computerized visual-search task
AS	absence seizures	CYP	cytochrome P-450
BCECTS	benign childhood epilepsy with centrotemporal spikes	DNET	dysembryoplastic neuroepithelial tumor
		DPT	diphtheria, pertussis and tetanus (vaccine)
BCEOP	benign childhood epilepsy with occipital paroxysms	DRPLA	dentato-rubral-pallido-luysian atrophy
		DSM	*Diagnostic and Statistical Manual*
BFIC	benign familial infantile convulsions	EA1	episodic ataxia type 1
BFNC	benign familial neonatal convulsions	EA2	episodic ataxia type 2
BH$_4$	tetrahydrobiopterin	EAR	epilepsy-associated repeat domain
BIPLED	bilateral independent periodic lateralized epileptiform discharge	EBV	Epstein-Barr virus
		ECD	ethyl cysteinate dimer
BLAST	basic local alignment search tool	ECG	electrocardiogram
BME	benign myoclonic epilepsy	EcoG	electrocorticography
BMEI	benign myoclonic epilepsy in infancy	EDE	electrodecremental event
BOLD	blood oxygenation level dependent	EEG	electroencephalogram
BPEA	benign partial epilepsy with affective symptomatology	EGTCSA	epilepsy with GTCS on awakening
		EIEE	early infantile epileptic encephalopathy with suppression burst
BPEAS	benign partial epilepsy with affective symptoms	EME	early myoclonic encephalopathy
		EMG	electromyelogram
BPERS	benign partial epilepsy with rolandic spikes	EMWA	eyelid myoclonia with absences
		EPC	epilepsia partialis continua
BPNH	bilateral periventricular nodular heterotopia	EPSP	excitatory postsynaptic potentials
		ERG	electroretinogram
BPP	bilateral perisylvian polymicrogyria	ERM	ezrin, radium and moesin
BPT	benign paroxysmal torticollis in infancy	ESAC	extra, structurally abnormal chromosome
Ca^{2+}	calcium		

ESR	erythrocyte sedimentation ratio	ICU	intensive care unit
EST	expressed sequence tag	IGE	idiopathic generalized epilepsy
ETS	euthosuximide	ILAE	International League Against Epilepsy
FAR	frontal arousal rhythm	ILS	isolated lissencephaly sequence
FC	febrile convulsions	IM	intramuscular
FCD	focal cortical dysplasia	IPES	Impact of Pediatric Epilepsy Scale
FCMD	Fukuyama congenital muscular dystrophy	IPS	intermittent photic stimulation
FDG-PET	2-deoxy-2[^{18}F]fluoro-D-glucose positron emission tomography	IPSP	inhibitory postsynaptic potentials
		IR	inversion recovery sequences
FHM	familial hemiplegic migraine	IRDA	intermittent rhythmic delta activity
FIME	familial infantile myoclonic epilepsy	ISA	intracarotid sodium amytal test
FIRDA	frontal intermittent rhythmic delta activity	ISS	infantile spasms
FISH	fluorescent *in situ* hybridization	ISSX	X-linked infantile spasms
FLAIR	fluid attenuated inversion recovery	JAE	juvenile absence epilepsy
fMRI	functional magnetic resonance imaging	JME	juvenile myoclonic epilepsy
FMZ	[^{11}C]flumazenil	K^+	potassium
FN	forced normalization	LCH	lissencephaly with cerebellar hypoplasia
FOS	fixation-off sensitivity	LD	linkage disequilibrium
FPEVF	familial partial epilepsy with variable foci	LGS	Lennox-Gastaut syndrome
FS	febrile seizures	LRR	leucine-rich repeat superfamily
GABA	γ-aminobutyric acid	LS	Leigh syndrome
GABA-T	GABA transaminase	LVA	low-voltage-activated
GAD	glutamic acid decarboxylase	MAs	myoclonic absences
GAMT	guanidinoacetate methyltransferase	MAC	membrane attack complex
GAP	GTPase-activating protein	MAE	myoclonic-astatic epilepsy
GAT	GABA transporter	MAM	methylazoxymethanol
GCS	Glasgow Coma Scale	MCD	malformations of cortical development
GCSE	generalized convulsive status epilepticus	MCT	medium chain triglycerides
Gd-DTPA	gadolinium diethylenetriamine pentaacetic acid	MDS	Miller-Dieker syndrome
		MEB	muscle-eye-brain disease
GEFS+	generalized epilepsy with febrile seizures plus	MEG	magnetoencephalography
GFAP	glial fibrillary acidic protein	MELAS	mitochondrial myopathy, encephalopathy, lactic acidosis and stroke-like episodes
G-proteins	GTP-coupled proteins		
GTCS	generalized tonic-clonic seizures	MEP	motor evoked potentials
HCN	hyperpolarization-activated, cyclic nucleotide-gated	MERRF	myoclonus epilepsy and ragged-red fibers
		MF	mixed features
HH	hemiconvulsions and hemiplegia syndrome	MHD	monohydroxy derivative
HHV	human herpesvirus	MMR	measles, mumps and rubella (vaccine)
5-HIAA	5-hydroxyindolacetic acid	MRI	magnetic resonance imaging
HIE	hypoxic-ischemic encephalopathy	MRR	magnetic resonance relaxometry
HIPDM	N,N,N′-trimethyl-N′2-Hydroxy-3-Methyl-5-iodobenzyl-1,3-propanediamine iodine-131	MRS	magnetic resonance spectroscopy
		MRSI	^{1}H-MRS imaging
HIV	human immunodeficiency virus	MS	myoclonic seizures
HLA	human lymphocyte antigens	MSI	magnetic source imaging
HME	hemimegalencephaly	MST	multiple subpial transection
HMPAO	hexamethyl propylene amine oxime	mtDNA	mitochondrial DNA
^{1}H-MRS	proton magnetic resonance spectroscopy	MTS	mesial temporal sclerosis
HS	hippocampal sclerosis	MVLGS	myoclonic variant of the Lennox-Gastaut syndrome
HS/AHS	hippocampal or Ammon's horn sclerosis		
5-HTP	5-hydroxytryptophan	Na$^+$	sodium
HVA	high-voltage-activated	NAA	N-acetylaspartate
HVA	homovanillic acid	NCL	neuronal ceroid lipofuscinoses
ICCA	infantile convulsions and choreoathetosis syndrome	NCPP	National Childhood Perinatal Project
		NCSE	nonconvulsive status epilepticus
ICD	International Classification of Diseases	NF1	neurofibromatosis 1

NKH	nonketotic hyperglycinemia	RCT	randomized controlled trial
NMDA	N-methyl-D-aspartate	RE	Rasmussen encephalitis
NMR	nuclear magnetic resonance	REM	rapid eye movement
OCT	ornithine transcarbamylase	RFLPs	restriction fragment length polymorphisms
OIRDA	occipital intermittent rhythmic delta activity	RMP	Resting membrane potential
OS	Ohtahara syndrome	SB	suppression-burst
PBDA	posterior bilateral delta activity	SBH	subcortical band heterotopia
PCR	polymerase chain reaction	SE	status epilepticus
PDC	paroxysmal dystonic choreoathetosis	SEP	somatosensory evoked potentials
PDHC	pyruvate dehydrogenase complex	SISCOM	subtraction ictal SPECT co-registered to MRI
PDR	posterior dominant rhythm		
PDS	paroxysmal depolarization shift	SLPE	schizophrenia-like psychoses of epilepsy
PE	phenytoin equivalent	SME	severe myoclonic epilepsy
PED	paroxysmal exercise-induced dyskinesia	SMEI	severe myoclonic epilepsy of infancy
PEHO	progressive encephalopathy with edema, hypsarrhythmia and optic atrophy	SNP	single-nucleotide polymorphisms
		SPECT	single photon emission computerized tomography
PEMA	phenylethylmalonamide		
PET	positron emission tomography	SQUID	superconducting quantum interference device
3-PGDH	3-phosphoglycerate dehydrogenase		
PGE	primary generalized epilepsy	SSCP	single strand conformational polymorphism
PGS	primary generalized seizures	SSPE	subacute sclerosing panencephalitis
PKD	paroxysmal kinesiogenic dyskinesia	SSRIs	selective serotonin reuptake inhibitors
PLED	periodic lateralized epileptiform discharge	SSW	slow spike-wave
PLP	pyridoxal-5′-phosphate	T_{max}	time to maximum concentration
PME	progressive myoclonus epilepsy	TCI	transient cognitive impairment
PMG	foci of polymicrogyria	TIRDA	temporal intermittent delta activity
^{1}P-MRS	phosphorus magnetic resonance spectroscopy	TLE	temporal lobe epilepsy
		TRH	thyrotropin releasing hormone
PNH	periventricular nodular heterotopia	TS	tuberous sclerosis
PNKD	paroxysmal nonkinesigenic dyskinesia (= PCD)	TSC	tuberous sclerosis complex
		UGT	uridine diphosphate gluguronosyltrasferase
POSTS	positive occipital sharp transients of sleep	V_d	volume of distribution
POTS	postural/orthostatic tachycardia syndrome	VDCCs	voltage-dependent calcium channels
PPR	photoparoxysmal responses	VFD	visual field defects
PPT	palmitoyl protein thioesterase	VGB	vigabatrin
PRDS	Pitt-Rogers-Danks syndrome	VGCC	voltage-gated calcium channels
PSW	polyspike waves	VIP	video-interface processor
PWS	Prader-Willi syndrome	VNS	vagal nerve stimulation
QOL	quality of life	WHS	Wolf-Hirschhorn syndrome
QOLIE-AD-48	Quality of Life in Epilepsy Inventory for Adolescents	WISC	Weschler Intelligence Scale for Children
		WS	West syndrome
RAKIT	Revised Amsterdam Child Intelligence Test	Xe-SPECT	xenon-133 single photon emission computed tomography
RAS	reflex anoxic seizures or reflex asystolic syncope		
		ZCA	zone of cortical abnormality
rCBF	regional cerebral blood flow	ZS	Zellweger syndrome

Definitions and classification of epileptic seizures and epilepsies

OLAF HENRIKSEN AND SHEILA J WALLACE

Variability in the clinical expressions of epileptic seizures was recognized by the Ancient Greeks, who described both generalized and focal seizures. However, more formal definitions and classifications were not published until the twentieth century, when it was recognized that these would advance the practice of epilepsy. Identification of seizure type is essential for correct management. Similarly, classification is necessary for communication and for comparing data. As such, it is important that the terminology is based on simple, well-defined facts that are retrievable and broadly acceptable. These aims led the International League Against Epilepsy (ILAE) to form Commissions on Classification. The need to include the EEG characteristics in addition to the clinical findings was recognized from the outset. Early discussions centered on defining the criteria for particular seizure types and a proposal for a clinical and electroencephalographic classification of epileptic seizures was published in 1981.[1] Consideration was then given to a classification based on age at onset, etiology, natural history and localization of the region of

Table 1.1 *Proposed diagnostic scheme for people with epileptic seizures and with epilepsy (Reproduced with the permission of Blackwell Publishing Ltd from Engel J Jr. Epilepsia 2001; 42: 796–803)*

Epileptic seizures and epilepsy syndromes are to be described and categorized according to a system that uses standardized terminology, and that is sufficiently flexible to take into account the following practical and dynamic aspects of epilepsy diagnosis:

1 Some patients cannot be given a recognized syndromic diagnosis.
2 Seizure types and syndromes change as new information is obtained.
3 Complete and detailed descriptions of ictal phenomenology are not always necessary.
4 Multiple classification schemes can, and should, be designed for specific purposes (e.g. communication and teaching, therapeutic trials, epidemiologic investigations, selection of surgical candidates, basic research, genetic characterizations).

This diagnostic scheme is divided into five parts, or axes, organized to facilitate a logical clinical approach to the development of hypotheses necessary to determine the diagnostic studies and therapeutic strategies to be undertaken in individual patients:

Axis 1 Ictal phenomenology, from the Glossary of Descriptive Ictal Terminology, can be used to describe ictal events with any degree of detail needed.
Axis 2 Seizure type, from the List of Epileptic Seizures. Localization within the brain and precipitating stimuli for reflex seizures should be specified when appropriate.
Axis 3 Syndrome, from the List of Epilepsy Syndromes, with the understanding that a syndromic diagnosis may not always be possible.
Axis 4 Etiology, from a Classification of Diseases Frequently Associated with Epileptic Seizures or Epilepsy Syndromes when possible, genetic defects, or specific pathologic substrates for symptomatic focal epilepsies.
Axis 5 Impairment: this optional, but often useful, additional diagnostic parameter can be derived from an impairment classification adapted from the WHO International Classification of Functioning and Disability (ICIDH-2).

Derby Hospitals NHS Foundation
Trust
Library and Knowledge Service

Table 1.2 *Definition of key terms (Reproduced with the permission of Blackwell Publishing Ltd from Engel J Jr. Epilepsia 2001; 42: 796–803)*

Epileptic seizure type

An ictal event believed to represent a unique pathophysiologic mechanism and anatomic substrate. This is a diagnostic entity with etiologic, therapeutic and prognostic implications. *[new concept]*

Epilepsy syndrome

A complex of signs and symptoms that define a unique epilepsy condition. This must involve more than just the seizure type: thus frontal lobe seizures *per se*, for instance, do not constitute a syndrome. *[changed concept]*

Epileptic disease

A pathologic condition with a single specific, well-defined etiology. Thus progressive myoclonus epilepsy is a syndrome, but Unverricht-Lundborg is a disease. *[new concept]*

Epileptic encephalopathy

A condition in which the epileptiform abnormalities themselves are believed to contribute to the progressive disturbance in cerebral function. *[new concept]*

Benign epilepsy syndrome

A syndrome characterized by epileptic seizures that are easily treated, or require no treatment, and remit without sequelae. *[clarified concept]*

Reflex epilepsy syndrome

A syndrome in which all epileptic seizures are precipitated by sensory stimuli. Reflex seizures that occur in focal and generalized epilepsy syndromes that also are associated with spontaneous seizures are listed as seizure types. Isolated reflex seizures also can occur in situations that do not necessarily require a diagnosis of epilepsy. Seizures precipitated by other special circumstances, such as fever or alcohol withdrawal, are not reflex seizures. *[changed concept]*

Focal seizures and syndromes

Replaces the terms partial seizures and localization-related syndromes. *[changed terms]*

Simple and complex partial epileptic seizures

These terms are no longer recommended, nor will they be replaced. Ictal impairment of consciousness will be described when appropriate for individual seizures, but will not be used to classify specific seizure types. *[new concept]*

Idiopathic epilepsy syndrome

A syndrome that is only epilepsy, with no underlying structural brain lesion or other neurologic signs or symptoms. These are presumed to be genetic and are usually age dependent. *[unchanged term]*

Symptomatic epilepsy syndrome

A syndrome in which the epileptic seizures are the result of one or more identifiable structural lesions of the brain. *[unchanged term]*

Probably symptomatic epilepsy syndrome

Synonymous with, but preferred to, the term cryptogenic, used to define syndromes that are believed to be symptomatic, but no etiology has been identified. *[new term]*

onset and this resulted in a proposal for a classification of epilepsies and epileptic syndromes in 1989.[2] More recently, attempts to correlate specific epilepsy syndromes with demonstrable changes in genotype have provided some unexpected results. For example, the clinical phenotype of generalized epilepsy with febrile seizures plus (GEFS+) (see Chapter 4A) embraces many different seizure types and a very variable natural history, and maps to more than one chromosomal site.

In 1997, the ILAE constituted a new Task Force on Classification, which formed four working groups concerned with (a) descriptive terminology for ictal events; (b) seizures; (c) syndromes and diseases; and (d) impairment.[3] The Proposed Diagnostic Scheme for People with Epileptic Seizures and with Epilepsy is reproduced (with permission) as Table 1.1[3] and the definitions of key terms as Table 1.2.[4]

The proposed diagnostic scheme classifies patients using four main axes: ictal phenomenology, seizure type, syndrome and etiology. A fifth axis, impairment, is considered to be often useful but has been proposed at this stage as an option.

KEY POINTS

- Definitions of seizure type are based on a purely descriptive phenomenological approach
- An **epilepsy syndrome** comprises a complex of signs and symptoms that define a unique epilepsy condition that may have different etiologies

- An **epileptic disease** is a pathologic condition with a single, well-defined etiology, e.g. Unverricht-Lundborg disease
- An **epileptic encephalopathy** is a condition in which the epileptiform abnormalities themselves are believed to contribute to the progressive disturbance in cerebral function
- It is proposed that the term **focal** replace **partial**
- It is proposed that impairment of consciousness not be used to classify a seizure and that the terms **simple** and **complex** be no longer used
- It is proposed that **probably symptomatic epilepsy syndrome** refer to those epilepsies previously described as **cryptogenic**
- The concept of **benign epilepsy syndrome** has been clarified and that of **reflex epilepsy syndrome** changed

REFERENCES

1. Commission on Classification and Terminology of the International League Against Epilepsy. Proposal for revised clinical and electroencephalographic classification of epileptic seizures. *Epilepsia* 1981; **22**: 489–501.
2. Commission on Classification and Terminology of the International League Against Epilepsy. Proposal for revised classification of epilepsies and epileptic syndromes. *Epilepsia* 1989; **30**: 389–399.
3. Engel J Jr. ILAE Commission Report. Proposed diagnostic scheme for people with epileptic seizures and with epilepsy: report of the ILAE task force on classification and terminology. *Epilepsia* 2001; **42**: 796–803.
4. Blume WT, Luders HO, Mizrahi E, Tassinari C, van Emde Boas, Engel J Jr. ILAE Commission Report. Glossary of descriptive terminology for ictal seminology: report of the ILAE task force on classification and terminology. *Epilepsia* 2001; **42**: 1212–1218.

Paroxysmal nonepileptic disorders: differential diagnosis of epilepsy

JOHN STEPHENSON, WILLIAM P WHITEHOUSE AND SAMEER ZUBERI

A significant proportion of children suspected of having epilepsy, and even those with a definite diagnosis of epilepsy or even refractory epilepsy, have never had an epileptic seizure. Misdiagnosis rates are high throughout the world, irrespective of the wealth and resources available to the health-care system. The principal reason for this is that the diagnosis of epilepsy will always be dependent on the difficult, lonely, art of history taking. The physician taking the history must have an expertise in recognizing the clinical features of all the myriad forms of epileptic seizures, but this must be combined with an equally expert knowledge of those paroxysmal disorders that may mimic epilepsy. Most of the patients presenting to a first seizure or epilepsy clinic will not have epilepsy, and this alone justifies the place of this chapter in a book on epilepsy.

The diversity of nonepileptic events is considerable and all of the variations have certainly not yet been described. The most common type of nonepileptic seizure leading to diagnostic confusion in clinical practice is the anoxic seizure, or syncopal convulsion.[1,2] The term seizure is used in this chapter to include nonepileptic events, such as fainting fits, in the same way that we use it when speaking of episodes with apparent psychological mechanism, the so-called pseudo-epileptic seizures.

It is our clinical impression that misdiagnoses of epilepsy are more likely to arise when a child has more than one paroxysmal nonepileptic disorder, for example

two or more of the following: psychological events, syncopes, migraine and sleep disorders. That said, syncope was a surprisingly uncommon diagnosis in recent video-EEG studies of paroxysmal nonepileptic events in children and adolescents from tertiary centres.[3,4] In the study of Bye et al.,[3] which included children with developmental delay and mental retardation, psychological and sleep phenomena predominated and the EEG frequently showed misleading 'epileptiform' discharges. Kotagal et al.[4] reported on 134 children and adolescents referred to a pediatric epilepsy monitoring unit at the Cleveland Clinic over a 6-year period. The most common diagnoses in children under 5 years of age were stereotypies, sleep jerks, parasomnias and Sandifer syndrome. The most common diagnoses in the 5–12-year age group were conversion disorder (psychogenic pseudo-epileptic seizures), inattention or day dreaming, stereotypies, sleep jerks and paroxysmal movement disorders. Finally, over 80 per cent in the 12–18-year age group had a diagnosis of conversion disorder (hysteria, or psychogenic pseudo-epileptic seizures). Why syncopes, the most common type of nonepileptic disorder misdiagnosed as epilepsy,[2,5] did not feature as highly in these studies is not clear, but might reflect an ascertainment bias in that these children had sufficiently frequent episodes to be admitted for video-EEG investigation and a significant proportion of the children studied had concomitant epilepsy.

We have somewhat arbitrarily divided nonepileptic events into the following categories:

- syncopes and anoxic seizures
- psychological disorders
- derangements of the sleep process
- paroxysmal movement disorders
- migraine and possibly related disorders
- miscellaneous neurological events
- anoxic-epileptic seizures. This is an important and under-recognized phenomenon in which provoked syncopes themselves trigger epileptic seizures in individuals who rarely have unprovoked epileptic seizures.[6]

SYNCOPES AND ANOXIC SEIZURES

An anoxic seizure is the consequence of a syncope, which occurs usually as a result of a sudden decrease in cerebral perfusion of oxygenated blood, either from a reduction in cerebral blood flow itself or from a drop in the oxygen content, or a combination of these.[1,6] Although we have categorized the syncopes, it must be recognized that overlaps occur. Indeed, it seems likely that what we call reflex anoxic seizures or reflex asystolic syncope (RAS), breath-holding spells or prolonged expiratory apnea, vasovagal syncope and neurocardiogenic syncope are all varieties of the same disorder, called by the adult cardiologists neurally mediated syncope. When parents or children are bewildered by these diagnoses, or annoyed when told that 'it's only breath holding' or 'only a simple faint', contact with a family support organization (such as http://www.stars.org.uk) may be very helpful.

Reflex anoxic seizures or reflex asystolic syncope (RAS)

Gastaut used the term **reflex anoxic cerebral seizure** to describe all the various syncopes, sobbing spasms and breath-holding spells which followed noxious stimuli in young children.[7] Since 1978, the term **reflex anoxic seizure** has been used more specifically to describe a particular type of nonepileptic convulsive event, most commonly induced in young children by an unexpected bump to the head.[8] Although other terminology, such as **pallid breath-holding** and **pallid infantile syncope** have been applied to such episodes,[9] the term **reflex anoxic seizure** is now widely recognized.[10,11]

The clinical picture has been extensively documented.[6] Previously, almost all the available information came from descriptions by parents who had witnessed their child's attack or from observations of episodes reproduced by ocular compression, and it is only in recent times that home video-recordings of reflex anoxic seizures have become available. The first video-recording of a 'natural' attack obtained by one of the authors occurred when a 4-year-old girl was having capillary blood taken. The accompanying convulsive syncope was more severe than that previously recorded in the same child after ocular compression. Although the duration of postictal stupor was also longer, other mothers who watched the videotape were surprised at how quickly the child recovered. Until the advent of cardiac loop recorders, there was very little direct evidence of the pathophysiology of natural attacks. In a child who had two episodes while connected to EEG and ECG recorders, cardiac asystole alone appeared to account for the resultant anoxic seizure.[6] At the time of the first edition of this book, only three further recordings had been obtained.[12] Observations of the anoxic seizure induced by ocular compression in one of these children help to explain the confusion between reflex anoxic seizures and breath-holding spells. When this particular girl had ocular compression, asystole was apparent from the moment the thumbs began the ocular pressure, which is the usual finding in such cases. In the first few seconds of the asystolic period, however, there were repeated expiratory grunts at about three grunts per second. The parents recognized these grunts as similar to those noticed in the natural events. Thus, the anoxic seizure in this case was clearly related to the cardiac asystole and the expiratory grunting was an epiphenomenon. In cyanotic breath-holding attacks resulting in syncope or even a convulsive syncope, the amount and duration of expiratory grunting is greater and longer and the latency between the stimulus and the nonepileptic motor seizure is undoubtedly greater. Since prolonged cardiac recording by loop recorders has become feasible in young children, many episodes of prolonged reflex asystole have been recorded and several examples published.[13–16]

Extracts from a letter from a consultant neurologist may give the reader some idea of the clinical diagnostic difficulties that were experienced before the phenomenon of reflex asystole was well known:

Thank you for asking me to see this seven-year-old young man. As a toddler he began to have attacks of loss of awareness, rigidity and eye rolling which would be induced by minor knocks. This has continued and recently an episode occurred in which he had an undoubted tonic/clonic seizure with incontinence of urine. Curiously, as far as I can tell from mother's account, every attack has been triggered by a minor bump on the head and he has never had an attack out of the blue. He had difficulties at birth. The family history is clear except for a convulsion in the mother when she was tiny, about which there is no further information. It seems to me that this boy is having a form of reflex epileptic seizure and my inclination would have been to start treatment with sodium valproate.

In fact mother told me that he is attending the paediatric department at ... and that he was started on Epilim just a couple of weeks ago. Even though two EEGs have been normal I do not doubt that he has an epileptic tendency and I am sure that he should be on treatment for at least a couple of years free from attacks.

When this boy was seen he was beginning to become an 'epileptic', his school knew about his 'epilepsy', his mother was in touch with an epilepsy association, and invalidity benefit had been applied for on the basis of epilepsy. Presumably the difficulty here was that neither the pediatrician nor the neurologist knew that this was precisely the description of a reflex anoxic seizure of the vagally mediated cardioinhibitory type, otherwise known as **reflex asystolic syncope**.

As children grow older reflex anoxic seizures may cease altogether or change to more obvious convulsive or nonconvulsive vasovagal syncope. Beyond the toddler stage, children may report sensory disturbances along with the syncopes. Most dramatic are out-of-body experiences with a dream-like quality,[15] which may include the child feeling as if they have floated up to the ceiling and are watching their body lying on the floor in a seizure.

Although it is often said that breath-holding spells or syncope caused by prolonged expiratory apnea may also occur in children who have reflex anoxic seizures, there are no good recordings that confirm this proposition. Rather, recordings of what may on history or observation be taken as 'breath-holding attacks' turn out to demonstrate primarily asystole. In one such case of a 4-year-old twin in whom the attack was triggered by her brother snatching a toy, the girl started to cry, made a few expiratory grunts, looked cross, and had an end-expiratory apnea and extensor axial spasm. The asystole lasted 25 s and started during the grunting. This child also had similar reflex anoxic seizures triggered by unexpected knocks to the head.

It is important to determine whether a convulsive syncope in a young child is cardiogenic or respiratory in origin. If it is cardiogenic, the main differential diagnosis of a reflex anoxic seizure (reflex asystolic syncope) is convulsive syncope from long QT syndrome or other cardiac cause. In contrast, the differential diagnosis of a respiratory syncope includes breath-holding spells and intentional suffocation (see below).

Vasovagal syncope

Vasovagal syncope is the most familiar and predominant form of neurally mediated syncope. Unlike classical reflex anoxic seizures, which represent a fairly pure vagal attack, vasovagal syncope involves a vasodepressor component with variable vagal accompaniment. Episodes may begin in infancy but are seen at all ages, becoming most dramatic perhaps in old age.[17] Tables in medical textbooks are extremely misleading and tend to perpetuate myths about factors that are useful in distinguishing vasovagal syncope from epileptic seizures. Contrary to what is often stated, vasovagal syncope may sometimes occur in the supine position, particularly in the case of episodes occurring during venepuncture. Similarly, pallor and sweating are not invariable features and the onset of the episode is not always gradual. There is no evidence that injury is less common in convulsive syncope than in a convulsive epileptic seizure. Convulsive jerks are certainly not rare and occur in perhaps 50 per cent of vasovagal syncopes[18] and more often in experimental syncope.[19] Urinary incontinence is common[20] and occurred in 10 per cent of cases in one experimental study.[6] Although consciousness is regained rapidly in mild syncope, it is often impaired initially and marked postictal confusion can occur.[1] Finally, vasovagal syncope may occur more than once a day in some individuals.

Stimuli maybe very subtle, but some sort of stimulus should be detected for at least some attacks in order to make this diagnosis. Indeed, the most reliable indicators of vasovagal syncope are the setting and stimulus, together with elicitation of the warning symptoms or aura that are often present. A seizure that occurs after a bath, while the child is having her hair blow-dried or brushed, is virtually certain to be a vasovagal nonepileptic convulsive syncope. Premonitory symptoms are usually present in older children, even if only for a second or two, but these may sometimes be forgotten and recalled only when syncope is reproduced by the head-up tilt test. Dizziness, graying out of vision and tinnitus are well-recognized symptoms of cerebral ischemia, but an important additional symptom is abdominal pain. Abdominal pain may be either a trigger of a vasovagal syncope or an actual intestinal symptom of a strong vagal discharge. The latter is more common than appreciated,[6] and is sometimes confused with the epigastic aura that may occur at the onset of a temporal lobe seizure. Almost all children with vasovagal syncope have an affected first-degree relative, commonly a parent.[21] It is unfortunately not uncommon to find that the patient, who now seems convincingly to have vasovagal convulsive syncope, has become irredeemably 'epileptic' and is too habituated (or too frightened of losing a precious driving license) to discontinue years of useless (and perhaps embryopathic) antiepileptic medication (histories are included in ref. 6).

Head-up tilt testing of children has now been reported by a number of authors.[22] We have used a technique of 60° head-up tilt with foot-plate support, recording simultaneous EEG and ECG on cassette tape linked to a video-camera through a video-interface processor (VIP). At the same time beat-to-beat blood pressure is measured noninvasively using the Finapres method. A witness to natural events, normally a parent, is always present during this tilt test to confirm that what is reproduced is identical to natural episodes. The child is also able to say whether premonitory symptoms are the same as those experienced 'in the field'. At the time of writing we have reproduced convulsive syncope in nine children aged 8–13 years using the head-up tilt test. In contrast to the adult situation,[23,24] there has been marked cardioinhibition with asystole varying from 4 to 30 s. We have been struck also by the high incidence of behaviors that resemble syncope but do not have the cardiovascular or cerebral features of true syncope. These emotional or psychogenic episodes have been described in adults also[24] and are discussed in the section on conversion disorder below. These events often occur in individuals who also have vasovagal syncope.

A case history illustrates the transition from reflex anoxic seizures in infancy through short latency pain-induced vasovagal syncope to blood-injury phobia in adolescence.[25,26] The mother gave the history when her affected daughter was aged 13 years. A consultation had been requested as soon as she saw the recording of a finger-prick-induced reflex anoxic seizure on television. Her daughter had been diagnosed previously at different times to have epilepsy, hypoglycemia and hysterical behavior.

> The first episode occurred at the age of 10 months after a very slight bump to the infant's head. The appearance of the attacks has been similar from then to now, except that severity has varied and tended to increase with the passage of time. Typically there is a latency of 10–20 s during which she may say 'oh mum I've hurt myself'. By this time the blood has drained from her face, she goes limp and falls as if dead, then going totally rigid making a noise like a cackle or gurgle, with her hands and feet turned in and her back sometimes forming the shape of an arc. Sometimes her arms and legs jerk, but not violently, as though pedaling her bicycle, but on occasion thrashing wildly like a full seizure (as her mother describes it). Again she looks like death and then wakes up as if coming out of a very deep sleep. She is then very disorientated, does not know what has happened or where she is, but within a couple of minutes she has come to herself and may then want to lie down again and have a proper sleep. Since about the age of 7 or 8 years she has described an aura. She hears a noise like a high-pitched screaming and sometimes hears a voice but cannot describe the voice precisely. Sometimes she sees red, a color she does not like.
>
> More recently she has had strange hallucinations during the warning period, such as seeing a train rushing towards her. The stimuli have modified over the years after the first head hump. All episodes in earlier years followed small pains like her finger being bent back. Then she developed the same reaction to seeing a minor injury such as a scab that had come off a wound, and then inevitable syncope at the sight of blood. Most recently merely the thought of self-injury was sufficient.
>
> On the evening before the intended consultation, she was told (wrongly) that her eyeballs would be pressed down and within 2 minutes she was stiff and snorting. Although a family history of syncope of any kind was denied, the mother later admitted to several faints in adolescence and in pregnancy but did not mention them because she did not have a 'fit'.

The results of a recent study suggest that adults with blood/injury phobia have a 'constitutional autonomic dysregulation' that predisposes them to neurally mediated syncope, even in the absence of any blood or injury stimulus, and that repeated syncopes resulting from such stimuli secondarily lead to the blood/injury phobia.[27]

Vagovagal syncope

In contrast to vasovagal syncope, convincing vagovagal syncope is rare. The reflex is usually triggered by swallowing or vomiting and the anoxic seizure occurs if the asystole is sufficiently prolonged. This is probably not a life-threatening disorder, but the symptoms can be troublesome, particularly if the patient also has migraine with associated vomiting. Pacemaker therapy has been used successfully in this situation.[6]

Hyperventilation syncope

Hyperventilation induces various symptoms in everyone. In certain individuals this may stimulate further hyperventilation and exacerbation of the original symptoms, and a degree of panic may result. Asking the child to hyperventilate (whether by getting them to repeatedly blow out a candle, blow soap bubbles, blow a tissue or to directly hyperventilate) may induce symptoms similar to those of which they complain. Continuation of hyperventilation once the directed hyperventilation has been stopped may be of additional diagnostic value. Hyperventilation may also lead to episodes that resemble absence seizures but are not associated with spike and wave discharges.[28]

Orthostasis

Syncope due to orthostatic hypotension secondary to autonomic failure is rare in childhood. Chronic orthostatic intolerance may be caused by dopamine β-decarboxylase deficiency.[29] Chronic orthostatic intolerance may also manifest in teenagers and young adults as the postural/orthostatic tachycardia syndrome (POTS).[30] Patients have symptoms of chronic orthostatic intolerance with significant daily disability, associated with a marked tachycardia on standing: a heart rate increase of >30 beats/min or a heart rate of >120 beats/min within 10 min of head-up tilt.[31] Chronic orthostatic intolerance is a treatable disorder and should be considered in the differential diagnosis of idiopathic chronic fatigue syndrome.

In addition to vasovagal syncope, chronic orthostatic intolerance can produce symptoms of light-headedness, dizziness, blurred vision, exercise intolerance, chronic fatigue, migrainous headache, nausea, abdominal discomfort, chest discomfort, palpitations, shortness of breath, hyperventilation, peripheral cyanosis, and sweating and flushing on standing.[31] The simplest way to demonstrate orthostatic intolerance is to stand the child on a foam mat (to avoid injury when falling) for 10 min with continuous blood pressure measurement, which is best done using Finapres recording from a finger with the hand secured at heart level. A similar method can also be used to provoke vasovagal syncope in young children, including those too young to tilt.[32]

Long QT disorders

The long QT syndromes are associated with genuinely life-threatening syncopes, which may be hypotonic or convulsive. The mechanism of the syncopes is a ventricular tachyarrhythmia, normally *torsades de pointes*. As a rule, there is no great difficulty in the diagnosis of the syndrome of Jervell and Lange-Nielsen,[33] in which congenital deafness is associated with an autosomal recessive inheritance. Much more difficult is the Romano-Ward syndrome,[34] which is dominantly inherited but with incomplete penetrance. There is a degree of overlap between the stimuli that induce the neurally mediated syncopes, and those that trigger the ventricular tachyarrhythmias of the long QT syndrome; for instance, head bumps may trigger long QT as well as RAS.[35] However, a history of convulsions triggered by fear or fright, particularly if they occur during exercise (especially when that exercise is emotionally charged) or during sleep is strongly suggestive of the long QT syndrome.

A personal example illustrates some of the diagnostic difficulties:

A 5-year-old girl presented with a history of convulsive syncope since the age of 2 years. At the first consultation the parents said that when she fell, not necessarily hurting herself and not necessarily falling on any particular part of her, she went gray or gray/purple around the mouth, looked faintish as if dead, went very, very rigid as her eyes rolled and her head flopped, she moaned and 'she was dead in my arms'. One of the episodes was said to have occurred as a splinter was being taken out of her finger by her mother. There was a positive family history in that the father had fainted on cutting his finger and the mother had faints in pregnancy. An interictal 24-h ambulatory cassette ECG of the child had been reported as normal. A diagnosis of reflex anoxic seizures (reflex asystolic syncope) was made and it was decided that it would not be necessary to do ocular compression as a confirmatory test. Three years later the consultant pediatrician wrote again:

'She had approximately one year without any episodes but has had two close episodes in the last few weeks both of which occurred during physical exertion during play. At least one of these episodes seemed to be associated with an olfactory aura, the child describing strange smells before the event. In both situations she was found unconscious, stiff and mottled gray but recovered fairly promptly. I guess this is still a vagally mediated event but the parents would value further assessment and reassurance'.

Review of the history revealed that although two of the episodes had originally been associated with falling when playing with a ball, other episodes had occurred when chasing a dog, trying to catch the waves at the edge of the sea, playing being chased on her bicycle and during a hopping race. The new historical details prompted immediate measurement of her QT interval, the corrected value of which (QTc) 479 ms (normal value less than 440 ms). A review of the original 24-h ECG from 3 years previously showed that the QTc was prolonged then also, at 470 ms. Her mother had a marginally prolonged QTc of 449 ms, whereas her father and sister had normal QTc measurements of 387 and 390 ms respectively.

Long QT disorders are very much less common than reflex anoxic seizures, but should be considered when the precipitants are not typical and particularly when exercise or sleep are triggers.

Other cardiac syncopes

Cardiac syncopes, other than those of the long QT syndromes, do not usually pose diagnostic difficulties. However, it is important for the clinician to obtain a sufficiently clear history to determine whether the event is an epileptic seizure or a nonepileptic convulsive syncope. Ventricular tachyarrhythmias may occur with normal QT intervals.[36–37] In patients with congenital heart disease, exercise can precipitate paroxysmal pulmonary hypertension, which may manifest as an anoxic seizure.[6] We have also seen a 10-year-old boy who presented with recurrent convulsions with pain or stress. A standard 12-lead ECG demonstrated third-degree heart block, for which he was successfully treated.

Breath–holding attacks

Breath-holding spells have been described for centuries[38] but controversy as to what they are remains.[39] The term breath-holding seems to imply some sort of voluntary 'I'll hold my breath until I get what I want' behavior, and many members of the public and even pediatricians appear to believe that breath-holding spells are a manifestation of a behavior disorder. Indeed, breath-holding attacks are described in the section on psychiatric or psychological disorders in some pediatric textbooks. However, behavioral disorders in those with breath-holding spells are not more common or different from those in control children.[40]

As with many paroxysmal disorders, there are very few precise detailed descriptions of what happens during an event. Cinematographic registration[41] and video-recordings have been obtained, predominantly of several episodes in a single child.[6,42] Southall, Samuels and Talbert[43] have made polygraphic recordings of a small number of children. There appears to be a pure respiratory 'breath-holding' spell or prolonged expiratory apnea,[44] which occurs without any change in cardiac rate or rhythm (albeit information on cardiac output is not available) and is associated with cyanosis, the so-called 'blue' breath-holding attack. However, there are also 'mixed' breath-holding episodes that are characterized by both expiratory apnea and also a degree of bradycardia or cardiac asystole.[6,42] Furthermore, we have seen a video with simultaneous ECG of a child with a prolonged expiratory apnea while crying who became unconscious and had an event typical of that seen in reflex asystolic syncopes. However, this child maintained sinus rhythm with a modest tachycardia throughout (personal communication, E Wylie, 2000). This illustrates that the clinical features of reflex anoxic seizures may also occasionally be provoked by crying and occur with pure 'breath-holding' or prolonged expiratory apnea.[6] The difficulty in distinguishing between these by history and video alone without simultaneous ECG emphasizes the importance of obtaining an ictal ECG recording if atropine or pacing is to be considered for treatment.[14]

Prolonged expiratory apnea (cyanotic breath-holding) attacks in neurodevelopmentally normal children are benign and have an excellent prognosis.[39,45] The reports of life-threatening episodes[46] reflect the fact that attacks with similar features may occur in children with other abnormalities. For example, infants with tracheal anomalies may have similar episodes.[41,47] In addition, severe cyanotic breath-holding spells resembling prolonged expiratory apnea may be seen in infants with structural malformations of the posterior fossa. We have also seen potentially life-threatening episodes in a variety of Joubert syndrome with supratentorial neuronal migration disorder.

Compulsive Valsalva maneuver

Children with abnormal neurological development, including those with autistic disorders, may compulsively self-induce their atonic or more dramatic syncopal seizures by something akin to a Valsalva or Weber maneuver.[1,48] Such episodes may be very severe and even have a fatal outcome.[49] If the episodes are very frequent, as is often the case, video-recording with polygraphic registration may be useful.[49] The episodes are characterized by 'breath-holding' for about 10 s in inspiration, reduction of the amplitude of the QRS complexes on ECG, and then a burst of high-voltage slow waves on EEG. Sometimes, hyperventilation precedes the Valsalva maneuver,[1] as in the experimental syncopes described by Lempert, Bauer and Schmidt.[19] It is likely that many of the reported seizures in Rett syndrome are of this nature.[50]

Gastroesophageal reflux

Much has been written about gastroesophageal reflux in infants, but video-recording or full polygraphic registration of a reflux-associated anoxic episode has not been reported, although a true reflux episode associated with an epileptic seizure has been described.[51] Nonetheless, a persuasively recognizable condition, the awake apnea syndrome, has been described.[52] The episodes occur within an hour of a feed and usually follow an imposed change of posture. The infant gasps, becomes apneic, stiffens, changes color and may then look startled.[6] What might be called a reflux (sic) anoxic seizure may well be an example of vagovagal syncope, but a respiratory cause such as laryngeal spasm may be responsible. Gastroesophageal reflux may also result in the Sandifer syndrome, mentioned under 'Miscellaneous neurological events' below.

Imposed upper airway obstruction: suffocation

Suffocation of a baby, usually by the mother,[53] is a rare but important cause of 'breath-holding spells'. This is a classic example of fabricated or induced illness.[54] The parent repeatedly suffocates the baby by pressing a hand or some material over the baby's mouth, or else the mother presses the baby's face against her bosom[6] with a resultant syncope and anoxic seizure. Unlike the reflex anoxic seizures that occur with reflex asystolic syncope or cyanotic breath-holding spells, the evolution is much longer, with a latency of approximately 2 min.[55] The diagnosis may be exceedingly difficult. A cardinal feature is that the episodes only begin in the presence of the mother and other observers see only the conclusion of the episodes.[56] The EEG and ECG demonstrate a particular sequence of abnormalities, including movement and muscle potentials[6] and features of hypoxemia.[57] Establishing a definite diagnosis may require covert video-recording.[54,58] It has been found helpful to involve another experienced pediatrician, a psychiatrist and child protection procedures before discussion of the mechanism of induction of these truly life-threatening anoxic seizures with the family.[6]

Hyperekplexia

Hyperekplexia is a rare disorder (or group of disorders), which may present dramatically in the neonatal period with nonepileptic convulsive syncopes that may prove fatal.[59] This is a treatable disorder and so diagnostic awareness should be high.[60] A major early paper on this topic[61] described a dominantly inherited disorder in which there was hypertonia in the neonatal period with later onset of pathologic startles. A consistent diagnostic sign of hyperekplexia is elicited by tapping the infant's nose.[62] Nose-tapping produces a minimal response in a normal infant, whereas there is an obvious and reproducible startle response including head retraction in affected children. This startle may be induced over and over again. The diagnosis is not too difficult in sporadic cases in which the baby is stiff and tends to startle. The diagnosis is more easily missed in the baby that is not stiff and has neonatal onset convulsions with severe syncope. The ability to precipitate these dramatic nonepileptic seizures using the nose-tap test is particularly helpful. It is very important for the parent (and the examining physician) to know that the episodes, which can be very dramatic and even life-threatening in some infants, can be aborted by neck flexion.[60] The EEG recording during an episode demonstrates characteristically a series of what superficially may appear to be spikes but are actually rapidly recurring muscle potentials from scalp muscle. The frequency of the 'spikes' decreases *pari passu* with slowing of both EEG and ECG in the resultant severe syncope. The genetic basis in both the dominantly inherited variety of hyperekplexia and the apparently sporadic cases is a defect in either the $\alpha(1)$[63] or β[64] subunits of the strychnine-sensitive glycine receptor. Clonazepam is the prophylactic treatment of choice.

Familial rectal pain syndrome

The curiously named familial rectal pain syndrome is very rare. However, we have seen three families and made or reviewed ictal video-recordings of three children and one adult, which suggests that this unpleasant disorder is also underdiagnosed.[65] Familial rectal pain syndrome is dominantly inherited, but apparently sporadic cases occur. The presenting feature is neonatal onset of dramatic seizures. These were initially considered to be epileptic seizures, in part because there was a favorable response to carbamazepine.[66] In our patients there were no other features that would suggest epilepsy, and no paroxysmal EEG discharges during many observed

seizures. There were two important clues to the diagnosis. First, there were frequent striking harlequin color changes. In particular, one side of the face would turn red while the other side would turn white. Secondly, the precipitating factor for the seizures was some sort of perineal stimulation, such as wiping or cleaning. We believe that the seizures are severe syncopal episodes, similar to those seen in neonatal hyperekplexia. There was bradycardia and sometimes asystole with slowing and then flattening of the EEG, and generally a life-threatening appearance. These episodes abated eventually, but the adults with a similar neonatal history described continuing attacks of excruciating pain that was maximum in the nether regions and precipitated by stimuli such as passing a constipated stool.

Other syncopes and presyncopes

Many varieties of syncope and pre-syncope have certainly not yet been described. In a study of 92 infants with apparently life-threatening events, 52 events were recorded in 34 patients. However, the precise mechanism of events could not be identified in 22 of the events, which were characterized by prolonged hypoxemia of entirely unexplained mechanism.[57]

PSYCHOLOGICAL DISORDERS

Some of the disorders listed in this section may not be fundamentally different from other disorders described above and elsewhere in this chapter. The disorders included in this section are those in which psychological mechanisms seem to play a significant role.

Daydreams

There is a general awareness that episodes referred to as daydreams may be mistaken for absence seizures. These may not differ fundamentally from that described in the next subsection as gratification, but the subsequent conditions are more likely to lead to diagnostic difficulties.

Gratification (including infantile masturbation) and stereotypies

More or less pleasurable behavior, apparently similar to masturbation, may be seen from infancy onwards, perhaps more in preschool girls.[67] Rhythmic hip flexion and adduction may be accompanied by a distant expression and perhaps somnolence thereafter. The relative frequency of events and occurrence in specific circumstances, such as when bored or in a car seat, lends this behavior to home video-recording.[67a] Parents understandably prefer the term **gratification** (or even **benign idiopathic infantile dyskinesia**) to **infantile masturbation**.

It is sometimes more difficult to diagnose a phenomenon that occurs in slightly older children, known as 'television in the sky'. Affected children appear to stare into space or have unvocalized speech with imaginary individuals. They sometimes seem to twitch or move one or more limbs for several minutes at a time (ref. 6, case 14.2, p. 144). When there are repeated jerks or spasms, there may be confusion with epileptic infantile spasms.

Benign nonepileptic infantile spasms (benign myoclonus of early infancy)

This important disorder is harmless only if it is not misdiagnosed as epileptic infantile spasms.[68] Although the original authors[69] and a more recent successor[70] favored the term **benign myoclonus of early infancy**, we prefer **benign nonepileptic infantile spasms**[71] because the movements are more sustained than those produced by the shock-like muscle contraction of myoclonus. We consider that this phenomenon is a special type of stereotypy (see previous section).

Out-of-body experiences

There are several situations in which children may describe experiences in which they appear to lose immediate contact with their bodies and perhaps see themselves from above. Such hallucinations have been described in epileptic seizures, anoxic seizures, migraine and as a 'normal' phenomenon. Some of these perceptual disorders have been described as the **Alice in Wonderland phenomenon**. Dissociated states have been well described by Mahowald and Schenck.[72]

Panic/anxiety

Panic attacks are well recognized in both adults and children, and criteria for their presence in children have been described.[73] However, it is important to recognize that panic attacks may also be manifestations of epileptic seizures.[74] As the latter authors emphasize, long-term video-EEG monitoring may be necessary to establish the correct diagnosis and prevent inappropriate psychiatric interventions.

Conversion disorder

Whether the term hysteria should be used is debatable, but self-induced nonepileptic and nonsyncopal episodes are not rare.[4] These have been termed **pseudo-seizures**, **pseudo-epileptic seizures**, **psychogenic nonepileptic seizures** and **nonepileptic attack disorder**, but none of these terms is satisfactory for every case. The psychiatric literature has used different terms over the years from **hysteria** to **conversion hysteria** to **conversion disorders** to **dissociative states**, without adding precision or clarity to the disorders. We strongly recommend to readers a clear and modern view of hysteria.[75] Whatever the mechanism, it is important to recognize these disorders so that they can be treated appropriately rather than with anticonvulsants. It is also important to appreciate that they can also occur in patients who have epilepsy.

The episodes may mimic epileptic seizures, particularly frontal lobe seizures, and can have prominent sexual and aggressive components. They can often be recognized readily by observation of an event or videotape. Some are characterized by a more or less graceful collapse without injury, often into a recovery position. There may be some rhythmic jerking of the head or one or more limbs, or thrusting of the trunk or pelvis may predominate.

The extent to which professional help is necessary depends on the severity and cause. A socio-medical model is useful for management, in which the illness is accepted as 'real' recognizing that it may be an inevitable response to a particular 'predicament'.[76,77] This allows the patient to recover while saving face.[78] Reassurance and encouragement, with or without simple behavioral techniques, is often effective. However, post-traumatic stress disorder, and in some cases incest or child sexual abuse, may be the etiology.[79,80] Psychiatric and/or psychologic consultation is important in patients who do not respond to a more simple approach but, even then, it is often difficult to identify underlying trauma or abuse.

What has been called a **psychosomatic syncope** has been described in adults who collapse on head-up tilt with normal vital signs.[24] This sort of response (**pseudo syncope**) can also be seen quite frequently in head-up tilt testing in children. One such child had been expelled from school because of frequent 'fainting'. Collapse occurred on head-up tilt without change in heart rate, blood pressure (continuously recorded by Finapres) or EEG. Simple psychotherapy was followed by prompt recovery. The differential diagnosis here includes hyperventilation syncope (see above).

Depression

Psychogenic pseudo-seizures have been described as a manifestation of depression in adults,[24] and depression is likely to be a factor in some children and adolescents with pseudo-seizures.

Schizophrenia

Alterations of behavior related to hallucinations in childhood may be due to schizophrenia and resemble certain types of epileptic seizure. Psychiatric evaluation may be necessary to clarify the diagnosis.

Fabricated illness or invention

In some families, episodes resembling seizures or syncopes are not induced but are invented.[81] These have been described in the section on suffocation above. This can be considered as a passive form of **Meadow syndrome** (**Munchausen by proxy**) and the diagnosis may require considerable professional collaboration. In one of our cases, the affected child was reported to be having daily seizures although these were no longer observed after admission to hospital. However, when adult psychiatrists at another hospital interviewed the mother during this time, she affirmed that the seizures were continuing with the same frequency as previously.

DERANGEMENTS OF THE SLEEP PROCESS

Parasomnias and neurological disorders of sleep such as narcolepsy may be confused with epilepsy because of their paroxysmal nature. The difficulty in distinguishing epileptic and nonepileptic events is compounded by the fact that paroxysmal nonepileptic sleep events are more common in children.[3] Sleep disorders in children remain a largely neglected and poorly understood area. With the use of video EEG and nocturnal polysomnography, many of these conditions are being classified and differentiated from epileptic seizures. However, if there are many 'funny turns' during the day that have not been described, there are even more types of sleep disturbance that fall into this category.

Parasomnias

A detailed history will distinguish most parasomnias from epileptic seizures. Parasomnias typically occur only once or twice a night. If events are occurring more often, they are more likely to be epileptic seizures, often arising from mesial/orbital frontal lobe structures. Epileptic seizures tend to occur more frequently in stage II sleep. In differentiating these events, video polysomnography and/or video-EEG are the most useful investigative tools.

Non–REM partial arousal disorders, arousal parasomnias and night terrors

Brief nocturnal arousals are normal in children. They occur typically in stage IV non-REM sleep, 1–2 h after sleep onset. They vary from normal events such as mumbling, chewing, sitting up and staring, to arousals, which can be thought of as abnormal because of the disruption they cause the family. These include calm and agitated sleepwalking, and a spectrum from confusional arousals to night terrors or *pavor nocturnus*.

The child may exhibit automatic behavior during night terrors, but the events are not truly stereotyped. Affected children appear very agitated and look frightened as if they do not recognize their parents. They look awake and may be partially responsive but in fact are still in deep slow-wave sleep (stage IV). These events typically occur only once a night, usually 1–2 h after falling asleep and nearly always in the first half of sleep. Children have no memory of the event, which typically lasts 10–15 min before the child either wakes or settles back to restful sleep. By contrast, nocturnal frontal lobe epileptic seizures typically last less than 2 min and will often occur in clusters. The distinction between non-REM arousal disorders and benign partial epilepsy with affective symptoms (BPEAS)[82] can be more difficult. In this disorder, children arouse and look similarly wild and combative. However, the epileptic seizures are brief, do not arise particularly from stage IV sleep, are more likely to occur towards the end of sleep, and may occur while awake.

Non-REM arousal disorders likely represent a disordered balance between the drive to wake and the drive to sleep. They are more common in toddlers who sleep very deeply, in children who are overtired because of insufficient sleep, and in those who are unwell or on certain medications. An increased drive to wake occurs if the child has an irregular sleep schedule, is unwell or needs environmental associations to fall asleep normally. These disorders are therefore primarily managed by reassurance, explanation and behavioral measures to establish stable sleep routines and ensure good sleep hygiene.

REM sleep disorders

Nightmares and sleep paralysis are the principal REM sleep disorders. Some 10–20 per cent of individuals will have some experience of sleep paralysis, which may be a frightening experience because it occurs when the person wakes from REM sleep without abolishing the physiological REM atonia that normally prevents us from 'acting out' our dreams. Nightmares are usually easier to distinguish from epileptic seizures than night terrors because the child will have a memory both of waking and of the dream, and will then move rapidly into normal wakefulness. In contrast to these disorders, nocturnal epileptic seizures rarely arise out of REM sleep. Behavioral management and treatment of any co-morbid medical conditions are the appropriate treatment strategies.

Sleep–wake transition disorders

Rhythmic movement disorders such as nocturnal head banging, body rocking and head rolling typically occur in infants and toddlers as they are trying to fall asleep. They can be present in deep sleep and in wakefulness. They will typically remit by 5 years of age but may persist into adult life. Management relies on good sleep hygiene and padding the headboard so the rest of the house is not woken.

Benign neonatal sleep myoclonus

The major importance of recognizing benign neonatal sleep myoclonus is to prevent the misdiagnosis of neonatal epileptic seizures,[83] which may result in inappropriate treatment that has even included admission to the intensive care unit and ventilation.[6] The baby exhibits repetitive, usually rhythmic, jerks of one or more limbs during sleep. There have been reports of the occasional jerk in the waking state. Slow (1/second) rocking of the infant's crib in a head-to-toe direction will often reproduce the myoclonus,[84] which – in contrast to the situation in jitteriness – does not stop if the limbs are restrained. These episodes are usually diagnosed easily from the history, but an EEG can be helpful if the diagnosis is uncertain.

Sleep starts

Vigevano's group have described the occurrence of repetitive sleep starts in children with epilepsy and cerebral palsy.[85] These jerks occurred repetitively at the onset of sleep in clusters lasting several minutes, with arousal appearance on EEG but no jerk-related spike discharges. These children already have epilepsy and so it is important to differentiate these sleep starts from epileptic seizures in order to avoid inappropriate dosage increases in the antiepileptic medication.

Restless legs syndrome

Although generally thought of as a condition of middle age, this disorder may present in childhood and be misdiagnosed as attention deficit disorder[86] or even absence epilepsy. Recognition is important in that it tends to be exquisitely sensitive to dopaminergic therapy.[87]

Narcolepsy–cataplexy syndrome

Narcolepsy is a disorder characterized by excessive daytime sleepiness, cataplexy, sleep paralysis, hypnagogic hallucinations and disturbed night-time sleep. The onset of narcolepsy occurs before 16 years of age in 33 per cent,

before 10 years in 10 per cent and under 5 years of age in 4 per cent of patients.[88] Deficiency of hypocretin (also known as orexin), a neurotransmitter produced in the hypothalamus, has been demonstrated in narcolepsy.[89] Hypocretins help mediate arousal and project to brainstem structures involved in muscle tone.

Cataplexy is a loss of tone in response to strong emotion, typically laughter. Consciousness is maintained during cataplexy, even though the eyes may be closed. Diagnostic confusion may arise if several attacks of cataplexy occur one after the other and the individual then falls asleep on the floor.[90] Typically the loss of tone spreads from the face down the body. The individual has a degree of control so that they will often collapse in a series of stages rather than a sudden fall. Narcolepsy is often misdiagnosed as epilepsy: four of the six children diagnosed by us between 1997 and 2000 had been given a diagnosis of epilepsy and one child had been treated with multiple antiepileptic medications. REM sleep characteristically occurs shortly after the onset of sleep and the diagnosis can be confirmed by a multiple sleep latency test, provided the child is 8 years or older.[91]

PAROXYSMAL MOVEMENT DISORDERS

The major distinguishing features between paroxysmal movement disorders and epileptic seizures are the frequent presence of precipitating factors and the retention of consciousness in the paroxysmal dyskinesias and ataxias. However, they share many symptoms and are frequently confused with each other. Indeed, the boundaries between epilepsy and movement disorders are increasingly difficult to define.[92] Recent reports have emphasized the co-occurrence of movement disorders and epilepsy within the same family, suggesting that they may share the same underlying mechanism.[92–96] The recognition that dysfunction of ion channels leads to cellular hyperexcitabilty, and that mutations in these channel proteins may be associated with both epilepsy and movement disorders, provides a possible mechanism of action.[97] It is possible that mutant ion channels are expressed in variable degrees in different central nervous system structures, and that this expression may also vary with brain development. Thus the phenotype of a genetic ion channelopathy might include partial epileptic seizures in infancy indicating a cortical abnormality, and an episodic ataxia in childhood and adolescence, suggesting cerebellar dysfunction. It may be relevant that many antiepileptic medications are effective in the treatment of paroxysmal movement disorders. The channelopathies affect the central nervous system in many ways and comprise a large group of paroxysmal disorders, including epilepsy, migraine, movement disorders and hyperekplexia.[94]

Various complex classifications have been proposed for the paroxysmal movement disorders (see Fahn[98] for a summary and a history of terminology). The most clinically relevant and simplest is used below. Most reports describe familial cases, which are easier to diagnose when more than one family member is affected, and are possibly more interesting to report than sporadic cases. However, it is our impression that most paroxysmal dyskinesias occur sporadically. Furthermore, many cases do not fit exactly into the classical descriptions outlined below.

Paroxysmal kinesigenic dyskinesia (PKD)

The onset is typically in early childhood or adolescence with episodes of choreoathetosis or dystonia. Attacks last seconds to 5 min and are precipitated by sudden movements, change in position or change in movement velocity.[99] Getting up from a chair and getting out of a car are frequent triggers. Some individuals may have a brief nonspecific warning or aura before an attack, and consciousness is retained. Interictal neurological examination is normal. Attacks tend to become less frequent in adult life or remit completely. Carbamazepine is often highly effective in small doses.

There is a family history of similar events in about a quarter of patients, and the most common pattern of inheritance is autosomal dominant. Linkage to several overlapping but distinct loci around the pericentromeric region of chromosome 16 has been reported but the genes involved have not been identified.[100,101] In some families the paroxysmal dyskinesia is associated with benign familial infantile convulsions.[93,95] This has been reported as the **infantile convulsions and choreoathetosis syndrome** (ICCA). However, the movement disorder may include paroxysmal dystonia and is therefore better classified as a paroxysmal dyskinesia.

Paroxysmal nonkinesigenic dyskinesia (PNKD)

In this disorder, sometimes referred to also as **paroxysmal dystonic choreoathetosis** (PDC), attacks are often longer than in kinesiogenic dystonia and may last up to several hours or even days. The attacks are often markedly dystonic and may be precipitated by alcohol, caffeine or stress. Treatment involves avoidance of precipitating factors. Antiepileptic medications are not very effective. Inheritance is usually autosomal dominant and linkage to chromosome 2 has been reported.[102,103]

Paroxysmal exercise-induced dyskinesia (PED)

The events occur usually after 10–15 min of exercise and not at the initiation of movement as in PKD.[104] Typically the part of the body that has been doing most exercise will become dystonic. The abnormal movement resolves gradually over 5–30 min after the exercise is stopped. Antiepileptic medications are not generally helpful, but acetazolamide has been effective in some families.[104]

Paroxysmal nocturnal (hypnogenic) dyskinesia

This condition is almost certainly a form of nocturnal frontal lobe epilepsy,[105–107] and this term will become obsolete. In a typical episode a child will rouse and exhibit mixed involuntary dyskinetic movements of the limbs often associated with a cry either before the event or after.[108] The events are typically brief, lasting 10 s to 2 min, and may occur multiple times a night. They may be confused with night terrors (see above). Carbamazepine is often effective in very low doses.

Benign paroxysmal torticollis in infancy (BPT)

Infants have attacks of retro-, latero- or torticollis, which may last from minutes to hours.[109] The attacks typically begin in early infancy and remit by 5 years of age. They may be triggered by movement and are heralded by irritability, pallor, vomiting, and in older children by ataxia. BPT is both a movement disorder and a migraine equivalent.[110] Two patients with BPT in a recent series came from a family with familial hemiplegic migraine linked to a mutation in the voltage-gated calcium channel gene *CACNA1A* on chromosome 19.[111]

Benign paroxysmal tonic upgaze of childhood

Benign paroxysmal tonic upgaze of childhood[112] typically presents in infants less than 3 months with prolonged periods (hours to days) of sustained or intermittent upgaze deviation. Ataxia may appear particularly during intercurrent illness. The episodes remit within a few years but are associated with psychomotor retardation or language delay in up to 80 per cent of cases.[113]

Episodic ataxias

Episodic ataxia type 1 (EA1) is a rare disorder caused by mutations in a voltage-gated potassium channel. Affected individuals have brief episodes of cerebellar ataxia lasting seconds or minutes.[114] Interictal myokymia detected clinically or by demonstration of continuous motor unit activity on EMG is the principal diagnostic feature. Paroxysmal ataxia may be mistaken as a partial epileptic seizure, but there is also an overrepresentation of epilepsy in families with EA1.[115,116] The potassium channel is expressed throughout the central and peripheral nervous system. Whether the phenotype comprises ataxia, myokymia (or neuromyotonia), or epilepsy or a combination of the above seems to relate to the functional consequences of the mutation and its tissue specific developmental expression.[116]

Episodic ataxia type 2 (EA2) is characterized by longer attacks, lasting minutes, and is less frequently mistaken for epilepsy. There may be interictal cerebellar signs including impairment of eye movement control. This disorder is associated with mutations in a voltage gated calcium channel gene CACNA1A located on chromosome 19.[117] It is allelic with familial hemiplegic migraine and spinocerebellar ataxia type 6. In their pure forms these are distinct disorders, but overlap syndromes do occur. Partial seizures have been documented in familial hemiplegic migraine families and there is a case report of a child with a *de novo* truncating mutation in CACNA1A who has EA2 and absence epilepsy.[118,119]

MIGRAINE AND POSSIBLY RELATED DISORDERS

Some authors regard migraine with aura as an important differential in the diagnosis of epilepsy.[120] Indeed, the similarity is close but distinct between migraine with visual aura and occipital epilepsy.[121] In this section we discuss disorders which are probably migraine equivalents, but also some that are only possibly related.

Familial hemiplegic migraine (FHM)

Insofar as virtually all attacks of FHM are associated with headache and a family history,[122] the differential diagnosis of this true migraine should not normally be difficult.

Benign paroxysmal vertigo of childhood

This is the most common migraine equivalent.[110] Although affected preschool children are often referred with a diagnosis of epilepsy, the characteristic history of anxious arrest of movement without loss of awareness and subjective vertigo or 'drunking' makes the diagnosis easy. A related migraine equivalent, benign paroxysmal torticollis of infancy, is discussed above.

Cyclical vomiting

Cyclical vomiting syndrome is clearly related to migraine,[123] but may be confused with epilepsy (or indeed EA2).

Benign nocturnal alternating hemiplegia of childhood

Benign nocturnal alternating hemiplegia of childhood is even rarer than the better-known alternating hemiplegia (described in the next section).[124] Neurodevelopmentally normal young children experience recurrent attacks of hemiplegia arising from sleep and lasting 5–20 min. Attacks begin between 4 months and 3½ years of age and the course is benign. There is often a family history of migraine.

Alternating hemiplegia

Alternating hemiplegia of childhood is fascinating neurologic disorder that is both underdiagnosed and underreported.[125–129] The attacks of flaccid hemiplegia affect one or other side, or both, begin at 6–18 months of life and are associated with autonomic phenomena. Nystagmus and strabismus are the earliest manifestation and may even be seen in the neonatal period. The nystagmus is paroxysmal and frequently unilateral. The strabismus may also be paroxysmal and is also associated with signs of transitory internuclear ophthalmoplegia.[130] Tonic and dystonic episodes may also appear early in infancy, well before the first hemiplegic attack. These consist of predominantly brief and perhaps clustered tonic attacks which may easily be mistaken for epileptic tonic seizures. These stiffenings are commonly unilateral, with some resemblance to the asymmetric tonic neck reflex. They may also be bilateral, with a degree of opisthotonus and up-deviation of the eyes. Pallor, crying or screaming, and general misery tend to accompany these attacks. The attacks may be unilateral or bilateral. Bilateral hemiplegia is associated particularly with autonomic phenomena and drooling. Some sort of trigger precedes attacks in most affected children. Emotional factors, excitement, bright lights and bathing, particularly in hot baths, have been described. The frequency of bathing as a precipitating factor is probably under-reported. Developmental delay, ataxia and persistent choreoathetosis develop in most of these children, and a few develop migraine with aura (ref. 126, case 3).[127]

MISCELLANEOUS NEUROLOGIC EVENTS

There are many paroxysmal neurologic disorders that may be mistaken for epileptic seizures. Some well-recognized examples are described briefly. Many disorders have surely yet to be described. Tics, whether simple, complex or as part of Tourette syndrome, do not usually pose diagnostic difficulty. Nonepileptic myoclonus occurs in many situations. Benign nonepileptic infantile spasms have been described above. If there is difficulty in diagnosis of these disorders, ictal EEG will determine whether the event is epileptic.

Cataplexy in other neurological disorders

Cataplexy has been described above in the narcolepsy–cataplexy syndrome. Cataplexy has also been described in association with acquired brainstem lesions, Niemann-Pick type C disease, Norrie disease, the Prader-Willi Syndrome,[131] and as an isolated familial trait. A cataplexy-like disorder is also seen in the Coffin-Lowry syndrome[132] and many of the early reports of epilepsy in this syndrome are probably describing the cataplexy-like disorder.

Nonepileptic head-drops

Nonepileptic head drops are characterized by repetitive head-nods that are not accompanied by generalized epileptiform discharges on EEG. The initial flexion of the neck and the subsequent extension occur at the similar velocity instead of the rapid head drop and slow recovery characteristic of epileptic head nods.[133]

Functional blinking

Functional blinking[134] should perhaps be included in the psychogenic section. Unlike the epileptic syndrome of eyelid myoclonia with absences, it is not associated with epileptiform EEG discharges. However, if drug treatment abolishes the absence seizures and photoparoxysmal response in patients with eyelid myoclonia and absences, they often continue to have eyelid myoclonia without EEG change, and may not be aware of the blinking.[135]

Jitteriness

Jitteriness[136] is a phenomenon of fullterm neonates and very young infants. In contrast to benign neonatal sleep myoclonus, the movements are suppressed by limb restraint.

Shuddering

Shuddering begins in infancy.[137] We agree with Kanazawa[138] that shuddering and benign myoclonus of early infancy or benign infantile spasms are the same condition. A child with shuddering may develop essential tremor, although this is not invariable.[139]

Craniocervical junction disorders – Chiari type 1

Disorders of the craniocervical junction, particularly congenital disorders such as type 1 Chiari malformation, may be responsible for apparent syncopes which are not associated with EEG or ECG change. Stimuli, such as coughing, which would be expected to increase downward brain herniation, may precipitate attacks. A definitive diagnosis can be established by brain MRI.

Raised intracranial pressure

Decorticate or decerebrate posturing may accompany brain swelling, for instance in *Hemophilus influenzae* meningitis, and are often misdiagnosed as tonic epileptic seizures and treated with repeated injections of diazepam, with disastrous results (ref. 6, case 15.46). Although immunization should now prevent serious *Hemophilus* infections, these episodes can be seen with any acute rise in intracranial pressure, such as with intracranial hemorrhage or decompensated hydrocephalus.

Tetany

Aside from metabolic derangements in which the diagnosis is obvious, tetany is most often seen with hyperventilation – see 'Vasovagal syncope', 'Hyperventilation syncope', 'Panic/anxiety' above. In hypoparathyroidism it is more usual to have some form of epileptic seizure than tetany.

Sandifer syndrome

Intermittent contortions of the neck with marked lateral flexion are occasionally seen with severe gastroesophageal reflux, particularly in children with dyskinetic cerebral palsy.

ANOXIC-EPILEPTIC SEIZURES

It is surprising that although there are many comments in the literature suggesting that it is 'common knowledge' that severe anoxia can cause a tonic-clonic epileptic seizure, there is no published, well-documented report of a generalized tonic-clonic epileptic seizure following acute anoxia either due to asphyxia or ischemia. In contrast, true epileptic seizures as an immediate consequence of syncope have been recorded and described.[6,140] We call this phenomenon of a syncope followed by an epileptic seizure an **anoxic-epileptic seizure** (AES).

Most anoxic-epileptic seizures have been reported in infants or young children who also had a history of reflex syncopes without an epileptic component. Most of these syncopes were reflex asystolic syncope, reflex expiratory apnea (cyanotic breath-holding spells), or mixed episodes. Compulsive Valsalva maneuvers have also caused AES.[141] The epileptic seizures precipitated by the syncopal episode have been predominantly clonic or absence seizures. Status epilepticus[142] is either common or a stimulus to the medical attendants to write a paper!

CONCLUDING DIAGNOSTIC REMARKS

A precise, detailed, consecutive, all-embracing history remains paramount in the diagnosis of nonepileptic paroxysmal disorders.[6] The introduction of home video-recording and, more recently, prolonged monitoring facilities have been major advances. Constraints on the physician's time contribute to misdiagnoses and unnecessary EEGs and brain imaging when the full story, with or without video evidence, would make all clear. A particularly useful addition to history gathering and home videotaping has been the practice of showing video-recordings of different epileptic and nonepileptic seizure examples to parents to discover which, if any, resemble their own child's attacks – the 'that's it!' phenomenon.[6] However, since every paroxysmal disorder is not yet on film, far less described, the ancient art of history taking must remain paramount. And the historian is you.

KEY POINTS

- Many children suspected of having epilepsy, and even those with a definite diagnosis of epilepsy, have **never had an epileptic seizure**
- Reflex anoxic seizures, breath-holding spells, vasovagal syncope and neurocardiogenic syncope may all be varieties of the same disorder, **neurally mediated syncope**
- **Reflex anoxic seizures** are nonepileptic convulsive episodes that are due to cardiac asystole that has been provoked by a noxious stimulus
- The most reliable indicators of **vasovagal syncope** are the setting of the event, the stimulus, and the warning symptoms or aura that are often present
- The major **distinguishing features** between paroxysmal movement disorders and epileptic seizures are the frequent presence of precipitating factors and the retention of consciousness in the paroxysmal dyskinesias and ataxias
- **Anoxic-epileptic seizures** are an important and under-recognized phenomenon in which triggered syncopes themselves provoke epileptic seizures. They usually occur in individuals who do not have epilepsy
- In the diagnosis of all paroxysmal disorders, **history** is all

REFERENCES

1. Stephenson JBP. Anoxic seizures: self-terminating syncopes. *Epileptic Disorders* 2001; **3**: 3–6.
2. Gomes MMM, Kropf LA, Beeck E, Eda S, Figueira, IL. Inferences from a community study about non-epileptic events. *Arquivos de Neuropsiquiatria* 2002; **60**(3-B): 712–716.
3. Bye AM, Kok DJ, Ferenschild FT, Vies JS. Paroxysmal non-epileptic events in children: a retrospective study over a period of 10 years. *Journal of Paediatrics and Child Health* 2000; **36**: 244–248.
4. Kotagal P, Costa M, Wyllie E, Wolgamuth B. Paroxysmal nonepileptic events in children and adolescence. *Pediatrics* 2002; **110**: E4–6.
5. Smith PE, Myson V, Gibbon F. A teenager epilepsy clinic: observational study. *European Journal of Neurology* 2002; **9**: 373–376.
6. Stephenson JBP. *Fits and Faints*. Cambridge: Cambridge University Press; New York: Mac Keith Press, 1990.
7. Gastaut H. A physiopathogenic study of reflex anoxic cerebral seizures in children (syncopes, sobbing spasms and breath-holding spells). In: Kellaway P, Petersen I (eds) *Clinical Electroencephalography of Children*. Stockholm: Almquist & Wiksell, 1968.
8. Stephenson JBP. Two types of febrile seizure – anoxic (syncopal) and epileptic mechanisms differentiated by oculocardiac reflex. *British Medical Journal* 1978; **2**: 726–728.
9. Lombroso CT, Lerman P. Breath-holding spells (cyanotic and pallid infantile syncope). *Pediatrics* 1967; **39**: 563–581.
10. Roddy SM, Ashwal S, Schneider S. Venepuncture fits: a form of reflex anoxic seizure. *Pediatrics* 1983; **72**: 715–718.
11. Appleton RE. Reflex anoxic seizures. *British Medical Journal* 1993; **307**: 214–215.
12. Wallace SJ. *Epilepsy in Children*. London: Chapman & Hall, 1996.
13. Sreeram N, Whitehouse W. Permanent cardiac pacing for reflex anoxic seizure. *Archives of Disease in Childhood* 1996; **75**: 462.
14. McLeod KA, Wilson N, Hewitt J, Norrie J, Stephenson JB. Cardiac pacing for severe childhood neurally mediated syncope with reflex anoxic seizures. *Heart* 1999; **82**: 721–725.
15. Stephenson JBP, McLeod KA. Reflex anoxic seizures. In: David TJ (ed.) *Recent Advances in Paediatrics 18*. Edinburgh: Churchill Livingstone, 2000.
16. Kelly AM, Porter CJ, McGoon MD, *et al.* Breath-holding spells associated with significant bradycardia: successful treatment with permanent pacemaker implantation. *Pediatrics* 2001; **108**: 698–702.
17. Fitzpatrick A, Sutton R. Tilting towards a diagnosis in recurrent unexplained syncope. *Lancet* 1989; **i**: 658–660.
18. Ziegler DK, Lin J, Bayer WL. Convulsive syncope: relationship to cerebral ischemia. *Transactions of the American Neurological Association* 1978; **103**: 150–154.
19. Lempert T, Bauer M, Schmidt D. Syncope: a videometric analysis of 56 episodes of transient cerebral hypoxia. *Annals of Neurology* 1994; **36**: 233–237.
20. Lempert T. Recognizing syncope: pitfalls and surprises. *Journal of the Royal Society of Medicine* 1996; **89**, 372–375.
21. Camfield PR, Camfield CS. Syncope in childhood: a case control clinical study of the familial tendency to faint. *Canadian Journal of Neurological Science* 1990; **17**: 306–308.

22. Seifer CM, Kenny RA. Head-up tilt testing in children. *European Heart Journal* 2001; **22**: 1968–1971.

23. Grossi D, Buonomo C, Mirizzi F, *et al.* Electroencephalographic and electrocardiographic features of vasovagal syncope induced by head-up tilt. *Functional Neurology* 1990; **5**: 257–260.

24. Linzer M, Varia I ,Pontinen M, *et al.* Medically unexplained syncope: relationship to psychiatric illness. *American Journal of Medicine* 1992; **92**(1A): 18S-25S.

25. Connolly J, Hallam RS, Marks IM. Selective association of fainting with blood-injury-illness fear. *Behaviour Therapy* 1976; **7**: 8–13

26. Marks I. Blood-injury phobia: a review. *American Journal of Psychiatry* 1988; **145**: 1207–1213.

27. Accurso V, Winnicki M, Shamsuzzaman AS, *et al.* Predisposition to vasovagal syncope in subjects with blood/injury phobia. *Circulation* 2001; **104**: 903–907.

28. North KN, Ouvrier RA, Nugent M. Pseudoseizures caused by hyperventilation resembling absence epilepsy. *Journal of Child Neurology* 1990; **5**: 288–294.

29. Mathias CJ, Bannister R, Cortelli P, *et al.* Clinical autonomic and therapeutic observations in two siblings with postural hypotension and sympathetic failure due to an inability to synthesize noradrenaline from dopamine because of a deficiency of dopamine betahydroxylase. *Quarterly Journal of Medicine* 1990; **75**: 617–633.

30. Stewart JM, Gewitz MH, Weldon A, Munoz J. Patterns of orthostatic intolerance: the orthostatic tachycardia syndrome and adolescent chronic fatigue. *Journal of Pediatrics* 1999; **135**: 218–225.

31. Stewart JM. Orthostatic intolerance in pediatrics. *Journal of Pediatrics* 2002; **140**: 404–411.

32. Oslizlok P, Allen M, Griffin M, Gillette P. Clinical features and management of young patients with cardioinhibitory response during orthostatic testing. *American Journal of Cardiology* 1992; **69**(16): 1363–1365.

33. Jervell A , Lange-Nielsen F. Congenital deaf-mutism, functional heart disease with prolongation of the Q–T interval and sudden death. *American Heart Journal* 1957; **54**: 59–67.

34. Ward OC. A new familial cardiac syndrome in children. *Journal of the Irish Medical Association* 1964; **54**: 103–106.

35. Breningstall GN. Breath-holding spells. *Pediatric Neurology* 1996; **14**: 91–97.

36. Shaw TR. Recurrent ventricular fibrillation associated with normal QT intervals. *Quarterly Journal of Medicine* 1981; **50**: 451–462.

37. Leenhardt A, Lucet V, Denjoy I, Grau F, Ngoc DD, Coumel P. Catecholaminergic polymorphic ventricular tachycardia in children. A 7-year follow-up of 21 patients. *Circulation* 1995; **91**: 1512–1519.

38. Culpepper N. *A Directory for Midwives; or a Guide for Women in their Conception, Bearing (etc.).* London: Bettersworth & Hitch, 1737.

39. Gordon N. Breath-holding spells. *Developmental Medicine and Child Neurology* 1987; **29**: 810–814.

40. DiMario FJ Jr, Burleson JA. Behaviour profile of children with severe breath-holding spells. *Journal of Pediatrics* 1993; **122**: 488–491.

41. Gauk EW, Kidd L, Prichard JS. Aglottic breath-holding spells. *New England Journal of Medicine* 1966; **275**: 1361–1362.

42. Stephenson JBP. Blue breath-holding is benign. *Archives of Disease in Childhood* 1991; **66**: 255–257.

43. Southall DP, Samuels MP, Talbert DG. Recurrent cyanotic episodes with severe arterial hypoxaemia and intrapulmonary shunting: a mechanism for sudden death. *Archives of Disease in Childhood* 1990; **65**: 953–961.

44. Southall DP, Johnson P, Morley CJ, *et al.* Prolonged expiratory apnoea: a disorder resulting in episodes of severe arterial hypoxaemia in infants and young children. *Lancet* 1985; ii: 571–577.

45. DiMario FJ Jr. Prospective study of children with cyanotic and pallid breath-holding spells. *Pediatrics* 2001; **107**: 265–269.

46. Samuels MP, Talbert DC, Southall DP. Cyanotic breath-holding and sudden death. *Archives of Disease in Childhood* 1991; **66**: 257–258.

47. Filler RM, Rossello PJ , Lebowitz RL. Life-threatening hypoxic spells caused by tracheal compression after repair of esophageal atresia: correction by surgery. *Journal of Pediatric Surgery* 1976; **11**: 739–748.

48. Gastaut H, Broughton R, de Leo G. Syncopal attacks compulsively self-induced by the Valsalva manoeuvre in children with mental retardation. *Electroencephalography and Clinical Neurophysiology* 1982; **35**(Suppl): 323–329.

49. Genton P, Dusserre A. Pseudo-absences atoniques par syncopes auto-provoquées (manoeuvre de Valsalva). *Epilepsies* 1993; **5**: 223–227.

50. Glaze DG, Schultz RJ, Frost JD. Rett syndrome: characterization of seizures versus non-seizures. *Electroencephalography and Clinical Neurophysiology* 1998; **106**: 79–83.

51. Navelet Y, Wood C, Robleux C, Tardieu M. Seizures presenting as apnoea. *Archives of Disease in Childhood* 1989; **64**: 357–359.

52. Spitzer AR, Boyle JT, Tuchman DN, Fox WW. Awake apnea associated with gastroesophageal reflux: a specific clinical syndrome. *Journal of Pediatrics* 1984; **104**: 200–205.

53. Meadow R. Suffocation, recurrent apnea, and sudden infant death. *Journal of Pediatrics* 1990; **117**: 351–357.

54. Royal College of Paediatrics and Child Health. *Fabricated or Induced Illness by Carers.* London: Royal College of Paediatrics and Child Health, 2002; 78.

55. Rosen CL, Frost JD, Bricker T, *et al.* Two siblings with recurrent cardiorespiratory arrest: Munchausen syndrome by proxy or child abuse? *Pediatrics* 1983; **71**: 715–720.

56. Rosen CL, Frost JD Jr, Glaze DG. Child abuse and recurrent infant apnea. *Journal of Pediatrics* 1986; **109**: 1065–1067.

57. Poets CF, Samuels MY, Noyes IP, *et al.* Home event recordings of oxygenation, breathing movements, and heart rate and rhythm in infants with recurrent life-threatening events. *Journal of Pediatrics* 1993; **123**: 693–701.

58. Southall DP, Plunkett MC, Banks MW, *et al.* Covert video recordings of life-threatening child abuse: lessons for child protection. *Pediatrics* 1997; **100**: 735–760.

59. Pascotto A, Coppola G. Neonatal hyperekplexia: a case report. *Epilepsia* 1992; **33**: 817–820.

60. Vigevano F, Di Capua M, Dalla Bernardina B. Startle disease: an avoidable cause of sudden infant death. *Lancet* 1989; i: 216.

61. Suhren O, Bruyn GW, Tuynman JA. Hyperexplexia: a hereditary startle syndrome. *Journal of the Neurological Sciences* 1966; **31**: 577–605.

62. Kurczynski TW. Hyperekplexia. *Archives of Neurology* 1983; **40**: 246–248.

63. Rees MI, Lewis TM, Vafa B, *et al.* Compound heterozygosity and nonsense mutations in the alpha(1)-subunit of the

inhibitory glycine receptor in hyperekplexia. *Human Genetics* 2001; **109**: 267–270.

64. Rees ML, Lewis TM, Kwok JB, *et al.* Hyperekplexia associated with compound heterozygote mutations in the beta-subunit of the human inhibitory glycine receptor (GLRB). *Human Molecular Genetics* 2002; **11**: 853–860.

65. Elmslie FV, Wilson J, Rossiter MA. Familial rectal pain: is it under-diagnosed? *Journal of the Royal Society of Medicine* 1996; **89**: 290–291P.

66. Schubert R, Cracco JB. Familial rectal pain: a type of reflex epilepsy? *Annals of Neurology* 1992; **32**: 824–826.

67. Fleisher DR, Morrison A. Masturbation mimicking abdominal pain or seizures in young girls. *Journal of Pediatrics* 1990; **116**: 810–814.

67a. Nechay A, Ross LM, Stephenson JBP, O'Regan M. Gratification disorder ("infantile masturbation"): a review. *Archives of Disease in Childhood.* In press.

68. Maydell BV, Berenson F, Rothner AD, *et al.* Benign myoclonus of early infancy: an imitator of West's syndrome. *Journal of Child Neurology* 2001; **16**: 109–112.

69. Lombroso CT, Fejerman N. Benign myoclonus of early infancy. *Annals of Neurology* 1977; **1**: 138–143.

70. Pachatz C, Fusco L, Vigevano F. Benign myoclonus of early infancy. *Epileptic Disorders* 1999; **1**: 57–61.

71. Dravet C, Giraud N, Bureau M, *et al.* Benign myoclonus of early infancy or benign non-epileptic infantile spasms. *Neuropediatrics* 1986; **17**: 33–38.

72. Mahowald MW, Schenck CH. Dissociated states of wakefulness and sleep. *Neurology* 1992; **42** (Suppl 6): 44–52.

73. Ollendick TH, Mattis SG, King NJ. Panic in children and adolescents: a review. *Journal of Child Psychology and Psychiatry* 1994; **35**: 113–134.

74. Huppertz HJ, Franck P, Korinthenberg R, Schulze-Bonhage A. Recurrent attacks of fear and visual hallucinations in a child. *Journal of Child Neurology* 2002; **17**: 230–233.

75. Jureidini J, Taylor DC. Hysteria. Pretending to be sick. *European Child and Adolescent Psychiatry* 2002; **11**: 123–128.

76. Taylor DC. The components of sickness: diseases, illnesses, and predicaments. *Lancet* 1979; **ii**(8150): 1008–1010.

77. Taylor DC. The sick child's predicament. *Australian and New Zealand Journal of Psychiatry* 1985; **19**: 130–137.

78. Gudmundsson O, Prendergast M, Foreman D, Cowley S. Outcome of pseudoseizures in children and adolescents: a 6-year symptom survival analysis. *Developmental Medicine Child Neurology* 2001; **43**: 547–551.

79. Goodwin DS, Simms M, Bergman R. Hysterical seizures: a sequel to incest. *American Journal of Orthopsychiatry* 1979; **49**: 698–703.

80. Alper K, Devinski O, Perrine K, *et al.* Non epileptic seizures and childhood sexual and physical abuse. *Neurology* 1993; **43**: 1950–1953.

81. Meadow R. Fictitious epilepsy. *Lancet* 1984; **ii**: 25–28.

82. Dalla Bernardina B, Colamaria V, Chiamenti C, *et al.* Benign partial epilepsy with affective symptoms (benign psychomotor epilepsy). In: Roger J, Bureau M, Dravet C, *et al.* (eds) *Epileptic Syndromes in Infancy, Childhood and Adolescence*, 2nd edn. London: John Libbey, 1992; 219–223.

83. Coulter DL, Allen RJ. Benign neonatal sleep myoclonus. *Archives of Neurology* 1982; **39**: 191–192.

84. Alfonso I, Papazian O, Aicardi J, Jeffries HE. A simple maneuver to provoke benign neonatal sleep myoclonus. *Pediatrics* 1995; **96**: 1161–1163.

85. Fusco L, Pachatz C, Cusmai R, Vigevano F. Repetitive sleep starts in neurologically impaired children: an unusual non-epileptic manifestation in otherwise epileptic subjects. *Epileptic Disorders* 1999; **1**: 63–67.

86. Walters AS, Picchietti DL, Ehrenberg BL, Wagner ML. Restless legs syndrome in childhood and adolescence. *Pediatric Neurology* 1994; **11**: 241–245.

87. Walters AS, Mandelbaum DE and Lewin DS, *et al.* Dopaminergic therapy in children with restless legs/periodic limb movements in sleep and ADHD. Dopaminergic Therapy Study Group. *Pediatric Neurology* 2000; **22**: 182–186.

88. Challamel MJ, Mazzola ME, Nevsmalova S, *et al.* Narcolepsy in children. *Sleep* 1994; **17**(Suppl 8): S17–20.

89. Nishino S, Ripley B, Overeem S, *et al.* Hypocretin (orexin) deficiency in human narcolepsy. *Lancet* 2000; **355**: 39–40.

90. Zeman A, Douglas N, Aylward R. Lesson of the week: Narcolepsy mistaken for epilepsy. *British Medical Journal* 2000; **322**: 216–218.

91. Guilleminault C, Pelayo R. Narcolepsy in children: a practical guide to its diagnosis, treatment and follow-up. *Paediatric Drugs* 2000; **2**: 1–9.

92. Guerrini R, Aicardi J, Andermann F, Hallett M (eds). *Epilepsy and Movement Disorders*. Cambridge: Cambridge University Press, 2002.

93. Szepotowski P, Rochette R, Berquin P *et al.* Familial infantile convulsions and paroxysmal choreoathetosis: A new neurological syndrome linked to the pericentromeric region of chromosome 16. *American Journal of Human Genetics* 1997; **61**: 889–898.

94. Zuberi SM, Hanna MG. Ion channels and neurology. *Archives of Disease in Childhood* 2001; **84**: 277–280.

95. Thiriaux A, de St Martin A, Vercueil L, *et al.* Co-occurrence of infantile epileptic seizures and childhood paroxysmal choreoathetosis in one family: clinical, EEG, and SPECT characterization of episodic events. *Movement Disorders* 2002; **17**: 98–104.

96. Guerrini R, Sanchez-Carpentiro R, Deonna T, *et al.* Early-onset absence epilepsy and paroxysmal dyskinesias. *Epilepsia* 2002; **43**: 1224–1229.

97. Singh R, Macdonnel RA, Scheffer IE, *et al.* Epilepsy and paroxysmal movement disorders in families: evidence for shared mechanisms. *Epileptic Disorders* 1999; **1**: 93–99.

98. Fahn S. The paroxysmal dyskinesias. In: Marsden CD, Fahn S (eds) *Movement Disorders 3*. Oxford: Butterworth-Heineman, 1994; 310–345.

99. Houser MK, Soland VL, Bhatia KP, Quinn MP, Marsden CD. Paroxysmal kinesigenic choreoathetosis: a report of 26 cases. *Journal of Neurology* 1999; **246**: 120–126.

100. Bennett LB, Roach ES, Bowcock AM. A locus for paroxysmal kinesigenic dyskinesia maps to human chromosome 16. *Neurology* 2000; **54**: 125–130.

101. Tomita H, Nagamitsu S, Wakui K, *et al.* A gene for paroxysmal kinesigenic choreoathetosis mapped to 16p11.2-q12.1. *American Journal of Human Genetics* 1999; **65**: 1688–1697.

102. Fink JK, Hedera P, Mathay JG, Albin R. Paroxysmal dystonic choreoathetosis linked to chromosome 2q: clinical analysis and proposed physiology. *Neurology* 1997; **49**: 177–183.

103. Fouad GT, Servidei S, Durcan S, Bertini E, Ptacek LJ. A gene for familial dyskinesia (FPDI) maps to chromosome 2q. *American Journal of Human Genetics* 1996; **59**: 135–139.

104. Bhatia KP, Soland VL, Bhatt MH, Quinn NP, Marsden CD. Paroxysmal exercise induced dystonia: eight new sporadic cases and a review of the literature. *Movement Disorders* 1997; **12**: 1007–1012.

105. Scheffer IE, Bhatia KP, Lopes-Cendes I, *et al.* Autosomal dominant nocturnal frontal lobe epilepsy diagnosed as sleep disorder. *Lancet* 1994; **343**: 515–517.

106. Scheffer IE, Bhatia KP, Lopes-Cendes I *et al.* Autosomal dominant nocturnal frontal lobe epilepsy. A distinctive clinical disorder. *Brain* 1995; **118**: 61–73.

107. Steinlein O, Mulley JC, Propping P, *et al.* A missense mutation in the neuronal nicotinic acetylcholine receptor α4 subunit is associated with autosomal dominant nocturnal frontal lobe epilepsy. *Nature Genetics* 1995; **11**: 201–203.

108. Lugaresi F, Cirignotta F. Hypnogenic paroxysmal dystonia: epileptic seizure or a new syndrome? *Sleep* 1981; **4**: 129–138.

109. Fernandez-Alvarez E. Transient movement disorders in children. *Journal of Neurology* 1998; **245**: 1–5.

110. Al-Twaijri WA, Shevell MI. Pediatric migraine equivalents: occurrence and clinical features in practice. *Pediatric Neurology* 2002; **26**: 365–368.

111. Giffin NJ, Benton S, Goadsby PJ. Benign paroxysmal torticollis of infancy: four new cases and linkage to CACNA1A mutation. *Developmental Medicine and Child Neurology* 2002; **44**: 490–493.

112. Ouvrier RA, Billson MD. Benign paroxysmal tonic upgaze of childhood. *Journal of Child Neurology* 1988; **3**: 177–180.

113. Hayman M, Harvey A, Hopkins IJ, *et al.* Paroxysmal tonic upgaze: a reappraisal of outcome. *Annals of Neurology* 1998; **43**: 514–520.

114. Browne DL, Gancher ST, Smith EA, *et al.* Episodic ataxia/ myokymia syndrome is associated with point mutations in the human potassium channel gene KCNA1. *Nature Genetics* 1994; **8**: 136–140.

115. Zuberi SM, Eunson LH, Spauschus A, *et al.* A novel mutation in the human voltage gated potassium channel gene (Kv1.1) associates with episodic ataxia and sometimes with partial epilepsy. *Brain* 1999; **122**: 817–825.

116. Eunson LH, Rea R, Zuberi SM, *et al.* Clinical, genetic, and expression studies of mutations in the human voltage-gated potassium channel KCNA1 reveal new phenotypic variability. *Annals of Neurology* 2000; **48**: 647–656.

117. Ophoff RA, Terwindt GM, Vergouwe MN, *et al.* Familial hemiplegic migraine and episodic ataxia type 2 are caused by mutations in the Ca^{2+} channel gene CACNL1A4. *Cell* 1996; **87**: 543–552.

118. Terwindt GM, Ophoff RA, Lindhout D, *et al.* Partial cosegregation of familial hemiplegic migraine and a benign familial epileptic syndrome. *Epilepsia* 1997; **38**: 915–921.

119. Jouvenceau A, Eunson LH, Spauschus A, *et al.* Human epilepsy associated with dysfunction of the brain P/Q-type calcium channel. *Lancet* 2001; **358**: 801–807.

120. Gibbs J, Appleton RE. False diagnosis of epilepsy in children. *Seizure* 1992; **1**: 15–18.

121. Panayiotopoulos CP. Visual phenomena and headache in occipital epilepsy: a review, a systematic study and differentiation from migraine. *Epileptic Disorders* 1999; **1**: 205–216.

122. Thomsen LL, Eriksen MK, Roemer SF, *et al.* A population-based study of familial hemiplegic migraine suggests revised diagnostic criteria. *Brain* 2002; **125**: 1389–1391.

123. Dignan F, Symon DNK, AbuArafeh I, Russell G. The prognosis of cyclical vomiting syndrome. *Archives of Disease in Childhood* 2001; **84**: 55–57.

124. Chaves-Vischer V, Picard F, Andermann E, *et al.* Benign nocturnal alternating hemiplegia of childhood: six patients and long-term follow-up. *Neurology* 2001; **57**: 1491–1493.

125. Verret S, Steele JC. Alternating hemiplegia in childhood: a report of eight patients with complicated migraine beginning in infancy. *Pediatrics* 1971; **47**: 675–680.

126. Casaer P. Flunarizine in alternating hemiplegia in childhood. An international study in 12 children. *Neuropediatrics* 1987; **18**: 191–195.

127. Silver K, Andermann F. Alternating hemiplegia of childhood: a study of 10 patients and results of flunarizine treatment. *Neurology* 1993; **43**: 36–41.

128. Bourgeois M, Aicardi J, Goutières F. Alternating hemiplegia of childhood. *Journal of Pediatrics* 1993; **122**: 673–679.

129. Mikati MA, Kramer U, Zupanc ML, Shanahan RJ. Alternating hemiplegia of childhood: clinical manifestations and long-term outcome. *Pediatric Neurology* 2000; **23**: 134–141.

130. Bursztyn J, Mikaeloff Y, Kaminska A, *et al.* Hémiplégies alternantes de l'enfant et leurs anomalies oculo-motrices [Alternating hemiplegia of childhood and oculomotor anomalies]. *Journal Français d'Ophthalmologie* 2000; **23**: 161–164.

131. Tobias ES, Tolmie JL, Stephenson JBP. Cataplexy in the Prader-Willi syndrome. *Archives of Disease in Childhood* 2002; **87**: 170.

132. Crow YJ, Zuberi SM, McWilliam R, *et al.* "Cataplexy" and muscle ultrasound abnormalities in Coffin-Lowry syndrome. *Journal of Medical Genetics* 1998; **35**: 94–98.

133. Brunquell P, McKeever M, Russman BS. Differentiation of epileptic from non-epileptic head drops in children. *Epilepsia* 1990; **31**: 401–405.

134. Vrabec TR, Levin AV, Nelson LB. Functional blinking in childhood. *Pediatrics* 1989; **83**: 967–970.

135. Kent L, Blake A, Whitehouse W. Eyelid myoclonus and absences: phenomenology in children. *Seizure* 1987; **7**: 193–199.

136. Parker S, Zuckerman B, Bauchner H, *et al.* Jitteriness in full-term neonates: prevalence and correlates. *Pediatrics* 1990; **85**: 17–23.

137. Holmes GL, Russman BS. Shuddering attacks. *American Journal of Diseases of Children* 1986; **140**: 72–74.

138. Kanazawa O. Shuddering attacks – report of four children. *Pediatric Neurology* 2000; **23**: 421–424.

139. Vanasse M, Bedard P, Andermann F. Shuddering attacks in children: an early clinical manifestation of essential tremor. *Neurology* 1976; **26**: 1027–1030.

140. Battaglia A, Guerrini R, Gastaut H. Epileptic seizures induced by syncopal attacks. *Journal of Epilepsy* 1989; **2**: 137–146.

141. Aicardi J, Gastaut H, Mises J. Syncopal attacks compulsively self-induced by Valsalva's manoeuvre associated with typical absence seizures. *Archives of Neurology* 1988; **45**: 923–925.

142. Kuhle S, Tiefenthaler M, Seidl R, Hauser E. Prolonged generalized epileptic seizures triggered by breath-holding spells. *Pediatric Neurology* 2000; **23**: 271–273.

3

Incidence and prevalence

LARS FORSGREN

DEFINITIONS

- The **incidence** of epilepsy is the number of new cases diagnosed annually per 100 000 population (or person-years), i.e. the annual incidence rate.
- The **prevalence** is the number of cases with epilepsy on a specific date (the prevalence day) per 1000 population.

For epidemiological studies to be comparable, the definition of epilepsy, and the sources from which the cases are identified, must be similar. International guidelines for epidemiological studies of epilepsy exist.[1] Usually, only 'active' cases are included. These are characterized by:

- the occurrence of at least two seizures
- seizures unprovoked by any immediate identified cause and
- the last unprovoked seizure occurred during the previous 5 years.

Many prevalence studies also include persons who are currently treated with antiepileptic drugs (AEDs), even if the last seizure occurred more than 5 years ago. The study population should be as representative as possible of the population to which the results are to be generalized. General life conditions differ widely throughout the world, and it is not feasible to identify a study population that is universally representative. Assessment of many populations is needed for an accurate picture of epidemiological characteristics shared between, or unique to, specific epilepsy populations to be obtained. Generally, the more sources of information are used, the more accurately will the epidemiological findings represent the true situation. Studies of children identified only from hospital clinics with a special interest in epilepsy underestimate overall incidence and prevalence and overestimate those with severe epilepsies and bad prognoses. Incidence and prevalence are affected by age. When epidemiological studies of epilepsy in children are compared awareness of the age groups included is important.

VALUE OF EPIDEMIOLOGICAL STUDIES

Epidemiological studies give important information on the magnitude, causes and consequences of epilepsy. Questions on impacts of etiological and other factors on prognostic variables of major clinical importance, such as: risks for further seizures, chances of remission, risks of dying from seizures, associations with low or high risks for intractable epilepsy, are best answered by incidence cohorts. These are especially valuable for planning, particularly for estimating the investigational resources needed. Hypotheses can be generated to assess possible risk factors and their potential prevention.

Prevalence studies in well-characterized populations also provide valuable information on: the totals with epilepsy; numbers with mild or severe epilepsy; frequencies in different age-ranges; numbers with, and types of, concomitant disorders, which can be used for planning purposes. Thus, the magnitude of and types of levels of care and support needed for the multiple subpopulations that make up the whole can be estimated and the costs calculated.

INCIDENCE

Eleven population-based studies on the incidence of childhood onset epilepsy have been published during the last 15 years (Table 3.1).[2–12] In less developed countries (Chile, Ethiopia, Tanzania, India), incidence rates range from figures comparable to those found in more developed countries up to considerably higher rates.[9–12] Studies on incidence that include provoked seizures are not discussed here. Based on available information on age-specific incidence, it can be estimated that, worldwide, 3.5 million people develop epilepsy annually. About 40 per cent of these are under the age of 15 years, and more than 80 per cent of them live in less developed countries.

Age-specific incidence

In Europe and North America the highest incidences of epilepsy are found in young children, and, also, particularly, in elderly people.[2,9,6,7] During childhood the incidence decreases from around 150/100 000 during the first year of life to around 60/100 000 at ages 5–9 years and 45–50/100 000 in older children (Figure 3.1, Europe and North America). The incidences in South America (Chile), Africa (Ethiopia, Tanzania) and Asia (India, Japan) are higher in children and adolescents than in any other age group (Figure 3.1).[9–13] The childhood part of the curve for Asia is mainly based on Japanese children,[13] which explains the similarity to that for Europe and North America, where economic standards are comparable. The higher incidence rates in economically less advanced countries are unexplained. Causes common to both

developed and developing countries, e.g. pre- and perinatal adverse events, head trauma and infections may be more frequent in poorer countries, where additional factors, such as neurocysticercosis, also occur. The roles of starvation or malnutrition in causation are not known: direct relationships have not been established in clinical studies.

Sex-specific incidence

There is no consistent difference in incidence rates between the sexes. Most studies report higher rates in boys,[7,8,10,12] but higher rates in girls[9] and no gender difference during childhood[2,3,5,6] have also been noted. Furthermore, where the crude rate (all childhood ages included) showed a gender difference, a shifting dominance by boys and girls for different specific age groups is invariably found.

Cumulative incidence

The cumulative incidence is the estimated proportion of a population which develops epilepsy over a specified time

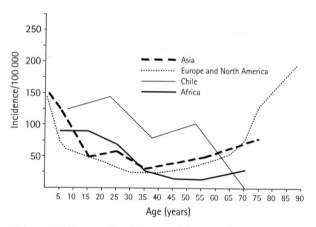

Figure 3.1 *Age-specific incidence of epilepsy in different parts of the world.*

Table 3.1 *Annual incidence (I)/100 000 of epilepsy/seizures in children. Studies published 1986 and later*

Country	Year	Study	Age group (years)	Incidence	No. of cases	Population
Canada	1996	2	0–15	41	693	>1 unprovoked seizure
UK	1992	3	0–10	43[a]	63	>1 unprovoked seizure
Sweden	1987	4	0–19	50	68	>1 unprovoked seizure
USA[b]	1993	5	0–19	50	90	>1 unprovoked seizure
India	1998	6	0–19	61	18	>1 unprovoked seizure
Iceland	1996	7	0–14	67	16	>1 unprovoked seizure
Faroe Islands	1986	8	0–19	71	121	>1 unprovoked seizure
Sweden	1993	9	0–15	73	61	Single seizures included
Ethiopia	1997	10	0–19	86	110	>1 unprovoked seizure
Tanzania	1992	11	0–19	93	94	>1 unprovoked seizure
Chile	1992	12	0–14	124	43	>1 unprovoked seizure

[a] Cumulative incidence.
[b] 1975–1984.

interval. Up to age 14–15 years, 1.0–1.7 per cent of children will have had at least one unprovoked seizure[5,9,13,14] and 0.7–0.8 per cent repeated unprovoked seizures, i.e. epilepsy.[5,13]

PREVALENCE

Most population-based studies in children include those up to ages 14, 15 or 19 years and exclude those who only had seizures during the first month of life. Others only include school age children. The prevalence rates are similar in both groups (Table 3.2). Studies from Europe and North America report rates from 3.6 to 6.5/1000, mostly 4–5/1000.[8,15–24] Those from Africa and South America give higher rates, from 6.6 to 17/1000.[11,12,25,26] Globally, 10.5 million children aged 0–14 years are estimated to have active epilepsy, constituting 25 per cent of the global epilepsy population.

Age-specific prevalence

The prevalence rate rises with increasing age.[8,11,12,15–20] Between 0 to 4–5 years, it is approximately 3.5/1000; between 5–6 and 9–10 years, 4.5/1000; and between 11 and 15–16 years, approximately 5/1000.

Sex-specific prevalence

Information on gender is provided in 13 of the 15 studies in Table 3.2. In 11 of them, the prevalence rate is higher for boys. Usually, the difference is minor and not statistically significant. Two studies report higher rates in girls.[18,19]

TIME TRENDS

During a 50-year period, from 1935 to 1984, the overall incidence of epilepsy was relatively stable in Rochester, USA.[5,27] However, the age-specific incidence decreased successively by 40–50 per cent between 1935 and 1984 in children younger than age 10 years, with a slight increase during the period 1975–1984.[5,27] Reasons for this decrease are unknown but improved ante- and perinatal care may be partly responsible. In the UK, the cumulative incidence by age 5 years declined from 4 per 1000 in children born in 1946[28] to 2.9 per 1000 in children born in 1958.[29]

TREATMENT GAP

Most patients in less developed countries do not receive pharmacological treatment. It is estimated that 85 per cent are either inappropriately treated or untreated.[30]

EPILEPSY IN OTHER DISORDERS

Mental retardation/learning disabilities

The commonest associated disorder is mental retardation (learning disability) (see Chapter 16).

Cerebral palsy

Cerebral palsy, occurring in 16–21 per cent, is the commonest associated motor disability.[19,23] Eighty-nine to

Table 3.2 *Prevalence of active epilepsy in children*

Country	Year	Study	Prevalence/1000	No. of children	Age (years)
Estonia	1999	15	3.6	560	0–19
Spain	1991	16	3.7	124	6–14
Finland	1997	17	3.9	329	0–15
USA[a]	1991	18	3.9	48	0–14
Sweden	1996	19	4.2	155	0–16
Lithuania	1997	20	4.3	378	0–15
Italy	1980	21	4.5	178	5–14
USA	1989	22	4.7	1159	0–19
Norway	2000	23	5.3	205	6–12
USA	1978	24	5.7	23	6–16
Faroe Islands	1986	8	6.5	106	0–19
Tanzania	1992	11	6.6	73	0–19
South Africa	2000	25	6.7	45	2–9
Bolivia	1999	26	8.4	43	0–14
Chile	1992	12	17.0	102	0–14

[a] Prevalence year 1980.

100 per cent of those with epilepsy and cerebral palsy are also mentally retarded.[19,23,31] Mental retardation with concurrent cerebral palsy increases the risk for epilepsy to 48 per cent, compared with 11 per cent when either of these disabilities presents alone.[32] Depending on the type of cerebral palsy present, epilepsy occurs in between 16 and 94 per cent.[33–35] In a cohort with cerebral palsy followed up to at least 4 years of age, or to death for those who died between ages 2–4 years, epilepsy occurred in 26 per cent and 36 per cent of children born preterm and term respectively.[36]

Hydrocephalus

In infantile hydrocephalus, defined as hydrocephalus manifested during the first year of life, unassociated with neural tube defects or intracranial malignant tumors, epilepsy occurred at 2–6 years of age in 33 per cent: 56 per cent in those with gestational ages <32 weeks, and 31 per cent of those born at term.[37] With shunted hydrocephalus, epilepsy occurs in 17–48 per cent.[38,39] The definitions of epilepsy, inclusion criteria, methods of ascertainment and lengths of follow-up vary between studies, but, overall, about one third of children with shunts are affected. Attributions to the shunt operations, shunt complications and shunt revisions also vary.[39] Seizures begin preoperatively in about one third.[39] The highest risks follow infections; lower risks accompany meningomyelocele.[39] Where seizures start after shunt operations the underlying encephalopathy seems more relevant than the surgery.[40]

Neurocutaneous syndromes

The prevalence of tuberous sclerosis is 4–8/100 000 and 60–90 per cent of patients have epilepsy:[41,42] 3–7/100 000 people have tuberous sclerosis and epilepsy. In the largest study of mutational analysis in tuberous sclerosis patients, 91 per cent had a history of epileptic seizures,[43] which were reported in 97 per cent of patients with mutations in the TSC2 gene, in 86 per cent with TSC1 mutations, and in 68 per cent with no identified mutation. Seizures occurred in 99 per cent of patients with and in 73 per cent without mental retardation. The various seizure types and syndromes reported in tuberous sclerosis are discussed further in Chapter 15. In Sturge-Weber syndrome, epilepsy is reported in 71–89 per cent, with onset between ages 0 and 23 years.[44,45] In neurofibromatosis 1, seizures are reported in 4–6 per cent: about 3 per cent fulfill criteria for epilepsy.[46] Although considerably lower than in tuberous sclerosis and Sturge-Weber syndrome, this figure is 3–4 times higher than that found in the general population.

KEY POINTS

- 40–70 children per 100 000 develop epilepsy yearly in **more developed countries**
- The yearly incidence is approximately 50 per cent higher in **less developed countries**
- Children constitute **25 per cent of new cases of epilepsy**, or globally 1.4 million annually
- The incidence is much higher **during the first year of life** than in other periods of childhood
- In the USA, the incidence of epilepsy in children younger than 10 years **decreased** by 40–50 per cent between 1935 and 1984
- In **more developed countries**, 4–5 children per 1000 have active epilepsy
- The prevalence is 50–100 per cent higher in **less developed countries**
- Children constitute **25 per cent of cases with established epilepsy**, or globally 10.5 million, of whom 85 per cent are estimated to get **inappropriate treatment or none at all**
- 1 in 5 children with epilepsy have **cerebral palsy**, and 1 in 3 children with cerebral palsy have epilepsy
- One in 3 children with **hydrocephalus** have epilepsy
- Epilepsy is found in approximately 80 per cent of patients with **tuberous sclerosis** and **Sturge-Weber syndrome**, and in 3 per cent with **neurofibromatosis 1**

REFERENCES

1. Commission on Epidemiology and Prognosis, International League Against Epilepsy. Guidelines for epidemiologic studies on epilepsy. *Epilepsia* 1993; **34**: 592–596.
2. Camfield, CS, Camfield PR, Gordon K, Wirrell E, Dooley JM. Incidence of epilepsy in childhood and adolescence: a population-based study in Nova Scotia from 1977 to 1985. *Epilepsia* 1996; **37**: 19–23.
3. Verity CM, Ross EM, Golding J. Epilepsy in the first 10 years of life: findings of the child health and education study. *BMJ* 1992; **305**: 857–861.
4. Brorson L-O, Wranne L. Long-term prognosis in childhood epilepsy: survival and seizure prognosis. *Epilepsia* 1987; **28**: 324–330.
5. Hauser WA, Annegers JF, Kurland LT. Incidence of epilepsy and unprovoked seizures in Rochester, Minnesota: 1935–1984. *Epilepsia* 1993; **34**: 453–468.
6. Mani KS, Rangan G, Srinivas HV, *et al*. The Yelandur study: a community-based approach to epilepsy in rural South India – epidemiological aspects. *Seizure* 1998; **7**: 281–288.
7. Olafsson E, Hauser WA, Ludvigsson P, Gudmundsson G. Incidence of epilepsy in rural Iceland – a population-based study. *Epilepsia* 1996; **37**: 951–955.

8. Joensen P. Prevalence, incidence, and classification of epilepsy in the Faroes. *Acta Neurologica Scandinavica* 1986; **74**: 150–155.

9. Sidenvall R, Forsgren L, Blomquist H.K. Heijbel J. A community-based prospective incidence study of epileptic seizures in children. *Acta Paediatrica* 1993; **82**: 62–65.

10. Tekle-Haimanot R, Forsgren L, Ekstedt J. Incidence of epilepsy in rural central Ethiopia. *Epilepsia* 1997; **38**: 541–546.

11. Rwiza HT, Kilonzo GP, Haule J, *et al.* Prevalence and incidence of epilepsy in Ulanga, a rural Tanzanian district: a community-based study. *Epilepsia* 1992; **33**: 1051–1056.

12. Lavados J, Germain L, Morales A, Campero M, Lavados P. A descriptive study of epilepsy in the district of El Salvador, Chile, 1984–1988. *Acta Neurologica Scandinavica* 1992; **85**: 249–256.

13. Tsuboi T. Prevalence and incidence of epilepsy in Tokyo. *Epilepsia* 1988; **29**: 103–110.

14. von Wendt L, Rantakallio P, Saukkonen A-L, Mäkinen H. Epilepsy and associated handicaps in a 1 year birth cohort in Northern Finland. *European Journal of Pediatrics* 1985; **144**: 149–151.

15. Beilmann A, Napa A, Sööt A, Talvik I, Talvik T. Prevalence of childhood epilepsy in Estonia. *Epilepsia* 1999; **40**: 1011–1019.

16. Sangrador CO, Luaces RP. Study of the prevalence of epilepsy among school children in Valladolid, Spain. *Epilepsia* 1991; **32**: 791–797.

17. Eriksson KJ, Koivikko MJ. Prevalence, classification, and severity of epilepsy and epileptic syndromes in children. *Epilepsia* 1997; **38**: 1275–1282.

18. Hauser WA, Annegers JF, Kurland LT. Prevalence of epilepsy in Rochester. Minnesota: 1940–1980. *Epilepsia* 1991; **32**: 429–445.

19. Sidenvall R, Forsgren L, Heijbel J. Prevalence and characteristics of epilepsy in children in Northern Sweden. *Seizure* 1996; **5**: 139–146.

20. Endziniene M, Pauza V, Miseviciene I. Prevalence of childhood epilepsy in Kaunas, Lithuania. *Brain Development* 1997; **19**: 379–387.

21. Cavazzuti GB. Epidemiology of different types of epilepsy in school age children of Modena, Italy. *Epilepsia* 1980; **21**: 57–62.

22. Cowan LD, Bodensteiner JB, Leviton A, Doherty L. Prevalence of the epilepsies in children and adolescents. *Epilepsia* 1989; **30**: 94–106.

23. Waaler PE, Blom BH, Skeidsvoll H, Mykletun A. Prevalence, classification, and severity of epilepsy in children in western Norway. *Epilepsia* 2000; **41**: 802–810.

24. Baumann RJ, Marx MB, Leonidakis MG. Epilepsy in rural Kentucky: prevalence in a population of school age children. *Epilepsia* 1978; **19**: 75–80.

25. Christianson AL, Zwane ME, Manga P, *et al.* Epilepsy in rural South African children – prevalence, associated disability and management. *South African Medical Journal* 2000; **90**: 262–266.

26. Nicoletti A, Reggio A, Bartoloni A, *et al.* Prevalence of epilepsy in rural Bolivia. A door-to-door survey. *Neurology* 1999; **53**: 2064–2069.

27. Annegers JF, Hauser WA, Lee JR, Rocca WA. Secular trends and birth cohort effects in unprovoked seizures in Rochester. Minnesota: 1935–1984. *Epilepsia* 1995; **36**: 575–579.

28. Britten N, Wadsworth M.EJ, Fenwick PB.C. Stigma in patients with early epilepsy: a national longitudinal study. *Journal of Epidemiology and Community Health* 1984; **38**: 291–295.

29. Kurtz Z, Tookey P, Ross E. Epilepsy in young people: 23 year follow up of the British national child development study. *BMJ* 1998; **316**: 339–342.

30. Meinardi H, Scott RA, Reis R, Sander JWAS. The treatment gap in epilepsy: the current situation and the way forward. *Epilepsia* 2001; **42**: 136–149.

31. Steffenburg U, Hagberg G, Viggedal G, Kyllerman K. Active epilepsy in mentally retarded children. I. Prevalence and additional neuroimpairments. *Acta Paediatrica* 1995; **84**: 1147–1152.

32. Hauser WA, Shinnar S, Cohen H, Inbar D, Benedetti MD. Clinical predictors of epilepsy among children with cerebral palsy and/or mental retardation. *Neurology* 1987; **37**(Suppl 1): 150.

33. Edebol-Tysk K. Epidemiology of spastic tetrapelgic cerebral palsy in Sweden. I. Impairment and disabilities. *Neuropediatrics* 1989; **20**: 41–5.

34. Uvebrant P. Hemiplegic cerebral palsy. Aetiology and outcome. *Acta Paediatrica Scandinavica* 1988; **345**(Suppl): 1–82.

35. Wallace SJ. Epilepsy in cerebral palsy. *Developmental Medicine and Child Neurology* 2001; **43**: 713–717.

36. Hagberg B, Hagberg G, Olow I, von Wendt L. The changing panorama of cerebral palsy in Sweden. VII. Prevalence and origin in the birth period 1987–90. *Acta Paediatrica* 1996; **85**: 954–960.

37. Fernell E, Hagberg G, Hagberg B. Infantile hydrocephalus – the impact of enhanced preterm survival. *Acta Paediatrica Scandinavica* 1990; **79**: 1080–1086.

38. Saukkonen A.L, Serlo W, von Wendt L. Epilepsy in hydrocephalic children. *Acta Paediatrica Scandinavica* 1990; **79**: 212–218.

39. Sato O, Yamguchi T, Kittaka M, Toyama H. Hydrocephalus and epilepsy. *Child's Nervous System* 2001; **17**: 76–86.

40. Keene DL, Ventureyra EC.G. Hydrocephalus and epileptic seizures. *Child's Nervous System* 1999; **15**: 158–162.

41. Shepherd CW, Beard CM, Gomez MR, Kurland LT, Whisnant JP. Tuberous sclerosis complex in Olmstead County, Minnesota, 1950–1989. *Archives of Neurology* 1991; **48**: 400–401.

42. Ahlsen G, Gillberg C, Lindblom R, Gillberg C. Tuberous sclerosis in Western Sweden. A population study of cases with early childhood onset. *Archives of Neurology* 1994; **51**: 76–81.

43. Dabora SL, Jozwiak S, Franz DN, *et al.* Mutational analysis in a cohort of 224 tuberous sclerosis patients indicates increased severity of TSC2, compared with TSC1, disease in multiple organs. *American Journal of Human Genetics* 2001; **68**: 64–80.

44. Kotagal P, Rothner AD. Epilepsy in the setting of neurocutaneous syndromes. *Epilepsia* 1993; **34**: S71–78.

45. Sujansky E, Conradi S. Outcome of Sturge-Weber syndrome in 52 adults. *American Journal of Medical Genetics* 1995; **57**: 35–45.

46. Kulkantrakorn K, Geller TJ. Seizures in neurofibromatosis 1. *Pediatric Neurology* 1998; **19**: 347–350.

4

Aspects of etiology

4A

Genetics

ROBERT ROBINSON AND R MARK GARDINER

The concept of a genetic predisposition to epilepsy was proposed over 40 years ago.[1] Twin studies have shown that genetic factors are particularly important in the generalized epilepsies but also play a role in the partial epilepsies.[2] The high frequency of monozygotic twins concordant with the same major syndrome suggests the existence of syndrome-specific determinants rather than a single broad predisposition to seizures.

Human genetic epilepsies can be categorized by mechanism of inheritance, whether they are idiopathic (primary) or symptomatic, whether they are generalized or partial and, where known, which class of gene is involved. The mechanism of inheritance identifies three major groups:

- **mendelian epilepsies:** mutations in a single gene can account for segregation of the disease trait
- **non-mendelian or 'complex' epilepsies:** several loci interact with environmental factors to produce the pattern of familial clustering. These include epilepsies which exhibit a maternal inheritance pattern due to mutations in mitochondrial DNA
- **chromosomal disorders:** in which the epilepsy results from a gross cytogenetic abnormality (see Chapter 4B).

The most commonly observed mendelian epilepsies are 'symptomatic'. Recurrent seizures result from one or more identifiable structural lesions, and are often one component of a diverse neurological phenotype. Over 200 mendelian diseases include epilepsy as part of the phenotype, but the mechanism of seizure generation is often indirect. The genetic bases of these disorders are considered in other chapters. The idiopathic epilepsies rarely display a mendelian inheritance pattern, but tend to show 'complex' inheritance and, often, age-dependant penetrance, with peak onset in childhood. Although rare, the idiopathic mendelian epilepsies have provided the major recent advances in the molecular basis of the epilepsies. Mutations have been identified in families segregating benign familial neonatal convulsions (BFNC), autosomal dominant nocturnal frontal lobe epilepsy (ADNFLE), generalized epilepsy with febrile seizures plus (GEFS+), childhood absence epilepsy with febrile seizures (CAE with FS), autosomal dominant partial epilepsy with auditory features (ADPEAF) and X-linked infantile spasms (ISSX) (Table 4A.1). Other than ADPEAF and ISSX, all mutations occur in genes encoding ion channels, identifying some idiopathic mendelian epilepsies as channelopathies. These also demonstrate both locus heterogeneity (mutations in more than one gene causing the same clinical phenotype) and phenotypic heterogeneity (mutations in the same gene causing different clinical phenotypes). Successful determination of the molecular genetic basis of the common familial epilepsies has been relatively slow. No gene identified in a mendelian epilepsy has been shown to act as a major locus in any non-mendelian epilepsy, and the extent of heterogeneity is likely to be far greater in the complex epilepsies.

STRATEGIES FOR MOLECULAR GENETIC ANALYSIS OF CHILDHOOD EPILEPSY

Strategies applied to mendelian diseases

A range of approaches to the investigation of the molecular basis of human inherited disease have been most successful in mendelian diseases. Positional cloning,

Table 4A.1 *Genes identified in idiopathic (primary) epilepsies*

Gene class	Gene	Gene location	Epilepsy syndrome(s)	Inheritance	Key references
Voltage-dependent ion channels					
Sodium channels	SCN1A	2q24	GEFS+	AD	44
			SMEI		45
	SCN2A	2q23-q24	GEFS+		47
	SCN1B	19q13			41
Potassium channels	KCNQ2	20q	BFNC	AD	10, 14
	KCNQ3	8q24			13, 18
	KCNA1	12p13	EA1 with partial epilepsy	AD	127
Ligand-gated ion channels					
Nicotinic acetylcholine receptors	CHRNA4	20q13.2	ADNFLE	AD	30, 31, 32
	CHRNB2	1p21			38
GABA_A receptor	GABRG2	5q34	GEFS+	AD	48
			FS with CAE		49
	GABRA1	5q34	ADJME	AD	84
Adhesive protein/receptor					
Leucine-rich, glioma inactivated protein	LGI1	10q24	ADPEAF	AD	52, 54
Transcription factor					
Aristaless-related, homeobox gene	ARX	Xp22.3-p21.1	ISSX	X-linked	63

GEFS+, generalized epilepsy with febrile seizures plus; SMEI, severe myoclonic epilepsy of infancy; BFNC, benign familial neonatal convulsions; EA1, episodic ataxia type 1; ADNFLE, autosomal dominant nocturnal frontal lobe epilepsy; FS, febrile seizures; CAE, childhood absence epilepsy; ADJME, autosomal dominant juvenile myoclonic epilepsy; ADPEAF, autosomal dominant partial epilepsy with auditory features; ISSX, X-linked infantile spasms.

candidate gene identification and mutational analysis have allowed the identification of several mendelian epilepsy genes. The complex epilepsies have generally proved resistant to these strategies.

POSITIONAL CLONING

This approach uses linkage analysis to map a gene locus to a small chromosomal region. Linkage analysis tests polymorphic genetic markers distributed across the genome (a 'genome-wide' scan) for co-segregation (linkage) with the disease phenotype. A single large pedigree or several small pedigrees are required. A 'linked' marker has undergone few recombinations with the causative gene during meiosis and therefore lies on the same chromosomal segment. A physical map of a linked chromosomal region can then be constructed, and coding DNA sequences identified for mutation screening. Linkage analysis as a method for mapping disease genes in humans was revolutionized by the development of methods for detecting polymorphism at the DNA level and a comprehensive genetic marker map of the human genome consisting of 5264 simple sequence length polymorphisms.[3]

Postitional cloning has led to the identification of disease genes for a large number of mendelian disorders including several epilepsies (Table 4A.1). There has recently been some limited success in a non-mendelian disorder, Crohn disease.[4,5] However, the statistical power of this approach is greatly reduced by genetic heterogeneity, uncertainty concerning the mode of inheritance and penetrance of disease alleles, and several other confounding factors. The family resource required is thus often unattainable, and linkage analysis has not yet led to the identification of a disease causing mutation in a non-mendelian epilepsy.

CANDIDATE GENE IDENTIFICATION

Classes of candidate gene for human epilepsies can be identified from studies on the mechanisms of seizure generation, isolation of genes causing seizures in animal models of human epilepsy, and linkage and association studies in humans. There is much evidence for the role of ion channels and related proteins in neuronal excitability and seizure generation, and ion channel genes have been identified in several murine and human epilepsies. Over 220 ion channel genes have now been identified, of which at least 100 are neuronally expressed. The neuronal ion channels are divided into those that are ligand-gated and those that are voltage-dependent (see Chapter 6). The former include the GABA_A receptors, glutamate receptors, neuronal nicotinic acetylcholine receptors and ligand-gated potassium channels, whilst the latter include the voltage-dependent sodium, potassium, calcium and chloride channels. Once identified, the role of a candidate gene in the etiology of a genetic epilepsy can be examined either by linkage analysis or by direct mutational analysis of the gene in affected individuals.

MUTATIONAL ANALYSIS

Several methodologies are now available for the identification of potential disease-causing mutations in candidate genes. These include single strand conformational polymorphism (SSCP), heteroduplex analysis, oligonucleotide arrays and direct sequencing. Functionally important regions of the gene are screened for mutations, and any identified sequence variant is then evaluated to determine its significance. The association of a mutation with the disease trait can be investigated both in family-based linkage studies and in population-based association studies. The functional consequences of a sequence variation depend in part on the location relative to the gene, pathogenic mutations usually occurring within the coding sequence of the gene but also occurring in intragenic noncoding sequences or regulatory sequences outside exons. Similarly, a functional variant is likely to alter a highly conserved amino acid or affect a splice site or stop codon. Ultimately, the effect of a mutation on gene expression and protein function may be investigated using a variety of *in vivo* and *in vitro* techniques.

Strategies applied to non–mendelian diseases

The methods of linkage analysis and positional cloning which are so powerful when applied to mendelian disorders are much less useful for those traits which display so-called 'complex' inheritance. Although there is increased familial clustering, segregation in families cannot be explained by the effect of a locus with dominant or recessive disease alleles. Interaction of several loci, each exerting a small effect, together with environmental factors is assumed. Such 'complex' traits include the common familial idiopathic generalized epilepsies.

VARIATION IN THE HUMAN GENOME

Two human genomes are, on average, 99.9 per cent identical. The 0.1 per cent which differs is mostly represented by so-called single-nucleotide polymorphisms (SNPs): single base pairs at which different alleles (bases) exist in normal individuals in some populations, with the minor allele frequency greater than 1 per cent. Most of these SNPs are 'neutral', but a subset with functional consequences is likely to include the allelic variation that accounts for common disease traits.

The second important issue is the nature and extent of linkage disequilibrium (LD) in the human genome. LD is the nonrandom occurrence of specific alleles at adjacent loci. Extensive blocks of LD are present, at least in the northern European population, which create haplotypes between 25 and 100 kb long.[6] It appears that a small number of SNPs in each gene will allow the most common haplotypes of that gene present in a given population to be determined.

GENETIC ARCHITECTURE OF 'COMPLEX' DISEASES

This has a major influence on the optimal strategy for detecting susceptibility loci responsible for 'complex' disease traits. Alleles at loci determining mendelian traits are rare (low frequency) and of major effect (highly penetrant). The same trait may be caused by rare, high-penetrance alleles at distinct loci (locus heterogeneity), and at a given locus many different disease alleles may occur (allelic heterogeneity).

Alleles at susceptibility loci are of small effect and likely to be of relatively high frequency (>1 per cent). The number of loci, the magnitude of their individual effect on risk, their mode of interaction and the number and population frequency of susceptibility alleles underlying any particular trait is unknown. Oligogenic traits with a few loci of significant effect represent one end of the spectrum, with truly polygenic traits caused by numerous loci of small effect at the other end. The 'common disease–common variant' hypothesis assumes that there is allelic homogeneity at each locus with the susceptibility allele present at high frequency (>5–10 per cent).[7]

LINKAGE OR ASSOCIATION

In linkage analysis co-segregation within pedigrees is sought between an anonymous polymorphism or candidate gene and a disease trait. Linkage can be carried out on large collections of nuclear pedigrees or affected sibling pairs. Unfortunately the power of linkage analysis is low if individual loci exert a small effect on the phenotype, or if there is extensive locus heterogeneity. Thus, adequate power to detect linkage can only be attained with numbers of pedigrees above the number it is practicable to ascertain. Numerous linkage analyses using a 'genome-wide' approach in other complex traits have failed to identify linked loci which have been highly significant (statistically), replicable or have led on to positional cloning of a susceptibility gene. Anyhow, in 'complex' traits, linkage cannot provide high-resolution localization and positive results usually cover very large chromosomal regions. Association studies detect nonrandom associations between a trait and either an allele or group of alleles in linkage disequilibrium (a haplotype). The control sample of chromosomes can be taken from a population, or, transmission of alleles from a heterozygous parent can be analyzed (intrafamilial association). Allelic association has greater power to detect susceptibility alleles of smaller effect, but is critically dependent on the 'common disease–common variant' hypothesis being true for a particular trait.[8] If a wide diversity of low-frequency alleles causes susceptibility, association would be difficult or impossible to detect.

CANDIDATE GENE OR GENOME–WIDE SEARCH

Both linkage and association can be used to evaluate the role of candidate genes or used to scan the entire genome without making assumptions about the genes likely to be involved. Candidate genes are identified on functional grounds, based on the likely biological pathways involved in the trait. For idiopathic epilepsies it is possible to identify about 150 candidate genes encoding ion channels and related molecules. Linkage analysis is undertaken using highly informative 'microsatellite' loci (usually dinucleotide repeats) either in or flanking the genes. Association analysis uses haplotype-tag SNPs, a set of 6–8 SNPs which identify the common haplotypes for the gene. These may or may not include the 'functional' SNPs which represent the actual disease-causing sequence variations.

For many 'complex' traits it is impossible to guess which genes are good candidates on functional grounds. The underlying biology is too obscure. Under these circumstances a 'genome-wide' scan is undertaken. For linkage this usually involves typing a grid of about 350 'microsatellite' loci which cover the entire genome at intervals of about 10 cM. In future, this will involve using a SNP-based HapMap, a map of haplotype 'blocks' in the genome-chromosomal regions within which a set of SNPs are in LD.

TECHNOLOGICAL FACTORS

These strategies involve making several million observations: typing large numbers of SNPs in hundreds or thousands of individuals. Current methods for doing this are both slow and expensive, but new high-throughput procedures are developing rapidly.

GENETICS OF CHILDHOOD EPILEPSIES

Mendelian epilepsies

Over 200 mendelian diseases include epilepsy as part of the phenotype. The small number of primary epilepsies which are inherited in a mendelian fashion are described here. Although they account for only a small number of epilepsy cases, recognition of the characteristic features and presence of a family history enable a correct diagnosis to be made. Identification of genes responsible for some of these disorders has provided valuable insights into the molecular mechanisms underlying epilepsy.

BENIGN FAMILIAL NEONATAL CONVULSIONS (See Chapter 7)

Benign familial neonatal convulsions (BFNC), a rare autosomal dominant idiopathic epilepsy, was the first epilepsy to be localized by linkage analysis.[9] Seizures occur in otherwise well neonates from day 2 or 3 of life and remit by week 2–3. BFNC is a good illustration of both clinical and genetic heterogeneity, the latter of which can be explained by the underlying molecular genetics. The first locus (EBN1) was identified on chromosome 20q by linkage analysis in a 4-generation family with 19 affected individuals.[10] Six other pedigrees confirmed this linkage.[11] However, another family which showed linkage to EBN1 included members with seizures persisting up to 2 years of age, and in one individual, into adolescence.[12] Another family, none of whose members had seizures after 2 months of age, could be excluded from linkage to EBN1, and was subsequently linked to a second locus (EBN2) on chromosome 8q.[13] The gene for EBN1, KCNQ2, was identified by characterization of a submicroscopic deletion on chromosome 20q13.3 and shows significant homology with a voltage-dependent delayed rectifying potassium channel gene, KCNQ1.[14] Members of the KCNQ potassium channel family comprise six transmembrane-spanning segments (S1–S6), a pore-forming loop linking S5 and S6, and intracellular N- and C-termini. These channels are involved in the repolarization of the action potential and thus in the electrical excitability of nerve and muscle. Mutations in KCNQ1 can cause the paroxysmal cardiac dysrhythmias long QT syndrome and Jervell-Lange-Nielson cardioauditory syndrome.[15,16] Six allelic variants of KCNQ2 segregate with the disease in families with BFNC, including one family whose affected members subsequently developed myokymia.[17] All mutations involve regions of the gene important for ion conduction.

Following identification of KCNQ2, a BLAST (basic local alignment search tool) search was made of the human expressed sequence tag (EST) database, to find cDNA sequences showing significant homology to KCNQ2. Rather fortuitously, a novel gene, KCNQ3, was identified with 69 per cent similarity to KCNQ2, which mapped to the EBN2 critical region on chromosome 8q24, and was found to be mutated in affected members of the BFNC/EBN2 family.[18] The missense mutation identified altered a conserved amino acid in the critical pore-forming region (the same amino acid found to be mutated in KCNQ1 in a patient with long QT syndrome).[15]

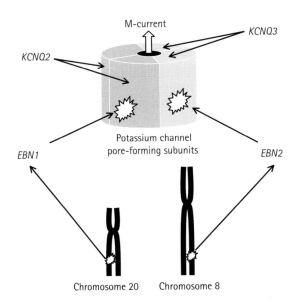

Figure 4A.1 *Mutations at either benign familial neonatal convulsions (BFNC) locus, EBN1 (KCNQ2) or EBN2 (KCNQ3) disrupt the heteromeric M-channel (potassium conductance) and result in an identical phenotype.*

KCNQ2 and KCNQ3 are co-expressed in most areas of the brain, especially the hippocampus, neocortex and cerebellum. They have been shown to co-assemble and form a heteromeric channel with essentially identical biophysical properties and pharmacologic sensitivities to the native neuronal M-channel.[19] The M-channel is a slowly activating and deactivating potassium conductance that plays a critical role in determining the subthreshold electroexcitability of neurons. Figure 4A.1 shows how mutations in either KCNQ2 or KCNQ3 disrupt the native M-current and result in an identical disease phenotype.

BENIGN FAMILIAL INFANTILE CONVULSIONS (BFIC)

This mendelian idiopathic epilepsy was first described as an autosomal dominant disorder in families of Italian origin,[20] and later in France and Singapore.[21,22] Partial or generalized seizures commenced between 3 and 12 months. Response to conventional antiepilepsy drugs was good, with resolution of seizures and no psychomotor retardation.

Gene mapping has demonstrated locus heterogeneity. A locus, BFIC1, was mapped to chromosome 19q.[23] A common haplotype was evident, suggesting a founder effect. A second locus, BFIC2, was mapped to 16p12-q12[24] and a third, BFIC3, to 2q24.[25] The disease genes have yet to be identified: it is possible that BFIC2 is an allelic variant of the gene causing infantile convulsions with choreoathetosis (ICCA) which maps to the same region.

FAMILIAL INFANTILE CONVULSIONS AND PAROXYSMAL CHOREOATHETOSIS (ICCA)

First described in four families from northwestern France, benign infantile convulsions was inherited as an autosomal dominant trait combined with paroxysmal choreoathetosis. A genome-wide screen gave evidence of linkage to the pericentromeric region of chromosome 16 encompassing a 10 cM interval 16p12-q12.[26] Confirmation of linkage to this region has subsequently been reported in a Chinese family.[27] Another phenotype, autosomal recessive rolandic epilepsy with paroxysmal exercise-induced dystonia and writer's cramp, maps to a region encompassed by the ICCA critical region.[28]

AUTOSOMAL DOMINANT NOCTURNAL FRONTAL LOBE EPILEPSY (ADNFLE)

First described in six families from Australia, Canada and the UK, ADNFLE is characterized by the occurrence of partial seizures almost exclusively during sleep.[29] There is a pronounced variation in severity among family members, and penetrance is incomplete (approximately 70 per cent). Seizures begin predominantly in childhood in individuals who are neurologically and intellectually normal, persist into adulthood, occur in clusters soon after falling asleep or before waking, and are characterized by brief tonic or hyperkinetic motor activity with retention of consciousness, although secondary generalization often occurs.

Linkage analysis in a single large Australian pedigree with 27 individuals assigned the gene to chromosome 20q13.2.[30] The gene for the α4 subunit of the neuronal nicotinic acetylcholine receptor (nAChR), CHRNA4, was known to map to the same chromosomal region, and also to be expressed in the frontal cortex. Mutational analysis of CHRNA4 identified a missense mutation that co-segregated with the disease in the chromosome 20-linked family.[31] The mutation converts a serine to phenylalanine in the M2 transmembrane domain, a crucial structure mediating ionic permeability, and is likely to be disease causing. Further site specific mutations in CHRNA4 affecting pore-forming amino acids have been associated with ADNFLE.[32–36]

In another family, a second locus was mapped to chromosome 15q24.[37] A cluster of nAChR genes (CHRNA3/CHRNA5/CHRNB4) in this region seemed good candidates, but no mutations were identified in the pore-forming regions. However, mutations have been identified in the gene for the β2 subunit of the nAChR, CHRNB2, on chromosome 1p21.[38,39] The main neuronal nAChR has a heteropentameric structure comprised of α4 and β2 subunits. Thus mutations in the pore-forming M2 domains of both CHRNA4 and CHRNB2 can produce similar functional effects causing the ADNFLE phenotype.

GENERALIZED EPILEPSY WITH FEBRILE SEIZURES PLUS SEVERE MYOCLONIC EPILEPSY OF INFANCY (GEFS+)

GEFS+ was first described in 1997.[40] Geneological information was obtained on 2000 family members dating back to the mid-1700s, and clinical information on 289 individuals, of whom 28 had seizures. The commonest phenotype comprised a childhood onset of multiple febrile seizures persisting beyond the age of 6 years, as well as a spectrum of afebrile seizures including absences, myclonic seizures, atonic seizures and rarely myoclonic-astatic epilepsy. Inheritance was autosomal dominant.

A second family with GEFS+ was linked to chromosome 19q13.1, and a point mutation identified in *SCN1B*, which encodes the β1 subunit of the voltage-gated sodium channel.[41]

Neuronal voltage-gated sodium channels contain a large α subunit associated with two smaller β subunits. The pore-forming α subunit contains four homologous domains each containing six membrane-spanning units. The β subunits contain a single transmembrane region, modulate the gating properties of the channel and are required for normal inactivation kinetics. Mutations in α subunit genes cause several paroxysmal disorders of muscle, including hyperkalemic periodic paralysis, paramyotonia congenita (*SCN4A*) and long QT syndrome (*SCN5A*).[42] Sodium channels are also modulated by AEDs such as phenytoin and carbamazepine.[43] They are thus good candidate genes for epilepsy.

The *SCN1B* mutation segregated with disease status in the 19q13.1-linked GEFS+ family. It changes a conserved cysteine residue that disrupts a disulfide bridge normally maintaining an extracellular immunoglobulin-like fold in the β subunit. After some intermediary effects, this results in persistent inward neuronal sodium currents, increased membrane depolarization, and neuronal hyperexcitability. This may also exaggerate the normal effects of temperature on both conductance and gating of neuronal sodium channels, explaining the apparent temperature dependence of the GEFS+ phenotype.

Two further families with GEFS+ showed linkage to chromosome 2q24, and mutations were identified in *SCN1A*, the gene encoding the sodium channel α1 subunit.[44] *De novo* mutations in this gene have also been identified in patients with severe myoclonic epilepsy of infancy (SMEI), which also involves fever-associated seizures.[45] Many patients with SMEI have a family history of seizures consistent with the spectrum of seizure phenotypes seen in GEFS+, suggesting that SMEI is the most severe phenotype in the GEFS+ spectrum.[46] A mutation in the gene encoding the α2 sodium channel subunit, *SCN2A*, has now been identified in a patient with febrile seizures associated with afebrile seizures, consistent with GEFS+. This mutation also slows channel inactivation, suggesting involvement in the epilepsy phenotype.[47]

The GEFS+ phenotype is not only caused by mutations in voltage-gated sodium channels. In one large GEFS+ family, mutations have been identified in the GABA$_A$ receptor γ subunit gene, *GABRG2*.[48] Binding of GABA opens an integral chloride channel, with resultant inhibition of neuronal activity. The GEFS+ mutation substitutes a serine for a methionine in the extracellular loop between transmembrane segments M2 and M3. Mutations in *GABRG2* also cause a phenotype of childhood absence epilepsy and febrile seizures.[49]

AUTOSOMAL DOMINANT PARTIAL EPILEPSY WITH AUDITORY FEATURES

Autosomal dominant partial epilepsy with auditory features (ADPEAF) was first described in a three-generation family with an idiopathic/cryptogenic epilepsy.[50] Starting between 8 and 19 years, infrequent, both simple and partial complex seizures progressed to secondarily generalized tonic-clonic seizures. Six of the 11 affected members reported auditory disturbances as a simple partial component of their seizures. A genome screen identified linkage over a 10-cM region on chromosome 10q23.3–24.[50] This region was narrowed to 3 cM by a genome screen in a large family segregating lateral temporal lobe epilepsy with auditory and visual features.[51] Construction of a physical map identified 28 putative genes of which 21 were sequenced in an affected individual from three families, and mutations subsequently checked in a further two families.[52] Mutations were identified in the leucine rich, glioma-inactivated 1 gene (*LGI1*) in all affected individuals and obligate carriers, as well as six unaffected members, consistent with a 71 per cent disease penetrance. The five mutations identified were not present in 123 unrelated controls.

LGI1 is a member of the leucine-rich repeat (LRR) superfamily, in particular the adhesive proteins and receptors. The *LGI1* protein consists of an extracellular domain with LRR repeat motifs, a transmembrane segment and an intracellular segment of unknown function.[53] The extracellular portion aligns most closely with a group of proteins involved in CNS development and in which the LRRs bind nerve growth factor and other neurotrophins. Interestingly, a C-terminal repeat motif, now referred to as the EAR (epilepsy-associated repeat) domain, has been identified in both *LGI1* and the *MASS1* gene, which is mutated in the Frings mouse model of audiogenic epilepsy.[54] This EAR domain is likely to play a role in the pathogenesis of epilepsy. *LGI1* is expressed predominantly in brain, muscle and spinal cord. Of the five mutations identified in ADPEA, three were missense mutations with predicted premature truncation of the *LGI1* protein, one was a nonsynonymous point mutation in the highly conserved extracellular and C-terminal region, and one was an intronic mutation predicted to alter a splice site. *LGI1* is therefore the first non-ion-channel gene identified as causing an idiopathic epilepsy in humans.

FAMILIAL PARTIAL EPILEPSY WITH VARIABLE FOCI (FPEVF) (See Chapter 6)

This idiopathic epilepsy displays autosomal dominant inheritance with reduced penetrance and locus heterogeneity. In an Australian pedigree, linkage with chromosome 2 was suggested,[55] and, subsequently, in two large French-Canadian families, with chromosome 22q11-q12.[56] Recurring partial seizures originate from different cortical areas, usually in the frontal or temporal lobes. The epileptic focus varies between family members.

INFANTILE SPASMS (WEST SYNDROME)

Infantile spasms are divided into those that are symptomatic and those that are cryptogenic or idiopathic. The majority (70–80 per cent) are symptomatic and may be attributed to a prenatal, perinatal or postnatal cause, of which prenatal etiologies are the most common (50 per cent). Many of these are genetically determined, including disorders of brain development, neurocutaneous syndromes, metabolic disorders and chromosomal abnormalities. These conditions are dealt with elsewhere.

Most cases of idiopathic infantile spasms are sporadic, and the recurrence risk is less than 1 per cent.[57] However, several familial cases have been identified consistent with X-linked inheritance. Feinberg and Leahy first reported five affected males in four sibships of a three-generation family.[58] Subsequently, five further families have been identified, some of which also include individuals with X-linked mental retardation without infantile spasms.[59–63] Linkage analysis in these families mapped the disease gene to chromosome Xp21.3-Xp22.1.[60–62] The *aristaless*-related homeobox gene, *ARX*, was considered a candidate on the basis of its expression pattern in fetal, infant and adult brain. Screening of this gene identified mutations in four of the five families with infantile spasms.[63] Mutations were also identified in five families with mental retardation together with myoclonic seizures or dystonia, but no infantile spasms. Two recurrent mutations identified in seven of the nine families result in expansion of polyalanine tracts of the ARX protein. These are likely to cause protein aggregation, as has been demonstrated in other human diseases caused by alanine expansions.[64] Homeobox-containing genes are known to be important in the regulation of key stages of development. ARX encodes one of a class of proteins incorporating a C-terminal *aristaless* domain thought to be particularly important in the differentiation and maintenance of specific neuronal subtypes in the cerebral cortex.[65]

Non-mendelian epilepsies

JUVENILE MYOCLONIC EPILEPSY (JME)
(see Chapter 12B)

JME accounts for 5–10 per cent of all epilepsy. It was first described as a distinct electroclinical syndrome in 1957.[66] In addition to myoclonic seizures, which occur predominantly in the morning, nearly all affected individuals have generalized tonic-clonic seizures, often following a series of myoclonic jerks, and about 20–40 per cent have absence seizures. Photosensitivity is common.

A genetic contribution to the etiology of JME is well established,[67–69] but the mode of inheritance is uncertain. Autosomal dominant,[70] autosomal recessive[71] and two-locus models have all been proposed.[72] Evidence for linkage of the JME trait to the serologic markers HLA and properdin factor B on chromosome 6p was first found in 1988,[73] and the locus designated *EJM1*. Subsequently confirmation was obtained in a separately ascertained group of 23 families using HLA serologic markers.[74] Analysis of a subset of these families, together with one new family, using HLA-DQ restriction fragment length polymorphisms (RFLPs), gave similar results.[75] Further work on a larger group of families confirmed linkage to the serologic markers HLA and properdin factor B, with a maximum lod score of 4.2 obtained at $\theta_{m,f}$ (recombination fraction) of 0.01.[76] Another study in a single large pedigree, using microsatellite markers on chromosome 6p, gave a maximum lod score of 3.67 ($\theta = 0$) between the marker D6S257 and a trait defined as the presence of clinical JME or an EEG showing diffuse 3.5–6 Hz multispike and slow wave complexes.[77] In addition, linkage analysis in 28 families ascertained through a JME patient in which family members with IGE were classified as affected gave a lod score for the *DQB1* locus of 4.2 at $\theta_{m,f} = 0.5, 0.1$. The linkage pattern observed suggested heterogeneity and an excess of transmission from mothers.[78]

Two studies from a single group have failed to find evidence for the existence of a locus on chromosome 6p.[79,80] These results suggest that genetic heterogeneity may exist within the JME phenotype.

Chromosomal regions harboring genes for subunits of the neuronal nicotinic acetylcholine receptor were tested for linkage to the JME trait in 35 pedigrees. Two-point lod scores were negative for all loci except *D15S128* and *D15S118* on chromosome 15q14. Seven additional marker loci encompassing a 20.1-cM region were selected in order to investigate this region further. A maximum multipoint lod score of 4.18 was obtained under the assumption of heterogeneity at $\alpha = 0.64$ (where α is the proportion of linked families). Analysis of recombinant events defined the 10-cM interval between *D15S144* and *D15S1012* as being the region in which the gene lies. The α7 subunit of the neuronal nicotinic acetylcholine receptor

(*CHRNA7*) maps within this interval and therefore represents an excellent candidate gene. These results indicate that a major susceptibility locus for JME may map to this region of chromosome 15q.[81]

More recently, linkage analysis with 7 microsatellite markers encompassing the *CHRNA7* region failed to replicate evidence of linkage in 11 families with at least two JME members. No evidence in favor of linkage to 15q14 was found under a broadened diagnostic scheme in 27 families of JME probands or in 30 families of probands with idiopathic absence epilepsy.[82] A subsequent study has clarified the linkage data in relation to the current map of the region under study.[83] The *CHRNA7* gene and its partial duplication *CHRFAM7A* were screened for mutations, but no causative sequence variants could be identified.

Linkage analysis in an extended autosomal dominant JME pedigree mapped the locus to 5q34, and a missense mutation (Ala 322 Asp) was identified in the *GABRA1* gene.[84]

CHILDHOOD ABSENCE EPILEPSY (CAE)
(Chapter 11A)

In CAE a genetic component is well established, but the mechanism of inheritance and the genes involved are unknown. Studies of familial clustering indicate that CAE has a 'complex' non-mendelian mode of inheritance.[85] Approximately 1.6 per cent of siblings of probands with CAE will have absence epilepsy, giving a λ_s (the risk to a sibling of an affected proband compared with the population risk) of at least 27.[86] However one segregation analysis was consistent with autosomal dominant inheritance with reduced penetrance.[87] From studies on the mechanism by which spike-wave seizures are generated; isolation of genes causing spike-wave seizures in rodents; and initial linkage and association studies in humans, a number of candidate genes and chromosomal regions can be identified for CAE.

Possible mechanisms for the generation of abnormal spike-wave activities in cortical and thalamic neurons include the loss of $GABA_A$ receptor-mediated inhibition between thalamic reticular cells, strong activation of thalamic GABAergic neurons by corticothalamic or thalamocortical afferents, or the enhancement of the low-threshold Ca^{2+} current.[88–92] Four mouse models of spike-wave epilepsy are caused by mutations in genes for different subunits of voltage-dependent calcium channels (VDCCs): tottering *tg*, *Cacna1a*;[93] lethargic *lh*, *Cacnb4*;[94] stargazer *stg*, *Cacng2*;[95] ducky *du*, *Cacna2d2*.[96] In addition, an association has been documented between polymorphisms in *CACNA1A* and IGE including CAE,[97] and novel *CACNA1A* mutations have been identified in a boy with episodic ataxia type 2 and absence epilepsy,[98] and in another boy with progressive and episodic ataxia, learning difficulties and absence epilepsy.[99]

Linkage analysis of a five-generation family in which affected patients had a persisting form of CAE provided evidence for a locus on chromosome 8q24.[100] The candidate region for this locus, designated *ECA1*, has been refined, but a gene remains to be identified.[101] Study of another extended pedigree in which affected individuals manifested both CAE and febrile seizures revealed a linked marker on chromosome 5 close to a cluster of genes encoding $GABA_A$ receptor subunits.[49] A mutation was found in *GABRG2* which changes a conserved amino acid and this appeared to contribute to the CAE phenotype. Mutations in this gene have also been identified in a family segregating GEFS+.[48] A possible association has also been documented between a polymorphism in *GABRB3* and patients with CAE,[102] and suggestive linkage to this gene found in eight families.[103] *GABRB3* maps to 15q11-q13, the region deleted in Angelman syndrome,[104] and mice with targeted disruption of the *GABRB3* gene have the epilepsy phenotype and behavioral characteristics of Angelman syndrome.[105]

The hypothesis that mutations in genes encoding $GABA_A$ receptor subunits, $GABA_B$ receptors or brain expressed voltage-dependent calcium channels, as well as unidentified candidate genes in the *ECA1* region on chromosome 8q24, may underlie CAE was tested by linkage analysis in 33 families.[106] Twenty-seven of 29 genes tested, as well as the *ECA1* region, were excluded as major loci in these families. One voltage-dependent calcium channel gene, *CACNG3* on chromosome 16p12-p13.1, and the cluster of $GABA_A$ receptor genes, *GABRA5*, *GABRB3*, and *GABRG3* on chromosome 15q11-q13, could not be excluded.

BENIGN CHILDHOOD EPILEPSY WITH CENTROTEMPORAL SPIKES (BCECTS)
(Chapter 11D)

BCECTS was first described in 1958.[107] Seizures begin between the ages of 3 and 13 in a child who is neurologically intact. Typically, they often occur at night and are preceded by a somatosensory aura around the mouth and followed by excessive salivation and speech arrest with retention of consciousness. Unilateral motor seizures of the face follow and can progress to a secondary generalization.[108] The pattern of the seizures varies diurnally, with nocturnal seizures more likely to generalize secondarily.[109] Seizures rarely persist beyond the age of 16 years. The EEG is characteristic. About 20 per cent of children who have Rolandic discharges on EEG will not have seizures.[110]

A family history of epilepsy is common, although the proportion varies from study to study, from 9 to 59 per cent.[111,112] In families of 40 patients with seizures and centrotemporal spikes, 36 per cent of siblings and 19 per cent of parents had focal epileptiform activity on the

EEG.[113] In a further 19 probands with BCECTS,[114] 15 of 34 siblings had Rolandic discharges and seizures, and a further 19 per cent had Rolandic discharges in isolation. These findings tend to support the suggestion of an autosomal dominant gene with age-dependent penetrance.

Generalized epileptiform activity has also been found in the EEGs of 26 out of 69 (38 per cent) siblings of 43 probands with BCECTS.[115] Among those siblings aged 5–12 years, 54 per cent had abnormal EEGs: the proportion declined in the younger and older age groups. This pattern of age-dependent penetrance and the finding of generalized EEG abnormalities in the siblings of patients has led to the suggestion that BCECTS and absence epilepsy may be linked.[116]

Twenty-two nuclear families segregating BCECTS were examined for linkage to chromosomal regions known to harbor neuronal nicotinic acetylcholine receptor (nAChR) subunit genes. Evidence was found for linkage with heterogeneity to a region on chromosome 15q14 in the vicinity of the α7 nAChR subunit gene, CHRNA7.[117]

FEBRILE SEIZURES (Chapter 8)

Susceptibility to febrile seizures clearly has a strong genetic basis, and a significant proportion of patients have a family history of febrile convulsions or other epilepsies. The proportion of probands with an affected first-degree relative has been estimated as between 8 per cent and 49 per cent.[118,119] The mode of inheritance seems to depend on the frequency of febrile seizures in the proband. Complex segregation analysis performed on 467 nuclear families, ascertained through probands with febrile seizures, showed clear evidence for polygenic inheritance in those families in which the proband had a single febrile seizure,[118] where the heritability of liability was estimated at 68 per cent. However, in the families of probands with more than three febrile seizures, there appeared to be a single major locus contributing to seizure susceptibility. Another study of the families of 52 probands with febrile seizures found that 40 families (77 per cent) had at least one further affected member, and this was consistent with an autosomal dominant mode of inheritance with reduced penetrance (64 per cent).[120]

The investigation of large pedigrees has led to the identification of several putative loci: FEB1 on chromosome 8q13-q21;[121] FEB2 on chromosome19p13.3;[122] FEB3 on chromosome 2q23–24;[123] and FEB4 on chromosome 5q14-q15.[124] A mutation in GABRG2 was identified in a family whose individuals manifested febrile seizures with or without CAE.[41] Febrile seizures occur as a part of the syndrome of GEFS+, for which several genes have been identified. The phenotype of the FEB2 family did resemble GEFS+, and FEB2 may correspond to one of the two GEFS+ loci on chromosome 2q.

Genetic counseling

The provision of genetic counseling requires knowledge of the mode of inheritance and recurrence risk of a particular epilepsy syndrome. The wide variety of conditions in which epilepsy can occur necessitates a completely accurate diagnosis. Any associated symptoms and signs must be considered and appropriate investigations arranged to differentiate a symptomatic from an idiopathic epilepsy, identify any underlying structural lesion and define the epilepsy syndrome involved. Construction of a pedigree may suggest the mode of inheritance, and in some cases help to diagnose a particular epilepsy syndrome.

For epilepsies displaying mendelian inheritance, the increasing availability of DNA-based diagnostics will allow presymptomatic diagnosis of individuals at risk. However, variable penetrance introduces an element of uncertainty. In the more common familial epilepsies displaying complex inheritance, the identification of susceptibility genes should help to delineate specific epilepsy syndromes and allow DNA analysis to improve the accuracy of recurrence risk calculation. However, at present, recurrence risks remain empirical.

The overall incidence of epilepsy in the offspring of epileptic parents is between 1.7 and 7.3 per cent, including febrile seizures and single seizures.[125] This compares with a cumulative incidence of epilepsy in the general population up to the age of 40 years of approximately 1.7 per cent.[126] However, unless the pedigree reveals a particular inheritance pattern, the recurrence risk quoted must depend on available information for the particular epilepsy concerned. Table 4A.2 provides a guide to recurrence risks to offspring or siblings for particular epilepsy diagnoses, although the diagnostic criteria used in the various studies are not always consistent.

The future

The major challenge is the identification of susceptibility genes for the common familial epilepsies. Publication of the draft version of the complete human genome sequence was a significant advance, but huge challenges remain in the field of human genomics. These include completion of the human genome sequence, annotation of the genome by assigning function to all genes, and characterization of the pattern and extent of human genetic variation. Approximately 50 per cent of putative gene products have been tentatively assigned functions, leaving almost 13 000 predicted proteins of unknown function. Similarly, the pattern and extent of LD across the human genes is only just beginning to emerge. Data indicate that extensive blocks of LD are present, often allowing the main haplotypes of a particular gene to be determined by a small number of SNPs. The current

Table 4A.2 *Risk of epilepsy in children and siblings of subjects with epilepsy[133,134]*

Epilepsy	Parent affected (%)	Sibling affected (%)	Reference
Juvenile myoclonic epilepsy	5.1–14.8	4.4–7	68, 125, 128
Childhood absence epilepsy	6.7–6.8	4.9–10	86, 125, 129, 130
Benign epilepsy with centrotemporal spikes	11 (incidence in parents of affected child)	15	114
Photosensitive epilepsy	7 (females)	9 (female)	131
	1.8 (males) (incidence in parents of affected child)	6.5 (male)	
Infantile spasms	0.7 (all first-degree relatives)	1.5–25	58, 59, 132

efforts to generate a SNP map of the human genome should allow the identification of susceptibility loci by association analysis, as long as the genetic architecture of the common epilepsies is favorable. However, DNA from large collections of well-characterized patients may be required to reveal small genetic contributions to diseases. Some encouragement is provided by the identification of a gene for another complex disease, Crohn's disease.[4,5] If the underlying biology is favorable, this could provide a model for the identification of susceptibility genes for the complex epilepsies.

Success in determining the molecular genetic basis of the common familial epilepsies will provide a greater understanding of the physiological defects involved. Improved diagnosis and the development of new targets for AEDs should follow. In the long term, microarray analysis of multiple susceptibility genes in an individual will allow a precise molecular diagnosis to be made, and a drug prescribed that is specifically designed for the particular electrophysiological dysfunction present.

KEY POINTS

- At least 40 per cent of all epilepsies are genetic in origin, with the proportion being higher in epilepsies of childhood onset
- Human genetic epilepsies may be categorized as mendelian epilepsies, non-mendelian or 'complex' epilepsies, and epilepsies associated with chromosomal disorders
- Twelve genes causing idiopathic mendelian epilepsies in humans have been identified, of which ten encode ion channels and cause idiopathic generalized epilepsies
- Novel strategies will be required for identification of susceptibility genes for the common familial epilepsies displaying complex inheritance
- Identification of susceptibility genes for epilepsy allows new approaches to diagnosis and treatment

REFERENCES

1. Lennox WG, Lennox MA. *Epilepsy and related disorders.* Boston: Little, Brown, 1960.
2. Berkovic SF, Howell RA, Hay DA, Hopper JL. Epilepsies in twins: genetics of the major epilepsy syndromes. *Annals of Neurology* 1998; **43**(4): 435–445.
3. Dib C, Faure S, Fizames C, *et al.* A comprehensive genetic map of the human genome based on 5,264 microsatellites. *Nature* 1996; **380**: 152–154.
4. Ogura Y, Bonen DK, Inohara N, *et al.* A frameshift mutation in NOD2 associated with susceptibility to Crohn's disease. *Nature* 2001; **411**(6837): 603–606.
5. Hugot JP, Chamaillard M, Zouali H, *et al.* Association of NOD2 leucine-rich repeat variants with susceptibility to Crohn's disease. *Nature* 2001; **411**(6837): 599–603.
6. Daly MJ, Rioux JD, Schaffner SF, *et al.* High-resolution haplotype structure in the human genome. *Nature Genetics* 2001; **29**(2): 229–232.
7. Reich DE, Lander ES. On the allelic spectrum of human disease. *Trends Genet* 2001; **17**(9): 502–510.
8. Wright AF, Hastie ND. Complex genetic diseases: controversy over the Croesus code. *Genome Biology* 2001; **2**(8).
9. Rett A, Teubel R. Neugeborenen Krampfe im Rahmen einer epileptisch belasten Familie. *Wiener Klinische Wochenschrift* 1964; **76**: 609–613.
10. Leppert M, Anderson VE, Quattlebaum T, *et al.* Benign familial neonatal convulsions linked to genetic markers on chromosome 20. *Nature* 1989; **337**(6208): 647–648.
11. Malafosse A, Leboyer M, Dulac O, *et al.* Confirmation of linkage of benign familial neonatal convulsions to D20S19 and D20S20. *Human Genetics* 1992; **89**: 54–58.
12. Ryan SG, Wiznitzer M, Hollman C, *et al.* Benign familial neonatal convulsions: evidence for clinical and genetic heterogeneity. *Annals of Neurology* 1991; **29**(5): 469–473.
13. Lewis TB, Leach RJ, Ward K, *et al.* Genetic heterogeneity in benign familial neonatal convulsions: identification of a new locus on chromosome 8q. *American Journal of Human Genetics* 1993; **53**: 670–675.
14. Singh NA, Charlier C, Stauffer D, *et al.* A novel potassium channel gene, *KCNQ2*, is mutated in an inhertied epilepsy of newborns. *Nature Genetics* 1998; **18**: 25–29.

15. Wang Q, Curran ME, Splawski I, *et al*. Positional cloning of a novel potassium channel gene: KVLQT1 mutations cause cardiac arrhythmias. *Nature Genetics* 1996; **12**(1): 17–23.

16. Neyroud N, Tesson F, Denjoy I, *et al*. A novel mutation in the potassium channel gene *KVLQT1* causes the Jervell and Lange-Nielsen cardioauditory syndrome [see comments]. *Nature Genetics* 1997; **15**(2): 186–189.

17. Dedek K, Kunath B, Kananura C, *et al*. Myokymia and neonatal epilepsy caused by a mutation in the voltage sensor of the KCNQ2 K+channel. *Proceedings of the National Academy of Sciences of the U S A* 2001; **98**(21): 12272–12277.

18. Charlier C, Singh NA, Ryan SG, *et al*. A pore mutation in a novel KQT-like potassium channel gene in an idiopathic epilepsy family [see comments]. *Nature Genetics* 1998; **18**(1): 53–55.

19. Wang HS, Pan Z, Shi W, *et al*. KCNQ2 and KCNQ3 potassium channel subunits: molecular correlates of the M-channel. *Science* 1998; **282**(5395); 1890–1893.

20. Vigevano F, Fusco L, Di Capua M, *et al*. Benign infantile familial convulsions. *European Journal of Pediatrics* 1992; **151**(8): 608–612.

21. Echenne B, Humbertclaude V, Rivier F, *et al*. Benign infantile epilepsy with autosomal dominant inheritance. *Brain and Development* 1994; **16**(2): 108–111.

22. Lee WL, Low PS, Rajan U. Benign familial infantile epilepsy. *Journal of Pediatrics* 1993; **123**(4): 588–590.

23. Guipponi M, Rivier F, Vigevano F, *et al*. Linkage mapping of benign familial infantile convulsions (BFIC) tochromosome 19q. *Human Molecular Genetics* 1997; **6**(3): 473–477.

24. Caraballo R, Pavek S, Lemainque A, *et al*. Linkage of benign familial infantile convulsions to chromosome 16p12- q12 suggests allelism to the infantile convulsions and choreoathetosis syndrome. *American Journal of Human Genetics* 2001; **68**(3): 788–794.

25. Malacarne M, Gennaro E, Madia F, *et al*. Benign familial infantile convulsions: mapping of a novel locus on chromosome 2q24 and evidence for genetic heterogeneity. *American Journal of Human Genetics* 2001; **68**(6): 1521–1526.

26. Szepetowski P, Rochette J, Berquin P, *et al*. Familial infantile convulsions and paroxysmal choreoathetosis: a new neurological syndrome linked to the pericentromeric region of human chromosome 16. *American Journal of Human Genetics* 1997; **61**(4): 889–898.

27. Lee WL, Tay A, Ong HT, *et al*. Association of infantile convulsions with paroxysmal dyskinesias (ICCA syndrome): confirmation of linkage to human chromosome 16p12-q12 in a Chinese family. *Human Genetics* 1998; **103**(5): 608–612.

28. Guerrini R, Bonanni P, Nardocci N, *et al*. Autosomal recessive rolandic epilepsy with paroxysmal exercise-induced dystonia and writer's cramp: delineation of the syndrome and gene mapping to chromosome 16p12-11.2. *Annals of Neurology* 1999; **45**(3): 344–352.

29. Scheffer IE, Bhatia KP, Lopes-Cendes I, *et al*. Autosomal dominant frontal epilepsy misdiagnosed as sleep disorder. *Lancet* 1994; **343**: 515–517.

30. Phillips HA, Scheffer IE, Berkovic SF, *et al*. Localization of a gene for autosomal dominant nocturnal frontal lobe epilepsy to chromosome 20q13.2. *Nature Genetics* 1995; **10**: 117–118.

31. Steinlein OK, Mulley JC, Propping P, *et al*. A missense mutation in the neuronal nicotinic acetylcholine receptor alpha 4 subunit is associated with autosomal dominant nocturnal frontal lobe epilepsy. *Nature Genetics* 1995; **11**(2): 201–203.

32. Steinlein O, Magnusson A, Stoodt J, *et al*. An insertion mutation of the CHRNA4 gene in a family with autosomal dominant nocturnal frontal lobe epilepsy. *Human Molecular Genetics* 1997; **6**(6): 943–947.

33. Steinlein OK, Stoodt J, Mulley J, *et al*. Independent occurrence of the CHRNA4 Ser248Phe mutation in a Norwegian family with nocturnal frontal lobe epilepsy. *Epilepsia* 2000; **41**(5): 529–535.

34. Hirose S, Iwata H, Akiyoshi H, *et al*. A novel mutation of CHRNA4 responsible for autosomal dominant nocturnal frontal lobe epilepsy. *Neurology* 1999; **53**(8): 1749–1753.

35. Saenz A, Galan J, Caloustian C, *et al*. Autosomal dominant nocturnal frontal lobe epilepsy in a Spanish family with a Ser252Phe mutation in the CHRNA4 gene. *Archives of Neurology* 1999; **56**(8): 1004–1009.

36. Phillips HA, Marini C, Scheffer IE, *et al*. A de novo mutation in sporadic nocturnal frontal lobe epilepsy. *Annals of Neurology* 2000; **48**(2): 264–267.

37. Phillips HA, Scheffer IE, Crossland KM, *et al*. Autosomal dominant nocturnal frontal-lobe epilepsy: genetic heterogeneity and evidence for a second locus at 15q24. *American Journal of Human Genetics* 1998; **63**(4): 1108–1116.

38. Phillips HA, Favre I, Kirkpatrick M, *et al*. CHRNB2 is the second acetylcholine receptor subunit associated with autosomal dominant nocturnal frontal lobe epilepsy. *American Journal of Human Genetics* 2001; **68**(1): 225–231.

39. Fusco M De, Becchetti A, Patrignani A, *et al*. The nicotinic receptor beta 2 subunit is mutant in nocturnal frontal lobe epilepsy. *Nature Genetics* 2000; **26**(3): 275–276.

40. Scheffer IE, Berkovic SF. Generalized epilepsy with febrile seizures plus. A genetic disorder with heterogeneous clinical phenotypes. *Brain* 1997; **120**: 479–490.

41. Wallace R, Wang D, Singh R, *et al*. Febrile seizures and generalized epilepsy associated with a mutation in the Na+-channel beta1 subunit gene SCN1B. *Nature Genetics* 1998; **19**(4): 366–370.

42. Bulman DE. Phenotype variation and newcomers in ion channel disorders. *Human Molecular Genetics* 1997; **6**(10): 1679–1685.

43. Macdonald RL, Kelly KM. Mechanisms of action of currently prescribed and newly developed antiepileptic drugs. *Epilepsia* 1994; **35**(Suppl 4): S41–50.

44. Escayg A, MacDonald BT, Meisler MH, *et al*. Mutations of SCN1A, encoding a neuronal sodium channel, in two families with GEFS+2. *Nature Genetics* 2000; **24**(4): 343–345.

45. Claes L. Del-Favero J, Ceulemans B, *et al*. De novo mutations in the sodium-channel gene SCN1A cause severe myoclonic epilepsy of infancy. *American Journal of Human Genetics* 2001; **68**(6): 1327–1332.

46. Singh R, Andermann E, Whitehouse WP, *et al*. Severe myoclonic epilepsy of infancy: extended spectrum of GEFS+? *Epilepsia* 2001; **42**(7): 837–844.

47. Sugawara T, Tsurubuchi Y, Agarwala KL, *et al*. A missense mutation of the Na+ channel alpha II subunit gene Na(v)1.2 in a patient with febrile and afebrile seizures causes channel dysfunction. *Proceedings of the National Academy of Sciences of the U S A* 2001; **98**(11): 6384–6389.

48. Baulac S, Huberfeld G, Gourfinkel-An I, *et al.* First genetic evidence of GABA(A) receptor dysfunction in epilepsy: a mutation in the gamma2-subunit gene. *Nature Genetics* 2001; **28**(1): 46–48.

49. Wallace RH, Marini C, Petrou S, *et al.* Mutant GABAA receptor gamma2-subunit in childhood absence epilepsy and febrile seizures. *Nature Genetics* 2001; **28**(1): 49–52.

50. Ottman R, Risch N, Hauser WA, *et al.* Localization of a gene for partial epilepsy to chromosome 10q. *Nature Genetics* 1995; **10**: 56–60.

51. Poza JJ, Saenz A, Martinez-Gil A, *et al.* Autosomal dominant lateral temporal epilepsy: clinical and genetic study of a large Basque pedigree linked to chromosome 10q. *Annals of Neurology* 1999; **45**(2): 182–1888.

52. Kalachikov S, Evgrafov O, Ross B, *et al.* Mutations in LGI1 cause autosomal-dominant partial epilepsy with auditory features. *Nature Genetics* 2002; **28**: 28.

53. Somerville RP, Chernova O, Liu S, *et al.* Identification of the promoter, genomic structure, and mouse ortholog of LGI1. *Mamm Genome* 2000; **11**(8): 622–627.

54. Scheel H, Tomiuk S, Hofmann K. A common protein interaction domain links two recently identified epilepsy genes. *Human Molecular Genetics* 2002; **11**(15): 1757–1762.

55. Scheffer IE, Phillips HA, O'Brien CE, *et al.* Familial partial epilepsy with variable foci: a new partial epilepsy syndrome with suggestion of linkage to chromosome 2. *Annals of Neurology* 1998; **44**: 890–899.

56. Xiong L, Labuda M, Li DS, *et al.* Mapping of a gene determining familial partial epilepsy with variable foci to chromosome 22q11-q12. *American Journal of Human Genetics* 1999; **65**(6): 1698–1710.

57. Dulac O, Feingold J, Plouin P, *et al.* Genetic predisposition to West syndrome. *Epilepsia* 1993; **34**(4): 732–737.

58. Feinberg AP, Leahy WR. Infantile spasms: case report of sex-linked inheritance. *Developmental Medicine and Child Neurology* 1977; **19**(4): 524–526.

59. Rugtveit J. X-linked mental retardation and infantile spasms in two brothers. *Developmental Medicine and Child Neurology* 1986; **28**(4): 544–546.

60. Claes S, Devriendt K, Lagae L, *et al.* The X-linked infantile spasms syndrome (MIM 308350) maps to Xp11.4-Xpter in two pedigrees. *Annals of Neurology* 1997; **42**(3): 360–364.

61. Stromme P, Sundet K, Mork C, *et al.* X linked mental retardation and infantile spasms in a family: new clinical data and linkage to Xp11.4-Xp22.11. *Journal of Medical Genetics* 1999; **36**(5): 374–378.

62. Bruyere H, Lewis S, Wood S, MacLeod PJ, Langlois S. Confirmation of linkage in X-linked infantile spasms (West syndrome) and refinement of the disease locus to Xp21.3-Xp22.1. *Clinical Genetics* 1999; **55**(3): 173–181.

63. Stromme P, Mangelsdorf ME, Shaw MA, *et al.* Mutations in the human ortholog of Aristaless cause X-linked mental retardation and epilepsy. *Nature Genetics* 2002; **30**(4): 441–445.

64. Calado A, Tome FM, Brais B, *et al.* Nuclear inclusions in oculopharyngeal muscular dystrophy consist of poly(A) binding protein 2 aggregates which sequester poly(A) RNA. *Human Molecular Genetics* 2000; **9**(15): 2321–2328.

65. Bienvenu T, Poirier K, Friocourt G, *et al.* ARX, a novel Prd-class-homeobox gene highly expressed in the telencephalon, is mutated in X-linked mental retardation. *Human Molecular Genetics* 2002; 11(8): 981–991.

66. Janz D, Christian W. Impulsiv-petit mal. *Otsch Z Nervenheik* 1957; **176**: 346–386. *Otsch Nerverheik,* Translation in English appears in Malafosse E, Gerton P, Hisch E, Marcesaux G, Broglin O, Bernasconi R eds *Idiopathic Generalized Epilepsies: Experimental and Genetic Aspects.* London: John Libbeig, 1994; 229–251.

67. Janz D. *Die Epilepsien.* Stuttgart: Thieme, 1969.

68. Tsuboi T, Christian W. On the genetics of primary generalised epilepsy with sporadic myoclonus of impulsive petit-mal type. *Humangenetik* 1973; **19**: 155–182.

69. Sundqvist A. Juvenile myoclonic epilepsy: events before diagnosis. *Journal of Epilepsy* 1990; **3**: 189–192.

70. Delgado-Escueta AV, Greenberg D, Weissbecker K. Gene mapping in the idiopathic generalised epilepsies. *Epilepsia* 1990; **31**(Suppl 3): S19–29.

71. Panayiotopoulos CP, Obeid T. Juvenile myoclonic epilepsy: an autosomal recessive disease. *Annals of Neurology* 1989; **25**: 440–443.

72. Greenberg DA, Delgado-Escueta AV, Widelitz H, *et al.* Strengthened evidence for linkage of juvenile myoclonic epilepsy to HLA and BF. *Cytogenetics and Cell Genetics* 1989; **51**: 1008.

73. Greenberg DA, Delgado-Escueta AV, Widelitz H, *et al.* Juvenile myoclonic epilepsy may be linked to the BF and HLA loci on human chromosome 6. *American Journal of Medical Genetics* 1988; **31**(1): 185–192.

74. Weissbecker KA, Durner M, Janz D, *et al.* Confirmation of linkage between juvenile myoclonic epilepsy locus and the HLA region on chromosome 6. *American Journal of Medical Genetics* 1991; **38**(1): 32–36.

75. Durner M, Sander T, Greenberg DA, *et al.* Localisation of idiopathic generalised epilepsy on chromosome 6p in families of juvenile myoclonic epilepsy patients. *Neurology* 1991; **41**(10): 1651–1655.

76. Greenberg DA, Delgado-Escueta AV. The chromosome 6p epilepsy locus: exploring mode of inheritance and heterogeneity through linkage analysis. *Epilepsia* 1993; **34**(Suppl 3): S12–8.

77. Liu AW, Delgado-Escueta AV, Serratosa JM, *et al.* Juvenile myoclonic epilepsy locus in chromosome 6p21.2-p11: linkage to convulsions and electroencephalography trait. *American Journal of Human Genetics* 1995; **57**: 368–381.

78. Greenberg DA, Durner M, Keddache M, *et al.* Reproducibility and complications in gene searches: linkage on chromosome 6, heterogeneity, association, and maternal inheritance in juvenile myoclonic epilepsy. *American Journal of Human Genetics* 2000; **66**(2): 508–516.

79. Whitehouse W, Diebold U, Rees M, *et al.* Exclusion of linkage of genetic focal sharp waves to the HLA region on chromosome 6p in families with benign partial epilepsy with centrotemporal spikes. *Neuropaediatrics* 1993; **24**: 208–210.

80. Elmslie FV, Williamson MP, Rees M, *et al.* Linkage analysis of juvenile myoclonic epilepsy and microsatellite loci spanning 61 cM of human chromosome 6p in 19 nuclear pedigrees provides no evidence for a susceptibility locus in this region. *American Journal of Human Genetics* 1996; **59**: 653–663.

81. Elmslie FV, Rees M, Williamson MP, *et al.* Genetic mapping of a major susceptibility locus for juvenile myoclonic epilepsy on

chromosome 15q. *Human Molecular Genetics* 1997; **6**(8): 1329–1334.

82. Sander T, Schulz H, Vieira-Saeker AM, *et al.* Evaluation of a putative major susceptibility locus for juvenile myoclonic epilepsy on chromosome 15q14. *American Journal of Medical Genetics* 1999; **88**(2): 182–187.

83. Taske NL, Williamson MP, Makoff A, *et al.* Evaluation of the positional candidate gene CHRNA7 at the juvenile myoclonic epilepsy locus (EJM2) on chromosome 15q13-14. *Epilepsy Research* 2002; **49**: 157–172.

84. Cossette P, Liu L, Brisebois K, *et al.* Mutation of GABRA1 in an autosomal dominant form of juvenile myoclonic epilepsy. *Nature Genetics* 2002; **31**(2): 184–9.

85. Gardiner RM. Genetics of human typical absence syndromes. In: Duncan JS, Panayiotopoulos CP (eds) *Typical Absences and Related Epileptic Syndromes.* London: Churchill Communications Europe, 1995.

86. Beck-Mannagetta G, Janz D. Syndrome-related genetics in generalised epilepsy. *Epilepsy Research* 1991; **4**: 105–111.

87. Buoni S, Grosso S, Di Cosmo G, *et al.* Segregation analysis in typical absence epilepsy. *Journal of Child Neurology* 1998; 13(2): 89–93.

88. Huguenard JR. Neuronal circuitry of thalamocortical epilepsy and mechanisms of antiabsence drug action. *Advances in Neurology* 1999; **79**: 991–999.

89. Leresche N, Parri HR, Erdemli G, *et al.* On the action of the anti-absence drug ethosuximide in the rat and cat thalamus. *J Neurosci* 1998; **18**(13): 4842–4853.

90. Pinault D, Leresche N, Charpier S, *et al.* Intracellular recordings in thalamic neurons during spontaneous spike and wave discharges in rats with absence epilepsy. *Journal of Physiology* 1998; **509**(2): 449–456.

91. Kim D, Song I, Keum S, *et al.* Lack of the burst firing of thalamocortical relay neurons and resistance to absence seizures in mice lacking alpha(1G) T-type Ca(2+) channels. *Neuron* 2001; **31**(1): 35–45.

92. Schuler V, Luscher C, Blanchet C, *et al.* Epilepsy, hyperalgesia, impaired memory, and loss of pre- and postsynaptic GABA(B) responses in mice lacking GABA(B(1)). *Neuron* 2001; **31**: 47–58.

93. Fletcher CF, Lutz CM, O'Sullivan TN, *et al.* Absence epilepsy in *tottering* mutant mice is associated with calcium channel defects. *Cell* 1996; **87**: 607–617.

94. Burgess DL, Jones JM, Meisler MH, Noebels JL. Mutation of the Ca^{2+} channel β subunit gene *Cchb4* is associated with ataxia and seizures in the lethargic (*lh*) mouse. *Cell* 1997; **88**: 385–392.

95. Letts VA, Felix R, Biddlecome GH, *et al.* The mouse stargazer gene encodes a neuronal Ca^{2+}-channel gamma subunit. *Nature Genetics* 1998; **19**: 340–347.

96. Barclay J, Balaguero N, Mione M, *et al.* Ducky mouse phenotype of epilepsy and ataxia is associated with mutations in the Cacna2d2 gene and decreased calcium channel current in cerebellar Purkinje cells. *Journal of Neuroscience* 2001; **21**(16): 6095–6104.

97. Chioza B, Wilkie H, Nashef L, *et al.* Association between the alpha(1a) calcium channel gene CACNA1A and idiopathic generalized epilepsy. *Neurology* 2001; **56**: 1245–1246.

98. Zuberi S, Eunson L, Hanna MJS, Ramesh V. The clinical phenotype of a child with a novel calcium channel gene

(CACNA1A) mutation associated with episodic ataxia type 2 and absence epilepsy. *European Journal of Paediatric Neurology* 1999; **3**(6): A55.

99. Hanna IM, Jouvenceau A, Eunson LH, *et al.* Human epilepsy – a possible role of the human voltage-gated P/Q type calcium channel. *Journal of the Neurological Sciences* 2001; **187**: S280.

100. Fong GC, Shah PU, Gee MN, *et al.* Childhood absence epilepsy with tonic-clonic seizures and electroencephalogram 3-4-Hz spike and multispike-slow wave complexes: linkage to chromosome 8q24. *American Journal of Human Genetics* 1998; **63**: 1117–1129.

101. Sugimoto Y, Morita R, Amano K, *et al.* Childhood absence epilepsy in 8q24: refinement of candidate region and construction of physical map. *Genomics* 2000; **68**: 264–272.

102. Feucht M, Fuchs K, Pichlbauer E, *et al.* Possible association between childhood absence epilepsy and the gene encoding GABRB3. *Biological Psychiatry* 1999; **46**: 997–1002.

103. Tanaka M, Castroviejo I, Medina M, *et al.* Linkage analysis between subsyndromes of childhood absence epilepsy and the GABA$_A$ receptor beta3 subunit on chromosome 15q11.2-12. *Epilepsia* 2000; **250**: 41.

104. Wagstaff J, Knoll JH, Fleming J, *et al.* Localization of the gene encoding the GABAA receptor beta 3 subunit to the Angelman/Prader-Willi region of human chromosome 15. *American Journal of Human Genetics* 1991; **49**: 330–337.

105. DeLorey TM, Handforth A, Anagnostaras SGA, *et al.* Mice lacking the beta3 subunit of the GABAA receptor have the epilepsy phenotype and many of the behavioral characteristics of Angelman syndrome. *Journal of Neuroscience* 1998; **18**: 8505–8514.

106. Robinson R, Taske N, Sander T, *et al.* Linkage analysis between childhood absence epilepsy and genes encoding GABA(A) and GABA(B) receptors, voltage-dependent calcium channels, and the ECA1 region on chromosome 8q. *Epilepsy Res* 2002; **48**: 169–179.

107. Nayrac P, Beaussart M. Les pointe-ondes prérolandique: expression EEG très particulière. *Revue Neurologique (Paris)* 1958; **99**: 201–206.

108. Panayiotopoulos CP. Benign childhood partial epilepsies: benign childhood seizure susceptibility syndromes. *Journal of Neurology, Neurosurgery and Psychiatry* 1993; **56**(1): 2–5.

109. Holmes GL. Benign focal epilepsies of childhood. *Epilepsia* 1993; **34**(Suppl 3): S49–61.

110. Beaussart M. Benign epilepsy of children with Rolandic (centro-temporal) paroxysmal foci. A clinical entity. Study of 221 cases. *Epilepsia* 1972; **13**(6): 795–911.

111. Lerman P, Kivity S. Benign focal epilepsy of childhood. A follow-up study of 100 recovered patients. *Archives of Neurology* 1975; **32**(4): 261–264.

112. Blom S, Heijbel J. Benign epilepsy of children with centro-temporal EEG foci. Discharge rate during sleep. *Epilepsia* 1975; **16**(1): 133–140.

113. Bray PF, Wiser WC. Hereditary characteristics of familial temporal-central focal epilepsy. *Paediatrics* 1965; **36**: 207–211.

114. Heijbel J, Blom S, Rasmuson M. Benign epilepsy of childhood with centrotemporal EEG foci: a genetic study. *Epilepsia* 1975; **16**: 285–293.

115. Degen R, Degen HE. Some genetic aspects of rolandic epilepsy: waking and sleeping EEGs in siblings. *Epilepsia* 1990; **31**: 795–801.

116. Bray PF, Wiser WC. A unifying concept of idiopathic epilepsy. *Postgraduate Medicine* 1969; **46**(1): 82–87.

117. Neubauer BA, Fiedler B, Himmelein B, *et al.* Centrotemporal spikes in families with rolandic epilepsy: linkage to chromosome 15q14. *Neurology* 1998; **51**(6): 1608–1612.

118. Rich SS, Annegers JF, Hauser WA, Anderson VE. Complex segregation analysis of febrile convulsions. *American Journal of Human Genetics* 1987; **41**: 249–257.

119. Wallace S. Genetic factors. In: Wallace S (ed) *The Child with Febrile Seizures.* London: John Wright, 1988: 24.

120. Johnson WG, Kugler SL, Stenroos ES, *et al.* Pedigree analysis in families with febrile seizures. *American Journal of Medical Genetics* 1996; **61**: 345–352.

121. Wallace RH, Berkovic SF, Howell RA, *et al.* Suggestion of a major gene for familial febrile convulsions mapping to 8q13-21. *Journal of Medical Genetics* 1996; **33**: 308–312.

122. Johnson EW, Dubovsky J, Rich SS, *et al.* Evidence for a novel gene for familial febrile convulsions, FEB2, linked to chromosome 19p in an extended family from the Midwest. *Human Molecular Genetics* 1998; **7**: 63–67.

123. Peiffer A, Thompson J, Charlier C, *et al.* A locus for febrile seizures (FEB3) maps to chromosome 2q23-24. *Annals of Neurology* 1999; **46**: 671–678.

124. Nakayama J, Hamano K, Iwasaki N, *et al.* Significant evidence for linkage of febrile seizures to chromosome 5q14-q15. *Human Molecular Genetics* 2000; **9**: 87–91.

125. Tsuboi T. Genetic risks in offspring of epileptic patients. In: Beck-Mannagetta G, Anderson V, Doose H, Janz D (eds) *Genetics of the Epilepsies.* Berlin: Springer, 1989; 111.

126. Anderson VE, Hauser WA, Rich SS. Genetic heterogeneity in the epilepsies. *Advances in Neurology* 1986; **44**: 59–75.

127. Spauschus A, Eunson L, Hanna MG, Kullmann DM. Functional characterization of a novel mutation in KCNA1 in episodic ataxia type 1 associated with epilepsy. *Annals of the New York Academy of Sciences* 1999; **868**: 442–446.

128. Janz D, Durner M, Beck-Mannagetta G. Family studies on the genetics of juvenile moclonic epilepsy (epilepsy with petit mal). In: Beck-Mannagetta G, Anderson V, Doose H, Janz D (eds) *Genetics of the Epilepsies.* Berlin: Springer, 1989: 43–52.

129. Beck-Mannagetta G, Anderson VE, Doose H, Janz D. *Genetics of the Epilepsies.* Berlin: Springer, 1989.

130. Doose H, Baier WK. Genetic factors in epilepsies with primarily generalised minor seizures. *Neuropaediatrics* 1987; **18**(Suppl 1): 1–64.

131. Doose H, Gerkern H, Horstman T, Volzke E. Genetic factors in spike-wave absences. *Epilepsia* 1973; **14**: 57–75.

132. Fleiszar KA, Daniel WL, Imrey PB. Genetic study of infantile spasm with hypsarrhythmia. *Epilepsia* 1977; **18**(1): 55–62.

133. Blandfort M, Tsuboi T, Vogel F. Genetic counselling in the epilepsies. *Human Genetics* 1987; **76**: 303–331.

134. Elmslie FV. Gardiner RM. The Epilepsies. In: Rimoin DL, Connor JM, Pyeritz RE (eds) *Emery and Rimoin's Principles and Practice of Medical Genetics*, 3rd edn. Edinburgh: Churchill Livingstone, 1997: 2177–2196.

4B

Chromosomal syndromes associated with epilepsy

DANIELA T PILZ AND DAVID RAVINE

The term **syndrome** is generally used for recurring and recognizable patterns of malformation. Many are due to chromosomal alterations. In a recent review, Singh *et al.* identified over 400 chromosomal imbalances associated with epilepsy or EEG abnormalities.[1] Recent advances in molecular cytogenetics have extended the number of detectable chromosomal syndromes.[2,3]

Epilepsy in isolation is rarely associated with an underlying chromosomal abnormality. An exception may be an apparently balanced translocation (see 'Chromosomal deletions and rearrangements' below) interrupting a specific epilepsy gene. Patient features that may point towards a chromosome abnormality include coexisting psychomotor retardation, pre- and postnatal growth retardation, congenital malformations and facial dysmorphism.

CHROMOSOMAL DELETIONS AND REARRANGEMENTS

Chromosomal deletions can arise within chromosomes (interstitial deletions) or at the ends of chromosomes (telomeric deletions). The telomeres of chromosomes are gene rich, and submicroscopic deletions may result in significant developmental abnormalities, including seizure disorders.[4] Deletions can arise *de novo* or be familial, often with a variable phenotype in deletion carriers. Balanced translocations, which involve exchange of chromosomal segments between different chromosomes without

apparent loss or gain of genetic material, or disruption of a functional gene, may lead to serious chromosomal imbalance among offspring.

Chromosome alterations larger than 2–3 Mb are usually detected microscopically using high-resolution banding. Fluorescent *in situ* hybridization (FISH), involving the hybridization (complementary base-pairing) of a fluorescently labeled DNA probe to a targeted chromosomal area, has been revolutionary for the detection of submicroscopic chromosome abnormalities and microdeletion syndromes.

Wolf–Hirschhorn syndrome

Wolf-Hirschhorn syndrome is due to deletions of the short arm of chromosome 4(pter-p15). Interestingly, the milder phenotype of Pitt-Rogers-Danks syndrome (PRDS) is due to smaller distal 4p deletions. The seizure types reported in Wolf-Hirschhorn syndrome are summarized by Singh *et al.*,[1] and epilepsy also occurs in PRDS.[5] Additional features of Wolf-Hirschhorn syndrome include intrauterine growth retardation, cardiac and renal malformations, characteristic 'Greek-helmet' facial appearance, cleft palate, cerebral anomalies and variable, but often profound, mental retardation.

INVESTIGATIONS

Karyotype, FISH of 4p.

Miller–Dieker syndrome

Miller-Dieker syndrome (MDS) is due to microscopic or submicroscopic deletions on the distal short arm of chromosome 17(p13.3), involving the *LIS1* gene. Hemizygosity involving *LIS1* is responsible for 'classical lissencephaly', the most prominent feature of MDS. Seizures in MDS usually occur within the first 6 months of life, often presenting as infantile spasms. The EEG is very abnormal, simulating hypsarrythmia.[6] MDS, associated with loss of several genes contiguous with *LIS1*, represents the most severe *LIS1*-associated syndrome. Most patients with 'classical lissencephaly' do not have the additional dysmorphic facial features and occasional visceral malformations associated with MDS, and may only develop seizures in later childhood. About 40 per cent of cases, termed **isolated lissencephaly sequence**, have a submicroscopic deletion involving the *LIS1* gene.[7] Mutations within the *LIS1* occur in a further 25 per cent of cases (see Chapter 4C).

INVESTIGATIONS

Karyotype, FISH of 17p13.3.

1p36 deletion syndrome

Seizures are reported in three quarters of cases of del(1) (p36.3), a microdeletion syndrome, that includes psychomotor retardation, cerebral abnormalities on imaging, facial dysmorphism and visceral anomalies.[1,8] Interestingly, a potassium channel β subunit gene, *KCNAB2*, is within the deleted region, raising the possibility that haploinsufficiency of this gene may be responsible for the occurrence of epilepsy in this condition.[9]

INVESTIGATIONS

Karyotype, FISH 1pter.

For another microdeletion syndrome commonly associated with epilepsy, Angelman syndrome, see below.

CHROMOSOMAL DUPLICATIONS

Duplication (dup) of a chromosomal segment results in three, rather than two copies of the genes located within the replicated region. **Direct duplications** are oriented the same way as the original segment; in **inverted duplication** the orientation is reversed.[10]

Inverted duplication 15 (inv dup 15)

Inverted chromosomal 15 duplications may be interstitial or present as an extra, structurally abnormal chromosome (ESAC). Larger inv dup 15s contain two or more copies of the Prader-Willi syndrome/Angelman syndrome region. They are associated with an abnormal phenotype, including autism, early onset seizures and ataxia, with a notable absence of dysmorphic features.[11]

INVESTIGATIONS

Karyotype, FISH with probes specific for Prader-Willi syndrome/Angelman syndrome.

RING CHROMOSOMES

Ring chromosomes are uncommon and usually sporadic, although there are rare instances of parent–child transmission. The amount of genetic material lost in the formation of the ring determines the phenotype.[10] Two ring chromosomes are particularly associated with epilepsy.

Ring chromosome 14 (r14)

Children with r14 have distinct facial features, psychomotor retardation, short stature, cutaneous dyspigmentation, retinal pigmentation, and neurological anomalies including hypo- or hypertonia, tremor and athetosis. Epilepsy beginning in infancy is a fairly constant feature, including myoclonic and tonic–clonic seizures.[1]

Ring chromosome 20 (r20)

The r20 syndrome includes epilepsy, mental retardation and microcephaly. Importantly, several patients have normal psychomotor development. Associated seizure and EEG patterns include prolonged complex partial seizures, and theta bursts on EEG.[12] Notably, genes for benign familial neonatal convulsions, *KCNQ2*, and for autosomal dominant nocturnal frontal lobe epilepsy, *CHRNA4*, are located on chromosome 20.

INVESTIGATIONS

Karyotype, chromosome painting (confirms chromosomal origin of the ring).

TRISOMIES

Seizures occur in 5–6 per cent of children with Down syndrome, due to the presence of an additional chromosome 21, also referred to as trisomy 21. Reflex epilepsies and infantile spasms may occur.[13] Seizures may also be a major clinical feature in the two other common viable trisomy syndromes: trisomy 13 (Patau syndrome) and trisomy 18 (Edward syndrome).

Library and Knowledge Service

MOSAISICM

As well as chromosomal abnormalities involving all body cells (constitutive anomalies), tissue-limited chromosomal abnormalities, or mosaicism, may present with a seizure disorder and other congenital anomalies.

Pallister–Killian syndrome

A distinctive dysmorphic syndrome associated with tetra-somy 12p mosaicism, this may present with seizures.[14]

Hypomelanomosis of Ito

A condition with hypopigmented lesions that may follow the lines of Blaschko, this is frequently associated with chromosomal mosaicism detectable in skin and blood. CNS malformations, seizures and mental retardation are common associations.

INVESTIGATIONS

Chromosomes from blood and from carefully positioned skin biopsy(ies). Inform cytogeneticist that mosaicism may be present.

IMPRINTED GENES

A gene may have a subtle modification or 'imprint' when inherited maternally or paternally. These imprinted genes are usually expressed only from the maternal or paternal allele. Absence of an expressed gene subject to imprinting cannot be compensated by its partner, because the inactivation arising from the imprinting process is irreversible. The resultant lack of gene product may result in a range of developmental anomalies, including the occurrence of epilepsy.

Angelman syndrome

Angelman syndrome is the best characterized of the imprinted disorders. Seizures occur in 80–90 per cent of cases. A deletion of 15q11–13 on the maternally derived chromosome is responsible for 70 per cent. Among the remainder, paternal uniparental disomy (2–3 per cent), imprinting center mutations within 15q11–13 (3 per cent) and mutations within the maternally derived UBE3A gene (7 per cent) result in critical lack of product from maternally expressed genes within this region of chromosome 15.[15] The EEG often shows characteristic generalized high amplitude slowing, which is posteriorly dominant with spike and sharp waves, often facilitated by eye closure.[16]

By contrast, seizures are uncommon in PWS, which arises from absence of a paternal derived 15q11–13 region.

INVESTIGATIONS

Karyotype. 15q11–13 methylation studies, FISH, UBE3A mutation analysis (Angelman syndrome).

Fragile X syndrome

Fragile X syndrome, mostly arising from an expanded tri-nucleotide repeat sequence within the FMR1 gene located at Xq28, is an important cause of mental retardation and seizures, particularly in boys. Often associated with a maternal family history of intellectual disability, 25–40 per cent of cases have seizures, generally with characteristic focal spikes during sleep, which improve with age.[17]

INVESTIGATIONS

FMR1 antibody analysis, methylation studies or direct sizing of CGG expansion. Karyotype.

KEY POINTS

- Over 400 **chromosomal imbalances** are associated with epilepsy
- Epilepsy is **rarely an isolated feature** of a chromosomal anomaly
- Coexisting **mental retardation**, pre- and postnatal **growth retardation**, **congenital malformations** and **facial dysmorphism** suggest the possibility of a chromosomal syndrome

---

REFERENCES

1. Singh R, McKinlay Gardner RJ, Crossland KM, et al. Chromosomal abnormalities and epilepsy: a review for clinicians and gene hunters. Epilepsia 2002; **43**: 127–140.
2. Schinzel A. Catalogue of Unbalanced Chromosome Aberrations in Man, 2nd edn. Berlin: de Gruyter, 2001.
3. Schinzel A, Niedrist D. Chromosome imbalances associated with epilepsy. American Journal of Medical Genetics 2001; **106**: 119–124.
4. de Vries BBA, White AO, Knight SJL, et al. Clinical studies on submicroscopic subtelomeric rearrangements: a checklist. Journal of Medical Genetics 2001; **38**: 145–150.
5. Kant SG, van Haeringen A, Bakker E, et al. Pitt-Rogers-Danks syndrome and Wolf-Hirschhorn syndrome are caused by a deletion in the same region on chromosome 4p16.3. Journal of Medical Genetics 1997; **34**: 569–572.

Derby Hospitals NHS Foundation
Trust
Library and Knowledge Service

6. Guerrini R, Carrozzo R. Epilepsy and genetic malformations of the cerebral cortex. *American Journal of Medical Genetics* 2001; **106**: 160–173.

7. Pilz DT, Macha ME, Precht KS, *et al.* Fluorescence in situ hybridization analysis with LIS1 specific probes reveals a high deletion mutation rate in isolated lissencephaly sequence. *Genetics in Medicine* 1998; **1**: 29–33.

8. Slavotinek A, Shaffer LG, Shapira SK. Monosomy 1p36. *Journal of Medical Genetics* 1999; **36:** 657–663.

9. Heilstedt HA, Burgess DL, Anderson AE, *et al.* Loss of the potassium channel beta-subunit gene, *KCNAB2*, is associated with epilepsy in patients with 1p36 deletion syndrome. *Epilepsia* 2001; **42**: 1103–1111.

10. Gardner RJM, Sutherland GR. *Chromosome Abnormalities and Genetic Counseling*, 2nd edn. New York: Oxford University Press, 1996.

11. Torrisi L, Sangiorgi E, Russo L, Gurrieri F. Rearrangements of chromosome 15 in epilepsy. *American Journal of Medical Genetics* 2001; **106**: 125–128.

12. Canevini MP, Sgro V, Zuffardi O, *et al.* Chromosome 20 ring: a chromosomal disorder associated with a particular electroclinical pattern. *Epilepsia* 1998; **39**: 942–951.

13. Stafstrom CE, Patxot OF, Gilmore HE, Wisniewski KE. Seizures in children with Down syndrome: etiology, characteristics and outcome. *Developmental Medicine and Child Neurology* 1991; **33**: 191–200.

14. Quarrell OWJ, Hamill MA, Hughes HE. Pallister-Killian mosaic syndrome with emphasis on the adult phenotype. *American Journal of Medical Genetics* 1988; **31**: 841–844.

15. Nichols RD. The impact of genomic imprinting for neurobehavioral and developmental disorders. *Journal of Clinical Investigation* 2000; **105**: 413–418.

16. Boyd SG, Harden A, Patton MA. The EEG in early diagnosis of the Angelman (happy puppet) syndrome. *European Journal of Pediatrics* 1988; **147**: 508–513.

17. Musemeci SA, Ferri R, Colognola RM , *et al.* Fragile-X syndrome: a particular epileptogenic EEG pattern. *Epilepsia* 1988; **29**: 41–47.

Abnormalities of brain development

RENZO GUERRINI AND LUCIO PARMEGGIANI

The malformations of cortical development (MCD)[1] most relevant in childhood epilepsy are usually characterized by malposition and faulty differentiation of gray matter. The epilepsy is usually severe, has onset during childhood and is associated with developmental delay. The incidence of epilepsy is variable in different malformations.[2] However, MCD are observed in up to 40 per cent of children with drug-resistant epilepsy[3] and in 50 per cent of children in surgical series that include very young patients.[4] MRI has played a major role in the diagnosis of MCD. Variations in distribution and depth of cortical sulci, cortical thickness, boundaries between gray and white matter, and signal intensity allow recognition of different malformation patterns, which may be restricted to discrete cortical areas or occur diffusely. Attempts at nosological subdivisions[1] and genetic linkage studies have led to the identification of several genes regulating brain development[5] (Table 4C.1) and mutations in these genes have been associated with specific malformations.

Table 4C.1 *Genes responsible for malformation of cortical development (modified from Barkovich et al.[1])*

Syndrome	Locus	Gene	Protein
ILS[DCX]	Xq22.3-q23	*DCX = XLIS*	DCX or doublecortin
SBH[DCX]	Xq22.3-q23	*DCX = XLIS*	DCX or doublecortin
MDS	17p13.3	Several contiguous	PAFAH1B1 and others
ILS[LIS1]	17p13.3	*LIS1*	PAFAH1B1
SBH[LIS1]	17p13.3	*LIS1*	PAFAH1B1
LCH[RELN]	7q22	*RELN*	Reelin
FCMD[FCMD]	9q31	*FCMD*	FCMD or fukutin
MEB	1p32	Unknown	Unknown
BPNH	Xq28	*FLM1*	Filamin-1
TSC1	9q32	*TSC1*	Hamartin
TSC2	16p13.3	*TSC2*	Tuberin

ILS, isolated lissencephaly sequence; SBH, subcortical band heterotopia; MDS, Miller-Dieker syndrome; LCH, lissencephaly with cerebellar hypoplasia; FCMD, Fukuyama congenital muscular dystrophy; MEB, muscle-eye-brain disease; BPNH, bilateral periventricular nodular heterotopia; TSC, tuberous sclerosis.

NORMAL DEVELOPMENT OF THE CORTEX

The cerebral cortex derives from telencephalic vesicles of the forebrain and starts to develop soon after the hemispheric vesicles form as diverticula of the primitive prosencephalon, in postovulatory week 4 of gestation. Early specification of the forebrain is related to the expression of several homeobox-containing and winged helix-containing genes. In animal models, loss of function of these genes produces abnormalities in forebrain specification and development.[6–12] At the early stages, the cerebral hemispheres consist of a single layer of pseudo-stratified columnar epithelium with frequent mitotic activity. The nuclei of these cells move up and down within the cytoplasm of the cell, undergoing mitotic division only at the ventricular surface. As the cerebral hemispheres grow in size, the initial columnar epithelium persists adjacent to the ependyma as the ventricular zone. Rapidly proliferating precursor cells in the ventricular zone generate many postmitotic but still immature neurons. The second or marginal layer is a sparsely cellular zone which forms superficial to the ventricular zone by week 5. The next major phase of cortical development begins at this time, when immature neurons start to migrate away from the proliferative zone, primarily by climbing radial glia fibers. The first wave of migrating cells forms the preplate during weeks 6 and 7, and begins formation of the cortical plate before slowing down by week 10. The second and larger wave begins generating neurons in week 10, peaks during weeks 12–14 and ends by week 16 when the ventricular zone is mostly depleted of cells.[13,14] These cells form the major portion of layers 2–6 of the mature cortex. Classical studies have shown that the cerebral cortex is formed by an 'inside-out' migration of ventricular zone cells, so neurons that are generated early during cortical development and migrate to the cortical plate first will occupy deeper layers, whereas later migrating neurons pass the established cells to occupy progressively more superficial positions.[15] By about week 22, the first distinctive layers begin to appear in the cortex. Further maturation consists of additional synaptogenesis, retraction of early axons which did not establish appropriate connections, neurotransmitter biosynthesis, and other processes. By week 27 of gestation, all six layers of the mature cortex are visible.[14]

CLASSIFICATION AND NOMENCLATURE OF CORTICAL MALFORMATIONS

Three distinct but overlapping processes are involved in development of the cerebral cortex, neuronal and glial proliferation, neuronal migration and cortical organization. Any or all of these processes can be altered, resulting in cortical malformations.[16,17] A classification system of cortical malformations, based on fundamental embryologic and genetic principles and a combination of neuroimaging, gross pathologic and histologic criteria, has been developed and subsequently updated (Table 4C.2).[1,18,19] The framework of this classification system is based on the three major embryological processes of cellular proliferation, neuronal migration and cortical organization. When more than one process was involved, classification was based on the earliest embryologic abnormality. The abnormalities that primarily affect proliferation are usually associated with an alteration in both neuronal and glial cell differentiation, producing abnormal cell size and morphology.[17] Disorders affecting neuronal migration are characterized by abnormal neuronal positioning.[17] When arrest of migration occurs early, heterotopic collections of immature neurons are found beneath the cortex, as in isolated subcortical nodular heterotopia and the agyria–pachygyria-band spectrum. When migration is arrested during later cortical development, abnormal cell position is more likely to be restricted to the cortex, as in unlayered polymicrogyria. In both of

Table 4C.2 *Classification of cortical malformations (modified from Barkovich et al.[1])*

I Malformations due to abnormal neuronal and glial proliferation or apoptosis
  A Decreased proliferation/increased apoptosis: microcephalies
    1 Microcephaly with normal to thin cortex
    2 Microlissencephaly (extreme microcephaly with thick cortex)
    3 Microcephaly with polymicrogyria/cortical dysplasia
  B Increased proliferation/decreased apoptosis (normal cell types): megalencephalies
  C Abnormal proliferation (abnormal cell types)
    1 Non-neoplastic
      a Cortical hamartomas of tuberous sclerosis
      b Cortical dysplasia with balloon cells
      c Hemimegalencephaly (HME)
    2 Neoplastic (associated with disordered cortex)
      a DNET (dysembryoplastic neuroepithelial tumor)
      b Ganglioglioma
      c Gangliocytoma

II Malformations due to abnormal neuronal migration
  A Lissencephaly/subcortical band heterotopia spectrum
  B Cobblestone complex
    1 Congenital muscular dystrophy syndromes
    2 Syndromes with no involvement of muscle
  C Heterotopia
    1 Subependymal (periventricular)
    2 Subcortical (other than band heterotopia)
    3 Marginal glioneuronal

III Malformations due to abnormal cortical organization (including late neuronal migration)
  A Polymicrogyria and schizencephaly
    1 Bilateral polymicrogyria syndromes
    2 Schizencephaly (polymicrogyria with clefts)
    3 Polymicrogyria with other brain malformations or abnormalities
    4 Polymicrogyria or schizencephaly as part of multiple congenital anomaly/mental retardation syndromes
  B Cortical dysplasia without balloon cells
  C Microdysgenesis

IV Malformations of cortical development, not otherwise classified
  A Malformations secondary to inborn errors of metabolism
    1 Mitochondrial and pyruvate metabolic disorders
    2 Peroxisomal disorders
  B Other unclassified malformations
    1 Sublobar dysplasia
    2 Others

these malformations, horizontal neuronal lamination is severely disrupted, but radial (vertical) organization is still recognizable. The best-known cortical malformation originating after neuronal migration is completed, during the stage of later cortical organization, is four-layered polymicrogyria, in which horizontal neuronal lamination usually persists.[17] This pattern of abnormality may result from damage to intermediate cortical layers which produces a difference in growth rate between outer and inner cortical layers, with consequent excessive folding of the cortical surface.[20]

MALFORMATIONS RELATED TO ABNORMAL PROLIFERATION OF NEURONS AND GLIA

Hemimegalencephaly (HME)

In HME one cerebral hemisphere is enlarged and presents with thick cortex, wide convolutions and reduced sulci (Figure 4C.1A). Although the abnormality is strictly unilateral in most cases,[21] postmortem examination showed minor abnormalities of the apparently unaffected hemisphere in two cases and mild cortical dysplastic abnormalities in another.[22,23] Laminar organization of the cortex is absent and gray–white matter demarcation is poor. There are giant neurons (up to 80 μm in diameter) throughout the cortex and the underlying white matter. In about 50 per cent of cases large, bizarre cells are observed, also called balloon cells.[21,22] HME is probably a heterogeneous condition. Localization of the abnormality to one cerebral hemisphere may indicate somatic mosaicism.[21] It has also been suggested that HME may result from a fault in programmed cell death (apoptosis).[24]

HME has been associated with many different disorders (Table 4C.3) but can occur in isolation. There is a broad clinical spectrum, ranging from severe epileptic encephalopathy beginning in the neonatal period[22] to patients with normal cognitive function.[25,26] Indeed, the milder end of the clinical spectrum in HME includes patients with well-controlled seizures or no seizures at all.[27] However, most patients have a severe structural abnormality and almost continuous seizures. The most common presentation is with asymmetric macrocrania, hemiparesis, hemianopia, mental retardation and seizures. The electroclinical features usually include partial motor seizures beginning in the neonatal period, infantile spasms and often a suppression burst pattern on sleep EEG.[27,29] Patients with early onset, severe epilepsy almost always develop major cognitive and motor impairment.[33] In addition, there is a high mortality rate in the first months or years of life with status epilepticus being the most important cause of death.[21,30–32] Seizure intractability in these patients can usually be established within the first year of life.[27,28] This is important because hemispherectomy may prevent both life-threatening seizures and permanent loss of functioning of the healthy hemisphere.[28,32] There are indications that the operation should be performed early.[34] Transfer of functions to the 'normal' hemisphere is greater in younger children and a better neuropsychological outcome is achieved in subjects operated on at an early age.

Focal cortical dysplasia (FCD)

FCD was originally described in 10 patients who were treated surgically for drug-resistant epilepsy.[36] The histologic abnormalities are restricted to one lobe or a small segment. Careful examination of brains with FCD may, however, show widespread minor dysplastic changes.[35] Histological abnormalities include (Figure 4C.2): local disorganization of laminar structure, large aberrant neurons, isolated neuronal heterotopia in subcortical white matter, balloon cells sharing histochemical characteristics of both neuronal and glial cells, giant and odd macroglia, and foci of demyelination and gliosis of adjacent white matter.[37] The abnormal area is not usually sharply delimited from adjacent tissue.[17,38] One or more of the above components may not be present and three main subtypes of FCD are recognized, which may correspond to the different times of embryologic origin. Type 1 is characterized by abnormal cortical lamination and ectopic neurons in white matter; type 2 presents with giant neurofilament-enriched neurons in addition to altered cortical lamination; and type 3 corresponds to Taylor-type FCD with giant dysmorphic neurons and balloon cells associated with cortical laminar disruption.[39] MR images show focal areas of cortical thickening, with simplified gyration, and rectilinear or blurred boundaries between gray and white matter (Figure 4C.1B).[40] Some cases present the involvement of an entire lobe (so-called partial HME). Normal brain MRI has been reported.[41,42]

FCD usually presents with intractable partial epilepsy, which may start at any age but generally before the end of adolescence. The focal features of the seizure depend on the location of the lesion and focal status epilepticus has frequently been reported.[41,43,44] Location in the precentral gyrus is often complicated by *epilepsia* partialis continua.[45–48] Unless the dysplastic area is large, patients do not suffer from severe neurological deficits. Interictal EEG shows focal, rhythmic epileptiform discharges in about half of the patients.[49] The ictal EEG abnormalities are highly specific for FCD, are located over the epileptogenic area and correlate with the continuous epileptiform discharges recorded during electrocorticography (EcoG).[43,50] ECoG seizure activity shows spatial co-localization with the lesion. At follow-up, most patients with complete resection of the tissue producing ictal ECoG discharges were seizure free or had over 90 per cent reduction in major seizures. None of the patients with persistence of discharging tissue had a favorable outcome.

Dysplastic tissue seems to have a peculiar tendency to produce epileptiform activity.[51,52] The mechanisms underlying the epileptiform activity generated by dysplastic

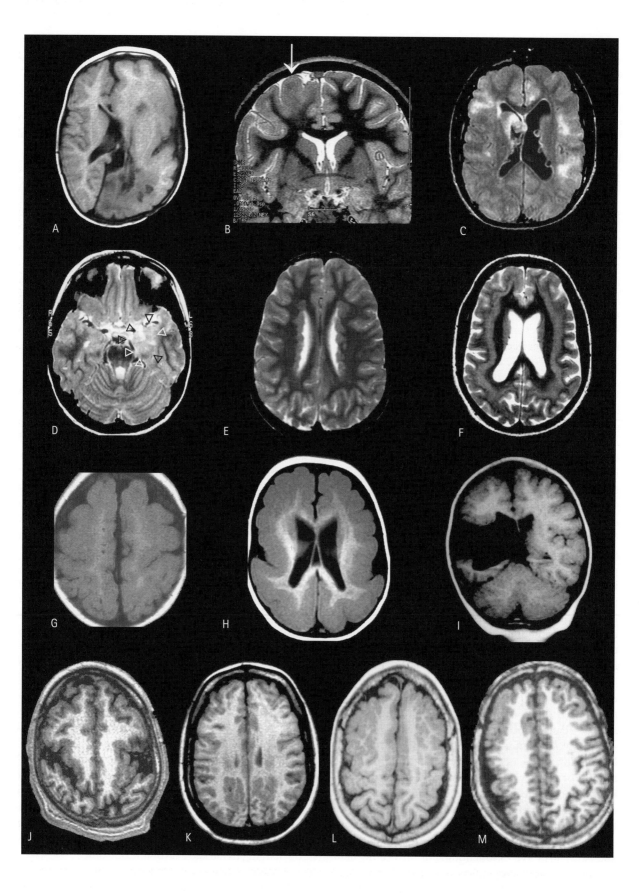

neocortex remain to be elucidated. In the abnormal cortical multilaminar organization typical of FCD, neurons are prevented from establishing normal synaptic connections with their neighbors and are dysfunctional. Intracellular recordings from neurons of dysplastic human neocortex have revealed no abnormalities in the membrane properties of single neurons.[53] However, a dysfunction of synaptic circuits seems to be responsible for the abnormal synchronization of neuronal populations underlying the genesis of epileptiform activity. Abnormalities

in the morphology and distribution of local-circuit GABAergic inhibitory neurons have been observed using immunocytochemistry.[46,54] Such abnormal circuitry may play an important role in originating and maintaining the epileptiform activity.

Most descriptions of FCD and HME are based on studies from epilepsy surgery centers, where histological

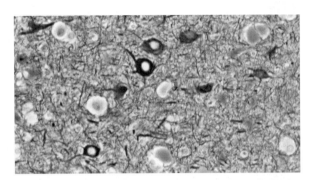

Figure 4C.2 *Focal cortical dysplasia. Silver-stained section showing irregular arrangement of large neurons and 'balloon cells'.*

Table 4C.3 *Conditions associated with hemimegalencephaly*

Epidermal nevus syndrome
Klippel-Trenaunay-Weber syndrome
Proteus syndrome
Neurofibromatosis
Ito hypomelanosis
Focal alopecia
Tuberous sclerosis
Dysembryoplastic neuroepithelial tumor

Opposite

Figure 4C.1 *A Hemimegalencephaly involving the left hemisphere. MRI, T1 weighted axial section. The architecture of the whole left hemisphere is severely impaired. Note the enlarged appearance of the hemisphere, bulging across the midline, with thickened and smooth cortex and blurred boundaries between gray and white matter, especially in the frontal lobe.*

B Right frontal focal cortical dysplasia (arrow) in a 14-year-old girl with intractable focal epilepsy. Coronal MRI scan. The cortex presents thickened gyri and is not clearly separated from the underlying white matter.

C Tuberous sclerosis in a 22-year-old male patient with symptomatic generalized epilepsy and mental retardation. PD weighted axial MRI scan. Several subependymal calcified nodules are present along the ventricular walls. At least three hyperintense, subcortical lesions are clearly visible, one in the right and two in the left frontal lobe. They represent cortical tubers. A fourth lesion (tumoral) involves the right thalamus.

D MRI, T2 weighted axial section. Left temporal DNET, visible as an area of enhanced signal is in the anteriomedial aspect of the left temporal lobe (arrows) in a 6-year-old boy with drug-resistant complex partial seizures.

E MRI, T2 weighted axial section. Bilateral periventricular nodular heterotopia. Nodules of gray matter, presenting the same signal as the normal cortex, are lining the lateral ventricles.

F Subcortical band heterotopia. MRI T2 weighted axial slice showing a thick diffuse band of heterotopic cortex. Twenty-year-old woman with drug-resistant partial epilepsy and DCX gene mutation.

G XLIS lissencephaly. T1 weighted axial section. A simplified gyral pattern with severely thickened cortex is observed with a prominent frontal involvement.

H LIS1 lissencephaly. T1 weighted axial section showing a simplified gyral pattern and a thick cortex that is completely smooth, especially in the posterior brain.

I Unilateral open lip schizencephaly. T1 weighted coronal MRI. A large cleft in the right hemisphere spans from the subarachnoid space to the lateral ventricle.

J Bilateral perisylvian polymicrogyria. T1 weighted axial section showing open sylvian fissures overlaid by an irregular and thick cortex. Sixteen-year-old male patient with facio-pharingo-glosso-masticatory diplegia, mild mental retardation and Lennox-Gastaut syndrome.

K Bilateral parasagittal parieto-occipital polymicrogyria. T1 weighted MRI showing irregular thickening and infolding of the cortex at mesial parieto-occipital junction.

L Bilateral frontal polymicrogyria. MRI, T1 weighted axial section. Polymicrogyric cortex with irregular, bumpy aspect involves all the gyral pattern anterior to the precentral gyri. A 10-year-old boy with spastic quadriparesis, moderate mental retardation and partial epilepsy. Seizures have been in remission for some years.

M Unilateral polymicrogyria. MRI, T1 weighted axial section. The right hemisphere is smaller than the left and the subarachnoid space overlying the right hemisphere is enlarged. The cortex on the right is irregular, with areas of thickening. Eight-year-old boy with left hemiparesis, moderate mental retardation, atypical absences and partial motor seizures.

diagnosis can be made during life. Thus, the clinical and electrophysiological features described are likely to be typical only of the most severe cases. Our experience indicates that there are some patients with well controlled seizures in whom MRI shows focal dysplastic lesions identical to those present in patients with histologically proven FCD.[55]

Tuberous sclerosis

Tuberous sclerosis or tuberous sclerosis complex (TSC) is a multisystem disorder involving primarily the central nervous system, the skin and the kidney.[56] The characteristic neuropathologic features are cortical tubers, subependymal nodules and giant cell tumors. The cortical tubers are characterized by their nodular appearance, firm texture, and variability in site, number and size and are the lesions that are most directly related to epileptogenesis. Microscopically, the tubers consist of subpial glial proliferation and an irregular neuronal lamination with giant multinucleated cells that are not clearly neuronal or astrocytic. These pathologic changes are similar to those seen in focal cortical dysplasia. The junction between gray and white matter is indistinct and may be partly demyelinated. Cortical tubers are usually well visualized by MRI scan as enlarged gyri with atypical shape and an abnormal signal intensity, involving mainly the subcortical white matter (Figure 4C.1C).[57] Tubers have a tendency to calcify, which increases with age. TSC is transmitted as an autosomal dominant trait, with variable expression. Recurrence in sibship of nonaffected parents has rarely been reported and is thought to be related to low expressivity or gonadal mosaicism. There is no clear evidence of nonpenetrance for TSC, so careful clinical and diagnostic evaluation of apparently unaffected parents is indicated before counseling the families. Between 50 and 75 per cent of all cases are sporadic. Linkage studies have allowed the identification of two loci for TSC, mapping to chromosome 9q34 (*TSC1*) and 16p13.3 (*TSC2*).[58] About 50 per cent of the families are linked to *TSC1*.[59] The *TSC1* gene consists of 23 exons and encodes for a predicted protein of 1164 amino acids called hamartin.[60] A mutation in this gene has been identified in about 80 per cent of the families linked to chromosome 9q34.[61] The identification of the gene mapping to 16p13.3 has been facilitated by the identification of interstitial deletions in five unrelated TSC patients.[62] A gene (*TSC2*) was found to be disrupted by all the deletions and was demonstrated to harbor intragenic mutations in other nondeleted TSC patients.[62] Both germline and somatic mutations in the *TSC2* genes have been demonstrated in tumors derived from patients with TS.

Epileptic seizures are frequent in TS, but it is not clear whether the epilepsy phenotype and long term seizure outcome of patients with *TSC1* and *TSC2* are different. However, sporadic patients with *TSC1* mutations usually have a milder disease than patients with *TSC2* mutations. They have a lower frequency of seizures and moderate to severe mental retardation, fewer subependymal nodules and cortical tubers, less severe kidney involvement, no retinal hamartomas, and less severe facial angiofibroma.[63] The seizures usually begin before the age of 15, with 70 per cent presenting before 2 years.[56] Infantile spasms are the most common manifestation of epilepsy in the first year of life, sometimes preceded by partial seizures.[64] In their study of 126 patients, Roger et al.[65] found 63 (50 per cent) with infantile spasms and 63 (50 per cent) with other types of epilepsy (35 partial, 11 Lennox-Gastaut syndrome, 4 symptomatic generalized, 6 occasional seizures and 7 unclassifiable). Two thirds of those patients without infantile spasms had their first seizure before the age of 2 years, and a poor prognosis was strongly related to early onset. Almost all patients were cognitively impaired, and the course of epilepsy was severe in about one third. The number and size of tubers seems to be correlated with the severity of epilepsy and of mental disturbances.[69] In children with partial epilepsy or with infantile spasms, the largest tuber was found in the area corresponding to the main EEG focus.[66] However, MRI may fail to show all the tubers in infants if myelination is not complete.[57] Patients with TS must be carefully investigated in order to determine whether there is a single epileptogenic area in that its surgical removal can yield good control of seizures.[67,68]

Gangliogliomas and dysembrioplastic neuroepithelial tumors (DNET)

These highly heterogeneous lesions are supratentorial tumours resembling gliomas, but characterized by a benign evolution and a distinct cortical topography. Gangliogliomas are histologically characterized by a glioma component intermixed with an atypical neuronal or ganglion cell component.[75] Atypical neuronal or ganglion cells are frequently binucleate. Cell proliferation studies show that the tumor growth rate is slow.[75] DNET are similar to gangliogliomas, but cytological atypia are rarer. The observation that dysplastic neurons are frequently adjacent to the neoplastic lesions[71,75] has suggested a maldevelopmental basis for the tumor origin.[70,71] In large series of patients with chronic drug-resistant epilepsy due to neoplastic lesions, gangliogliomas and DNET represent the majority (50–75 per cent) of histopathologically diagnosed lesions after surgery.[71–74] Any lobe can be affected, but the temporal lobe is the most frequent for both gangliogliomas and DNET.[71]

Neuroradiological studies typically show an hypodense lesion on CT scan, with possible associated hyperdense calcified lesions. The overlying skull can be deformed in superficially located lesions.[71] A cystic component is frequently observed. MRI scan (Figure 4C.1D) shows an hyperintense T1 lesion, with peripheral enhancement after gadolinium administration. Gray and white matter are both involved.[71] A well-demarcated, multilocular appearance is typically seen.

The typical clinical presentation is with a drug-resistant partial epilepsy with onset before age 20.[71] In a population of 89 patients presenting with DNET, partial seizures were the first clinical signs in 75 per cent of patients; only 9 per cent had neurological deficits consisting of quadrantanopia.[71] Epilepsy started at a mean age of 9 years (range 1–20 years) and proved resistant to different antiepileptic medications. Complete surgical removal of the lesion is associated to remission of epilepsy in all patients.[71]

MALFORMATIONS DUE TO ABNORMAL NEURONAL MIGRATION

Scattered and rare heterotopic neurons are occasionally found in subcortical white matter of normal subjects, but a density exceeding 8 neurons/2 mm^2 is considered neuronal heterotopia,[77] and a density visible to the naked eye is considered gray matter heterotopia.[78] Histologically, these neurons have a normal morphology but lack normal synaptic connections.[76] The most common type of heterotopia is nodular heterotopia located in either a subependymal or subcortical location. Other minor forms of heterotopia include leptomeningeal neuronal heterotopia,[24] subpial neuronal heterotopia, and ectopic neurons scattered throughout the molecular layer. Gray matter heterotopia has the same signal characteristics as normal cortex on MRI and the same metabolic activity as normal gray matter on FDG-PET imaging.[79] Gray matter heterotopia can occur diffusely or be localized. Diffuse involvement occurs as subcortical band (or laminar) heterotopia[80] and as bilateral periventricular nodular heterotopia. Localized forms can be unilateral or bilateral subependymal, unilateral subcortical (nodular, laminar), or may extend from the subependymal region to the subcortex unilaterally.

Bilateral periventricular nodular heterotopia (BPNH)

BPNH consists of confluent and symmetric subependymal nodules of gray matter located along the lateral ventricles particularly along the ventricular body (Figure 4C.1E). The extent of the heterotopia and associated clinical symptoms are heterogeneous. BPNH occurs much more frequently in females, as part of the syndrome of X-linked BPNH, which is associated with prenatal lethality in almost all males[81] and a 50 per cent recurrence risk in the female offspring of affected women. X-linked BPNH and BPNH occurring sporadically have been associated with mutations of the filamin A gene (*FLNA*).[82–84] BPNH is an X-linked dominant disorder and heterozygous females have epilepsy and coagulopathy. The disease has been mapped to Xq28 by linkage analysis, and mutations in *FLNA* have been demonstrated in both familial and sporadic patients with BPNH.[82,83] Other unidentified genes may cause bilateral periventricular heterotopia in both sexes, with slightly different anatomic characteristics. *FLNA* promotes orthogonal branching of actin filaments and links actin filaments to membrane glycoproteins.

Approximately 88 per cent of patients with BPNH have epilepsy,[88] which can begin at any age. Seizure intractability is common. Female patients with BPNH usually have normal to borderline intelligence and epilepsy of variable severity. The only two living male patients reported both have features similar to those described in females.[83] Several other syndromes characterized by BPNH and mental retardation have also been described. These always occur sporadically and almost exclusively in boys.[85–87]

Classical lissencephaly and subcortical band heterotopia (the agyria–pachygyria–band spectrum)

Lissencephaly (smooth brain) is a severe abnormality of neuronal migration characterized by absent (agyria) or decreased (pachygyria) convolutions, producing a smooth cerebral surface.[89] Although there are several types of lissencephaly,[16] the most frequent and best-characterized forms are caused by mutations of the *LIS1* gene[90] and of the *XLIS* (or *DCX*) gene.[91,92] Subcortical band heterotopia (SBH) is at the mild end of the agyria–pachygyria–band spectrum of malformations.[81] In SBH, the gyral pattern is usually simplified with broad convolutions and increased cortical thickness. Just beneath the cortical ribbon, a thin band of white matter separates the cortex from a heterotopic band of gray matter of variable thickness and extension (Figure 4C.1F).[93] In general, the thicker the heterotopic band, the higher the chances of finding a pachygyric cortical surface.[80] *XLIS* lissencephaly (Figure 4C.1G) and SBH have been observed in different individuals within the same family.[94,95] Pathological studies of both lissencephaly and SBH demonstrate incomplete neuronal migration. In classical lissencephaly, the cerebral cortex is abnormally thick. The cytoarchitecture consists of four primitive layers including an outer marginal layer, a superficial cellular layer which corresponds to the true cortex, a variable cell sparse layer and a deep cellular layer composed of heterotopic neurons.[89]

As neuropathological studies were carried out before the distinction between *LIS1* (Figure 4C.1H) and *XLIS* lissencephaly was made, it is not known whether these two forms have distinctive histologic findings. SBH consists of symmetric and circumferential bands of gray matter, which may extend from the frontal to occipital regions but show regional predominance in many patients. The cortex overlying the bands appears either normal or pachygyric. Pathologic study of the brains of three women with SBH[76] revealed that the cerebral cortex had normal cell density and laminar organization. Neurons in the heterotopic band were either arranged haphazardly or organized in a pattern suggestive of columnar organization. Several malformation syndromes associated with classical lissencephaly have been described. The best known of these is Miller-Dieker syndrome, which is caused by large deletions of *LIS1* gene and contiguous genes.[96] The most frequent form, X-linked dominant lissencephaly and SBH, is characterized by classical lissencephaly in hemizygous males and SBH in heterozygous females.

The *DCX* gene is located on chromosome Xq22.3-q24.[92,97-99] Mutations of the coding region of *DCX* were found in all reported pedigrees[95] and in 38–91 per cent of sporadic female patients.[98,100,101] Whereas all women with *DCX* mutations have anteriorly predominant band/pachygyria, about one fourth of those with anterior band and all those with posteriorly predominant band or with unilateral band have not shown *DCX* mutations, suggesting that other loci or mosaicism may be responsible for these variable phenotypes.[101,102] Maternal germline or mosaic *DCX* mutations may occur in about 10 per cent of cases of either SBH or *XLIS*.[102] The rare cases of SBH reported in boys have been associated with missense mutations of *DCX* or *LIS1*.[103] The genetics and function of *DCX* are discussed extensively by Gleeson in a recent review.[93] *LIS1* (approved gene symbol *PAFAH1B1*) is the gene responsible for Miller-Dieker lissencephaly and maps to chromosome 17p13.3.[90] In addition, approximately 65 per cent of patients with classic lissencephaly who lack the facial changes of Miller-Dieker syndrome, isolated lissencephaly (ILS), show a mutation involving the *LIS1* gene. Among all the patients with ILS, 40 per cent exhibit a deletion involving the entire gene,[104] and 25 per cent show an intragenic mutation (4 per cent gross rearrangement, 17 per cent deletion/truncating mutations, 4 per cent missense mutations).[105] Patients with missense mutations generally have milder malformations than those with truncating/deletion mutations.[105, 106]

Classical lissencephaly appears to be quite rare, with a prevalence of 11.7 per million births (1 in 85 470).[107] Affected children have early developmental delay and eventual profound mental retardation and spastic quadriparesis. Some children with lissencephaly have lived more than 20 years, but life span is often much shorter. Seizures occur in over 90 per cent of children, with onset before 6 months in about 75 per cent. About 80 per cent of children have infantile spasms, although the EEG may not show typical hypsarrhythmia. Most children subsequently have multiple seizure types including persisting spasms, focal motor and generalized tonic seizures,[25,108-110] complex partial seizures, atypical absences, atonic and myoclonic seizures. In this severe malformation the physiological processes of postnatal cortical maturation are lacking as shown by the absence of any age- or localization-related changes in regional cerebral blood flow using SPECT.[111] The EEG in many children with lissencephaly demonstrates diffuse high-amplitude fast rhythms[112] and this pattern is considered to be highly specific for this malformation.[113]

The main clinical manifestations of SBH are mental retardation and epilepsy. Cognitive function ranges from normal to severe retardation and correlates with the width of the band and degree of pachygyria.[80] Epilepsy is common, although very early seizure onset is uncommon. About 85 per cent of patients have epilepsy[25,80,114-118] and 65 per cent have an intractable form. Among patients with epilepsy, about 50 per cent have partial epilepsy and 50 per cent have a generalized form, often Lennox-Gastaut syndrome. Those with more severe MRI abnormalities have significantly earlier seizure onset and are more likely to develop Lennox-Gastaut syndrome or other generalized symptomatic epilepsy. Using depth electrodes, Morrell *et al.*[117] demonstrated that epileptiform activity may originate directly from the heterotopic neurons, independently of the activity of the overlying cortex. Callosotomy has been associated with worthwhile improvement in drop attacks in a few patients.[115,118]

Autosomal recessive lissencephaly with cerebellar hypoplasia

Two recessive pedigrees, each with three affected sibs showing moderately severe pachygyria and severe cerebellar hypoplasia, have been associated with mutations of the reelin gene.[119] Affected children in one family had congenital lymphedema, hypotonia, severe developmental delay and generalized seizures that were controlled by drugs. Severe hypotonia, delay and seizures were reported also in the other pedigree.

MALFORMATIONS DUE TO ABNORMAL CORTICAL ORGANIZATION

Aicardi syndrome

Aicardi syndrome[120,121] has been reported only in females, except for two males who each had two X chromosomes.[122] There has been a report of two affected sisters.[123]

It may be caused by an X-linked gene with lethality in the hemizygous male. Eye abnormalities and agenesis of the corpus callosum are frequently associated with translocations involving Xp22.3, suggesting a possible linkage of Aicardi syndrome to the short arm of chromosome X. The neuropathological findings include a thin unlayered cortex, diffuse unlayered polymicrogyria with fused molecular layers, and nodular heterotopias in the periventricular region and in the centrum semiovale.[125,126] No laminar organization is recognizable in the cortex beyond the molecular layer, and neurons have a radial disposition. As a result of the fusion of the molecular layers, the microgyri are packed and not visible on MRI. Less frequent malformations include agenesis of the anterior commissure, the fornix, or both, choroid plexus cysts, colobomata, and vertebral and costal abnormalities.

The clinical picture includes severe mental retardation, infantile spasms, chorioretinal lacunae and agenesis of the corpus callosum. There is often an early onset of infantile spasms and partial seizures. Spasms were the only seizure type in 47 per cent and were accompanied by partial seizures in 35 per cent of 184 patients.[127] The partial seizures involved mainly the eyes and face, and often began in the first days of life. Hypsarrhythmia is observed in only about 18 per cent of patients.[122] Interictal EEG abnormalities are typically asymmetric and asynchronous and may include suppression bursts during wakefulness and sleep. The seizures are almost always resistant to medication and the seizure types and EEG patterns change little over time. Life expectancy is shortened, with an estimated survival rate of 75 per cent at 6 years and 40 per cent at 15 years.[124]

Schizencephaly

Schizencephaly (cleft brain) consists of a unilateral or bilateral full-thickness cleft of the cerebral hemispheres with communication between the ventricle and extra-axial subarachnoid spaces (Figure 4C.1I). The walls of the clefts may be widely separated (open-lip schizencephaly) or closely adjacent (closed-lip schizencephaly). The clefts may be located in any region of the hemispheres, but are most often found in the perisylvian area.[128] Bilateral clefts are usually symmetric in location, but not necessarily in size. Septo-optic dysplasia (agenesis of the septum pellucidum and optic nerve hypoplasia) is seen in up to one third of patients.[129] Schizencephaly is a malformation that is difficult to classify. This disorder may be due to a regional absence of proliferation of neurons and glia or to defective cortical organization.[16] The cortex surrounding the cleft consists of polymicrogyric convolutions with a stellate aspect.[130,131] Yakovlev and Wadsworth[130] suggested that the pathogenesis involved a local failure of induction of neuronal migration. In contrast, Barkovich

and Kjos[128] considered that ischemic damage during early gestation could cause focal necrosis with destruction of the radial glial fibers and consequent abnormalities of neuronal migration, such as unlayered polymicrogyria and gray matter heterotopia. However, recent reports from the same group indicate that familial occurrence[132] and a specific genetic origin due to germline mutations in the homeobox gene EMX2 (human), may be responsible in rare cases.[133,134] Severe mutations were associated with severe bilateral schizencephaly, whereas missense mutations were associated with a milder cortical abnormality.[135]

The broad range of clinical findings mirrors the wide spectrum of anatomic abnormalities in schizencephaly. Unilateral clefts and closed-lip clefts are associated with a less severe clinical phenotype. Small, unilateral closed-lip clefts may be demonstrated on MRI scans performed after the onset of seizures in otherwise normal individuals.[128] Patients with bilateral clefts usually have microcephaly, severe developmental delay and spastic quadriparesis.[128,136] Partial seizures occur in 81 per cent of patients and usually begin before 3 years of age. The incidence of seizures is similar in those with unilateral and bilateral clefts but seizures are more often intractable when the malformation is bilateral.[136]

Polymicrogyria

Polymicrogyria is characterized by an excessive number of small and prominent convolutions spaced out by shallow and enlarged sulci, giving the cortical surface a lumpy aspect.[89] Cortical infolding and secondary, irregular, thickening due to packing of microgyri are quite distinctive MRI characteristics of polymicrogyria (Figure 4C.1J–M).[16,137] However, polymicrogyria may be difficult to recognize on MRI because the microconvolutions are often packed and merged.[44] Two histologic types of polymicrogyria are recognized. In unlayered polymicrogyria, the external molecular layer is continuous and does not follow the profile of the convolutions, and the underlying neurons have radial distribution but no laminar organization.[131] These features suggest an early disruption of normal neuronal migration with subsequent disordered cortical organization. In contrast, four-layered polymicrogyria is believed to result from perfusion failure, occurring between weeks 20 and 24 of gestation, which leads to intracortical laminar necrosis with consequent late migration disorder and postmigratory disruption of cortical organization.[138] The two types of polymicrogyria may co-occur in contiguous cortical areas (Figure 4C.3),[139] indicating that they may comprise a single spectrum. The extent of polymicrogyria varies greatly and there is a broad range of clinical manifestations from severe encephalopathy with intractable epilepsy to individuals with only selective impairment of cognitive functions.[140]

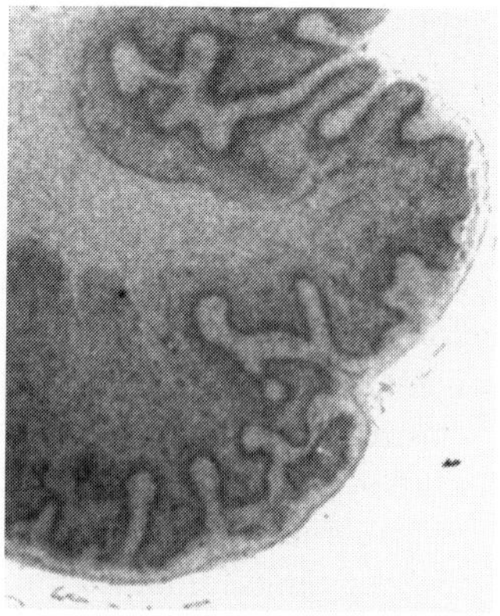

Figure 4C.3 *Specimen of the right frontal lobe from postmortem brain examination in a newborn with diffuse polymicrogyria. Areas of typical four-layered polymicrogyria with abnormal cortical infolding and packing of microgyri border with zones of cortical thickening with loss of layering (Cresyl violet).*

Several syndromes featuring bilateral polymicrogyria have been described, including bilateral perisylvian polymicrogyria (BPP – Figure 4C.1J),[141] bilateral parasagittal parietooccipital polymicrogyria (Figure 4C.1K),[142] bilateral frontal polymicrogyria (Figure 4C.1L)[143] and unilateral perisylvian or multilobar polymicrogyria (Figure 4C.1M).[44] These may represent distinct entities that reflect the influence of regionally expressed developmental genes. However, consistent familial recurrence has been reported only for BPP,[144] which is sporadic in the great majority of patients. Genetic factors may also play a role in the pathogenesis of unilateral polymicrogyria, at least in some cases.[145]

Bilateral perisylvian polymicrogyria (BPP)

This malformation involves the gray matter bordering the sylvian fissure bilaterally. Neuropathologic studies in four sporadic cases demonstrated four-layered polymicrogyria in three[141,146] and unlayered polymicrogyria in one.[147] It is unclear whether these cases represent a spectrum of changes within a single malformation with the same etiology or different malformations with the same topography. Several families with multiple affected members have been reported, indicating genetic heterogeneity with possible autosomal recessive,[144] X-linked dominant[148] and X-linked recessive[149] inheritance. Recently a locus for X-linked BPP was mapped to Xq28.[150] Polymicrogyria, including BPP, has been reported in association with a deletion at 22q11.2,[151–153] although most patients with 22q11.2 deletion do not have any brain abnormality.[154] BPP has also been reported in children born from monochorionic biamniotic twin pregnancies which were complicated by twin–twin transfusion syndrome,[155,156] indicating causal heterogeneity.

Patients with BPP have facio-pharyngo-glosso-masticatory diplegia[47,157] and dysarthria. Most have mental retardation and epilepsy. Seizures usually begin between age 4 and 12 years and are poorly controlled in about 65 per cent of patients. The most frequent seizure types are atypical absence, tonic, atonic drop attacks and tonic-clonic seizures, often occurring as Lennox-Gastaut-like syndromes.[3,158] A minority of patients (26 per cent) have partial seizures.

KEY POINTS

- Malformations of the cerebral cortex are the cause of some of the most severe forms of childhood epilepsy, but there is a **broad range of seizure severity**
- Early onset severe epilepsy in children with **cortical dysplasia** significantly reduces the potential for an independent adult life. Seizure improvement is possible, but long-lasting remission is exceptional
- MRI has demonstrated that **brain malformations are common in children with epilepsy**. However, MRI is often normal in patients with malformations and often fails to demonstrate the full extent of the abnormality
- **Abnormally connected neurons in malformations have a high intrinsic epileptogenicity** and some electrographic patterns are highly suggestive of an underlying area of cortical dysplasia
- Co-localization of the abnormality on neuroimaging with epileptogenic EEG activity may help considerably in planning a surgical resection. **Functional neuroimaging**, particularly PET and ictal SPECT, may also help to establish the location of the epileptogenic dysplastic cortex

---

REFERENCES

1. Barkovich AJ, Kuzniecky RI, Jackson GD, Guerrini R, Dobyns WB. Classification system for malformations of cortical development. Update 2001. *Neurology* 2001; **57**: 2168–2178.
2. Guerrini R, Holthausen H, Parmeggiani L, Chiron C. Epilepsy and malformations of the cerebral cortex. In: Roger J, Bureau M, Dravet C, *et al.* (eds) *Epileptic Syndromes in Infancy, Childhood and Adolescence*, 3rd edn. London, John Libbey, 2002.
3. Kuzniecky RI. Magnetic resonance imaging in developmental disorders of the cerebral cortex. *Epilepsia* 1994; **35**(Suppl. 6): S44–56.
4. Tuxhorn I, Holthausen H, Boenigk H (eds). *Paediatric Epilepsy Syndromes and their Surgical Treatment*. London: John Libbey, 1997; 749–773.

5. Walsh CA. Genetic malformations of the human cerebral cortex. *Neuron* 1999; **23**: 19–29.

6. Acampora D, Mazan S, Lallemand Y, *et al.* Forebrain and midbrain regions are deleted in Otx2−/− mutants due to a defective anterior neuroectoderm specification during gastrulation. *Development* 1995; **121**: 3279–3290.

7. Matsuo I, Kuratani S, Kimura C, Takeda N, Aizawa S. Mouse Otx2 functions in the formation and patterning of rostral head. *Genes and Development* 1995; **9**: 2646–2658.

8. Qiu M, Bulfone A, Martinez S, *et al.* Null mutation of Dlx-2 results in abnormal morphogenesis of proximal first and second branchial archderivatives and abnormal differentiation in the forebrain. *Genes and Development* 1995; **9**: 2523–2538.

9. Labosky PA, Winnier GE, Jetton TL, *et al.* The winged helix gene, Mf3, is required for normal development of the diencephalon and midbrain, postnatal growth and the milk-ejection reflex. *Development* 1997; **124**: 1263–1274.

10. Porter FD, Drago J, Xu Y, *et al.* Lhx2, a LIM homeobox gene, is required for eye, forebrain, and definitive erythrocyte development. *Development* 1997; **124**: 2935–2944.

11. Szucsik JC, Witte DP, Li H, *et al.* Altered forebrain and hindbrain development in mice mutant for the Gsh-2 homeobox gene. *Developmental Biology* 1997; **191**: 230–242.

12. Yoshida M, Suda Y, Matsuo I, *et al.* Emx1 and Emx2 functions in development of dorsal telencephalon. *Development* 1997; **124**: 101–111.

13. Sidman RL, Rakic P. Development of the human central nervous system. In: Haymaker W, Adams RD (eds) *Histology and Histopathology of the Nervous System*. Springfield: Charles Thomas, 1982; 3–145.

14. Norman MG, McGillivray BC, Kalousek DK, Hill A, Poskitt KJ. *Congenital Malformations of the Brain: Pathological, Embryological, Clinical, Radiological and Genetic Aspects*. New York: Oxford University Press, 1995.

15. Rakic P. Mode of cell migration to the superficial layers of fetal monkey neocortex. *Journal of Comparative Neurology* 1972; **145**: 61–83.

16. Barkovich AJ. Magnetic resonance imaging of lissencephaly, polymicrogyria, schizencephaly, hemimegalencephaly, and band heterotopia. In: Guerrini R, Andermann F, Canapicchi R, *et al.* (eds) *Dysplasias of Cerebral Cortex and Epilepsy*. Philadelphia: Lippincott-Raven, 1996; 115–129.

17. Robain O. Introduction to the pathology of cerebral cortical dysplasia. In: Guerrini R, Andermann F, Canapicchi R, *et al.* (eds) *Dysplasias of Cerebral Cortex and Epilepsy*. Philadelphia: Lippincott-Raven, 1996; 1–9.

18. Guerrini R, Andermann F, Canapicchi R, *et al.* (eds) *Dysplasias of Cerebral Cortex and Epilepsy*. Philadelphia: Lippincott-Raven, 1996.

19. Barkovich AJ, Kuzniecky RI, Dobyns WB, *et al.* A classification scheme for malformations of cortical development. *Neuropediatrics* 1996; **27**: 59–63.

20. Richman DP, Stewart RM, Caviness VS Jr. Cerebral microgyria in a 27-weeks fetus: an architectonic and topographic analysis. *Journal of Neuropathology and Experimental Neurology* 1974; **33**: 374–384.

21. Robain O, Gelot A. Neuropathology of hemimegalencephaly. In: Guerrini R, Andermann F, Canapicchi R, *et al.* (eds) *Dysplasias of Cerebral Cortex and Epilepsy*. Philadelphia: Lippincott-Raven, 1996; 89–92.

22. Robain O, Floquet J, Heldt N, Rozemberg F. Hemimegalencephaly: a clinicopathological study of four cases. *Neuropathology and Applied Neurobiology* 1988; **14**: 125–135.

23. Jahan R, Mischel PS, Curran JG, *et al.* Bilateral neuropathologic changes in a child with hemimegalencephaly. *Pediatric Neurology* 1997; **17**: 344–349.

24. Sarnat HB. *Cerebral Dysgenesis: Embryology and Clinical Expression*. New York: Oxford University Press, 1992.

25. Guerrini R, Dravet C, Bureau M, *et al.* Diffuse and localized dysplasias of cerebral cortex: clinical presentation, outcome, and proposal for a morphologic MRI classification based on a study of 90 patients. In: Guerrini R, Andermann F, Canapicchi R, *et al.* (eds) *Dysplasias of Cerebral Cortex and Epilepsy*. Philadelphia: Lippincott-Raven, 1996; 255–269.

26. Fusco L, Ferracuti S, Fariello G, Manfredi M, Vigevano F. Hemimegalencephaly and normal intellectual development. *Journal of Neurology, Neurosurgery and Psychiatry* 1992; **55**: 720–722.

27. Vigevano F, Fusco L, Granata T, *et al.* Hemimegalencephaly: clinical and EEG characteristics. In: Guerrini R, Andermann F, Canapicchi R, *et al.* (eds) *Dysplasias of Cerebral Cortex and Epilepsy*. Philadelphia: Lippincott-Raven, 1996; 285–294.

28. Vigevano F, Bertini E, Boldrini R, *et al.* Hemimegalencephaly and intractable epilepsy: benefits of hemispherectomy. *Epilepsia* 1989; **30**: 833–843.

29. Paladin F, Chiron C, Dulac O, Plouin P, Ponsot G. Electroencephalographic aspects of hemimegalencephaly. *Developmental Medicine and Child Neurology* 1989; **31**: 377–383.

30. Bignami A, Palladini G, Zappella M. Unilateral megalencephaly with cell hypertrophy. An anatomical and quantitative histochemical study. *Brain Research* 1968; **9**: 103–114.

31. Tjiam AT, Stefanko S, Shenk VWD, de Vlieger M. Infantile spasms associated with hemihypsarrhythmia and hemimegalencephaly. *Developmental Medicine and Child Neurology* 1978; **20**: 779–789.

32. King M, Stephenson JB, Ziervogel M, Doyle D, Galbraith S. Hemimegalencephaly. A case for hemispherectomy? *Neuropediatrics* 1985; **16**: 46–55.

33. Trounce JQ, Rutter N, Mellor DH. Hemimegalencephaly: diagnosis and treatment. *Developmental Medicine and Child Neurology* 1991; **33**: 257–266.

34. Di Rocco C. Surgical treatment of hemimegalencephaly. In: Guerrini R, Andermann F, Canapicchi R, *et al.* (eds) *Dysplasias of Cerebral Cortex and Epilepsy*. Philadelphia: Lippincott-Raven, 1996: 295–304.

35. Janota I, Polkey CE. Cortical dysplasia in epilepsy. A study of material from surgical resections for intractable epilepsy. In: Pedley TA, Meldrum BS (eds) *Recent Advances in Epilepsy*. New York: Churchill Livingstone, 1992; 37–49.

36. Taylor DC, Falconer MA, Bruton CJ, Corsellis JAN. Focal dysplasia of the cerebral cortex in epilepsy. *Journal of Neurology, Neurosurgery and Psychiatry* 1971; **34**: 369–387.

37. Jay V, Becker LE, Otsubo H, Hwang PA, Hoffman HJ, Harwood-Nash D. Pathology of temporal lobectomy for refractory seizures in children. Review of 20 cases including some unique malformative lesions. *Journal of Neurosurgery* 1993; **79**: 53–61.

38. Mischel PS, Nguyen LP, Vinters HV. Cerebral cortical dysplasia associated with pediatric epilepsy. Review of neuropathologic features and proposal for a grading system. *Journal of Neuropathology and Experimental Neurology* 1995; **54**: 137–153.

39. Tassi L, Colombo N, Garbelli R, *et al*. Focal cortical dysplasia: neuropathological subtypes, EEG, neuroimaging and surgical outcome. *Brain* 2002; **125**: 1719–1732.

40. Kuzniecky RI. MRI in focal cortical dysplasia. In: Guerrini R, Andermann F, Canapicchi R, *et al*. (eds) *Dysplasias of Cerebral Cortex and Epilepsy*. Philadelphia: Lippincott-Raven, 1996; 145–150.

41. Desbiens R, Berkovic SF, Dubeau F, *et al*. Life-threatening focal status epilepticus due to occult cortical dysplasia. *Archives of Neurology* 1993; **50**: 695–700.

42. Fogarasi A, Janszky J, Faveret E, Pieper T, Tuxhorn I. A detailed analysis of frontal lobe seizure semiology in children younger than 7 years. *Epilepsia* 2001; **42**: 80–85.

43. Palmini A, Gambardella A, Andermann F, *et al*. Intrinsic epileptogenicity of human dysplastic cortex as suggested by corticography and surgical results. *Annals of Neurology* 1995; **37**: 476–487.

44. Guerrini R, Dravet C, Raybaud C, Roger J, *et al*. Epilepsy and focal gyral anomalies detected by magnetic resonance imaging: electroclinico-morphological correlations and follow-up. *Developmental Medicine and Child Neurology* 1992; **34**: 706–718.

45. Kuzniecky R, Berkovic S, Andermann F, *et al*. Focal cortical myoclonus and rolandic cortical dysplasia: clarification by magnetic resonance imaging. *Annals of Neurology* 1988; **23**: 317–325.

46. Ferrer I, Pineda M, Tallada M, *et al*. Abnormal local circuit neurons in epilepsia partialis continua associated with focal cortical dysplasia. *Acta Neuropathologica* 1992; **83**: 647–652.

47. Kuzniecky R, Powers R. Epilepsia partialis continua due to cortical dysplasia. *Journal of Child Neurology* 1993; **8**: 386–388.

48. Aicardi J. The place of neuronal migration abnormalities in child neurology. *Canadian Journal of Neurological Science* 1994; **21**: 185–193.

49. Gambardella A, Palmini A, Andermann F, *et al*. Usefulness of focal rhythmic discharges on scalp EEG of patients with focal cortical dysplasia and intractable epilepsy. *Electroencephalography and Clinical Neurophysiology* 1996; **98**: 243–249.

50. Palmini A, Gambardella A, Andermann F, *et al*. The human dysplastic cortex is intrinsically epileptogenic. In: Guerrini R, Andermann F, Canapicchi R, *et al*. (eds) *Dysplasias of Cerebral Cortex and Epilepsy*. Philadelphia: Lippincott-Raven, 1996: 43–52.

51. Avoli M, Mattia D, Siniscalchi A, Perreault P, Tomaiuolo F. Pharmacology and electrophysiology of a synchronous GABA-mediated potential in the human neocortex. *Neuroscience* 1994; **62**: 655–666.

52. Mattia D, Oliver A, Avoli M. Seizures-like discharges recorded in the human dysplastic neocortex maintained *in vitro*. *Neurology* 1995; **45**: 1391–1395.

53. Avoli M, Hwa GGC, Lacaille JC, Olivier A, Villemeure JG. Electrophysiological and repetitive firing properties of neurons in the superficial/middle layers of the human neocortex. *Experimental Brain Research* 1994; **98**: 135–144.

54. Spreafico R, Battaglia G, Arcelli P, *et al*. Cortical dysplasia: an immunocytochemical study of three patients. *Neurology* 1998; **50**: 27–36.

55. Dravet C, Guerrini R, Mancini J, *et al*. Different outcomes of epilepsy due to cortical dysplastic lesions. In: Guerrini R, Andermann F, Canapicchi R, *et al*. (eds) *Dysplasias of Cerebral Cortex and Epilepsy*. Philadelphia: Lippincott-Raven, 1996; 323–328.

56. Gomez MR. *Tuberous Sclerosis*. New York: Raven Press, 1979.

57. Barkovich AJ. *Pediatric Neuroimaging*. New York: Raven Press, 1995.

58. Povey S, Burley MW, Attwood J, *et al*. Two loci for tuberous sclerosis: one on 9q34 and one on 16p13. *Annals of Human Genetics* 1994; **58**: 107–127.

59. Van Bakel I, Sepp T, Ward S, Yates JRW, Green AJ. Mutations in the TSC2 gene: analysis of the complete coding sequence using the protein truncation test [PTT]. *Human Molecular Genetics* 1997; **6**: 1409–1414.

60. Curatolo P, Cusmai R. MRI in Bourneville disease: relationship with EEG findings. *Neurophysiologie Clinique* 1988; **18**: 149–157.

61. Van Slegtenhorst M, de Hoogt R, Hermans C, *et al*. Identification of the tuberous sclerosis gene TSC1 on chromosome 9q34. *Science* 1997; **277**: 805–808.

62. Jones AC, Shyamsundar MM, Thomas MW, *et al*. Comprehensive mutation analysis of TSC1 and TSC2 and phenotypic correlations in 150 families with tuberous sclerosis. *American Journal of Human Genetics* 1999; **64**: 1305–1315.

63. European Chromosome 16 Tuberous Sclerosis Consortium. Identification and characterization of the tuberous sclerosis gene on chromosome 16. *Cell* 1993; **75**: 1305–1315.

64. Dabora SL, Jozwiak S, Franz DN, *et al*. Mutational analysis in a cohort of 224 tuberous sclerosis patients indicates increased severity of TSC2, compared with TSC1, disease in multiple organs. *American Journal of Human Genetics* 2001; **68**: 64–80.

65. Dulac O, Lemaitre A, Plouin P. Maladie de Bourneville: aspects cliniques et électroencéphalographiques de l'épilepsie dans la première année. *Bollettino della Lega Italiana contro l'Epilessia* 1984; **45/46**: 39–42.

66. Roger J, Dravet Ch, Boniver C, *et al*. L'épilepsie dans la sclérose tubéreuse de Bourneville. *Bollettino della Lega Italiana contro l'Epilessia* 1984; **45/46**: 33–38.

67. Bebin EM, Kelly PJ, Gomez M. Surgical treatment in cerebral tuberous sclerosis. *Epilepsia* 1993; **34**: 651–657.

68. Sivelle G, Kahane P, de Saint-Martin A, *et al*. La multilocalité des lésions dans la sclérose tubéreuse de Bourneville contre-indique-t-elle une approche chirurgicale? *Epilepsies* 1995; **7**: 451–464.

69. Jambaqué I, Cusmai R, Curatolo P, *et al*. Neuropsychological aspects of tuberous sclerosis in relation to epilepsy and MRI findings. *Developmental Medicine and Child Neurology* 1991; **33**: 698–705.

70. Prayson RA, Estes ML, Morris HH. Coexistence of neoplasia and cortical dysplasia in patients presenting with seizures. *Epilepsia* 1993; **34**: 609–615.

71. Daumas-Duport C. Dysembryoplastic neuroepithelial tumors in epilepsy surgery. In: Guerrini R, Andermann F, Canapicchi R, *et al*. (eds) *Dysplasias of Cerebral Cortex and Epilepsy*. Philadelphia: Lippincott-Raven, 1996; 71–80.

72. Pasquier B, Bost F, Peoc'h M, Barnoud R, Pasquier D. Neuropathologic data in drug-resistant partial epilepsy. Report of a series of 195 cases. *Annals of Pathology* 1996; **16**: 174–181.

73. Morris HH, Estes ML, Prayson RA, *et al.* Frequency of different tumor types encountered in the Cleveland Clinic epilepsy surgery program. *Epilepsia* 1996; **37**(suppl. 5): S96.

74. Zentner J, Hufnagel A, Wolf HK, Ostertun B, *et al.* Surgical treatment of neoplasms associated with medically intractable epilepsy. *Neurosurgery* 1997; **41**: 378–386.

75. Prayson RA. Pathology of neoplastic lesions causing epilepsy. In: Luders HO, Comair YG. *Epilepsy Surgery*, 2nd edn. Philadelphia: Lippincott Williams and Wilkins 2001: 915–926.

76. Harding B. Gray matter heterotopia. In: Guerrini R, Andermann F, Canapicchi R, *et al.* (eds) *Dysplasias of Cerebral Cortex and Epilepsy*. Philadelphia: Lippincott-Raven, 1996; 81–88.

77. Hardiman O, Burke T, Phillips J, *et al.* Microdysgenesis in resected temporal neocortex: incidence and clinical significance in focal epilepsy. *Neurology* 1988; **38**: 1041–1047.

78. Raymond AA, Fish DR, Sisodya SM, *et al.* Abnormalities of gyration, heterotopias, focal cortical dysplasia, microdysgenesis, dysembryoplastic neuroepithelial tumour and dysgenesis of the archicortex in epilepsy. Clinical, EEG and neuroimaging features in 100 adult patients. *Brain* 1995; **118**: 629–660.

79. Falconer J, Wada J, Martin W, Li D. PET, CT, and MRI imaging of neuronal migration anomalies in epileptic patients. *Canadian Journal of Neurological Science* 1990; **17**: 35–39.

80. Barkovich AJ, Guerrini R, Battaglia G, *et al.* Band heterotopia: correlation of outcome with magnetic resonance imaging parameters. *Annals of Neurology* 1994; **36**: 609–617.

81. Dobyns WB, Andermann E, Andermann F, *et al.* X-linked malformations of neuronal migration. *Neurology* 1996; **47**: 331–339.

82. Fox JW, Lamperti ED, Eksioglu YZ, *et al.* Mutations in filamin 1 prevent migration of cerebral cortical neurons in human periventricular heterotopia. *Neuron* 1998; **21**: 1315–1325.

83. Sheen VL, Dixon PH, Fox JW, *et al.* Mutations in the X-linked filamin 1 gene cause periventricular nodular heterotopia in males as well as in females. *Human Molecular Genetics* 2000; **10**: 1775–1783.

84. Moro F, Carrozzo R, Veggiotti P, *et al.* Familial periventricular heterotopia: missense and distal truncating mutations of the FLN1 gene. *Neurology* 2002; **58**: 916–921.

85. Dobyns WB, Guerrini R, Czapansky-Beilman DK, *et al.* Bilateral periventricular nodular heterotopia (BPNH) with mental retardation and syndactyly in boys: a new X-linked mental retardation syndrome. *Neurology* 1997; **49**: 1042–1047.

86. Guerrini R, Dobyns WB. Bilateral periventricular nodular heterotopia with mental retardation and frontonasal malformation. *Neurology* 1998; **51**: 499–503.

87. Guion-Almeida ML, Richieri-Costa A. Frontonasal dysplasia, macroblepharon, eyelid colobomas, ear anomalies, macrostomia, mental retardation, and CNS structural anomalies. A new syndrome? *Clinical Dysmorphology* 1999; **81**: 1–4.

88. Dubeau F, Tampieri D, Lee N, *et al.* Periventricular and subcortical nodular heterotopia. A study of 33 patients. *Brain* 1995; **118**: 1273–1287.

89. Friede RL. *Developmental Neuropathology*, 2nd edn. New York: Springer-Verlag, 1989.

90. Reiner O, Carrozzo R, Shen Y, *et al.* Isolation of a Miller-Dieker lissencephaly gene containing G protein beta-subunit-like repeats. *Nature* 1993; **364**: 717–721.

91. Des Portes V, Pinard JM, Billuart P, *et al.* Identification of a novel CNS gene required for neuronal migration and involved in X-linked subcortical laminar heterotopia and lissencephaly syndrome. *Cell* 1998; **92**: 51–61.

92. Gleeson JG, Allen KM, Fox JW, *et al.* Doublecortin, a brain-specific gene mutated in human X-linked lissencephaly and double cortex syndrome, encodes a putative signaling protein. *Cell* 1998; **92**: 63–72.

93. Gleeson JG. Classical lissencephaly and double cortex (subcortical band heterotopia): LIS1 and doublecortin. *Current Opinion in Neurology* 2000; **13**: 121–125.

94. Pinard JM, Motte J, Chiron C, *et al.* Subcortical laminar heterotopia and lissencephaly in two families: a single X linked dominant gene. *Journal of Neurology, Neurosurgery and Psychiatry* 1994; **7**: 914–920.

95. Matsumoto N, Leventer RJ, Kuc JA, *et al.* Mutation analysis of the DCX gene and genotype/phenotype correlation in subcortical band heterotopia. *European Journal of Human Genetics* 2001; **9**: 5–12.

96. Dobyns WB, Reiner O, Carrozzo R, Ledbetter DH. Lissencephaly: a human brain malformation associated with deletion of the LIS1 gene located at chromosome 17p13. *JAMA* 1993; **1270**: 2838–2842.

97. Ross ME, Allen KM, Srivastava AK, *et al.* Linkage and physical mapping X-linked lissencephaly/SBH [XLIS]: a novel gene causing neuronal migration defects in human brain. *Human Molecular Genetics* 1997; **6**: 555–562.

98. Des Portes V, Francis F, Pinard JM, *et al.* Doublecortin is the major gene causing X-linked subcortical laminar heterotopia (SCLH). *Human Molecular Genetics* 1998; **7**: 1063–1070.

99. Sossey-Alaoui K, Hartung AJ, Guerrini R, *et al.* Human doublecortin (DCX) and the homologous gene in mouse encode a putative Ca2-dependent signaling protein which is mutated in human X-linked neuronal migration defects. *Human Molecular Genetics* 1998; **7**: 1327–1332.

100. Gleeson JG, Minnerath SR, Fox JW, *et al.* Characterization of mutations in the gene doublecortin in patients with double cortex syndrome. *Annals of Neurology* 1999; **45**: 146–153.

101. Gleeson JG, Luo RF, Grant PE, *et al.* Genetic and neuroradiological heterogeneity of double cortex syndrome. *Annals of Neurology* 2000; **47**: 265–269.

102. Gleeson JG, Minnerath S, Kuzniecky RI, *et al.* Somatic and germline mosaic mutations in the doublecortin gene are associated with variable phenotypes. *American Journal of Human Genetics* 2000; **67**: 574–581.

103. Pilz DT, Kuc J, Matsumoto N, *et al.* Subcortical band heterotopia in rare affected males can be caused by missense mutations in DCX [XLIS] or LIS1. *Human Molecular Genetics* 1999; **8**: 1757–1760.

104. Pilz DT, Macha ME, Precht KS, *et al.* Fluorescence *in situ* hybridization analysis with LIS1 specific probes reveals a

high deletion mutation rate in isolated lissencephaly sequence. Genetics in Medicine 1998; **1**: 29–33.

105. Cardoso C, Leventer RJ, Matsumoto N, et al. The location and type of mutation predict malformation severity in isolated lissencephaly caused by abnormalities within the LIS1 gene. *Human Molecular Genetics* 2000; **9**: 3019–3028.

106. Dobyns WB, Truwit CL. Lissencephaly and other malformations of cortical development: 1995 update. *Neuropediatrics* 1995; **26**: 132–147.

107. De Rijk-van Andel JF, Arts WFM, et al. Epidemiology of lissencephaly type I. *Neuroepidemiology* 1991; **10**: 200–204.

108. Dulac O, Plouin P, Perulli L, et al. Aspects électroencéphalographiques de l'agyrie-pachygyrie classique. *Revue d'Electroencéphalolgraphie et Neurophysiologie Clinique* 1983; **13**: 232–239.

109. Guerrini R, Robain O, Dravet Ch, Canapicchi R, Roger J. Clinical, electrographic and pathological findings in the gyral disorders. In: Fejerman N, Chamoles NA (eds) *New Trends in Pediatric Neurology*, Amsterdam: Elsevier, 1993: 101–107.

110. Fogli A, Guerrini R, Moro F, et al. Intracellular levels of the LIS1 protein correlate with clinical and neuroradiological findings in patients with classical lissencephaly. *Annals of Neurology* 1999; **45**: 154–156.

111. Chiron C, Nabbout R, Pinton F, et al. Brain functional imaging SPECT in agyria-pachygyria. *Epilepsy Research* 1996; **24**: 109–117.

112. Hakamada S, Watanabe K, Hara K, Miyazaki S. The evolution of electroencephalographic features in lissencephaly syndrome. *Brain Development* 1979; **4**: 277–283.

113. Quirk JA, Kendall B, Kingsley DPE, Boyd SG, Pitt MC. EEG features of cortical dysplasia in children. *Neuropediatrics* 1993; **24**: 193–199.

114. Livingston J, Aicardi J. Unusual MRI appearance of diffuse subcortical heterotopia or 'double cortex' in two children. *Journal of Neurology, Neurosurgery and Psychiatry* 1990; **53**: 617–620.

115. Palmini A, Andermann F, Aicardi J, et al. Diffuse cortical dysplasia, or the double cortex syndrome: the clinical and epileptic spectrum in 10 patients. *Neurology* 1991; **41**: 1656–1662.

116. Ricci S, Cusmai R, Fariello G, Fusco L, Vigevano F. Double cortex. A neuronal migration disorder as a possible cause of Lennox-Gastaut syndrome. *Archives of Neurology* 1992; **49**: 61–64.

117. Morrell F, Whisler WW, Hoeppner TJ, et al. Electrophysiology of heterotopic gray matter in the 'double cortex' syndrome. *Epilepsia* 1992; **33**(suppl. 3): 76.

118. Landy HJ, Curless RG, Ramsay RE, et al. Corpus callosotomy for seizures associated with band heterotopia. *Epilepsia* 1993; **34**: 79–83.

119. Hong SE, Shugart YY, Huang DT, et al. Autosomal recessive lissencephaly with cerebellar hypoplasia is associated with human RELN mutations. *Nature Genetics* 2000; **26**: 93–96.

120. Aicardi J, Lefebvre J, Lerique-Koechlin A. A new syndrome: spasms in flexion, callosal agenesis, ocular abnormalities. *Electroencephalography and Clinical Neurophysiology* 1965; **19**: 609–610.

121. Aicardi J, Chevrie JJ, Rousselie F. Le syndrome agénésie calleuse, spasmes en flexion, lacunes choriorétiniennes. *Archive Française de Pédiatrie* 1969; **26**: 1103–1120.

122. Aicardi J. Aicardi syndrome. In: Guerrini R, Andermann F, Canapicchi R, et al. (eds) *Dysplasias of Cerebral Cortex and Epilepsy*. Philadelphia: Lippincott-Raven, 1996; 211–216.

123. Molina JA, Mateos F, Merino M, Epifanio JL, Gorrono M. Aicardi syndrome in two sisters. *Journal of Pediatrics* 1989; **115**: 282–283.

124. MacGregor DL, Menezes A, Buncic JR. Aicardi syndrome (AS): natural history and predictors of severity. *Canadian Journal of Neurological Science* 1993; **20**(Suppl. 2): S36.

125. Billette de Villemeur T, Chiron C, Robain O. Unlayered polymicrogyria and agenesis of the corpus callosum: a relevant association? *Acta Neuropathologica* 1992; **83**: 265–270.

126. Ferrer I, Cusi MV, Liarte A, Campistol J. A Golgi study of the polymicrogyric cortex in Aicardi syndrome. *Brain Development* 1986; **8**: 518–525.

127. Chevrie JJ, Aicardi J. The Aicardi syndrome. In: Pedley TA, Meldrum BS (eds) *Recent Advances in Epilepsy*, Vol. 3. Edinburgh: Churchill Livingston, 1986: 189–210.

128. Barkovich AJ, Kjos BO. Nonlissencephalic cortical dysplasias: correlation of imaging findings with clinical deficits. *AJNR* 1992; **3**: 95–103.

129. Barkovich AJ, Norman D. MR of schizencephaly. *AJNR* 1988; **9**: 297–302.

130. Yakovlev PL, Wadsworth RC. Schizencephalies: a study of congenital clefts in the cerebral mantle, II. Clefts with hydrocephalus and lips separated. *Journal of Neuropathology and Experimental Neurology* 1946; **5**: 169–206.

131. Ferrer I. A Golgi analysis of unlayered polymicrogyria. *Acta Neuropathologica*. 1984; **65**: 69–76.

132. Hosley MA, Abroms IF, Ragland RL. Schizencephaly: case report of familial incidence. *Pediatric Neurology* 1992; **8**: 148–150.

133. Brunelli S, Faiella A, Capra V, et al. Germline mutations in the homeobox gene EMX2 in patients with severe schizencephaly. Nature Genetics 1996; **12**: 94–96.

134. Granata T, Farina L, Faiella A, et al. Familial schizencephaly associated with EMX2 mutation. *Neurology* 1997; **48**: 1403–1406.

135. Faiella A, Brunelli S, Granata T, et al. A number of schizencephaly patients including 2 brothers are heterozygous for germline mutations in the homeobox gene EMX2. *European Journal of Human Genetics* 1997; **5**: 186–190.

136. Granata T, Battaglia G, D'Incerti L, et al. Schizencephaly: clinical findings. In: Guerrini R, Andermann F, Canapicchi R, et al. (eds) *Dysplasias of Cerebral Cortex and Epilepsy*. Philadelphia: Lippincott-Raven 1996: 407–415.

137. Barkovich AJ, Hevner R, Guerrini R. Syndromes of bilateral symmetrical polymicrogyria. *AJNR* 1999; **20**: 1814–1821.

138. Evrard P, De Saint-Georges P, Kadhim H, Gadisseux JF. Pathology of prenatal encephalopathies. In: French J (ed) *Child Neurology and Developmental Disabilities*. Baltimore: Brookes, 1990: 153–176.

139. Harding B, Copp A. Malformations of the nervous system. In: Graham JG, Lantos PL. (eds) *Greenfield's Neuropathology*. London: Edward Arnold, 1997: 521–638.

140. Galaburda AM, Sherman GF, Rosen GD, Aboitiz F, Geschwind N. Developmental dyslexia: four consecutive patients with cortical anomalies. *Annals of Neurology* 1985; **18**: 222–233.

141. Kuzniecky R, Andermann F, Guerrini R and CBPS Multicenter Collaborative Study. Congenital bilateral perisylvian syndrome: study of 31 patients. *Lancet* 1993; **341**: 608–612.

142. Guerrini R, Dubeau F, Dulac O, *et al.* Bilateral parasagittal parietooccipital polymicrogyria and epilepsy. *Annals of Neurology* 1997; **41**: 65–73.

143. Guerrini R, Barkovich AJ, Sztriha L, Dobyns WB. Bilateral frontal polymicrogyria: a newly recognized brain malformation syndrome. *Neurology* 2000; **54**: 909–913.

144. Guerreiro MM, Andermann E, Guerrini R, *et al.* Familial perisylvian polymicrogyria: a new familial syndrome of cortical maldevelopment. *Annals of Neurology* 2000; **48**: 39–48.

145. Bartolomei F, Gavaret M, Dravet C, Guerrini R. Familial epilepsy with unilateral and bilateral malformations of cortical development. *Epilepsia* 1999; **40**: 47–51.

146. Ruton MC, Expert-Bezançon MC, Bursztyn J, Mselati JC, Robain O. Polymicrogyrie bioperculaire associée a une ophtalmoplégie congénitale par atteinte du noyau du nerf moteur oculaire commun. *Revue Neurologique* 1994; **150**: 363–369.

147. Becker PS, Dixon AM, Troncoso JC. Bilateral opercular polymicrogyria. *Annals of Neurology* 1989; **25**: 90–92.

148. Borgatti R, Triulzi F, Zucca C, *et al.* Bilateral perisylvian polymicrogyria in three generations. *Neurology* 1999; **52**: 1910–1913.

149. Yoshimura K, Hamada F, Tomoda T, Wakiguchi H, Kurashige T. Focal pachypolymicrogyria in three siblings. *Pediatric Neurology* 1998; **18**: 435–438.

150. Villard L, Nguyen K, Cardoso C, *et al.* A Locus for bilateral perisylvian polymicrogyria maps to Xq28. *American Journal of Human Genetics* 2002; **70**: 1003–1008.

151. Bingham PM, Lynch D, McDonald-McGinn D, Zackai E. Polymicrogyria in chromosome 22 deletion syndrome. *Neurology* 1998; **51**: 1500–1502.

152. Kawame H, Kurosawa K, Akatsuka A, Ochiai Y, Mizuno K. Polymicrogyria is an uncommon manifestation in 22q11.2 deletion syndrome. *American Journal of Medical Genetics* 2000; **94**: 77–78.

153. Worthington S, Turner A, Elber J, Andrews PI. 22q11 deletion and polymicrogyria – cause or coincidence? *Clinical Dysmorphology* 2000; **9**: 193–197.

154. Ryan AK, Goodship JA, Wilson DI, *et al.* Spectrum of clinical features associated with interstitial chromosome 22q11 deletions: a European collaborative study. *Journal of Medical Genetics* 1997; **34**: 798–804.

155. Van Bogaert P, Donner C, David P, *et al.* Congenital bilateral perisylvian syndrome in a monozygotic twin with intra-uterine death of the co-twin. *Developmental Medicine and Child Neurology* 1996; **38**: 166–171.

156. Baker EM, Khorasgani MG, Gardner-Medwin D, Gholkar A, Griffiths PD. Arthrogryposis multiplex congenita and bilateral parietal polymicrogyria in association with the intrauterine death of a twin. *Neuropediatrics* 1996; **27**: 54–56.

157. Guerrini R, Dravet C, Raybaud C, *et al.* Neurological findings and seizure outcome in children with bilateral opercular macrogyric-like changes detected by MRI. *Developmental Medicine and Child Neurology* 1992; **34**: 694–705.

158. Guerrini R, Genton P, Bureau M, *et al.* Multilobar polymicrogyria, intractable drop attack seizures, and sleep-related electrical status epilepticus. *Neurology* 1998; **51**: 504–512.

Epilepsy following acute brain injury

KEVIN FARRELL

Epileptic seizures can occur as an acute symptom of brain injury or as a consequence of permanent brain injury. This chapter discusses their occurrence following accidental and nonaccidental traumatic brain injury, and following stroke.

ACCIDENTAL HEAD TRAUMA

Early seizures

Early seizures occur within 1 week of the injury and are nearly always acute symptomatic seizures, caused by the head injury directly or by systemic factors such as electrolyte abnormalities. Approximately 95 per cent of early seizures occur within 24 hours of the injury.[1] They happen more often in children, particularly those under 5 years of age,[2,3] and have been reported in 3–10 per cent of children with a head injury.[1,2,4] The lowest incidence is reported in population studies,[4] which are probably more accurate.

The incidence of early seizures is threefold higher in children with severe head injuries[4] except in children under 5 years of age, in whom early seizures often follow relatively trivial head trauma.[3] Approximately one-third of children with a Glasgow Coma Scale (GCS) score <8 develop early seizures. Focal neurologic signs, depressed skull fracture, diffuse cerebral edema and acute subdural hematoma are associated with the greatest risk of early seizures in children with severe head injury.[1,3] Early seizures may be focal or generalized. Status epilepticus occurs more often in children under 5 years of age than in older children.[3]

Both phenytoin and carbamazepine have been demonstrated to be effective in reducing the risk of early seizures.[5–7] Patients with early seizures are usually treated with phenytoin, which can be administered intravenously to achieve a level in the therapeutic range within a reasonable time. It is important not to overtreat seizures occurring after relatively trivial head injuries. These tend to occur in younger children and have an excellent prognosis. Children are also often treated prophylactically during the first weeks following severe head injury.[1] However, neither phenytoin nor carbamazepine prevents the development of late epilepsy and neither has any effect on mortality rate or long-term neurologic disability.[5–7] Thus, there appears little rationale for the maintenance of anticonvulsant treatment after the acute neurological symptoms have resolved.

The occurrence of early seizures, particularly focal seizures, in children is less predictive of late seizures than in adults.[3] Indeed, the incidence of late seizures had no relation to the occurrence of early seizures in children in one population study.[4] In contrast, Appleton[8] reported that tonic-clonic seizures in the first week and a low initial GCS score were significantly associated with later epilepsy. This difference may relate to the relatively high incidence of early seizures in those less than 5 years of age following trivial head trauma in Annegers population study.[4] EEG abnormalities around the time of the acute brain injury have also not been demonstrated to predict the later onset of seizures, and EEG is of limited value in the assessment of early seizures.[9]

Late seizures

The mechanisms underlying trauma-induced epileptogenesis are poorly understood. Intracortical injection of iron in animals is associated with focal epileptiform discharges and seizures.[10] This may explain the increased risk of epilepsy in humans following intracerebral hemorrhage. Studies in rats have demonstrated a selective loss of hilar interneurons in the dentate gyrus[11] and a chronic network defect in the hippocampal formation[12] following a single traumatic event. These mechanisms may play an important role in post-traumatic epilepsy in humans, in whom damage to the hippocampus is common following severe head injury.

Children have a lower incidence of late seizures following head injury than adults.[3] The risk of children developing late seizures is influenced most by the severity of the brain injury. The incidence of epilepsy after mild head injuries is not much greater than in the normal population.[4,13] The incidence after 5 years was 0.2 per cent after mild head trauma, 1.6 per cent after moderate head trauma and 7.4 per cent after severe head trauma.[4] Similarly, whereas late epilepsy occurred in only 0.9 per cent of 1000 children admitted to hospital with head trauma and followed for 19 months to 7 years, 3.4 per cent of 262 children referred for rehabilitation and 9 per cent of the 102 children who received inpatient rehabilitation developed epilepsy.[8] Eight of the nine children who developed post-traumatic epilepsy also had motor, cognitive and/or behavioral sequelae and only one was otherwise neurologically normal.[8] MRI head scans demonstrated abnormalities in seven of the nine children.[8] The contribution of different risk factors following traumatic brain injury has been analyzed in a study involving all ages.[14] The risk of developing seizures was increased as follows:[14]

- brain contusion and subdural hematoma: ×12.1
- subdural hematoma alone: ×6.7
- brain contusion alone: ×5.0
- linear or depressed fracture in patients older than 5 years: ×2.0
- loss of consciousness >24 hours or post-traumatic amnesia for greater than 24 hours: ×1.9.

A positive family history of epilepsy is also more common in children who develop late epilepsy.[3] The EEG during the acute illness does not contribute usefully to the prediction of post-traumatic epilepsy.[9]

Late seizures are nearly always partial onset seizures.[8] When the seizure focus is in the frontal lobe, the seizures are often secondarily generalized and status epilepticus is more common.[15] Multiple minor seizures associated with generalized sharp and slow waves have been described in children following traumatic brain injury.[16] The onset of late epilepsy occurs later in children than in adults; 42 per cent of children have onset by the end of the first year and 71 per cent by the fourth year after the injury.[3] A seizure occurring more than 1 week after a head injury is likely to recur. Thus, treatment with antiepileptic drugs (AEDs) should be considered after a first late seizure.

There are limited data on the natural history of post-traumatic epilepsy in children, but approximately 50 per cent remit within 5 years.

Not all paroxysmal events following head trauma are epileptic seizures. A history of head trauma is commonly obtained in both adults and children with nonepileptic seizures.[17–19] Thus, patients with intractable seizures after head injury, particularly a mild head injury, should be carefully evaluated for nonepileptic seizures.[17]

NONACCIDENTAL HEAD TRAUMA

Early post-traumatic seizures are common in nonaccidental head injury and occurred in 73 per cent and 79 per cent of children in two studies.[20,21] Late epilepsy occurred in 22 per cent of the survivors followed for a median of 3 years in one study.[20] The high incidence of both early and late seizures probably reflects the greater severity of brain injury that tends to occur in this type of head trauma.[20]

STROKE

Stroke may be complicated by acute symptomatic seizures during the days after the event, or by the development of late seizures more than 1 week after the event. In a population-based study of the natural history of stroke in adults, 6 per cent developed early seizures, most within the first 24 h.[22] The cumulative risk of developing epilepsy was 3 per cent by 1 year and 9 per cent by 10 years. Stroke in children has been associated with a much higher incidence of late seizures. At least one seizure occurred in 49 per cent and recurrent seizures occurred in 29 per cent of 73 children with stroke in one study that excluded stroke due to trauma, malignancy and infection, and those in the neonatal period.[23] The incidence of seizures is much higher in those children with stroke, who demonstrate cortical involvement on neuroradiologic studies.[23] Similarly, in a study of 37 children at a median of 7 years following stroke, 4 had died, 2 were lost to follow-up and 9 developed seizures.[24] Finally, seizures were an acute manifestation of cerebral sinovenous thrombosis in 48 per cent of 91 consecutive children older than 4 weeks.[25]

KEY POINTS

- **Early seizures** occur within 1 week of the injury and are acute symptomatic seizures
- **Late seizures** occur more than 1 week after the injury and most recur

- Early seizures are **more common in children than in adults** and are less predictive of late seizures
- **Phenytoin** and **carbamazepine** reduce the risk of early seizures but not of late seizures
- An **EEG** in the period immediately after the trauma is of little value in predicting the risk of late seizures
- Depressed skull fracture, intracranial hematoma, diffuse cerebral edema and focal neurologic signs are **risk factors for late seizures**
- 40 per cent of children who will **develop late seizures** do so within 1 year and 70 per cent within 4 years
- Patients with intractable seizures after head injury, particularly a mild head injury, should be carefully evaluated for **nonepileptic seizures**
- Approximately half of the patients with post-traumatic epilepsy will eventually achieve **remission**
- Early post-traumatic seizures occur in approximately three-quarters of children with **nonaccidental head injury**
- Acute symptomatic seizures occur commonly in **stroke**. Later epilepsy is more common in those with cortical involvement on neuroimaging

REFERENCES

1. Hahn YS, Fuchs S, Flannery AM, Barthel MJ, McLone DG. Factors influencing post-traumatic seizures in children. *Neurosurgery* 1988; **22**: 864–867.
2. Desai BT, Whitman S, Coonley-Hoganson R, *et al.* Seizures and civilian head injuries. *Epilepsia* 1983; **24**: 289–296.
3. Jennett B. *Epilepsy after Non-missile Head Injuries*, 2nd edn. Chicago: Year Book Medical Publishers, 1975.
4. Annegers JF, Grabow JD, Groover RV, *et al.* Seizures after head trauma; a population study. *Neurology* 1980; **30**: 683–689.
5. Temkin NR, Dikmen SS, Wilensky AJ, Keihm J, Chabal S. A randomized, double-blind study of phenytoin for the prevention of post-traumatic seizures. *New England Journal of Medicine* 1990; **323**: 497–502.
6. Schierout G, Roberts I. Prophylactic anti-epileptic drugs after head injury: a systematic review. *Journal of Neurology, Neurosurgery and Psychiatry* 1998; **70**: 350–358.
7. Temkin NR. Antiepileptogenesis and seizure prevention trials with antiepileptic drugs; meta-analysis of controlled trials. *Epilepsia* 2001; **42**: 515–524.
8. Appleton RE, Demellweek C. Post-traumatic epilepsy in children requiring inpatient rehabilitation following head injury. *Journal of Neurology, Neurosurgery and Psychiatry* 2002; **72**: 669–672.
9. Jennett B, van de Sande J. EEG prediction of post-traumatic epilepsy. *Epilepsia* 1975; **16**: 251–256.
10. Willmore LJ, Sypert GW, Munson JB. Recurrent seizures induced by cortical iron injection: a model of post-traumatic epilepsy. *Annals of Neurology* 1978; **4**: 329–336.
11. Lowenstein DH, Thomas MJ, Smith DH, McIntosh TK. Selective vulnerability of dentate hilar neurons following traumatic brain injury: a potential mechanistic link between head trauma and disorders of the hippocampus. *Neuroscience* 1992; **12**: 4846–4853.
12. Santhakumar V, Ratzliff AD, Jeng J, Toth Z, Soltesz I. Long-term hyperexcitability in the hippocampus after experimental head trauma. *Annals of Neurology* 2001; **50**: 708–717.
13. Singer RB. Incidence of seizures after traumatic brain injury – a 50 year population survey. *Journal of Insurance Medicine* 2001; **33**: 42–45.
14. Annegers JF, Coan SP. The risks of epilepsy after traumatic brain injury. *Seizure* 2000; **9**: 453–457.
15. Aicardi J. *Epilepsy in Children*, 2nd edn. New York: Raven Press, 1994.
16. Niedermeyer E, Walker AE, Burton C. The slow spike-wave complex as a correlate of frontal and fronto-temporal post-traumatic epilepsy. *European Neurology* 1970; **3**: 330–346.
17. Barry E, Krumholz A, Bergey GK, *et al.* Nonepileptic posttraumatic seizures. *Epilepsia* 1998; **39**: 427–431.
18. Westbrook LE, Devinsky O, Geocadin R. Nonepileptic seizures after head injury. *Epilepsia* 1998; **39**: 978–982.
19. Pakalnis A, Paolicchi J. Psychogenic seizures after head injury in children. *Journal of Child Neurology* 2000; **15**: 78–80.
20. Barlow KM, Spowart JJ, Minns RA. Early post-traumatic seizures in non-accidental head injury: relation to outcome. *Developmental Medicine and Child Neurology* 2000; **42**: 591–594.
21. Gilles EE, Nelson MD. Cerebral complications of nonaccidental head injury in childhood. *Pediatric Neurology* 1998; **19**: 119–128.
22. So EL, Annegers JF, Hauser WA, O'Brien PC, Whisnant JP. Population-based study of seizure disorders after cerebral infarction. *Neurology* 1996; **46**: 350–355.
23. Yang JS, Park YD, Hartlage PL. Seizures associated with stroke in childhood. *Pediatric Neurology* 1995; **12**: 136–138.
24. De Schryver EL, Kappelle LJ, Jennekens-Schinkel A, Boudewyn Peters AC. Prognosis of ischemic stroke in childhood: a long-term follow-up study. *Developmental Medicine and Child Neurology* 2000; **42**: 313–318.
25. De Veber AM, Canadian Pediatric Ischemic Stroke Study Group. Cerebral sinovenous thrombosis in children. *New England Journal of Medicine* 2001; **345**: 417–423.

Disorders of metabolism and neurodegenerative disorders associated with epilepsy

BWEE TIEN POLL-THE

Epileptic seizures play a variable part in inherited disorders of metabolism and neurodegenerative disorders. The epilepsy may be nonspecific or take such a typical course that its clinical pattern or EEG features, or both, act as significant aids in early diagnosis. In order to present the most important disorders in detail, a selection is made of those where:

- Epilepsy is seen early in the course of the disease and plays a significant role in the diagnostic process.
- Specific seizure types such as myoclonus, infantile spasms, or neonatal seizures are present.
- Management of seizures causes special problems.
- Considerations of clinical diagnosis and of treatment make it necessary to take the age at onset into account. This applies especially to the neonatal period.

DISORDERS WITH NEONATAL ONSET

Inborn errors of metabolism may present with neonatal seizures; may have alarming symptoms such as progressive drowsiness and 'irritability' before convulsions appear; or drowsiness and irritability may start coincidentally with a series of seizures. The presence of neurological symptoms as well as seizures suggests that the underlying disorder is destructive.

In any newborn with seizures, hypoglycemia, hypocalcemia, infection and hemorrhage should first be excluded. Antepartum fetal hypoxia/ischemia, meconium-stained amniotic fluid and low Apgar scores do not exclude inborn errors, particularly if further deterioration takes place. Non-optimal adaptation to the birth process may be the first indication of an inborn error.

Amino acid disorders, including disorders of neurotransmitters

VITAMIN B₆ DEPENDENCY

Vitamin B_6 is present in various dietary products. The phosporylated active compound, pyridoxal-5′-phosphate, is required as a cofactor to glutamic acid decarboxylase, which catalyzes the formation of GABA (γ-amino-butyric acid) from glutamate (Figure 4E.1). In vitamin B_6 dependency, seizures are due to an inherited autosomal recessive disorder. Typically, they occur within hours after birth, are difficult to control by conventional antiepileptic therapy, and respond promptly to administration of a high

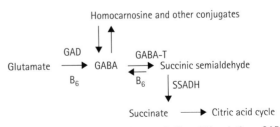

Figure 4E.1 *Disorders of GABA metabolism. Abbreviations: GAD, glutamic acid decarboxylase; GABA, γ-aminobutyric acid; SSADH, succinic semialdehyde dehydrogenase.*

dose of pyridoxine intramuscularly or intravenously. They may be felt prenatally as hiccup-like fetal movements. However, sometimes seizures begin as late as 2 years of age, and additional clinical features occur.[1] The pathogenesis of vitamin B_6-dependent seizures is still unknown, but genetic analysis suggests linkage to chromosome 5q31. Diagnosis depends on demonstration that the seizures are controlled with pharmacologic doses of pyridoxine and recur when it is withdrawn. In any child who presents with refractory seizures with an onset before 2 years of age, or has seizures known to be familial, pyridoxine should be tried. The amount needed is not clear, but 100 mg (intravenously or intramuscularly) is recommended, and, if no improvement is observed within 10 min, additional 100 mg doses should be administered to a total of 500 mg, before excluding the diagnosis.[2] However, in general, the response will be quick. Facilities for resuscitation should be available: there is a possible danger of respiratory depression following the first large dose.

FOLINIC ACID RESPONSIVE SEIZURES

Folinic acid (formyl-tetrahydrofolate)-dependent seizures are probably due to an inherited disease. In the cases reported,[3] treatment with folinic acid stopped the seizures within 1–5 days. All three confirmed inherited diseases of folate absorption and metabolism have been excluded. Folinic acid responsive seizures should be added to the list of possibilities when infants present with seizures within the first few weeks.

GABA TRANSAMINASE (GABA–T) DEFICIENCY

GABA-T deficiency (Figure 4E.1) is another disorder in the metabolic routes of GABA which leads to neonatal seizures.[4] A single causative mutation has been identified in one of two siblings. Patients have accelerated somatic growth, megalencephaly, severe psychomotor retardation, and spongiform degeneration of myelin. Levels of GABA and β-alanine are increased in plasma, CSF and urine; and concentrations of homocarnosine and other GABA conjugates are increased in CSF. The fasting plasma growth hormone is elevated. GABA-T activity is decreased in liver biopsy specimens.

NONKETOTIC HYPERGLYCINEMIA

This is an autosomal recessive disorder leading to excess glycine in CSF, blood and urine. Affected babies are usually asymptomatic at birth, but become obtunded, with apneic spells which progress to coma, and respiratory failure, between 7 h and 8 days.[5] Myoclonia, often stimulus-evoked, as well as generalized seizures have been observed: these become difficult to manage with routine anticonvulsants. The EEG in nonketotic hyperglycinemia, although highly characteristic with brief high-voltage paroxysms, predominantly over the vertex in a burst-suppression pattern, is not pathognomonic. However, in an initially normal neonate with a rapidly progressive encephalopathy, such a recording should always arouse the suspicion of nonketotic hyperglycinemia. Affected babies may die in the neonatal period or may spontaneously improve in vital functions and survive with severe brain damage. Their epilepsy may proceed to West syndrome. In nonketotic hyperglycinemia, glycine is relatively more elevated in CSF than in plasma. The highest CSF/plasma ratios are associated with the poorest outcomes. Prenatal onset of the cerebral damage is indicated by the occasional finding of dysgenesis of the corpus callosum.[6] No therapy has proved effective so far, though a promising EEG response to dextromethorphan has been described.[7] High-dose benzoate reduces the glycine concentration to normal in plasma, and substantially in CSF, and dextromethorphan combined with benzoate has been effective in some patients.[8] Valproic acid must be avoided, since it tends to increase glycine levels. Otherwise, routine antiepileptic medication is appropriate.

SULFITE OXIDASE DEFICIENCY AND MOLYBDENUM COFACTOR DEFICIENCY

Sulfite oxidase deficiency occurs in two forms: as an isolated enzyme defect and as part of a general deficiency of the molybdenum cofactor-containing enzymes. Both conditions lead to the accumulation of sulfite, and share the same clinical symptomatology. Severe and irreversible cerebral damage starts immediately after birth. Both deficiencies have autosomal recessive inheritance. Patients with either defect may display abnormal facial features: enophthalmy, microcephaly and palatoschisis have been described. Association with a Dandy-Walker complex has also been reported.[9] Convulsions usually start in the first week. Neuroimaging displays early signs of severe brain damage, which may appear very similar to the effects of perinatal asphyxia, with universal hypodensity and loss of distinction between cortex and central and subcortical white matter (Figure 4E.2). Later, generalized shrinkage and cortical and thalamic calcification may continue to suggest that perinatal asphyxia is causative. Early central hypoventilation and ventilator dependency may precede death in the neonatal period. Later symptoms include spastic quadriplegia and severe cognitive impairment. Neuropathologic descriptions suggest a severe destructive process is operating on both the cerebral cortex and the subcortical deep white matter.[10,11] Loss of neurons, especially in the cerebral cortex, is extreme, and is more severe than is usually encountered in perinatal hypoxic-ischemic encephalopathy (Figure 4E.3). Sulfite oxidase deficiency should be suspected in any neonate where unexpected encephalopathy and seizures follow normal birth. Urine specimens screened for the presence of sulfite must be

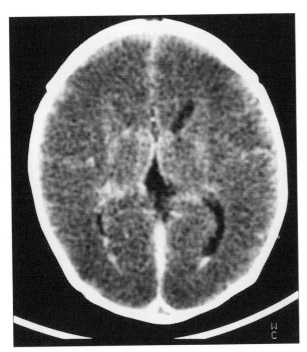

Figure 4E.2 *CT scan of neonate with molybdenum cofactor deficiency (contrast enhanced). Loss of distinction between neocortex and central white matter suggests cytotoxic edema. Hypodensity of neocortex and thalamus. Minor hemorrhage in the posterior horns. The picture is similar to severe hypoxic/ischemic damage.*

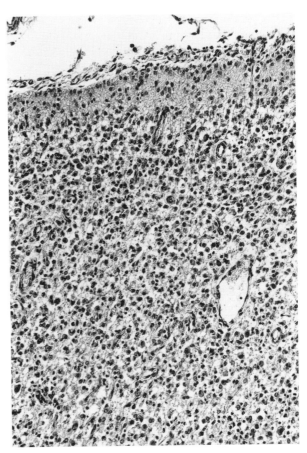

Figure 4E.3 *Neocortex of 9-day-old neonate with molybdenum cofactor deficiency displays severe destruction. Loss of normal distinction between cortical layers is caused by severe loss of neurons and dense infiltration with macrophages.*

fresh: sulfite in the urine is oxidized to sulfate on standing. In both disorders, increased levels of sulfite, S-sulphocysteine, thiosulfate, taurine, and decreased cystine are found in urine. In addition, in molybdenum cofactor deficiency, elevated levels of xanthine and hypoxanthine are found. No effective specific treatment is available.

Disorders of the urea cycle (hyperammonemias)

Inherited deficiency of an urea cycle enzyme may result in a severe neonatal encephalopathy, with coma and epileptic seizures. Carbamyl phosphate synthetase, argininosuccinic acid synthetase, argininosuccinate lyase, and ornithine transcarbamylase are most frequently affected. Ornithine transcarbamylase deficiency is X-linked, and although female carriers may be clinically affected, usually only males suffer the severe neonatal form. The other enzyme deficits are inherited by autosomal recessive modes. Patients with neonatal hyperammonemia behave normally initially. After birth, ammonia starts to accumulate, leading to poor feeding and drowsiness, usually after the first 24 h. Focal or generalized seizures may occur, together with abnormal posturing and diaphoresis. Levels of ammonia above 400 μmol/L result in coma, and above

500 μmol/L in brain swelling and irreversible brain damage (Figure 4E.4).[12] Prompt diagnosis and treatment are needed, with strategies designed to reduce protein intake, enhance anabolism, utilize alternative pathways of nitrogen excretion and replace nutrients that are deficient. When an overwhelming illness presents in the newborn period, the prognosis is usually very poor, even with the most aggressive treatment.

Peroxisomal disorders

The biochemistry of these disorders is summarized in Figure 4E.5. Enzymes contained within the peroxisomal membrane act in tandem as metabolic pathways in the β-oxidation system which contains two sets of enzymes with high affinity for very long straight-chain fatty acids, dicarboxylic acids, bile acid precursors, docosahexanoic acid precursor and very long branched-chain fatty acids, such as phytanic acid, and the latter's α-oxidation product, pristanic acid.[13] The regular turnover of very long chain polyenoic fatty acids is mandatory for the

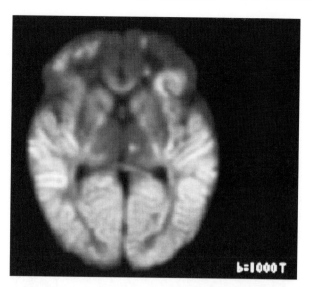

Figure 4E.4 *Diffusion weighted MR image of a 12-day-old neonate with urea cycle defect (blood ammonia normalized on day 8). High signal intensity of the temporal, parietal and occipital cortex and in both caudate nuclei, thalami, internal capsules and globus pallidus, suggesting cytotoxic edema. MRI at age 4 months showed extensive tissue loss in these cerebral regions.*

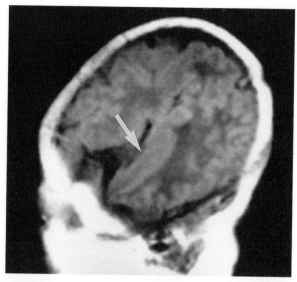

Figure 4E.6 *Neocortical dysplasia in a newborn with Zellweger syndrome. Lateral sagittal T1 weighted magnetic resonance image shows patch of thickened cortex adjacent to Sylvian fissure (arrow). In Zellweger syndrome this abnormal image represents crowded microgyri, rather than true pachygyria.*

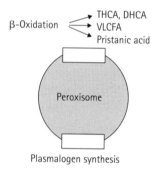

Figure 4E.5 *β-Oxidation and plasmalogen synthesis represent different enzyme systems, each within the peroxisomal membrane. Impairment of both systems results from a peroxisomal assembly disorder (generalized peroxisomal disorder). Abbreviations: THCA, trihydroxycholestanoic acid; DHCA, dihydroxycholestanoic acid; VLCFA, very long chain fatty acid.*

maintenance of myelin and requires intact peroxisomes. Other peroxisomal metabolic pathways include part of the synthetic machinery for plasmalogens that constitute a quantitatively important part of complex lipids in the brain. Generalized peroxisomal diseases are peroxisomal assembly disorders: at least 12 genes are involved. Only those peroxisomal disorders that express abnormalities in the oxidation of very long chain fatty acids give rise to neonatal seizures. These include disorders of peroxisomal biogenesis assembly and isolated deficiencies of one peroxisomal β-oxidation enzyme with intact peroxisomes.

PEROXISOMAL BIOGENESIS DISORDERS

Three clinical phenotypes are recognized. Zellweger syndrome presents with severe hypotonia, paresis, dystrophy and swallowing disorders: death occurs early. Infantile phytanic acid storage or infantile Refsum's disease is a moderate expression, and neonatal adrenoleukodystrophy lies in between these two.[14] All three are inherited as autosomal recessive disorders. Neonatal seizures occur in Zellweger syndrome and neonatal adrenoleukodystrophy. In Zellweger syndrome, characteristic external features and severe hypotonia are associated in all patients with neocortical dysplasia and clusters of neuronal heterotopia,[15] some of which show on MRI, but often they are of minute size and below the threshold of resolution.[16] The most characteristic, although not pathognomonic, sign in Zellweger syndrome is a steep parietal cleft which joins the Sylvian fissure to the superior part of the cerebral hemisphere. Pachymicrogyria, patches of apparently thickened cortex, are also present, especially around the Sylvian fissure and its abnormal extension (Figure 4E.6). Outside the CNS, there are renal cortical cysts and periarticular calcification, especially visible around the knees, may be seen on radiologic skeletal survey. Pigmentary retinopathy, hepatic fibrosis or cirrhosis, and fatty changes in astrocytes also occur.[17] Initially status epilepticus is unusual in Zellweger syndrome, but seizures characterized by apneic spells, blinking, and generalized and partial clonic movements may be difficult to control. On EEG, continuous negative sharp waves and spikes are considered characteristic.[18]

In neonatal adrenoleukodystrophy, facial dysmorphism is less typical and neither renal cortical cysts nor periarticular calcifications are found. Malformations in the brain are limited to polymicrogyric patches of neocortex. Degenerative changes of progressive myelin breakdown with perivascular cuffing, are not unlike those in X-linked adrenoleukodystrophy. Late-onset cerebral white matter disease may occur in peroxisome biogenesis disorders.[19] Pigmentary retinopathy, sensory deafness and liver pathology are also found.

SINGLE DEFECTS OF PEROXISOMAL β-OXIDATION

Phenocopies of Zellweger syndrome and neonatal adrenoleukodystrophy exist as isolated peroxisomal β-oxidation defects with intact peroxisomes. The β-oxidation cycle requires an activating enzyme and three other enzymes for the repeating cycle to octanoic acid, which is further oxidized in the mitochondria.[13] Deficiency of peroxisomal acyl-CoA synthetase leads to X-linked adrenoleukodystrophy/adrenomyeloneuropathy in childhood or adulthood. Deficiency of acyl-CoA oxidase, or D-bifunctional protein or peroxisomal thiolase will cause neurological symptoms, including seizures in the neonatal period. In any neonate with seizures and severe generalized hypotonia that cannot be otherwise explained, a peroxisomal disorder should be suspected. Determination of very long chain fatty acids in plasma or serum is the first step in diagnosis. Definite elevation of C26 (hexacosanoic acid) is proof of a disorder of peroxisomal β-oxidation. Measurements of the concentrations of plasmalogens in erythrocytes and levels of bile acids in plasma are also important for more precise diagnosis. Fibroblasts should be sampled in any case of very long chain fatty acid elevation for final studies and as a reference for future prenatal diagnosis. There are no objections to giving standard antiepileptic medication to children with peroxisomal disorders, but dosages should be adjusted according to plasma levels when there is hepatic disease. Renal excretion is usually unimpaired, even in the presence of renal cortical cysts.

DISORDERS ARISING IN INFANTS AND CHILDREN

Amino acid and organic acid disorders, including GABA-related disorders

GLUTARIC ACIDEMIA TYPE 1

Glutaric acidemia type 1 is due to an autosomal recessive deficiency of the enzyme glutaryl-CoA dehydrogenase.

Infants and children have megalencephaly, and on imaging a characteristic wide gap is seen between the frontal and parietal opercula, without initial signs of a destructive process. Starting acutely between 6 and 18 months, and often provoked by mild infection, episodes of decreased consciousness and hypotonia may be accompanied by seizures. Recovery is frequently incomplete, and severe incapacitating dystonia is usual.[20]

DISORDERS OF THE UREA CYCLE WITH LATE ONSET

Inherited urea cycle disorders may present after the neonatal period with intermittent hyperammonemia leading to episodes of metabolic encephalopathy. Acute episodes are rarely accompanied by seizures. However, in arginase deficiency, a progressive spastic paraparesis may develop, together with epileptic seizures, even when hyperammonemia is well controlled.

BIOTINIDASE DEFICIENCY

Biotin is a water-soluble vitamin which becomes part of four carboxylases. These are involved in fatty acid synthesis and incorporate and recycle their biotin component with holocarboxylase synthetase and biotinidase. Deficiency of one of these latter enzymes leads to functional deficiency of all the carboxylases. Holocarboxylase synthetase deficiency mainly manifests before 3 months of age, and biotinidase deficiency at later ages. A small proportion of synthetase-deficient patients have seizures, but a majority of the biotinidase-deficient patients have seizures both as initial manifestations and as major neurologic problems. Recognition may be delayed since the characteristic skin rash and alopecia only develop in a minority, and metabolic acidosis and ketosis are not seen initially. Seizures in unrecognized biotinidase deficiency are difficult to control by conventional anticonvulsants, but biotin therapy is effective.[21] Outside periods of crisis, abnormal metabolic abnormalities in the urine may be minimal, though CSF/plasma ratios for lactate and 3-hydroxy-isovaleric acid may be elevated.[22] Biotinidase levels can be determined in plasma. Early recognition is important, because there is an excellent response to treatment. The pathology is similar to that of Leigh syndrome.[23]

POSTNEONATAL VITAMIN B6 DEPENDENCY

The initial impression that B_6 dependency is limited to neonatal seizures had to be modified following several reports on postneonatal onset of therapy-refractory epilepsy with generalized, focal, myoclonic, partial motor, or partial complex types[24,25] due to vitamin B_6 dependency.

SUCCINIC SEMIALDEHYDE DEHYDROGENASE DEFICIENCY

Succinic semialdehyde dehydrogenase deficiency, or 4-hydroxybutyric aciduria (Figure 4E.1), is another inborn error of GABA-related metabolism which may be associated with epilepsy in almost 50 per cent of patients.[26] The clinical features vary from mild to severe, and include developmental delay, hypotonia, hyporeflexia, ataxia and behavioral problems. 4-Hydroxybutyric acid accumulates in plasma, urine and CSF. Therapeutic intervention with vigabatrin is clinically beneficial in only about one third of patients.

DISORDERS OF SERINE METABOLISM

The recognition of serine deficiency disorders depends on detection of low concentrations of amino acids in plasma and CSF. 3-Phosphoglycerate dehydrogenase (3-PGDH) deficiency is characterized by congenital microcephaly, severe delayed psychomotor development presenting in the first months of life and the onset of intractable epilepsy soon after. EEGs show either hypsarrhythmia or severe multifocal epileptic abnormalities with poor background activity.[27,28] Brain MRI may demonstrate profound reduction in the white matter volume and cerebral hypotrophy. Treatment with oral L-serine and glycine has beneficial effects on the epilepsy and brain white matter abnormalities.[29] EEG abnormalities can persist for some months after clinically manifest seizures have stopped. Plasma amino acids must be measured in the fasting state, because serine and glycine can be normal after feeding. In CSF, serine concentrations are always decreased in 3-PGDH deficiency.

DISORDERS OF AMINE METABOLISM

Disorders of tetrahydrobiopterin metabolism ('malignant phenylketonuria')

At least five enzyme deficiencies lead to disordered tetrahydrobiopterin (BH$_4$) homeostasis.[30] Typically the patient suffers from neurological deterioration despite excellent dietary control of the hyperphenylalaninemia. The deterioration may include seizures, although the main symptoms are extrapyramidal.

AROMATIC AMINO ACID DECARBOXYLASE DEFICIENCY

Serotonin and dopamine are depleted because the common decarboxylase which acts on L-DOPA and on 5-hydroxytryptophan (5-HTP) is deficient[31] (Figure 4E.7). Since phenylalanine is not elevated, biogenic amines must be determined. If untreated, the symptoms are very similar to those in the defects of BH$_4$ metabolism: hypotonia,

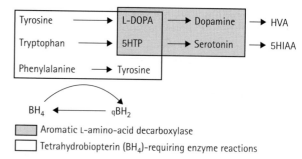

Figure 4E.7 *Disorders of biogenic amine metabolism. Tetrahydrobiopterin (BH$_4$) deficiency results in the loss of activity of three enzyme activities depicted in the unshaded rectangle. Resulting deficiency of L–DOPA and 5HTP in turn causes deficiency of the neurotransmitters dopamine and serotonin. Aromatic L–amino-acid decarboxylase catalyzes the reactions indicated in the shaded rectangle. Deficiency also results in deficiency of dopamine and serotonin. Abbreviations: L–DOPA, L-dihydroxyphenylalanine; 5HTP, 5-hydroxytryptophan; HVA, homovanillic acid; 5HIAA, 5-hydroxyindolic acid; qBH$_2$, quinonoid form of dihydrobiopterin.*

oculogyric crises, extrapyramidal symptoms, defective temperature regulation and later hypotension.

DISORDERS OF PYRIMIDINE METABOLISM

Dihydropyrimidine dehydrogenase deficiency

Uracil and thymine accumulate. Affected patients may have mental retardation, microcephaly and epilepsy,[32] though some have only epilepsy.

Glucose transporter deficiency[33]

Repeated generalized seizures, with normal EEG, start within a few months after birth. The CSF/blood ratio for glucose is decreased and CSF lactate is low, suggesting that there is diminished availability of blood glucose to the brain. A glucose transporter deficiency in red blood cells has been proven. An identical transporter, which is encoded by the *GLUT1* gene, exists in brain endothelial cells and astroglia. Patients improve dramatically with the provision of an alternative energy source to the brain, i.e. a ketogenic diet.

Creatine deficiency

Creatine biosynthesis involves arginine:glycine amidinotransferase and guanidinoacetate methyltransferase (GAMT) as enzymes, and glycine arginine and *S*-adenosylmethionine as substrates. The clinical presentation in GAMT deficiency[34] may be severe or moderate.

Patients with severe phenotypes have intractable epilepsy, early developmental delay and extrapyramidal symptoms.[35] Characteristic biochemical findings include brain creatine deficiency (seen on *in vivo* proton magnetic resonance scanning), and accumulation of guanidinoacetate in brain and in body fluids. Systemic depletion of creatine and creatine phosphate leads to low urinary creatine excretion, and low creatine concentrations in plasma and CSF.[35] Clinical, biochemical and neuroradiologic improvement follows creatine supplementation. X-linked creatine transporter defect has been described with early developmental delay, seizures, a region of T2-weighted hyperintense signal in the right posterior white matter, and brain creatine depletion detected by proton MRS.[36] In contrast to GAMT deficiency, brain creatine deficiency is not reversible by oral creatine substitution, guanidinoacetate concentrations in plasma and urine are normal, and creatine values are elevated in urine and plasma. Arginine:glycine amidinotransferase deficiency is associated with a response similar to that observed in patients with GAMT deficiency when treated with oral supplements of creatine monohydrate.[37]

Disorders of the respiratory chain and pyruvate dehydrogenase complex

Seizures caused by mitochondrial disorders are mainly related to deficiencies of the respiratory chain and the pyruvate dehydrogenase complex (PDHC). Less frequently a deficiency of the citric acid (Krebs) cycle or pyruvate carboxylase may be involved. Disorders of mitochondrial β-oxidation affect the brain indirectly by causing hypoglycemic episodes. Point mutations in nuclear or mitochondrial DNA (mtDNA), large deletions in mtDNA, and variable tissue distribution of mutant mtDNA cause many different disorders. Depletion of mtDNA or intergenomic signaling defects are possible.[38] Leigh syndrome; Alpers' disease; mitochondrial myopathy, encephalopathy, lactic acidosis and stroke-like episodes (MELAS); and myoclonus epilepsy and ragged-red fibers (MERRF) are caused by respiratory chain deficiency. Leigh syndrome may also be caused by deficiency of PDHC. Defined by its pathologic features, clinically Leigh syndrome is highly variable, with a remitting course and exacerbations often provoked by intercurrent infections. Hypotonia, vomiting and brainstem symptoms predominate. Leigh syndrome has become firmly linked to various sites of the respiratory chain and PDHC.[39] Lactic acidemia and elevated lactic acid in the CSF are usual. Seizures were seen at onset in 8 per cent of 173 proven cases.[40] Therapy-resistant epilepsy and status epilepticus are less frequent.

In Alpers' disease, there is severe degeneration of the cortex, basal ganglia and nuclear systems in the brainstem.[41] Especially in infants, cortical atrophy is extreme and devastating, so that cortical layers become indistinct. After normal early development, convulsions and myoclonia appear before 2 years, with coincident arrest in motor development. A special type is combined with diffuse liver disease.[42] All affected children develop seizures, often with an explosive onset. Frequently, these consist of isolated twitching of one or other limb, sometimes continuing incessantly for weeks.[43] The EEG is characterized by focal very high voltage, very slow waves, alternating with low voltage superimposed polyspikes, usually contralateral to the focal seizures. The electroretinogram is normal. An association between Alpers' disease, ragged-red muscle fibres and elevation of lactic acid in blood, urine and CSF may be found.[44] In addition, complex I deficiency, complex IV deficiency and a defect in the citric acid cycle between succinyl-CoA and fumarate have been reported. In the hepatocerebral form of Alpers' disease, there is an apparent specific vulnerability to toxic effects of valproic acid.

MELAS syndrome[45] can start at any time from age 3 to 40 years. Progressive encephalopathy is typically accompanied by migraine-like headache, dementia, seizures and stroke-like episodes.[46] Lactic acidosis is usual, and ragged-red fibers are seen in muscle biopsies. The inheritance is matrilinear.[38]

MERRF can start in childhood with bursts of myoclonus, seizures, intention tremor, ataxia, mental deterioration, muscular weakness and pes cavus. Lactic acidemia is usual. Neuropathologic findings show degeneration of cerebellar cortex, dentate and red nuclei, globus pallidus and subthalamic nucleus.[47] MERRF is transmitted by maternal inheritance. It should be distinguished from Ramsey-Hunt disease.

PEROXISOMAL DISORDERS

The most important peroxisomal disease with onset after the neonatal period is X-linked adrenoleukodystrophy. Seizures are the presenting symptom in a small minority, and can be secondary to hypoglycemia, associated with the adrenal insufficiency.

LYSOSOMAL DISORDERS

Lysosomal disorders are typically storage disorders with a progressive course. The propensity to epileptic seizures varies, but is reported as 34 per cent in fucosidosis,[48] and prominent in α-N-acetylgalactosaminidase deficiency (Schindler's disease).[49] Both sialidosis and galactosialidosis may present as the cherry-red spot-myoclonus syndrome. Early-onset sialidosis presents between 0 and 10 months, and the late-onset type between 8 and 25 years. Galactosialidosis presents between birth and 6 years: symptoms largely overlap with those of pure sialidosis. Sphingolipidoses that preferentially affect metabolism of myelin (lysosomal leukodystrophies), such as metachromatic leukodystrophy and Krabbe's disease, eventually cause epilepsy, but only some time after the onset of functional regression: they usually respond to antiepileptic medication.

Neuronal ceroid lipofuscinoses

The neuronal ceroid lipofuscinoses, a 'new' group of lysosomal disorders, are a large group of autosomal recessive neurodegenerative disorders with clinically and genetically different features. All of these disorders are characterized by accumulation of autofluorescent storage material, ceroid, in lysosomes of neurons and other tissues. Previously, diagnoses of neuronal ceroid lipofuscinoses were based on clinicopathologic findings and age of onset, and the main types were known by eponymous names: Santavuori-Hagberg (infantile type), Jansky-Bielschowsky (late infantile type) and Spielmeyer-Vogt (juvenile type). However, reports on variant types, new entities and knowledge about the genes necessitated another delineation (Table 4E.1). The adult neuronal ceroid lipofuscinoses, Kufs disease, is not included in this review. The known gene products appear to be lysosomal enzymes (NCL1 and NCL2) or lysosomal membrane proteins (NCL3 and NCL5). All types of NCL cause progressive visual and mental decline, motor disturbance and epilepsy.[50] Except for Northern epilepsy, all childhood neuronal ceroid lipofuscinoses belong to the group of myoclonic epilepsies and have retinal degeneration with extinguished electroretinogram.[51]

INFANTILE NEURONAL CEROID LIPOFUSCINOSIS (SANTAVUORI-HAGBERG TYPE, CLN1)

After normal early development, decline starts between 8 and 24 months with ataxia, muscle hypotonia followed by spasticity, visual loss, loss of interest, prominent myoclonus, epileptic seizures and 'knitting' hyperkinesia. Microcephaly, usually present at onset, is progressive. A vegetative state is reached by 3 years. EEG shows progressive diminution of voltage until the third year, after which the recording becomes isoelectric. Electroretinography is of lowered amplitude, even at an early stage.[52] Optic atrophy with brown discoloration of the macular region is seen later. Death is mostly between 5 and 10 years. Extreme cerebral atrophy is seen at autopsy, when microscopy shows disappearance of cortical neurons, with storage of autofluorescent material in any which remain. The storage material is also seen widely in reticuloendothelial and other cell types outside the CNS. Diagnosis by biopsies (skin, conjunctiva, skeletal muscle, lymphocytes) should be possible, but is confirmed by finding deficiency of palmitoyl protein thioesterase activity. Mutations in the CLN1 gene can be associated with five different phenotypes.

LATE INFANTILE NEURONAL CEROID LIPOFUSCINOSIS (JANSKY-BIELSCHOWSKY DISEASE, CNL2)

Onset is between 2 and 4 years of age, with rapidly progressing epilepsy, ataxia and blindness. Spastic paresis follows. Epilepsy takes the form of generalized tonic-clonic seizures, drop attacks and massive myoclonus. Progression of myoclonus ultimately leads to a permanent myoclonic state. Patients usually die before 8 years. Optic atrophy and retinopathy develop early in the disease. The electroretinogram, which is negative at an early age, is a highly suggestive test at the beginning of the disease. A grossly enlarged visual evoked potential and short generalized discharges in the EEG following each flash at low frequency stroboscopy[53] are also helpful in diagnosis. Storage and atrophy occur in the brain, but are much less severe than in the infantile type. So-called curvilinear and other profiles within lysosomal membranes are found widely in

Table 4E.1 *Neuronal ceroid lipofuscinoses in childhood*

Disease	Gene	Diagnostics
Infantile, classic (Santavuori-Hagberg) and later ages of onset up to adulthood	CLN1	Palmitoyl protein thioesterase activity Mutation analysis
Late infantile, classic (Jansky-Bielschowsky) and later ages of onset up to juvenile	CLN2	Tripeptidyl peptidase I activity Mutation analysis
Finnish variant late infantile	CLN5	Transmembrane CLN5 protein Mutation analysis
Variant late infantile	CLN6	Transmembrane CLN6 protein Mutation analysis
Variant late infantile, Turkish	CLN7	?
Northern epilepsy	CLN8	Transmembrane CLN8 protein Mutation analysis
Juvenile, classic (Spielmeyer-Vogt)	CLN3	Transmembrane CLN3 protein Mutation analysis

cerebral neurons, and in eccrine sweat glands, striated muscle cells, and Schwann cells. Lymphocytes may also display storage material, in some cases. The diagnosis can be confirmed by analysis of tripeptidyl peptidase I activity in lymphocytes, fibroblasts, and brain. The same *CLN2* gene may cause juvenile, as well as late-infantile, disease.

JUVENILE NEURONAL CEROID LIPOFUSCINOSIS (SPIELMEYER–VOGT, *CLN3*)

Onset is between 4 and 8 years with retinal blindness, later followed by dementia, generalized seizures, regression of motor functions with a Parkinsonian syndrome and death after 20 years. Although present, epilepsy is not a major problem. The lysosomal protein battenin is defective in juvenile NCL. However, no biochemical assay is currently available for the diagnosis.

OTHER TYPES OF NEURONAL CEROID LIPOFUSCINOSIS IN CHILDREN

- **Finnish variant late-infantile (CLN5).** The clinical features mostly reflect the late-infantile type, but the onset is at a later age and the electronmicroscopic findings differ from those in *CLN2*.[54] Biochemical diagnosis is not yet available.
- **Variant late-infantile/atypical NCL (CLN6)** and the **Turkish variant late-infantile NCL (CLN7)** resemble the classic late-infantile NCL.
- **Northern epilepsy** or **progressive epilepsy with mental retardation (CLN8)** becomes apparent between 5 and 10 years.[55] All patients have generalized tonic-clonic or complex partial seizures. Mental retardation begins 2–5 years after the onset of seizures.

SEIZURES IN SOME INHERITED NEURODEGENERATIVE DISORDERS

Rett syndrome

Typical Rett syndrome in girls is characterized by an initial 6–18-month period of apparently normal development followed by loss of learned language and motor skills. In the more advanced stages, epilepsy is usual, but occasionally seizures, or even status epilepticus, are the initial events, and may obscure the otherwise clear symptoms. Generalized tonic-clonic seizures are most common, with partial complex seizures next commonest.[56] Neuroimaging suggests that the decreased brain volume results from global reductions in both gray and white matter.[57] The identification of the causative gene, X-linked methyl-CpG binding protein 2 (*MECP2*), provides a diagnostic test.[58] Mutations

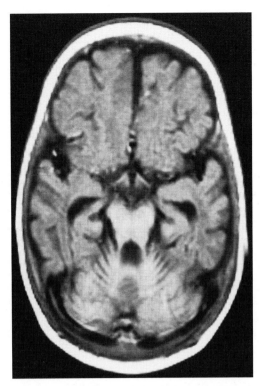

Figure 4E.8 *1-year-old patient with PEHO syndrome. Transverse proton-density MRI shows atrophy of temporal lobes and folial atrophy of the cerebellum.*

in the *MECP2* gene have been found in 70–90 per cent of classic Rett patients. Recently atypical variants and affected males have been identified, making the spectrum of associations with the *MECP2* mutation wide, ranging from males with early-onset lethal encephalopathy to adults with severe mental retardation. Depending, at least in part, on the patterns of X-chromosome inactivations[59] female cases can range from asymptomatic or mildly mentally retarded cases to severe variants with congenital onset.

PEHO syndrome

Progressive encephalopathy with oedema, hypsarrhythmia and optic atrophy (PEHO), also known as infantile cerebello-optic atrophy, is an autosomal recessive disorder which presents as an early-onset neurodegenerative disorder with therapy-refractory infantile spasms, profound psychomotor retardation, hypotonia, absent visual contact and optic atrophy. Microcephaly and subcutaneous edema of the limbs and face follow. There is severe and generalized cerebellar atrophy, and some macroscopic atrophy and myelination delay in the cerebral hemispheres. Neuropathologic, EEG, neuroradiologic, and ophthalmologic findings give a fairly consistent and recognizable pattern (Figure 4E.8).[60,61]

KEY POINTS

- In disorders of metabolism and neurodegenerative disorders, epilepsy is usually part of a **generalized encephalopathy**
- In the neonate, the following conditions should be considered: **vitamin B$_6$ dependency, folinic acid responsive seizures, GABA-T deficiency, nonketotic hyperglycinemia, sulfite oxidase deficiency, hyperammonemia** and **peroxisomal disorders**
- Seizures in infants and children can be secondary to disturbances of **amino- and organic acid metabolism**, disorders of the **urea cycle** with late onset, **biotinidase deficiency**, postneonatal **vitamin B$_6$ dependency**, disorders of **amine metabolism**, **glucose transporter deficiency**, disorders of the **respiratory chain** and **pyruvate dehydrogenase complex, peroxisomal** and **lysosomal disorders, neuronal ceroid lipofuscinosis, Rett** and **PEHO syndromes**
- In some conditions, e.g. biotinidase deficiency and vitamin B$_6$ dependency, **correction of the metabolic disturbances** can control otherwise resistant seizures
- **Valproic acid should not be given** in the cerebrohepatic form of Alpers' disease, or in hyperglycinemia

REFERENCES

1. Baxter P. Pyridoxine-dependent and pyridoxine-responsive seizures. *Developmetal Medicine and Child Neurology* 2001; **43**: 416–420.
2. Gospe SM Jr. Current perspectives on pyridoxine-dependent seizures. *Journal of Pediatrics* 1998; **132**: 919–923.
3. Hyland K, Buist NR, Powell BR, *et al*. Folinic acid responsive seizures: a new syndrome? *Journal of Inherited Metabolic Disease* 1995; **18**: 177–181.
4. Jaeken J, Casaer P, de Cock, *et al*. Gamma-aminobutyric acid-transaminase deficiency: a newly recognized inborn error of neurotransmitter metabolism. *Neuropediatrics* 1984; **15**: 165–169.
5. Gitzelmann R, Steinmann B. Clinical and therapeutic aspects of non-ketotic hyperglycinemia. *Journal of Inherited Metabolic Disease* 1982; **25**(Suppl 2): 113–116.
6. Dobyns WB. Agenesis of the corpus callosum and gyral malformations are frequent manifestations of nonketotic hyperglycinemia. *Neurology* 1989; **39**: 817–820.
7. Schmitt B, Steinmann B, Gitzelmann R, *et al*. Nonketotic hyperglycinemia: clinical and electrophysiologic effects of dextromethorphan, an antagonist of the NMDA receptor. *Neurology* 1993; **43**: 421–424.
8. Hamosh A, Maher JF, Bellus GA, *et al*. Long-term use of high-dose benzoate and dextromethorphan for the treatment of nonketotic hyperglycinemia. *Journal of Pediatrics* 1998; **132**: 709–713.
9. Arslanoglu S, Yalaz M, Göksen D, *et al*. Molybdenum cofactor deficiency associated with Dandy-Walker complex. *Brain and Development* 2001; **23**: 815–818.
10. Rosenblum WI. Neuropathologic changes in a case of sulfite oxidase deficiency. *Neurology* 1968; **18**: 1187–1196.
11. Barth PG, Beemer FA, Cats BP, *et al*. Neuropathological findings in a case of combined deficiency of sulphite oxidase and xanthine dehydrogenase. *Virchow's Arch. Pathol. [A]* 1985; **408**: 105–106.
12. Breningstall GN. Neurologic syndromes in hyperammonemic disorders. *Pediatric Neurology* 1986; **2**: 253–262.
13. Wanders RJA, Barth PG, Heymans HS. Single peroxisomal enzyme deficiencies. In: Scriver CR, Baudet AL, Valle D, Sly WS (eds). *The Metabolic and Molecular Bases of Inherited Disease*, 8th edn. New York: McGraw-Hill, 2001; 3219–5326.
14. Poll-The BT, Saudubray JM, Ogier HAM, *et al*. Infantile Refsum disease: an inherited peroxisomal disorder. Comparison with Zellweger syndrome and neonatal adrenoleukodystrophy. *European Journal of Pediatrics* 1987; **146**: 477–483.
15. Powers JM, Moser HW, Moser AB, *et al*. Fetal cerebro-hepato-renal (Zellweger) syndrome: dysmorphic, radiologic, biochemical, and pathologic findings in four affected fetuses. *Human Pathology* 1985; **16**: 610–620.
16. Van der Knaap MS, Valk J. The MR spectrum of peroxisomal disorders. *Neuroradiology* 1991; **33**: 30–37.
17. Aubourg P, Robain O, Rocchiccioli F, *et al*. The cerebro-hepato-renal (Zellweger) syndrome: lamellar lipid profiles in adrenocortical, hepatic mesenchymal, astrocyte cells and increased levels of very long chain fatty acids and phytanic acid in the plasma. *Journal of the Neurological Sciences* 1985; **69**: 9–25.
18. Govaerts L, Colon E, Rotteveel J, Monnens LA. Neurophysiological study of children with the cerebro-hepato-renal syndrome of Zellweger. *Neuropediatrics* 1985; **16**: 185–190.
19. Barth PG, Gootjes J, Bode H, *et al*. Late onset white matter disease in peroxisome biogenesis disorder. *Neurology* 2001; **57**: 1949–1955.
20. Hoffmann GF, Athanassopoulos S, Burlina A, *et al*. Clinical course, early diagnosis, treatment and prevention of disease in glutaryl-CoA dehydrogenase deficiency. *Neuropediatrics* 1996; **27**: 115–123.
21. Salbert BA, Pellock JM, Wolf B. Characterization of seizures associated with biotinidase deficiency. *Neurology* 1993; **43**: 1351–1355.
22. Duran M, Baumgartner ER, Suormala TM, *et al*. Cerebrospinal fluid organic acids in biotinidase deficiency. *Journal of Inherited Metabolic Disease* 1993; **16**: 513–516.
23. Honavar M, Janota I, Neville BGR, Chalmers RA. Neuropathology of biotinidase deficiency. *Acta Neuropatholica (Berlin)* 1992; **84**: 461–464.
24. Goutières F, Aicardi J. Atypical presentations of pyridoxine dependent seizures: a treatable cause of intractable epilepsy in infants. *Annals of Neurology* 1985; **17**: 117–120.
25. Coker SB. Postneonatal vitamin-B$_6$-dependent epilepsy. *Pediatrics* 1992; **90**: 221–223.
26. Gibson KM, Christensen E, Jakobs C, *et al*. The clinical phenotype of succinic semialdehyde dehydrogenase deficiency (4-hydroxybutyric aciduria): case reports of 23 new patients. *Pediatrics* 1997; **99**: 567–574.

27. De Koning TJ, Duran M, Dorland L, *et al.* Beneficial effects of L-serine and glycine in the management of seizures in 3-phosphoglycerate dehydrogenase deficiency. *Annals of Neurology* 1998; **44**: 261–265.

28. Pineda M, Vilaseca MA, Artuch R, *et al.* 3-Phosphoglycerate dehydrogenase deficiency in a patient with West syndrome. *Developmetal Medicine and Child Neurology* 2000; **42**: 629–633.

29. De Koning TJ, Jaeken J, Pineda M, *et al.* Hypomyelination and reversible white matter attenuation in 3-phosphoglycerate dehydrogenase deficiency. *Neuropediatrics* 2000; **31**: 287–292.

30. Thöny B, Auerbach G, Blau N. Tetrahydrobiopterin biosynthesis, regeneration and functions. Biochemical Journal 2001; **347**: 1–16.

31. Hyland K. Abnormalities of biogenic amine metabolism. *Journal of Inherited Metabolic Disease* 1993; **16**: 676–690.

32. Braakhekke JP, Renier WO, Gabreëls FJM, *et al.* Dihydropyrimidine dehydrogenase deficiency. Neurological aspects. *Journal of the Neurological Sciences* 1987; **78**: 71–77.

33. De Vivo DC, Trifiletti RR, Jacobson RI, *et al.* Defective glucose transport across the blood-brain barrier as a cause of persistent hypoglycorrhachia, seizures, and developmental delay. *New England Journal of Medicine* 1991; **325**: 703–709.

34. Stöckler S, Holzbach U, Hanefeld F, *et al.* Creatine deficiency in the brain: a new treatable inborn error of metabolism. *Pediatric Research* 1994; **36**: 409–413.

35. Schulze A, Hess T, Wevers R, *et al.* Creatine deficiency syndrome caused by guanidinoacetate methyltransferase deficiency: diagnostic tools for a new inborn error of metabolism. *Journal of Pediatrics* 1997; **131**: 626–631.

36. Cecil KM, Salomons GS, Ball WS, *et al.* Irreversible brain creatine deficiency with elevated serum and urine creatine: a creatine transporter defect? *Annals of Neurology* 2001; **49**: 401–404.

37. Bianchi MC, Tosetti M, Fornai F, *et al.* Reversible brain creatine deficiency in two sisters with normal blood creatine level. *Annals of Neurology* 2000; **47**: 511–513.

38. De Vivo DC. The expanding clinical spectrum of mitochondrial diseases. *Brain and Development* 1993; **15**: 1–22.

39. Wallace DC. Mitochondrial defects in neurodegenerative disease. *MRDD Research Reviews* 2001; **7**: 158–166.

40. Van Erven PMM, Gillessen JPM, Eekhoff EMW, *et al.* Leigh syndrome. A mitochondrial encephalo(myo)pathy. *Clinical Neurology and Neurosurgery* 1987; **89**: 217–230.

41. Jellinger K, Seitelberger F. Spongy glio-neuronal dystrophy in infancy and childhood. *Acta Neuropathologica (Berlin)* 1979; **16**: 125–140.

42. Blackwood W, Buxton PH, Cumings JN, *et al.* Diffuse cerebral degeneration in infancy (Alpers' disease). *Archives of Disease in Childhood* 1963; **38**: 193–204.

43. Boyd SG, Harden A, Egger J, Pampiglione G. Progressive neuronal degeneration of childhood with liver disease ('Alpers' disease'): characteristic neurophysiological features. *Neuropediatrics* 1986; **17**: 75–80.

44. Shapira Y, Cederbaum SD, Cancilla PA, *et al.* Familial poliodystrophy, mitochondrial myopathy, and lactate acidemia. *Neurology* 1975; **25**: 614–621.

45. Pavlakis SG, Phillips PC, DiMauro, S, *et al.* Mitochondrial myopathy, encephalopathy, lactic acidosis and strokelike episodes: a distinctive clinical syndrome. *Annals of Neurology* 1984; **16**: 481–488.

46. Montagna P, Gallassi R, Medori R, *et al.* MELAS syndrome: characteristic migrainous and epileptic features and maternal transmission. *Neurology* 1988; **38**: 751–754.

47. Takeda S, Wakabayashi K, Ohama E, Ikuta F. Neuropathology of myoclonus epilepsy associated with ragged-red fibers (Fukuhara's disease). *Acta Neuropathologica (Berlin)* 1988; **75**: 433–440.

48. Willems PJ, Gatti R, Darby JK, *et al.* Fucosidosis revisited: A review of 77 patients. *American Journal of Medical Genetics* 1991; **38**: 111–131.

49. Desnick RJ, Wang AM. Schindler disease: an inherited neuroaxonal dystrophy due to a-N-acetylgalactosaminidase deficiency. *Journal of Inherited Metabolic Disease* 1990; **13**: 549–559.

50. Hofman SL, Peltonen L. The neuronal ceroid lipofuscinoses. In: Scriver CR, Baudet AL, Valle D, Sly WS (eds) *The Metabolic and Molecular Bases of Inherited Disease*, 8th edn. New York: McGraw-Hill, 2001: 3877–3894.

51. Veneselli E, Biancheri R, Buoni S, Fois A. Clinical and EEG findings in 18 cases of late infantile neuronal ceroid lipofuscinosis. *Brain and Development* 2001; **23**: 306–311.

52. Santavuori P, Haltia M, Rapola J, Raitta C. Infantile type of so-called neuronal ceroid-lipofuscinosis. Part 1. A clinical study of 15 patients. *Journal of the Neurological Sciences* 1973; **18**: 257–267.

53. Harden A, Pampiglione G, Picton-Robinson N. Electroretinogram and visual evoked response in a form of 'neuronal lipidosis' with diagnostic EEG features. *Journal of Neurology, Neurosurgery and Psychiatry* 1973; **36**: 61–67.

54. Santavuori P, Rapola, J, Raininko R, *et al.* Early juvenile neuronal ceroid-lipofuscinosis or variant Jansky-Bielschowsky disease: Diagnostic criteria and nomenclature. *Journal of Inherited Metabolic Disease* 1993; **16**: 230–232.

55. Hirvasniemi A, Lang H, Lehesjoki A-E, Leisti J. Northern epilepsy syndrome: an inherited childhood onset epilepsy with associated mental deterioration. *Journal of Medical Genetics* 1994; **31**: 177–182.

56. Steffenburg U, Hagberg G, Hagberg B. Epilepsy in a representative series of Rett syndrome. *Acta Paediatrica* 2001; **90**: 34–39.

57. Naidu S, Kaufmann WE, Abrams MT, *et al.* Neuroimaging studies in Rett syndrome. *Brain and Development* 2001; **23**: S62–71.

58. Amir RE, Van den Veyver IB, Wan M, *et al.* Rett syndrome is caused by mutations in X-linked *MECP2*, encoding methyl-CpG-binding protein 2. *Nature Genetics* 1999; **23**: 185–188.

59. Hoffbuhr K, Devaney JM, La Fleur B, *et al.* *MECP2* mutations in children with and without the phenotype of Rett syndrome. *Neurology* 2001; **56**: 1486–1495.

60. Haltia M, Somer M. Infantile cerebello-optic atrophy. Neuropathology of the progressive encephalopathy syndrome with edema, hypsarrhythmia and optic atrophy (the PEHO syndrome). *Acta Neuropathologica (Berlin)* 1993; **85**: 241–247.

61. Somer M, Sainio K. Epilepsy and the electroencephalogram in progressive encephalopathy with edema, hypsarrhythmia, and optic atrophy (the PEHO syndrome). *Epilepsia* 1993; **34**: 727–731.

Infection and postinfective causes of epilepsy

ANNA LECTICIA RIBEIRO PINTO AND PAULO ROGÉRIO M DE BITTENCOURT

Infections are an important cause of epilepsy in many parts of the world, and early treatment of the cause may prevent long-term neurologic sequelae. Infections are the commonest cause of status epilepticus and the second commonest cause of seizures of recent onset in children in tropical countries.[1] Some 5 per cent of all patients have epilepsy as a long-term complication of CNS infection. In the neonatal period infections account for 10 per cent of seizure disorders, a percentage varying with social and environmental factors.[2] The types of infection and their prevalence vary widely in different geographical regions. Only 3 per cent of 495 cases of brain damage in Finland were related to bacterial or viral disease and none were ascribed to parasitic disease, but the opposite is true in tropical regions where malaria is possibly the commonest cause of febrile seizures and acute bacterial meningitis is responsible for 20 per cent of acute symptomatic seizures in children.[1]

Seizures may occur during the acute infection or as a remote complication. In acute bacterial meningitis this distinction is clear. In contrast, neurocysticercosis and HIV encephalopathy do not have clear-cut acute and chronic phases, and seizures can occur throughout the course of the disease. Acute seizures due to infection can be of particular prognostic value. A severe acute symptomatic seizure disorder during cerebral malaria is a risk factor for chronic neurologic sequelae, including hemiplegia, cortical blindness, aphasia and ataxia. Similarly, Annegers et al.[3] showed that the 20-year risk for remote symptomatic epilepsy after viral encephalitis was 22 per cent in those with seizures and 10 per cent in those with no seizures, and after acute bacterial meningitis was 13 per cent in those with seizures and 2.4 per cent in those without seizures.

PATHOPHYSIOLOGY

Most seizures associated with acute bacterial, parasitic and viral diseases are partial or secondarily generalized.[1] In cysticercosis, seizures may occur when the parenchyma around a cysticercus is disturbed by inflammation, as when it degenerates. In patients with chronic calcified lesions, the seizures and encephalopathy may be due to microscopic permanent damage not detected by the low-field MR scanners that have been used in most studies.[4] In tuberculosis, cryptococcosis and toxoplamosis, localized vasculitis and inflammation are the cause of focal-onset seizures. In cerebral, malignant or falciparum malaria there is a widespread immune-mediated vascular disturbance, which results in tonic-clonic seizures. The seizures observed in subacute sclerosing panencephalitis (SSPE) and HIV are due to diffuse cortical neuronal damage.[2] In herpes simplex encephalitis, there is localized neuronal destruction. Shigellosis and common vivax malaria are associated with a toxemia, characterized by fever and other systemic effects, which cause generalized tonic-clonic seizures. Similarly, the multiple organ dysfunction seen in advanced forms of schistosomiasis, toxocariasis and filariasis is associated with generalized tonic-clonic seizures.[1] Nervous system complications of measles and pertussis vaccines have been reported to be linked to genetic predisposition and an immune pathogenesis.[5] Pertussis immunization in infants with recent seizures should be deferred until a progressive neurologic disorder is excluded or the cause of the earlier seizure has been determined.[6]

DIAGNOSIS

In patients with seizures and acute infections, the only other signs may be fever and malaise. In subacute or chronic diseases such as tuberculosis and cryptococcal meningitis, the neurological signs may include intracranial hypertension, meningismus, disturbances of behaviour and consciousness, and focal signs. The erthyrocyte sedimentation ratio (ESR) can help to distinguish between different types of infection. The ESR is high in bacterial and a few viral diseases, but normal in parasitic and most viral infections.[1] CT shows focal areas of low attenuation, with peripheral enhancement, in a variety of granulomatous disorders, including toxoplasmosis, neurocysticercosis and tuberculosis.[1] There may be signs of vasculitis, varying from irregular 'fluffy' enhancement to frank infarction. Cerebral infarction and edema predict a poor outcome. Obstructive hydrocephalus may also be demonstrated by CT head scan. MR imaging may permit a more definite diagnosis of certain disorders, e.g. venous sinus thrombosis.

The question of when CSF should be obtained in children presenting with seizures and fever has been the object of much discussion.[7] An algorithm for diagnosis and therapy in patients with seizures and infections is shown in Figure 4F.1. When there are clinical signs of raised intracranial pressure or a focal abnormality, a CT scan should always be performed before the lumbar puncture. Most other children with a first seizure with fever should have a lumbar puncture, unless a typical benign febrile seizure is highly likely and the physical examination shows no neurologic or meningeal signs. When a lumbar puncture is performed, a simultaneous blood sugar should always be measured in order to interpret the significance of the CSF glucose, which can be particularly important in infections. EEG may demonstrate focal abnormalities in patients with generalized seizures without other signs of localization, and also may have prognostic value in acute bacterial[8] and tuberculous meningitis.[9]

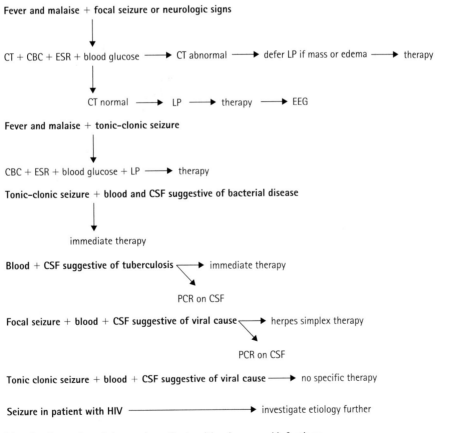

Figure 4F.1 *Algorithm for diagnosis and therapy in patients with seizures and infections.*

BACTERIAL DISEASES OF THE CNS

Although the incidence of community-acquired bacterial meningitis has decreased by 55 per cent over a period of 10 years in the USA,[10] this has not been the case in the developing world. The most common organism varies with age and environmental factors. *Haemophilus influenza* type B conjugate vaccine has been dramatically effective in certain countries, and the most common bacterial cause of meningitis is now *Streptococcus pneumoniae* (Table 4F.1), with an increasing frequency of penicillin- and cephalosporin-resistant strains.[11]

In one of the few published reports of the characteristics of seizures and epilepsy in acute bacterial meningitis,[8] 31 per cent of the 185 children had acute seizures, of which two thirds were partial seizures. Remote epilepsy occurred in 5.4 per cent of the children evaluated up to 9 years after the acute bacterial meningitis; typically patients had partial-onset seizures, were refractory to therapy and had a neurological deficit. In patients evaluated between 3 and 40 years after surgery for cerebral abscess,[12] 11 of 21 who were under 15 years of age at the time of surgery developed epilepsy after surgery, most in the first 2 years. Seizures were tonic-clonic in 60 per cent, simple partial in 14 per cent and complex partial in 21 per cent of cases. Epilepsy was refractory to therapy in one third of the patients, and 2 of the 11 had had status epilepticus.

Acute symptomatic seizures in patients with tuberculosis may be due to metabolic abnormalities, inappropriate secretion of antidiuretic hormone, cerebral tuberculomata or arteritis.[13] Seizures associated with tuberculomata or arteritis occur particularly during the acute illness,[2] and generalized tonic-clonic seizures are the commonest seizure type.[13] Focal seizures are associated usually with EEG and CT scan abnormalities.[13] The role of tuberculosis as a cause of remote symptomatic epilepsy is not clear.

PARASITIC DISEASES

The commonest worldwide cause of the febrile illness in febrile seizures may well be common malaria, caused by

Table 4F.1 *Frequency of etiology of acute bacterial meningitis in children worldwide*[11]

Etiologic agent	% of cases	Case fatality rate (%)
Streptococcus pneumoniae	30–50	19–46
Neisseria meningitidis	15–40	3–17
Haemophilus influenzae	2–7	3–11
Listeria monocytogenes	1–3	15–40
Other bacteria	<5	–

Plasmodium vivax. In contrast, the acute symptomatic seizures that occur in cerebral malaria, caused by *P. falciparum*, are a consequence of sequestration and hemolysis of blood cells, which results in decreased cerebral blood flow, hypoxia, infarction and hemorrhage. Remote symptomatic epilepsy is less common.

Congenital toxoplasmosis may be asymptomatic or result in remote symptomatic epilepsy. Toxoplasmosis is a frequent cause of localized symptomatic seizures in adults with HIV infection.[1] Neurocysticercosis may occur in children, and frequently manifests with seizures.[1,2] Seizures tend to be more severe during the active disease but may also occur during the inactive lifelong period of calcification. Acute symptomatic seizures are as common as remote symptomatic epilepsy. Seizures are partial-onset, and simple partial status is common. Generalized tonic-clonic seizures occur in 28–68 per cent of patients, despite the presence of a focal lesion.[14] Relatively good control of seizures is often achieved in adults following the active phase of the disease, when calcification has developed.[1]

VIRAL DISEASES

Herpes simplex encephalitis is a severe illness associated with acute symptomatic seizures and remote symptomatic epilepsy.[1] Partial seizures occur frequently in the acute phase, and simple or complex partial seizures, which are often intractable, are a common sequela. In neonates, herpes simplex encephalitis often manifests with partial motor seizures in the first week of life after initial lethargy and low-grade fever.

CNS HIV infection in children presents with developmental delay, cognitive decline, microcephaly and corticospinal tract signs. Seizures have been observed in 10–20 per cent of children with HIV encephalopathy. Neurological damage is secondary to strokes, neoplasia and opportunistic infections of the CNS. Cerebral infarction and hemorrhage may complicate the course of congenital HIV-1 infection and present with neurological deficits and sometimes seizures.[15] Thrombocytopenia, arteritis, intratumor bleeding and cardiomyopathy are causes of stroke in these patients. Primary CNS B-cell lymphoma and systemic lymphoma metastases to the CNS are the commonest neoplastic lesions, and both may present with focal neurologic deficits, seizures and changes of mental status. The immune deficiency evolves more rapidly in children than in adults and neurologic deterioration may be rapidly progressive and fulminant.

Congenital cytomegalovirus (CMV) infection may cause epilepsy, mental retardation, microcephaly and deafness. Patients with neurological abnormalities at birth have a significant risk of developing West syndrome. In patients with HIV infection, it may be difficult to distinguish the encephalopathies caused by HIV and CMV, which is the most common opportunistic viral agent to cause meningoencephalitis in HIV patients.[1]

Although acute symptomatic seizures occur in approximately 50 per cent of patients with measles encephalitis, only 10 per cent develop remote symptomatic seizures.[1] Focal seizures during the acute illness are of poor prognostic significance for the development of subsequent epilepsy.

Exanthem subitum, due to human herpes virus 6, may be complicated by encephalitis.[16] In a study of 21 cases, all had seizures in the febrile pre-eruptive phase of the disease. Acute symptomatic generalized tonic or tonic-clonic seizures were observed in 15 and lateralized seizures in 6. One of four patients who developed encephalopathy or encephalitis defined by CT and EEG abnormalities developed remote symptomatic epilepsy, and one died.

There is a strong correlation between nonpolio enteroviral CNS infection and seizures, particularly coxsackie virus group A.[17] The enteroviruses can be detected in the CSF. The neurological complications of Epstein-Barr virus (EBV) infection include encephalitis, acute inflammatory polyneuropathy, cerebellitis, aseptic meningitis and cranial neuropathy. The striking clinical abnormalities are seizures, hemiparesis and coma. Direct viral involvement is responsible for immune complex deposition and for the postinfectious inflammatory reaction.[18]

SYSTEMIC INFECTION

Tonic-clonic seizures may occur in a multitude of systemic infections that are not associated with damage to the CNS, as in septicemia or disorders leading to hepatic or renal failure. When seizures are focal, imaging studies are more likely to show cerebral involvement of one of the previously described specific diseases. *Mycoplasma pneumoniae*, a major cause of respiratory infection, may present with meningoencephalitis, seizures, psychosis and Guillain-Barré syndrome, probably as a manifestation of an autoimmune encephalomyelitis,[5] a monophasic illness that has also been associated with rubella, varicella, herpes zoster and mumps infection or immunization.[19]

NEWLY RECOGNIZED INFECTIONS

Prions have become a major topic of interest, first with the discovery of kuru, the progressive cerebellar syndrome of females and children in Papua New Guinea, and subsequently of Creutzfeld-Jakob disease, a subacute disease presenting usually in adults with dementia, myoclonus and periodic complexes in the EEG, that has been shown to be causally related to prions.[20] A disease similar to Creutzfeldt-Jakob has been described in much younger patients in the UK,[21] and a child of 12 years of age has been reported with this variant of Creutzfeld-Jakob disease.[22] Unlike the classical form, psychiatric symptoms are the most common early manifestation of variant Creutzfeld-Jakob disease and seizures occur much later.

KEY POINTS

- Infections are the **commonest cause of status epilepticus** in children, especially in tropical countries
- Seizures may occur **acutely or as a remote complication of a CNS infection**; in some diseases, such as HIV and neurocysticercosis, the distinction between acute and chronic phases is less definite
- Some 5 per cent of all patients with CNS infections develop remote **symptomatic epilepsy**
- **Seizures during the acute disease** increase the risk of remote symptomatic epilepsy
- **Acute bacterial meningitis** is complicated by remote symptomatic epilepsy in 5 per cent of patients, often in association with mental or motor deficits
- Acute seizures do not indicate failure of antibiotic treatment in acute bacterial meningitis, but are associated with a worse **prognosis**
- The **essential investigations** in a patient with seizures and a severe febrile illness are the ESR, CT and CSF analysis
- **Seizures can be due to the systemic illness** associated with acute infections, such as shigellosis, toxocariasis, tuberculosis or benign vivax malaria

REFERENCES

1. Bittencourt PRM, Sander JW, Mazer S. Viral, bacterial and parasitic infections associated with seizure disorder. In: Meinardi H (ed) *Handbook of Clinical Neurology*, vol. 72. Amsterdam: Elsevier Science, 1999; 145–174.
2. Commission on Tropical Disease of the International League Against Epilepsy. Epilepsy in the Tropics I. Epidemiology, socioeconomic risk factors and etiology. *Epilepsia* 1996; **37**: 1128–1137.
3. Annegers JF, Hauser W, *et al*. The risk of unprovoked seizures after encephalitis and meningitis. *Neurology* 1988; **38**: 1407–1410.
4. Goldsmith P, Sandmann MC, Souza DS, *et al*. The relationship between parasite location and epileptogenic region in neurocysticercosis. *Neurological Infections and Epidemiology* 1996; **1**: 127–133.

5. Hewlett EL. *Bordetella pertussis.* In: Scheld WM, Whitley RJ, Durak DT (eds) *Infections of the Central Nervous System.* Philadelphia, Pa.: Lippincott-Raven, 1997; 655–666.

6. American Academy of Pediatrics. *2000 Red Book: Report of the committee on infectious diseases,* 25th edn. Elk Grove Village, Ill.: American Academy of Pediatrics, 2000.

7. Wallace SJ. Convulsions and lumbar puncture. *Developmental Medicine and Child Neurology* 1985; **27**: 69–75.

8. Pomeroy SL, Holmes SJ, *et al.* Seizures and other neurologic sequelae of bacterial meningitis in children. *New England Journal of Medicine* 1990; **323**: 1651–1657.

9. Kalita J, Misra UK. EEG changes in tuberculous meningitis: a clinicoradiological correlation. *Electroencephalography and Clinical Neurophysiology* 1998; **107**: 39–43.

10. Schuchat A, Robinson K, Wenger JD, *et al.* Bacterial meningitis in the United States in 1995. *New England Journal of Medicine* 1997; **337**: 970–976.

11. Roos KL. Acute bacterial meningitis. *Seminars in Neurology* 2000; **20**: 293–306.

12. Nielsen H, Harmsen A, Gyldensted C. Cerebral abscess: A long-term follow-up. *Acta Neurologica Scandinavica* 1983; **67**: 330–337.

13. Patwari AK, Aneja S, Ravi RN, *et al.* Convulsions in tuberculous meningitis. *Journal of Tropical Pediatrics* 1996; **42**: 91–97.

14. Pal DK, Carpio A, Sander JWAS. Neurocysticercosis and epilepsy in developing countries. *Journal of Neurology, Neurosurgery and Psychiatry* 2000; **68**: 137–143.

15. Belman AL. AIDS and pediatric neurology. In: Bodensteiner J. (ed) *Pediatric Neurology. Neurologic Clinics of North America* 1990; **8**: 571–603.

16. Suga S, Yoshikawa T, Asano Y, *et al.* Clinical and virological analyses of 21 infants with exanthem subitum (roseola infantum) and central nervous system complications. *Neurology* 1993; **33**: 597–603.

17. Hosoya M, Sato M, Konzumi K, *et al.* Association of nonpolio enteroviral infection in the central nervous system of children with febrile seizures. *Pediatrics* 2001; **107**: E12.

18. Caruso JM, Tung GA, Gascon GG, *et al.* Persistent preceding focal neurologic deficits in children with chronic Epstein-Barr virus encephalitis. *Journal of Child Neurology* 2000; **15**: 791–796.

19. Hung KL, Liao HT, Tsai ML. Postinfectious encephalomyelitis: etiologic and diagnostic trends. *Journal of Child Neurology* 2000; **15**: 666–670.

20. Brown P, Preece M, Brandel J, *et al.* Iatrogenic Creutzfeldt-Jakob disease at the milennium. *Neurology* 2000; **55**: 1075–1081.

21. Will RG, Zeidler M, Stewart GE, *et al.* Diagnosis of new variant of Creutzfeldt-Jakob disease. *Annals of Neurology* 2000; **47**: 575–582.

22. Verity CM, Nicoll A, Will RG, Devereux G, Stellitano L. Variant Creutzfeldt-Jakob disease in UK children: a national surveillance study. *Lancet* 2000; **356**: 1224–1227.

Derby Hospitals NHS Foundation
Trust
Library and Knowledge Service

Pathology of childhood epilepsies

HAJIME MIYATA AND HARRY V VINTERS

ROLE OF THE NEUROPATHOLOGIST IN ASSESSING 'EPILEPTOGENIC' TISSUE

This chapter deals with clinicopathologic tissues relevant to 'infantile/pediatric epilepsy', and describes neuropathologic findings of non-neoplastic lesions in the brains of infants and children who have intractable seizure disorders. Recent advances in the molecular biological aspects of tuberous sclerosis-associated cortical tubers will also be briefly described. Until recently, these abnormalities (including malformative and inflammatory lesions) were usually assessed at necropsy,[1] by which time 'secondary' changes (brain structural abnormalities resulting from a protracted seizure disorder, rather than contributing to its cause) were likely to have complicated the neuropathologic findings. In recent years the surgical treatment of pediatric epilepsy has evolved into an acceptable alternative to the medical management of intractable seizures in children.[2,3] The result has been that neuropathologists have had the opportunity to assess brain lesions (associated with seizures in infants and children) in a relatively pristine state, allowing for more reasonable clinicopathologic correlations than were possible in the past using only autopsy tissues.

Modern immunohistochemical, ultrastructural, molecular, biochemical and pharmacologic techniques can also be applied more accurately and reproducibly to surgical specimens than to autopsy materials, allowing for analyses of human (in this case pediatric) brain tissues comparable in sophistication to those previously possible only in experimental animal studies. This frequently allows for rapid extrapolation of novel findings in experimental paradigms to the comparable human situation, and in general more meaningful communication between basic neuroscientists interested in pediatric epilepsy and neurologists, neurosurgeons and neuropathologists involved in the treatment of childhood seizure disorders. Examples will be provided below of how this interaction has shed light on basic mechanisms in the pathophysiology of pediatric epilepsy.

As long as care is taken to standardize tissue-processing parameters, surgically resected 'epileptic' brain can provide a wealth of neurobiologic information that may not be available in necropsy material. Immunostaining of tissues can be carried out to search for novel antigens, e.g. structural (cytoskeletal) proteins or those associated with cell proliferation.[4,5] Using the polymerase chain reaction (PCR), unique genes can be isolated, amplified and further studied, sometimes even using paraffin-embedded tissue blocks as a starting material.[6] PCR and *in situ* hybridization methodology have been combined to allow for gene and mRNA amplification and visualization within tissue sections.[7] All these molecular techniques can be applied to the study of single cells of interest within immunostained sections of surgically resected tissue from patients with intractable epilepsy.[8,9] mRNA isolated from freshly resected brain tissue as well as single cells in immunostained specimens can be used to construct cDNA libraries that may then be used to look for new genes (including epilepsy-associated genes)

Derby Hospitals NHS Foundation
Trust
Library and Knowledge Service

in the CNS.[8] Epileptic brain tissue can be used for electrophysiologic measurements and subsequently studied morphologically[10] by injecting tracer dyes into the cell bodies of neurons from which recordings have been made. Whole-cell voltage clamp recordings can be performed in combination with infrared videomicroscopy to distinguish abnormal cells within malformative lesions from normal-appearing neurons in the resected tissue from the same patient.[11]

Morphologic studies of brain tissue from epileptic patients (examined either at the time of surgery or at autopsy) are recognized as being inherently valuable in helping to understand the pathogenesis of human seizures, but care must be taken not to overinterpret brain lesions as being causal, rather than simply associated with a given epileptic disorder.[12] For example, in brain tissue from patients with cortical dysplasia (CD)/malformation of cortical development (MCD), the finding of severely disorganized cortex, though it suggests deranged movement of neurons from the germinal matrix to their normal location in the neocortex during intrauterine life and thus extremely abnormal cortical 'wiring', does not necessarily explain the genesis of the abnormal electrical activity within the brain that presumably underlies the generation of the seizures.

UNIQUE FEATURES OF NEUROPATHOLOGIC FINDINGS IN INFANTS OR CHILDREN WITH EPILEPSY

Pediatric epilepsy, particularly in its most severe manifestations in infants and children with intractable and catastrophic forms of seizure disorder such as infantile spasms, is associated with unique types of neuropathologic abnormality[13–16] that in general are hypothesized to reflect either abnormal migration of neurons to their 'usual' location in the neocortex (i.e. MCD), or sequelae of destructive brain lesions that occur *in utero* or in the perinatal period. The patterns of neuropathologic change identified are different than those seen in the brains of patients with primary generalized seizures or temporal lobe epilepsy.

There is debate about the significance of subtle cortical cytoarchitectural abnormalities such as 'microdysgenesis' identified in the CNS of patients with primary generalized seizures, i.e. seizures not associated with a structural lesion such as a neoplasm or encephalitis. Some authors believe that regional microdysgenesis is a lesion of possible etiologic importance for the genesis of seizures,[17] whereas others contend that such abnormalities are so commonly identified in neurologically normal controls that they do not have a causal role in producing primary generalized seizures.[18] Nevertheless, extratemporal corticectomies,

lobectomies and functional hemispherectomies performed for the treatment of chronic drug-resistant epilepsy in the second and third decades of life show a variety of less subtle structural abnormalities, including glioneuronal and vascular malformations (with or without hamartomas), lesions suggestive of pre- or perinatal brain necrosis (e.g. ulegyria, porencephaly), low-grade glial neoplasms or infectious/inflammatory disorders.[19,20] Though these abnormalities occur or become symptomatic somewhat later in life than those associated with catastrophic infantile or pediatric seizure disorders, they clearly overlap with morphologic alterations noted in resected brain tissues from infants and younger children with intractable epilepsy, and highlight the importance of common pathophysiologic mechanisms.

Temporal lobe epilepsy is commonly associated with hippocampal or Ammon's horn sclerosis (HS/AHS) or neoplasms, including ganglioglioma and dysembryoplastic neuroepithelial tumor (DNET), though other types of neuropathologic change observed include metabolic diseases and neurocutaneous syndromes; focal cortical dysplasia (FCD) and other MCDs; vascular malformations; and sequelae of cerebrovascular disease, trauma, or infectious/inflammatory disorders.[21–23] Even in patients whose resected temporal lobe shows the expected lesion of HS/AHS, extrahippocampal lesions may often be present ('dual pathology'),[24] emphasizing the need to precisely define the 'true epileptogenic area' before surgical treatment of temporal lobe epilepsy is undertaken. Low-grade tumors are commonly encountered in temporal lobectomy specimens from children with temporal lobe epilepsy.[25]

CEREBRAL LESIONS ASSOCIATED WITH INFANTILE OR PEDIATRIC EPILEPSY

In young patients studied as part of the UCLA Pediatric Epilepsy Surgery Program, the **zone of cortical abnormality** putatively linked to a given seizure disorder is defined by a combination of methodologies, including MRI, EEG and PET. Following tissue resection, it becomes the task of the neuropathologist to further define the cellular and (when possible) molecular substrates of the lesion(s).

Destructive lesions

The developing CNS is at risk of structural damage caused by inadequate oxygenation of the fetus *in utero*, in the intrapartum and early perinatal periods, the latter particularly if a baby is born prematurely.[26–30] The lesions that result can be envisioned simplistically as infantile 'strokes', though the range of resultant infarcts and hemorrhages seen by the neuropathologist is even greater than the spectrum of 'stroke' in the adult or aging brain, possibly because the 'insult' producing a structural anomaly will produce different results depending on the developmental stage of the affected CNS. The descriptive terms applied to the involved brain reflect the heterogeneity of the lesions encountered. The best characterized (though still poorly understood) of these include germinal matrix hemorrhages, multicystic gliotic encephalopathy, periventricular leukomalacia and hydranencephaly.[29]

That these lesions, variable though they are, can produce epilepsy in infants and children is suggested by the experience of encountering them in cerebral cortical resection specimens from infants and children with a history of infantile spasms or West syndrome.[15,16] In our initial experience with specimens from 13 such patients, destructive brain lesions were encountered in 4. We have used the generic term **cystic encephalomalacia** to describe these, though the spectrum of neuropathologic change has been broad, ranging from cortical and white matter infarcts identical in appearance to those seen in adults with large-vessel occlusions, to large cysts lined by astrocytes that are confined to the white matter.[31] Hemosiderin at the edges of some foci of encephalomalacia reflects a hemorrhagic component. In some instances, only intense cortical astrogliosis of apparent anoxic-ischemic origin is identified.[14]

Figure 5.1 illustrates an example of one lesion from this category, with glial cysts involving the cortex and underlying white matter, and 'mushroom-like' gyri best described by the term **ulegyria**. Many of the encephalomalacic lesions have been extensively calcified, reflecting the propensity of infant brain to show dystrophic calcification in areas of injury, often regardless of the inciting event.

Malformative–hamartomatous lesions

These are among the more biologically intriguing anomalies observed in a surgical neuropathologic practice.[32,33] The variability of the precise nature and severity of the morphologic alterations in the CNS fails to obscure the fact that certain neuropathologic 'themes' pointing to deranged histogenesis of the neocortex recur upon review of the clinicopathologic material. Furthermore, the cellular and molecular pathologic changes seen in some forms of neocortical malformation, best characterized by the terms **focal cortical dysplasia** (FCD) initially described by Taylor et al.,[34] or MCD, often bear a striking resemblance to brain lesions seen in patients with tuberous sclerosis complex (TSC). Among cortical resections (including hemispherectomies) performed as part of the therapy of intractable childhood epilepsy at the UCLA Medical Center, malformations (with or without associated hamartomas) have recently been encountered more frequently than encephalomalacic lesions,[14] and are

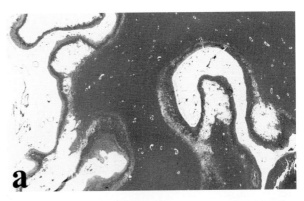
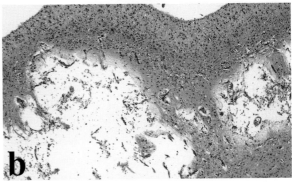

Figure 5.1 *Cystic gliotic encephalopathy: (a) An autopsy specimen from a child shows multiple cysts involving both cortex and underlying white matter. Tissue destruction has resulted in some of the gyri taking on a 'mushroom-like' appearance. (b) Microscopic appearance of the lesions in panel (a) showing cystic cavities surrounded by densely packed fibrillary gliosis. (Hematoxylin & eosin, original magnification (a) × 4.3; (b) × 40.)*

especially common in infants and very young children who present with West syndrome.[16,35]

Here, somewhat arbitrarily, cortical/white matter malformations have been subclassified into three main types, accepting the fact that in a given cortical resection specimen there may be a mix of the specific neuropathologic features. These are best characterized as:

- polymicrogyria[1]
- heterotopic collections of neurons and single heterotopic neurons in the subcortical white matter
- cortical dysplasia (with severe disorganization of the normal hexalaminar neocortical pattern).

The lesions in the last subcategory most closely resemble those of TSC. In its most severe form CD shows bizarre, enlarged, cytomegalic neurons with concomitant cytoskeletal abnormalities, and 'balloon cells' that resemble gemistocytic astrocytes with oval, pale, glassy, eosinophilic cytoplasm. This change is variably severe throughout a corticectomy specimen. Neuronal cytoskeletal abnormalities and balloon cells are commonly situated in the deep cortex or the superficial subcortical white matter, though

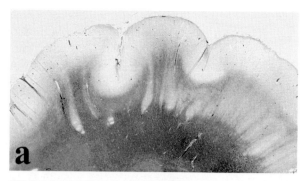

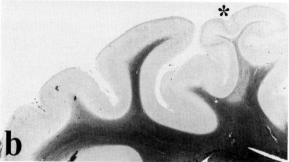

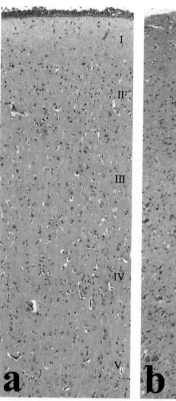

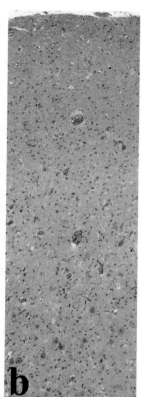

Figure 5.2 *Patterns of CD/MCD from pediatric cortical resection specimens: (a) Poorly demarcated cortex-white matter junction, with obvious heterotopic collections of 'gray matter' within the subcortical white matter. (b) Relatively well-defined cortex-white matter junction, but hyperconvoluted cortex (*) in one region indicative of focal polymicrogyria. (Klüver-Barrera, original magnification (a) ×3; (b) ×3.5.)*

they may be present throughout the involved cerebral hemisphere.

Cortical malformations can often be seen on cut sections of the fixed brain, where they may be quite focal and thus most easily appreciated in contrast to the adjacent uninvolved neocortical ribbon and underlying homogeneous white matter.[14] Even in a grossly normal cortical resection specimen, the presence of different patterns of CD will become readily apparent on superficial inspection of whole mount sections, especially those stained with a technique (e.g., Klüver-Barrera) that highlights differences between cortical gray matter and underlying myelinated fibers (Figure 5.2).

The cellular pathology of CD can further be stratified depending on whether or not certain specific microscopic abnormalities are noted in a given specimen (Figure 5.3). In a review of over 70 examples of CD from young patients who underwent lobectomy or hemispherectomy,[36] eight major histopathologic features were scored as being present or absent in each specimen. The specific light microscopic changes sought (and the relative percentage of cases in which they were found) were:

- cortical laminar disorganization (a defining feature of CD and hence present in all specimens)

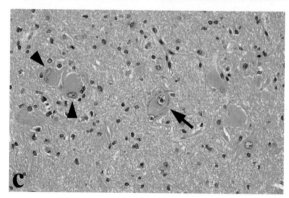

Figure 5.3 *Microscopic features of cortical dysplasia: (a) Normal cerebral cortex (middle temporal gyrus) from a patient with intractable temporal lobe epilepsy. Note well-organized cortex with five out of six cortical layers clearly identified. (b) Surgically resected cortical dysplasia from a pediatric patient with intractable epilepsy. Note severely disorganized cortical tissue without a laminar substructure. (c) A high-power view of the disorganized tissue shown in panel (b). Note a large/giant dysplastic cytomegalic neuron (arrow) with a large nucleolated nucleus and scattered Nissl substance at the periphery of pale cytoplasm, and large gemistocytic astrocyte-like 'balloon cells' (arrowheads). (Hematoxylin & eosin, original magnification (a),(b) ×50; (c) ×240.) (See Plate 1.)*

- single heterotopic neurons within the deep white matter or molecular layer (layer I) of cortex (98.7 per cent)
- neuronal cytomegaly (55.8 per cent)

- neuronal cytoskeletal abnormalities[5] (51.9 per cent)
- macroscopically visible neuronal heterotopias, usually in the subcortical white matter (41.6 per cent)
- neuroglial excrescences in the subarachnoid space (29.9 per cent)
- balloon cell change, consisting of gemistocytic astrocyte-like cells with variable glial fibrillary acidic protein (GFAP) cytoplasmic immunoreactivity (22.1 per cent)
- foci of polymicrogyria (14.3 per cent).

On the basis of the presence or absence of various combinations of these histologic features, individual cases could be subclassified as being mild, moderate or severe, and mean preoperative seizure frequency correlated well with the histologic grade. Children with moderate or severe degrees of CD were more likely to have shown a preoperative neurologic deficit.[36]

Many of the cells in FCD show morphological and immunohistochemical features suggesting the existence of an indeterminate or 'uncommitted' phenotype, with both neuronal and glial features. For example, a cell may possess a characteristic nucleolated nucleus (typical of neurons) but show glassy, eosinophilic cytoplasm, a feature more suggestive of astrocytic differentiation, expressing both GFAP and neurofilament.[14,15,37,38] Furthermore, recent novel techniques including cellular, electrophysiologic and molecular strategies are likely to provide answers to the most vexing and important question about MCD: why is it so strongly associated with epilepsy? Intracranial grid recordings have clearly demonstrated that the ictal onset zone is within the malformation in patients with MCDs.[39,40] Periventricular nodular heterotopias have been recognized as causing intractable epilepsy in some but not all patients, as demonstrated by depth electrode recording.[41] Field potential and intracellular recordings within surgically resected FCD/MCD have shown that dysplastic cortex itself is hyperexcitable[11,42] and that a subset of dysplastic neurons generate repetitive ictal discharges.[43] Some studies suggest selective reduction of GABAergic interneurons in MCD[44,45] and loss of $GABA_A$ receptor subunits in FCD,[46] and increased expression of several glutamate receptor subunits including NR2B, GluR1, GluR2 has also been reported.[46-48] More recently an increased number of excitatory neurons has been found in TSC tubers[45] and in FCD.[49]

A large and rapidly growing body of literature deals with the spectrum of CD/MCD and its role in pediatric and adult epilepsy, including descriptions of modern neuroimaging techniques.[50,51] Even lesions involving eloquent brain areas may be successfully resected,[52] although satisfactory seizure control in MCD patients may be particularly difficult to attain even with antiepileptic drug (AED) polytherapy and surgical resection.[53] An understanding of the basic neurobiology that underlies the pathogenesis of

CD/MCD is likely to emerge as the mysteries of normal human brain development are unraveled using modern immunohistochemical and molecular techniques[54] that, in turn, illuminate key events in neuronal precursor migration from the germinal matrix to the neocortex and synaptogenesis.

In addition, over the past 10 years, there has been an explosion of information on the genetics of MCD. At least eight genes responsible for MCDs have been cloned. These include TSC1[55] and TSC2[56] for TSC, FLN1 for periventricular nodular heterotopia[57] and others (for review, see ref. 58). This permits important mechanistic studies to be carried out with the purpose of understanding how mutations within these genes result in abnormal cortical cytoarchitecture and anomalous neuroglial differentiation. Even with our present level of knowledge about human brain embryogenesis and maturation, hypotheses can be formulated about when 'insults' must impact the developing brain to produce specific types of CD/MCD.[58,59] One of the key questions that will require a coherent answer is: why are manifestations of CD/MCD so often strikingly unilateral?

An example of the latter phenomenon is encountered in a subset of CD/MCD, best described as **hemimegalencephaly**. In this rare malformation (Figure 5.4), which may be amenable to surgical treatment by hemispherectomy,[60] a malformed cerebral hemisphere shows various combinations of neuropathologic change that range from hemilissencephaly to polymicrogyria to hamartomatous malformation.[61,62] Most of the eight cellular features of CD described above are seen in various combinations in hemimegalencephaly. Morphometric data[61] have shown significant increases (above autopsy controls) in neuronal profile area and (sometimes) increase in neuronal cell density in hemimegalencephalic brain.

Tuberous sclerosis complex (TSC)

TSC is a syndrome, components of which include regions of malformed/dysplastic cerebral neocortex (tubers) with hamartomatous proliferation of neuroectodermal (undifferentiated/dedifferentiated) cells, subependymal giant cell astrocytomas, cutaneous and visceral manifestations, the latter usually hamartomas or neoplasms of the heart (rhabdomyomas) and kidneys (angiomyolipomas), though other organ systems are frequently involved.[63] Tubers apparently causing epilepsy may be removed neurosurgically, though they constitute a relatively rare type of specimen in comparison to the large numbers of destructive lesions and CD/MCD operated on in infants and children with intractable seizures. CD/MCD often shows the cellular features of cerebral TSC, i.e. disorganized cortex with enlarged dysmorphic neuronal cell bodies sometimes showing marked cytoskeletal and cytoplasmic

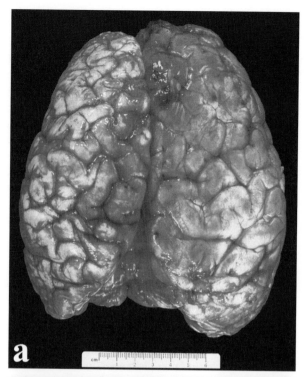

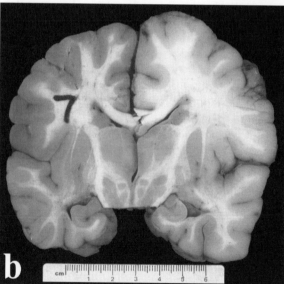

Figure 5.4 *Hemimegalencephaly. (a),(b) Autopsy specimen from a 7-month-old child with severe seizures, viewed from the convexities. Note diffuse enlargement of the right cerebral hemisphere, widening of the gyri and blurring of the cortex-white matter junction throughout the affected hemisphere. Deep central gray structures are relatively well preserved in a representative coronal section (b).*

abnormalities[5] (Figure 5.3). The balloon cells seen with severe CD are identical to their variably GFAP-immunoreactive counterparts in neocortical tubers of TSC.[64] Ultrastructural and immunocytochemical features of the cells seen in tubers support the view that they are

'uncommitted' cells that have features of both neurons and astrocytes.[64,65] In this regard, they are similar to some of the cell types seen in CD cortex (from patients without visceral manifestations of TSC).[15] Studies using markers of cellular proliferation[4,58] show that balloon cells in both FDC and tuber of TSC constitute a largely nonproliferating cell population.

TSC may be seen in very young children and even premature infants.[66–68] It is a bigenic autosomal dominant disorder caused by mutations in one of two nonhomologous tumor suppressor genes, *TSC1*[55] on chromosomes 9 (9q34) encoding a 130-kDa protein, hamartin, and *TSC2*[56] on chromosome 16 (16p13.3) encoding a 200-kDa protein, tuberin. Recent studies have suggested that hamartin and tuberin interact with each other to regulate cell proliferation and cell cycle progression.[55,69,70] Hamartin may also interact with other proteins including the ERM (ezrin, radixin, and moesin) family of actin-binding proteins to activate Rho GTPases.[71] Tuberin contains a conserved C-terminal region that exhibits sequence homology to the catalytic domain of a GTPase-activating protein (GAP) for Rap1[72] and for Rab5.[73] In several cell lines tuberin and Rap1 co-localize in the Golgi apparatus.[74] Tuberin is thought to be involved in the regulation of neuronal differentiation.[75] Mutations in *TSC2* may result in constitutive activation of Rap1 leading to enhanced proliferation or incomplete cellular differentiation. *Tsc1* and *Tsc2*, *Drosophila* homologs of *TSC1* and *TSC2*, function together *in vivo* to negatively regulate cell size, cell proliferation and organ size in the insulin signaling pathway (PI3Kinase-Akt/PKB-mTOR-S6K) at a position downstream of *dAkt* (*Drosophila* Akt) and upstream of *dS6k* (*Drosophila* S6kinase), although the precise positioning of these genes relative to this pathway is still uncertain.[76] Recent studies of animal models suggest possible treatment of TSC-associated lesions by targeting downstream components of the insulin signaling pathway.[77]

Rho GTPases regulate actin cytoskeleton, and are thought to be involved in neuronal developmental processes including neuronal migration, establishment of polarity, axon growth and guidance, dendrite elaboration and plasticity, and synapse formation.[78] ERM proteins function in multiple different fashions according to their interaction with various membrane proteins, Ras superfamily GTPases and the actin cytoskeleton, and appear to be involved in the formation of microvilli, cell–cell adhesion, maintenance of cell shape, cell motility and membrane trafficking.[79] The fact that hamartin binds to ezrin *in vivo* and can modulate the activity of RhoA (Ras homologous member A)[71] suggests that tuberin and hamartin may be attached to the membrane-cytoskeletal cortex through activated ERM proteins.[80] Evidence from several reports suggests that ERM proteins function at a position upstream and downstream of Rho GTPases to regulate cellular adhesion and motility[81,82] as well as neuronal developmental processes as mentioned above. In fact, ezrin and moesin are expressed in germinal matrix cells, migrating cells, and radial glial fibers in the developing human brain.[80] This specific expression correlates with the RhoA expression in proliferating and migrating cells (but not in cells already positioned in the cortical plate) in developing rat brain.[83]

Mutations in the *filamin1* (*FLN1*) gene encoding filamin1, another F-actin-binding protein whose activity is regulated by the phosphorylation of RhoA, result in periventricular nodular heterotopia.[57,84] In a similar way, dysfunction of tuberin and hamartin in response to gene mutations may perturb communication between ERM proteins and Rho GTPase to cause abnormal neuronal migration, polarity and morphology, resulting in the formation of dysplastic cortex. Abnormalities of radial glia have also been implicated in the pathogenesis of brain lesions of TSC.[68]

Immunohistochemical studies have demonstrated that TSC gene products and ERM proteins are co-expressed within a subpopulation of abnormal neuroglial cells in TSC-associated cortical tubers.[80,85] This suggests that ERM proteins are upregulated within these cells in response to TSC gene mutation, possibly as a compensatory mechanism. More recently, it has also been demonstrated that hamartin *per se* has the ability to modulate cell proliferation independent of the presence of functional tuberin, suggesting that binding to hamartin is not always essential for tuberin to affect cell proliferation.[86]

As noted above, CD is one of the major neuropathologic abnormalities encountered in pediatric patients who undergo cortical resection or hemispherectomy to treat infantile spasms and related intractable seizure disorders of infancy or childhood.[15,35,87–89] Given the essentially identical morphologic features of FCD among patients of different ages, however, it is enigmatic that they give rise to both infantile spasms and, in others, intractable epilepsy with onset in adolescence or even adulthood. To date, specific protein expressions patterns in FCD tissue correlated with age of seizure onset are not available, although many studies on the expression of various kinds of proteins in CD brains have been reported.[5,37,38,58,90–94]

Chronic (Rasmussen type) encephalitis

Though the clinicopathologic features of this syndrome, first recognized by Rasmussen in the late 1950s, are remarkably stereotyped, its etiology is still unknown.[95–98] It produces seizures in young children who have, until the time of onset of the epileptic disorder, usually developed normally, with onset in 85 per cent of cases occurring before the age of 10 years.[99] Rasmussen encephalitis is characterized by clinically intractable epilepsy, epilepsia

partialis continua,[100] and a progressive deterioration of neurologic functions related to the affected hemisphere, finally resulting in hemiplegia, hemianopia and aphasia. Hemispherectomy has become one of the standard treatments in childhood-onset Rasmussen encephalitis, since the seizures are usually unresponsive to standard antiepileptic medications.[101,102] The pathologic change encountered within the 'epileptogenic' hemisphere includes features of a chronic, patchy and severe encephalitis, with evidence of chronic inflammation (perivascular lymphocytic cuffing and microglial nodules), neuronal loss, astrocytic gliosis, microcystic change and a prominent microvascularity[103,104] (Figure 5.5; see also Plate 2).

Despite the 'inflammatory' neuropathologic features of Rasmussen encephalitis, which strongly suggest that the cause of the syndrome is viral infection of the CNS, no consistent data implicating a single pathogen or group of pathogens had, until recently, emerged. For instance, no viral inclusions could consistently be identified in brains from patients with Rasmussen encephalitis. However, several reports over the past decade have implicated herpesviruses, especially cytomegalovirus (CMV) and Epstein-Barr virus (EBV), in the pathogenesis of Rasmussen encephalitis,[105,106] though molecular probe studies attempting to localize these viral genes in Rasmussen encephalitis brain tissue were not consistently positive.[107] The results of a study using PCR to examine DNA extracted from Rasmussen encephalitis tissues for genes specific to human herpesviruses[6] suggest that herpesvirus infection of the CNS does not result directly in Rasmussen encephalitis, though the possibility that it triggers an autoimmune response that is of pathogenetic importance cannot be ruled out. Autoantibodies against the glutamate receptor, GluR3, found in a rabbit experimental model of Rasmussen encephalitis, as well as in some affected children, has suggested an autoimmune mechanism for Rasmussen encephalitis.[108] There has, however, been debate about the precise role of the autoantibodies in the etiology and pathogenesis of Rasmussen encephalitis. Serum anti-GluR3 antibodies raised in rabbits have been shown to destroy primary mixed neuronal-glial cultures in a complement (C′)-dependent manner.[109] Immunohistochemical detection of human IgG, C′ components (C4, C8), and the membrane attack complex (MAC) in neurons has been demonstrated in surgically resected cerebral cortex from a subset of Rasmussen encephalitis patients.[110] Immunohistochemical labeling of rat neurons by anti-GluR3 IgG from two Rasmussen encephalitis patients has also been demonstrated.[111] Another study, however, suggests that astrocytes rather than neurons are the principal target of anti-GluR3 antisera-mediated cytotoxic effects, as demonstrated in primary mixed neuronal-glial cultures of rat cortex.[112] A more recent study suggests that neuronal death in Rasmussen encephalitis is directly induced by a

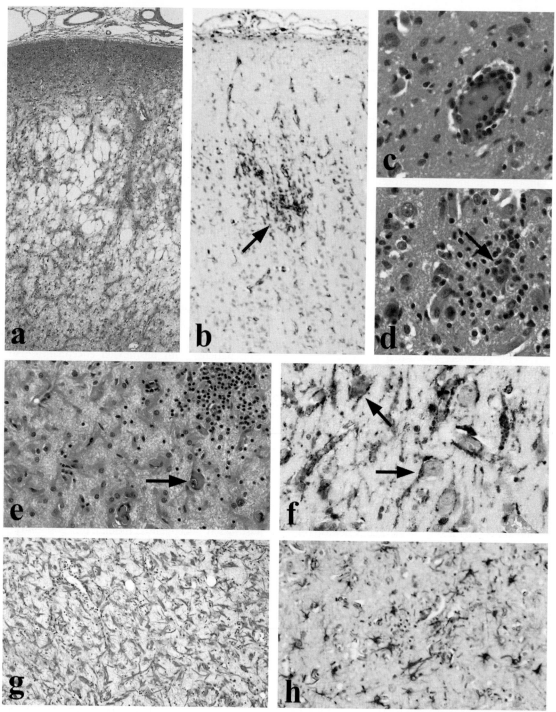

Figure 5.5 *Rasmussen encephalitis. (a) Extensive loss of neurons with microcystic change or 'status spongiosus', accompanied by capillary proliferation, but relatively minimal inflammation. Leptomeningeal infiltration of mononuclear inflammatory cells is also seen. (Hematoxylin & eosin, ×50.) (b) In contrast to (a), this panel shows a relatively intact cortex with a single inflammatory (microglial) nodule (arrow) in mid-cortex. (CD68 immunostain, ×125.) (c) Mononuclear inflammatory cells infiltrating the wall of a cortical microvessel ('perivascular cuffing'). (Hematoxylin & eosin, ×400.) (d) Mononuclear inflammatory cells and microglial cells surrounding a single neuron showing 'neuronophagia', indicated by an arrow. (Hematoxylin & eosin, ×400.) (e) Higher magnification of (a) showing severe neuronal loss with rarefaction of neuropil totally replaced by gemistocytic reactive astrocytes, and capillary proliferation. A focus of mononuclear cell infiltration (right upper corner) and a single chromatolytic neuron (arrow) remain. (Hematoxylin & eosin, ×200.) (f) High-power view of (b) showing CD68-positive microglial cells surrounding each neuronal profile (arrows). (CD68 immunostain, ×400.) (g) Severely affected area shown in panel (a) containing numerous GFAP-positive reactive astrocytes. (GFAP immunostain, ×100.) (h) Relatively well-preserved cortex showing rather less but definite astrogliosis as opposed to more severely affected area shown in panel (g). (GFAP immunostain, ×200.) (All immunostains were performed by the avidin–biotin–peroxidase complex (ABC) method and counterstained with hematoxylin, original magnifications shown.) (See Plate 2).*

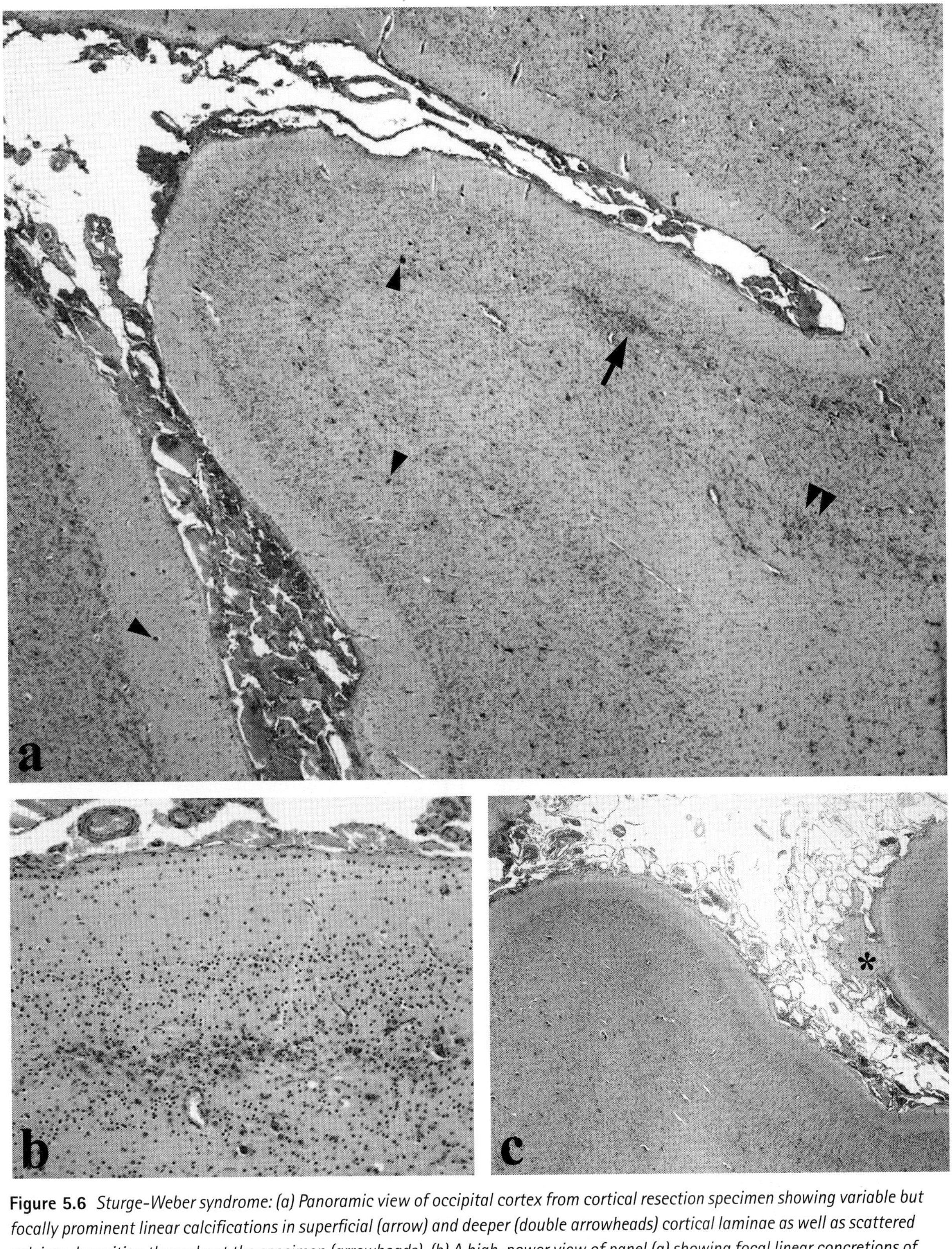

Figure 5.6 *Sturge-Weber syndrome: (a) Panoramic view of occipital cortex from cortical resection specimen showing variable but focally prominent linear calcifications in superficial (arrow) and deeper (double arrowheads) cortical laminae as well as scattered calcium deposition throughout the specimen (arrowheads). (b) A high-power view of panel (a) showing focal linear concretions of calcium. (c) Leptomeningeal angiomatosis continuous with a leptomeningeal glioneuronal heterotopia or excrescence (asterisk). (Hematoxylin & eosin, original magnifications (a) × 40; (b) × 100; (c) × 20.) (See Plate 3).*

T-cell-mediated cytotoxic reaction.[98] These new data obtained from human Rasmussen encephalitis and its animal models indicate that immune factors may play a central role in the pathogenesis of this disorder and may lead to a better understanding of its pathogenesis, as well as that of other seizure disorders with immunological concomitants.

Sturge–Weber syndrome (encephalotrigeminal angiomatosis)

This is encountered in surgical specimens from infants and children with intractable epilepsy much less commonly than the destructive and malformative/hamartomatous lesions already described at length. Clinicopathologic reports describe the association of the cerebral lesion, usually localized to the occipital cortex, with facial capillary hemangioma (port wine stain) in the distribution of the trigeminal nerve, and provide excellent accounts of the natural history of the disorder.[113–115] Visceral angiomas may be encountered in some patients.[116]

Neuropathologic abnormalities in cortical resection specimens are easily appreciated at low magnification (Figure 5.6; see also Plate 3), and soft tissue radiographs of the sliced specimen may show the characteristic 'tramtrack' pattern of neocortical calcification. The leptomeninges show a dense angiomatosis, characterized by some authors as a venous angioma.[113] The cortex itself shows calcifications often centered on microvessels, with associated neuronal loss and astrocytic gliosis that is assumed to result from ischemic phenomena secondary (at least in part) to the meningeal angiomatosis. Ultrastructural studies of the parenchymal calcifications in Sturge-Weber brain have suggested that the earliest calcium deposits occur within perithelial cells of small blood vessels, and that the underlying cause of the calcification may be anoxic injury to endothelial, perithelial, and glial mitochondria due to stasis and abnormally increased vascular permeability of vessels in the hemangioma.[117,118]

FUTURE DIRECTIONS

Neuropathologists, especially in collaboration with their clinical and basic research colleagues, are in a unique position to contribute to an understanding of the morphologic substrates of basic cellular mechanisms of epilepsy.[119] Investigations into the etiology and pathogenesis of each of the subtypes of neuropathologic change encountered will require distinctive neurobiologic approaches, but the tools of immunocytochemistry, pharmacology and molecular biology can be brought to bear on a more complete understanding of how and why the structurally abnormal brain generates seizures. An even more pertinent question might

be: why do seizures occur in one individual with a given type of brain lesion, but not in another patient with the otherwise identical abnormality? A neuropathologist who deals with lesions discovered in the course of hemispherectomy or unihemispheral cortical resections cannot help but be struck by another peculiarity of these lesions – their occurrence predominantly or exclusively on one side of the brain. The latter observation suggests a very specific insult that 'scars' one cerebral hemisphere in utero (in the case of CD/MCD and encephalomalacic lesions) or during later brain development (in Rasmussen encephalitis). Attempting to understand these peculiarities of 'epileptogenic' brain will be certain to yield insights into the most basic questions of human neurobiology. The discovery of genes responsible for many MCDs permits further analyses of the encoded proteins, and this may subsequently lead to better understanding of the pathogenesis of these disorders and also to designing effective therapeutic strategies.

KEY POINTS

- **Malformative/hamartomatous lesions** and **encephalomalacic lesions** are the most common abnormalities encountered among cortical resections from pediatric patients with intractable epilepsy, including infantile spasms
- There is substantial evidence that **dysplastic lesions themselves are epileptogenic**
- The discovery of genes responsible for many MCDs allows further mechanistic studies to be carried out with the purpose of understanding how **mutations** within these genes result in abnormal cortical cytoarchitecture and anomalous neuroglial differentiation
- Molecular pathomechanisms of **TSC-related brain lesions** are among the best studied among MCDs
- **Immunological factors (including autoimmunity)** may play important roles in the pathogenesis of Rasmussen encephalitis and of other seizure disorders with immunological concomitants

---

ACKNOWLEDGMENTS

Long-term collaborators in this work include Dr. Michael Farrell (Dublin, Ireland), Dr. Robin Fisher (UCLA) and Dr. Gary Mathern (UCLA). Outstanding technical assistance was provided by Diana Lenard Secor, Laurel Reed, Alex Brooks and Beth Johnson. We are indebted to the clinicians involved with the UCLA Pediatric Epilepsy Surgery Program.

REFERENCES

1. Friede RL. (ed.) *Developmental Neuropathology*, 2nd revised and expanded edition. Berlin: Springer-Verlag, 1989.
2. Chugani HT, Shewmon DA, Shields WD, *et al.* Surgery for intractable infantile spasms: neuroimaging perspectives. *Epilepsia* 1993; **34**: 764–771.
3. Shields WD, Duchowny MS, Holmes GL. Surgically remediable syndromes of infancy and early childhood. In: Engel J Jr. (ed.) *Surgical Treatment of the Epilepsies*, 2nd edn. New York: Raven Press, 1993: 35–48.
4. De Rosa MJ, Farrell MA, Burke MM, Secor DL, Vinters HV. An assessment of the proliferative potential of 'balloon cells' in focal cortical resections performed for childhood epilepsy. *Neuropathology and Applied Neurobiology* 1992; **18**: 566–574.
5. Duong T, De Rosa MJ, Poukens V, Vinters HV, Fisher RS. Neuronal cytoskeletal abnormalities in human cerebral cortical dysplasia. *Acta Neuropathologica* 1994; **87**: 493–503.
6. Vinters HV, Wang R, Wiley CA. Herpesviruses in chronic encephalitis associated with intractable childhood epilepsy. *Human Pathology* 1993; **24**: 871–879.
7. Nuovo GJ, Forde A, MacConnell P, Fahrenwald R. *In situ* detection of PCR-amplified HIV-1 nucleic acids and tumor necrosis factor cDNA in cervical tissues. *American Journal of Pathology* 1993; **143**: 40–48.
8. Crino PB, Trojanowski JQ, Dichter MA, Eberwine J. Embryonic neuronal markers in tuberous sclerosis: single-cell molecular pathology. *Proceedings of the National Academy of Sciences of the USA* 1996; **93**: 14152–14157.
9. Kacharmina JE, Crino PB, Eberwine J. Preparation of cDNA from single cells and subcellular regions. *Methods in Enzymology* 1999; **303**: 3–18.
10. Wuarin JP, Kim YI, Cepeda C, *et al.* Synaptic transmission in human neocortex removed for treatment of intractable epilepsy in children. *Annals of Neurology* 1990; **28**: 503–511.
11. Mathern GW, Cepeda C, Hurst RS, Flores-Hernandez J, Mendoza D, Levine MS. Neurons recorded from pediatric epilepsy surgery patients with cortical dysplasia. *Epilepsia* 2000; **41** (Suppl 6): S162–167.
12. Vinters HV, Armstrong DL, Babb TL, *et al.* The neuropathology of human symptomatic epilepsy. In: Engel J Jr. (ed.) *Surgical Treatment of the Epilepsies*, 2nd edn. New York: Raven Press, 1993: 593–608.
13. Vinters HV, Mah V, Shields WD. Neuropathologic correlates of pediatric epilepsy. *Journal of Epilepsy* 1990; **3** (Suppl): 227–235.
14. Farrell MA, DeRosa MJ, Curran JG, *et al.* Neuropathologic findings in cortical resections (including hemispherectomies) performed for the treatment of intractable childhood epilepsy. *Acta Neuropathologica* 1992; **83**: 246–259.
15. Vinters HV, Fisher RS, Cornford ME, *et al.* Morphological substrates of infantile spasms: studies based on surgically resected cerebral tissue. *Child's Nervous System* 1992; **8**: 8–17.
16. Robain O, Vinters HV. Neuropathologic studies in West syndrome. In: Dulac O, Chugani HT, Dalla Bernardina B. (eds) *Infantile Spasms and West syndrome*. London: W.B. Saunders, 1994: 99–117.
17. Meencke HJ, Janz D. Neuropathological findings in primary generalized epilepsy: a study of eight cases. *Epilepsia* 1984; **25**: 8–21.
18. Lyon G, Gastaut H. Considerations on the significance attributed to unusual cerebral histological findings recently described in eight patients with primary generalized epilepsy. *Epilepsia* 1985; **26**: 365–367.
19. Robitaille Y, Rasmussen T, Dubeau F, Tampieri D, Kemball K. Histopathology of nonneoplastic lesions in frontal lobe epilepsy. Review of 180 cases with recent MRI and PET correlations. *Advances in Neurology* 1992; **57**: 499–513.
20. Wolf HK, Zentner J, Hufnagel A, *et al.* Surgical pathology of chronic epileptic seizure disorders: experience with 63 specimens from extratemporal corticectomies, lobectomies and functional hemispherectomies. *Acta Neuropathologica* 1993; **86**: 466–472.
21. Armstrong DD. The neuropathology of temporal lobe epilepsy. *Journal of Neuropathology and Experimental Neurology* 1993; **52**: 433–443.
22. Plate KH, Wieser HG, Yasargil MG, Wiestler OD. Neuropathological findings in 224 patients with temporal lobe epilepsy. *Acta Neuropathologica* 1993; **86**: 433–438.
23. Wolf HK, Campos MG, Zentner J, *et al.* Surgical pathology of temporal lobe epilepsy. Experience with 216 cases. *Journal of Neuropathology and Experimental Neurology* 1993; **52**: 499–506.
24. Levesque MF, Nakasato N, Vinters HV, Babb TL. Surgical treatment of limbic epilepsy associated with extra-hippocampal lesions: the problem of dual pathology. *Journal of Neurosurgery* 1991; **75**: 364–370.
25. Adelson PD, Peacock WJ, Chugani HT, *et al.* Temporal and extended temporal resections for the treatment of intractable seizures in early childhood. *Pediatric Neurosurgery* 1992; **18**: 169–178.
26. Norman MG. Perinatal brain damage. *Perspectives in Pediatric Pathology* 1978; **4**: 41–92.
27. Fenichel GM. Hypoxic-ischemic encephalopathy in the newborn. *Archives of Neurology* 1983; **40**: 261–266.
28. Guzzetta F. Ischemic and hemorrhagic cerebral lesions of the newborn. Current concepts. *Child's Nervous System* 1991; **7**: 417–424.
29. Rorke LB. Anatomical features of the developing brain implicated in pathogenesis of hypoxic-ischemic injury. *Brain Pathology* 1992; **2**: 211–221.
30. Younkin DP. Hypoxic-ischemic brain injury of the newborn – statement of the problem and overview. *Brain Pathology* 1992; **2**: 209–10.
31. Vinters HV. Vascular diseases. In: Duckett S. (ed.) *Pediatric Neuropathology*. Baltimore: Williams & Wilkins, 1994: 302–333.
32. Cochrane DD, Poskitt KJ, Norman MG. Surgical implications of cerebral dysgenesis. *Canadian Journal of Neurological Science* 1991; **18**: 181–195.
33. Hirabayashi S, Binnie CD, Janota I, Polkey CE. Surgical treatment of epilepsy due to cortical dysplasia: clinical and EEG findings. *Journal of Neurology, Neurosurgery and Psychiatry* 1993; **56**: 765–770.
34. Taylor DC, Falconer MA, Bruton CJ, Corsellis JA. Focal dysplasia of the cerebral cortex in epilepsy. *Journal of Neurology, Neurosurgery and Psychiatry* 1971; **34**: 369–387.

35. Vinters HV, De Rosa MJ, Farrell MA. Neuropathologic study of resected cerebral tissue from patients with infantile spasms. *Epilepsia* 1993; **34**: 772–779.

36. Mischel PS, Nguyen LP, Vinters HV. Cerebral cortical dysplasia associated with pediatric epilepsy. Review of neuropathologic features and proposal for a grading system. *Journal of Neuropathology and Experimental Neurology* 1995; **54**: 137–153.

37. Crino PB, Trojanowski JQ, Eberwine J. Internexin, MAP1B, and nestin in cortical dysplasia as markers of developmental maturity. *Acta Neuropathologica* 1997; **93**: 619–627.

38. Duggal N, Iskander S, Hammond RR. Nestin expression in cortical dysplasia. *Journal of Neurosurgery* 2001; **95**: 459–465.

39. Palmini A, Gambardella A, Andermann F, *et al.* Intrinsic epileptogenicity of human dysplastic cortex as suggested by corticography and surgical results. *Annals of Neurology* 1995; **37**: 476–487.

40. Preul MC, Leblanc R, Cendes F, *et al.* Function and organization in dysgenic cortex. Case report. *Journal of Neurosurgery* 1997; **87**: 113–121.

41. Kothare SV, VanLandingham K, Armon C, Luther JS, Friedman A, Radtke RA. Seizure onset from periventricular nodular heterotopias: depth-electrode study. *Neurology* 1998; **51**: 1723–1727.

42. Mattia D, Olivier A, Avoli M. Seizure-like discharges recorded in human dysplastic neocortex maintained *in vitro*. *Neurology* 1995; **45**: 1391–1395.

43. Avoli M, Bernasconi A, Mattia D, Olivier A, Hwa GG. Epileptiform discharges in the human dysplastic neocortex: *in vitro* physiology and pharmacology. *Annals of Neurology* 1999; **46**: 816–826.

44. Spreafico R, Battaglia G, Arcelli P, *et al.* Cortical dysplasia: an immunocytochemical study of three patients. *Neurology* 1998; **50**: 27–36.

45. White R, Hua Y, Scheithauer B, Lynch DR, Henske EP, Crino PB. Selective alterations in glutamate and GABA receptor subunit mRNA expression in dysplastic neurons and giant cells of cortical tubers. *Annals of Neurology* 2001; **49**: 67–78.

46. Crino PB, Duhaime AC, Baltuch G, White R. Differential expression of glutamate and GABA-A receptor subunit mRNA in cortical dysplasia. *Neurology* 2001; **56**: 906–913.

47. Kerfoot C, Vinters HV, Mathern GW. Cerebral cortical dysplasia: giant neurons show potential for increased excitation and axonal plasticity. *Developmental Neuroscience* 1999; **21**: 260–270.

48. Mikuni N, Babb TL, Ying Z, *et al.* NMDA-receptors 1 and 2A/B coassembly increased in human epileptic focal cortical dysplasia. *Epilepsia* 1999; **40**: 1683–1687.

49. Crino PB, Jin H, Shumate MD, Robinson MB, Coulter DA, Brooks-Kayal AR. Increased expression of the neuronal glutamate transporter (EAAT3/EAAC1) in hippocampal and neocortical epilepsy. *Epilepsia* 2002; **43**: 211–218.

50. Kuzniecky R, Garcia JH, Faught E, Morawetz RB. Cortical dysplasia in temporal lobe epilepsy: magnetic resonance imaging correlations. *Annals of Neurology* 1991; **29**: 293–298.

51. Simone IL, Federico F, Tortorella C, *et al.* Metabolic changes in neuronal migration disorders: evaluation by combined MRI and proton MR spectroscopy. *Epilepsia* 1999; **40**: 872–879.

52. Marusic P, Najm IM, Ying Z, *et al.* Focal cortical dysplasia in eloquent cortex: functional characteristics and correlation with MRI and histopathologic changes. *Epilepsia* 2002; **43**: 27–32.

53. Mathern GW, Giza CC, Yudovin S, *et al.* Postoperative seizure control and antiepileptic drug use in pediatric epilepsy surgery patients: the UCLA experience, 1986–1997. *Epilepsia* 1999; **40**: 1740–1749.

54. Rakic P. Molecular and cellular mechanisms of neuronal migration: relevance to cortical epilepsies. *Advances in Neurology* 2000; **84**: 1–14.

55. van Slegtenhorst M, de Hoogt R, Hermans C, *et al.* Identification of the tuberous sclerosis gene *TSC1* on chromosome 9q34. *Science* 1997; **277**: 805–808.

56. The European Chromosome 16 Tuberous Sclerosis Consortium. Identification and characterization of the tuberous sclerosis gene on chromosome 16. *Cell* 1993; **75**: 1305–1315.

57. Fox JW, Lamperti ED, Eksioglu YZ, *et al.* Mutations in filamin 1 prevent migration of cerebral cortical neurons in human periventricular heterotopia. *Neuron* 1998; **21**: 1315–1325.

58. Crino PB, Miyata H, Vinters HV. Neurodevelopmental disorders as a cause of seizures: Neuropathologic, genetic and mechanistic considerations. *Brain Pathology* 2002; **12**: 212–233.

59. Palmini A, Andermann F, de Grissac H, *et al.* Stages and patterns of centrifugal arrest of diffuse neuronal migration disorders. *Developmental Medicine and Child Neurology* 1993; **35**: 331–339.

60. King M, Stephenson JB, Ziervogel M, Doyle D, Galbraith S. Hemimegalencephaly – a case for hemispherectomy? *Neuropediatrics* 1985; **16**: 46–55.

61. De Rosa MJ, Secor DL, Barsom M, Fisher RS, Vinters HV. Neuropathologic findings in surgically treated hemimegalencephaly: immunohistochemical, morphometric, and ultrastructural study. *Acta Neuropathologica* 1992; **84**: 250–260.

62. Robain O, Floquet C, Heldt N, Rozenberg F. Hemimega-lencephaly: a clinicopathological study of four cases. *Neuropathology and Applied Neurobiology* 1988; **14**: 125–135.

63. Critchley M, Earl CJC. Tuberous sclerosis and allied conditions. *Brain* 1932; **55**: 311–346.

64. Bender BL, Yunis EJ. Central nervous system pathology of tuberous sclerosis in children. *Ultrastructal Pathology* 1980; **1**: 287–299.

65. Dumas JL, Poirier J, Escourolle R. Ultrastructural study of cerebral lesions in tuberous sclerosis. *Acta Neuropathologica* 1973; **25**: 259–270.

66. Thibault JH, Manuelidis EE. Tuberous sclerosis in a premature infant. Report of a case and review of the literature. *Neurology* 1970; **20**: 139–146.

67. Probst A, Ohnacker H. Sclérose tubereuse de Bourneville chez un prématuré. Ultrastructure des cellules atypiques: présence de microvillosités. *Acta Neuropathologica* 1977; **40**: 157–161.

68. Park SH, Pepkowitz SH, Kerfoot C, *et al.* Tuberous sclerosis in a 20-week gestation fetus: immunohistochemical study. *Acta Neuropathologica* 1997; **94**: 180–186.

69. Catania MG, Mischel PS, Vinters HV. Hamartin and tuberin interaction with the G2/M cyclin-dependent kinase CDK1 and its regulatory cyclins A and B. *Journal of Neuropathology and Experimental Neurology* 2001; **60**: 711–723.

70. Hengstschläger M, Rodman DM, Miloloza A, Hengstschläger-Ottnad E, Rosner M, Kubista M. Tuberous sclerosis gene products in proliferation control. *Mutation Research* 2001; **488**: 233–239.

71. Lamb RF, Roy C, Diefenbach TJ, *et al.* The *TSC1* tumour suppressor hamartin regulates cell adhesion through ERM proteins and the GTPase Rho. *Nature Cell Biology* 2000; **2**: 281–287.

72. Wienecke R, König A, DeClue JE. Identification of tuberin, the tuberous sclerosis-2 product. Tuberin possesses specific Rap1GAP activity. *Journal of Biological Chemistry* 1995; **270**: 16409–16414.

73. Xiao GH, Shoarinejad F, Jin F, Golemis EA, Yeung RS. The tuberous sclerosis 2 gene product, tuberin, functions as a Rab5 GTPase-activating protein (GAP) in modulating endocytosis. *Journal of Biological Chemistry* 1997; **272**: 6097–6100.

74. Wienecke R, Maize JC Jr, Shoarinejad F, *et al.* Co-localization of the TSC2 product tuberin with its target Rap1 in the Golgi apparatus. *Oncogene* 1996; **13**: 913–923.

75. Soucek T, Holzl G, Bernaschek G, Hengstschläger M. A role of the tuberous sclerosis gene-2 product during neuronal differentiation. *Oncogene* 1998; **16**: 2197–2204.

76. Potter CJ, Huang H, Xu T. *Drosophila Tsc1* functions with *Tsc2* to antagonize insulin signaling in regulating cell growth, cell proliferation, and organ size. *Cell* 2001; **105**: 357–368.

77. Kwiatkowski DJ, Zhang H, Bandura JL, *et al.* A mouse model of TSC1 reveals sex-dependent lethality from liver hemangiomas, and up-regulation of p70S6 kinase activity in Tsc1 null cells. *Human Molecular Genetics* 2002; **11**: 525–534.

78. Luo L. Rho GTPases in neuronal morphogenesis. *Nat Rev Neurosci* 2000; **1**: 173–180.

79. Louvet-Vallée S. ERM proteins: from cellular architecture to cell signaling. *Biology of the Cell* 2000; **92**: 305–316.

80. Johnson MW, Miyata H, Vinters HV. Ezrin and moesin expression within the developing human cerebrum and tuberous sclerosis-associated cortical tubers. *Acta Neuropathologica* 2002; **104**: 188–196.

81. McKay DJG, Esch F, Furthmayr H, Hall A. Rho- and rac-dependent assembly of focal adhesion complexes and actin filaments in permeabilized fibroblasts: an essential role for ezrin/radixin/moesin proteins. *Journal of Cell Biology* 1997; **138**: 927–938.

82. Takahashi K, Sasaki T, Mammoto A, *et al.* Direct interaction of the Rho GDP dissociation inhibitor with ezrin/radixin/moesin initiates the activation of the Rho small G protein. *Journal of Biological Chemistry* 1997; **272**: 23371–23375.

83. Olenik C, Aktories K, Meyer DK. Differential expression of the small GTP-binding proteins RhoA, RhoB, Cdc42u and Cdc42b in developing rat neocortex. *Brain Research. Molecular Brain Research* 1999; **18**: 9–17.

84. Lambert de Rouvroit C, Goffinet AM. Neuronal migration. *Mechanisms of Development* 2001; **105**: 47–56.

85. Johnson MW, Emelin JK, Park SH, Vinters HV. Co-localization of *TSC1* and *TSC2* gene products in tubers of patients with tuberous sclerosis. *Brain Pathology* 1999; **9**: 45–54.

86. Miloloza A, Kubista M, Rosner M, Hengstschläger M. Evidence for separable functions of tuberous sclerosis gene products in mammalian cell cycle regulation. *Journal of Neuropathology and Experimental Neurology* 2002; **61**: 154–163.

87. Vinters HV. Histopathology of brain tissue from patients with infantile spasms. *International Review of Neurobiology* 2002; **49**: 63–76.

88. Peacock WJ, Wehby-Grant MC, Shields WD, *et al.* Hemispherectomy for intractable seizures in children: A report of 58 cases. *Child's Nervous System* 1996; **12**: 376–384.

89. Prayson RA. Clinicopathological findings in patients who have undergone epilepsy surgery in the first year of life. *Pathology International* 2000; **50**: 620–625.

90. Yamanouchi H, Jay V, Otsubo H, Kaga M, Becker LE, Takashima S. Early forms of microtubule-associated protein are strongly expressed in cortical dysplasia. *Acta Neuropathologica* 1998; **95**: 466–470.

91. Arai Y, Edwards V, Becker LE. A comparison of cell phenotypes in hemimegalencephaly and tuberous sclerosis. *Acta Neuropathologica* 1999; **98**: 407–413.

92. Nishio S, Morioka T, Hamada Y, Hisada K, Fukui M. Immunohistochemical expression of trk receptor proteins in focal cortical dysplasia with intractable epilepsy. *Neuropathology and Applied Neurobiology* 1999; **25**: 188–195.

93. Vinters HV, Park SH, Johnson MW, Mischel PS, Catania M, Kerfoot C. Cortical dysplasia, genetic abnormalities and neurocutaneous syndromes. *Developmental Neuroscience* 1999; **21**: 248–259.

94. Kyin R, Hua Y, Baybis M, *et al.* Differential cellular expression of neurotrophins in cortical tubers of the tuberous sclerosis complex. *American Journal of Pathology* 2001; **159**: 1541–1554.

95. Rasmussen T, Olszewski J, Lloyd-Smith D. Focal seizures due to chronic localized encephalitis. *Neurology* 1958; **8**: 435–445.

96. Aguilar MJ, Rasmussen T. Role of encephalitis in pathogenesis of epilepsy. *Archives of Neurology* 1960; **2**: 663–676.

97. Rasmussen T. Further observations on the syndrome of chronic encephalitis and epilepsy. *Applied Neurophysiology* 1978; **41**: 1–12.

98. Bien CG, Bauer J, Deckwerth TL, *et al.* Destruction of neurons by cytotoxic T cells: A new pathogenic mechanism in Rasmussen's encephalitis. *Annals of Neurology* 2002; **51**: 311–318.

99. Villani F, Spreafico R, Farina L, *et al.* Positive response to immunomodulatory therapy in an adult patient with Rasmussen's encephalitis. *Neurology* 200; **56**: 248–250.

100. Zupanc ML, Handler EG, Levine RL, *et al.* Rasmussen encephalitis: epilepsia partialis continua secondary to chronic encephalitis. *Pediatric Neurology* 1990; **6**: 397–401.

101. Honavar M, Janota I, Polkey CE. Rasmussen's encephalitis in surgery for epilepsy. *Developmental Medicine and Child Neurology* 1992; **34**: 3–14.

102. Vining EP, Freeman JM, Pillas DJ, *et al.* Why would you remove half a brain? The outcome of 58 children after hemispherectomy – the Johns Hopkins experience: 1968 to 1996. *Pediatrics* 1997; **100**: 163–171.

103. Robitaille Y. Neuropathologic aspects of chronic encephalitis. In: Andermann F. (ed.) *Chronic Encephalitis and Epilepsy, Rasmussen's Syndrome.* Oxford: Butterworth-Heinemann, 1991: 79–110.

104. Gordon N. Chronic progressive epilepsia partialis continua of childhood: Rasmussen syndrome. *Developmental Medicine and Child Neurology* 1992; **34**: 182–185.

105. Walter GF, Renella RR, Hori A, Wirnsberger G. Nachweis von Epstein-Barr-Viren bei Rasmussen's Enzephalitis. *Nervenarzt* 1989; **60**: 168–170.

106. Power C, Poland SD, Blume WT, Girvin JP, Rice GP. Cytomegalovirus and Rasmussen's encephalitis. *Lancet* 1990; **336**: 1282–1284.

107. Farrell MA, Cheng L, Cornford ME, Grody WW, Vinters HV. Cytomegalovirus and Rasmussen's encephalitis. *Lancet* 1991; **337**: 1551–1552.

108. Rogers SW, Andrews PI, Gahring LC, *et al.* Autoantibodies to glutamate receptor GluR3 in Rasmussen's encephalitis. *Science* 1994; **265**: 648–651.

109. He XP, Patel M, Whitney KD, Janumpalli S, Tenner A, McNamara JO. Glutamate receptor GluR3 antibodies and death of cortical cells. *Neuron* 1998; **20**: 153–163.

110. Whitney KD, Andrews PI, McNamara JO. Immunoglobulin G and complement immunoreactivity in the cerebral cortex of patients with Rasmussen's encephalitis. *Neurology* 1999; **53**: 699–708.

111. Frassoni C, Spreafico R, Franceschetti S, *et al.* Labeling of rat neurons by anti-GluR3 IgG from patients with Rasmussen encephalitis. *Neurology* 2001; **57**: 324–327.

112. Whitney KD, McNamara JO. GluR3 autoantibodies destroy neural cells in a complement-dependent manner modulated by complement regulatory proteins. *Journal of Neuroscience* 2000; **20**: 7307–7316.

113. Wohlwill FJ, Yakovlev PI. Histopathology of meningo-facial angiomatosis (Sturge-Weber's disease). *Journal of Neuropathology and Experimental Neurology* 1957; **16**: 341–364.

114. Venes JL, Linder S. Sturge-Weber-Dimitri syndrome. Encephalotrigeminal angiomatosis. In: Edwards MSB, Hoffman HJ. (eds) *Cerebral Vascular Disease in Children and Adolescents.* Baltimore: Williams & Wilkins, 1989: 337–341.

115. Oakes WJ. The natural history of patients with the Sturge-Weber syndrome. *Pediatric Neurosurgery* 1992; **18**: 287–290.

116. Bentz MS, Towfighi J, Greenwood S, Zaino R. Sturge-Weber syndrome. A case with thyroid and choroid plexus hemangiomas and leptomeningeal melanosis. *Archives of Pathology and Laboratory Medicine* 1982; **106**: 75–78.

117. Guseo A. Ultrastructure of calcification in Sturge-Weber Disease. *Virchows Archiv A Pathological Anatomy and Histopathology* 1975; **366**: 353–356.

118. Norman MG, Schoene WC. The ultrastructure of Sturge-Weber disease. *Acta Neuropathologica* 1977; **37**: 199–205.

119. Najm I, Ying Z, Janigro D. Mechanisms of epileptogenesis. *Neurologic Clinics* 2001; **19**: 237–250.

6

Pathophysiology of childhood epilepsies

RÜDIGER KÖHLING AND JOHN GR JEFFERYS

Our aim in this chapter is to discuss the neuronal basis of epileptic discharges, how this is affected by developmental processes, and finally what kinds of problems during development can lead to epilepsy in infants and children. First, however, we outline how bioelectric activity is generated. Bioelectricity refers to the ability of cells to generate the membrane potential, i.e. an electric gradient across the membrane, which can undergo sudden changes that will allow for information coding. The principles underlying these phenomena have mainly been discovered in animal experiments, but also in human tissue obtained from surgical resections, showing that they are virtually identical across a wide range of species, including humans.

BASIS OF BIOELECTRIC ACTIVITY

The cellular membrane potential results from the concentration gradient of K^+ and Na^+ ions across the membrane (arising from work performed by Na^+/K^+ ATPase pumping Na^+ out of and K^+ into the cells) and the fact that, at least at rest, the membrane is selectively permeable to K^+. Whole-cell recordings from neurons at rest typically reveal a small leak current ($\sim$100 pA) of K^+ driven by the concentration gradient. In accordance with Ohm's law, this leak across the high resistance ($\sim$1 GΩ) of the membrane generates the membrane potential of approximately -100 mV (in fact biologically realistic resting membrane potentials are closer to -80 mV, but these round numbers illustrate the point). Obviously, if the concentration gradient for K^+ changes, e.g. due to a rise of

extracellular K^+ such as can occur during epileptic activity (see below), the driving force for the leak current is diminished and the membrane potential is reduced to more positive values. The Nernst equation allows us to calculate this driving force:

$$E_K = \frac{R \times T}{z \times F} \times \text{Ln} \frac{\text{(extracellular concentration)}}{\text{(intracellular concentration)}}$$

where R is the gas constant (8.3 VA s K^{-1} mol^{-1}), T is the temperature in Kelvin, z is the ionic charge and F is the Faraday constant (96 500 A s mol^{-1}). The value E_K is termed the equilibrium potential of K^+ (given in volts); i.e. the force driving the ions across the membrane. At rest the K^+ conductance is much larger than all other conductances, so the resting membrane potential usually is close to E_K.

Function of voltage-gated channels

Information coding in excitable cells such as neurons and muscles is brought about by rapid and reversible changes of the membrane potential – the **action potential**. This is carried by a sodium current, which is transiently switched on and dominates the ever-present leak conductance. During the action potential, Na^+ flows into the cell, across voltage-gated channels selectively permeable for Na^+, causing a drop of membrane potential (**depolarization**). The opening of these channels is gated by a small depolarization (usually caused by synaptic activation; see below) to a threshold value (usually around -55 mV). Once threshold is reached, virtually all sodium channels are opened for a short period of time ($\sim 1\,\mathrm{ms}$), provided they had been kept inactive at negative potentials. This leads to a sharp, transient depolarization of the membrane, even overshooting zero, to reach $\sim +20\,\mathrm{mV}$. All parts of the neuronal membrane – somatic, axonal and dendritic – possess voltage-gated sodium channels, so the action potential can propagate throughout the cell. Neurons carry many other kinds of voltage-gated channels, notably those selectively permeable to Ca^{2+} (depolarizing) or K^+ (re- and hyperpolarizing). The opening of these channels modulate action potential generation. For example, additional activation of calcium channels leads to a more pronounced and prolonged depolarization, or rebound depolarizations, and can result in the firing of bursts of action potentials mediated by Na^+. Conversely, activation of voltage-gated potassium channels (which are unrelated to leak channels) will cause fast repolarizations after the action potential, or prolonged after-hyperpolarizations, but also a rise in extracellular K^+ with strong (e.g. epileptic) neuronal activity. In effect, these modulations will govern the overall firing properties of neurons, and these properties may be altered in epileptic tissue, as described below.

Mechanisms of network synchronization

In order to communicate information coded as firing sequences of individual neurons to neighbouring ones, within the neuronal network, synaptic transmission has to occur. This mainly happens in two ways:

- transmission of **electrical signals** across specialized intracellular pores, so called **gap junctions**, which convey membrane potential changes more or less similar to an ohmic resistor (which can be modulated by intracellular Ca^{2+}, pH and other factors)
- transmission of **chemical signals** by diffusion across intercellular gaps, the **synaptic clefts**, and binding of the chemical transmitters to specialized receptors on the postsynaptic membrane.

Communication via gap junctions is common in certain brain nuclei, such as the olive, but also occurs in other brain regions, including the hippocampus or neocortex, especially during development. The more important form of intercellular communication in these neo- and archi-cortical areas is the chemical synapse. Here, binding of the different transmitters (e.g. glutamate, γ-aminobutyric acid (GABA), adenosine, glycine, serotonin, acetylcholine, dopamine, noradrenaline) leads to either the gating of an associated ion channel causing de- or hyperpolarization in so-called **ionotropic receptors**, or to intracellular metabolic changes in so-called **metabotropic receptors**

generally via activation of GTP-coupled proteins (G-proteins). The latter often induce conductance changes in ionic channels, e.g. by phosphorylation, which in turn result in de- or hyperpolarizations via this metabolic detour.

The most important receptors causing depolarizations or excitatory postsynaptic potentials (EPSP) are glutamatergic. They are subdivided into major groups by their preferred ligands: α-amino-3-hydroxy-5-methyl-4-isoxazolepropionic acid (AMPA), kainate and N-methyl-D-aspartate (NMDA). NMDA receptors differ markedly from AMPA and kainate in their kinetic and permeability properties (Figure 6.1).[1] Metabotropic glutamate receptors (mGluR) also exist and mediate a variety of reactions. The most prominent inhibitory receptor causing hyperpolarizations or inhibitory postsynaptic potentials (IPSP) is GABAergic, which again is subdivided functionally into the ionotropic GABA$_A$ and metabotropic GABA$_B$ receptors (Figure 6.1). Additionally, an ionotropic GABA$_C$ type can been found particularly in the retina, which is pharmacologically distinct from the GABA$_A$ type. Although glutamate and GABA appear to predominate as transmitters in the brain, substances such as adenosine or acetylcholine extensively modulate activity, usually via metabotropic receptors. These modulatory influences can be of special importance in epilepsy; for instance, adenosine is thought to act as an endogenous antiepileptic transmitter.[2] The level of network excitation found at any one moment is a function of the temporal and spatial summation of the many synaptic inputs on to each of the many neurons in the network. These complex interactions are further modified, at least under certain conditions, by nonsynaptic mechanisms of synchronization, such as activity-dependent increases in extracellular K^+ leading to membrane depolarizations (see above), or so-called **ephaptic interactions**, where activity in one cell depolarizes the membrane of its neighbour as current flow is directed not only extracellularly but also across cells, particularly in regions of high extracellular resistance. This can be found in densely packed regions such as the hippocampus, or under conditions of cell swelling induced for example by epileptic activity.

The 'epileptic' discharge

Animal experiments have been widely used to analyze the elementary mechanisms underlying epileptic activity. Some epilepsy models are genetic, such as strains of epilepsy-prone rats, mice and primates. Examples include photosensitive baboons, Genetic Absence Epilepsy Rat from Strasbourg (GAERS), DBA2 mice with sound-induced seizures, Reeler and Tottering mice. Other models use experimental epileptogenic treatments that result in chronic pro-epileptic changes in the brain, such as kindling (repetition of subconvulsive electrical or chemical

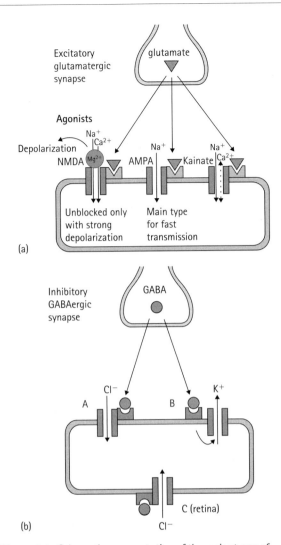

Figure 6.1 *Schematic representation of the major types of excitatory glutamatergic (a) and inhibitory GABAergic (b) receptors in the brain. Receptors are classified according to their selective agonists, and they differ in ionic permeability of the associated channels as well as their kinetics. NMDA receptors in adult tissue are usually blocked by Mg^{2+} and become unblocked with membrane depolarization e.g. during intense activity; juvenile NMDA receptors lack the Mg^{2+} block (see text). AMPA receptors are thus the main glutamate receptor for fast transmission. Kainate receptors are found in spinal cord, and also in several brain regions where they may play an important role in epileptogenesis. $GABA_A$ and $GABA_C$ receptors are ionotropic receptors directly associated with chloride channels; the $GABA_B$ receptor is metabotropic, which indirectly acts on associated potassium channels.*

stimulation until seizures arise), systemic convulsant injection (e.g. kainate or pilocarpine) or focal epileptogenesis using topical epileptogenic substances (e.g. alumina cream, kainate or tetanus toxin). Finally, acute models (strictly speaking these are of convulsions rather than epilepsy) use electrical stimulation or chemical convulsants such as

bicuculline, penicillin or strychnine. Brain slices maintained *in vitro* have played a crucial role in developing ideas on epileptic activity, initially focusing on the acute models, but more recently being exploited in unraveling the mechanisms of chronic models.

In all of these models, as in human epilepsy, epileptic activity differs sharply from normal neuronal activity. This is reflected in changes of the network behavior which can be monitored by EEG or field potential recordings. In the case of absence seizures, the abnormal EEG is a widely synchronous 3-Hz spike and wave discharge. On the other hand, focal epilepsies typically exhibit interictal spikes, polyspikes and full-blown ictal discharges. A combination of experimental and theoretical work, mainly on animal models, has resulted in rather detailed accounts of how the abnormal synchronization of epileptic discharges occurs, at least for the early stages of focal seizures and for primary generalized absence seizures.[3]

Basic mechanisms of focal epilepsy

A key early observation was the detection of abnormal activity in single neurons associated with interictal spikes. This was the characteristic epileptic discharge called paroxysmal depolarization shift (PDS), first described by Goldensohn and Purpura,[4] and subsequently found in all focal epilepsy models and animal tissues (including human), albeit with lower probability in chronic neocortical models.[5] It consists of an initial action potential, which is followed by a barrage of further action potentials, triggered by a prolonged plateau depolarization lasting tens to hundreds of milliseconds, and a steep repolarization (Figure 6.2). A multitude of experiments suggests the following processes are essential. The PDS is generally initiated by large synaptic depolarizations, or EPSPs (Figure 6.2). This is followed by a voltage-gated calcium inward current, superimposed by fast action potentials mediated by fast, voltage-gated sodium currents. The plateau phase is mediated by calcium-activated unspecific cation inward currents, and possibly supported by continued synaptic activation. Lastly, voltage- and calcium-activated potassium currents mediate repolarization and termination of the PDS (Figure 6.2).[6–9] As a consequence of this massively prolonged discharge (in comparison to normal action potentials), barrages of action potentials are generated in the neuronal axons, leading to excessive release of transmitters and synchronization of synaptically coupled neurons.

The pathological synchronization of this synaptically coupled network depends on its rather complex nonlinear dynamics,[10,11] but several key aspects can be identified in qualitative terms:

- The connectivity must be divergent; each neuron needs to excite more than one postsynaptic neuron

PDS

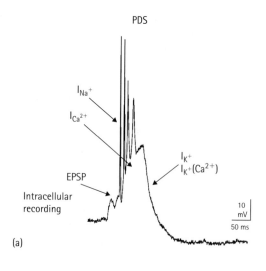

I_{Na^+}

$I_{Ca^{2+}}$

I_{K^+}
$I_{K^+(Ca^{2+})}$

EPSP

Intracellular
recording

10
mV
50 ms

(a)

BURST

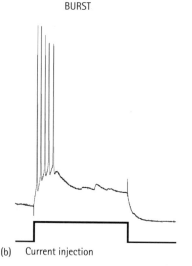

(b)   Current injection

Figure 6.2 *Recordings of an epileptic discharge (a; paroxysmal depolarization shift, PDS) in chronically epileptic human neocortical tissue slice excised during epilepsy surgery and exposed to an epileptogenic agent (bicuculline), and a burst discharge (b) in the CA3 subfield of a rat hippocampal slice elicited by current injection. Whereas the PDS arises spontaneously out of an excitatory postsynaptic potential (EPSP), the burst discharge in normal rat tissue can be provoked only with strong artificial depolarization. Various voltage-gated and Ca^{2+}-activated currents support the different phases of PDS generation as indicated.*

in the same population. This produces a network of recurrent or mutually excitatory connections which allows excitation to spread as a chain reaction throughout the population under the right conditions.

- The synapses must be strong, i.e. they must have a high probability of bringing their targets to threshold. This is helped by the tendency of certain

neurons to fire bursts of action potentials, as a consequence of having relatively slow voltage-gated calcium or persistent sodium currents, which boosts the temporal summation of the repeated synaptic potentials.

- The population must be large enough so that all the neurons can be connected by polysynaptic pathways. In practice about 1000 neurons suffice in the rodent hippocampus.[12]

Of course these networks do not exist to cause epilepsy, but to sustain whatever function the particular brain region serves – associative memory, sensory feature detection and many other operations depend on interactions between excitatory neurons. Synchronization is normally held in check by the operation of inhibitory neurons which dampen the excessive build-up of excitation long before it becomes epileptic, which of course is why blocking inhibitory receptors is a good way of triggering seizures.

The prolongation of these brief events into full seizures depends on other mechanisms that are far from clear, although some progress has been made in the crucial area, with ideas on the roles of extracellular potassium accumulation, abnormal properties of axonal excitability, inhibitory transmission, clearance of transmitters, and so on.[13–15]

Basic mechanisms of absence seizures

Very different mechanisms have been implicated in absence seizures. These seizures are quite distinctive with their characteristic generalized 3-Hz spike and wave discharge, symptoms and pharmacology. They depend on the interplay between circuits within the thalamus and cortex. The 'fast spiking' neurons of the nucleus reticularis within the thalamus are interconnected into an inhibitory network. They also inhibit the thalamocortical projection neurons of the specific thalamic nuclei, and when synchronized this inhibition can be strongly hyperpolarizing. This is important because the thalamocortical neurons have special intrinsic properties that mean they fire 'rebound' bursts after periods of hyperpolarization, due to well-developed low-threshold calcium currents. As a result the thalamocortical neurons fire synchronous bursts after they have been subjected to synchronous inhibition. This sends a strong excitatory input to the corresponding neocortical region, producing the 'spike' on the EEG. Inhibitory neurons within the cortex are activated both by the thalamic input and the local cortical circuitry, producing the slower 'wave' in the EEG. Finally the activity of the cortical circuitry excites the corticothalamic neurons, which excite the thalamic network to initiate the next cycle.[16] The whole network seems to be required, and the rather regular rhythm of this kind of epileptic discharge appears to be set by the kinetics of the $GABA_B$ in the thalamus. This is a compelling model, although important questions do remain to be resolved.[17] Nevertheless, the dependence on both thalamus and cortex working together, and the prominent role of inhibitory circuits, is clear, as is the marked difference from the circuitry implicated in focal epilepsies.

Processes responsible for epileptogenesis

Although the PDS has been identified as the characteristic focal epileptic discharge on the cellular level, the special features of epileptic tissue that lead to the generation of PDS are still not fully understood, nor indeed is the relationship between the PDS and the much more prolonged seizure discharge. Similarly the specific features of the thalamus and/or cortex in absence epilepsy that lead to the generation of the 3 per second spike are not clear. In general, intrinsic and synaptic properties of epileptic tissue have to be considered as possible 'epileptogenicity' candidates.

One of the most intriguing properties of neurons is the ability that some have to fire bursts rather than single action potentials. Neuronal bursts have similarities to PDS (Figure 6.2): they consist of a burst of sodium action potentials riding on a prolonged underlying relatively slow depolarization carried by a calcium[18] or a noninactivating sodium inward current.[19–22] Such bursting neurons can be found in distinct areas of the brain (CA regions of the hippocampus, and layer V, but possibly also II/III, of the neocortex).[19,20,23,24] In epileptic tissue the incidence of bursting neurons is markedly increased,[18] indicating that they may indeed promote the network synchronization necessary for epileptic seizures. Voltage-gated calcium[25] and persistent sodium currents[26,27] are enhanced in epileptic tissue, supporting a role for their promotion of epileptic activity, presumably as a result of increasing intrinsic bursts.

Synaptic mechanisms also play a crucial role in epileptogenesis, in terms both of changes in receptor properties and of connectivity. There are examples of epilepsy models with increases in the density or conductance of glutamate NMDA[28] or non-NMDA receptors.[29,30] Recently there have been reports of functional mutations of $GABA_A$ receptors in rare epilepsies in humans,[31,32] mutations that depress responses either to GABA or to presumed endogenous ligands for the benzodiazepine site. There also is considerable evidence of abnormal connectivity in epileptic tissue, which will tend to strengthen recurrent excitation, or even create it in areas where it is normally absent. Perhaps the best-known example is in the dentate gyrus of the hippocampus. These neurons have properties that make it relatively easy to see that their axons aberrantly grow into their dendritic zones.[33,34]

There is also evidence this occurs in the CA1 region of the hippocampus, and it is likely that it occurs in CA3 too, where recurrent excitation is normally rather prominent.

Functional modulation of synaptic signalling may aggravate the situation and further increase the tendency to synchronize: intense activity has been demonstrated to lead to both short-term (so-called post-tetanic) and long-term potentiation of excitatory synapses. Both the short- and long-term effects are due to a rise in intracellular calcium, which raises the probability of transmitter release in the short term and leads to structural changes of the synapses in the long run, for example by incorporating more receptors, and of different types, in the postsynaptic membrane. Although these changes can also be observed in healthy tissue, it is conceivable that they take place abundantly in tissue which repeatedly exhibits massive and prolonged activation in the form of epileptic discharges,[35] although protective mechanisms such as increased intracellular calcium buffering may partly prevent them.[36] Interestingly, inhibitory synapses often lose effectivity with prolonged activation, in part due to desensitization of the receptors in continued presence of the transmitter.[37] Electrical synapses may also play a role; electrical coupling among neurons has been been demonstrated to increase after chronic epilepsy.[38]

Finally, nonsynaptic mechanisms may contribute to epileptic neuronal synchronization. As already mentioned, prolonged neuronal activity induces rises in extracellular K^+ due to the activation of voltage-gated and calcium-dependent K^+ conductances and K^+-dependent transporters. With epileptic activity, K^+ levels reach 10–16 mmol/L, approximately five times the normal value,[39,40] which will lead to depolarization of neighbouring neurons, possibly over large distances because the syncytial network of glial cells takes up and extensively redistributes K^+ in a process fittingly termed **spatial buffering**.

In summary, several intrinsic, synaptic and nonsynaptic processes can be seen to change with epileptogenesis which might account for the increased synchronization encountered in epileptic tissue. During the course of ontogenetic brain maturation, several physiological changes occur in neurons and their interconnections which may have deep implications for the development of epileptic activity in immature brain. The following section reviews these changes and discuss their relevance for epileptogenicity.

NEONATAL PHYSIOLOGY

As already mentioned, studies on mechanisms of epileptogenesis are usually performed in animal models, most commonly using the rat. This raises the challenge of how to compare developmental stages in rats and humans. A very rough estimate of correlation of stages in brain development between the species suggests that a 5-day-old rat is equivalent to a fullterm infant, and the second and third brain growth spurts in rat, occurring on postnatal days (PN) 8–12 and PN 17–24, correspond to growth periods terminating around the first and fifth year in human. Periadolescence in rats is reached by PN 30–35.[41,42] Thus, in ontogenetic studies in rodents, most authors concentrate on three periods: week 1 (PN 0–6), week 2–3 (PN 8–21), and week 4 (PN 22–28). On PN 30 and beyond, rats are usually considered young adults.

Although epileptic activity in immature tissue is also characterized by the appearance of PDS, typical and concomitant field potential discharges and intracellular rises of Ca^{2+}, one clear result of ontogenetic sudies on epilepsy showed that, in all models tested, there are developmental differences in seizure susceptibility, which can be summarized as follows: Directly after birth, epileptogenicity is low (PN 0–7 in rat). After this, a period of raised susceptibility follows, both regarding severity and spread of discharges (PN 8–21 in rat). These changes subside during periadolescence (PN 22–28) to reach adult levels (by PN 30–35 in rat).[42–56] These changes in seizure susceptibility can be related to different developmental features, in particular changes in neuronal excitability and synaptic properties, and the following paragraphs will summarize crucial findings, most pertaining to experiments made on rats (Figures 6.3 and 6.4).

Excitability of neurons

This is substantially governed by membrane properties and voltage-gated channels, as well as external factors such as ionic microenvironment regulating some of these properties. During ontogenesis, marked changes of these factors take place (Figures 6.3 and 6.4).

MEMBRANE PROPERTIES

Resting membrane potential of neurons is low and rises to adult levels during PN 0–14. Input resistance is high and drops about threefold during PN 0–21.[49,50,57] Thus, the threshold for action potential generation may be reached more easily in young neurons.

VOLTAGE–GATED INWARD CURRENTS

These currents lead to depolarization and contribute to action potential generation. The major currents to be considered are sodium currents and calcium currents. Sodium current density increases steadily 5–6 fold during PN 0–20, and consequently, action potentials in very young

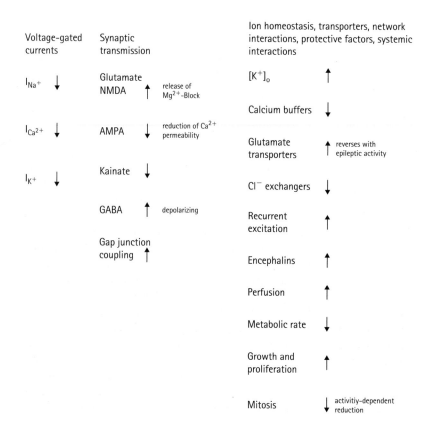

Figure 6.3 *Functional differences in voltage- and ligand-gated processes and metabolic and systemic factors which might account for differences in seizure susceptibility of juvenile compared with adult brain tissue. Arrows indicate relative level in juveniles.*

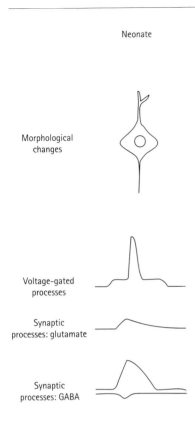

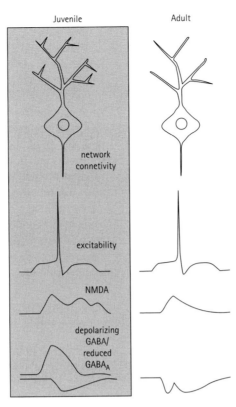

Neonate   Juvenile   Adult

Morphological changes

Voltage-gated processes

Synaptic processes: glutamate

Synaptic processes: GABA

network connetivity

excitability

NMDA

depolarizing GABA/ reduced GABA$_A$

Figure 6.4 *Time window of increased epileptogenicity of juvenile tissue explained by changes in morphological features, in cellular excitability and in synaptic mechanisms. Although additional factors will equally play a role, the coincidence of high network connectivity, virtually fully expressed neuronal excitability, prolonged excitatory synaptic potentials (presumably mediated via NMDA) and continued appearance of depolarizing GABA$_A$ currents in conjunction with little or no early hyperpolarizing GABA$_A$ function (note biphasic GABA response in adult tissue brought about by initial GABA$_A$ and subsequent GABA$_B$ receptor activation) is particularly suited to raise overall network excitability.*

tissue are broad and of low amplitude. Likewise high-voltage-activated calcium currents, which are activated at strongly depolarized potentials, also mature slowly until PN20. Consequently, in immature tissue they seem to play a less important role in the generation of epileptiform activity.[49] Tissue differences exist, for instance maturation of high-voltage-activated calcium currents occurs faster in the hippocampus than in the neocortex. By contrast, low-voltage-activated calcium currents operating near, or just hyperpolarized to, resting membrane potential appear to diminish with increasing age in most tissues, or move from somatic to dendritic regions. There, they may play an important role in boosting of synaptic potentials which by themselves might not reach threshold.[58–60] On the whole, these properties would favor decreased excitability in early ontogenesis. The situation is more complex, however. For instance, sodium channel density is lower in immature than adult tissue, but slowly-inactivating sodium currents (which will support bursting in neurons) are more abundant.[61,62]

VOLTAGE–GATED OUTWARD CURRENTS

These currents (mainly potassium) contribute to repolarization. The transient, inactivating I_A, and the delayed, noninactivating I_K responsible for longer lasting repolarization, and consequently favoring low firing rates in neurons, are particularly interesting. Whereas I_A seems to dominate in young neurons (PN 0–8), I_K develops to

adult levels around PN 9–14,[57,63,64] so that after hyperpolarizations in juvenile neurons can be relatively weak, tending to favour excitation.

Excitatory and inhibitory synaptic mechanisms

These follow different time courses during ontogenesis in a pattern which favours excitation via Ca^{2+}-permeable (and thus potentially plasticity-mediating; see above) NMDA receptors, and possibly by GABA receptors, which, of course, normally are inhibitory (Figures 6.3 and 6.4):

Excitatory synapses operating with glutamate mature quickly (within the first week) and show prolonged depolarizations in young animals. Specific types of glutamate receptors – the NMDA receptors, which are probably involved in different forms of synaptic plasticity – seem to be more strongly expressed during PN 8–21 than in adult animals. Furthermore, in young neurons these receptors display significantly less Mg^{2+}-dependent block (Figure 6.1) and are therefore also active close to resting membrane potential; their slower kinetics may explain why young neurons generate prolonged EPSPs, which are not normally found in adult tissue.[50,65–71] The Ca^{2+}-permeable NMDA receptors are prominently active during early developmental stages, but the largely Ca^{2+}-impermeable kainate receptors are less active, and AMPA receptors show reduced permeability to Ca^{2+}, or are not functional.[29,72]

Functional receptors for GABA, the main inhibitory transmitter in the brain, are present during embryonic stages or shortly after birth, but hyperpolarizing inhibitory postsynaptic potentials (IPSP) only mature later. Specifically, during PN 0–16, responses mediated by $GABA_A$ receptors, are either absent or weak, or are depolarizing rather than hyperpolarizing. They may occur spontaneously, generating 'giant depolarizing potentials' which can unblock NMDA receptors,[73] and can even trigger action potentials.[74] $GABA_A$-mediated hyperpolarizing potentials appear around PN 28. In adult tissue depolarizing GABAergic potentials are found only under abnormal, often epileptogenic, conditions.[14,75] Long-lasting inhibiton mediated by the metabotropic $GABA_B$ receptors also have delayed maturation, appearing around PN 20 in neocortical neurons, and somewhat earlier in hippocampal neurons,[73,76–79] so that on the whole, in early development GABA-mediated depolarization is favored.

Electrical synapses also show postnatal maturation: gap junctions which enable electrotonic contacts between neurons (and glia) are also possibly involved in synapse formation, sprouting phenomena or second-messenger diffusion.[80] They are very common in embryonic and early postnatal brain tissue – supporting synchronous network activity – and decrease to adult levels around PN 14.[81,82]

Morphological features, specifically the degree of functional connectivity, actually determine whether and how many receptors can be synaptically activated by any given neuron. Morphological and electrophysiological evidence shows during the seizure-susceptible period of approximately PN 7–12, that neuronal processes are extensively ramified to a degree possibly exceeding adult stages.[83] This, in conjunction with other factors, e.g. prolonged NMDA-mediated synaptic excitation, reduced or depolarizing GABAergic transmission, and gradually normalizing neuronal excitability, appears to favour a time window during which seizure susceptibility is markedly enhanced (Figure 6.4).

Other factors

Various other factors, such as changes in the ionic microenvironment leading to increases in extracellular potassium concentration ($[K^+]_o$) occurring during epileptiform activity can contribute to heightened excitability (Figure 6.3). Ontogenetic differences can be found regarding such seizure-associated rises in $[K^+]_o$. In adult brain, elevations of $[K^+]_o$ during epileptiform activity seldom exceed a 'ceiling' of 10–14 mmol/L. By contrast, juvenile animals, up to around PN 20, can sustain much larger increases, to 20 mmol/L or more, possibly due to late maturation of glial spatial buffering capacities, of the Na^+/K^+ exchanger, or due to specific properties of excitatory

synaptic transmission as discussed above,[39,84–88] but there is some evidence against this change in potassium homeostasis during development.[89] Further factors contributing to excitability, network synchronization or neuronal plasticity properties specific to immature tissue are a decrease in calcium buffering capacity,[90] reverse operation of glutamate-uptake transporters during epileptic activity,[91] low efficacy of chloride extrusion mechanisms (which will promote depolarizing actions of GABA[92]) and increased recurrent excitation.[83] Immature brain appears to be more vulnerable, partly due to the cell proliferation and growth necessarily in progress, and partly due to factors such as an increased susceptibility to oxidative stress.[93] On the other hand, the developing brain does have features that tend to protect it from seizure activity and its consequences, for instance neonatal brain has a lower metabolic rate and different responses to seizures.[94–96]

CORTICAL DYSPLASIA (See Chapter 4C)

So far aspects of the normal course of brain development that are relevant to epilepsy have been considered. It has become increasingly clear that pathological changes during development may be associated with, or even causal for, the manifestation of epilepsy. A developmental condition which has attracted much interest in recent years is cortical dysplasia (CD). Thus, clinical data suggest that CD, which includes migrational disorders and abnormalities of cell proliferation, differentiation and death, is often associated with intractable epilepsies[97–99] that are particularly resistant to pharmacotherapy. Increasing evidence from animal experiments supports the hypothesis that dysplastic tissue has raised seizure susceptibility, either native or when exposed to epileptogenic conditions,[100] although spontaneous seizures were only rarely observed in animal models.[101–104] Several models are used to mimic migration disorders in animals, the most common of which are postnatal freeze lesion resulting in polymicrogyria, or prenatal treatments such as γ-radiation, exposure to methylazoxymethanol, application of BCNU (carmustine) or exposure to cocaine. All of these result in nodular heterotopia and cortical dyslamination, thus mimicking two major conditions found in patients, namely malformations due to abnormal cortical organization (microgyria) or to abnormal neuronal migration (heterotopias). In addition, several mutant rodent strains exist with abnormal cortical development. These include the *reeler* mouse, which lacks the extracellular matrix protein reelin (resulting in an upside-down organization of the cortex, and, indeed, spontaneous seizures) and the TISH rat, which shows multiple heterotopias with different degrees of dysplasia.

In virtually all of these models, indications of neuronal hyperexcitability have been found, usually consisting of excessive responses to external stimulation, both on the cellular and the network level.[102,103,105–108] As with epilepsy in general, several mechanisms for raised excitability and the inherent epileptogenicity in dysplasias are discussed:

- changes of cellular firing properties with a high incidence of bursting neurons[109] possibly due to loss of the fast repolarizing potassium current I_A[101]
- alterations of synaptic mechanisms, and in particular widespread changes of receptor distribution and subunit composition[30,110–113] which may result in an overall loss of inhibition in some[108] but not all models[114]
- glial changes which suggest decreased spatial buffering capacity (and hence larger increases in K^+)[115]
- an extensive reorganization of network connectivity,[115,116] also seen in human tissue,[117] which may underlie the hyperexcitability particularly of the paradysplastic zones.[113]

Although not all models show all of the alterations listed above, it is entirely conceivable that singly, or in conjunction, some of the peculiarities of dysplastic tissue result in its striking epileptogenicity. Pathological changes resulting in dysplasia may thus play a key role in a number of childhood epilepsies.

NEONATAL PATHOPHYSIOLOGY

Although juvenile tissue is undoubtedly on the whole more susceptible to seizure generation, it was long thought that continued epileptic activity was less damaging to immature tissue than to adult brain. This apparent paradox was explained by an inherently larger potential for plasticity and repair mechanisms in young animals. Indeed, in several studies dealing with repetitive or prolonged status epilepticus induced by various agents such as pilocarpine, kainate, flurothyl, PTZ or electrical stimuli in juvenile animals (usually rats), in the majority of cases, no cell death was observed in the regions found most vulnerable to such conditions in adult animals, i.e. the hippocampus (Table 6.1). Yet, some authors did report cell damage, especially with models other than kainate injection (kainate receptors are thought to be expressed later in development, so that receptor-mediated actions of kainate before PN 12 are unlikely; Table 6.1). Furthermore, extrahippocampal regions do undergo cell damage under these conditions, even though the hippocampus may be spared.[118] The picture becomes even more complicated when morphological criteria other than cell death are considered. Profound changes become apparent, particularly irreversible growth retardation, brain weight loss and extensive sprouting with the establishment of aberrant

Table 6.1 *Status epilepticus-induced brain lesions in different models applied at various stages of maturation (cell death)*

Model	Age (days)	Number of seizures	Duration (min)	Lesion	Reference
Kainate	≤18	1	120	None	140
Kainate	≤30	1		None	141
Kainate	≤15	1	>30	None	142
Kainate	10	1		None	143, 144
Kainate	≤26	4		None	145
Kainate	≤14	1	>60	None	94
Pilocarpine	12	1		None	44
Pilocarpine	10	1	>180	None	146
Pilocarpine	≤14	1		None	147
Pilocarpine	10	1	>180	None	148
Tetanus toxin	10	100		None	121
PTZ	21	1		None	149
Flurothyl	≤10	50		None	150
Flurothyl	≤23	50		None	151
Flurothyl	≤14	1	60	None	152
Kainate	≤10	1		Cell death	153
Pilocarpine	7–21	1		Cell death	147
Pilocarpine	14–21	1		Cell death	154
Electrical stimuli	14–15	1	960	Cell death	155
Febrile convulsions	10	1	30	Altered inhibition	61
Pilocarpine	≤9	3		Cognitive deficit Seizure threshold↓	166
Kainate	14	1	210	Learning deficits Altered inhibition	167

Table 6.2 *Status epilepticus-induced brain lesions in different models applied at various stages of maturation (morphology)*

Model	Age (days)	Number of seizures	Duration (min)	Change	Reference
Kainate	14	1	>30	None	142
Kainate	20	1	240	None	156
Florothyl	14	1	60	None	152
Flurothyl	4	1	120	RNA↓, DNA↓, protein↓ Brain weight↓	157, 158
Pilocarpine	21	1		Mossy fibre sprouting	154
Tetanus toxin	10	100		Mossy fibre sprouting Dendritic spine loss	121
Flurothyl	≤10	50		Mossy fibre sprouting	150
Flurothyl	11–16	25		Mossy fibre sprouting	151
Bicuculline	≤20			Brain weight↓	158
CRH	10–13			Mossy fibre sprouting	159, 160
Electrical stimuli	2–11	20		Brain weight↓	161
Stargazer mutant (mouse)	17–18	>50		Mossy fibre sprouting	162
PTZ (after flurothyl)	10	15		Mossy fibre sprouting	163

Table 6.3 *Status epilepticus-induced brain lesions in different models applied at various stages of maturation (functional alterations)*

Model	Age (days)	Number of seizures	Duration (min)	Change	Reference
Kainate	≤10	1		None	143, 164
Kainate	15	1	>30	None	142
Kainate	20	4	120	None	145
Kainate	20	1	240	None	156
Flurothyl	14	1	60	None	152
Kainate	10	1		Learning deficits	165
Pilocarpine	21	1		Spontaneous seizures	154
Flurothyl	10	50		Seizure threshold↓ Learning deficits	150
Electrical stimuli	15	1	960	Seizure threshold↓	155
Febrile convulsions	10	1	30	Altered inhibition	61
Pilocarpine	≤9	3		Cognitive deficit Seizure threshold↓	166
Kainate	14	1	210	Learning deficits Altered inhibition	167

connectivities that persist throughout life (Table 6.2). These morphological changes apparently also have functional consequences. With the possible exception of kainate-induced status epilepticus, early seizures result in an increased seizure-susceptibility, functional changes in neurotransmission and neuronal plasticity and learning and memory deficits (Table 6.3). The learning deficits shown in Table 6.3 are for models with an initial status epilepticus, which are often, but not always, associated with substantial cell loss. Indeed, gross cell loss is not necessary for learning deficits, because intrahippocampal injection of tetanus toxin causes permanent deficits in learning and memory without causing status epilepticus or any major losses of neurons,[119,120] whether administered to adults or neonates at PN 10. These two stages differ in the much higher incidence of seizures 6 months after the injection made at PN 10[121] than at adult stages.[122] Considering the full range of experimental models, it is clear that intense seizure activity early in life can be functionally as damaging as status epilepticus is in more mature tissue.

Febrile seizures

These are a fairly common problem in children. Some of them seem to have a genetic basis, but elevated core temperature will trigger seizures in many patients without obvious predisposition. In most cases there appears to be no long-term consequence. However, patients with

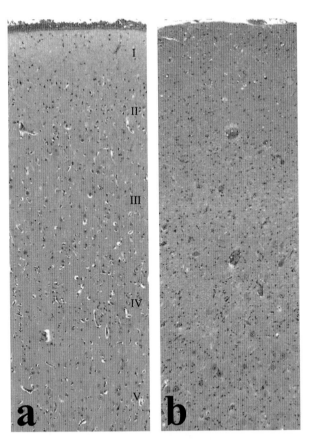

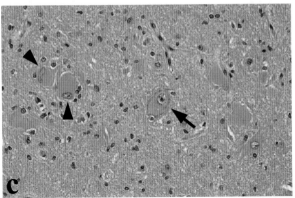

Plate 1 *Microscopic features of cortical dysplasia:
(a) Normal cerebral cortex (middle temporal gyrus) from a patient
with intractable temporal lobe epilepsy. Note well-organized
cortex with five out of six cortical layers clearly identified.
(b) Surgically resected cortical dysplasia from a pediatric patient
with intractable epilepsy. Note severely disorganized cortical
tissue without a laminar substructure. (c) A high-power view of
the disorganized tissue shown in panel (b). Note a large/giant
dysplastic cytomegalic neuron (arrow) with a large nucleolated
nucleus and scattered Nissl substance at the periphery of pale
cytoplasm, and large gemistocytic astrocyte-like 'balloon cells'
(arrowheads). (Hematoxylin & eosin, (a),(b) × 50; (c) × 240.)
See also Figure 5.3.*

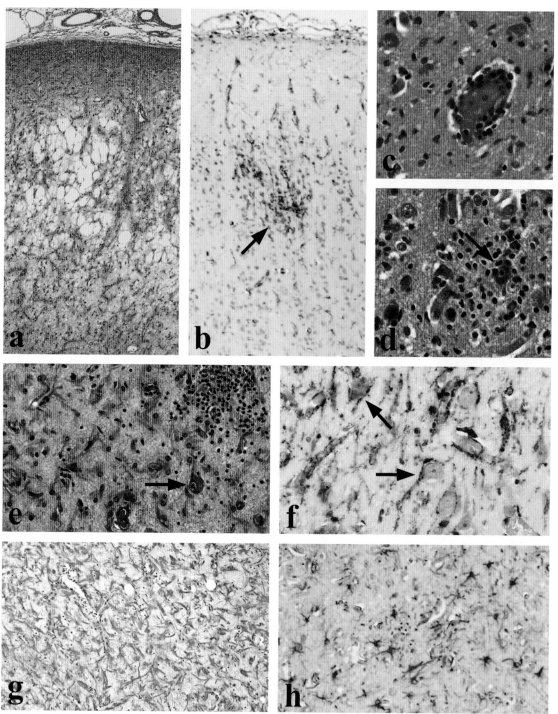

Plate 2 *Rasmussen encephalitis. (a) Extensive loss of neurons with microcystic change or 'status spongiosus', accompanied by capillary proliferation, but relatively minimal inflammation. Leptomeningeal infiltration of mononuclear inflammatory cells is also seen. (Hematoxylin & eosin, ×50.) (b) In contrast to (a), this panel shows a relatively intact cortex with a single inflammatory (microglial) nodule (arrow) in mid-cortex. (CD68 immunostain, ×125.) (c) Mononuclear inflammatory cells infiltrating the wall of a cortical microvessel ('perivascular cuffing'). (Hematoxylin & eosin, ×400.) (d) Mononuclear inflammatory cells and microglial cells surrounding a single neuron showing 'neuronophagia', indicated by an arrow. (Hematoxylin & eosin, ×400.) (e) Higher magnification of (a) showing severe neuronal loss with rarefaction of neuropil totally replaced by gemistocytic reactive astrocytes, and capillary proliferation. A focus of mononuclear cell infiltration (right upper corner) and a single chromatolytic neuron (arrow) remain. (Hematoxylin & eosin, ×200.) (f) High-power view of (b) showing CD68-positive microglial cells surrounding each neuronal profile (arrows). (CD68 immunostain, ×400.) (g) Severely affected area shown in panel (a) containing numerous GFAP-positive reactive astrocytes. (GFAP immunostain, ×100.) (h) Relatively well-preserved cortex showing rather less but definite astrogliosis as opposed to more severely affected area shown in panel (g). (GFAP immunostain, ×200.) (All immunostains were performed by the avidin–biotin–peroxidase complex (ABC) method and counterstained with hematoxylin.) See also Figure 5.5.*

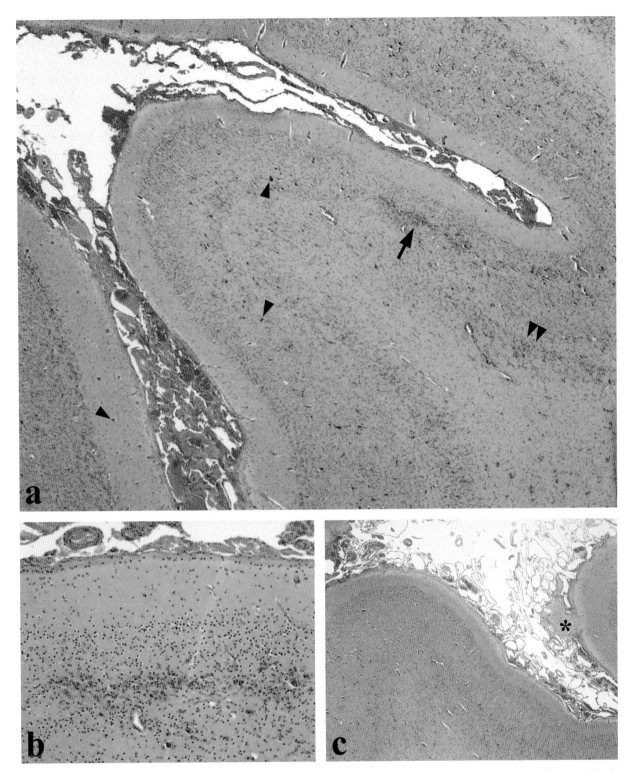

Plate 3 *Sturge-Weber syndrome: (a) Panoramic view of occipital cortex from cortical resection specimen showing variable but focally prominent linear calcifications in superficial (arrow) and deeper (double arrowheads) cortical laminae as well as scattered calcium depositions throughout the specimen (arrowheads). (b) A high-power view of panel (a) showing focal linear concretions of calcium. (c) Leptomeningeal angiomatosis continuous with a leptomeningeal glioneuronal heterotopia or excrescence (asterisk). (Hematoxylin & eosin, (a) ×40; (b) ×100; (c) ×20.) See also Figure 5.6.*

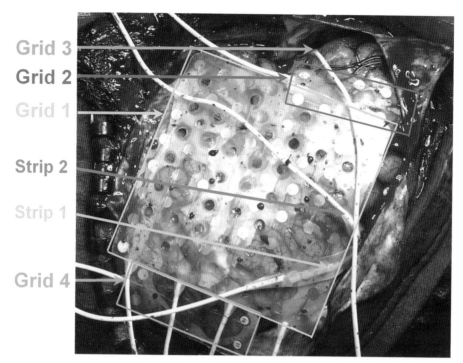

Plate 4 *Subdural electrodes covering the frontal parietal area. See also Figure 18.25.*

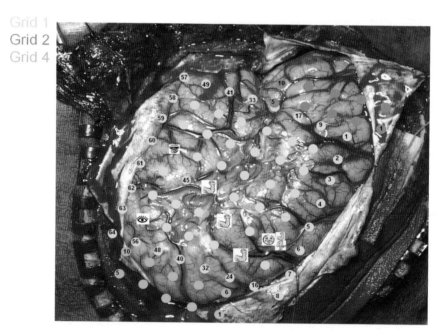

Plate 5 *Mapping of eloquent brain function using cortical stimulation. See also Figure 18.26.*

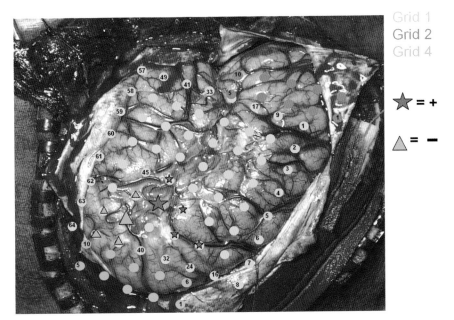

Grid 1
Grid 2
Grid 4

☆ = +

△ = –

Plate 6 *Median nerve somatosensory evoked potential demonstrating area of maximum positivity and negativity on the cortical grid electrodes. Stars indicate positive areas, triangles negative. See also Figure 18.27.*

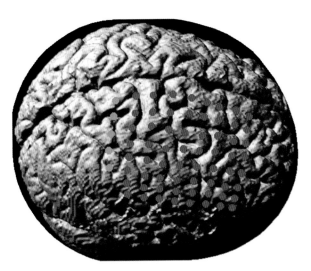

Plate 7 *Segmentation result of the patient's brain after removal of extracranial tissue. Dots denote the superimposed subdural grid electrode positions. See also Figure 18.28*

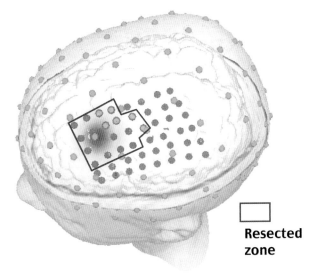

Resected zone

Plate 8 *Same patient, with scalp/skull tissues rendered semi-transparent. Scalp and subdural grid electrodes are displayed. The resection zone is indicated by the black line. See also Figure 18.29.*

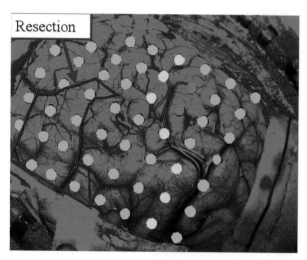

Resection

Plate 9 *Digital photograph of exposed craniotomy site, showing cortical features with resection zone marked. Dots denote subdural grid electrodes. See also Figure 18.30.*

temporal lobe epilepsy have a higher than chance incidence of febrile seizures, suggesting that febrile seizures can increase the risk of subsequent epilepsy, at least in vulnerable individuals. Rat pups 10–11 days old made hyperthermic (core temperature >39.5°C) for 30 min have a high risk of subsequently developing limbic seizures and are used to explore the possible mechanisms for this linkage.[123] One remarkable result is that inhibition appears to be strengthened, which is not an obvious mechanism for epileptogenesis. However there is a parallel long-term enhancement of an membrane current known as I_h,[124] which is activated by hyperpolarization, mediated by cations and is depolarizing. The effect of this change in intrinsic properties may have the effect of increasing the variability of activity in many classes of interneuron, and this could play a key role in promoting excessive synchronization amongst the pyramidal cells.[125]

GENETIC MUTATIONS IN CHILDHOOD EPILEPSY (See Chapter 4A)

One of the scientifically most exciting discoveries is the observation that distinct epileptic syndromes are definitely linked to certain genetic mutations. The clinical syndromes involved in this are benign familial neonatal convulsions (BFNC), generalized epilepsy with febrile seizures plus (GEFS+), juvenile myoclonic epilepsy and autosomal dominant nocturnal frontal lobe epilepsy. One of the first epilepsy syndromes recognized to be associated with a distinct genetic defect was BFNC. In this autosomal dominantly inherited syndrome, a mutation of potassium channels was identified on chromosome 20 which resulted in a particularly slowly activating potassium current and hence less effective repolarization.[126–128] GEFS+ type 1 has been linked to a mutation of the sodium channel subunit gene SCN1b on chromosome 19q. Sodium channels with an amino acid substitution corresponding to the above mutation yield currents with much longer inactivation kinetics than normal channels.[129] Polymorphism of the disease is likely, because further sodium channel mutations with GEFS+ have since been discovered on the SCN1a gene on chromosome 2q (GEFS+ type 2).[130,131] Also, SCN2 or SCN3 genes, in addition to SCN1, have been linked to GEFS+,[132] with a mutation on the SCN2a gene recently being identified.[133] When the major SCN1a and SCN2a mutations were introduced experimentally into cell expression systems they appeared to result in a shift towards a slowly inactivating sodium current.[26,133,134]

A word of caution is appropriate here. Finding a mutation linked to a specific disease is very exciting, especially when it alters cellular function in a manner potentially relevant to the symptoms of that disease. However, in most, if not all, of the genetically linked epilepsies, the link between the gene defect and specific epileptic symptoms is far from clear. In fact, although the symptoms appear clearly delineated, different pathomechanisms may share the same phenotype. For instance, the phenotype GEFS+ is also brought about by a mutation of the γ2 subunit of the GABA$_A$ receptor, resulting in a weakened response to GABA,[31] showing that this kind of epilepsy is not strictly linked to altered functions of voltage-gated channels. Similarly, both nocturnal frontal lobe epilepsy and juvenile myclonic epilepsy are associated with other mutations of ligand-gated channels at variable gene loci, in these cases of acetylcholine receptors.[135,136] The situation is made even more complex by gene mutations that result in more than one kind of disease. Thus, another mutation of the γ2 subunit of the GABA$_A$ receptor, which abolishes the response to diazepam (and presumably to whatever is the endogenous ligand for this site), results in two distinct epilepsy phenotypes, childhood absence epilepsy and febrile seizures.[32] Similarly mutations of the sodium channel α1 subunit gene, SCN1a, which has been implicated in GEFS+, has recently been shown to produce diverse seizure types, including partial seizures, prompting the proposal that GEFS+ be renamed **autosomal dominant epilepsy with febrile seizures plus**.[137] Other mutations can result in ataxia as well as epilepsy; for instance, a mutation of the calcium channel β4 subunit results in idiopathic generalized epilepsy in one family, but in episodic ataxia in another,[138] while a mutation in one of the voltage-gated potassium channels results in episodic ataxia, with the additional problem of partial epilepsy in some of the affected individuals.[139]

In summary, although the detailed mechanisms have yet to be elucidated, there is thus increasing and compelling evidence that at least some epilepsy syndromes constitute channelopathies. However, these examples remain a small minority of all epilepsies. Even among the genetic epilepsies, in most cases the functional significance of the mutations and how they relate to epileptogenesis remain obscure.

KEY POINTS

- Basic mechanisms of **focal and absence seizures** are different
- Several intrinsic synaptic and nonsynaptic **processes change with epileptogenesis**
- Physiological changes which occur in neurons and their interconnections during ontogenetic **brain maturation** may have deep implications for the development of epileptic activity in the immature brain
- **Pathological changes resulting in CD** may play a key role in many childhood epilepsies

- **Intense seizure activity in early life** can be functionally as damaging as status epilepticus is in mature tissue
- **Genetic defects in ion channel functioning** have been identified in some epilepsies

REFERENCES

1. Lees GJ. Pharmacology of AMPA/kainate receptor ligands and their therapeutic potential in neurological and psychiatric disorders. *Drugs* 2000; **59**: 33–78.

2. Haas HL, Selbach O. Functions of neuronal adenosine receptors. *Naunyn Schmiedebergs Archiv für Pharmacologie* 2000; **362**: 375–381.

3. McCormick DA, Contreras D. On the cellular and network bases of epileptic seizures. *Annual Review of Physiology* 2001; **63**: 815–846.

4. Goldensohn ES, Purpura DP. Intracellular potentials of cortical neurons during focal epileptogenic discharges. *Science* 1963; **139**: 840–842.

5. Prince DA, Futamachi KJ. Intracellular recordings in chronic focal epilepsy. *Brain Research* 1968; **11**: 681–684.

6. Empson RM, Jefferys JGR. Ca^{2+} entry through L-type Ca^{2+} channels helps terminate epileptiform activity by activation of a Ca^{2+} dependent after hyperpolarisation in hippocampal CA3. *Neuroscience* 2001; **102**: 297–306.

7. Alger BE, Williamson A. A transient calcium-dependent potassium component of the epileptiform burst after hyperpolarization in rat hippocampus. *Journal of Physiology* 1988; **399**: 191–205.

8. Johnston D, Brown TH. Control theory applied to neural networks illuminates synaptic basis of interictal epileptiform activity. *Advances in Neurology* 1986; **44**: 263–274.

9. Traub RD, Miles R, Jefferys JGR. Synaptic and intrinsic conductances shape picrotoxin-induced synchronized after-discharges in the guinea-pig hippocampal slice. *Journal of Physiology* 1993; **461**: 525–547.

10. Traub RD, Miles R. *Neuronal Networks in the Hippocampus.* Cambridge: Cambridge University Press, 1991.

11. Traub RD, Jefferys JGR. Epilepsy in vitro: electrophysiology and computer modeling. In: Engel J Jr, Pedley TA, Aicardi J, *et al.* (eds) *Epilepsy: A Comprehensive Textbook.* Philadelphia: Lippincott-Raven, 1997: 405–418.

12. Wong RKS, Traub RD, Miles R. Cellular basis of neuronal synchrony in epilepsy. *Advances in Neurology* 1986; **44**: 583–592.

13. Finnerty GT, Whittington MA, Jefferys JGR. Altered dentate filtering during the transition to seizure in the rat tetanus toxin model of epilepsy. *Journal of Neurophysiology* 2001; **86**: 2748–2753.

14. Köhling R, Vreugdenhil M, Bracci E, Jefferys JGR. Ictal epileptiform activity is facilitated by hippocampal GABA$_A$ receptor-mediated oscillations. *Journal of Neuroscience* 2000; **20**: 6820–6829.

15. Traub RD, Borck C, Colling SB, Jefferys JGR. On the structure of ictal events *in vitro. Epilepsia* 1996; **37**: 879–891.

16. Destexhe A, McCormick DA, Sejnowski TJ. Thalamic and thalamocortical mechanisms underlying 3 Hz spike-and-wave discharges. *Progress in Brain Research* 1999; **121**: 289–307.

17. Pinault D, Leresche N, Charpier S, *et al.* Intracellular recordings in thalamic neurones during spontaneous spike and wave discharges in rats with absence epilepsy. *Journal of Physiology* 1998; **509**: 449–456.

18. Sanabria ER, Su H, Yaari Y. Initiation of network bursts by Ca^{2+}-dependent intrinsic bursting in the rat pilocarpine model of temporal lobe epilepsy. *Journal of Physiology* 2001; **532**: 205–216.

19. Alkadhi KA, Tian LM. Veratridine-enhanced persistent sodium current induces bursting in CA1 pyramidal neurons. *Neuroscience* 1996; **71**: 625–632.

20. Deisz RA. A tetrodotoxin-insensitive sodium current initiates burst firing of neocortical neurons. *Neuroscience* 1996; **70**: 341–351.

21. Franceschetti S, Guatteo E, Panzica F, Sancini G, Wanke E, Avanzini G. Ionic mechanisms underlying burst firing in pyramidal neurons: intracellular study in rat sensorimotor cortex. *Brain Research* 1995; **696**: 127–139.

22. Su H, Alroy G, Kirson ED, Yaari Y. Extracellular calcium modulates persistent sodium current-dependent burst-firing in hippocampal pyramidal neurons. *Journal of Neuroscience* 2001; **21**: 4173–4182.

23. Azouz R, Jensen MS, Yaari Y. Ionic basis of spike after-depolarization and burst generation in adult rat hippocampal CA1 pyramidal cells. *Journal of Physiology (London)* 1996; **492**: 211–223.

24. Connors BW, Gutnick MJ. Intrinsic firing patterns of diverse neocortical neurons. *Trends in Neuroscience* 1990; **13**: 99–104.

25. Vreugdenhil M, Wadman WJ. Enhancement of calcium currents in rat hippocampal CAl neurons induced by kindling epileptogenesis. *Neuroscience* 1992; **49**: 373–381.

26. Kearney JA, Plummer NW, Smith MR, *et al.* A gain-of-function mutation in the sodium channel gene *Scn2a* results in seizures and behavioral abnormalities. *Neuroscience* 2001; **102**: 307–317.

27. Sashihara S, Yanagihara N, Kobayashi H, *et al.* Overproduction of voltage-dependent Na^+ channels in the developing brain of genetically seizure-susceptible E1 mice. *Neuroscience* 1992; **48**: 285–291.

28. Köhr G, De Koninck Y, Mody I. Properties of NMDA receptor channels in neurons acutely isolated from epileptic (kindled) rats. *Journal of Neuroscience* 1993; **13**: 3612–3627.

29. Friedman LK, Pellegrini-Giampietro DE, Sperber EF, *et al.* Kainate-induced status epilepticus alters glutamate and GABA$_A$ receptor gene expression in adult rat hippocampus: an in situ hybridization study. *Journal of Neuroscience* 1994; **14**: 2697–2707.

30. Zilles K, Qu M, Schleicher A, Luhmann HJ. Characterization of neuronal migration disorders in neocortical structures: quantitative receptor autoradiography of ionotropic glutamate, GABA$_A$ and GABA$_B$ receptors. *European Journal of Neuroscience* 1998; **10**: 3095–3106.

31. Baulac S, Huberfeld G, Gourfinkel-An I, *et al.* First genetic evidence of GABA$_A$ receptor dysfunction in epilepsy: a mutation in the γ2-subunit gene. *Nature Genetics* 2001; **28**: 46–48.

32. Wallace RH, Marini C, Petrou S, *et al.* Mutant GABA$_A$ receptor γ2-subunit in childhood absence epilepsy and febrile seizures. *Nature Genetics* 2001; **28**: 49–52.

33. Parent JM, Yu TW, Leibowitz RT, *et al.* Dentate granule cell neurogensis is increased by seizures and contributes to aberrant network reorganization in the adult rat hippocampus. *Journal of Neuroscience* 1997; **17**: 3727–3738.

34. Sutula T, He XX, Cavazos J, Scott G. Synaptic reorganization in the hippocampus induced by abnormal functional activity. *Science* 1988; **239**: 1147–1150.

35. Morgan SL, Teyler TJ. Epileptic-like activity induces multiple forms of plasticity in hippocampal area CA1. *Brain Research* 2001; **917**: 90–96.

36. Lowenstein DH, Gwinn RP, Seren MS, Simon RP, McIntosh TK. Increased expression of mRNA encoding calbindin-D28K, the glucose-regulated proteins, or the 72 kDa heat-shock protein in three models of acute CNS injury. *Brain Research. Molecular Brain Research* 1994; **22**: 299–308.

37. Thompson SM, Gähwiler BH. Activity-dependent disinhibition. III. Desensitization and $GABA_B$ receptor-mediated presynaptic inhibition in the hippocampus in vitro. *Journal of Neurophysiology* 1989; **61**: 524–533.

38. Colling SB, Man WDC, Draguhn A, Jefferys JGR. Dendritic shrinkage and dye-coupling between rat hippocampal CA1 pyramidal cells in the tetanus toxin model of epilepsy. *Brain Research* 1996; **741**: 38–43.

39. Avoli M, Louvel J, Kurcewicz I, Pumain R, Barbarosie M. Extracellular free potassium and calcium during synchronous activity induced by 4-aminopyridine in the juvenile rat hippocampus. *Journal of Physiology* 1996; **493**: 707–717.

40. Heinemann U, Konnerth A, Pumain R, Wadman WJ. Extracellular calcium and potassium concentration changes in chronic epileptic brain tissue. *Advances in Neurology* 1986; **44**: 641–661.

41. Gottlieb A, Keydar I, Epstein HT. Rodent brain growth stages: an analytical review. *Biology of the Neonate* 1977; **32**: 166–176.

42. Moshe SL, Cornblath M. Developmental aspects of epileptogenesis. In: Wyllie E (ed.) *The Treatment of Epilepsy: Principles and Practice.* Philadelphia: Lea & Febiger, 1993: 99–110.

43. Albrecht D, Heinemann U. Low calcium-induced epileptiform activity in hippocampal slices from infant rats. *Brain Research. Developmental Brain Research* 1989; **48**: 316–320.

44. Cavalheiro EA, Silva DF, Turski WA, *et al.* The susceptibility of rats to pilocarpine-induced seizures is age-dependent. *Brain Research* 1987; **465**: 43–58.

45. Gloveli T, Albrecht D, Heinemann U. Properties of low Mg^{2+} induced epileptiform activity in rat hippocampal and entorhinal cortex slices during adolescence. *Brain Research. Developmental Brain Research* 1995; **87**: 145–152.

46. Hablitz JJ. Spontaneous ictal-like discharges and sustained potential shifts in the developing rat neocortex. *Journal of Neurophysiology* 1987; **58**: 1052–1065.

47. Hablitz JJ, Heinemann U. Extracellular K^+ and Ca^{2+} changes during epileptiform discharges in the immature rat neocortex. *Brain Research* 1987; **433**: 299–303.

48. Hoffman SN, Prince DA. Epileptogenesis in immature neocortical slices induced by 4-aminopyridine. *Brain Research. Developmental Brain Research* 1995; **85**: 64–70.

49. Köhling R, Straub H, Speckmann E-J. Differential involvement of L-type calcium channels in epileptogenesis of rat hippocampal slices during ontogenesis. *Neurobiology of Disease* 2000; **7**: 471–482.

50. Kriegstein AR, Suppes T, Prince DA. Cellular and synaptic physiology and epileptogenesis of developing rat neocortical neurons in vitro. *Brain Research* 1987; **431**: 161–171.

51. Michelson HB, Lothman EW. An ontogenetic study of kindling using rapidly recurring hippocampal seizures. *Brain Research. Developmental Brain Research* 1991; **61**: 79–85.

52. Prince DA, Gutnick MJ. Neuronal activities in epileptogenic foci of immature cortex. *Brain Research* 1972; **45**: 455–468.

53. Purpura DP. Stability and seizure susceptibility of immature brain. In: Jasper HH, Ward AA Jr, Pope A, (eds) *Basic Mechanisms of the Epilepsies.* Boston: Little Brown, 1969: 481–505.

54. Swann JW, Brady RJ. Penicillin-induced epileptogenesis in immature rat CA3 hippocampal pyramidal cells. *Brain Research. Developmental Brain Research* 1984; **12**: 243–254.

55. Mares P, Makal V, Velisek L. Increased epileptogenesis in the immature brain. *Epilepsy Research Supplement* 1992; **9**: 127–129.

56. Vilagi I, Tarnawa I, Banczerowski-Pelyhe I. Changes in seizure activity of the neocortex during the early postnatal development of the rat: an electrophysiological study on slices in Mg^{2+}-free medium. *Epilepsy Research* 1991; **8**: 102–106.

57. Spigelman I, Zhang L, Carlen PL. Patch-clamp study of postnatal development of CA1 neurons in rat hippocampal slices: membrane excitability and K^+ currents. *Journal of Neurophysiology* 1992; **68**: 55–69.

58. Huguenard JR. Low-threshold calcium currents in central nervous system neurons. *Annual Review of Physiology* 1996; **58**: 329–348.

59. Karst H, Joels M, Wadman WJ. Low-threshold calcium current in dendrites of the adult rat hippocampus. *Neuroscience Letters* 1993; **164**: 154–158.

60. Huguenard JR, Hamill OP, Prince DA. Developmental changes in Na^+ conductances in rat neocortical neurons: appearance of a slowly inactivating component. *Journal of Neurophysiology* 1988; **59**: 778–795.

61. Chen K, Baram TZ, Soltesz I. Febrile seizures in the developing brain result in persistent modification of neuronal excitability in limbic circuits. *Nature Medicine* 1999; **5**: 888–894.

62. Felts PA, Yokoyama S, Dib-Hajj S, Black JA, Waxman SG. Sodium channel alpha-subunit mRNAs I, II, III, NaG, Na6 and hNE (PN1): different expression patterns in developing rat nervous system. *Brain Research. Molecular Brain Research* 1997; **45**: 71–82.

63. Beck H, Ficker E, Heinemann U. Properties of two voltage-activated potassium currents in acutely isolated juvenile rat dentate gyrus granule cells. *Journal of Neurophysiology* 1992; **68**: 2086–2099.

64. Klee R, Ficker E, Heinemann U. Comparison of voltage-dependent potassium currents in rat pyramidal neurons acutely isolated from hippocampal regions CA1 and CA3. *Journal of Neurophysiology* 1995; **74**: 1982–1995.

65. Burgard EC, Hablitz JJ. Developmental changes in NMDA and non-NMDA receptor-mediated synaptic potentials in rat neocortex. *Journal of Neurophysiology* 1993; **69**: 230–240.

66. Carmignoto G, Vicini S. Activity-dependent decrease in NMDA receptor responses during development of the visual cortex. *Science* 1992; **258**: 1007–1011.

67. Hestrin S. Developmental regulation of NMDA receptor-mediated synaptic currents at a central synapse. *Nature* 1992; **357**: 686–689.

68. Insel TR, Miller LP, Gelhard RE. The ontogeny of excitatory amino acid receptors in rat forebrain—I. N-methyl-D-aspartate and quisqualate receptors. *Neuroscience* 1990; **35**: 31–43.

69. Kirson ED, Schirra C, Konnerth A, Yaari Y. Early postnatal switch in magnesium sensitivity of NMDA receptors in rat CA1 pyramidal cells. *Journal of Physiology* 1999; **521**(1): 99–111.

70. Kleckner NW, Dingledine R. Regulation of hippocampal NMDA receptors by magnesium and glycine during development. *Brain Research. Molecular Brain Research* 1991; **11**: 151–159.

71. Morrisett RA, Mott DD, Lewis DV, Wilson WA, Swartzwelder HS. Reduced sensitivity of the N-methyl-D-aspartate component of synaptic transmission to magnesium in hippocampal slices from immature rats. *Brain Research. Developmental Brain Research* 1990; **56**: 257–262.

72. Campochiaro P, Coyle JT. Ontogenetic development of kainate neurotoxicity: correlates with glutamatergic innervation. *Proceedings of the National Academy of Sciences of the USA* 1978; **75**: 2025–2029.

73. Holmes GL, Khazipov R, Ben Ari Y. New concepts in neonatal seizures. *NeuroReport* 2002; **13**: A3–A8.

74. Ben-Ari Y, Cherubini E, Corradetti R, Gaiarsa J-L. Giant synaptic potentials in immature rat CA3 hippocampal neurones. *Journal of Physiology* 1989; **416**: 303–325.

75. Avoli M, Barbarosie M, Lucke A *et al.* Synchronous GABA-mediated potentials and epileptiform discharges in the rat limbic system in vitro. *Journal of Neuroscience* 1996; **16**: 3912–3924.

76. Fukuda A, Mody I, Prince DA. Differential ontogenesis of presynaptic and postsynaptic GABA$_B$ – inhibition in rat somatosensory cortex. *Journal of Neurophysiology* 1993; **70**: 448–452.

77. Gaiarsa JL, McLean H, Congar P, *et al.* Postnatal maturation of gamma-aminobutyric acid A and B-mediated inhibition in the CA3 hippocampal region of the rat. *Journal of Neurobiology* 1995; **26**: 339–349.

78. Luhmann HJ, Prince DA. Postnatal maturation of the GABAergic system in rat neocortex. *Journal of Neurophysiology* 1991; **65**: 247–263.

79. Sutor B, Luhmann HJ. Development of excitatory and inhibitory postsynaptic potentials in the rat neocortex. *Perspectives on Developmental Neurobiology* 1995; **2**: 409–419.

80. Jefferys JGR. Non-synaptic modulation of neuronal activity in the brain: electric currents and extracellular ions. *Physiological Reviews* 1995; **75**: 689–723.

81. Connors BW, Benardo LS, Prince DA. Coupling between neurons of the developing rat neocortex. *Journal of Neuroscience* 1983; **3**: 773–782.

82. Rörig B, Sutor B. Regulation of gap junction coupling in the developing neocortex. *Molecular Neurobiology* 1996; **12**: 225–249.

83. Gomez-Di Cesare CM, Smith KL, Rice FL, Swann JW. Axonal remodeling during postnatal maturation of CA3 hippocampal pyramidal neurons. *Journal of Comparative Neurology* 1997; **384**: 165–180.

84. Connors BW, Ransom BR, Kunis DM, Gutnick MJ. Activity-dependent K$^+$ accumulation in the developing rat optic nerve. *Science* 1982; **216**: 1341–1343.

85. Hablitz JJ, Heinemann U. Alterations in the microenvironment during spreading depression associated with epileptiform activity in the immature neocortex. *Brain Research. Developmental Brain Research* 1989; **46**: 243–252.

86. Haglund MM, Schwartzkroin PA. Role of Na-K pump potassium regulation and IPSPs in seizures and spreading depression in immature rabbit hippocampal slices. *Journal of Neurophysiology* 1990; **63**: 225–239.

87. Heinemann U, Albrecht D, Beck H *et al.* Delayed K$^+$ regulation and K$^+$ current maturation as factors of enhanced epileptogenicity during ontogenesis of the hippocampus of rats. *Epilepsy Research* 1992 (Suppl 9): 107–114.

88. Swann JW, Smith KL, Brady RJ. Extracellular K$^+$ accumulation during penicillin-induced epileptogenesis in the CA3 region of immature rat hippocampus. *Brain Research* 1986; **395**: 243–255.

89. Stringer JL, Lothman EW. During after discharges in the young rat in vivo extracellular potassium is not elevated above adult levels. *Brain Research. Developmental Brain Research* 1996; **91**: 136–139.

90. Hof PR, Glezer II, Conde F, *et al.* Cellular distribution of the calcium-binding proteins parvalbumin, calbindin, and calretinin in the neocortex of mammals: phylogenetic and developmental patterns. *Journal of Chemical Neuroanatomy* 1999; **16**: 77–116.

91. Katsumori H, Baldwin RA, Wasterlain CG. Reverse transport of glutamate during depolarization in immature hippocampal slices. *Brain Research* 1999; **819**: 160–164.

92. Rivera C, Voipio J, Payne JA, *et al.* The K$^+$/Cl$^-$ co-transporter KCC2 renders GABA hyperpolarizing during neuronal maturation. *Nature* 1999; **397**: 251–255.

93. Ferriero DM. Oxidant mechanisms in neonatal hypoxia-ischemia. *Developmental Neuroscience* 2001; **23**: 198–202.

94. Friedman LK. Developmental switch in phenotypic expression of preproenkephalin mRNA and ^{45}Ca^{2+} accumulation following kainate-induced status epilepticus. *Brain Research. Developmental Brain Research* 1997; **101**: 287–293.

95. Pereira DV, Boyet S, Koziel V, Nehlig A. Effects of pentylenetetrazol-induced status epilepticus on local cerebral blood flow in the developing rat. *Journal of Cerebral Blood Flow and Metabolism* 1995; **15**: 270–283.

96. Vannucci RC, Vannucci SJ. Glucose metabolism in the developing brain. *Seminars in Perinatology* 2000; **24**: 107–115.

97. Crino PB, Miyata H, Vinters HV. Neurodevelopmental disorders as a cause of seizures: neuropathologic, genetic, and mechanistic considerations. *Brain Pathology* 2002; **12**: 212–233.

98. Porter BE, Brooks-Kayal A, Golden JA. Disorders of cortical development and epilepsy. *Archives of Neurology* 2002; **59**: 361–365.

99. Kuzniecky RI, Barkovich AJ. Malformations of cortical development and epilepsy. *Brain Development* 2001; **23**: 2–11.

100. Avoli M, Bernasconi A, Mattia D, Olivier A, Hwa GG. Epileptiform discharges in the human dysplastic neocortex: in vitro physiology and pharmacology. *Annals of Neurology* 1999; **46**: 816–826.

101. Castro PA, Cooper EC, Lowenstein DH, Baraban SC. Hippocampal heterotopia lack functional Kv4.2 potassium channels in the methylazoxymethanol model of cortical malformations and epilepsy. *Journal of Neuroscience* 2001; **21**: 6626–6634.

102. Luhmann HJ, Karpuk N, Qu M, Zilles K. Characterization of neuronal migration disorders in neocortical structures.

II. Intracellular in vitro recordings. *Journal of Neurophysiology* 1998; **80**: 92–102.

103. Luhmann HJ, Raabe K, Qu M, Zilles K. Characterization of neuronal migration disorders in neocortical structures: extracellular in vitro recordings. *European Journal of Neuroscience* 1998; **10**: 3085–3094.

104. Roper SN, King MA, Abraham LA, Boillot MA. Disinhibited in vitro neocortical slices containing experimentally induced cortical dysplasia demonstrate hyperexcitability. *Epilepsy Research* 1997; **26**: 443–449.

105. Baraban SC, Wenzel HJ, Hochman DW, Schwartzkroin PA. Characterization of heterotopic cell clusters in the hippocampus of rats exposed to methylazoxymethanol in utero. *Epilepsy Research* 2000; **39**: 87–102.

106. Jacobs KM, Hwang BJ, Prince DA. Focal epileptogenesis in a rat model of polymicrogyria. *Journal of Neurophysiology* 1999; **81**: 159–173.

107. Redecker C, Lutzenburg M, Gressens P, *et al*. Excitability changes and glucose metabolism in experimentally induced focal cortical dysplasias. *Cerebral Cortex* 1998; **8**: 623–634.

108. Zhu WJ, Roper SN. Reduced inhibition in an animal model of cortical dysplasia. *Journal of Neuroscience* 2000; **20**: 8925–8931.

109. Baraban SC, Schwartzkroin PA. Electrophysiology of CA1 pyramidal neurons in an animal model of neuronal migration disorders: prenatal methylazoxymethanol treatment. *Epilepsy Research* 1995; **22**: 145–156.

110. Hablitz JJ, DeFazio RA. Altered receptor subunit expression in rat neocortical malformations. *Epilepsia* 2000; 41 Suppl **6**: S82–585.: S82–S85.

111. DeFazio RA, Hablitz JJ. Alterations in NMDA receptors in a rat model of cortical dysplasia. *Journal of Neurophysiology* 2000; **83**: 315–321.

112. Jacobs KM, Gutnick MJ, Prince DA. Hyperexcitability in a model of cortical maldevelopment. *Cerebral Cortex* 1996; **6**: 514–523.

113. Redecker C, Luhmann HJ, Hagemann G, Fritschy JM, Witte OW. Differential downregulation of GABA$_A$ receptor subunits in widespread brain regions in the freeze-lesion model of focal cortical malformations. *Journal of Neuroscience* 2000; **20**: 5045–5053.

114. Hagemann G, Redecker C, Witte OW. Intact functional inhibition in the surround of experimentally induced focal cortical dysplasias in rats. *Journal of Neurophysiology* 2000; **84**: 600–603.

115. Bordey A, Lyons SA, Hablitz JJ, Sontheimer H. Electrophysiological characteristics of reactive astrocytes in experimental cortical dysplasia. *Journal of Neurophysiology* 2001; **85**: 1719–1731.

116. Rosen GD, Burstein D, Galaburda AM. Changes in efferent and afferent connectivity in rats with induced cerebrocortical microgyria. *Journal of Comparative Neurology* 2000; **418**: 423–440.

117. Köhling R, Qu M, Zilles K, Speckmann EJ. Current-source-density profiles associated with sharp waves in human epileptic neocortical tissue. *Neuroscience* 1999; **94**: 1039–1050.

118. Kubova H, Druga R, Lukasiuk K, *et al*. Status epilepticus causes necrotic damage in the mediodorsal nucleus of the thalamus in immature rats. *Journal of Neuroscience* 2001; **21**: 3593–3599.

119. Brace HM, Jefferys JGR, Mellanby J. Long-term changes in hippocampal physiology and in learning ability of rats after intrahippocampal tetanus toxin. *Journal of Physiology* 1985; **368**: 343–357.

120. Lee CL, Hannay J, Hrachovy R, *et al*. Spatial learning deficits without hippocampal neuronal loss in a model of early-onset epilepsy. *Neuroscience* 2001; **107**: 71–84.

121. Anderson AE, Hrachovy RA, Antalffy BA, Armstrong DL, Swann JW. A chronic focal epilepsy with mossy fiber sprouting follows recurrent seizures induced by intrahippocampal tetanus toxin injection in infant rats. *Neuroscience* 1999; **92**: 73–82.

122. Milward AJ, Meldrum BS, Mellanby JH. Forebrain ischaemia with CA1 cell loss impairs epileptogenesis in the tetanus toxin limbic seizure model. *Brain* 1999; **122**: 1009–1016.

123. Baram TZ, Gerth A, Schultz L. Febrile seizures: an appropriate-aged model suitable for long-term studies. *Brain Research. Developmental Brain Research* 1997; **98**: 265–270.

124. Chen K, Aradi I, Thon N, *et al*. Persistently modified h-channels after complex febrile seizures convert the seizure-induced enhancement of inhibition to hyperexcitability. *Nature Medicine* 2001; **7**: 331–337.

125. Aradi I, Soltesz I. Modulation of network behaviour by changes in variance in interneuronal properties. *Journal of Physiology* 2002; **538**: 227–251.

126. Lerche H, Biervert C, Alekov AK, *et al*. A reduced K$^+$ current due to a novel mutation in KCNQ2 causes neonatal convulsions. *Annals of Neurology* 1999; **46**: 305–312.

127. Biervert C, Schroeder BC, Kubisch C, *et al*. A potassium channel mutation in neonatal human epilepsy. *Science* 1998; **279**: 403–406.

128. Castaldo P, del Giudice EM, Coppola G, *et al*. Benign familial neonatal convulsions caused by altered gating of KCNQ2/KCNQ3 potassium channels. *Journal of Neuroscience* 2002; **22**: RC199.

129. Wallace RH, Wang DW, Singh R, *et al*. Febrile seizures and generalized epilepsy associated with a mutation in the Na$^+$-channel β1 subunit gene SCN1B. *Nature Genetics* 1998; **19**: 366–370.

130. Escayg A, Heils A, MacDonald BT, *et al*. A novel SCN1A mutation associated with generalized epilepsy with febrile seizures plus – and prevalence of variants in patients with epilepsy. *American Journal of Human Genetics* 2001; **68**: 866–873.

131. Escayg A, MacDonald BT, Meisler MH, *et al*. Mutations of SCN1A, encoding a neuronal sodium channel, in two families with GEFS +2. *Nature Genetics* 2000; **24**: 343–345.

132. Baulac S, Gourfinkel-An I, Picard F, *et al*. A second locus for familial generalized epilepsy with febrile seizures plus maps to chromosome 2q21–q33. *American Journal of Human Genetics* 1999; **65**: 1078–1085.

133. Sugawara T, Tsurubuchi Y, Agarwala KL, *et al*. A missense mutation of the Na$^+$ channel alpha II subunit gene Na(v)1.2 in a patient with febrile and afebrile seizures causes channel dysfunction. *Proceedings of the National Academy of Sciences of the USA* 2001; **98**: 6384–6389.

134. Alekov A, Rahman MM, Mitrovic N, Lehmann-Horn F, Lerche H. A sodium channel mutation causing epilepsy in man exhibits subtle defects in fast inactivation and activation in vitro. *Journal of Physiology* 2000; **529**: 533–539.

135. Phillips HA, Scheffer IE, Crossland KM, *et al*. Autosomal dominant nocturnal frontal-lobe epilepsy: genetic heterogeneity and evidence for a second locus at 15q24. *American Journal of Human Genetics* 1998; **63**: 1108–1116.

136. Steinlein OK. Neuronal nicotinic receptors in human epilepsy. *European Journal of Pharmacology* 2000; **393**: 243–247.

137. Ito M, Nagafuji H, Okazawa H, *et al.* Autosomal dominant epilepsy with febrile seizures plus with missense mutations of the Na$^+$-channel alpha 1 subunit gene, *SCN1A*. *Epilepsy Research* 2002; **48**: 15–23.

138. Escayg A, De Waard M, Lee DD, *et al.* Coding and noncoding variation of the human calcium-channel β4-subunit gene *CACNB4* in patients with idiopathic generalized epilepsy and episodic ataxia. *American Journal of Human Genetics* 2000; **66**: 1531–1539.

139. Zuberi SM, Eunson LH, Spauschus A, *et al.* A novel mutation in the human voltage-gated potassium channel gene (Kv1.1) associates with episodic ataxia type 1 and sometimes with partial epilepsy. *Brain* 1999; **122**: 817–825.

140. Nitecka L, Tremblay E, Charton G, *et al.* Maturation of kainic acid seizure-brain damage syndrome in the rat. II. Histopathological sequelae. *Neuroscience* 1984; **13**: 1073–1094.

141. Holmes GL, Thompson JL, Marchi T, Feldman DS. Behavioral effects of kainic acid administration on the immature brain. *Epilepsia* 1988; **29**: 721–730.

142. Sperber EF, Haas KZ, Stanton PK, Moshé SL. Resistance of the immature hippocampus to seizure-induced synaptic reorganization. *Brain Research. Developmental Brain Research* 1991; **60**: 88–93.

143. Stafstrom CE, Thompson JL, Holmes GL. Kainic acid seizures in the developing brain: status epilepticus and spontaneous recurrent seizures. *Brain Research. Developmental Brain Research* 1992; **65**: 227–236.

144. Stafstrom CE, Tandon P, Hori A, *et al.* Acute effects of MK801 on kainic acid-induced seizures in neonatal rats. *Epilepsy Research* 1997; **26**: 335–344.

145. Sarkisian MR, Tandon P, Liu Z, *et al.* Multiple kainic acid seizures in the immature and adult brain: ictal manifestations and long-term effects on learning and memory. *Epilepsia* 1997; **38**: 1157–1166.

146. Hirsch E, Baram TZ, Snead OC, III. Ontogenic study of lithium-pilocarpine-induced status epilepticus in rats. *Brain Research* 1992; **583**: 120–126.

147. Sankar R, Shin DH, Wasterlain CG. Serum neuron-specific enolase is a marker for neuronal damage following status epilepticus in the rat. *Epilepsy Research* 1997; **28**: 129–136.

148. Dube C, Andre V, Covolan L, *et al.* C-Fos, Jun D and HSP72 immunoreactivity, and neuronal injury following lithium-pilocarpine induced status epilepticus in immature and adult rats. *Brain Research. Molecular Brain Research* 1998; **63**: 139–154.

149. Motte JE, Silva Fernandes MJ, Marescaux C, Nehlig A. Effects of pentylenetetrazol-induced status epilepticus on c-Fos and HSP72 immunoreactivity in the immature rat brain. *Brain Research. Molecular Brain Research* 1997; **50**: 79–84.

150. Huang L, Cilio MR, Silveira DC, *et al.* Long-term effects of neonatal seizures: a behavioral, electrophysiological, and histological study. *Brain Research. Developmental Brain Research* 1999; **118**: 99–107.

151. Liu Z, Yang Y, Silveira DC, *et al.* Consequences of recurrent seizures during early brain development. *Neuroscience* 1999; **92**: 1443–1454.

152. Sperber EF, Haas KZ, Romero MT, Stanton PK. Flurothyl status epilepticus in developing rats: behavioral, electrographic histological and electrophysiological studies. *Brain Research. Developmental Brain Research* 1999; **116**: 59–68.

153. Cook TM, Crutcher KA. Extensive target cell loss during development results in mossy fibers in the regio superior (CA1) of the rat hippocampal formation. *Brain Research* 1985; **353**: 19–30.

154. Sankar R, Shin DH, Liu H, Mazarati A, Pereira D, V, Wasterlain CG. Patterns of status epilepticus-induced neuronal injury during development and long-term consequences. *Journal of Neuroscience* 1998; **18**: 8382–8393.

155. Thompson K, Holm AM, Schousboe A, Popper P, Micevych P, Wasterlain C. Hippocampal stimulation produces neuronal death in the immature brain. *Neuroscience* 1998; **82**: 337–348.

156. Tandon P, Yang Y, Das K, Holmes GL, Stafstrom CE. Neuroprotective effects of brain-derived neurotrophic factor in seizures during development. *Neuroscience* 1999; **91**: 293–303.

157. Dwyer BE, Wasterlain CG, Fujikawa DG, Yamada L. Brain protein metabolism in epilepsy. *Advances in Neurology* 1986; **44**: 903–918.

158. Wasterlain CG, Dwyer BE. Brain metabolism during prolonged seizures in neonates. *Advances in Neurology* 1983; **34**: 241–260.

159. Baram TZ, Ribak CE. Peptide-induced infant status epilepticus causes neuronal death and synaptic reorganization. *NeuroReport* 1995; **6**: 277–280.

160. Ribak CE, Baram TZ. Selective death of hippocampal CA3 pyramidal cells with mossy fiber afferents after CRH-induced status epilepticus in infant rats. *Brain Research. Developmental Brain Research* 1996; **91**: 245–251.

161. Wasterlain CG. Effects of neonatal status epilepticus on rat brain development. *Neurology* 1976; **26**: 975–986.

162. Qiao X, Noebels JL. Developmental analysis of hippocampal mossy fiber outgrowth in a mutant mouse with inherited spike-wave seizures. *Journal of Neuroscience* 1993; **13**: 4622–4635.

163. Holmes GL, Sarkisian M, Ben Ari Y, Chevassus-au-Louis N. Mossy fiber sprouting after recurrent seizures during early development in rats. *Journal of Comparative Neurology* 1999; **404**: 537–553.

164. Stafstrom CE, Chronopoulos A, Thurber S, Thompson JL, Holmes GL. Age-dependent cognitive and behavioral deficits after kainic acid seizures. *Epilepsia* 1993; **34**: 420–432.

165. de Feo MR, Mecarelli O, Palladini G, Ricci GF. Long-term effects of early status epilepticus on the acquisition of conditioned avoidance behavior in rats. *Epilepsia* 1986; **27**: 476–482.

166. Santos NF, Marques RH, Correia L, *et al.* Multiple pilocarpine-induced status epilepticus in developing rats: a long-term behavioral and electrophysiological study. *Epilepsia* 2000; **41**(Suppl 6): S57–63.

167. Lynch M, Sayin U, Bownds J, Janumpalli S, Sutula T. Long-term consequences of early postnatal seizures on hippocampal learning and plasticity. *European Journal of Neuroscience* 2000; **12**: 2252–2264.

Seizures in the neonate

ELI M MIZRAHI

The occurrence of seizures in the neonate raises a number of concerns relating both to the neuroscience of epileptogenesis in the immature and to clinical issues of diagnosis and management. Although seizures in the neonate have been the topic of considerable basic and clinical investigations for some time and more intensively in recent years, there still remain considerable gaps in knowledge that require the clinician to develop management strategies with limited established data. These areas relate to diagnosis, pathophysiology, etiology, therapy and prognosis.

Neonatal seizures may be the first, and perhaps the only, clinical sign of the presence of a CNS disorder in the neonate. Thus, they may indicate the presence of a potentially treatable etiology and should prompt an immediate search for seizure cause and institution of appropriate therapy. The seizures themselves may require emergent therapy, since they may, either directly or indirectly, disrupt the infant's homeostasis or they may contribute to further brain injury. Seizure occurrence, and particularly the type of seizures, may have predictive value in determination of outcome.

INCIDENCE

The incidence of seizure occurrence is greatest in childhood compared to other periods of life,[1] and within the first few years of life, greatest in the neonatal period.[2] The incidence rate of seizures has been reported to be 1.5–5.5/1000 neonates,[3–8] depending on various study methodologies. Most seizures occur within the first week of life[6] (Figure 7.1). It has also been reported that seizure

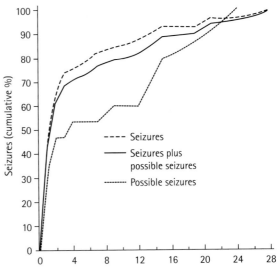

Figure 7.1 *Cumulative incidence of neonatal seizures within the first month of life. Reproduced with permission from Lippincott, Williams & Wilkins, from Lanska et al.[6]*

incidence varies with some specific risk factors. Occurrence increases in those with younger gestational age or lower birthweight. Lanska and colleagues[6] found an incidence of seizures in all neonates to be 3.5/1000 but 57.5/1000 in very low birthweight infants (<1500 g), 4.4/1000 in low birthweight infants (1500–2499 g) and 2.8/1000 in infants of normal birthweight (2500–3999 g). Scher and colleagues[9,10] reported that seizures occurred in 3.9 per cent of neonates of less than 30 weeks conceptional age and 1.5 per cent of those older than 30 weeks conceptional age.

Although the incidence of neonatal seizures may be relatively high, the occurrence of specific neonatal epileptic syndromes is quite rare. These are **benign neonatal convulsions, benign familial neonatal convulsions, early myoclonic encephalopathy** and **early epileptic encephalopathy**.[11–13]

CLINICAL FEATURES

Seizures in the neonate have clinical features that are unique when compared to those that occur in older infants and children. These differences are based on mechanisms of epileptogenesis and state of early development in the immature brain and on the relative importance of nonepileptic mechanism of seizure generation in this age group. Neonatal seizures have been classified according to clinical manifestations, the relationship between clinical seizures and electrical seizure activity on the EEG, or seizure pathophysiology.

There have been a number of clinical classifications of neonatal seizures.[14–20] Early classifications focused on the differences between neonatal seizures and those of older children: neonatal seizures were reported to be either clonic or tonic, not tonic-clonic and when focal, they were either unifocal or multifocal. Later classifications included myoclonus. A important distinction between seizures of the neonate and older children is the occurrence of events initially described as 'anarchic',[14] then 'minimal'[21] or 'subtle'.[17] These characterizations included events of oral-buccal-lingual movements such as sucking and chewing; movements of progression, such as bicycling of the legs and swimming movements of the arms; and random eye movements. These events were initially considered to be epileptic in origin, but others later suggested that they were exaggerated reflex behaviors and thus referred to them as **brain stem release phenomena** or **motor automatisms**.[19] Table 7.1 lists the clinical characteristics of neonatal seizures according to a current classification scheme.[19] This scheme can be applied through clinical observation of the infant.

Neonatal seizures may also be classified according to the temporal relationship of clinical events to the occurrence

Table 7.1 *Clinical characteristics, classification and presumed pathophysiology of neonatal seizures*

Classification	Characterization
Focal clonic	Repetitive, rhythmic contractions of muscle groups of the limbs, face or trunk
	May be unifocal or multifocal
	May occur synchronously or asynchronously in muscle groups on one side of the body
	May occur simultaneously, but asynchronously on both sides
	Cannot be suppressed by restraint
	Pathophysiology: epileptic
Focal tonic	Sustained posturing of single limbs
	Sustained asymmetrical posturing of the trunk
	Sustained eye deviation
	Cannot be provoked by stimulation or suppressed by restraint
	Pathophysiology: epileptic
Generalized tonic	Sustained symmetrical posturing of limbs, trunk and neck
	May be flexor, extensor or mixed extensor/flexor
	May be provoked or intensified by stimulation
	May be suppressed by restraint or repositioning
	Presumed pathophysiology: nonepileptic
Myoclonic	Random, single, rapid contractions of muscle groups of the limbs, face or trunk
	Typically not repetitive or may recur at a slow rate
	May be generalized, focal or fragmentary
	May be provoked by stimulation
	Presumed pathophysiology: may be epileptic or nonepileptic
Spasms	May be flexor, extensor, or mixed extensor/flexor
	May occur in clusters
	Cannot be provoked by stimulation or suppressed by restraint
	Pathophysiology: epileptic
Motor automatisms	
Ocular signs	Random and roving eye movements or nystagmus (distinct from tonic eye deviation)
	May be provoked or intensified by tactile stimulation
	Presumed pathophysiology: nonepileptic
Oral-buccal-lingual movements	Sucking, chewing, tongue protrusions
	May be provoked or intensified by stimulation

(table continued)

(table 7.1 continued)

Classification	Characterization
Progression movements	Presumed pathophysiology: nonepileptic
	Rowing or swimming movements
	Pedalling or bicycling movements of the legs
	May be provoked or intensified by stimulation
	May be suppressed by restraint or repositioning
	Presumed pathophysiology: nonepileptic
Complex purposeless movements	Sudden arousal with transient increased random activity of limbs
	May be provoked or intensified by stimulation
	Presumed pathophysiology: nonepileptic

of electrical seizure activity recorded on EEG. When the clinical event overlaps in time with electrographic seizure activity, the seizure can be described as **electroclinical**. Some clinical events that are characterized as neonatal seizures may occur in the absence of any EEG seizure activity. These events are referred to as '**clinical only**' events. Electrical seizures may occur in the absence of any clinical events and are referred to 'electrical only' seizures.

Seizures may also be classified according to their pathophysiology: epileptic or nonepileptic in origin (Table 7.2). Some seizures are clearly of epileptic origin. They occur in close association with EEG seizure activity and the clinical event cannot be provoked by stimulation of the infant and cannot be suppressed by restraint of the infant. At a basic and at a systems level they are generated by hypersynchronous cortical neuronal discharges and there are properties of the developing brain that enhance seizure initiation, maintenance and propagation: enhanced cellular excitation, enhanced synaptic excitation and tendency to enhance propagation of an epileptic discharge.[22–27] The clinical events that are most clearly epileptic in origin are: focal clonic, focal tonic, some types of myoclonic and the rare spasms (Tables 7.1 and 7.2). The electrical only seizures are, of course, also epileptic in origin.

Other seizures are best considered nonepileptic in origin.[19,28] These events occur in the absence of electrical seizure activity, but more importantly have clinical characteristics similar to reflex behaviors. These clinical events can be provoked by stimulation of the infant, and both the provoked and spontaneous events can be suppressed by restraint of the infant or by repositioning the infant during the event. In addition, the clinical events may increase in intensity with the increase in the repetition rate of stimulation (temporal summation) or the sites of simultaneous stimulation (spatial summation). The clinical events that can be classified as nonepileptic in origin are some types of myoclonic events, generalized tonic posturing and motor automatisms (Tables 7.1 and 7.2).

It has been suggested that changes related to the autonomic nervous system may also be manifestations of seizures. These include alterations in heart rate, respiration and blood pressure.[18,29–30] It has also been reported

Table 7.2 *classification of neonatal seizures based on electroclinical findings*

Clinical seizures with a consistent electrocortical signature (pathophysiology: epileptic)
Focal clonic
    Unifocal
    Multifocal
    Hemiconvulsive
    Axial
Focal tonic
    Asymmetrical truncal posturing
    Limb posturing
    Sustained eye deviation
Myoclonic
    Generalized
    Focal
Spasms
    Flexor
    Extensor
    Mixed extensor/flexor

Clinical seizures without a consistent electrocortical signature (pathophysiology: presumed nonepileptic)
Myoclonic
    Generalized
    Focal
    Fragmentary
Generalized tonic
    Flexor
    Extensor
    Mixed extensor/flexor
Motor automatisms
    Oral-buccal-lingual movements
    Ocular signs
    Progression movements
    Complex purposeless movements
Electrical seizures without clinical seizure activity

that flushing, salivation and pupil dilatation may also be signs of seizures. However, any of these findings as isolated epileptic events are rare. When they do occur, they do so most consistently in association with other clinical manifestations of seizures.[19]

Table 7.3 *Comparison* of early myoclonic encephalopathy (EME) and early infantile epileptic encephalopathy (EIEE)*

	EME	EIEE
Age of onset	Neonatal period	Within first 3 months
Neurologic status at onset	Abnormal at birth or at seizure onset	Always abnormal, even before seizure onset
Characteristic seizure type	Erratic or fragmentary myoclonus	Tonic spasm
Additional seizure types	Massive myoclonus, simple partial seizures, infantile spasms (tonic)	Focal motor seizures, hemiconvulsions, myoclonus (rare)
Background EEG	Suppression-burst	Suppression-burst
Etiology	Inborn errors of metabolism, familial, cryptogenic	Cerebral dysgenesis, anoxia, cryptogenic
Natural course	Progressive impairment	Static impairment
Incidence of death	Very high, occurring in infancy	High, occurring in infancy, childhood or adolescence
Status of survivors	Vegetative state	Severe mental retardation, quadraplegia and bed-ridden
Long-term seizure evolution	Infantile spasms	West syndrome, Lennox-Gastaut syndrome

*Based on data from Aicardi[63] and Ohtahara *et al.*[32] Reprinted with permission from Neonatal seizures: early-onset seizure syndromes and their consequences for development. Mizrahi and Clancy[12], *Mental Retardation and Developmental Disabilities Research Reviews,* © 2000. Reprinted by permission of Wiley-Liss, Inc., a subsidiary of John Wiley & Sons, Inc.

The application of a syndromic classification to neonatal seizure is somewhat limited when considered in the light of the International League Against Epilepsy classification.[11] Almost all neonatal seizures are thought to be symptomatic – occurring as a consequence of a specific etiology. Four specific syndromes occur in the neonatal period. Benign neonatal convulsions and benign familial neonatal convulsions are discussed below. Early myoclonic encephalopathy (EME)[31] and early infantile epileptic encephalopathy (EIEE)[32] are forms of catastrophic epilepsy with onset in the neonatal period, characteristic seizure types, EEG findings and etiology[33] (Table 7.3).

ELECTRODIAGNOSIS

Clinical observation is critical to the diagnosis of neonatal seizures, but the EEG is the most important laboratory examination in diagnosis. The degree of abnormality of the interictal background activity may provide information about the extent and type of CNS dysfunction associated with seizures and may also suggest the relative risk individual infants may have in eventually experiencing a seizure;[34] infants with normal background activity are less likely to eventually experience seizures than those with persistent diffuse background abnormalities. Persistent focal sharp waves may suggest focal injury; multifocal sharp waves may suggest diffuse dysfunction; and spikes may have uncertain diagnostic significance.[35] Interictal focal sharp waves and spikes typically are not considered to be indicators of epileptogenesis in the same way they are in older children and adults. Thus, this interictal finding may not be as useful in predicting which patients may eventually experience seizures as neonates rather than later in childhood.

Electrical seizure activity in the neonatal may have varied manifestations and is thought to be rare before 34–35 weeks conceptional age. Frequency, voltage and morphology of the discharges may change within an individual seizure and between seizures in an individual infant. The duration of seizure discharges may also vary; they can be quite long although the minimum duration has been designated as 10 s.[36] The electrical events are typically focal and well circumscribed, most often arising in the central or centrotemporal region of one hemisphere and less commonly in the occipital, frontal or midline central regions. The seizures may arise focally and remain confined to that region, or may spread by a gradual widening of the focal area; by abrupt changes from a small regional focus to involvement of the entire hemisphere (so-called **hemiconvulsive seizure**); by migration of the electrical seizure from one area of a hemisphere to another (Figure 7.2); or from one hemisphere to another.[37]

Some ictal patterns are unique to the neonatal period and are typically associated with severe encephalopathies. Electrical seizures of the depressed brain[35] are typically low in voltage, long in duration and highly localized (Figure 7.3). They may be unifocal or multifocal and show little tendency to spread or modulate. They are typically not associated with clinical seizures, occur when the EEG background is depressed and undifferentiated, and suggest a poor prognosis. Alpha seizure activity[38–40] is characterized by a sudden, but transient appearance of rhythmic activity of the α frequency (8–12 Hz) typically in the temporal or central region. Clinical events usually do not occur with these discharges. The presence of an alpha seizure discharge usually indicates the presence of a severe encephalopathy and poor prognosis (Figure 7.4).

EEG-video monitoring of neonates has been the basis of clinical investigations that have addressed classification, therapy and prognosis.[19,41–45] Although it is a powerful tool in diagnosis, it is not available at most centers for routine use. Thus, attended EEG with simultaneous observation by trained electroneurodiagnostic technologists who can carefully observe infants and characterize events remains the standard of care.

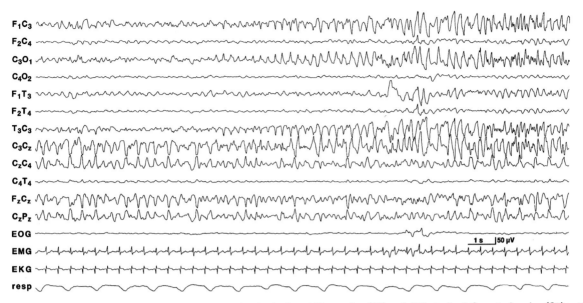

Figure 7.2 *Migration of electrical seizure activity that begins in the midline region (CZ) and shifts to the left central region (C3) as the CZ region becomes less involved. This EEG was recorded from a 4-day-old, 40-week gestational age female infant with hypoxic-ischemic encephalopathy and suppression-burst EEG background. No clinical seizures were present during the electrical seizure activity. From Mizrahi and Kellaway.*[37]

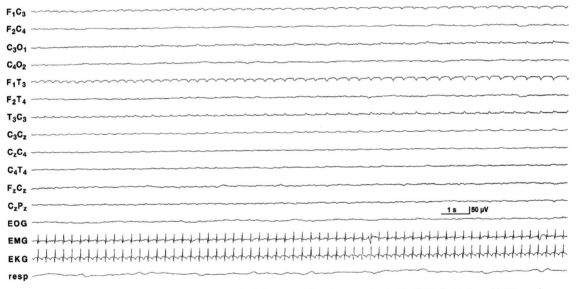

Figure 7.3 *Seizure discharge of the depressed brain in the left temporal region occuring in the EEG of a 2-day-old, 38-week gestational aged female infant with hypoxic-ischemic encephalopathy. The EEG background is depressed and undifferentiated. No clinical seizures accompanied the electrical seizure activity. From Mizrahi and Kellaway.*[37]

ETIOLOGY

There is a wide range of possible etiologic factors of neonatal seizures. This, in association with the predisposition of the immature brain towards epileptogenesis, may account for the high incidence of seizures in the neonate. Most etiologic factors can be broadly categorized as: hypoxia-ischemia, metabolic disturbances, CNS or systemic infections and structural brain lesions. Table 7.4 lists the most frequently identified etiologies of neonatal seizures; more comprehensive lists can be found elsewhere.[37]

The diagnosis of **hypoxic-ischemic encephalopathy** is fraught with difficulty because criteria may vary among institutions and because established criteria may be too restrictive or may not predict the occurrence of long-term neurologic sequelae.[46–48] The American College of

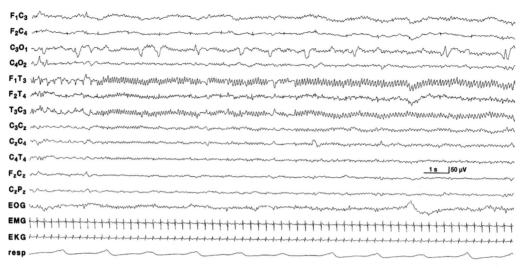

Figure 7.4 *Alpha seizure discharge in the left temporal region is characterized by sinusoidal 10–11-Hz rhythmic activity that evolved from rhythmic sharp-wave activity. There is also an independent, repetitive, slow, sharp transient in the left occipital region. The EEG background activity is depressed and undifferentiated. This EEG was recorded from a 4-week-old, 38-week gestational aged male infant with pneumococcal meningitis. No clinical seizures occurred with these electrical seizure discharges. From Mizrahi and Kellaway.[37]*

Obstetricians and Gynecologists, in association with the American Academy of Pediatrics, has provided guidelines for the diagnosis of hypoxic-ischemic encephalopathy.[49] At some centers, current practice is directed towards the identification of measures of asphyxia that have predictive value in the occurrence of long-term sequelae[50] and that have less restrictive criteria for hypoxic-ischemic encephalopathy. Both approaches include the tabulation of delivery room Apgar scores and need for resuscitation, recognition of clinical aspects of encephalopathy, and indication of multisystem involvement.

Metabolic disturbances may also be associated with neonatal seizures and represent an important group of potentially treatable etiologies. These include **hypocalcemia**, **hypomagnesemia** and **hypoglycemia**. Much less frequent is the finding of an inborn error of metabolism such as an aminoaciduria, urea cycle defect or organic aciduria. Other rare causes of medically refractory neonatal seizures that are potentially treatable include pyridoxine deficiency (which is exceedingly rare) and biotinidase deficiency (also a rare disorder) (see Chapter 4E).

Both bacterial and viral agents can be causes of **CNS infection** in the neonate that are associated with seizures. In addition, prenatal infections can also be risk factors for seizures. **Structural brain lesions** associated with neonatal seizures include hemorrhage (intracerebral, subarachnoid, intraventricular), infarctions, and congenital anomalies of the brain. Brain malformations may range from highly localized focal dysplasias to catastrophic defects.

Genetically determined neonatal seizures have received considerable attention since benign familial neonatal convulsions were shown to have a pattern of autosomal

Table 7.4 *Most frequently occurring etiologies of neonatal seizures[a]*

Hypoxia-ischemia
Intracranial hemorrhage
   Intraventricular
   Intracerebral
   Subdural
   Subarachnoid
Infection – CNS
   Meningitis
   Encephalitis
   Intrauterine
Infarction
Metabolic
   Hypoglycemia
   Hypocalcemia
   Hypomagnesemia
Chromosomal anomalies
Congenital abnormalities of the brain
Neurodegenerative disorders
Inborn errors of metabolism
Benign neonatal convulsions
Benign familial neonatal convulsions
Drug withdrawal or intoxication

[a] Listed in relative order of frequency. Not listed is 'unknown' etiology, which is encountered in approximately 10 per cent of cases (although some in this category may be benign neonatal convulsions). From Mizrahi and Kellaway.[37]

transmission based at a locus on chromosome 20.[51,52] Singh and colleagues[53] identified a submicroscopic deletion of chromosome 20q13.3 and encoded a novel voltage-gated potassium channel, KCNQ2, as the basis of this disorder. This disorder is now considered to be one of several

Table 7.5 *Etiology-specific therapy for neonatal seizures of metabolic origin*

	Acute therapy	Maintenance therapy
Glucose, 10% solution	2 mL/kg, IV	Up to 8 mg/kg/min, IV
Calcium gluconate, 10% solution (9.4 mg of elemental Ca/mL)	2 mL/kg IV over 10 min (18 mg of elemental Ca/kg)	8 m/kg/day IV[a] (75 mg of elemental Ca/k per day)
Magnesium sulfate, 50% solution (50 mg of elemental Mg/mL)	0.25 mL/kg, IM	0.25 ml/kg IM repeated every 12 h until normomagnesemia
Pyridoxine	100 mg, IV	

[a] After restoration of normocalcemia, tapering dosage may help in preventing rebound hypocalcemia.
Diagnosis of hypoglycemia, hypocalcemia and hypomagnesium may vary between laboratories and is dependent on a neonate's gestational age (with preterm infants tending to tolerate lower physiologic levels). Administration of metabolic correcting solutions requires careful monitoring of infant's systemic homeostasis, including ECG monitoring during administration of calcium.[66,67] From Mizrahi and Kellaway.[37]

epileptic disorders characterized as a channelopathy.[54–58] Benign familial neonatal convulsions had been considered to be benign because initial reports suggested no long-term neurologic sequelae. However subsequent studies indicate that not all affected infants have a normal outcome.[59]

Some neonatal seizures are considered **idiopathic** since no cause can be identified and there are no long-term sequelae. Some such affected infants are thought to have benign neonatal convulsions.[60–62] The infants are typically full term and products of normal pregnancy and delivery. The seizures are usually brief, most often clonic, and have their onset between days 4 and 6 of life.

THERAPY

Comprehensive therapy of neonatal seizures begins with the application of the principles of general management since some seizures may be associated with changes in respiration, heart rate and blood pressure. In addition, antiepileptic drug (AED) therapy may also be associated with these types of changes. Thus strategies to ensure airway and obtain access to the circulatory system are considered early in the course of treatment.

If specific causes of seizures are identified that have specific treatment, such therapy is initiated. This may be critical in seizure management since some seizures may not be controlled effectively with AEDs unless their underlying cause is treated. This is particularly evident when seizures are caused by metabolic disturbances such as hypocalcemia, hypomagnesemia and hypoglycemia. Etiologic-specific therapies for these disorders are listed in Table 7.5. Although the treatment of some etiologies may not immediately affect seizure occurrence, therapy is still critical since it may limit the degree of CNS injury; for example in cases of CNS infection.

Before considering specific AED agents, factors that may prompt the institution of AED therapy are typically considered. AEDs are used to treat neonatal seizures of epileptic origin. Thus, initial considerations are given to the clinical and EEG features of the events. In addition, there has been discussion concerning the need to treat all neonatal seizures of epileptic origin since some are brief, infrequent and self-limited, occurring only in reaction to an acute CNS insult. In these instances, no AED may be warranted and the infant need not be exposed to acute and chronic AED therapy. On the other hand, some neonatal epileptic seizures are long in duration, frequent and not self-limited. These are treated acutely and vigorously with AEDs. The clinical difficulty arises in the management of those infants whose seizures have characteristics that fall between these two extremes. Currently, almost all neonatal epileptic seizures within this intermediate category are treated with AEDs.

First-line AEDs and dosing schedules are listed in Table 7.6. The individual drugs have been well studied in neonates, but there have been few comprehensive clinical trials conducted to specify the most effective regimen, with notable exceptions.[68] The traditional strategy is to acutely treat seizures with an AED that can be subsequently given as maintenance therapy. Phenobarbital is most frequently used as the initial drug, followed by phenytoin. As an alternative to phenytoin, fosphenytoin may be used because of reports of reduced adverse effects with acute administration.[69] An alternative strategy of seizure management is acute treatment with repeated doses of short-acting benzodiazepines until seizures are controlled, thus avoiding chronic AED therapy.

The decision to institute acute therapy is accompanied by recognition of criteria to determine whether the therapy has been successful. However, this may be difficult. A typical response by electroclinical seizures to acute AED therapy is the initial control of the clinical seizures with the persistence of the electrical seizure activity.[19,70] With additional doses the electrical seizures may be controlled. However, there are also instances in which the EEG seizures cannot be controlled despite increasing doses of the initial AED and addition of others. Current practice consists of acute AED therapy until clinical seizures are controlled, with the first AED given to serum levels in the

Table 7.6 *Dosages of first-line and second-line AEDs in the treatment of neonatal seizures*

Drug	Dose Loading	Maintenance	Average therapeutic range	Apparent half-life
Diazepam	0.25 mg/IV (bolus) 0.5 mg/kg (rectal)	May be repeated 1–2 times		31–54 h
Lorazepam	0.05 mg/kg (IV) (over 2–5 min)	May be repeated		31–54 h
Phenobarbital	20 mg/kg IV (up to 40 mg)	3–4 mg/kg in 2 doses	20–40 µg/ml/ (85–170 µmol/L)	100 h after day 5–7
Phenytoin	20 mg/kg IV (over 30–45 min)	3–4 mg/kg in 2–4 doses	15–25 µg/ml (60–100 µmol/L)	100 h (40–200)

Based on data from Aicardi[63], Fenichel[64] and Volpe.[65] From Mizrahi and Kellaway.[37]

high theraputic range or maximum tolerated dose followed by the second – benzodiazepines are also given is needed. If EEG is utilized, the same AED strategy is followed, although the AEDs are only given to high therapeutic range – since the electrical seizure discharges are most often resistant to further AED therapy, additional drugs are not given in order to avoid adverse effects without significant benefit.

The use of phenobarbital and phenytoin in the neonate require additional knowledge concerning their pharmacologic characteristics that are summarized here but described in detail elsewhere.[71–74] Phenobarbital is a weak acid and is protein bound. Thus infants with acidosis may have less active AED available and those with hypoalbuminemia may have greater unbound or active drug available. Both conditions may be found in sick neonates. Phenobarbital is eliminated by the liver and kidney, so infants with impaired hepatic or renal function, such as those with HIE, will have a reduced rate of elimination and potential for toxicity with standard dosing. There is a greater half-life of phenobarbital in premature compared to term infants and in term infants it is reduced with chronologic age in the first month of life. Thus in premature infants there is a potential for higher serum levels with standard doses and the potential for toxicity; as the infant becomes older there is the potential for identical doses to result in lower serum levels and creating the potential for breakthrough seizures with no other change in the infants clinical condition. Overall, monitoring trends of serum levels rather than day-to-day fluctuations is more useful in management of phenobarbital therapy.[65,74–77]

The most significant pharmacologic characteristic of phenytoin is its nonlinear pharmacokinetics: steady-state plasma concentrations at one dosing schedule do not directly predict the steady-state concentrations at another schedule[78,79] There is also a variable rate of hepatic metabolism, a decrease in elimination rates during the first weeks of life and a variable bioavailability of the drug with various generic preparations. In addition, there is a redistribution of the AED after the initial dose, resulting in a drop in brain concentrations after the first dose. Thus, phenytoin use requires individualization of dosing after initiation therapy.

Second-line, alternative or adjuvant AEDs have been utilized either intravenously or orally with limited success in the control of other medically refractory neonatal seizures. Those given intravenously include clonazepam,[80] lidocaine,[81] midazolam[82] and paraldehyde.[83] Those given orally include carbamazepine,[84] primidone,[85] valproic acid,[86] vigabatrin[87] and lamotrigine.[88]

Not all neonates will require chronic therapy after acute seizures have been controlled, although there are no well-defined criteria for maintenance AED treatment. When chronic therapy is selected maintenance doses of either phenobarbital or phenytoin are given of 3–4 mg/kg per day and serum levels are monitored. There are also no well-established criteria for discontinuation of maintenance AED therapy. Reported schedules range from 1 week up to 12 months after the last seizure,[89] although a currently utilized schedule is to withdraw AEDs 2 weeks after the infant's last seizure.[90]

PROGNOSIS

The outcome of infants with neonatal seizures has been assessed in terms of survival, neurological disability, developmental delay and postneonatal epilepsy. Ortibus and colleagues reported that 28 per cent of those with neonatal seizures died; 22 per cent of survivors were neurologically normal at an average of 17 months of age; 14 per cent had mild abnormalities and 36 per cent had severe abnormalities.[91] In a prospective study of full-term infants 2 years after neonatal seizures, Mizrahi and colleagues found that 25 per cent died and 25 per cent of the survivors had abnormal neurological examinations; 25 per cent had developmental delay (Bayley Developmental Assessment of Mental Development Index and Psychomotor Developmental Index <80) and 25 per cent had postneonatal epilepsy.[92] Brunquell and colleagues found that 30 per cent of those with neonatal seizures died and 59 per cent of survivors had abnormal neurological examinations, 40 per cent were mentally retarded, 43 per cent had cerebral palsy and 21 per cent had postneonatal epilepsy when followed up to a mean of 3.5 years.[93]

Postneonatal epilepsy is of particular interest. Ellenberg and colleagues found approximately 20 per cent of those who survived neonatal seizures experienced one or more seizures up to 7 years of age, nearly two thirds occurring within the first 6 months of life.[94] Similar rates were found by Ortibus and colleagues (28 per cent);[91] Bye and colleagues (21 per cent);[44] Scher and colleagues (17–30 per cent);[9] Mizrahi and colleagues (25 per cent);[92] and Brunquell *et al.* (21 per cent).[93] Clancy and Legido found a higher rate of postneonatal epilepsy (56 per cent) although their study population had relatively high risk factors for CNS dysfunction.[95] Both partial and generalized seizures characterize postneonatal epilepsy. Watanabe and colleagues considered in detail a selected population of infants with neonatal seizures that persisted and could be classified as epilepsy of neonatal onset.[96] For most of those infants with severe encephalopathy syndromes such as early epileptic encephalopathy and early myoclonic encephalopathy, their initial epileptic syndrome evolved to West syndrome with a fewer number evolving to symptomatic localization-related epilepsy.

The goals of acute management of neonatal seizures are rapid diagnosis, identification of etiology, institution of etiologic-specific therapy and successful AED treatment in order to prevent adverse sequelae and to improve long-term outcomes. However, both basic science and clinical investigations have yet to conclude which of these goals is the critical factor that will improve prognosis. There has been controversy, based on basic research, about the degree to which seizure activity may effect the developing brain.[27] Immature animals are more resistant than older animals to some seizure-induced injury.[26] Although the immature brain may be resistant to acute seizure-induced cell loss, there are functional abnormalities that follow seizures such as impairment of visual-spatial memory and reduced seizure threshold, and there are seizure-induced changes in brain development including altered synaptogenesis and reduction in neurogenesis.[97,98]

Clinical studies are more difficult to interpret in order to determine whether seizures adversely affect the developing brain. It may appear that seizure duration may influence outcome, since infants who experience brief and infrequent seizures may have a relatively good long-term outcomes, whereas those with prolonged seizures may not do as well. However, seizures that are easily controlled or self-limited may be the result of transient, successfully treated or benign CNS disorders of neonates whereas medically refractory neonatal seizures may be the result of more sustained, less treatable or more severe brain disorders. However, it has been demonstrated that there is a relationship between a greater amount of electrographic seizure activity and subsequent, relative increased mortality and morbidity in at-risk infants in general and in infants with perinatal asphyxia.[99] In addition, other investigators, using proton MRS in neonates, found an association of seizure severity with impaired cerebral metabolism measured by lactate/choline and compromised neuronal intergrity measured by *N*-acetylaspartate/choline and suggested this

Table 7.7 *Prognosis of neonatal seizures according to neurologic disorder*

Neurologic disorder	Normal development (%)[a]
Hypoxic-ischemic encephalopathy	50
Intraventricular hemorrhage[b]	10
Primary subarachnoid hemorrhage	90
Hypocalcemia	
Early onset	50[c]
Late onset	100
Hypoglycemia	50
Bacterial meningitis	50
Developmental brain defect	0

Prognosis is for those with the stated neurologic disease when seizures are a manifestation (thus, value usually differs from overall prognosis).
[a] Values are rounded to the nearest 5 per cent.
[b] Usually severe intraventricular hemorrhage associated with major periventricular hemorrhagic infarction.
[c] Represents primarily the prognosis of complicating illness; prognosis approaches that of later onset hypocalcemia if no or only minor neurologic illness present.
Reprinted from Volpe[65] with permission from Elsevier.

to be evidence of brain injury not limited to structural damage detected by MRI.[100]

However, the dominant factor that appears to predict outcome may be the underlying cause of the seizures rather than the presence, duration or degree of brain involvement of the epileptic seizures themselves. Mizrahi and Kellaway[37] analyzed a number of clinical studies that indicated that normal outcomes occurred with increasing frequency in association with the following etiologies: HIE, infection, hemorrhage, hypoglycemia and hypocalcemia.[4,9,15,16,101–103] In discussing prognosis, Volpe[65] emphasized the factors of gestational age and etiology on outcome (Table 7.7). Mortality increases with the greater degree of prematurity and specific etiologies are associated with varying degrees of developmental delay.

It has also been suggested that seizure type may also predict outcome.[37] Focal clonic and focal tonic seizures are suggested to have a relatively good outcome primarily because these are typically associated with relatively confined brain injury and spared CNS function. Generalized tonic posturing and motor automatisms suggest a poor outcome since they are associated with diffuse CNS dysfunction. Brunquell and colleagues have demonstrated similar findings in long-term studies.[93]

Multivariant analysis has been applied in attempts to more precisely define predictors of outcome of those who have experienced neonatal seizures. Factors considered have been features of the interictal EEG from one or serial recordings; the ictal EEG; the neurological examination at the time of seizures; the character or duration of the seizures; etiology; findings on neuroimaging; conceptional age and birthweight. Multiple rather than single factors appear to be most accurate in predicting outcome. For example, Ortibus and colleagues found that the predicted outcome is less reliable when based solely on EEG variables from a single recording obtained at seizure onset than when based on a combination of imaging findings, clinical and EEG data.[91] However, all variables related to a single factor – the degree of brain injury at the time of seizure occurrence, and this, in turn, related to etiology.

KEY POINTS

- Neonatal seizures may be the only clinical sign of a **CNS disorder** in the neonate and should prompt an immediate search for the seizure cause and institution of appropriate therapy
- Neonatal seizures themselves may contribute to further brain injury and require **emergent therapy**
- Neonatal seizure occurrence, particularly the type of seizure, may have **predictive value** in determination of outcome
- Although the incidence of neonatal seizures is relatively high, the occurrence of specific **neonatal epileptic syndromes** is quite rare. These syndromes are **benign neonatal convulsions, benign familial neonatal convulsions, early myoclonic encephalopathy**, and **early epileptic encephalopathy**
- The most common etiologies of neonatal seizures are **hypoxia-ischemia, metabolic disturbances, CNS or systemic infections** and **structural brain lesions**
- The goals of **acute management of neonatal seizures** are rapid diagnosis, identification of etiology, institution of etiologic-specific therapy and successful AED treatment

---

ACKNOWLEDGMENTS

Supported in part by Contract Number NS-0-1234, National Institutes of Neurological Disorders and Stroke, National Institutes of Health, Bethesda, MD, USA and the Peter Kellaway Research Endowment, Baylor College of Medicine, Houston, Texas, USA.

REFERENCES

1. Hauser WA, Hesdorffer DC. *Epilepsy: Frequency, Causes and Consequences.* New York, Demos Publications, 1990, 378.
2. Kellaway P, Hrachovy RA. Status epilepticus in newborns: a perspective on neonatal seizures. In: Delgado-Escueta AV, Wasterlain CG, Treiman DM, Porter RJ (eds) *Advances in Neurology*, Vol. 34: *Status Epilepticus.* New York: Raven Press, 1983: 93–99.
3. Eriksson M, Zetterström R. Neonatal convulsions. Incidence and causes in the Stockholm area. *Acta Paediatrica Scandinavica* 1979; **68**: 807–811.
4. Bergman I, Painter MJ, Hirsch RP, Crumrine PK, David R. Outcome in neonates with convulsions treated in an intensive care unit. *Annals of Neurology* 1983; **14**: 642–647.
5. Spellacy WN, Peterson PQ, Winegar A, *et al.* Neonatal seizures after cesarean delivery: higher risk with labor. *American Journal of Obstetrics and Gynecology* 1987; **157**: 377–379.
6. Lanska MJ, Lanska DJ, Baumann RJ, *et al.* A population-based study of neonatal seizures in Fayette County, Kentucky. *Neurology* 1995; **45**: 724–732.
7. Ronen GM, Penney S. The epidemiology of clinical neonatal seizures in Newfoundland, Canada: A five-year cohort. *Annals of Neurology* 1995; **38**: 518–519.
8. Saliba RM, Annegers JF, Waller DK, Tyson JE, Mizrahi EM. Incidence of neonatal seizures in Harris County, Texas, 1992–1994. *American Journal of Epidemiology* 1999; **150**(7): 763–769.
9. Scher MS, Aso K, Beggarly M, *et al.* Electrographic seizures in preterm and full-term neonates: Clinical correlates, associated brain lesions, and risk for neurologic sequelae. *Pediatrics* 1993; **91**: 128–134.
10. Scher MS, Hamid MY, Steppe DA, Beggarly ME, Painter MJ. Ictal and interictal electrographic seizure durations in preterm and term neonates. *Epilepsia* 1993; **34**: 284–288.
11. Commission on Classification and Terminology of the International League Against Epilepsy. Proposal for revised clinical and classification of epilepsies and epileptic syndromes. *Epilepsia* 1989; **30**: 389–399.
12. Mizrahi EM, Clancy RR. Neonatal seizures: early-onset seizure syndromes and their consequences for development. *Mental Retardation and Developmental Disabilities Research Reviews* 2000: **6**: 229–241.
13. Tharp, BR. Neonatal seizures and syndromes. *Epilepsia* 2002; **43**(Suppl 3): 2–10.
14. Dreyfus-Brisac C, Monod N. Electroclinical studies of status epilepticus and convulsions in the newborn. In: Kellaway P, Petersén I (eds) *Neurological and Electroencephalographic Correlative Studies in Infancy.* New York: Grune and Stratton, 1964: 250–272.
15. Rose AL, Lombroso CT. A study of clinical, pathological, and electroencephalographic features in 137 full-term babies with a long-term follow-up. *Pediatrics* 1970; **45**: 404–425.
16. Lombroso CT. Prognosis in neonatal seizures. *Advances in Neurology* 1983; **34**: 101–113.
17. Volpe JJ. Neonatal seizures. *New England Journal of Medicine* 1973; **289**: 413–416.
18. Watanabe K, Hara K, Miyazaki S, *et al.* Electroclinical studies of seizures in the newborn. *Folia Psychiatrica et Neurologica Japonica* 1977; **31**: 383–392.
19. Mizrahi EM, Kellaway P. Characterization and classification of neonatal seizures. *Neurology* 1987; **37**: 1837–1844.
20. Volpe JJ. Neonatal seizures: Current concepts and revised classification. *Pediatrics* 1989; **84**: 422–428.
21. Lombroso CT. Seizures in the newborn. In: Vinken PJ, Bruyn GW (eds), *The Epilepsies. Handbook of Clinical Neurophysiology, Vol 15.* Amsterdam: North-Holland, 1974: 189–218.

22. Hablitz JJ, Lee WL, Prince DA, *et al*. III. Excitatory amino acids NMDA receptor involvement in epileptogenesis in the immature neocortex. In: Avanzini G, Engel J, Fariello R. *et al*. (eds), *Neurotransmitters in Epilepsy (Epilepsy Research Suppl 8)*. New York: Elsevier Science, 1992.

23. Prince DA. Basic mechanisms of focal epileptogenesis. In: Avanzini G, Fariello R, Heinemann U, Mutani R (eds), *Epileptogenic and Excitotoxic Mechanisms*. London, John Libbey, 1993: 17–27.

24. Moshé SL. Seizures in the developing brain. *Neurology* 1993; **43**: S3–7.

25. Schwartzkroin PA. Plasticity and repair in the immature central nervous system. In: Schwartzkroin PA, Moshé SL, Noebels JL, Swann JW (eds), *Brain Development and Epilepsy*. New York: Oxford University Press, 1995: 234–267.

26. Swann JW. Synaptogenesis and epileptogenesis in developing neural networks. In: Schwartzkroin PA, Moshé SL, Noebels JL, Swann JW (eds), *Brain Development and Epilepsy*. New York: Oxford University Press, 1995: 195–233.

27. Holmes GL. Epilepsy in the developing brain: Lessons from the laboratory and clinic. *Epilepsia* 1997; **38**: 12–30.

28. Kellaway P, Hrachovy RA. Status epilepticus newborns; A perspective on neonatal seizures. *Adv Neurol* 1983; **34**: 93–99.

29. Lou HC, Friis-Hansen B. Arterial blood pressure elevations during motor activity and epileptic seizures in the newborn. *Acta Paediatrica Scandinavica* 1979; **68**: 803–806.

30. Goldberg RN, Goldman SL, Ramsay RE, *et al*. Detection of seizure activity in the paralyzed neonate using continuous monitoring. *Pediatrics* 1982; **69**: 583–586.

31. Aicardi J, Goutiéres F. Encéphalopathie myoclonique néonatale. *Revue d'Electroencephalographie et Neurophysiologie Clinique* 1978; **8**: 99–101.

32. Ohtahara S, Ohtsuka Y, Yamatogi Y, Oka E, Inoue H. Early-infantile epileptic encephalopathy with suppression-bursts. In: Roger J, Bureau M, Dravet Ch, Dreifuss FE, Perret A, Wolf P (eds), *Epileptic Syndromes in Infancy, Childhood and Adolescence*, 2nd edn. London: John Libbey, 1992: 25–34.

33. Aicardi J, Ohtara S. Severe neonatal epilepsies with suppression-burst pattern. In: Roger J, Bureau M, Dravet C. *et al*. (eds), *Epileptic Syndromes in Infancy, Childhood and Adolescence*, 3rd edn. London: John Libbey 2002: 33–44.

34. Laroia N, Guillet R, Burchfiel J, McBride MC. EEG background as predictor of electrographic seizures in high-risk neonates. *Epilepsia* 1998; **39**: 545–551.

35. Hrachovy RA, Mizrahi EM, Kellaway P. Electroencephalography of the newborn. In: Daly D, Pedley TA (eds), *Current Practice of Clinical Electroencephalography*, 2nd edn. New York: Raven Press, 1990: 201

36. Clancy RR, Legido A. The exact ictal and interictal duration of electroencephalographic neonatal seizures. *Epilepsia* 1987; **28**: 537–541.

37. Mizrahi EM, Kellaway P. *Diagnosis and Management of Neonatal Seizures*. Philadelphia: Lippincott-Raven, 1998: 181.

38. Knauss TA, Carlson CB. Neonatal paroxysmal monorhythmic alpha activity. *Archives of Neurology* 1978; **35**: 104–107.

39. Willis J, Gould JB. Periodic alpha seizures with apnea in a newborn. *Developmental Medicine and Child Neurology* 1980; **22**: 214–222.

40. Watanabe K, Hara K, Miyazaki S, Hakamada S, Kuroyanagi M. Apneic seizures in the newborn. *American Journal of Disease of Children* 1982; **136**: 980–984.

41. Mizrahi EM. Electroencephalographic-video monitoring in neonates, infants, and children. *Journal of Child Neurology* 1994; **9**(Suppl): S46–56.

42. Boylan GB, Pressler RM, Rennie JM, *et al*. Outcome of electroclinical, electrographic, and clinical seizures in the newborn infant. *Developmental Medicine and Child Neurology* 1999; **41**: 819–825.

43. Boylan, GB, Rennie, JM, Pressler RM, *et al*. Phenobarbitone, neonatal seizures, and video-EEG. *Archives of Disease in Childhood. Fetal and Neonatal Edition* 2002; **86F**: 165–170.

44. Bye AM, Cunningham CA, Chee KY, Flanagan D. Outcome of neonates with electrographically identified seizures, or at risk of seizures. *Pediatric Neurology* 1997; **16**(3): 225–231.

45. Rennie, JM. Neonatal seizures. *European Journal of Pediatrics* 1997; **156**: 83–87.

46. Nelson KB, Leviton A. How much of neonatal encephalopathy is due to birth asphyxia? *American Journal of Diseases of Children* 1991; **145**: 1325–1331.

47. Paneth N. The causes of cerebral palsy. Recent evidence. *Clinical and Investigative Medicine* 1993; **16**: 95–102.

48. Leviton A, Nelson KB. Problems with definitions and classifications of newborn encephalopathy. *Pediatric Neurology* 1992; **8**: 85–90.

49. Committee on Obstetric Practice and American Academy of Pediatrics: Committee on Fetus and Newborn. ACOG committee opinion. Use and abuse of the Apgar score. Number 174, July 1996. American College of Obstetricians and Gynecologists. *International Journal of Gynaecology and Obstetrics* 1996; **54**: 303–305.

50. Perlman JM. Intrapartum hypoxic-ischemic cerebral injury and subsequent cerebral palsy: Medicolegal issues. *Pediatrics* 1997; **99**: 851–859.

51. Quattlebaum TG. Benign familial convulsions in the neonatal period and early infancy. *Journal of Pediatrics* 1979; **95**: 257–259.

52. Leppert M, Anderson VE, Quattlebaum TG, *et al*. Benign familial neonatal convulsions linked to genetic markers on chromosome 20. *Nature* 1989; **337**: 647–648.

53. Singh NA, Charlier C, Stauffer D, *et al*. A novel potassium channel gene, KCNQ2, is mutated in an inherited epilepsy of newborns. *Nature Genetics* 1998 **18**(1): 25–29.

54. Noebels JL. Ion channelopathies and heritable epilepsy. *News in Physiological Sciences* 1998; **13**(Oct) 255–256.

55. Noebels J. Exploring new gene discoveries in idiopathic generalized epilepsy. *Epilepsia* 2003; **44**(Suppl 2): 16–21.

56. Leppert M. A novel potassium channel gene, KCNQ2, is mutated in an inherited epilepsy of newborns. *Nature Genetics* 1998; **18**(1): 25–29.

57. Leppert M. Novel K$^+$ channel genes in benign familial neonatal convulsions. *Epilepsia* 2000; **41**(8): 1066–1067.

58. Leppert M, Singh N. Benign familial neonatal epilepsy with mutations in two potassium channel genes. *Current Opinion in Neurology* 1999; **12**(2): 143–147.

59. Ronen GM, Rosales TO, Connolly M, *et al*. Seizure characteristics in chromosome 20 benign familial neonatal convulsions. *Neurology* 1993; **43**: 1355–1360.

60. Plouin P. Benign neonatal convulsions. In: Wasterlain CG, Vert P (eds) *Neonatal Seizures*. New York: Raven Press, 1990, pp. 51–59.

61. Plouin P. Benign idiopathic neonatal convulsions. In Roger J, Bureau M, Dravet C, *et al*. (eds), *Epileptic Syndromes in Infancy, Childhood and Adolescence*, 2nd edn. London: John Libbey, 1992: 3–11.

Derby Hospitals NHS Foundation
Trust
Library and Knowledge Service

62. Plouin P, Anderson VE. Benign familial and non-familial neonatal seizures. In: Roger J, Bureau M, Dravet C, *et al.* (eds) *Epileptic Syndromes in Infancy, Childhood and Adolescence*, 3rd edn. London: John Libbey, 2002: 3–13.

63. Aicardi J. Neonatal seizures. In: *Epilepsy in Children*, 2nd edn. International Review of Child Neurology Series. New York: Raven Press, 1994: 217–252.

64. Fenichel GM. *Neonatal Neurology.* New York: Churchill Livingstone, 1990, 261.

65. Volpe JJ. *Neurology of the Newborn,* Chapter 5, Neonatal Seizures. Philadelphia: W.B. Saunders, 1995: 172–207.

66. Kalhan S, Saker F. Metabolic and endocrine disorders. In Fanaroff AA, Martin RJ (eds), *Neonatal-Perinatal Medicine: Diseases of the Fetus and Infant.* New York: Mosby, 1997: 1439–1563.

67. Koo WW, Tsang RC. Calcium and magnesium homeostasis. In: Avery GB, Fletcher MA, MacDonald MB (eds), *Neonatal: Pathophysiology and Management of the Newborn.* Philadelphia: Lippincott, 1994: 585–604.

68. Painter MJ, Scher MS, Stein AD, *et al.* Phenobarbital compared with phenytoin for the treatment of neonatal seizures. *New England Journal of Medicine* 1999; **341**: 485–489.

69. Pellock JM Fosphenytoin use in children. *Neurology* 1996; **46**(6)(Suppl 1): S14–16.

70. Mizrahi EM, Kellaway P. The response of electroclinical neonatal seizures to antiepileptic drug therapy. *Epilepsia* 1992; **33**(Suppl 3): 114.

71. Levy RA, Mattson RH, Meldrum (eds) *Antiepileptic Drugs*, 4th edn. New York: Raven Press, 1995.

72. DeLorenzo RJ. Phenytoin. Mechanisms of action. In: Levy RH, Mattson RH, Meldrum BS (eds), *Antiepileptic Drugs*, 4th edn. New York: Raven Press, 1995: 271–282.

73. Macdonald RL. Benzodiazepines. In: Levy RH, Mattson RH, Meldrum BS (eds), *Antiepileptic Drugs*, 4th edn. New York: Raven Press, 1995: 695–703.

74. Painter MJ, Gaus LM. Phenobarbital: Clinical use. In: Levy H, Mattson RH, Meldrum BS (eds), *Antiepileptic Drugs*, 4th edn. New York: Raven Press, 1995: 401–407.

75. Painter MJ, Pippenger C, MacDonald H, Pitlick W. Phenobarbital and diphenylhydantoin levels in neonates with seizures. *Journal of Pediatrics* 1978; **92**: 315–319.

76. Gal P, Toback J, Boer HR, Erkan NV, Wells TJ. Efficacy of phenobarbital monotherapy in treatment of neonatal seizures – relationship to blood levels. *Neurology* 1982; **32**: 1401–1404.

77. Donn SM, Grasela TH, Goldstein GW. Safety of a higher loading dose of phenobarbital in the term newborn. *Pediatrics* 1985; **75**: 1061–64.

78. Bourgeois BFD, Dodson WE. Phenytoin elimination in newborns. *Neurology* 1983; **33**: 173–178.

79. Dodson WE. Antiepileptic drug utilization in pediatric patients. *Epilepsia* 1984; **25**: S132–139.

80. André M, Boutray MJ, Dubruc O, *et al.* Clonazepam pharmacokinetics and therapeutic efficacy in neonatal seizures. *European Journal of Clinical Pharmacology* 1986; **305**: 585–589.

81. Hellström-Westas L, Westgren U, Rosen I, Svenningsen NW. Lidocaine for treatment of severe seizures in newborn infants. I. Clinical effects and cerebral electrical activity monitoring. *Acta Paediatrica Scandinavica* 1988; **77**: 79–84.

82. Sheth RD, Buckley DJ, Gutierrez AR *et al* Midazolam in the treatment of refractory neonatal seizures. *Clinical Neuropharmacology* 1996; **19**: 165–170.

83. Koren G, Warwick B, Rajchgot R, *et al.* Intravenous paraldehyde for seizure control in newborn infants. *Neurology* 1986; **36**: 108–111.

84. Mackintosh DA, Baird-Lampert J, Buchanan N. Is carbamazepine an alternative maintenance therapy for neonatal seizures. *Developments in Pharmacological Therapy* 1987; **10**: 100–106.

85. Sapin JI, Riviello JJ Jr, Grover WD. Efficacy of primidone for seizure control in neonates and young infants. *Pediatric Neurology* 1988; **4**: 292–295.

86. Gal P, Otis K, Gilman J, Weaver R. Valproic acid efficacy, toxicity and pharmacokinetics in neonates with intractable seizures. *Neurology* 1988; **38**: 467–471.

87. Aicardi J, Mumford JP, Dumas C *et al.* Vigabatrin as initial therapy for infantile spasms: a European retrospective survey. *Epilepsia* 1996; **37**: 638–642.

88. Barr PA, Buettiker VE, Antony JH. Efficacy of lamotrigine in refractory neonatal seizures. *Pediatric Neurology* 1999; **20**(2): 161–163.

89. Boer HR, Gal P. Neonatal seizures: A survey of current practice. *Clinical Pediatrics* 1982; **21**: 453–457.

90. Fenichel GM. Paroxysmal disorders. In: Fenichel GM. *Clinical Pediatric Neurology*, 3rd edn. Philadelphia: W.B. Saunders, 1997: 1–43.

91. Ortibus EL, Sum JM, Hahn JS. Predictive value of EEG for outcome and epilepsy following neonatal seizures. *Electroencephalography and Clinical Neurophysiology* 1996; **98**: 175–185.

92. Mizrahi EM, Clancy RR, Dunn JK, *et al.* Neurologic impairment, developmental delay and postnatal seizures 2 years after EEG-video documented seizures in near-term and term neonates: report of the clinical research centers for neonatal seizures. *Epilepsia* 2001; **42**(Suppl 7): 102.

93. Brunquell PJ, Glennon CM, DiMario FJ Jr, Lerer T, Eisenfeld L. Prediction of outcome based on clinical seizure type in newborn infants. *Journal of Pediatrics* 2002; **140**(6): 707–712.

94. Ellenberg JH, Hirtz DG, Nelson KB. Age at onset of seizures in young children. *Annals of Neurology* 1984; **15**: 127–134.

95. Clancy RR, Legido A. Postnatal epilepsy after EEG-confirmed neonatal seizures. *Epilepsia* 1991; **32**: 69–76.

96. Watanabe K, Miura K, Natsume J, *et al.* Epilepsies of neonatal onset: seizure type and evolution. *Developmental Medicine and Child Neurology* 1999; **41**(5): 318–322.

97. Holmes GL, Ben-Ari Y. The neurobiology and consequences of epilepsy in the developing brain. *Pediatric Research* 2001: **49**: 320–325.

98. Holmes GL. Seizure-induced neuronal injury: animal data. *Neurology* 2002; **59**(Suppl.5): S3–6.

99. McBride, MC, Laroia, N., Guillet, R. Electrographic seizures in neonates correlate with poor neurodevelopmental outcome *Neurology* 2000; **55**: 506–513.

100. Miller SP, Weiss J, Barnwell A, *et al.* Seizure-associated brain injury in term newborns with perinatal asphyxia. *Neurology* 2002; **58**(4): 542–548.

101. McInerny TK, Schubert WK. Prognosis of neonatal seizures. *American Journal of Disease of Children* 1969; **117**: 261–264.

102. Mannino FL, Trauner DA. Stroke in neonates. *Journal of Pediatrics* 1983; **10**: 605–610.

103. Clancy R, Malin S, Laraque D, Baumgart S, Younkin D. Focal motor seizures heralding stroke in full-term neonates. *American Journal of Disease of Children* 1985; **139**: 601–606.

Febrile seizures

SHEILA J WALLACE

Seizures associated with a febrile illness are usually transient, age-related responses to noxious stimuli. Nevertheless, they can be an indication of an acute neurologic disorder. Furthermore, some children with febrile seizures are at higher risk of long-term educational and behavioral disorders and of epilepsy. For reviews of earlier literature, see Wallace.[1]

DEFINITION

The most recent International League Against Epilepsy (ILAE) report on classification and terminology lists febrile seizures as conditions with epileptic seizures that do not require a diagnosis of epilepsy. Febrile seizures are invariably associated with a rise in body temperature, which is usually at least 38°C. A previous area of contention related to seizures which were a complication of an intracranial infection, particularly bacterial meningitis. Some authors[2,3] excluded children with meningitis and/or encephalitis from their studies, whereas others[4,5] suggested that the actual seizure was no different. However, the Consensus Conference defined febrile seizures as 'an event in infancy or childhood, usually occurring between 3 month and 5 years of age, associated with fever but without evidence of intracranial infection or defined cause'[6] and this has been generally accepted. Febrile seizures are considered 'simple' when they are generalized, do not recur within a defined illness, and are of less than 15 min duration. Complex, complicated or severe febrile seizures have focal features, are repeated within the same illness and/or are prolonged.

EPIDEMIOLOGY

Between 2 and 4 per cent of children have at least one febrile seizure before the age of 5 years. In a study of 21 544 children aged up to 6 years, 115 newly diagnosed cases were identified over a period of 20 months.[7] In the same period, district nurses, physicians and the neurophysiology laboratory identified 128 children.[8] The risk rate in the age group up to 4 years was 500/100 000 and the annual incidence rate 460/100 000. The cumulative incidence was 4.1 per cent. Factors that influence the prevalence are listed in Table 8.1.

AGE

Febrile seizures occur most often between 6 and 36 months of age and are particularly common during the second year. A temporary age-related imbalance between

Table 8.1 *Risk factors for febrile seizures*

Social class	Not relevant
Race	Not relevant
Child of parent(s) with febrile seizures	Increased risk ($\times$4)
Child of parent(s) with epilepsy	Risk slightly raised (to 5 per cent)
Sibling of child with febrile seizures	Increased risk ($\times$3.5)
Male sex:female sex	1.72:1

Table 8.2 *Factors associated with an early age at onset of febrile seizures*

Negative family history of febrile seizures
Greater risk of complex febrile seizures, but not necessarily febrile status epilepticus
Recurrence of febrile seizures
Later non-febrile seizures
Later cognitive problems

Table 8.3 *Familial factors and febrile seizures*

Epilepsies with proven genetic relationship to febrile seizures
  Generalized epilepsy with febrile seizures plus (GEFS+)
  Absence epilepsy and febrile seizures
  Febrile seizures and hippocampal sclerosis
  Febrile seizures and non-febrile partial seizures
Patients with positive family histories for febrile seizures
  Complex features less likely[15]
  Recurrence risk of febrile seizures increased

Table 8.4 *Pre- and perinatal factors that predispose to febrile seizures*[1,3,19,20]

Chronic maternal ill-health, often associated with reduced fertility
Smoking and alcohol
Early, repeated, slight vaginal bleeding
Toxemia
Maternal therapeutic drug use
Maternal seizures
Delivery other than by the vertex
Relative reduction of birthweight for gestation
Neonatal sepsis
Errors of metabolism in the neonatal period

the normal development of excitatory and inhibitory mechanisms of brain function seems likely. The demonstration of age-dependent spatiotemporal evolution of hyperpolarization-activated, cyclic nucleotide-gated channels in rat hippocampus[9] could lead to better understanding of the functioning of ion channels in critical periods of human brain development. Factors associated with an early age at onset are listed in Table 8.2. The age at each recurrence has predictive value for subsequent episodes.[10]

GENETIC FACTORS

Inheritance of febrile seizures is complex in most children. Advances in molecular genetics (see Chapter 4A) have clarified some of the inheritance patterns and facilitated our understanding of the place of febrile seizures within a number of epilepsies.[11] Table 8.3 lists the epilepsies with proven genetic relationships to febrile seizures. In families with autosomal dominant inheritance, genes for febrile seizures have been mapped to chromosomes 19p and 5q and possibly 8q. Another locus, found on chromosome 2q, is considered to be identical to one of those for generalized epilepsy with febrile seizures plus (GEFS+). Both this and the other gene for GEFS+ on 19q are involved in sodium channel regulation, with mutations in one of them also reported in severe myoclonic epilepsy in infancy (SMEI). Such mutations have also been found in individuals with febrile seizures and nonfebrile partial seizures.[12] A mutation has also been identified in the benzodiazepine binding domain of the GABA receptor subunit GABRG2 in a large family with absence epilepsy and febrile seizures,[13] and in some families with GEFS+.[14]

Significant increases have been observed in the incidences of febrile seizures in mothers ($p < 0.001$) and fathers ($p < 0.002$), but not in siblings ($p < 0.49$), although the risk to siblings was increased by 3.5 times.[7,8] In the same study,[7] 24 per cent of children with febrile seizures, but only 5 per cent of controls, had a parent or sibling with febrile seizures ($p < 0.001$). Both patients with febrile seizures and controls had a similar incidence of afebrile seizures in parents and siblings. Intrapair similarity is much greater in monozygotic than dizygotic twins. The genetic influences on the characteristics of febrile seizures are summarized in Table 8.3.

Members of families with febrile seizures and hippocampal sclerosis may have brief and bilateral febrile seizures,[16] but preceding febrile seizures are often complex where there is heterogeneity in familial temporal lobe epilepsy.[17] Interestingly, some completely seizure-free members of families with febrile seizures and subsequent hippocampal sclerosis demonstrate a unilateral small hippocampus with a blurred internal pattern.[15] Digenic inheritance could be the explanation.[18]

PREDISPOSING FACTORS FROM THE PRE- AND PERINATAL PERIODS

Some factors predispose children to febrile seizures (Table 8.4), including maternal renal disease, thyrotoxicosis, mental disorders, epilepsy, hypertension and autoimmune disorders.[1,19] A positive family history for seizures

Table 8.5 *Postnatal factors found more commonly prior to febrile seizures*[1,2,4,6,8,22]

Upper and lower respiratory tract infections, otitis media
'Soft' neurological signs
Delay in walking
Delay in talking
Mental retardation
Larger or smaller than usual occipitofrontal head
 circumferences

Table 8.6 *Illnesses associated with febrile seizures*

Commonest clinical diagnosis
 Upper respiratory tract infection
Less common clinical diagnoses
 Otitis media
 Bronchopneumonia
 Pertussis
 Gastroenteritis
 Pyuria
 Measles
 Exanthem subitum
 Scarlet fever

Table 8.7 *Factors associated with complex initial febrile seizure*[1,16,21,22,26,47]

Young age
Negative family history
Adverse perinatal events
Neonatal seizures
Prior neurologic dysfunction
Abnormal neurologic development
Infection with malaria or HHV-6
Short duration of fever prior to seizure
Relatively low fever

adds to the risk of febrile seizures if perinatal problems have occurred.[1] Birth order, durations of gestation and labor, and prolonged rupture of the membranes and fetal distress are unimportant.[1,3,20] Children with adverse pre- and perinatal events have increased risks of complex initial febrile seizures, and of later afebrile seizures. Neonatal seizures predispose to febrile status epilepticus.[21]

POSTNATAL DEVELOPMENT BEFORE THE FIRST SEIZURE

Most children with febrile seizures are healthy and their prior neurologic development is normal. Table 8.5 lists factors found more commonly than expected. Fewer than 5 per cent have seriously disabling conditions and prior mental retardation is rare. Later cognitive impairment correlates with earlier onset of febrile seizures but it is not always easy to determine whether the development was delayed before the initial seizure if the seizure occurs at an early age. Prior neurologic abnormality predisposes to complex febrile seizures,[1,20,21] recurrence of febrile seizures, development of afebrile seizures, cognitive delay and later EEG abnormalities. Death, albeit extremely rare, is commoner in those with prior neurological abnormalities.

PRECIPITATING FACTORS

The ultimate height of the fever seems more important than the rate of rise of the temperature.[1] The commoner underlying illnesses associated with febrile seizures are listed in Table 8.6. Viral invasion of the CNS can be implied from CSF immunoglobulin estimations and confirmed by demonstration of viral DNA in CSF cell pellets.[1,5,23,24] Primary human herpesvirus (HHV)-6 infection has been found in 10–20 per cent of patients with febrile seizures, of whom the majority had exanthem subitum clinically.[23] HHV-7 may also precipitate febrile seizures. Both HHV-6 and HHV-7 can invade the CNS[24] and it has been postulated that reactivated latent infections may be the cause of further seizures. Following vaccination, a significantly increased risk of seizures exists only within 24 h for

diphtheria, pertussis and tetanus (DPT) vaccine, and only from 8–14 days later for measles, mumps and rubella (MMR):[25] the numbers of febrile seizures attributable to DPT are 6–9 per 100 000 children and to MMR 25–34 per 100 000 children.

THE INITIAL SEIZURE

A complex febrile seizure is either focal, repeated within the same illness or prolonged.[27] The criteria of the National Collaborative Perinatal Project (NCPP)[2] considered a seizure lasting more than 15 min as prolonged. Table 8.7 lists factors associated with complex febrile seizures. Careful characterization of the initial seizure is important because complex febrile seizures are associated with a poorer prognosis than simple febrile seizures. Although approximately 30 per cent of febrile seizures are considered to be focal, a higher incidence is found when focal features are specifically sought. In a study of 100 febrile seizures, inter-rater agreement on classification was only fair to good on focality.[28] Difficulties related to lateral eye deviation, staring episodes and motor asymmetries in bilateral seizures. All observers agreed that 60 of 100 seizures were completely generalized. Subsequent partial epilepsy and neurologic and cognitive problems occur in at least one third of children who have complex febrile seizures.

ACUTE NEUROLOGIC PROBLEMS

Prolonged disturbance of consciousness occurs in 31 per cent of children and can be secondary to the underlying infection, related to the pyrexia or a consequence of a prolonged seizure. Where careful examination is conducted and minor asymmetries are included, about one third of children show neurologic abnormalities when examined following a febrile seizure, usually asymmetric pyramidal tract signs.[1] Cerebellar ataxia and upper motor neuron facial palsies may also occur. Acute, transient hemiparesis following a prolonged, lateralized febrile seizure is associated with a significantly higher risk of subsequent complex partial seizures.

INVESTIGATION AT PRESENTATION

Investigation aims to identify the underlying illness and highlight features that might lower the seizure threshold. In children under 3 years of age with fever more than 39°C and no obvious cause, a complete blood count, blood culture and urinalysis should be performed unless the child looks well and can be monitored carefully. Routine blood studies are not helpful.

It has been suggested that signs other than seizures are always present in bacterial meningitis,[29] but there are difficulties with establishing absolute clinical criteria in younger children. Lumbar puncture is considered essential when there is meningism or when the child is less than 18 months at presentation.

Plain skull radiographs are unhelpful. A CT head scan should be performed before lumbar puncture in children with seizures associated with fever when the child has a prolonged postictal focal deficit or does not recover consciousness within several hours of the seizure.

The EEG is of no benefit in the management of children with simple febrile convulsions and is not helpful in prognosis. Paroxysmal abnormalities tend to be age-related.

ACUTE THERAPY

Prevention of prolonged seizures is paramount. Ninety per cent of febrile seizures are self-limiting but those lasting more than 5–10 min are unlikely to stop spontaneously within the next few minutes. Thus, seizures lasting longer than 10 min should be treated in a similar fashion to status epilepticus (Chapter 17). Intramuscular phenobarbital followed by oral phenobarbital and rectal diazepam have been used in the prevention of repeated attacks during the same illness.[30]

Treatment of the fever and the underlying illness are also important. Antipyretic medication, preferably with paracetamol, is better than physical cooling. Underlying infections should be treated appropriately.

PATHOLOGIC AND PATHOPHYSIOLOGIC FEATURES

Table 8.8 lists the biochemical abnormalities observed in the CSF of patients following a febrile seizure. Similar CSF histamine levels are observed in afebrile, nonconvulsing children, children with afebrile seizures and those with febrile seizures. This is consistent with the hypothesis that the central histaminergic neuron system may be involved in inhibition of seizures associated with febrile illnesses. Children in whom the CSF histamine does not rise when they become febrile may be more susceptible to febrile seizures.[31]

A well-recognized association exists between prolonged or lateralized febrile seizures and later mesial temporal sclerosis.[32–35] Diffusion-weighted MRI within 2 days of a prolonged febrile seizure has demonstrated unilateral acute edema of the head, body and tail of the hippocampus.[36] MRI demonstrated changes consistent with acute unilateral hippocampal edema in 4 of 15 children with complex febrile convulsions within several days of the seizure.[37] Those with hippocampal edema had prolonged lateralized convulsions. Hippocampal atrophy has been demonstrated within 2 months in patients with hippocampal edema following a prolonged febrile seizure.[36] Reduced N-acetyl aspartate levels in the hippocampus within 2 days of a febrile seizure also suggest the occurrence of irreversible damage to the hippocampus following a febrile seizure.[36] Complex febrile seizures can occur in association with pre-existing temporal lobe anomalies[33,37] and extratemporal heterotopias.[35,38] MRI confirms loss of mesial temporal structures when seizures of temporal lobe origin occur following febrile seizures.

Table 8.8 *Chemical constituents of cerebrospinal fluid in febrile seizures*

Lactate raised with complex febrile seizures
γ-Aminobutyric acid reduced with prolonged febrile seizures
5-Hydroxyvaleric acid: transient reduction, a secondary phenomenon
Prostaglandin E-2 raised secondary to the fever, not seizure
Purine metabolites unchanged
Pyrimidine bases unchanged
Free amino acid findings equivocal
Arginine vasopressin: no significant change
Histamine: expected rise not observed

RECURRENCE OF FEBRILE SEIZURES: PROPHYLACTIC THERAPY

The overall recurrence risk of a recurrent febrile convulsion is approximately 30–40 per cent.[1,8,10,39–41] Table 8.9 describes factors known to influence the recurrence risk. The risk of recurrence increases with the number of factors present.[42] Having a first-degree relative with a history of a febrile seizure increases the risk of a recurrent febrile seizure from 27 to 52 per cent.[41] A multivariate analysis has found children at most risk (48 per cent risk) had a temperature of less than 40°C, a positive family history of febrile seizures, or multiple seizures at the time of the first febrile seizure, whereas those at least risk (15 per cent) had a fever of more than 40°C, a negative family history or a simple initial febrile seizure.[10] In a meta-analysis of the predictors of recurrent febrile seizures, age at onset less than or equal to 1 year and a family history of febrile seizures were the most useful predictors and were each associated with a 50 per cent risk of recurrence.[39] Following initial complex febrile seizures, the risk that any further episodes will be complex rises to 40 per cent as the number of recurrences increases.[27]

Drug therapy may aim to prevent recurrent febrile seizures or to ensure that they are not prolonged. There is no evidence that drugs used to prevent recurrent febrile seizures reduce the risk of later epilepsy. A meta-analysis of preventive treatment demonstrated that both continuous oral phenobarbital and valproic acid are effective in preventing recurrent febrile seizures but that their potential side-effects limited their use.[43] Intermittent use of rectal or oral diazepam, rectal or oral clonazepam and oral clobazam at times of fever have all been described, although failure to recognize pyrexia before the seizure and the sedation associated with these drugs are potential complications of intermittent therapy. Patients in whom the initial febrile seizure was prolonged are at greater risk of prolonged febrile seizures if there is a recurrence. The preferred management in these children is to treat with rectal diazepam at the onset of the seizure. Intranasal or buccal midazolam may replace this regime in the future. The child should be placed in the recovery position, and excessive heating and cooling avoided.

DEVELOPMENT OF AFEBRILE SEIZURES AND EPILEPSY

The risk of subsequent afebrile seizures is significantly increased. Between 2–3 per cent of children with febrile seizures have an afebrile seizure by 7 years of age[2] and 7 per cent do so by 25 years of age.[44] However, afebrile seizures may present between 1 month and 28 years after the initial febrile seizure. The most common afebrile seizure types are generalized tonic-clonic, absence and partial seizures with automatisms and other motor symptomatology.[1,22,45] Complex partial seizures occurring in patients with mesial temporal lobe sclerosis are the most classical seizure type following febrile convulsions. Hippocampal malformations[15] have been demonstrated in patients with familial febrile convulsions and temporal lobe epilepsy.[18] A mutation in the GABA_A receptor has been demonstrated in a large family in which affected individuals had childhood absence epilepsy and febrile seizures.[13] In GEFS+, the seizure phenotype can be very variable[46] and may even include SMEI.[47]

LONG-TERM NEUROLOGIC OUTLOOK

The neurologic status following a febrile seizure is influenced mainly by the neurologic development prior to the attack. New neurologic deficits are uncommon even following febrile status epilepticus. Most patients with neurologic impairment following a prolonged febrile seizure have a pre-existing neurologic deficit.[48]

Long-term EEG changes

Generalized paroxysmal EEG abnormalities may be observed later in childhood in children with febrile seizures. Some 20–50 per cent patients who have serial EEGs starting at least 2 years after the initial febrile seizure demonstrate spikes or spike-waves.[1] Eight to ten years after single febrile seizures, 60 per cent had paroxysmal theta activity, asymmetries or intermittent focal slow waves although only 5 per cent had spikes or spike-wave on their EEGs. Those with prolonged, lateralized febrile seizures were more likely to show early asymmetries or focal slow waves, with or without spikes, which persisted and evolved into frank epileptic foci in some patients. In a separate

Table 8.9 *Factors known to influence risk of recurrent febrile seizures*

Increased risk
  Age less than 1 year
  Family history of febrile seizure in first-degree relative
  Low social class
  Persistent neurologic abnormality
  Complex febrile seizure initially

Decreased risk
  Fever of >40°C

No relevance
  EEG findings
  Proven viral infection

study of children with febrile convulsions followed up to the age of 11–13 years with on average 12 EEG records per individual, a genetically determined EEG pattern was observed in 81 per cent of patients:[49] Theta rhythms were observed in 54 per cent, spikes and waves in 49 per cent and photosensitivity in 42 per cent. The occurrence of these abnormalities peaked at 5–6 years of age. Centrotemporal spikes are much more frequent than expected, but do not necessarily imply clinical epilepsy.[50]

Cognitive abilities

Cognitive abilities of children with febrile seizures are generally comparable to those of unaffected children. Hospital-based studies have demonstrated poor speech and language abilities, problems with short-term memory and difficulties with copying shapes and/or drawing pictures of people. Hospital-based studies have also demonstrated that 12–19 per cent have specific difficulties with reading accuracy and/or comprehension when tested 8–10 years later and that attention deficits are significantly increased. Poor cognitive abilities correlated with low social class, repeated febrile seizures, continuing neurologic handicap and later nonfebrile seizures. However, population-based studies have demonstrated that children with simple, complex or recurrent febrile seizures did not differ significantly from controls at 10 years of age in measures of academic progress, intelligence and behavior.[51] Special schooling was required slightly more often for children who had febrile seizures in the first year of life.[51]

Behavioral problems

A higher incidence of behavioral difficulties has been described in hospital-based studies,[20] but behavioral outcome at 10 years was similar to that of the general childhood population in a population-based study.[51]

Social aspects

Although febrile seizures have an excellent medical prognosis, they often have a profound emotional effect on the parents. They occur unexpectedly when parents are likely to be relatively young and inexperienced. Seventy-seven per cent of parents think that their child is dead or dying, and 15 per cent imagine that their child has suffocated or has meningitis.[52] Only 21 per cent position the child correctly. They may subsequently sit and watch the child at night and during fevers, and suffer from restless sleep and/or dyspepsia. These parental behaviors and symptoms do not relate to the child's sex or age, the seizure characteristics, the presence of cyanosis, previous

knowledge of febrile seizures, their thoughts during the seizure or the appropriateness of their management. Further seizures cause a significant exacerbation of the parental symptoms. It is important therefore to educate parents on the excellent prognosis, and on how to manage subsequent episodes of fever.

KEY POINTS

- Febrile seizures occur in a **minority of children who have acute infections** in the first 5 years of life
- Febrile seizures occur most often **between 6 and 42 months of age**
- **Genetic factors are important**, and sodium channel and GABA-receptor mutations have been identified in studies of large families
- The **precipitating infection is usually viral**
- **Recurrences** of simple febrile seizures occur in 30–50 per cent of children and are more common in those with a first degree relative who has had febrile seizures and in those with a first febrile seizure under 1 year of age
- A **complex febrile seizure** is one that lasts longer than 15 min, is focal, or is repeated in the same illness. Approximately 30–40 per cent of febrile seizures are complex
- A complex febrile seizure and abnormal neurologic development are **risk factors for the subsequent development of epilepsy**. Children with no risk factors have approximately a 2 per cent risk of developing epilepsy and those with two risk factors have approximately a 15 per cent risk of developing epilepsy
- **Long-term prognosis** for neurologic development, educational achievement and behavior is generally good

REFERENCES

1. Wallace S. *The Child with Febrile Seizures*. London: Butterworth, 1988.
2. Nelson KB, Ellenberg JH. Predictors of epilepsy in children who have experienced febrile seizures. *New England Journal of Medicine* 1976; **295**: 1029–1033.
3. Verity CM, Butler NR, Golding J. Febrile convulsions in a national cohort followed up from birth. I – Prevalence and recurrence in the first five years of life. *BMJ* 1985; **290**: 1307–1310.
4. Wallace SJ. Neurological and intellectual deficits: convulsions with fever viewed as acute indications of life-long developmental defects. In: Brazier MAB, Coceani F (eds) *Brain Dysfunction in Infantile Febrile Convulsions*. New York: Raven Press, 1976: 259–277.

5. Lewis HM, Parry JV, Parry RP, *et al.* Role of viruses in febrile convulsions. *Archives of Disease in Childhood* 1979; **54**: 869–876.

6. Consensus Development Panel. Febrile seizures: Long term management of children with fever-associated seizures. *Pediatrics* 1980; S**66**: 1009–1012.

7. Forsgren L, Sidenvall R, Blomquist HK, *et al.* An incident case-referrent study of febrile convulsions in children: genetical and social aspects. *Neuropediatrics* 1990; **21**: 153–159.

8. Forsgren L, Sidenvall R, Blomquist HK, Heijbel J. A prospective incidence study of febrile convulsions. *Acta Paediatrica Scandinavica* 1990; **79**: 550–557.

9. Bender RA, Brewster A, Santoro B, Baram TZ. Differential and age-dependent expression of hyperpolarization-activated, cyclic nucleotide-gated cation channel isoforms 1–4 suggests evolving roles in the rat hippocampus. *Epilepsia* 2001; **42**(Suppl 7): 107.

10. Offringa M, Derksen-Lubsen C, Bossuyt PM, Lubsen J. Seizure recurrence after a first febrile seizure: a multivariate approach. *Developmental Medicine and Child Neurology* 1992; **34**: 15–24.

11. Berkovic SF, Scheffer IE. Genetics of the epilepsies. *Epilepsia* 2001; **42**(Suppl 5): 16–23.

12. Fukama G, Sugawara T, Ho M *et al.* Two novel missense mutations of the voltage-gated Na$^+$ channel alpha-1 subunit gene NAvL1 (SCN1A) found in individuals with febrile seizures (FS) associated with afebrile partial seizures. *Epilepsia* 2001; **42**(Suppl 7): 18–19.

13. Wallace RH, Marini C, Petrou S *et al.* Mutant GABA$_A$ receptor beta 2-subunit in childhood absence epilepsy and febrile seizures. *Nature Genetics* 2001; **28**: 49–52.

14. Baulac S, Huberfeld G, Gourfinkel-Au I, *et al.* First genetic evidence of GABA$_A$ receptor dysfunction in epilepsy: a mutation in the gamma 2-subunit gene. *Nature Genetics* 2001; **28**: 46–48.

15. van Stuijvenberg M, van Beijeren E, Wils NH, *et al.* Characteristics of the initial seizure in familial febrile seizures. *Archives of Disease in Childhood* 1999; **80**: 178–180.

16. Fernandez G, Effenberger O, Vinz B, *et al.* Hippocampal malformation as a cause of familial febrile convulsions and subsequent hippocampal sclerosis. *Neurology* 1998; **50**: 909–917.

17. Cendes F, Lopes-Cendes I, Andermann E, Andermann F. Familial temporal lobe epilepsy: A clinically heterogenous syndrome. *Neurology* 1998; **50**: 554–557.

18. Baulac S, Picard F, Herman A, *et al.* Evidence for digenic inheritance in a family with both febrile convulsions and temporal lobe epilepsy implicating chromosomes 18qter and 1q25-q31. *Annals of Neurology* 2001; **49**: 786–792.

19. Nelson KB, Ellenberg JH. Prenatal and perinatal antecedents of febrile seizures. *Annals of Neurology* 1990; **27**: 127–131.

20. Madge N, Diamond J, Miller D, *et al.* The National Childhood Encephalopathy Study: a 10 year follow-up. *Developmental Medicine and Child Neurology* 1993; **35**(Suppl): 68.

21. Shinnar S, Pellock JM, Berg AT, *et al.* Short term outcomes of children with febrile status epilepticus. *Epilepsia* 2001; **42**: 47–53.

22. Verity CM, Butler NR, Golding J. Febrile convulsions in a national cohort followed up from birth. II – Medical history and intellectual ability at five years of age. *BMJ* 1985; **290**: 1307–1310.

23. Suga S, Suzuki K, Ihara M, *et al.* Clinical characteristics of febrile convulsions during primary HHV-6 infection. *Archives of Disease in Childhood* 2000; **82**: 62–66.

24. Yoshikawa T, Ihira M, Suzuki K, *et al.* Invasion by human herpesvirus 6 and human herpesvirus 7 of the central nervous system in patients with neurological signs and symptoms. *Archives of Disease in Childhood* 2000; **83**: 170–171.

25. Barlow WE, Davis RL, Glasser JW, *et al.* The risk of seizures after receipt of whole-cell pertussis or measles, mumps and rubella vaccine. *New England Journal of Medicine* 2001; **345**: 656–661.

26. Crawley J, Smith S, Muthinji P, *et al.* Electroencephalographic and clinical features of cerebral malaria. *Archives of Disease in Childhood* 2001; **84**: 247–253.

27. Berg AT, Shinnar S. Complex febrile seizures. *Epilepsia* 1996; **37**: 126–133.

28. Berg AT, Steinschneider M, Kang H, Shinnar S. Classification of complex features of febrile seizures; inter-rater agreement. *Epilepsia* 1992; **33**: 661–666.

29. Green SM, Rothrock SG, Clem KJ, *et al.* Can seizures be the sole manifestation of meningitis in febrile children? *Pediatrics* 1993; **92**: 527–534.

30. Sopo SM, Pesarei MA, Celestini E, Stabile A. Short-term prophylaxis of febrile convulsions. *Acta Paediatrica Scandinavica* 1991; **80**: 248–249.

31. Kiviranta T, Tuomisto L, Airaksinen EM. Histamine in cerebrospinal fluid of children with febrile convulsions. *Epilepsia* 1995; **36**: 276–280.

32. Abou-Khalil B, Andermann E, Andermann F, *et al.* Temporal lobe epilepsy after prolonged febrile convulsions: Excellent outcome after surgery. *Epilepsia* 1993; **34**: 878–883.

33. Cendes F, Andermann F, Gloor P, *et al.* Atrophy of mesial temporal structures in patients with temporal lobe epilepsy: cause or consequence of repeated seizures? *Annals of Neurology* 1993; **34**: 795–801.

34. Hamati-Haddad A, Abou-Khalil B. Epilepsy diagnosis and localization in patients with antecedent childhood febrile convulsions. *Neurology* 1998; **50**: 917–922.

35. Lawson JA, Vogrin S, Bleasel AF, *et al.* Predictors of hippocampal, cerebral, and cerebellar volume reduction in childhood epilepsy. *Epilepsia* 2000; **41**: 1540–5154.

36. Zimmerman RA. New methods in pediatric neuroradiology. Lecture, 7th Mediterranean Child Neurology Meeting, Turkey, 2001.

37. van Landringham KE, Heinz ER, Cavazas JE, Lewis DV. Magnetic resonance imaging evidence of hippocampal injury after prolonged focal febrile convulsions. *Annals of Neurology* 1998; **43**: 413–426.

38. Sisodiya SM, Moran N, Free SL, *et al.* Correlation of widespread preoperative magnetic resonance imaging changes with unsuccessful surgery for hippocampal sclerosis. *Annals of Neurology* 1997; **41**: 490–496.

39. Berg AT, Shinnar S, Hauser WA, Leventhal JM. Predictors of recurrent febrile seizures: a meta-analytic review. *Journal of Pediatrics* 1990; **116**: 329–337.

40. Berg AT, Shinnar S, Hauser WA, *et al.* A prospective study of recurrent febrile seizures. *New England Journal of Medicine* 1992; **327**: 1122–1127.

41. van Esch A, Steyerberg EW, Berger MY, *et al.* Family history and recurrence of febrile seizures. *Archives of Disease in Childhood* 1994; **70**: 395–399.

42. Knudsen FU. Recurrence risk after first febrile seizure and effect of short term diazepam prophylaxis. *Archives of Disease in Childhood* 1985; **60**: 1045–1049.

43. Rantala H, Tarkka R, Uhari M. A meta-analytic review of the preventive treatment of recurrences of febrile seizures. *Journal of Pediatrics* 1997; **131**: 922–925.

44. Annegers JF, Hauser WA, Shirts SB *et al*. Factors prognostic of unprovoked seizures after febrile convulsions. *New England Journal of Medicine* 1987; **316**: 493–498.

45. Berg AT, Shinnar S, Levy SR, Testa FM. Childhood epilepsy with and without preceding febrile seizures. *Neurology* 1999; **53**: 1742–1748.

46. Scheffer IE, Berkovic SF. Generalized epilepsy with febrile seizures plus. A genetic disorder with heterogeneous clinical phenotypes. *Brain* 1997; **120**: 479–490.

47. Singh R, Andermann E, Whitehouse WPA, *et al*. Severe myoclonic epilepsy of infancy: Extended spectrum of GEFS+? *Epilepsia* 2001; **42**: 837–844.

48. Camfield P, Camfield C, Gordon K, Dooley J. What types of epilepsy are preceded by febrile seizures? A population-based study of children. *Developmental Medicine and Child Neurology* 1994; **36**: 887–892.

49. Doose H, Ritter K, Vlzke E. EEG longitudinal studies in febrile convulsions. *Neuropediatrics* 1983; **14**: 81–87.

50. Kajitani T, Kimura T, Sumita M, Kaneko M. Relationship between benign epilepsy of childhood with centro-temporal EEG foci and febrile convulsions. *Brain Development* 1992; **14**: 230–234.

51. Verity CM, Ross EM, Golding J. Outcome of childhood status epilepticus and lengthy febrile convulsions: findings of a national cohort. *BMJ* 1993; **307**: 225–228.

52. Balslev T. Parental reactions to a child's first febrile convulsion. A follow-up investigation. *Acta Paediatrica Scandinavica* 1991; **80**: 466–469.

9

Epilepsies with onset in the first year of life

Early epileptic encephalopathies

SHUNSUKE OHTAHARA, YASUKO YAMATOGI AND YOKO OHTSUKA

In childhood, there are several epileptic encephalopathies in which excessive neuronal activity may not only cause clinical seizures but also lead to a stagnation or regression in the development of cognitive and motor function. Early-infantile epileptic encephalopathy with suppression-burst, Ohtahara syndrome and early myoclonic encephalopathy (EME) present in the neonatal or early infantile period, a time when seizure-susceptibility is low and only a few epileptic syndromes are observed.[1–3] Both syndromes are characterized by a suppression-burst pattern on EEG and by frequent intractable seizures. They are inclusively called **early infantile epileptic syndromes** or **encephalopathies with suppression-burst**.[4,5]

Ohtahara syndrome has the earliest presentation of the three age-dependent epileptic encephalopathies, which include Ohtahara syndrome, West syndrome and Lennox-Gastaut syndrome. Although each of these three syndromes has specific clinical and electroencephalographic features, they have the following common characteristics:

- occurrence in a specific age group
- particular seizure types that occur frequently
- severe and continuous epileptic EEG abnormalities
- heterogeneous etiology
- intractability to medications
- poor prognosis for mental development.[6,7]

Transition is often observed with age between these syndromes; approximately three-quarters of patients with Ohtahara syndrome develop West syndrome in middle infancy, and more than half of patients with West syndrome develop Lennox-Gastaut syndrome, usually in early childhood.[8–10] Their common characteristics and the frequent transition between syndromes led Ohtahara to inclusively name each of these three syndromes as an **age-dependent epileptic encephalopathy**.[6,7] Despite their common features, each of the three syndromes usually presents at a certain age and has particular clinical and EEG features. In that each syndrome may be due to a wide variety of etiologies, the age at presentation is probably a major factor in the manifestation of the specific electroclinical features of each. Thus, these syndromes may be the age-specific epileptic response to various brain insults.

EPIDEMIOLOGY OF OHTAHARA SYNDROME AND EME

An epidemiologic study on childhood epilepsy carried out in Okayama Prefecture, Japan, detected 1 case of Ohtahara syndrome (0.04 per cent) and 4 cases of EME (0.168 per cent) among 2378 epileptic children younger than 10 years of age in 1980.[11] Compared to the 40 cases (1.68 per cent) of West syndrome observed in the same study, the prevalence of Ohtahara syndrome is low. The prevalence of these syndromes was also low in a more recent study performed using the same method.[12] Thus, there were no cases of Ohtahara syndrome, 2 cases (0.09 per cent) of EME and 57 cases (2.57 per cent) of West syndrome in 2222 children with epilepsy younger than 13 years of age in 1999. Similarly, Kramer described 1 case of Ohtahara syndrome (0.2 per cent) and 40 cases of West syndrome (9.1 per cent) in a cohort of 440 consecutive children with epilepsy under 15 years of age in Tel Aviv.[13] Thus, the relative prevalence of Ohtahara syndrome to West syndrome is approximately 1 in 40 and that of EME to West syndrome is approximately 1 in 10. In a study of 75 infants with epilepsies of neonatal onset, which were monitored intensively, 8 cases (10.7 per cent) of Ohtahara syndrome, 2 cases (2.7 per cent) of EME and none of West syndrome were observed.[14]

EARLY-INFANTILE EPILEPTIC ENCEPHALOPATHY WITH SUPPRESSION-BURST: OHTAHARA SYNDROME

Outline

Ohtahara syndrome presents in the first few months of life and often in the newborn period. It is characterized by frequent tonic spasms, which can be isolated or occur in clusters. The EEG demonstrates a suppression-burst pattern in both the waking and sleep states. The seizures are intractable to medications and the prognosis for neurologic development is very poor. This syndrome was described first by Ohtahara,[15] who mentioned particularly the differences from West syndrome.

Clinical seizures

The onset of the seizures occurs within the first 3 months after birth, usually in the first month.[2,6–10,15–19] The cardinal seizure type is the tonic spasm, usually emprosthotonic, which may be isolated or occur in clusters. The spasms occur not only in waking but also in the sleeping state in most patients. The duration of each tonic spasm is up to 10 s and the seizure frequency is very high, ranging from 10 to 300 spasms or 10–20 series of clusters daily. In addition to tonic spasms, partial seizures such as erratic focal motor seizures and hemiconvulsions are observed in one third to one half of cases. In contrast to EME, myoclonic seizures are rare.

EEG findings

The most characteristic EEG feature is the suppression-burst pattern, which is consistently observed in both waking and sleeping states (Figure 9A.1). The suppression-burst pattern is characterized by high-voltage bursts alternating with nearly flat patterns at an approximately regular rate. Bursts of 1–3 s duration comprise 150–350 μV high-voltage slow waves intermixed with multifocal spikes. The duration of the suppression phase is 2–5 s. The burst-burst interval, measured from beginning to beginning of bursts, ranges from 5 to 10 s. Some asymmetry in suppression-burst is noted in approximately two thirds of cases, presumably reflecting the underlying brain lesions.

The ictal EEG of tonic spasms shows principally desynchronization with or without evident initial fast activity.[8,17]

Neuroimaging and laboratory findings

CT and MRI demonstrate abnormalities that are often asymmetric, even at a young age. SPECT and PET often show corresponding abnormalities. Abnormalities may also be observed in auditory brainstem and visual evoked potentials,[2] but are not usually observed in metabolic investigations, e.g. levels of amino acids and organic acids, or lysosomal enzyme assays. Cytochrome oxidase deficiency[20] and Leigh encephalopathy[21,22] have been reported rarely.

Underlying pathologies and presumptive causes

The etiologies of Ohtahara syndrome are heterogeneous and include brain malformations, such as hemimegalencephaly,[23–25] porencephaly, Aicardi syndrome,[26] olivary-dentate dysplasia,[27,28] agenesis of mamillary bodies,[29] linear sebaceous naevus syndrome,[30,31] cerebral dysgenesis[2] and focal cortical dysplasia.[32,33] In a neuropathologic comparison of Ohtahara syndrome with EME and West syndrome, Itoh et al.[34] observed that Ohtahara syndrome patients had the most widespread and severe lesions, which were in the putamen, thalamus and hippocampus as well as the tegmentum of the brainstem. Reduced expression of tyrosine hydroxylase and trytophan hydroxylase was noted particularly in patients with Ohtahara syndrome, which may indicate dysfunction of the catecholaminergic and serotonergic systems.[34] Cytochrome c oxidase deficiency[20] and Leigh encephalopathy[21,22] have been reported rarely. A patient with cytochrome c oxidase deficiency was demonstrated to have a transient deficiency and it was postulated that this might have resulted in abnormal neuronal migration or demyelination by depletion of energy during a critical period of brain development.[20] Postmortem pathologic examination has sometimes disclosed dysgenetic abnormalities not demonstrated on neuroimaging,[35] and it is possible that many cryptogenic cases may also have an undetectable migration disorder or microdysgenesis.[2,18] No familial case has been reported, excepting for those with Leigh encephalopathy.[22]

Pathophysiology of suppression-burst pattern

The pathophysiological mechanism of suppression-burst is not clear. Its similarity to tracé alternant in neonatal quiet sleep and to burst-suppression in brain-damaged neonates may indicate an excessive subcortical neuronal discharge modified by subcortico–cortical dysregulation or by cortical lesions.[15] Spreafico et al.[36] demonstrated in the white matter the persistence of early generated neurons, which are necessary for neocortical histogenesis but programmed to die near the end of gestation or soon

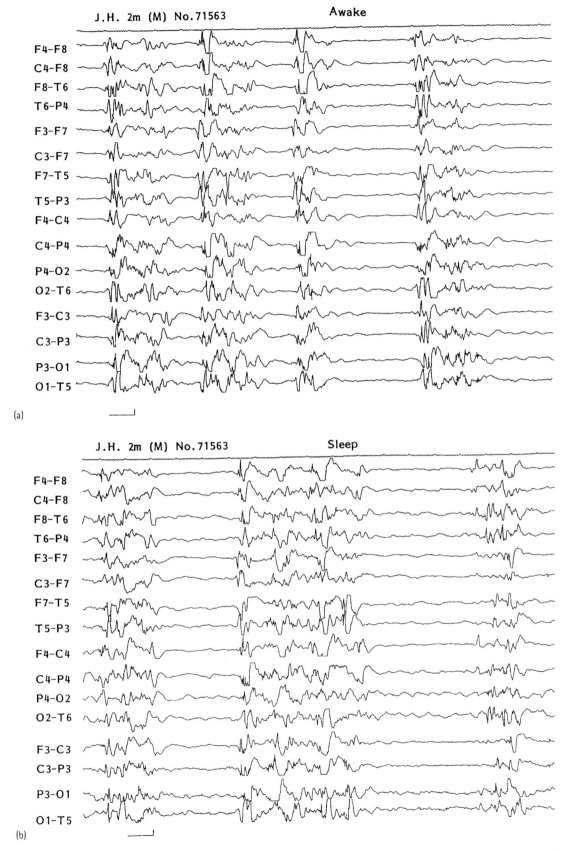

Figure 9A.1 *Suppression-burst pattern in a 2-month-old boy with Ohtahara syndrome: (a) awake, (b) natural sleep. Horizontal calibration mark 1 s; vertical 50 μV.*

Table 9A.1 *Early encephalopathies with suppression-bursts. Transitional change with age*

	First year of life				Late infancy, childhood
	Neonatal	Early	Middle	Late	
Organic/static encephalopathy					
Type of epilepsy	OS	OS	WS, (SPE)	WS, SPE	LGS, SE-MISF, SPE
EEG	SB	SB	SB ~ Hyps, MISF, SF	Hyps, (MISF, SF)	DSSW, MISF, SF
Metabolic encephalopathy					
Type of epilepsy	EME	EME	WS, EME	WS, EME	EME
EEG	SB (BS type)	MISF, SB	Hyps, MISF, SB	Hyps, MISF, SB	MISF, SB

BS, burst-suppression; DSSW, diffuse slow spike-waves; EME, early myoclonic encephalopathy; Hyps, hypsarrhythmia; LGS, Lennox-Gastaut syndrome; MISF, multiple independent spike foci; OS, Ohtahara syndrome; SB, suppression-burst; SE-MISF, severe epilepsy with multiple independent spike foci; SF, spike foci, SPE, symptomatic partial epilepsy; WS, West syndrome.

after birth, in two children with EME. He postulated that they provided an anatomic basis for subcortico–cortical disconnection, providing a pathophysiologic basis for burst-suppression in EME. The markedly asymmetric and sometimes unilateral suppression-burst pattern reported in hemimegalencephaly suggests the significance of extensive cortical lesions which influence subcortico–cortical regulation and modify subcortical discharges to generate suppression-burst pattern.[24,25]

Treatment and prognoses

Ohtahara syndrome is the most intractable age-dependent epileptic encephalopathy. Pyridoxal phosphate, valproate, benzodiazepines, adrenocorticotropic hormone (ACTH) and steroids, including liposteroid,[37] have been used but their efficacy is limited. Thyrotropin releasing hormone (TRH), a TRH analog,[38] the ketogenic diet[18,39] and gamma-globulin[22] have been reported to have a partial effect. More recently, vigabatrin[40] and zonisamide[41] have been reported to be of some value. Successful resection has been described in those with focal cortical dysplasia and was associated with relatively improved neurological development postoperatively.[32,33]

Although seizures may be suppressed by school age in approximately half of the patients, the prognosis for neurological development is very poor. All survivors are severely handicapped, both mentally and physically. Furthermore, the mortality rate is high, especially in the early stage of the disorder. One quarter of our patients had died before 2 years of age.

Evolution of clinical and EEG features

The characteristic evolution is from Ohtahara syndrome to West syndrome in infancy in most cases, and from West syndrome to Lennox-Gastaut syndrome in early childhood in some cases (Table 9A. 1). The transition from Ohtahara syndrome to West syndrome of the clinical ictal symptoms is less clear than the change in the EEG features. Evolution from suppression-burst to hypsarrhythmia is observed at around 3–6 months of age, and from hypsarrhythmia to diffuse slow spike-waves at around 1 year of age. Timing of transition corresponds to the critical age at onset of each syndrome and EEG pattern.

Transition of suppression-burst to hypsarrhythmia starts with a gradual increase in the amplitude of the suppression phase. Disappearance of the suppression-burst in waking precedes that in sleep. In the course of evolution from hypsarrhythmia to diffuse slow spike-waves, the earliest changes occur in the waking EEG and the changes in the sleeping EEG occur later. Thus, the changing process from a suppression-burst pattern to hypsarrhythmia and further to a diffuse slow spike-wave pattern successively proceeds in a close relation with the waking and sleeping cycle.

Differential diagnosis

The differential diagnoses include EME, early onset West syndrome or West syndrome with the periodic hypsarrhythmia, severe epilepsy with multiple independent spike foci[42] and neonatal hypoxic-ischemic encephalopathy with burst-suppression pattern. The age of onset tends to be in the neonatal period or early infancy for Ohtahara syndrome and in middle to late infancy for West syndrome, although West syndrome may occasionally present in early infancy. Although the tonic spasm is the main seizure type in both syndromes, the tonic spasms in Ohtahara syndrome usually appear not only during waking but also during sleep, and may also occur as isolated spasms. Partial seizures also occur in some Ohtahara syndrome cases, but are rare in West syndrome. Furthermore, most patients with Ohtahara syndrome have markedly abnormal cerebral cortex and asymmetric lesions can often be demonstrated on neuroimaging.

EEG is particularly useful in discriminating Ohtahara syndrome from West syndrome. The suppression-burst pattern differs from the periodic type of hypsarrhythmia in which periodicity becomes evident during sleep, and sleep spindles may be observed in the suppressed phase after 2 months of age. Finally, the seizures are more intractable in Ohtahara syndrome than in West syndrome and adrenocorticotropic hormone (ACTH) therapy is usually not as effective. Similarly, the prognosis for neurological development is less favorable in Ohtahara syndrome.

EARLY MYOCLONIC ENCEPHALOPATHY (EME)

Outline

EME is a rare epileptic syndrome of very early onset characterized by frequent myoclonias and partial seizures and by a suppression-burst pattern in the EEG. It was first described by Aicardi and Goutières in 1978[43] and has been variously named neonatal myoclonic epileptic encephalopathy, myoclonic encephalopathy with neonatal onset, neonatal epileptic encephalopathy with periodic EEG bursts and early myoclonic epileptic encephalopathy.[44] No sex difference has been described.

Clinical features

The seizure onset is confined to the first 3 months of age and occurs mostly within 1 month of birth. Fragmentary myoclonias are the essential symptom, appearing initially in most cases.[3] The myoclonias are usually associated with no ictal EEG change, although some occur coincidentally with epileptiform bursts of suppression-burst. The myoclonias are mostly fragmentary and are characterized by only a slight twiching of the distal ends of the extremities, eyelids or corners of the mouth. Frequent partial seizures, massive myoclonias, and tonic spasms are also seen. Dalla Bernardia et al.[44,45] reported that partial seizures following erratic myoclonias were particularly characteristic of EME. Partial seizures are the cardinal epileptic seizure type throughout the course of the disorder. Those include complex partial seizures with eye-deviation or autonomic symptoms such as apnea and facial flushing, clonic seizures in various parts of the body, and asymmetric tonic posturing with or without generalization. Massive myoclonia and tonic spasms may be observed in some patients. Tonic spasms usually appear, either in series or isolated, at 3–4 months of age, suggesting an atypical form of West syndrome. The period of atypical West syndrome is, however, transient and the features of EME recur and persist for a long period thereafter.

EEG findings

The interictal EEG characteristically shows a suppression-burst pattern, which consists of bursts lasting 1–5 s alternating with almost isoelectric periods lasting 3–10 s. The suppression-burst pattern of EME becomes more distinct during sleep, especially during deep sleep.[44,46] (Figure 9A. 2). The suppression-burst pattern tends to be replaced by atypical hypsarrhythmia or by multifocal paroxysms after 3–5 months of age. However, in most cases, the appearance of atypical hypsarrhythmia is transient,[46] and subsequently the suppression-burst pattern returns and persists characteristically for a long period thereafter.[44,46]

Underlying pathologies

The most striking feature is the high incidence of familial cases.[3,44,45] This suggests that genetic factors and/or inborn errors of metabolism play a prominent role. Non-ketotic hyperglycinemia,[47–49] propionic aciduria, methylmalonic acidemia, D-glyceric acidemia, sulfite and xanthine oxidase deficiency, Menkes disease and Zellweger syndrome have all presented with EME,[3,50] but the underlying cause is not demonstrated in the majority of cases. As the gene locations of these metabolic errors vary widely, it is more likely that EME is not due to specific genes but rather to extensive cortico–subcortical dysfunction as a consequence of metabolic disorders.

In contrast to Ohtahara syndrome, CT and MRI imaging rarely demonstrate abnormalities in the early stage of the disorder. However, progressive cortical and periventricular atrophy develop in some cases.[3,46]

Treatment and prognosis

Conventional antiepileptic drugs, ACTH, corticosteroids and pyridoxine have all been ineffective. Both partial seizures and myoclonias, however, decrease gradually with age. Mortality is high and most deaths occur before 2 years of age. Almost all survivors show progressive psychomotor deterioration and eventually are in a vegetative state.

DIFFERENTIAL DIAGNOSIS BETWEEN OHTAHARA SYNDROME AND EME

Ohtahara syndrome and EME share common clinical and electrical characteristics, such as onset in the first few months of life and a suppression-burst pattern on EEG. Thus, it is important to recognize the features that distinguish these disorders (Table 9A.2).[2,17]

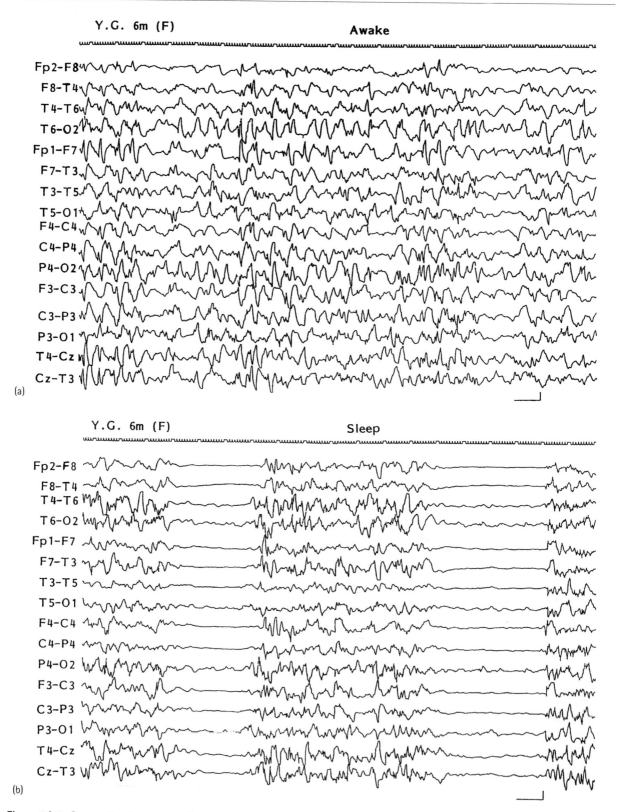

Figure 9A.2 *Suppression-burst pattern in a 6-month-old girl with EME: (a) awake, (b) natural sleep. Horizontal calibration mark 1 s; vertical 50 μV.*

Table 9A.2 *Differential characteristics of early epileptic encephalopathies*

Characteristics	Ohtahara syndrome	EME
Age of onset	Early infancy	Early infancy
Etiology	Polyetiology; mainly organic, malformative brain lesion (organic/static encephalopathy)	Some metabolic disorders (metabolic encephalopathy)
Clinical seizure		
Initial seizure type	Tonic spasms, partial seizures	Myoclonia, partial seizures
Nonepileptic myoclonia	+ (erratic)	+++ (erratic, fragmentary)
Tonic spasms	Main seizure type (single/in series)	Transiently in middle or late infancy (single/in series)
PS	+	+++ (main seizure type)
Circadian cycle	Diffuse	Diffuse
EEG		
Interictal	Suppression-burst (SB)	SB (BS type in neonate)
Burst-burst interval	Relatively regular	Irregular (shorter burst and longer suppression in neonatal period)
Circadian cycle	Consistently, regardless of sleep-wake cycle	Enhanced by sleep (after neonate)
Course of SB	Transition to hypsarrhythmia or focal spike after middle infancy	Persist even after 1 year of age
Ictal EEG	Desynchronization (tonic spasm)	Focal rhythmic discharge (PS), myoclonia sometimes concordant with burst
Treatment	Intractable; ACTH, ZNS, etc.	Extremely intractable
Evolution	To WS, LGS, SE-MISF, SPE	Long-term persistence with regression
Prognosis	Poor	Extremely poor

BS, burst-suppression; LGS, Lennox-Gastaut syndrome; PS, partial seizure; SB, suppression-burst; SE-MISF, severe epilepsy with multiple independent spike foci; SPE, symptomatic partial epilepsy; WS, West syndrome; ZNS, zonisamide.

- The main seizure type in Ohtahara syndrome is the tonic spasm; myoclonias are rarely seen. In contrast, myoclonias, especially erratic myoclonias, and frequent partial seizures predominate in EME.
- Although the suppression-burst pattern is common to both syndromes, its relation to the circadian cycle, the time of its appearance and the time of its disappearance differ considerably. In Ohtahara syndrome, suppression-burst occurs consistently during both waking and sleeping states, whereas in EME, suppression-burst is enhanced by sleep and often not manifest in the waking state. In addition, the suppression-burst pattern appears at the beginning of the disease and disappears within the first 6 months of life in Ohtahara syndrome, whereas it becomes distinct at 1–5 months of age in some cases of EME and persists for a long period in most patients.[44,46]
- In Ohtahara syndrome, the EEG paroxysms characteristically evolve from a suppression-burst pattern to hypsarrhythmia in many cases and further from hypsarrhythmia to diffuse slow spike-waves in some cases.[2,17] In EME, atypical hypsarrhythmia may occur transiently in some cases but the suppression-burst pattern reappears and persists for a prolonged period.[46] Similarly, whereas Ohtahara syndrome shows a specific pattern of evolution into other age-dependent epileptic encephalopathies, EME has no age-related evolution.
- Ohtahara syndrome is usually due to obvious static brain lesions, including brain malformations, and neuroimaging discloses abnormal findings in many patients, even at the early stage. In addition, no familial cases have been reported. In EME, brain anomalies are rarely demonstrated on MRI and the high incidence of familial cases suggests that inborn metabolic disorders are a common cause.

These observations suggest that there are fundamental differences between Ohtahara syndrome and EME. It is highly likely that they constitute different electroclinical entities, and that Ohtahara syndrome occurs in patients with organic/static abnormalities whereas EME appears to occur most in patients with metabolic disorders.[4]

KEY POINTS

Ohtahara syndrome:

- The syndrome presents in the **first 3 months of life and often in the newborn period**

- It is characterized by frequent **tonic spasms**, which can be isolated or occur in clusters, and occur in both the waking and sleep state
- Partial seizures are observed in one-third to one half of cases but **myoclonic seizures are rare**
- The EEG demonstrates a **suppression-burst pattern** in both the waking and sleep states. This evolves into **hypsarrhythmia** at around 3–6 months of age in many infants
- **Neuroimaging** commonly demonstrates abnormalities that are often asymmetric
- The seizures are **intractable** to medications and the prognosis for neurologic development is very poor

Early myoclonic encepahalopathy (EME):

- The seizure onset is confined to **the first 3 months of age and occurs mostly within 1 month of birth**
- **Fragmentary myoclonias** are the essential symptom, but are associated usually with no ictal EEG change
- **Partial seizures** are the cardinal epileptic seizure type
- Tonic spasms may appear transiently, either in series or isolated and usually at 3–4 months of age, suggesting an **atypical form of West syndrome**
- The characteristic EEG is a **suppression-burst pattern** that, unlike in Ohtahara syndrome, is enhanced by sleep and often not manifest in the waking state. In EME, atypical hypsarrhythmia may occur transiently in some cases but the **suppression-burst pattern reappears and persists for a prolonged period**
- There is a high incidence of familial cases and **inborn errors of metabolism** rather than congenital malformations are the most commonly demonstrated etiology
- The seizures are **intractable** to medications, the **prognosis** for neurologic development is very poor and the mortality rate is high

REFERENCES

1. Commission on Classification and Terminology of the International League Against Epilepsy. Proposal for revised classification of epilepsies and epileptic syndromes. *Epilepsia* 1989; **30**: 389–399.
2. Ohtahara S, Ohtsuka Y, Yamatogi Y, Oka E, Inoue H. Early-infantile epileptic encephalopathy with suppression-bursts. In: Roger J, Bureau M, Dravet C *et al.* (eds) *Epileptic Syndromes, in Infancy, Childhood and Adolescence*, 2nd edn. London: John Libbey, 1992; 25–34.
3. Aicardi J. Early myoclonic encephalopathy (neonatal myoclonic encephalopathy). In: Roger J, Bureau M, Dravet C *et al.* (eds) *Epileptic Syndromes, in Infancy, Childhood and Adolescence*, 2nd edn. London: John Libbey, 1992; 13–23.
4. Schlumberger E, Dulac O, Plouin P. Early infantile epileptic syndrome(s) with suppression-burst: nosological considerations. In: Roger J, Bureau M, Dravet C *et al.* (eds) *Epileptic Syndromes, in Infancy, Childhood and Adolescence*, 2nd edn. London: John Libbey, 1992; 35–42.
5. Shields WD. Catastrophic epilepsy in childhood. *Epilepsia* 2000; **41**(Suppl. 2); S2–6.
6. Ohtahara S. A study on the age-dependent epileptic encephalopathy. *No To Hattatsu* (Tokyo)1977; **9**: 2–21 (in Japanese).
7. Ohtahara S. Clinico-electrical delineation of epileptic encephalopathies in childhood. *Asian Medical Journal* 1978; **21**: 499–509.
8. Yamatogi Y, Ohtahara S. Age-dependent epileptic encephalopathy: a longitudinal study. *Folia Psychiatrica et Neurologica Japonica* 1981; **35**: 321–331.
9. Ohtsuka Y, Ogino T, Murakami N, *et al.* Developmental aspects of epilepsy with special reference to age-dependent epileptic encephalopathy. *Japanese Journal of Psychiatry and Neurology* 1986; **40**: 307–313.
10. Ohtahara S, Yamatogi Y. Evolution of seizures and EEG abnormalities in childhood onset epilepsy. In: Wada JA, Ellingson RJ. (eds) *Clinical Neurophysiology of Epilepsy.* Handbook of Electroencephalography and Clinical Neurophysiology, Revised Series, vol. 4, Amsterdam: Elsevier, 1990; 457–477.
11. Oka E, Ishida S, Ohtsuka Y, Ohtahara S. Neuroepidemiological study of childhood epilepsy by application of international classification of epilepsies and epileptic syndromes (ILAE, 1989). *Epilepsia* 1995; **36**: 658–661.
12. Oka E. Childhood epilepsy in Okayama Prefecture, Japan; a neuroepidemiological study. *No To Hattatsu* (Tokyo) 2002; **34**: 95–102 (in Japanese).
13. Kramer U, Nevo Y, Neufeld MY, *et al.* Epidemiology of epilepsy in childhood: a cohort of 440 consecutive patients. *Pediatric Neurology* 1998; **18**: 46–50.
14. Watanabe K, Miura K, Natsume J, *et al.* Epilepsies of neonatal onset: seizure type and evolution. *Developmental Medicine and Child Neurology* 1999; **41**: 318–322.
15. Ohtahara S, Ishida T, Oka E, Yamatogi Y, Inoue H. On the specific age dependent epileptic syndrome: the early-infantile epileptic encephalopathy with suppression-bursts. *No To Hattatsu* (Tokyo) 1976; **8**: 270–280 (in Japanese).
16. Donat JF. The age-dependent epileptic encephalopathies. *Journal of Child Neurology* 1992; **7**: 7–21.
17. Yamatogi Y, Ohtahara S. Early-infantile epileptic encephalopathy with suppression-bursts, Ohtahara syndrome; its overview referring to our 16 cases. *Brain Development* 2002; **24**: 13–23.
18. Clarke M, Gill J, Noronha M, McKinlay I. Early infantile epileptic encephalopathy with suppression burst: Ohtahara syndrome. *Developmental Medicine and Child Neurology* 1987; **29**: 520–528.
19. Konno K, Miura Y, Suzuki H, Karahashi M, Takagi T. A study on clinical features of the early infantile epileptic encephalopathy with suppression burst or Ohtahara syndrome. *No To Hattatsu* (Tokyo) 1982; **14**: 395–404 (in Japanese).
20. Williams AN, Gray RG, Poulton K, Ramani P, Whitehouse WPA. A case of Ohtahara syndrome with cytochrome oxidase

deficiency. *Developmental Medicine and Child Neurology* 1998; **40**: 568–570 (refer to 2000; **42**: 785–787).

21. Tatsuno M, Hayashi M, Iwamoto H, *et al.* Leigh's encephalopathy with wide lesions and early infantile epileptic encephalopathy with burst-suppression: an autopsy case. *No To Hattatsu* (Tokyo) 1984; **16**: 68–75 (in Japanese).

22. Miyake S, Yamashita S, Yamada M, Iwamoto H. [Therapeutic effect of ACTH and gamma-globulin in 8 cases with the early-infantile epileptic encephalopathy with suppression-burst (EIEE).] (in Japanese) *Shonika Rinsho* (Tokyo) 1987; **40**: 1681–1688.

23. Bermejo AM, Martin VL, Arcas J, *et al.* Early infantile epileptic encephalopathy: a case associated with hemimegalencephaly. *Brain Development* 1992; **14**: 425–428.

24. Ogihara M, Kinoue K, Takamiya H, *et al.* A case of early infantile epileptic encephalopathy (EIEE) with anatomical cerebral asymmetry and myoclonus. *Brain Development* 1993; **15**: 133–139.

25. Ohtsuka Y, Ohno S, Oka E. Electroclinical characteristics of hemimegalencephaly. *Pediatric Neurology* 1999; **20**: 390–393.

26. Ohtsuka Y, Oka E, Terasaki T, Ohtahara S. Aicardi syndrome: a longitudinal clinical and electroencephalographic study. *Epilepsia* 1993; **34**: 627–634.

27. Harding BN, Boyd SG. Intractable seizures from infancy can be associated with dentato-olivary dysplasia. *J Neurological Sciences* 1991; **104**: 157–165.

28. Robain O, Dulac O. Early epileptic encephalopathy with suppression bursts and olivary-dentate dysplasia. *Neuropediatrics* 1992; **23**: 162–164.

29. Trinka E, Rauscher C, Nagler M, *et al.* A case of Ohtahara syndrome with olivary-dentate dysplasia and agenesis of mamillary bodies. *Epilepsia* 2001; **42**: 950–953.

30. Kurokawa T, Sasaki K, Hanai T, Goya N, Komaki S. Linear nevus sebaceous syndrome. Report of a case with Lennox-Gastaut syndrome following infantile spasms. *Archives of Neurology* 1981; **38**: 375–377.

31. Hirata Y, Ishikawa A, Somiya K. A case of linear nevus sebaceous syndrome associated with early-infantile epileptic encephalopathy with suppression burst (EIEE). *No To Hattatsu* (Tokyo) 1985; **17**: 577–582 (in Japanese).

32. Pedespan JM, Loiseau H, Vital A, *et al.* Surgical treatment of an early epileptic encephalopathy with suppression-bursts and focal cortical dysplasia. *Epilepsia* 1995; **36**: 37–40.

33. Komaki H, Sugai K, Maehara T, Shimizu H. Surgical treatment of early-infantile epileptic encephalopathy with suppression-bursts associated with focal cortical dysplasia. *Brain Development* 2001; **23**: 727–731.

34. Itoh M, Hanaoka S, Sasaki M, Ohama E, Takashima S. Neuropathology of early-infantile epileptic encephalopathy with suppression-bursts; comparison with those of early myoclonic encephalopathy and West syndrome. *Brain Development* 2001; **23**: 721–726.

35. Miller SP, Dilenge M-E, Meagher-Villemure K, O'Gorman AM, Shevell MI. Infantile epileptic encephalopathy (Ohtahara syndrome) and migrational disorder. *Pediatric Neurology* 1998; **19**: 50–54.

36. Spreafico R, Angelini L, Binelli S, *et al.* Burst suppression and impairment of neocortical ontogenesis: electroclinical and neuropathologic findings in two infants with early myoclonic encephalopathy. *Epilepsia* 1993; **34**: 800–808.

37. Yoshikawa H, Ikeda S, Watanabe T. Trial of liposteroid treatment in a case of early infantile epileptic encephalopathy with suppression burst. *No To Hattatsu* (Tokyo) 1998; **30**: 551–554 (in Japanese).

38. Ishii M, Tamai K, Sugita K, Tanabe Y. Effectiveness of TRH analog in a case of early infantile epileptic encephalopathy. *No To Hattatsu* (Tokyo) 1990; **22**: 507–511 (in Japanese).

39. Takusa Y, Ito M, Kobayashi A, *et al.* [Effect of the ketogenic diet for West syndrome into which early infantile epileptic encephalopathy with suppression-burst was evolved.] (in Japanese) *No To Hattatsu* (Tokyo) 1995; **27**: 383–387.

40. Dulac O. Epileptic encephalopathy. *Epilepsia* 2001; **42**(Suppl. 3): 23–26.

41. Ohno M, Shimotsuji Y, Abe J, Shimada D, Tamiya H. Zonisamide treatment of early infantile epileptic encephalopathy. *Pediatric Neurology* 2000; **23**: 341–344.

42. Ohtsuka Y, Amano R, Mizukawa M, Maniwa S, Ohtahara S. Long-term prognosis of the Lennox-Gastaut syndrome: Consideration in its evolutional change. In: Fukuyama Y, Kamoshita S, Ohtsuka C, Suzuki Y (eds) *Modern Perspectives of Child Neurology*. Tokyo: The Japan Society of Child Neurology, 1991; 215–222.

43. Aicardi J, Goutières F. Encéphalopathie myoclonique néonatale. *Revue d'Electroencephalographie et Neurophysiologie* 1978; **8**: 99–101.

44. Dalla Bernardina B, Dulac O, Fejerman N, *et al.* Early myoclonic epileptic encephalopathy (EMEE). *European Journal of Pediatrics* 1983; **140**: 248–252.

45. Dalla Bernardina B, Dulac O, Bureau M, *et al.* Encéphalopathie myoclonique précoce avec épilepsie. *Revue d'Electroencephalographie et Neurophysiologie* 1982; **12**: 8–14.

46. Murakami N, Ohtsuka Y, Ohtahara S. Early infantile epileptic syndromes with suppression-bursts: early myoclonic encephalopathy vs Ohtahara syndrome. *Japanese Journal of Psychiatry and Neurology* 1993; **47**: 197–200.

47. Dalla Bernardina B, Aicardi J, Goutières F, Plouin P. Glycine encephalopathy. *Neuropädiatrie* 1979; **10**: 209–225.

48. Terasaki T, Yamatogi Y, Ohtahara S, *et al.* A long-term follow-up study on a case with glycine encephalopathy. *No To Hattatsu* 1988; **20**: 15–22.

49. Chen P-T, Young C, Lee W-T, Wang P-J, Peng SS, Shen Y-Z. Early epileptic encephalopathy with suppression burst electroencephalographic pattern: an analysis of eight Taiwanese patients. *Brain Development* 2001; **23**: 715–720.

50. Lombroso C.T. Early myoclonic encephalopathy, early infantile epileptic encephalopathy, and benign and severe infantile myoclonic epilepsies: a critical review and personal contributions. *Journal of Clinical Neurophysiology* 1990; **7**: 380–408.

9B

West syndrome

RAILI RIIKONEN

West syndrome consists of infantile spasms, hypsarrhythmia and intellectual disability. The typical syndrome begins between 3 and 7 months of age, and virtually never after the age of 1 year. West syndrome is estimated to occur in between 1.6 and 4.3 of each 10 000 live births. There has been no change in incidence over the past 30 years.[1]

SPASMS

According to the International Classification (Chapter 1), the spasms are generalized epilepsies. They may be flexor, extensor or, most commonly, mixed flexor and extensor. Individual children may have various types of spasms. Subtle, asymmetric or asynchronous spasms and focal neurological signs suggest a symptomatic etiology. Partial seizures may precede or coincide with infantile spasms in up to 40 per cent of cases.[2,3] Spasms occur in series. They are commonly associated with drowsiness and occur at arousal, or soon thereafter. Comparison with video-recordings shows that a vast number of spasms are missed by parents. When typical, the diagnosis is easy. However, erroneous diagnoses of colic, startle responses or normal infant behavior are often made. Repetitive, stereotyped characterization of any movements in infancy should suggest the possibility of infantile spasms and lead to an immediate EEG. Infants with symptomatic etiology may show only subtle spasms: video-EEG studies are necessary in these cases.

EEG

Hypsarrythmia is characterized by irregular, diffuse, asymmetric, high-voltage slow waves, interspersed with sharp waves and spikes, distributed randomly throughout scalp recordings. There is a total disorganization of cortical electrogenesis. 'Modified hypsarrhythmia' occurs in about 40 per cent of cases and implies the presence of some preservation of background rhythms, synchronous bursts of spike-wave activity, significant asymmetry, or a burst-suppression appearance. A constant focus of abnormal discharges may also precede, accompany and/or follow hypsarrhythmia.[4,5] With long duration of untreated spasms, multifocal spikes may evolve into hypsarrhythmia.[6,7] A generalized slow wave, usually followed by attenuation of background activity, is the commonest ictal pattern associated with symmetrical spasms.[3,8] Sometimes the infant ceases to take any interest in the surroundings, and blindness is suspected. This functional amaurosis is associated with absent or grossly abnormal visual evoked potentials and probably corresponds to perfusion defects involving the parieto-occipital areas.[9,10] In infants under the age of 1 year, behavioral regression should be considered a strong indication for an EEG: hypsarrhythmia may reveal the cause of the regression. Constantly normal tracings, including sleep recordings, effectively rule out the possibility of infantile spasms.

DIFFERENTIAL DIAGNOSIS

Benign myoclonus of early infancy may closely mimic infantile spasms, but the EEG is normal.[11] Benign myoclonic epilepsy with favorable outcome (Chapter 10D) is often misdiagnosed as West syndrome, but the EEG shows generalized spike-waves occurring in brief bursts during the early stages of sleep. Other early-onset syndromes include early myoclonic encephalopathy and early infantile epileptic encephalopathy: both have burst-suppression patterns on EEG, and include infants with very serious brain pathologies and outcomes (Chapter 10A). Early infantile encephalopathy often evolves to West syndrome. In about one quarter of those with West syndrome evolution to Lennox-Gastaut syndrome occurs: this is an important differential diagnosis in patients aged more than 1 year.

ETIOLOGY

West syndrome has many etiologies, but two main groups are recognized: symptomatic and cryptogenic. Within these groups, the prognoses and responses to treatment differ and they seem to have different levels of some biochemical and endocrine parameters.[12,13] Classification depends to a great extent on the investigations performed. The cryptogenic group comprises patients with no known or suspected etiology, other than possible hereditary predispositions. They are considered to have the idiopathic form. Various pre- and postnatal insults are responsible for the majority of symptomatic cases. The findings in a recent large population-based cohort including 102 children[1] are given in Table 9B.1. Infants who are small for gestational age seem more liable than preterm babies of appropriate size to develop infantile spasms,[1] but increased survival of infants of very low birthweight seems not to increase the overall numbers. Although malformations are reported in 18–20 per cent of patients in clinical and neuroradiological series, two thirds of those who come to autopsy are considered to have epilepsy of embryofetal origin.[14] Microdysgenesis is also often found in surgical specimens.[15]

GENETICS

Recurrence of West syndrome in families is considered to result from either genetically determined syndromes, encephalopathy, or persisting factors predisposing to brain damage during pregnancy and delivery. Tuberous sclerosis is the most important genetically defined disorder. Other conditions associated with West syndrome are Aicardi syndrome, Miller-Dieker syndrome (type I lissencephaly) and PEHO syndrome (progressive encephalopathy, hypsarrhythmia, optic atrophy). Rarely, West syndrome is symptomatic of single-gene metabolic disorders (see Chapter 4D). The empirical recurrence risks are estimated at 1.5 per cent for siblings and 0.7 per cent for all first-degree relatives.[16] However, some families may have higher risks, related to as yet unidentified autosomal recessive disorders.[17] Familial cases are recorded in 4–5 per cent of patients.[18,19] In addition, familial idiopathic West syndrome has recently been reported.[20] Compared with prenatal and perinatal etiologies of 10 per cent and 9 per cent, respectively, a positive family history of epilepsy has been found in 40 per cent of those with spasms: genetic links to both febrile seizures and idiopathic generalized epilepsies have been noted.[21] It seems that heritable factors could play an important role in idiopathic, but not symptomatic, groups.

ETIOLOGICAL INVESTIGATIONS

In order to formulate both accurate prognoses and the need for genetic counseling, a careful search for etiological factors is essential in all cases. Comprehensive histories, with special regard to familial disorders and pre- and perinatal events, should be taken, and a thorough clinical examination performed, e.g. to check for signs of tuberous sclerosis. The importance of neuro-ophthalmogical, neuroradiological (especially MRI), virological (IgG index, viral antibody index[22]) and neurometabolic studies is further stressed. Chromosomal analysis is indicated where structural anomalies of the brain or other evidence of dysmorphism are apparent.

Table 9B.1 *Etiological factors in a population-based study including 102 patients[1]*

Symptomatic causes	Per cent
Brain malformations and tuberous sclerosis	35
Perinatal insults	9
Undetermined pre/perinatal factors	19
Early infections	2
Symptomatic neonatal hypoglycaemia	8
Familial or metabolic causes	9
Cryptogenic	18

PATHOPHYSIOLOGICAL MECHANISMS

Problems with modulation of neurotransmitters at a specific period of brain maturation are believed to be fundamental to the development of infantile spasms. The latter usually appear at the age which corresponds to the critical period of maximal cerebral development.[23] The discrepancy between brain development and age is supported as follows:

- infantile spasms and hypsarrythmia tend to disappear spontaneously with age
- defective dendritic development, suggesting possible developmental arrest, has been shown in autopsy specimens
- glucocorticoids have an accelerating effect on some physiological events (enzymes, myelination, neuroblast growth).[24–27]

It has recently been suggested that early stress (injury or insult) during a critical pre- and perinatal period of high corticotrophin (CRF) abundance may increase CRF synthesis and activity, with resultant long-term effects.[28] Other pathogenetic theories relate to dysfunction of the brainstem[29] and abnormal cortical–subcortical interaction.[30]

TREATMENT

Steroids and vigabatrin are the first-line drugs for infantile spasms.

Steroids

Following the good response reported 40 years ago, ACTH or glucocorticoids have remained the therapy of choice. The efficacy of high-dose ACTH has been considered better than that of prednisone in a single-blind prospective study,[31] but a small prospective double-blind investigation found otherwise,[32] and follow-up data was similar in the two studies. ACTH has been given in daily dosages varying from 3–14 IU in Japan,[33,34] through 18–36 IU in Finland[35] up to 80 IU in USA,[31] and for periods varying from 3 weeks to 6 months or longer. Daily dosages of corticosteroids are hydrocortisone 15 mg/kg[36] or prednisone 2 mg/kg.[31] Although prolonged high-dose ACTH is favored by some authors,[37] a large retrospective study[4] and a blind prospective investigation[38] have shown that this is no more effective than lower doses of ACTH or hydrocortisone[36] given for shorter periods. In addition, the long-term cognitive outcome was better after low-dose ACTH.[1,4] I recommend that treatment is started with oral pyridoxine 150 mg daily for 3–4 days, to exclude the possibility of underlying pyridoxine dependency or deficiency. If there is no response, corticotrophin, preferably natural ACTH, is commenced and used in a stepwise manner based on etiology and response, as suggested in Table 9B.2. Subsequently, appropriate cortisol supplementation is provided during periods of stress. With this regime, adverse aspects of ACTH treatment are kept to a

Table 9B.2 *Regime for the use of IM natural ACTH * in infantile spasms*

All cases
Weeks 1 and 2:   ACTH 3 iu/kg/day
Cryptogenic responders
Week 3:   ACTH 1.5 iu/kg/day
Week 4:   ACTH 0.75 iu/kg/day
Symptomatic responders
Weeks 3 and 4:   ACTH 3 iu/kg/day
                              Hydrocortisone 1 mg/kg/day
Week 5 on: Half dose of ACTH at weekly intervals
                              Withdraw hydrocortisone once ACTH response normal
Cryptogenic and symptomatic non-responders
Weeks 3 and 4:   ACTH 6 iu/kg/day
                              Hydrocortisone 1 mg/kg/day
Week 5 on: Half dose of ACTH at weekly intervals
                              Withdraw hydrocortisone once ACTH response normal

Add nitrazepam/valproic acid/vigabatrin if ACTH not effective

Prophylactic trimethoprim-sulfazole therapy is recommended for infants with a history of frequent respiratory infections. Blood pressure should be monitored and significant hypertension treated.

*Zn tetracosactrin (synthetic analog of ACTH) 0.03 mg/kg on alternate days is equivalent to natural ACTH 3 iu/kg/day.

Table 9B.3 *Effects of ACTH and corticosteroids on the brain*

- Acceleration of physiological events during critical stages of brain development, through action as a trophic hormone[23]
- Amelioration of cortisol releasing hormone overactivity[28]
- Potentiation of nerve growth factor stimulating effect,[39] leading to balance of inhibitory (nerve growth factor) and excitatory (glutamate and/or nitrite/nitrate) factors[13]
- Decrease in cortisol releasing factor via melanotropic receptors[40]

minimum.[35] A summary of the effects of ACTH/steroids on the brain is given in Table 9B.3. Although ACTH acts directly on melanotropic receptors, and not through effects on cortisol releasing factor (CRF), to decrease excitability in the limbic system,[40] steroids themselves, which do not have downregulating effects on CRF, have clear clinical influences in West syndrome. The reasons for the efficacies of ACTH and steroids in West syndrome require further elucidation.

Vigabatrin

Vigabatrin (VGB) has gained popularity rapidly because of its efficacy and initial favorable adverse event profiles. In Europe, opinion is divided in regard to VGB as initial treatment. The dose has ranged from 50 to 120 mg/kg per day, with 40–60 mg/kg usually given, administered in two daily doses. In the only open, randomized prospective study which has compared ACTH and VGB,[41] the two drugs were of equal efficacy, with similar relapse rates. In a prospective study, VGB was given as the first drug to all patients for 7–20 days and the response rate, measured by video-EEG in all patients, was 26 per cent.[42] A multicenter VGB study in Europe[43] found an initial response rate of 68 per cent, but this study lacked EEG evaluation and the drop-out rate was high. In comparing the two drugs further, when data from seven separate trials was pooled, VGB was effective in 49 per cent of 426 patients;[44,45] and, with combined data from eight separate trials, ACTH was effective in 58 per cent of 451 patients. Thus, overall, ACTH seems to be somewhat more effective than VGB, but it is difficult to compare the trials because of their nonhomogeneity. In tuberous sclerosis, VGB seems to be effective. However, the reports on high initial response rates are comparable with those for ACTH, varying from 100 per cent for VGB[36] to 74 per cent for ACTH.[46] The mean response rate for VGB was 74 per cent in eight studies.[44] The rates of relapse after VGB are not yet well established. In a study which reported the highest rate of response,[47] the relapse rate was also highest, new seizures were more frequent in young patients with tuberous sclerosis, and VGB was subsequently not recommended as monotherapy. A serious concern has arisen in relation to the use of VGB. Concentric visual field defects (VFD), which occur in about 40 per cent of adult patients on VGB, have now also been reported in 49 per cent of children.[48,49] In short, VGB would be an ideal drug for infantile spasms if it could be shown that it does not cause VFD in infants. However, this seems unlikely. Vigabatrin is administered to young children at high dosage over long periods of time and there are currently no methods available which can identify young children at risk of developing VFD. Therefore, steroids should be used as first choice for the treatment of infantile spasms: their side-effects are well-known and treatable, and can be reversed by discontinuation. Furthermore, the long-term outcome following ACTH is known, but after VGB therapy it remains uncertain.

As alternatives to ACTH and VGB, high-dose valproic acid,[50] nitrazepam,[51] pyridoxine,[52] zonisamide,[53] lamotrigine[54] and topiramate[55] have been used, but are less effective than ACTH or VGB.

Surgery

Some children with medically refractory infantile spasms have localized brain defects. Focal abnormalities can be seen in up to 30 per cent of patients in the initial EEG, in 57 per cent at some time,[4] and in 65 per cent when studied by EEG and neuroimaging.[56] Control of the spasms following removal of structural abnormalities, such as tumors, porencephaly or hemimegalencephalic changes, has been reported for many years. Increasingly, resective surgery is being used to treat children with intractable infantile spasms. When a single lesion is identified on MRI, and there is good correlation with EEG localization, surgical treatment is quite favorable in terms of both seizure control and cognitive development.[57,58] However, PET is the preferred imaging modality: it provides a very unique and important assessment of the integrity of the brain regions outside the area of potential resection (see Chapter 19B). Postoperatively, the best cognitive outcome is achieved if the entire zone of cortical abnormality, rather than just the seizure focus, is resected.[56] Surgery should be considered early in medically refractory cases. However, the term 'intractability' is difficult to define in a very young child; epileptic focal abnormalities tend to disappear spontaneously, or migrate, and the long-term effects of surgery on cognitive functioning need further evaluation. Removal of hypometabolic areas seen on PET, in the presence of normal CT or MRI scans, remains controversial.[59] Nevertheless, the development of newer, more specific PET probes for epilepsy has led to improved and more accurate localization of seizure foci, and is likely to improve the outcome following surgery.

PROGNOSIS

The presence or absence of structural abnormalities and their nature strongly influence prognosis. Normal development is recorded in 12–25 per cent of cases overall, and in 40–44 per cent of those with cryptogenic etiology. After cessation of spasms, other seizures, starting as early as 3–4 months, are seen after both ACTH and VGB treatment. In 214 Finnish patients followed up for 20–35 years, or until death,[60] one third had died, with one third of these dying before the age of 3 years. Of the survivors, intellectual outcome was normal or slightly impaired in a quarter: they completed their education in normal schools, or in schools for educationally impaired children. Nine of them attended secondary schools; seven had professional occupations; ten were married and five had children. Another 25 per cent were in special training schools, and the remaining 50 per cent were uneducable. A third of the patients were seizure-free. Psychiatric disorders, such as infantile autism and hyperkinetic behavior, occurred in a quarter of the cases. In patients with autism after infantile spasms, 71 per cent had temporal focal abnormalities on EEG,[61] and bitemporal pathology has been shown using PET.[62] In tuberous sclerosis, autism follows after infantile spasms in 26–58 per cent.[63]

In three large series of patients with longer follow-up times, shorter, rather than longer, periods between the onset of spasms and the start of treatment correlated with more favorable outcomes in both symptomatic and cryptogenic groups.[4,60,64]

KEY POINTS

In West syndrome, many crucial problems remain unresolved. Nevertheless, many advances have been achieved:

- **Identification** is more precise, using time-synchronized video and polygraphic recordings
- More accurate **etiological diagnoses** can be made by clinical, neuroimaging, virological, biochemical and pathological methods. Various **genetic patterns** are recognized
- **Side-effects of the main drugs** in clinical use, ACTH and vigabatrin, are better known
- In some patients, a **surgical approach** seems of benefit in achieving seizure control
- **PET has proved useful** in assisting selection for surgery

On the other hand:

- There is a **lack of consensus on the drug of first choice** for infantile spasms. An open, prospective study is necessary to compare the efficacy, relapse rate and outcome after steroids and vigabatrin

Important goals are:

- Understanding of brain maturation through focus on studies which attempt to elucidate the **metabolic and pathophysiological mechanisms of West syndrome** which currently remain unclear
- Identification of the frequency of VFD after vigabatrin; prediction of which patients could be less susceptible to vigabatrin-induced retinal toxicity; and quantification of long-term effects of vigabatrin in general

---

REFERENCES

1. Riikonen R. Decreasing perinatal mortality – unchanged infantile spasms morbidity. *Developmental Medicine and Child Neurology* 1995; **37**: 232–238.
2. Ohtsuka Y, Murashima I, Asano, T, *et al.* Partial seizures in West syndrome. *Epilepsia* 1996; **37**: 1060–1067.
3. Gaily E, Shewman D, Chugani, H, *et al.* Asymmetric and asynchronous infantile spasms, *Epilepsia* 1995; **36**: 873–882.
4. Riikonen R. A long-term follow-up study of 214 children with the syndrome of infantile spasms. *Neuropediatrics* 1982; **13**: 14–23.
5. Yamamoto N, Watanabe K, Negoro T, *et al.* Partial seizures evolving to infantile spasms. *Epilepsia* 1988; **29**: 34–40.
6. Watanabe K, Iwase, K, Hara K. The evolution of EEG features in infantile spasms: a prospective study. *Developmental Medicine and Child Neurology* 1973; **15**: 584–596.
7. Kotagal P. Multifocal independent spike syndrome: relationship to hypsarrhythmia and slow spike-wave (Lennox-Gastaut) syndrome. *Clinical Electroencephalography* 1995; **26**: 23–29.
8. Fusco L, Vigevano F. Ictal clinical electroencephalographic findings of spasms in West syndrome. *Epilepsia* 1993; **34**, 671–678.
9. Chugani HT, Phelps ME, Mazziotta JC. Positron emission tomography study of human brain functional development. *Annals of Neurology* 1987; **22**: 22, 487–497.
10. Jambaqué I, Chiron C, Dulac O, *et al.* Visual inattention in West Syndrome: a neuropsychological and neurofunctional imaging study. *Epilepsia* 1993; **34**: 692–700.
11. Lombroso CT, Fejerman N. Benign myoclonus of early infancy. *Annals of Neurology* 1977; **1**: 38–148.
12. Riikonen R. How do cryptogenic and symptomatic infantile spasms differ? A review of biochemical studies in Finnish patients. *Journal of Child Neurology* 1996; **11**: 383–388.
13. Vanhatalo S, Riikonen R. Nitric oxide metabolites, nitrites and nitrates in the cerebrospinal fluid in children with West syndrome. *Epilepsy Research* 2001; **46**: 3–13.
14. Jellinger K. Neuropathological aspects of infantile spasms. *Brain Development* 1987; **9**: 349–357.
15. Vinters HV, Fisher RS, Cornford ME, *et al.* Morphological substrates of infantile spasms: studies based on surgically resected cerebral tissue. *Child's Nervous System* 1992; **8**: 8–17.
16. Fleiszar K, Daniel W, Imrey P. Genetic study of infantile spasms with hypsarrhythmia. *Epilepsia* 1977; **18**: 55–62.
17. Sugai K, Fukuyama Y, Yasuda K, *et al.* Clinical and pedigree study of familial cases of West syndrome in Japan. *Brain Development* 2001; **23**: 558–564.
18. Riikonen R. Infantile spasms in siblings. *Journal of Pediatric Neuroscience* 1987; **3**: 235–244.
19. Dulac O, Feingold J, Plouin P, *et al.* Genetic predisposition to West syndrome. *Epilepsia* 1993; **34**: 732–737.
20. Reiter E, Tiefenthaler M, Freilinger M, *et al.* Familial idiopathic West syndrome. *Journal of Child Neurology* 2000; **15**: 249–252.
21. Vigevano F, Fusco L, Cusmai R, *et al.* The idiopathic form of West syndrome. *Epilepsia* 1993; **34**: 743–746.
22. Riikonen R. Infantile spasms: infectious disorders. *Neuropediatrics* 1993; **24**: 274–280.
23. Riikonen R. Infantile spasms: some new theoretical aspects. *Epilepsia* 1983; **24**: 159–168.
24. Palo J, Savolainen H. Effect of high doses of synthethic ACTH on the rat brain. *Brain Research* 1974; **70**: 313–320.
25. Dunn A, Gispen W. How ACTH acts on the brain. *Biobehavioral Reviews* 1977; **1**: 15–23.
26. Lindholm D, Castren M, Hengerer B, *et al.* Glucocorticoids and neurotrophin gene regulation in the nervous system. *Ann NY Acad Sci* 1994; **746**: 195–202.

27. Mochetti I, Spiga G, Hayes V, Isackson PJ, Colangelo A. Glucocorticoids differentially increase nerve growth factor and basic fibroblast growth factor expression in the rat brain. *Journal of Neuroscience*; 1996; **16**: 2141–2148.

28. Baram TZ. Pathophysiology of massive infantile spasms: perspective on the putative role of the brain adrenal axis. *Annals of Neurology* 1993; **33**: 231–236.

29. Satoh J, Mizutani T, Horimatsu Y, *et al.* Neuropathology of the brain-stem in age-dependent epileptic encephalopathy – especially in cases with infantile spasms. *Brain Development* 1986; **8**: 443–449.

30. Chugani HT, Shewmon A, Sankar R, *et al.* Infantile spasms: II. Lenticular nuclei and brain stem activation on positron emission tomography. *Annals of Neurology* 1992; **131**: 212–219.

31. Baram TZ, Mitchell WG, Tournay A, *et al.* High-dose corticotropin (ACTH) versus prednisone for infantile spasms: a prospective, randomized, blinded study. *Pediatrics* 1996; **97**: 375–379.

32. Hrachovy R, Frost J, Kellaway P, Zion T. Double-blind study of ACTH vs prednisone for infantile spasms. *Journal of Pediatrics* 1983; **103**: 641–645.

33. Ito M, Okuno T, Fuji T, *et al.* ACTH therapy in infantile spasms: Relationship between dose of ACTH and initial effect or long-term prognosis. *Pediatric Neurology* 1990; **6**: 240–244.

34. Watanabe K. Medical treatment of West syndrome in Japan. *Journal of Child Neurology* 1995; **10**: 143–147.

35. Heiskala H, Riikonen R, Santavuori P, *et al.* Infantile spasms: individualized ACTH therapy. *Brain Development* 1996; **18**: 456–460.

36. Chiron C, Dumas C, Jambaque I, *et al.* Randomized trial comparing vigabatrin and hydrocortisone in infantile spasms due to tuberous sclerosis. *Epilepsy Research* 1997; **26**: 389–395.

37. Lerman P, Kivity S. The efficacy of corticotrophin in primary infantile spasms. *Journal of Pediatrics* 1982; **101**: 294–296.

38. Hrachovy R, Frost J, Glaze D. High-dose, long-duration versus low-dose, short-duration corticotrophin therapy for infantile spasms. *Journal of Paediatrics* 1994; **124**: 803–806.

39. Riikonen R, Söderström S, Vanhala R, *et al.* West's syndrome: Cerebrospinal fluid nerve growth factor and effect of ACTH. *Pediatric Neurology* 1997; **17**: 224–229.

40. Brunson K, Khan N, Eghbal-Ahmadi M, Baram T. Corticotropin (ACTH) acts directly on amygdala neurons to down-regulate corticotropin-releasing hormone gene expression. *Annals of Neurology* 2001; **49**: 304–312.

41. Vigevano F, Cilio MR. Vigabatrin versus ACTH as first-line treatment for infantile spasms: a randomized, prospective study. *Epilepsia* 1997; **38**: 1270–1274.

42. Granström M-L, Gaily E, Liukkonen E. Treatment of infantile spasms: results of a population-based study with vigabatrin as the first drug for infantile spasms. *Epilepsia* 1999; **40**: 950–957.

43. Aicardi J, Mumford JP, Dumas C, *et al.* Vigabatrin as initial therapy for infantile spasms: a European retrospective survey. *Epilepsia* 1996; **37**: 638–642.

44. Riikonen R. Steroids or vigabatrin in the treatment of infantile spasms? *Pediatric Neurology* 2000; **23**: 403–408.

45. Elterman RD, Shields WD, Mansfield KA, *et al.* Randomized trial of vigabatrin in patients with infantile spasms. *Neurology* 2001; **57**: 1416–1421.

46. Riikonen R, Simell O. Tuberous sclerosis and infantile spasms. *Developmental Medicine and Child Neurology* 1990; **32**: 203–209.

47. Nabbout R, Chiron C, Mumford C, *et al.* Vigabatrin in partial seizures in children *Journal of Child Neurology* 1977; **12**: 172–177.

48. Gross-Tsur V, Banin E, Shahar E, *et al.* Visual impairment in children with epilepsy treated with vigabatrin. *Annals of Neurology* 2000; **48**: 60–64.

49. Russell-Eggitt I, Mackey D, Taylor D, *et al.* Vigabatrin-associated visual field defects in children. *Eye* 2000; **14**: 334–339.

50. Siemens H, Spohr H, Michael T, *et al.* Therapy of infantile spasms with valproate: results of a prospective study. *Epilepsia* 1988; **29**: 553–560.

51. Dreifuss F, Farwell JN, Holmes G, *et al.* Infantile spasms, comparative trial of nitrazepam and corticotropin. *Archives of Neurology* 1986; **37**: 379–385.

52. Ohtsuka Y, Matsuda M, Ogino T, *et al.* Treatment of West syndrome with high-dose pyridoxal phosphate. *Brain Development* 1987; **9**: 418–421.

53. Yanai S, Hanai T, Narazaki O. Treatment of infantile spasms with zonisamide. *Brain Development* 1999; **21**: 157–161.

54. Veggiotti P, Cieta C, Rey E, *et al.* Lamotrigine in infantile spasms. *Lancet* 1994; **344**: 1375–1376.

55. Glauser TA, Clark PO, McGee K. Long-term response to topiramate in patients with West-syndrome. *Epilepsia* 2000; **41**(Suppl. 1): S91–94.

56. Shields D, Shewmon A, Chugani HT, *et al.* Treatment of infantile spasms: medical or surgical? *Epilepsia* 1992; **33**(Suppl. 4): S26–31.

57. Asano E, Chugani D, Juhasz C, *et al.* Surgical treatment of West syndrome. *Brain Development* 2001; **23**: 668–676.

58. Asarnow RF, LoPresti C, Guthrie D, *et al.* Developmental outcomes in children receiving resection surgery for medical intractable infantile spasms. *Developmental Medicine and Child Neurology* 1997; **39**: 430–440.

59. Snead OC, Nelson M. PET does not eliminate need for extraoperative, intracranial monitoring in pediatric epilepsy surgery. *Pediatric Neurology* 1993; **5**: 409–410.

60. Riikonen R. Long-term outcome of West syndrome: A study of adults with a history of infantile spasms. *Epilepsia* 1996; **37**: 369–372.

61. Riikonen R, Amnell G. Psychiatric disorders in children with earlier infantile spasms. *Developmental Medicine and Child Neurology* 1981; **23**: 747–60.

62. Chugani H, Da Silva F, Chugani D. Infantile spasms: III. Prognostic implications of bitemporal hypometabolism on positron emission tomography. *Annals of Neurology* 1996; **39**: 643–649.

63. Hunt A, Dennis J. Psychiatric disorder among children with tuberous sclerosis. *Developmental Medicine and Child Neurology* 1987; **29**: 190–198.

64. Koo B, Hwang P, Logan W. Infantile spasms: outcome and prognostic factors of cryptogenic and symptomatic groups. *Neurology* 1993; **43**: 2322–2327.

Partial epilepsies in infancy

OLIVIER DULAC AND JEAN-PAUL RATHGEB

In infancy, the term 'partial epilepsy' was first recognized as recently as 1978.[1] Subsequent literature includes the proceedings of a symposium on partial epilepsies.[2]

INCIDENCE

An incidence of partial seizures in the first year of life of 15/100 000 is reported in the single available study.[3]

CLINICAL AND EEG FEATURES

Ictal clinical manifestations

Motor and vegetative features are most frequent. Tonic or clonic movements may involve the face, one or both arms, or one side of the body. The involved arm is typically elevated, with abduction of the shoulder and flexion of the elbow, wrist and fingers.[4] Bilateral eyelid jerking and lateral deviation of the mouth are frequent. Lateral deviation of the head and/or eyes is usually tonic. Lateral jerks of the eyes, 'epileptic nystagmus', occur occasionally. Vegetative manifestations include apnea, either respiratory pause or tonic contraction of the respiratory muscles. Flushing or pallor may involve the whole body, the face or only the lips. Tachypnea and mydriasis are sometimes reported. Automatisms consist of swallowing, chewing and tongue-smacking or licking of the lips, purposeless hand movements, extension and/or flexion of limbs, and head shaking.[5] Other seizures incorporate motion arrest,

decreased responsiveness, staring and blank eyes.[6] Lack of reaction to stimulation affects over three-quarters of the cases. An aura of fear is occasionally reported in the second year of life. Tonic-clonic secondary generalization affects 25–100 per cent of cases. Postictal confusion, disorientation, lethargy or focal motor defects are frequent. Vegetative manifestations usually precede motor activity, whereas alimentary automatisms tend to be seen more often after convulsive movements. Infrequently, generalized tonic seizures may evolve to partial clonic manifestations. In 25 per cent of individual patients, there is a trend towards more focal manifestations with increasing age. Durations range from 30 s to 4 min. with secondary generalization lasting 1–2 min. Seizure classification criteria[7] distinguish three types, simple partial seizures, complex partial seizures (CPS) with striking motor manifestations, and CPS with impaired consciousness at onset. The combination of a partial seizure intermingled with a cluster of spasms is well recognized. Focal features may precede spasms, as though the spasms are 'triggered' by the focal discharge,[8,9] occur at the end or appear during the course of the cluster.[10] The focal seizure then consists of arrest of activity, staring or lateral deviation of head or eyes, oculoclonia,[11] hemitonia, or it may be entirely subclinical.

Ictal EEG manifestations

There is resemblance to recruiting rhythms with low-voltage fast waves, or rhythmic sharp waves or spikes, in the theta or beta ranges. Additional slow waves, later in the discharge, can produce a pattern of spikes and sharp waves. The discharge is focal, spreading to adjacent or contralateral areas; or may remain in the same area throughout; or may involve a whole hemisphere; or is generalized from the onset, and it is only later in the course of the disease that a clear focal onset emerges.

Clinical EEG correlations

The ictal discharge may involve any area of the cerebral cortex, sometimes with loose correlation to clinical manifestations,[5] but usually, motor features are contralateral to the EEG discharge, and ocular clonus contralateral to the occipital discharge.[12] Versive phenomena can be ipsilateral or contralateral, and chewing movements result from a temporal discharge. Frontal lobe seizures consist of arrest of activity with eyelid clonias eventually followed by either hypertonia or pedaling movements; Rolandic seizures of clonic jerks, which eventually proceed to tonic contraction, of one or all four limbs; and temporal seizures of eye-opening with cessation of activities, and turning of the head to one side with oral automatisms. In occipital seizures, there is eye-opening, lateral rotation of the eyes and head, lateral clonic jerks of the eyes and jerks of the eyelids, with eventual propagation to frontal or temporal lobes.

Status epilepticus and HH syndrome

Repeated focal seizures without recovery of consciousness and prolonged hemiclonic seizures followed by hemiplegia, features that define the HH syndrome,[13] may occur.

Interictal EEG activity

Focal spikes are recorded in 25–50 per cent of cases.[14] In most instances, only the background activity is abnormal. The tracing is normal in 12–50 per cent.

PARTIAL SEIZURES AND ONTOGENY OF THE BRAIN

The ontogeny of the brain clearly contributes to the clinical signs of partial seizures.[15] The frequencies of auras, limb automatisms, dystonic posturing, secondary generalization and unresponsiveness, and, the relative incidence of frontal as compared with occipital seizures increases with age. No case affecting the leg has been reported in the first year of life. Partial epilepsy involving the occipital areas seems to begin mostly in the first

2 months of life, constituting a cryptogenic condition that combines very frequent intractable seizures and major and prolonged disorders of vision and interpersonal contact.[16] Age of onset is determined by topography of the epileptogenic zone since maturation of the cerebral cortex, as shown by functional imaging[17,18] (see also Chapters 4C, 19), starts in the occipital areas in the first 2 months, and occurs later and in the frontal and temporal areas.

ETIOLOGY AND COURSE

General considerations

Delayed development prior to seizures and abnormal interictal EEG correlate with poor seizure and developmental outcome, and imaging abnormalities with poor seizure outcome.[19] Neonatal seizures and lack of familial antecedents correlate with poor development. The age of occurrence correlates with etiology, perinatal causes having later onset than prenatal.[20] Uncontrolled partial seizures may affect psychomotor development.[21]

Identifiable causes

Among neurocutaneous disorders, Sturge-Weber disease often results in status epilepticus, when seizures begin in the first year of life, particularly between 3 and 6 months of age. In incontinentia pigmenti, the first seizure often consists of an episode of focal status epilepticus.[22] In both instances, focal ischaemia causes status epilepticus. In tuberous sclerosis, partial seizures may precede the occurrence of infantile spasms, from the very first weeks of life. They may also start after 6 months of life without previous infantile spasms. Cases with hemiconvulsions and hemiplegia (HH syndrome) have been reported. Major malformations, i.e. Aicardi's syndrome, agyria and hemimegalencephaly often produce focal seizures at onset, before the age of 3 months and before the occurrence of infantile spasms. In focal dysplasia, the incidence of focal seizures is more problematic since the lesion may be overlooked until myelination is completed.[23] In these cases, Ohtahara or West syndrome may precede partial seizures, or partial seizures precede West syndrome, or infantile spasms evolve to Lennox-Gastaut syndrome. However, most cases combine focal seizures with infantile spasms: this pattern remaining unchanged until the end of follow-up, and without evolution to Lennox-Gastaut syndrome.[24] In prepeduncular hamartomata, focal motor seizures may occur very early in life, before gelastic seizures become the characteristic ictal hallmark.[25] The size[26] and anatomical aspects of the hamartomata determine clinical expression, with sessile hamartomas producing epilepsy.[27] Surgical approach was considered impossible, but disconnection with ventriculoscopy has been successful.[28] Radionecrosis has also been advised.[29] Tumors underlie 1–2 per cent of epilepsy beginning in infancy. They usually have benign histologic characteristics – astrocytomata, gangliogliomata, or dysembryoplastic neuroepithelial tumors – and it may be difficult to distinguish some benign tumors from dysplasia: occasionally both are found in an individual patient.[30] Due to bleeding in infancy, both arteriovenous and cavernous angiomas may produce occasional seizures before chronic epilepsy develops. Sequelae of pre-, peri- or postnatal circulatory failure, including porencephaly or ulegyria, may be involved, often producing infantile spasms before focal epilepsy.[26] The same applies to neonatal bacterial meningitis, and to neo- or postnatal herpetic encephalitis. The latter may be overlooked in the newborn and recognized later, based on neuroradiological findings and the characteristics of the epilepsy that often consists of late onset, intractable infantile spasms. Epilepsia partialis continua can suggest Alpers disease (Chapter 4D). Infants with daily seizures rarely develop hippocampal atrophy,[31,32] and this is by no means a cause of infantile epilepsy. Various chromosomal aberrations may be associated with partial epilepsy (Chapter 4B).

Migrating partial seizures

Onset is before the 6 months, usually between 2 and 4 months, in previously normal infants with negative neuroradiologic investigations.[31] Patients first suffer rare focal seizures for a few weeks. Then seizures become more or less continuous, and have random topography of onset, involving both hemispheres. The ictal EEG pattern is similar, although the site of onset varies from one seizure to the next. There is rhythmic activity of decreasing frequency and increasing amplitude, with progressive recruitment of adjacent areas of the cortex: discharges involving different areas may overlap. Each discharge lasts 1–4 min. Frontal involvement may be delayed until 6 months of age. Video-EEG shows clear correlation with the topography.[12] Very frequent seizures cause loss of all skills. The head circumference stops growing and severe hypotonia develops. After a few months, seizures occur in clusters of a few days, more or less regularly. Three of a series of 14 reported patients died but neuropathology failed to determine the cause. This recognizable, nonfamilial epilepsy of unknown etiology[32–34] may benefit from bromide.

Benign infantile partial epilepsy

Benign partial epilepsy in infancy has been described by Japanese authors.[6,35,36] Seizures often occur in clusters,

between 3 and 20 months of age, with motor arrest, staring eyes and, eventually, secondary generalization. The EEG shows focal recruiting rhythms, later mixed with slow waves of decreasing frequency, then spikes, polyspikes and sharp wave complexes, originating in the rolandic, occipital, temporal or parietal areas of both hemispheres. Investigations are negative, and seizures easily controlled. Focal seizures after 4 weeks of life, with normal development, interictal EEG, and imaging, predict a benign outcome in over 75 per cent.[37] One variant with onset at 13–30 months and vertex spikes and waves in sleep is reported.[38]

Benign familial infantile convulsions

Benign familial infantile convulsions (BFIC) begin between 4 and 6 months of age with partial seizures, occurring in clusters of 4–10 a day, for 2–4 days.[39–41] Seizures consist of arrest of activity, slow lateral deviation of the head and eyes, loss of consciousness, diffuse hypertonia and unilateral clonic jerks becoming secondarily generalized. The side of lateral deviation may vary from one seizure to the next. Sei-zures last a few minutes. The ictal EEG pattern is similar to that of nonfamilial cases. The interictal EEG is normal. Seizures are easily controlled by antiepileptic drugs. Linkage to chromosome 16 has been shown in affected patients, who late in the first decade, develop paroxysmal dystonia.[42]

TREATMENT

In practice, the difficulties reaching a reliable diagnosis of partial epilepsy, except where a single focal epileptogenic lesion shows imaging, must be emphasized: only in these latter cases should carbamazepine be administered. In all others, the risk of secondary generalization, either with spasms or worsening of an overlooked generalized epilepsy, contraindicates the use of carbamezepine. Valproic acid is a better choice, provided the parents are aware that vomiting and increased seizures may be the first signs of intolerance. Vigabatrin may be a preferable option for patients at risk of later infantile spasms.

Epilepsy surgery may be performed from the first months of life. Hemispherotomy, a procedure developed for the treatment of diffuse unilateral brain damage, can be successful from the age of 4 months.[43] Focal surgery requiring intracranial grids, although technically more difficult, and even more dangerous, because of the risks of infection, is also possible in infancy. Bilateral resection has been performed in one patient with tuberous sclerosis.[44]

KEY POINTS

- Infants can suffer from **partial epilepsy**
- Partial seizures may be the only expression of a **diffuse involvement of the cortex**, probably as a consequence of immature pathways
- Therapeutically, **the distinction between partial and generalized seizures is very important:** drugs effective in partial epilepsy may worsen some patients with generalized epilepsy, i.e. severe myoclonic epilepsy in infancy, which often begins with focal seizures in the first year of life

REFERENCES

1. Di Cagno L, Ravetto F, Rigardetto R, Capizzi G. Aspetti clinici ed evolutivi a medio termine delle crisi partiali dei primi due anni. *Bollettino della Lega Italiana contro l'Epilessia* 1978; **22/23**: 145–152.
2. Roger J. Introduction: partial epilepsies symposium. *Epilepsia* 1989; **30**: 797.
3. Luna D, Chiron C, Pajot N, *et al. Epidémiologie des épilepsies de l'enfant dans le département de l'Oise (France).* In: *Epidémiologie des Epilepsies.* London: J. Libbey; Paris: Eurotext, 1988; 41–53.
4. Luna D, Dulac O, Plouin P. Ictal characteristics of cryptogenic partial epilepsies in infancy. *Epilepsia* 1989; **30**: 827–832.
5. Yamamoto N, Watanabe K, Negoro T, *et al.* Complex partial seizures in children: ictal manifestations and their relation to clinical course. *Neurology* 1987; **37**: 1379–1382.
6. Watanabe K, Negoro T, Aso K. Benign partial epilepsy with secondary generalised seizures in infancy. *Epilepsia* 1993; **34**: 635–638.
7. Commission on Classification and Terminology of the International League Against Epilepsy. Proposal for revised clinical and electroencephalographic classification of epileptic seizures. *Epilepsia* 1981; **22**: 489–501.
8. Dalla Bernardina B, Colamaria V, Capovilla G, *et al.* Sindromi epilettiche precoci e malformation bi cerebrali. Studio multicentrico. *Bollettino della Lega Italiana contro l'Epilessia* 1984; **45/46**: 65–67.
9. Bour F, Chiron C, Dulac O, Plouin P. Caractères électrocliniques des crises dans le syndrome d'Aicardi. *Revue d'Electroencephalographie et de Neurophysiologie Clinique* 1986; **16**: 341–353.
10. Carrazzana EJ, Lombroso CT, Mikati M, *et al.* Facilitation of infantile spasms by partial seizures. *Epilepsia* 1993; **34**: 97–109.
11. Shewmon DA. Ictal aspects, with emphasis on unusual variants. In: Dulac O, Chugani H, Dalla Bernardina B. (eds) *Infantile Spasms and West syndrome.* London: Saunders, 1995; 36–57.
12. Chiron C, Soufflet C, Pollack C, Cusmai R. Semiology of cryptogenic multifocal partial seizures in infancy. *Electroencephalography and Clinical Neurophysiology* 1988; **70**: 9–16P.
13. Gastaut H, Poirier F, Payan H, *et al.* HHE syndrome: hemiconvulsions-herniplegia-epilepsy. *Epilepsia* 1960; **1**: 418–447.
14. Dravet C, Catani C, Bureau M, Roger J. Partial epilepsies in infancy – a study of 40 cases. *Epilepsia* 1989; **30**: 807–812.
15. Nordli DR Jr, Kuroda MM, Hirsch LJ. The ontogeny of partial seizures in infants and young children. *Epilepsia* 2001; **42**: 986–990.
16. Lortie A, Plouin P, Pinard JM, Dulac O. In: Beaumanoir A *et al.* (eds) *Occipital Epilepsy in Neonates and Infants.* London: J. Libbey and Co, 1995 121–132.
17. Chugani HT, Phelps ME, Mazziotta JC. Positron emission tomography study of human brain functional development. *Annals of Neurology* 1987; **22**: 487–497.
18. Chiron C, Raynaud C, Maziere B, *et al.* Changes in regional cerebral blood flow during brain maturation in children and adolescents. *Journal of Nuclear Medicine* 1991; **33**: 696–703.
19. Okumura A, Hayakawa F, Kato T, *et al.* Five-year follow-up of patients with partial epilepsies in infancy. *Pediatric Neurology* 2001; **24**: 290–296.
20. Okumura A, Hayakawa F, Kato T, *et al.* Early recognition of benign partial epilepsy in infancy. *Epilepsia* 2000; **41**: 714–717.
21. Kramer U, Fattal A, Nevo Y, Leitner Y, Harel S. Mental retardation subsequent to refractory partial seizures in infancy. *Brain Development* 2000; **22**: 31–34.
22. Avrahami E, Harel S, Jurgehson U, *et al.* Computed tomographic demonstration of brain changes in incontinentia pigmenti. *American Journal of Diseases of Children* 1985; **139**: 372–374.
23. Bogaert P Van, Chiron C, Andamsbaum C, *et al.* Value of magnetic resonance imaging in West syndrome of unknown etiology. *Epilepsia* 1993; **34**: 701–706.
24. Kobayashi K, Ohtsuka Y, Ohno S, *et al.* Clinical spectrum of epileptic spasms associated with cortical malformation. *Neuropediatrics* 2001; **32**: 236–244.
25. Plouin P, Ponsot C, Dulac O, *et al.* Hamartomes hypothalamiques et crises de rire. *Revue d'Electroencephalographie et de Neurophysiol Clinique* 1983; **13**: 312–316.
26. Diebler C, Dulac O. Pediatric neurology and neuroradiology. In: *Cerebral and Cranial Diseases.* Berlin: Springer, 1987; 408.
27. Debeneix C, Bourgeois M, Trivin C, Sainte-Rose C, Brauner R. Hypothalamic hamartoma: comparison of clinical presentation and magnetic resonance images. *Hormone Research* 2001; **56**: 12–18.
28. Delalande O, Rodriguez D, Chiron C, Fohlen M. Successful surgical relief of seizures associated with hamartoma of the floor of the fourth ventricle in children: report of two cases. *Neurosurgery* 2001; **49**: 726–730.
29. Regis J, Bartolomei F, de Toffol B, *et al.* Gamma knife surgery for epilepsy related to hypothalamic hamartomas. *Neurosurgery* 2000; **47**: 1343–1351.
30. Prayson RA, Estes ML, Morris HH. Coexistence of neoplasia and cortical dysplasia in patients presenting with seizures. *Epilepsia* 1993; **34**: 609–615.
31. Coppola C, Plouin P, Chiron C, *et al.* Migrating partial seizures in infancy: a malignant disorder with developmental arrest. *Epilepsia* 1995; **36**: 1017–1024.

32. Wilmshurst JM, Appleton DB, Grattan-Smith PJ. Migrating partial seizures in infancy: two new cases. *Journal of Child Neurology* 2000; **15**: 717–722.

33. Okuda K, Yasuhara A, Kamei A, *et al.* Successful control with bromide of two patients with malignant migrating partial seizures in infancy. *Brain Development* 2000; **22**: 56–59.

34. Veneselli E, Perrone MV, Di Rocco M, Gaggero R, Biancheri R. Malignant migrating partial seizures in infancy. *Epilepsy Research* 2001; **46**: 27–32.

35. Watanabe K, Yamamoto N, Negoro T, *et al.* Benign complex partial epilepsies in infancy. *Pediatric Neurology* 1987; **3**: 208–211.

36. Watanabe K, Yamamoto N, Negoro T, *et al.* Benign infantile epilepsy with complex partial seizures. *Journal of Clinical Neurophysiology* 1990; **7**: 409–416.

37. Okumura A, Watanabe K, Negoro T, *et al.* MRI findings in patients with symptomatic localization-related epilepsies beginning in infancy and early childhood. *Seizure* 2000; **9**: 566–571.

38. Capovilla G, Beccaria F. Benign partial epilepsy in infancy and early childhood with vertex spikes and waves during sleep: a new epileptic form. *Brain Development* 2000; **22**: 93–98.

39. Vigevano F, Fusco L, di Capua M, *et al.* Benign infantile familial convulsions. *European Journal of Pediatrics* 1992; **151**: 608–612.

40. Echenne B, Rivier F, Humbertclaude V, *et al.* Benign familial infantile convulsions. *Archives of Pediatrics* 2000; **6**: 54–58.

41. Nagase T, Takahashi Y, Iida S, *et al.* Ictal and interictal single photon emission computed tomography in a patient with benign familial infantile convulsions. *Journal of Neuroimaging* 2002; **12**: 75–77.

42. Szepetowski P, Rochette J, Berquin P, *et al.* Familial infantile convulsions and paroxysmal choreoathetosis: a new neurological syndrome linked to the pericentric region of human chromosome 16. *American Journal of Human Genetics* 1997; **61**: 889–898.

43. Villemure JG, Vernet O, Delalande O. Hemispheric disconnection: callosotomy and hemispherotomy. *Adv Tech Stand Neurosurg* 2000; **26**: 25–78.

44. Romanelli P, Weiner HL, Najjar S, Devinsky O. Bilateral resective epilepsy surgery in a child with tuberous sclerosis: case report. *Neurosurgery* 2001; **49**: 732–734.

Benign myoclonic epilepsy in infancy

NATALIO FEJERMAN

The classification of the myoclonic epilepsies in infancy and childhood has been controversial.[1–7] The International League Against Epilepsy (ILAE) classification[8] includes benign myoclonic epilepsy in infancy (BMEI) among the idiopathic generalized epilepsies and considers it to be an early presentation of idiopathic myoclonic epilepsy. The high incidence of educational difficulties in these children raises questions about the use of the term 'benign', which is reserved usually for epilepsies associated with normal neuropsychologic development. Since its description in 1981, 67 cases of BMEI had been reported by 2002.[9,10] We have followed 25 cases (Fejerman and Caraballo, unpublished report, 2002).

Epidemiologic data about prevalence of this syndrome are limited. Myoclonic seizures (not only BMEI) were present in 2.2 per cent of 440 consecutive pediatric patients with epilepsy.[11] In a separate study, BMEI was diagnosed in 2 per cent of infants less than 3 years of age with epilepsy.[1] We diagnosed BMEI in 6 of 471 patients (1.3 per cent) with epilepsy in the first year of life.[12]

Myoclonic seizures occurring as a reflex to acoustic or tactile stimuli have been reported as a separate clinical entity in a small series of otherwise normal infants, and termed reflex myoclonic epilepsy.[13–15] However, it has been suggested that this disorder is probably a variant of BMEI[10] and the issue is not fully resolved.[16] Reflex myoclonic epilepsy has not been included as a separate syndrome in the most recent report of the ILAE Task Force on Classification and Terminology.[17] An infantile myoclonic epilepsy syndrome occurring in otherwise normal children has been described recently in a large kindred with autosomal recessive inheritance,[18] and the gene mapped to chromosome 16.[19]

CLINICAL AND EEG FEATURES

A family history of epilepsy has been reported in 25–30 per cent of the patients.[10,20,21] In our 25 cases, there was a history of epilepsy in 4 relatives and of febrile seizures in a further 4 (Fejerman and Caraballo, unpublished report 2002).

Febrile seizures were reported initially in 4 of 37 affected children.[20] Subsequently, the same authors reported that simple febrile seizures preceded the onset of myoclonia in 20 per cent of the cases.[20] Similarly, febrile seizures were observed in 5 of our 25 cases (Fejerman and Caraballo, unpublished report 2002) and in 5 of the 10 patients reported by Lin.[22]

The usual sequence is the onset of brief bilateral myoclonic seizures in a neurologically normal infant aged between 6 months and 2 years. Jerks are more prominent in the upper part of the body, manifesting as a head drop and upward and outward extension of upper limbs. Polygraphic recordings have shown that the head drops in BMEI are associated with myoclonic jerks and that absences or tonic seizures are never detected.[20] The jerks may be single and very brief or repetitive with a pseudo-rhythmic pattern, lasting several seconds. The eyes may roll up but consciousness is never completely lost; and, only very rarely, when the lower limbs are moved involved, does the child fall. The myoclonic seizures can occur at any time of the day.

Neurophysiologic studies have demonstrated a rostro-caudal muscle activation of symmetric myoclonus. A negative spike precedes the myoclonic jerks by 30 ± 2 ms. The duration of the myoclonic jerk is approximately

100 ms.[23] Every seizure is associated with a discharge of generalized spike-waves or polyspike-waves. It is rare to find subclinical discharges in the waking EEG. On the other hand, drowsiness and the early stages of sleep activate the discharges, some of which are unaccompanied by a clinical expression. A photosensitive response is seen in the EEG in approximately 20 per cent of the cases. It is important to appreciate that the interictal EEG is usually normal in the waking state. The EEG may also be normal when the child is pharmacologically sedated and the recording omits the drowsy state and the early stages of sleep.

Valproic acid has been reported to be the drug of choice and gives excellent control of seizures. In some cases generalized tonic-clonic seizures have appeared later in childhood or adolescence upon stopping medication.[20,22]

Approximately 21–41 per cent of patients with BMEI have educational difficulties. The suggestion that early treatment might prevent occurrence of these difficulties has not been verified,[3,10,20,24] raising questions as to the appropriateness of the term 'benign'. The educational progress of children with BMEI should be monitored carefully, and assistance given to those with specific difficulties.

DIFFERENTIAL DIAGNOSIS

The major nonepileptic and epileptic conditions which should be considered in the differential diagnosis of BMEI are listed in Table 9D.1. More detailed analyses of these nonepileptic and epileptic paroxysmal disorders or episodic symptoms with onset during the first year of life are given in Chapters 2, 9B, 9E and elsewhere.[25,26]

It is important to stress the difference between benign myoclonic epilepsy of infancy and benign myoclonus of early infancy,[5–31] a nonepileptic condition for which the same abbreviation (BMEI) is often used. In both syndromes, myoclonias appear at similar ages in babies with previously normal development, mostly in the awake state, and affect predominantly the head and upper limbs. Brief jerks tend to be repeated for some seconds, without loss of consciousness. In a proportion of cases of

Table 9D.1 *Differential diagnosis of benign myoclonic epilepsy in infancy*

Nonepileptic conditions
  physiologic myoclonus (sleep jerks)
  hyperekplexia
  benign myoclonus of early infancy

Epileptic syndromes
  West syndrome
  severe myoclonic epilepsy in infancy
  early-onset Lennox-Gastaut syndrome
  epilepsy with myoclonic-astatic seizures
  familial infantile myoclonic epilepsy

benign nonepileptic myoclonus, the jerks resemble shuddering attacks,[32] or may simulate infantile spasms, which led to the term 'benign nonepileptic infantile spasms'.[33] The clinical evolution, however, is different. The non-epileptic benign myoclonia tend to disappear during the second and third year of life. In addition, antiepileptic drugs (AEDs) have no clear effect on them. The EEG shows no abnormality during a benign myoclonus. In contrast, an ictal record or one capturing drowsiness and the early stages of sleep should confirm a diagnosis of benign myoclonic epilepsy of infancy.

The possibility of West syndrome is undoubtedly the main concern when a baby has brief repetitive seizures affecting axial and upper limb musculature. The EEG is clearly an important method for differentiating these conditions, in that the spike-wave or polyspike-wave discharges observed on a normal background rhythm in patients with BMEI differs markedly from hypsarrhythmia.

Differentiating BMEI from Dravet syndrome (severe myoclonic epilepsy of infancy)[34,35] is usually not difficult. However, it has been suggested that these syndromes may only reflect different degrees of severity in a single condition, described as infantile myoclonic epilepsy following febrile convulsions.[4] The clinical and EEG features can usually distinguish between the two disorders:

- Febrile seizures are always prolonged in Dravet syndrome and brief in BMEI; febrile seizures occur in only 10–20 per cent of the cases of BMEI.
- Myoclonic seizures are very rare during the first year of life in Dravet syndrome and are the unique seizures in BMEI.
- The EEG is usually normal during the first year of life in Dravet syndrome.
- The arrest of neurologic development appears earlier and is more severe in Dravet syndrome, whereas only 20–40 per cent of patients with BMEI have cognitive problems and these usually become evident at an older age.

Early-onset Lennox-Gastaut syndrome may be associated with myoclonic seizures. However, different seizure types, mainly atonic, tonic and atypical absences, characterize Lennox-Gastaut syndrome. In contrast, the seizures in BMEI are usually myoclonic-atonic or atonic. Furthermore, the EEG during drowsiness in Lennox-Gastaut syndrome is characterized by slow spike-waves in the interictal state, and a recruiting rhythm is associated with brief tonic seizures.[36]

Epilepsy with myoclonic-astatic seizures (MAE) may start in early childhood and pose difficulties for nosologic identification. The course and outcome of MAE are quite variable[8,37] and MAE probably encompasses syndromes that many authors consider as separate, ranging from BMEI to the myoclonic variant of Lennox-Gastaut syndrome[3,5,38] (see Chapter 11C). Nevertheless, the main features of MAE are the association of myoclonic-astatic seizures leading to drop attacks with absences and tonic-clonic seizures; the frequent occurrence of absence status; and the presence of 4–7-Hz rhythms in the EEG, in addition to numerous spike-wave and polyspike-wave discharges. These features are not shared by BMEI.

Advances in our understanding of the genetics of epilepsies are likely to influence our understanding of the myoclonic epilepsies. Dravet syndrome has been recognized to be a phenotype within the spectrum of the febrile seizures plus (FS+) syndrome.[39–43] If FS+ syndrome may include some patients with febrile seizures, MAE and Dravet syndrome, it seems logical to consider that it may also include some patients with BMEI, since 10–20 per cent of BMEI have a history of febrile seizures.

Finally, two new entities with myoclonic seizures have been mapped to specific chromosomes. De Falco et al.[18] have described a large kindred in which myoclonic epilepsy affected 8 patients and a locus was mapped to chromosome 16p13.[19] The seizures in this familial infantile myoclonic epilepsy (FIME) appeared between 5 and 36 months of age and persisted to adulthood in all patients. All affected individuals had normal psychomotor development and had no signs of cognitive deterioration. All patients developed generalized tonic-clonic seizures between 12 and 16 years of age, which showed a good response to valproic acid. Interestingly, afebrile generalized seizures preceded the appearance of myoclonic seizures in 4 of the 8 patients. The family descended from the intermarriage of two pairs of siblings, suggesting an autosomal recessive inheritance, and the mapping of a locus to chromosome 16p13 in this kindred may provide some clues as to the mechanisms of some of the myoclonic epilepsies.[18,19] In addition, a familial form of adult myoclonic epilepsy has been reported, which maps to chromosome 8q24.[44,45]

KEY POINTS

- **Bilateral myoclonic seizures** are seen first between 6 months and 2 years in neurologically normal infants
- A **family history of epilepsy and/or febrile seizures** is obtained in 20–25 per cent of patients
- A **preceding history of febrile seizures** is present in approximately 20 per cent of children
- Ictal **EEG** shows generalized spike-waves. Interictal EEG is normal in the waking state but there may be interictal spike-wave discharges in drowsiness and light sleep
- **Photosensitivity** is observed in approximately 20 per cent of patients
- **Valproic acid** is the most effective drug

- **Educational difficulties** are encountered by 20–40 per cent of patients

REFERENCES

1. Dalla Bernardina B, Colamaria V, Capotilla G, Bonavalli S. Nosological classification of epilepsias in the first three years of life. In: Nistico G et al. (eds) Epilepsy: An Update in Research and Therapy. New York: Alan Liss, 1983; 165–183.
2. Dravet C, Bureau M, Roger J. Benign myoclonic epilepsy in infants. In: Roger J et al. (eds) Epileptic Syndromes in Infancy, Childhood and Adolescence. London: John Libbey; Paris: Eurotext, 1985; 51–57.
3. Aicardi J, Levy-Gomes AL. The myoclonic epilepsies of childhood. Cleveland Clinic Journal of Medicine 1989; 56(Suppl. 1): 534–539.
4. Lombroso CT. Early myoclonic encephalopathy, early infantile epileptic encephalopathy, and benign and severe infantile myoclonic epilepsies: a critical review and personal contributions. Journal of Clinical Neurophysiology 1990; 7: 380–408.
5. Fejerman N. Myoclonies et epilepsies chez l'enfant. Revue Neurologique (Paris) 1991; 147: 782–797.
6. Dulac O, Plouin P, Shewmon A. Myoclonus and epilepsy in childhood. 1996 Royaumont meeting. Epilepsy Research 1998; 30: 91–106.
7. Oguni H, Fukuyama Y, Tanaka T, et al. Myoclonic-astatic epilepsy of early childhood-clinical and EEG analysis of myoclonic-astatic seizures, and discussions on the nosology of the syndrome. Brain Development 2001; 23(7): 757–764.
8. Commission on Classification and Terminology of the International League Against Epilepsy. Proposal for revised classification of epilepsies and epileptic syndromes. Epilepsia 1989; 30: 389–399.
9. Dravet C, Bureau M. L'epilepsie myoclonique benigne du nourrisson. Revue d'Electroencephalographie et Neurophysiologie 1981; 11: 438–444.
10. Dravet C, Bureau M. Benign myoclonic epilepsy in infancy. In: Engel J, Fejerman N. (eds) MedLink Neurology. San Diego: MedLink Corporation, 2002; www.medlink.com.
11. Kramer U, Nevo Y, Neufeld MY, et al. Epidemiology of epilepsy in childhood: a cohort of 440 consecutive patients. Pediatric Neurology 1998; 18(1): 46–50.
12. Caraballo R, Cersosimo R, Galicchio S, Fejerman N. Epilepsias en el primer año de vida. Revue Neurologique 1997; 25(146): 1521–1524.
13. Ricci S, Cusmai R, Fusco L, Vigevano F. Reflex myoclonic epilepsy in infancy: a new age-dependent idiopathic epileptic syndrome related to startle reaction. Epilepsia 1995; 36(4): 342–348.
14. Vigevano F, Cusmai R, Ricci S, Watanabe K. Benign epilepsy of infancy. In: Engel J, Pedley TA (eds) Epilepsy: A Comprehensive Textbook. Philadelphia: Lippincott-Raven, 1997; 2267–2276.
15. Caraballo HR, Yepez I, Ledesma D, Donari J, Fejerman N. Epilepsia mioclónica refleja del lactante. Revista Ecuatoriana de Neurologia 1998; 7: 62–65.

16. Guerrini R, Bonanni P, Rothwell J, Hallett M. Myoclonus and epilepsy. In: Guerrini R *et al.* (eds) *Epilepsy and Movement Disorders.* Cambridge: Cambridge University Press, 2002; 165–210.

17. Engel J. A proposed diagnostic scheme for people with epileptic seizures and with epilepsy: report of the ILAE Task Force on Classification and Terminology. *Epilepsia* 2001; **42**(6): 796–803.

18. de Falco FA, Majello L, Santangelo R, *et al.* Familial infantile myoclonic epilepsy: clinical features in a large kindred with autosomal recessive inheritance. *Epilepsia* 2001; **42**: 1541–1548.

19. Zara F, Gennaro E, Stabile M, *et al.* Mapping of a locus for a familial autosomal recessive idiopathic myoclonic epilepsy of infancy to chromosome 16p13. *American Journal of Human Genetics* 2000; **66**: 1552–1557.

20. Dravet C, Bureau M, Roger J. Benign myoclonic epilepsy in infants. In: Roger J *et al.* (eds) *Epileptic Syndromes in Infancy, Childhood and Adolescence*, 2nd edn. London: John Libbey, 1992; 67–74.

21. Giovanardi Rossi P, Parmeggiani A, Posar A, *et al.* Benign myoclonic epilepsy: long-term follow-up of 11 new cases. *Brain Development* 1997; **19**: 473–479.

22. Lin Y, Itomi K, Takada H, *et al.* Benign myoclonic epilepsy in infants: video-EEG features and long-term follow-up. *Neuropediatrics* 1998; **29**(5): 268–271.

23. Guerrini R, Parmeggiani L, Volzone A, Bonanni P. Cortical myoclonus in early childhood epilepsy. In: Majkowski J, Owczarek K, Zwolinski P (eds) *3rd European Congress of Epileptology.* Bologna: Monduzzi editore, 1998; 99–105.

24. Todt H, Muller D. The therapy of benign myoclonic epilepsy in infants. In: Degen R, Dreifuss F (eds) *Benign Localized and Generalized Epilepsies in Early Childhood, Epilepsy Research.* Amsterdam: Elsevier, 1992.

25. Fejerman N. Differential diagnosis. In: Dulac O *et al.* (eds) *Infantile Spasms and West Syndrome.* London: W.B. Saunders, 1994; 88–98.

26. Fejerman N. Nonepileptic neurologic paroxysmal disorders and episodic symptoms in infants. In: Engel J, Pedley TA (eds) *Epilepsy: A Comprehensive Textbook.* Philadelphia: Lippincott-Raven, 1998; 2745–2754.

27. Fejerman N. Mioclonías benignas de la infancia temprana. Comunicación preliminar. In: *Actas IV Jornadas Rioplatenses de Neurología Infantil 1976. Neuropediatría Latinoamericana.* Montevideo: Delta, 1977; 131–134.

28. Fejerman N. Mioclonías benignas de la infancia temprana. *Annales Espanoles de Pediatria* 1984; **21**: 725–731.

29. Lombroso CT, Fejerman N. Benign myoclonus of early infancy. *Annals of Neurology* 1977; **1**: 138–148.

30. Fejerman N, Medina CS. *Convulsiones en la infancia,* 2nd edn. Buenos Aires: El Ateneo, 1986.

31. Fejerman N, Caraballo R. Appendix to 'Shuddering and benign myoclonus of early infancy' (Pachatz C, Fusco L, Vigevano F).

In: Guerrini J *et al.* (eds) *Epilepsy and Movement Disorders.* Cambridge: Cambridge University Press, 2002; 343–351.

32. Vanasse M, Bedard P, Andermann F. Shuddering attacks in children: an early clinical manifestation of essential tremor. *Neurology* 1976; **26**: 1027–1030.

33. Dravet C, Giraud N, Bureau M, *et al.* Benign myoclonus of early infancy or benign non epileptic infantile spasms. *Neuropediatrics* 1986; **1**(17): 33–38.

34. Dravet C. Les epilepsies graves de l'enfance. *Vie Médicale* 1978; **8**: 543–548.

35. Dravet C, Bureau M. Severe myoclonic epilepsy in infants. In: Roger J *et al.* (eds) *Epileptic Syndromes in Infancy, Childhood and Adolescence.* London: John Libbey; Paris, Eurotext, 1985; 58–67.

36. Beaumanoir A. The Lennox-Gastaut syndrome. In: Roger J *et al.* (eds) *Epileptic Syndromes in Infancy, Childhood and Adolescence.* London: John Libbey; Paris, Eurotext, 1985; 89–99.

37. Doose H. Myoclonic astatic epilepsy of early childhood. In: Roger J *et al.* (eds) *Epileptic Syndromes in Infancy, Childhood and Adolescence.* London: John Libbey; Paris, Eurotext, 1985; 78–88.

38. Delgado-Escueta AV, Greenberg D, Weissbecker K, *et al.* Gene mapping in the idiopathic generalizad epilepsias: juvenile myoclonic epilepsy, childhood absence epilepsy, epilepsy with grand mal seizures, and early childhood myoclonic epilepsy. *Epilepsia* 1990; **31**(Suppl. 3): S19–29.

39. Scheffer IE, Berkovic SF Generalized epilepsy with febrile seizures plus. A genetic disorder with heterogeneous clinical phenotypes. *Brain* 1997; **120**: 479–490.

40. Wallace RH, Wang DW, Singh R, *et al.* Febrile seizures and generalized epilepsy associated with a mutation in the Na$^+$ channel B1 subunit gene SCN1B. *Nature Genetics* 1998; **19**: 366–370.

41. Singh R, Scheffer IE, Crossland K, Berkovic SF. Generalised epilepsy with febrile seizures plus (GEFS): a common, childhood onset, genetic epileptic syndrome. *Annals of Neurology* 1999; **45**: 75–81.

42. Singh R, Andermann E, Whitehouse WP, *et al.* Severe myoclonic epilepsy of infancy: extended spectrum of GEFS+? *Epilepsia* 2001; **42**(7): 837–844.

43. Claes L, Del-Favero J, Ceulemans B, *et al.* De novo mutations in the sodium-channel gene SCN1A cause severe myoclonic epilepsy of infancy. *American Journal of Human Genetics* 2001; **68**(6): 1327–1332.

44. Mikami M, Yasuda T, Terao A, *et al.* Localization of a gene for benign adult familial myoclonic epilepsy to chromosome 8q23.3-q24.1. *American Journal of Human Genetics* 1999; **65**(3): 745–751.

45. Plaster NM, Uyama E, Uchino M, *et al.* Genetic localization of the familial adult myoclonic epilepsy (FAME) gene to chromosome 8q24. *Neurology* 1999; **53**(6): 1180–1183.

Severe myoclonic epilepsy in infancy (Dravet syndrome)

NATALIO FEJERMAN

Severe myoclonic epilepsy in infancy (SMEI) is an epileptic syndrome with distinctive electroclinical features described first by Dravet[1] and subsequently by many authors.[2–7] The occurrence in a significant number of patients of a similar electroclinical picture except for the absence of myoclonic seizures prompted the term 'severe polymorphic epilepsy of infancy'.[8,9] The Task Force on Classification of the International League Against Epilepsy (ILAE) has more recently recommended the name **Dravet syndrome**.[10] The prevalence of Dravet syndrome has been estimated to be 1/20 000–1/40 000 infants,[11,12] and boys are more often affected than girls.

CLINICAL AND EEG FEATURES

Neurological development is normal before the onset of the seizures. The first seizure is often a prolonged clonic or tonic-clonic seizure, either generalized or unilateral, and occurs between 2 and 9 months of age. It is usually associated with fever and, when afebrile, a recent history of vaccination or infectious disease is often obtained. Further clonic seizures occur after an interval of weeks or a few months with or without fever. It has been suggested that hot water immersion may also trigger these seizures.[7] Tonic-clonic convulsions, either generalized or unilateral, are generally seen throughout the course of the disease.[3,7] Conventional antiepileptic drugs (AEDs) do not prevent recurrence of these seizures.

Myoclonic seizures usually appear in the second year of life. These may vary from mild and occasional segmentary myoclonus causing only jerks of a limb, facial muscles or axial muscles, to generalized, massive and frequent myoclonic seizures resulting in drop attacks. Myoclonic seizures occur particularly on awakening and can be triggered by variations in light intensity, closure of the eyes or hot baths.[2,13,14] A clear increase in their frequency often precedes generalized seizures.[12] Some authors have described cases with all of the other features of Dravet syndrome but without myoclonic seizures.[7,15]

Status epilepticus is common and can be either convulsive (often associated with fever and occurring in the first years) or nonconvulsive status with myoclonias.[2,7,12,16] Other afebrile seizure types may occur between 1 and 4 years of age, including versive seizures and complex partial seizures. Absences are less frequent, very rarely typical, and consist of brief isolated loss of consciousness or an arrest of activity with a myoclonic component. There are disagreements in the literature as to whether absences form part of repeated myoclonic attacks.[2,12,17,18] Tonic seizures are not usually seen in Dravet syndrome and their occurrence suggests a different diagnosis.

Neurological development is normal before the onset of the seizures. As the seizures become more frequent, the rate of development slows. Language acquisition is usually delayed and intellectual development becomes progressively more delayed. Some degree of hyperactivity, which may also be influenced by AEDs, is common. There may be mild cerebellar and pyramidal signs associated with clumsiness and ataxia of gait.

The EEG is usually normal during the first year of life[2,12,19] but spontaneous or photic-induced spike-wave discharges were described by this age in 4 of 63 cases[2] and in 13 of 40 patients.[19] Epileptiform EEG abnormalities appear more often between the second and third years of life and include short bursts of generalized polyspikes, polyspikes and waves, or spikes and waves, which occur with or without myoclonic jerks. The background rhythms probably remain normal in many patients, although there are limited data available. A particular theta (4–5 Hz) monomorphic activity, maximal in the frontocentral and lateral regions, has been described in the waking state.[12,17,20]

ETIOLOGY

An underlying neurologic disease has not been demonstrated in these patients. A history of a remote neurologic insult is very uncommon and extensive metabolic investigations and neuroimaging studies have consistently been negative. In one autopsied case, microdysgenetic lesions were found in the spinal cord and cerebellum.[21] Focal PET abnormalities were described in 6 out of 8 children with Dravet syndrome, resulting in the speculation that there might be a unifocal origin for the seizures in some patients.[22] However, the unilateral seizures often occur on either side in the same patient.

Genetic factors play a significant role in this epilepsy. There have been isolated reports of Dravet syndrome in siblings and two pairs of affected monozygotic twins have been described.[14,23] A positive family history of epilepsy and/or febrile seizures is common, occurring in 20–54 per cent of cases.[2,5–8,18–20,24] Patients with Dravet syndrome had a significantly increased incidence of febrile convulsions (FCs) and of epilepsy in their relatives compared with a control group. The epilepsy in relatives of patients with SMEI had the characteristics of idiopathic generalized epilepsy.[6] Dravet syndrome has also been reported to occur in some families with the generalized epilepsy with febrile seizures plus (GEFS+) syndrome,[25–28] and it has been suggested that Dravet syndrome may represent the severe end of the spectrum of GEFS+ syndrome.[26] Missense mutations in the gene that codes for a neuronal voltage-gated sodium-channel α-subunit (SCN1A) have been identified in families with GEFS+. Similarly, seven unrelated probands with Dravet syndrome were shown to have de novo mutations in the gene that codes for SCN1A.[29]

TREATMENT AND OUTCOME

The seizures rarely respond to standard AEDs. Valproic acid[30] and the benzodiazepines (clobazam, clonazepam, lorazepam) seem to be the most useful drugs. Status epilepticus is common, and an important early therapeutic measure is to teach the parents to use rectal diazepam at the onset of a clonic seizure. The addition of stiripentol to valproic acid and clobazam was shown to be effective in a randomized double-blind, placebo controlled study in children with Dravet syndrome. Fifteen of the 21 patients who received stiripentol had more than 50 per cent reduction in the frequency of clonic or tonic-clonic seizures.[31] Vigabatrin achieved fairly good seizure control in four children in the second year of life treated by the author, but a better indication for this drug may be those cases without myoclonic seizures.[32] Nine of 18 patients with Dravet syndrome achieved a 75–100 per cent reduction of seizures when treated with topiramate as adjunctive therapy, but the period of control only ranged from 6 to 18 months.[33] Zonisamide[7,15,34] and bromides[7] have also been reported to be useful in this condition. Lamotrigine has been reported to exacerbate seizures in Dravet syndrome.[32] Phenytoin was reported to cause choreoathetosis in three patients with SMEI.[35]

The ketogenic diet has been reported to be effective, and it is our practice to start the ketogenic diet as soon as possible after the first year of life in children with Dravet syndrome.[7,36] Seven of 13 children with Dravet syndrome had good seizure control and continued on the diet for 1–3 years, five of them achieving a 75–100 per cent reduction in seizures and a significant improvement in quality of life.[36]

Generalized or secondary generalized tonic-clonic seizures tend to persist, but complex partial seizures seem to disappear after a few years.[2,7] The frequency of myoclonia decreases progressively over the course of time.[2,7,8,12,13,19,20] The prognosis for intellectual development is always poor. In the largest series of patients, all the patients aged 10 years or over were dependent and institutionalized.[2] The prognosis may be less severe in those patients with Dravet syndrome without myoclonic seizures.[7,15] A high mortality rate has been reported in several series. Thus, death in childhood was described in 3 of 40,[19] 10 of 63,[2] and 7 of 39 patients with Dravet syndrome.[7]

DIFFERENTIAL DIAGNOSIS

The occurrence of recurrent prolonged seizures in the first year of life, either febrile or associated with vaccinations or infectious diseases,[2,5] is suggestive of this diagnosis. A definite diagnosis is possible, however, only when enough time has elapsed to allow the full picture to evolve.[17,37–40] Myoclonic seizures are the most obvious next clinical feature. However, cases with similar features and evolution but without myoclonic seizures have been reported.[7,12,15,24] Consequently, the absence of myoclonic seizures is not considered to exclude the diagnosis of Dravet syndrome in patients who demonstrate all of the other features.[41]

The differential diagnosis of Dravet syndrome includes several early-onset epileptic syndromes. Benign myoclonic epilepsy in infancy (Chapter 9D) is also associated with myoclonic seizures in infancy but prolonged febrile seizures are not a feature. The criteria for the diagnosis of epilepsy with myoclonic-astatic seizures (Chapter 10A) are less precise, and some of the patients reported initially with myoclonic-astatic seizures might have been cases of Dravet syndrome.[42] Cryptogenic Lennox-Gastaut syndrome[43] may also start in infancy, may be associated with myoclonic seizures, and may not show its typical EEG pattern in the first few months (Chapter 10B). However, febrile seizures are an uncommon initial feature in Lennox-Gastaut syndrome. Only one case of Lennox-Gastaut syndrome was reported in 369 children with febrile seizures followed for at least 2 years.[44] Dravet syndrome has certain clinical features in common with myoclonic-astatic seizures and Lennox-Gastaut syndrome such as presence of different types of seizures, intractability to medication and the development of intellectual disability over time.[45] Thus, it can be difficult to classify certain patients and intermediate cases straddling the boundaries between myoclonic-astatic seizures, Lennox-Gastaut syndrome and Dravet syndrome have been reported.[7,9,12,15,40] Finally, mesial temporal lobe epilepsy following prolonged febrile seizures may be in the differential diagnosis of some patients in the early stages of Dravet syndrome.[46] Thus, both conditions may be associated with antecedent febrile seizures, the appearance of complex partial seizures and secondary generalized clonic or tonic-clonic seizures, and an initially normal interictal EEG. However, the later clinical and EEG features are quite distinct.

KEY POINTS

- Dravet syndrome is **one of the most severe epileptic syndromes** with onset in infancy
- Prolonged **unilateral or generalized febrile clonic seizures** are usually the initial seizure type, presenting in the first year of life
- **Myoclonic seizures** are the most common second seizure type and start usually after the first year. Other seizure types may include complex partial and absence seizures
- The **absence of myoclonic seizures** does not preclude the diagnosis of Dravet syndrome if all other features are present
- The seizures are **highly intractable to AED treatment**
- **Prognosis is very poor** in terms of intellectual abilities
- There is often a **family history** of febrile seizures and of idiopathic generalized epilepsy
- **Mutations in a gene** that codes for a neuronal voltage-gated sodium-channel α-subunit (SCN1A) have been described in patients with Dravet syndrome
- Patients with Dravet syndrome have been described in **families with GEFS+**

REFERENCES

1. Dravet C. Les epilepsies graves de l'enfance. *Vie Médicale* 1978; **8**: 543–548.
2. Dravet C, Bureau M Guerrini R, *et al*. Severe myoclonic epilepsy in infancy, childhood and adolescence. In: Roger J *et al*. (eds) *Epileptic Syndromes in Infancy*, 2nd edn. London: John Libbey, 1992; 75–88.
3. Ohki T, Watanabe K Negoro T, *et al*. Severe myoclonic epilepsy in infancy: evolution of seizures. *Seizure* 1997; **6**(3): 219–224.
4. Fernandez-Jaen A, Leon MC, Martinez-Granero MA, *et al*. Diagnosis in severe myoclonic epilepsy in childhood: study of 13 cases. *Revue Neurologique* 1998; **26**(153): 759–762.
5. Nieto Barrera M, Lillo MM, Rodriguez-Collado C, *et al*. Epilepsia mioclónica severa de la infancia. Estudio epidemiológico analítico. *Revue Neurologique* 2000; **30**: 620–624.
6. Benlounis A, Nabbout R, Feingold J, *et al*. Genetic predisposition to severe myoclonic epilepsy in infancy. *Epilepsia* 2001; **42**(2): 204–209.
7. Oguni H, Fukuyama Y, Tanaka T, *et al*. Myoclonic-astatic epilepsy of early childhood – clinical and EEG analysis of myoclonic-astatic seizures, and discussions on the nosology of the syndrome. *Brain Development* 2001; **23**(7): 757–764.
8. Aicardi J, Levy-Gomes AL. The myoclonic epilepsies of childhood. *Cleveland Clinic Journal of Medicine* 1989; **56**(Suppl. 1): 534–539.
9. Aicardi J (ed). *Epilepsy in Children*, 2nd edn. New York: Raven Press, 1994.
10. Engel J. A proposed diagnostic scheme for people with epileptic seizures and with epilepsy: report of the ILAE Task Force on Classification and Terminology. *Epilepsia* 2001; **42**(6): 796–803.
11. Hurst DL. Epidemiology of severe myoclonic epilepsy in infancy. *Epilepsia* 1990; **31**: 297–400.
12. Yakoub M, Dulac O, Jambaqué I, *et al*. Early diagnosis of severe myoclonic epilepsy in infancy. *Brain and Development* 1992; **14**: 209–303.
13. Ogino T. Severe myoclonic epilepsy in infancy – a clinical and electroencephalographic study. *Journal of the Japanese Epileptic Society* 1986; **4**: 114–126. (Summary in English).
14. Fujiwara T, Nakamura H, Watanabe M, *et al*. Clinicoelectrographic concordance between monozygotic twins with severe myoclonic epilepsy in infancy. *Epilepsia* 1990; **31**: 281–286.

15. Kanazawa O. Refractory grand mal seizures with onset during infancy including severe myoclonic epilepsy in infancy. *Brain Development* 2001; **23**(7): 749–756.

16. Wakai S, Ikehata M, Nihira H, *et al*. 'Obtundation status (Dravet)' caused by complex partial status epilepticus in a patient with severe myoclonic epilepsy in infancy. *Epilepsia* 1996; **37**(10): 1020–1022.

17. Dalla Bernardina B, Capovilla G, Gattoni MB, *et al*. Epilepsie myoclonique grave de la premiere annee. *Revue d'Electroencephalographie et de Neurophysiologie Clinique* 1982; **12**: 21–25.

18. Dulac O, Arthuis M. Epilepsie myoclonique sévere de l'enfant. In: *Journées Parisiennes de Pédiatrie*. Paris: Flammarion, 1982: 259–268.

19. Dalla Bernardina B, Capovilla G, Chiamenti C, *et al*. Cryptogenetic myoclonic epilepsies of infancy and early childhood: nosological and prognostic approach. In: Wolf P, *et al*. (ed.) *Advances in Epileptology*, vol. 16. New York: Raven Press, 1987; 175–179.

20. Giovanardi Rossi P, Santucci M, Gobbi G, *et al*. Long-term follow-up of severe myoclonic epilepsy in infancy. In: Fukuyama Y *et al*. (ed.) *Modern Perspectives of Child Neurology*. Tokyo: Japanese Society of Child Neurology, Asahi Daily News Co., 1991; 205–213.

21. Renier WO, Renkawek K. Clinical and neuropathological findings in a case of severe myoclonic epilepsy in infancy. *Epilepsia* 1990; **31**: 287–291.

22. Ferrie CD, Maisey M, Cox T, *et al*. Focal abnormalities detected by 18FDG PET in epileptic encephalopathies. *Archives of Disease in Childhood* 1996; **75**(2): 102–107.

23. Woo Y, Choi B, Park K. Monozygotic twins with severe myoclonic epilepsy in infancy. In: Fukuyama Y (ed.) *Program and Abstracts, International Symposium on the West Syndrome and Other Infantile Epileptic Encephalopathies* 2001: 74.

24. Ogino T, Ohtsuka Y, Yamatogi Y, *et al*. The epileptic syndromes sharing common characteristics during early childhood with severe myoclonic epilepsy in infancy. *Japanese Journal of Psychiatric Neurology (Tokyo)* 1989; **43**: 479–481.

25. Singh R, Scheffer IE, Crossland K, Berkovic SF. Generalised epilepsy with febrile seizures plus (GEFS): a common, childhood onset, genetic epileptic syndrome. *Annals of Neurology* 1999; **45**: 75–81.

26. Singh R, Andermann E, Whitehouse WP, *et al*. Severe myoclonic epilepsy of infancy: extended spectrum of GEFS+? *Epilepsia* 2001; **42**(7): 837–844.

27. Veggiotti P, Cardinali S, Montalenti E, *et al*. Generalized epilepsy with febrile seizures plus and severe myoclonic epilepsy in infancy: a case report of two Italian families. *Epileptic Disorders* 2001; **3**(1): 29–32.

28. Scheffer IE, Wallace R, Mulley JC, Berkovic SF. Clinical and molecular genetics of myoclonic-astatic epilepsy and severe myoclonic epilepsy in infancy (Dravet syndrome). *Brain Development* 2001; **23**(7): 732–735.

29. Claes L, Del-Favero J, Ceulemans B, *et al*. De novo mutations in the sodium-channel gene SCN1A cause severe myoclonic epilepsy of infancy. *American Journal of Human Genetics* 2001; **68**(6): 1327–1332.

30. Hurst DL. Severe myoclonic epilepsy in infancy. *Pediatric Neurology* 1987; **3**: 269–272.

31. Chiron C, Marchand MC, Tran A, *et al*. Stiripentol in severe myoclonic epilepsy in infancy: a randomised placebo-controlled syndrome-dedicated trial. STICLO study group. *Lancet* 2000; **11**(356): 1638–1642.

32. Guerrini R, Dravet C, Genton P, *et al*. Lamotrigine and seizure aggravation in severe myoclonic epilepsy. *Epilepsia* 1998; **39**(5): 508–512.

33. Nieto Barrera M, Candau R, Nieto-Jimenez M, *et al*. Topiramate in the treatment of severe myoclonic epilepsy in infancy. *Seizure* 2000; **9**(8): 590–594.

34. Kanazawa O, Shirane S. Can early zonisamide medication improve the prognosis in the core and peripheral types of severe myoclonic epilepsy in infants? *Brain Development* 1999; **21**: 503.

35. Saito Y, Oguni H, Awaya Y, Hayashi K, Osawa M. Phenytoin-induced choreoathetosis in patients with severe myoclonic epilepsy in infancy. *Neuropediatrics* 2001; **32**(5):231–235.

36. Caraballo R, Cersosimo R, Yépez I, Fejerman N. Severe myoclonic epilepsy in infancy treated with ketogenic diet (abstract). *Epilepsia* 1999; **40**(Suppl. 2): 170.

37. Commission on Classification and Terminology of the International League Against Epilepsy. Proposal for revised classification of epilepsies and epileptic syndromes. *Epilepsia* 1989; **30**: 389–399.

38. Dravet C, Bureau, M, Roger J. Benign myoclonic epilepsy in infants. In: Roger J *et al*. (eds) *Epileptic Syndromes in Infancy, Childhood and Adolescence*. London: John Libbey; Paris: Eurotext, 1985; 51–57.

39. Fejerman N, Medina CS. *Convulsiones en la Infancia*, 2nd edn. Buenos Aires: El Ateneo, 1986.

40. Fejerman N. Myoclonus and epilepsies in children. *Revue Neurologique, Paris* 1991; **147**(12): 782–797.

41. Engel J. A proposed diagnostic scheme for people with epileptic seizures and with epilepsy: Report of the ILAE Task Force on Classification and Terminology. *Epilepsia* 2001; **42**(6): 796–803.

42. Doose H. Myoclonic astatic epilepsy of early childhood. In: Roger J *et al*. (eds) *Epileptic Syndromes in Infancy, Childhood and Adolescence*. London: John Libbey; Paris: Eurotext, 1985; 78–88.

43. Boniver C, Dravet C, Bureau M, Roger J. Idiopathic Lennox-Gastaut syndrome. In: Wolf P *et al*. (eds) *Advances in Epileptology*, vol. 16. New York: Raven Press, 1987;195–200.

44. Wallace SJ. Epileptic syndromes linked with previous history of febrile seizures. In: Fukuyama Y *et al*. (eds) *Modern Perspectives of Child Neurology*. Tokyo: Japanese Society of Child Neurology, Asahi Daily News Co., 1991; 175–81.

45. Beaumanoir A. The Lennox-Gastaut syndrome. In: Roger J *et al*. (eds) *Epileptic Syndromes in Infancy, Childhood and Adolescence*. London: John Libbey; Paris: Eurotext, 1985; 89–99.

46. Wallace SJ. *The Child with Febrile Seizures*. London: John Wright, 1988.

Epileptic syndromes with onset in early childhood

Myoclonic-astatic epilepsy

JEAN AICARDI

There is considerable confusion regarding myoclonic-astatic epilepsy (MAE). The varying definitions and criteria used by different investigators have contributed to this problem. Doose, who described MAE initially[1,2] did not set out to describe a limited 'rigidly defined syndrome', but rather to draw attention to a group of patients with epilepsies of early onset characterized by myoclonic and atonic seizures in which no lesional cause could be demonstrated and in which genetic factors appeared to be a major factor. He emphasized the occurrence of fast spike-wave or polyspike-wave complexes and the absence of organic brain damage, in contrast to the slow spike-wave complexes and symptomatic nature of the Lennox-Gastaut syndrome. Doose and colleagues also highlighted the biparietal theta activity on EEG and the importance of genetic factors. Thus, Doose considered MAE to include the primary generalized epilepsies of childhood whose main clinical manifestation were myoclonic and/or astatic seizures. The inclusion of MAE under the heading of 'cryptogenic and symptomatic epilepsy syndromes' in the 1989 ILAE classification[3] was not consistent with this concept. However, the recent ILAE proposal for a new classification scheme lists MAE as an idiopathic or cryptogenic epilepsy syndrome.[4]

The main seizure types are myoclonic and astatic seizures. The latter are characterized by falls attributed to lapses of muscle tone. However, falls can result from several causes[5] including the myoclonic jerk itself, loss of muscle tone resulting in atonia, brief tonic seizures or a combination of these mechanisms. Determination of the mechanism of the falls is clinically very difficult and requires simultaneous recording of EMG and EEG.

There have been very few such studies.[6–11] Recent articles appear to agree that the essential features include (a) the occurrence of frequent falls, which can be associated with myoclonic jerks but are mostly due to atonia (when this precision is given) and (b) bursts of mostly >3-Hz generalized spike wave complexes; and there may be other seizure types. The recent proposal of the ILAE Task Force for a new classification scheme[4] has recommended that 'epilepsy with myoclonic astatic seizures' be included in the list of recognized or accepted syndromes. In our present state of knowledge, it may be reasonable to include all cases of myoclonic epilepsy that do not satisfy the strict criteria for benign myoclonic epilepsy or severe myoclonic epilepsy in the MAE category. Whether the benign myoclonic epilepsy group is a different entity from MAE or represents only the more benign part of a spectrum remains uncertain. MAE is clearly a heterogeneous disorder, and some of the cases reported as MAE with a severe course are at least closely related, if not identical to, the so-called myoclonic variant of Lennox-Gastaut syndrome.[12,13] Genetic studies will probably clarify some of the above issues with time.

ETIOLOGIC AND EPIDEMIOLOGIC DATA

MAE is relatively uncommon. However, the variable classification criteria used make quantitative estimates unreliable. Acquired factors are demonstrated infrequently and neuroimaging is usually normal. In contrast, genetic factors are common and were found in 32 per cent of

Doose's patients. A previous history of febrile convulsions or other epileptic seizures is found in a substantial proportion of patients. In addition, the frequency of EEG markers, such as photosensitivity, parietal theta rhythms, and spike-waves is markedly increased in siblings and parents.[14] The marked predominance of boys (73–79 per cent) in most series is remarkable.[15–17] Interestingly, the proportion of boys was also high (68 per cent) in the cases of 'benign myoclonic epilepsy' reviewed by Dravet et al.[18]

CLINICAL AND EEG PRESENTATION

The age of onset is usually between 7 months and 8 years of age, with a peak incidence between 2 and 6 years, but onset as early as 1 month has been described.[16] Neurologic development is normal before the first seizures in most patients.

The seizures are often frequent and may occur several dozen times daily. Approximately two thirds of children have drop attacks.[11] In a series of 29 children studied polygraphically, the seizures were myoclonic in 17, atonic with or without a previous minor myoclonus in 11, and myoclonic-atonic in 3.[11] A change in facial expression and/or a brief twitch of the extremities may precede an atonic event and probably indicates a brief positive phenomenon. Myoclonic-atonic seizures consist of brief massive or axial symmetrical jerk, involving the neck, shoulders and arms, and often resulting in head-nodding and abduction of arms. When the lower limbs are involved the myoclonus can precipitate a fall. The jerk is immediately followed by an abrupt loss of muscle tone that seems to be the commonest cause of the fall.[5,19] Violent myoclonus followed by an abrupt fall may result in severe injuries especially of the nose and face. The duration of a seizure is usually less than 2–3 s. The jerks may be isolated or occur in short series at a rhythm of about 3 Hz, resulting in saccadic flexion of the head and/or abduction of the arms.

The EEG during myoclonic-atonic seizures shows bursts of spike wave complexes or polyspike waves at a rhythm of 2–4 Hz. The electromyogram shows that the muscle contraction responsible for the myoclonic jerk is usually followed by a brief period of EEG silence during which tonic muscle activity disappears for a duration of up to 120 ms. The silent period sometimes occurs without a preceding jerk, although it is difficult to exclude the possibility of a mild contraction in muscles that are not being sampled.[10,20] In many patients, however, loss of muscle tone appears to be a primary pnenomenon. In such cases, the silent period tends to be longer, lasting up to 400 ms.[21] Atonia is usually associated with the slow wave of a single or multiple spike-wave complex,[5,20] although the relationship with the spike may be variable. Bonanni et al.[22] have shown that the myoclonic seizures that occur in

Lennox-Gastaut syndrome and myoclonic astatic epilepsy differ neurophysiologically. They are synchronous on both hemispheres in MAE, whereas in Lennox-Gastaut syndrome one side consistently leads, preceding the EEG activity of the contralateral hemisphere by 20 ± 10 ms. They interpreted this difference as indicating that myoclonic attacks were primary generalized seizures in MAE, whereas in Lennox-Gastaut syndrome they probably represented the secondary generalization of an initial focal discharge.

Other seizure types are common and include generalized tonic-clonic seizures and atypical absences. Nonconvulsive status epilepticus has been described by all authors and is characterized by variable changes in consciousness often associated with drooling, brief head nods and/or erratic twitches of facial and perioral and hand muscles. These episodes can begin insidiously, may be difficult to recognize and may last from minutes to weeks. Repeated and prolonged episodes are associated with a poor cognitive outcome.[16,23] Long trains of slow-waves, fast spike-waves and slow spike-wave complexes characterize the EEG during these episodes. The irregular, polymorphous paroxysmal abnormalities may be so severely disorganized as to simulate a hypsarrhythmic pattern.[24] Neurological signs, particularly ataxia and pseudo-cerebellar signs, may be seen during nonconvulsive status and can suggest a degenerative condition. However, these signs fluctuate and disappear after the status resolves.[25,26]

Although tonic seizures are classically absent in MAE,[27–29] Kaminska et al. described these seizures in 38 per cent of cases.[16] Tonic seizures occurred even in those with a favorable outcome, although the tonic seizures tended to be less frequent and shorter in these patients. Tonic seizures are considered by some investigators to indicate a transition from MAE to Lennox-Gastaut syndrome.[30] The cases that feature frequent tonic attacks after a variable period of myoclonic activity appear to be similar to the so-called **myoclonic variant of the Lennox-Gastaut syndrome** (MVLGS).

The interictal EEG in MAE may be normal at onset.[24] Bursts of 3-Hz spike-waves, which may be activated by sleep, may occur without apparent clinical manifestations. Characteristic features are 4–7-Hz theta rhythms with parietal accentuation and occipital 4-Hz rhythms, blocked by eye opening.[11,15,24] Variable lateralization of paroxysmal bursts may be seen, but a consistently localized focus is distinctly unusual. Intermittent photic stimulation often induces a paroxysmal response.

COURSE AND OUTCOME

The course of MAE is variable and unpredictable. The disorder may be self-limited and the seizures abate after a few years, even in children with frequent seizures of multiple types. This pattern was reported in 54–89 per cent of patients.[11,15–17] The mean duration of the active phase was under 3 years in this group. Cognitive and behavioral outcome appears satisfactory in this group but some have residual mild cognitive and behavioral problems, especially hyperactivity.[11,16,17] Other children run a more severe course. Their epilepsy remains intractable and cognitive and behavioral deterioration becomes evident, even though the seizures may eventually disappear. Intellectual disability of variable degree becomes apparent in these patients after several years and can be severe.

The factors that influence different outcomes are not well understood. Doose and his collaborators[15,23] emphasized the association of a poor mental outcome with repeated, prolonged episodes of nonconvulsive status epilepticus, a finding confirmed by other investigators.[16,30,31] The acquired dementia may, perhaps, be regarded as a form of 'epileptic encephalopathy', in which the epileptic activity itself plays an important role in the loss of mental abilities.[4] Prompt treatment of these episodes might improve cognitive outcome, but this has not yet been demonstrated. Children with a poor outcome cannot be distinguished at an early stage from those with a more favorable course on the basis of age, antecedents, or clinical presentation.[16]

Other factors thought to be associated with an unfavorable outcome include the occurrence of atypical absences, repeated generalized tonic-clonic seizures, and repeated falls. The occurrence of nocturnal tonic seizures has been classically considered to be indicative of a poor outcome. However, some investigators have observed them in 'benign' cases and they may be compatible with a favorable outcome.[16] Persistence of rhythmic EEG slowing until adolescence, without development of a stable alpha rhythm, may be an indicator of an unfavorable course.[32]

DIAGNOSTIC AND NOSOLOGICAL ASPECTS

The lack of agreement on the criteria for classification complicates the distinguishing MAE from Lennox-Gastaut syndrome, benign myoclonic epilepsy, severe myoclonic epilepsy and other syndromes featuring falls or myoclonic jerks. The distinction between Lennox-Gastaut syndrome, severe myoclonic epilepsy and myoclonic-astatic epilepsy, however, may be of both therapeutic and genetic importance. Myoclonic seizures may be exacerbated by drugs, such as vigabatrin, which have been recommended in the treatment of Lennox syndrome.[33] In addition, the familial recurrence risk of epilepsy is probably higher in MAE than in Lennox-Gastaut syndrome.

Atypical partial benign epilepsy and the progressive myoclonic epilepsies (Chapter 14) such as myoclonus epilepsy and ragged-red fibers (MERRF), Unverricht-Lundborg or Lafora disease can be difficult to distinguish clinically from MAE at the onset of these disorders. Neurologic signs, especially ataxia and apparent cognitive deterioration, may occur in MAE as a result of episodes of nonconvulsive status.[25,26] Similar episodes can be induced in various myoclonic epilepsies by the administration of carbamazepine,[34] phenytoin, phenobarbital or vigabatrin.[35] Other epilepsies, such as absence, can be associated with prominent myoclonic activity and distinction from MAE may be difficult initially. Non-epileptic myoclonus is rarely an important diagnostic consideration. However, some degenerative disorders may be associated with erratic non-epileptic myoclonus and may initially mimic MAE.

Benign myoclonic epilepsy is characterized by the exclusive occurrence of brief myoclonic seizures, has a good prognosis, and is regarded as a different entity from MAE.[3] In contrast, the seizures of MAE feature both myoclonic jerks and astatic falls and the outcome is often less favorable. However, the myoclonic seizures in children with benign myoclonic epilepsy can occasionally provoke falls. Moreover, falls seem not to have been considered as a necessary criterion for inclusion in MAE in several series.[11,16] Similarly, the contrast between the favorable course of benign myoclonic epilepsy and that of MAE is not always obvious. In the series of Kaminska et al.,[16] half the cases of MAE had an excellent outcome. Similarly, Oguni et al.[11] reported spontaneous remission of seizures in 25 per cent of patients. In addition, 89 per cent of patients were free of myoclonic-astatic attacks within 3 years, and approximately 60 per cent of the children had a normal IQ level. Thus, the distinction between benign myoclonic epilepsy and MAE can be difficult.

Severe myoclonic epilepsy has several features that are clearly different from MAE. The onset is nearly always in the first year of life, with febrile convulsions that are often prolonged and unilateral. In addition, the myoclonus in severe myoclonic epilepsy seldom appears before the second or third year of life. The myoclonic and drop seizures and episodes of nonconvulsive status that can be observed at that stage can wrongly suggest MAE if the significance of the early febrile seizures is not appreciated. However, even the criteria for the diagnosis of severe myoclonic epilepsy have been disputed (see Chapter 9E).[36] Severe myoclonic epilepsy has recently been linked genetically to the generalized epilepsy with febrile seizures plus (GEFS+) syndrome, and probably with the other forms of myoclonic epilepsies.[37]

Differentiation of MAE from Lennox-Gastaut syndrome is usually straightforward. The main types of seizures in Lennox-Gastaut syndrome are atonic, tonic and atypical absence and the EEG characteristically demonstrates interictal slow spike-waves and fast (ictal) rhythms. However, the electroclinical features of Lennox-Gastaut syndrome may not appear until after an initial phase of predominantly myoclonic attacks. This pattern, which has been described by some as the 'myoclonic variant of the Lennox-Gastaut syndrome',[13,18,30] presents at 3–4 years of age. Myoclonic seizures and episodes of nonconvulsive status are prominent and 2–3-Hz spike-wave complexes characterize the EEG. However, tonic seizures appear much later. The outcome of the myoclonic variant of Lennox-Gastaut syndrome is less severe than that of the tonic-atonic type of the syndrome. In these patients, the syndrome is indistinguishable initially from MAE and subsequently fulfils the criteria for Lennox-Gastaut syndrome.[30] This variant may be more closely related to MAE than to Lennox-Gastaut syndrome in the usual absence of brain lesions and the frequency of genetic antecedents.

Although there are well-recognized syndromes with myoclonic seizures, many children with myoclonic seizures are difficult to classify. Dravet et al.[12] were unable to classify 34 of 142 cases of myoclonic epilepsy, and other investigators have also encountered similar problems.[28] The absence of precise criteria for delineation of some of the syndromes contributes to these difficulties. For example, the proportion of tonic seizures that rules out the diagnosis of MAE has never been proposed. Similarly, it is not clear that the occurrence of a few other seizure types, such as absences or occasional generalized tonic-clonic seizures, fundamentally modifies the good outcome in benign myoclonic epilepsy, which classically should feature only myoclonic seizures. One group[17,38] has found a similarly favorable outcome in a group of 19 patients defined by the predominance of myoclonic seizures but not excluding cases in which a few other generalized seizure types were observed. Furthermore, those patients with MAE who had epilepsy for less than 3 years and an excellent cognitive outcome, frequently had several types of seizures, including even nocturnal tonic attacks and brief episodes of nonconvulsive status epilepticus.[16] Thus, it might perhaps be more realistic to accept that the epilepsies of early childhood that feature prominent myoclonic activity, with the exception of severe myoclonic epilepsy, Lennox-Gastaut syndrome and the progressive myoclonic epilepsies, are probably part of a continuum of cases with different degrees of severity but probably closely related in terms of clinical presentation, idiopathic etiology and perhaps even genetics.

TREATMENT

There have been very few systematic studies of the management of MAE. Most articles deal with the treatment of myoclonic epilepsies in general. Many consider valproic acid a first-choice drug, although no comparative study is currently available. The drug is often effective as monotherapy and approximately half the cases respond to moderate doses. Some patients may respond to doses of up to 80 mg/kg per day. Other drugs that can also be useful include ethosuximide, benzodiazepines (especially clobazam and clonazepam), acetazolamide and sometimes phenobarbital.[24] Ethosuximide[39] is often effective, as a monotherapy or in combination with valproic acid. Indeed, Oguni et al.[11] considered ethosuximide to be the most effective drug and reported a 'good response' in 64 per cent of patients, a response rate almost equal to that of ACTH. These investigators also found the ketogenic diet to be very effective, with 58 per cent of patients demonstrating an excellent result, regardless of whether the classical or MCT (medium chain triglyceridos) diet was used. Lamotrigine[40,41] is probably effective but has been reported to exacerbate seizures in some patients with severe myoclonic epilepsy.[33] It is not clear whether this adverse effect is specific for this syndrome or may also occur in patients with other myoclonic seizures. The combination of lamotrigine and valproic acid is often used. In that situation, the addition of lamotrigine to valproic acid should be done very slowly because of the pharmacokinetic interaction between these two agents and the increased risk of serious drug rash when lamotrigine dosage escalation is rapid (see Chapters 21, 22A). The roles of topiramate and of levetiracetam are not yet defined although they seem to have some efficacy. Treatment of the episodes of status epilepticus is probably highly desirable, given their suspected role in cognitive and developmental deterioration. Unfortunately, these episodes are very refractory to treatment. Ethosuximide is sometime successful and deserves to be systematically tried. Other possibly effective agents include high-dose pulses of diazepam,[42] sulthiame[43,44] and corticosteroids or ACTH.

KEY POINTS

- MAE is relatively uncommon and **usually starts between 2 and 6 years of age**
- MAE is **characterized by myoclonic seizures and drop-attacks**. Other types of seizures often occur, of which nonconvulsive status epilepticus is associated with a poor prognosis. It is probably an **idiopathic** epilepsy
- There is no strong consensus on the definition or criteria of the syndrome. Most investigators separate MAE from severe myoclonic epilepsy of infants and from Lennox-Gastaut syndrome. However, **intermediate and transitional forms exist** and the myoclonic epilepsies might constitute a spectrum of related cases rather than a collection of distinct syndromes.
- The **prognosis of MAE is variable**, but 50–90 per cent have a good outcome. Frequent episodes of nonconvulsive status epilepticus are associated with a poor prognosis.

REFERENCES

1. Doose H, Gerken H, Leonhardt R, Volzke E, Volz C. Centrencephalic myoclonic-astatic petit mal. Clinical and genetic investigation. *Neuropëdiatrie* 1970; **2**: 59–78.

2. Doose H, Baier WK. Epilepsy with primarily generalized myoclonic-astatic seizures: a genetically determined disease. *European Journal of Pediatrics* 1987; **146**: 550–554.

3. Commission on Classification and Terminology of the International League Against Epilepsy. Proposal for revised classification of epilepsies and epileptic syndromes. *Epilepsia* 1989; **30**: 389–399.

4. Engel J Jr. Classification of epileptic disorders. *Epilepsia* 2001; **42**: 317–320.

5. Tassinari CA, Michelucci R, Shigematsu H, Seino M. Atonic and falling seizures. In: Engel J Jr, Pedley TA (eds) *Epilepsy: A Comprehensive Textbook*. Philadelphia: Lippincott-Raven, 1998; 605–616.

6. Dravet C, Bureau M, Tassinari CA, Roger J. Different types of epileptic drop seizures in children. *Neurology and Psychiatry* 1988; **11**(Suppl. 1): 7–16.

7. Egli M, Mothersill I, O'Kane M, *et al.* The axial spasm-the predominant type of drop seizure in patients with secondary generalized epilepsy. *Epilepsia* 1985; **26**: 401–415.

8. Gastaut H, Broughton R. *Epileptic Seizures*. Springfield, IL: CC Thomas, 1972.

9. Ikeno T, Shigematsu H, Miyakashi M, *et al.* An analytical study of epileptic falls. *Epilepsia* 1985; **26**: 612–621.

10. Oguni H, Fukuyama Y, Imaizumi Y, Uehara T. Video analysis of drop seizures in myoclonic-astatic epilepsy of early childhood (Doose syndrome). *Epilepsia* 1993; **33**: 805–813.

11. Oguni H, Tanaka T, Hayashi K, *et al.* Treatment and long-term prognosis of myoclonic-astatic epilepsy of early childhood. *Neuropediatrics* 2002; **33**: 122–132.

12. Dravet C, Roger J, Bureau M, Dalla Bernardina B. Myoclonic epilepsies in childhood. In: Akimoto A, Kazamatsuri A, Seino M, Ward A (eds) *Advances in Epileptology: XIIIth Epilepsy International Symposium* New York: Raven Press, 1982; 135–140.

13. Chevrie JJ, Aicardi J. Childhood epileptic encephalopathy with slow spike-wave. A statistical study of 80 cases. *Epilepsia* 1972; **13**: 259–271.

14. Doose H , Baier W. Genetic aspects of childhood epilepsy. *Cleveland Clinic Journal of Medicine* 1989; **56**(Suppl. 1): S105–110.

15. Doose H. Myoclonic-astatic epilepsy. *Epilepsy Research* (Suppl.). 1992; **6**: 163–168.

16. Kaminska A, Ickowicz A, Plouin P, *et al.* Delineation of cryptogenic Lennox-Gastaut syndrome and myoclonic-astatic epilepsy using multiple correspondence analysis. *Epilepsy Research* 1999; **36**: 15–29.

17. Aicardi J, Levy-Gomes A. The myoclonic epilepsies of childhood. *Cleveland Clinic Journal of Medicine* 1989; **59**: S9–34.

18. Dravet C, Bureau M, Roger J. Benign myoclonic epilepsy in infants. In: Roger J, Bureau M, Dravet C *et al.* (eds) *Epileptic Syndromes in Infancy, Childhood and Adolescence*. London: John Libbey, 1992; 67–74.

19. Janz D, Inoue Y, Seino M. Myoclonic seizures. In: Engel J Jr, Pedley TA (eds) *Epilepsy: A Comprehensive Textbook*. Philadelphia: Lippincott-Raven, 1998; 591–603.

20. Shewmon DA, Erwin RJ. Focal spike-induced cerebral dysfunction is related to the after-coming slow wave. *Annals of Neurology* 1988; **23**: 131–137.

21. Guerrini R, Dravet C, Genton P, *et al.* Epileptic negative myoclonus. *Epilepsia* 1993; **43**: 1078–1093.

22. Bonanni P, Parmeggiani L, Guerrini R. Different neurophysiologic patterns of myoclonus characterize Lennox-Gastaut syndrome and myoclonic astatic epilepsy. *Epilepsia* 2002; **43**: 609–615.

23. Doose H, Volzke E. Petit mal status in early childhood and dementia. *Neuropadiatrie* 1979; **10**: 10–14.

24. Genton P, Dravet C. Lennox-Gastaut syndrome and other childhood epileptic encephalopathies. In: Engel J Jr, Pedley TA (eds) *Epilepsy: A Comprehensive Textbook*. Philadelphia: Lippincott-Raven, 1998; 2355–2366.

25. Bennett HS, Selman JE, Rapin I, Rose A. Nonconvulsive epileptiform activity appearing as ataxia. *American Journal of Disease of Children* 1982; **136**: 30–32.

26. Aicardi J, Chevrie JJ. Myoclonic epilepsies of childhood. *Neuropadiatrie* 1971; **3**: 177–190.

27. Dravet C, Natale O, Magaudda A, *et al.* Les états de mal dans le syndrome de Lennox-Gastaut. *Revue d'Electroencéphalographie et de Neurophysiologie Clinique* 1985; **15**: 361–368.

28. Giovanardi Rossi P, Gobbi G, Melideo A, *et al.* Myoclonic manifestations in the Lennox-Gastaut syndrome and other childhood epilepsies. In: Niedermeyer E, Degen R (eds) *The Lennox-Gastaut Syndrome*. New York: Alan Liss, 1988; 137–158.

29. Dravet C. Myoclonic-astatic epilepsy. Paper presented at the *Marseille Meeting on Myoclonic Epilepsies*, June 1992.

30. Hoffmann-Riem M, Diener W, Benninger C, *et al.* Nonconvulsive status epilepticus: a possible cause of mental retardation in patients with Lennox-Gastaut syndrome. *Neuropediatrics* 2000; **31**: 169–174.

31. Dulac O, Plouin P, Chiron C. Forme 'bénigne' d'épilepsie myoclonique chez l'enfant. *Revue de Neurophysiologie Clinique* 1990; **20**: 115–129.

32. Gundel A, Baier W, Doose H. Spedtral analysis of EEG in the late course of primary generalized myoclonic-astatic epilepsy. II. Cluster analysis of the power spectrum. *Neuropediatrics* 1981; **12**: 110–118.

33. Guerrini R, Dravet C, Genton P. Lamotrigine and seizure aggravation in severe myoclonic epilepsy. *Epilepsia* 1998; **39**: 508–512.

34. Snead OC, Hosey LC. Exacerbation of seizures in children by carbamazepine. *New England Journal of Medicine* 1985; **313**: 916–921.

35. Marciani MG, Maschio M, Spanedda F, Iani C, Gigli GL, Bernardi G. Development of myoclonus in patients with partial epilepsy during treatment with vigabatrin: an electroencephalographic study. *Acta Neurol Scand* 1995; **91**: 1–5.

36. Lombroso CT. Early myoclonic encephalopathy, early infantile epileptic encephalopathy, and benign and severe infantile myoclonic epilepsies: a critical review and personal contributions. *Journal of Clinical Neurophysiology* 1990; **7**: 380–408.

37. Claes L, Del-Favero J, Ceulemans B, *et al.* De novo mutations in the sodium-channel gene SCN1A cause severe myoclonic epilepsy of infancy. *American Journal of Human Genetics* 2001; **68**(6): 1327–1332.

38. Dravet C, Bureau M, Guerrini R, *et al.* Severe myoclonic epilepsy in infants. In: Roger J *et al.* (eds) *Epileptic Syndromes in Infancy, Childhood and Adolescence.* New York: Raven Press, 1992; 75–88.

39. Schneider S. Clinical use of ethosuximide, methosuximide and trimethadione. In: Pellock JM, Dodson WE, Bourgeois BF (eds) *Pediatric epilepsy: diagnosis and therapy,* 2nd edn. New York: Demos, 2001; 447–52.

40. Schlumberger E, Chavez F, Palacios L, *et al.* Lamotrigine in treatment of 120 children with epilepsy. *Epilepsia* 1998; **35**: 359–367.

41. Ericksson AS, Nergardh A, Hoppu K. Lamotrigine in children and adolescents with refractory generalized epilepsy: a randomized, double blind, crossover study. *Epilepsia* 1998; **39**: 495–501.

42. De Negri M, Baglietto MG, Battaglia FM, Gaggero R, Pessagno A, Recarati L. Treatment of electrical status epilepticus by short diazepam (DZP) cycles after DZP rectal bolus test. *Brain Dev* 1995; **17**: 330–333.

43. Lerman P, Nussbaum E. The use of sulthiame in myoclonic epilepsy of childhood and adolescence. *Acta Neurol Scand* Suppl 1975; **60**: 7–12.

44. Lerman P, Lerman-Sagie T. Sulthiame revisited. *Journal of Child Neurology* 1995; **10**: 241–242.

Lennox-Gastaut syndrome

JEAN AICARDI

The definition of the Lennox-Gastaut syndrome remains controversial. It is most often defined as an epilepsy syndrome characterized by multiple seizure types, including brief tonic, atonic, myoclonic and atypical absence seizures, associated with an interictal EEG pattern of diffuse, slow (<2.5 Hz) spike-wave complexes.[1] Intellectual disability is a very frequent but not a constant feature.[2] Episodes of nonconvulsive status epilepticus occur frequently. Some authors[3,4] consider that two additional criteria are necessary for the diagnosis: the occurrence of generalized tonic seizures, and runs of fast (10 Hz) rhythms, which occur especially during non-REM sleep, with or without tonic seizures.

The situation is complicated by the occurrence of these seizure types and EEG features in other epilepsy syndromes. In addition, other seizure types, e.g. focal and myoclonic seizures, may occur long before the more typical seizures.[5–7] Furthermore, not all of the typical features are found in every case. In recent studies, tonic seizures were present in only 80–92 per cent of patients[3,8] and fast rhythms during slow sleep in only 55 per cent of those patients who had whole-night sleep recordings. As a result, investigators have used different criteria to define Lennox-Gastaut syndrome and some of the differences between reports of Lennox-Gastaut syndrome reflect the differences in the populations studied. Lennox-Gastaut syndrome is usually considered as a secondary generalized epilepsy.

INCIDENCE AND ETIOLOGY

Lennox-Gastaut syndrome has been variously estimated to account for 1–10 per cent of childhood epilepsies,[9,10] with the former figure being probably closer to reality. Epidemiological studies show that the proportion of Lennox-Gastaut syndrome seems relatively consistent across various populations. The prevalence of Lennox-Gastaut syndrome in mentally retarded children was reported as 0.06/1000,[11] and the percentage of Lennox-Gastaut syndrome in institutionalized patients with intellectual disability may be as high as 16.3 per cent.[12] Boys are affected slightly more often than girls. The onset of the seizures is between 1 and 7 years of age in the vast majority. The peak age of onset is between 3 and 5 years of age but is before 2 years in up to 20 per cent of cases. Onset in late childhood, adolescence and even adulthood has been reported.[13]

Two thirds to three-quarters of cases result from demonstrable brain abnormality or occur in patients with previous developmental delay[5,14] and are considered symptomatic. The remainder occur in children with previous normal development, no neurologic abnormality, and with no abnormalities on brain imaging. Thus, the term **idiopathic Lennox-Gastaut syndrome** was proposed for such cases[15,16] The term **cryptogenic** was subsequently adopted in the 1989 Classification of

Epilepsies and Epileptic Syndromes[1] because intellectual disability usually became apparent. However, this may be the consequence not of the underlying brain lesion but of the epileptic activity itself.

The etiology of Lennox-Gastaut syndrome is heterogeneous. Brain abnormalities play a major role and genetic factors are generally less important. The frequency of a family history of epilepsy has varied considerably, from 2.5 per cent[5] to 48 per cent.[17] This discrepancy probably reflects the different diagnostic criteria used. Most brain lesions are abnormalities of brain development. Many types of cortical malformation have been reported, although Lennox-Gastaut syndrome has never been described in the Aicardi syndrome. The cortical abnormalities include bilateral perisylvian and central dysplasia,[18–21] diffuse subcortical laminar heterotopias[22] and focal cortical dysplasias.[23,24] Rare cases are due to Sturge-Weber syndrome[25,26] or tumors, especially of the frontal lobes.[27] Lennox-Gastaut syndrome has also been reported in cases of hypothalamic hamartomas following a long period of focal gelastic seizures.[28] Roger and Gambardelli-Dubois[26] described abnormalities of cortical development in 10 of 30 autopsy cases studied. There is limited information on the pathologic correlate of Lennox-Gastaut syndrome in cases not due to macroscopic lesions. Biopsy studies[29,30] have shown only relatively minor changes, such as poor dendritic arborization and disturbed synaptic development of pyramidal cells in the inners layers of the cortex. Acquired destructive lesions are less common. Lennox-Gastaut syndrome has been associated with hypoxic brain damage[16,26] and with large porencephalic defects.[16,31] Post-traumatic epilepsy may occasionally manifest with the characteristic Lennox-Gastaut syndrome seizures and diffuse slow spike-wave complexes.[32]

Lennox-Gastaut syndrome can follow other epilepsy syndromes. The most common is West syndrome, which has been reported to precede Lennox-Gastaut syndrome in 18–41 per cent of cases.[2,16,33] Lennox-Gastaut syndrome following infantile spasms tends to have an earlier onset, predominance of tonic seizures occurring in clusters and a particularly poor prognosis.[2,14,33] Tonic seizures may emerge as a prominent feature in some patients late in the course of myoclonic astatic epilepsy.[7] Such cases then fulfil the criteria for the Lennox-Gastaut syndrome and have been reported by some under the term 'myoclonic variant of the Lennox-Gastaut syndrome',[5,6] whereas other authors have regarded the later onset of tonic seizures as an occasional feature of myoclonic-astatic epilepsy.

Focal seizures, unilateral seizures, generalized tonic-clonic seizures and episodes of convulsive status epilepticus may occur before the appearance of Lennox-Gastaut syndrome. Focal seizures are relatively common,[5,8,34] but primary generalized seizures, including typical absences, have been observed only rarely.[3,4] Some cases with myoclonic absences have been reported to evolve into Lennox-Gastaut syndrome.[35]

CLINICAL AND EEG ICTAL MANIFESTATIONS

The seizures usually occur many times daily and are particularly frequent during sleep. However, the frequency of seizures can vary considerably with alternating 'bad' and 'good' periods. Not all of the characteristic seizures are present in all children. One type may predominate (e.g. the 'myoclonic variant') and occasionally only one type of seizure, usually tonic seizures, occurs in association with slow spike-waves. Other seizure types, including generalized tonic-clonic seizures, partial seizures, and unilateral clonic seizures often occur, and can precede the characteristic seizures.

Tonic seizures

Tonic seizures are the most characteristic type.[4,5] The axial subtype consists of a brief, but sustained, bilateral symmetric contraction of the axial muscles that results in a flexor movement of the head and trunk. Clouding of consciousness and autonomic manifestations are usually associated. The seizures may be quite mild, especially in sleep, when they are often limited to a brief apnea, an upwards deviation of the eyes or minimal stiffening. In axorhizomelic seizures there is associated abduction and elevation of the arms, while global tonic attacks involve most muscles. Tonic seizures can be very brief (2–4 s) and precipitate falls if the child is standing.[36,37] In infants, tonic seizures tend to occur in clusters and be followed by atonia, which makes them difficult to distinguish from infantile spasms.[4,33] In older patients, episodes of automatic behavior may follow the tonic phase or alternate with tonic contractions.[38] Such tonic-automatic seizures were found in 16 per cent of cases.[4]

The ictal EEG of tonic seizures is a 10-Hz or faster discharge, usually of increasing amplitude, which may be followed by a brief discharge of spike-wave complexes. These last 4–10 s in most cases but may last up to 30–60 s.

Atypical absence seizures

These are the second most common type of seizure in Lennox-Gastaut syndrome.[8,39] They may resemble typical absence seizures, but their onset and termination are less abrupt. They may be mild and hard to detect clinically because the incomplete loss of consciousness allows the child to continue ongoing activities, albeit slowly and imperfectly. They are often associated with some loss of muscle tone, erratic myoclonic jerks, sialorrhea or mild hypertonia of neck and back muscles.

The ictal EEG pattern of atypical absence seizures is variable. It is often a 10-Hz discharge, similar to that recorded during tonic seizures. Other ictal patterns include a burst of spike-waves, usually at 2.5 Hz or less, which are sometimes preceded by a brief phase of fast rhythm; and a sudden voltage attenuation, sometimes with superimposed 20-Hz low-amplitude activity.

Myoclonic and atonic seizures

Myoclonic and atonic (or myo-atonic) seizures are usually less frequent than tonic or atypical absence seizures, but may be quite prominent in some patients (so-called **myoclonic variant**). The myoclonic jerk, which may be very mild, is often followed by a brief period of decreased muscle tone. These seizures are probably the most common cause of the falls that constitute a major problem for children with Lennox-Gastaut syndrome.

The ictal EEG demonstrates bursts of generalized polyspike-waves often with a frontal predominance during most myoclonic or myo-atonic seizures. In patients with Lennox-Gastaut syndrome, unlike patients with an idiopathic myoclonic epilepsy, the generalized spike waves during myoclonic seizures are not bilateral and synchronous. In a small group of patients, Bonanni et al.[40] showed that the discharge was always generated in one hemisphere with rapid generalization consistent with callosal transmission, which suggests that the origin of the myoclonic seizures may be focal in at least some patients with Lennox-Gastaut syndrome. In some purely atonic attacks, the ictal EEG has shown runs of spike-waves or rapid rhythms similar to those that accompany tonic seizures. The electromyogram of affected muscles during a myoclonic seizure shows of a muscular spike lasting less than 100 ms, followed by a period of electrical silence of variable duration, which corresponds to clinical atonia that is responsible for a fall if its duration is sufficient.

Nonconvulsive status epilepticus

Fifty to 75 per cent of patients with Lennox-Gastaut syndrome have episodes of nonconvulsive status. The most typical form consists of subcontinuous atypical absences with variable degrees of altered consciousness, interrupted periodically by recurring brief tonic seizures. The absences are marked by the occurrence of slow spike-wave complexes, and the tonic attacks are associated with a 10 Hz rhythm.[41,42] In episodes of pure tonic status, the intensity of tonic contractions decreases with time and becomes difficult to detect. Pure tonic status can be accompanied by major autonomic disturbances including apnea and bronchial hypersecretion, which may become life-threatening when the status is prolonged. Another common manifestation of nonconvulsive status is mental slowing, which may vary in severity from mild obtundation to coma, and may be associated with drooling and erratic myoclonus involving the perioral and/or distal limb muscles.

Episodes of nonconvulsive status often last hours or days and exceeded 1 week in half the cases in one series.[41] Their exact duration is often difficult to determine because they can closely resemble the 'bad' periods that often occur in Lennox-Gastaut syndrome.

INTELLECTUAL DISABILITY

This is the third component of the classical Lennox-Gastaut syndrome triad, but 7–10 per cent of children with Lennox-Gastaut syndrome remain within the accepted limits of normality.[3–5,16,39,43] However, even those with normal intelligence often have difficulties in everyday life and have slowing of some aspects of mental processing. In the 25–30 per cent who appear to develop normally before the first seizure, it is not entirely clear whether cognitive deterioration occurs after onset of the seizures or whether there is slowing of the rate of mental development. There has been no longitudinal study of neuropsychologic function, but the clinical impression is that loss of skills occurs in some children.[44] Deterioration is self-limited, not associated with neurologic signs and may be partially reversible if the epileptic activity is better controlled. It seems likely that the epileptic activity itself plays a role in the pathogenesis of the cognitive and behavioral difficulties. This supports inclusion of Lennox-Gastaut syndrome in the group of **epileptic encephalopathies**, as defined in the new International League Against Epilepsy proposal for classification of the epilepsies.[45]

The ultimate degree of intellectual disability is often severe: in one series 48 of 89 patients had an IQ of less than 25,[46] and in another 21 of 40 children had an IQ of less than 50.[2] In addition, many patients have psychiatric problems, are hyperactive and aggressive[47] or have autistic features.[8] The overall disability markedly limits normal school learning and social integration, even when the cognitive deficit is of a lesser degree.

INTERICTAL EEG FEATURES

The classical interictal EEG feature of Lennox-Gastaut syndrome is the slow spike-wave (SSW) pattern. The SSW complex consists of a spike (<80 ms) or sharp wave (80–200 ms) followed by a sinusoidal electronegative slow wave of 350–400 ms duration. A prominent positive trough is present between the fast and the slow components.[48,49] The SSW complexes may appear singly or in runs, with a repetition rate of 1–2.5 Hz. They are bilateral and roughly symmetric, though shifting asymmetries are often evident. They are diffuse but usually predominate over the frontocentral part of the scalp.[50] They may occasionally be more obvious over the occipitotemporal area.[48] The SSW complexes are usually abundant but may occasionally only be visible during slow wave sleep, which increases their frequency in all cases.[4,51] They are not always symmetric and consistent lateral predominance may occasionally be present. The SSW complexes are not precipitated by photic stimulation and rarely, if ever, by hyperventilation.

Bursts of diffuse or bilateral fast (10-Hz) rhythms (or polyspikes), originally termed 'grand mal pattern', are frequently recorded during slow wave sleep but disappear during REM sleep. They usually last a few seconds but tend to recur at relatively brief intervals. These bursts are identical to those associated with clinical tonic seizures, although they are often of shorter duration. Polygraphic sleep recording has demonstrated that some are associated with brief apnea and/or mild axial contraction, indicating that some are subtle tonic seizures.[3,43,51] They are not pathognomonic of Lennox-Gastaut syndrome and have been recorded in cases of focal epilepsy.[4,52] However, such discharges are highly suggestive of Lennox-Gastaut syndrome and are considered necessary for the diagnosis by some[4,13] but not all authors. Thus, Baldy-Moulinier et al.[51] found them in only 44 of 80 patients diagnosed with Lennox-Gastaut syndrome who had all-night EEG recording.

Polyspike-wave complexes are also frequent in slow wave sleep,[4,53] possibly even more than the 10-Hz bursts. Slowing of the background rhythms is present in the waking state in most but not all patients. Focal paroxysmal activity (sharp waves or spikes) and focal slow activity are not infrequently seen.

COURSE AND PROGNOSIS

The overall outcome of Lennox-Gastaut syndrome is very poor. Seizure remission rates of 0 per cent,[3] 4 per cent[13] and 6.7 per cent[8] have been reported. The severity of the cognitive delay roughly parallels that of the seizures. Studies that use the strict inclusion criteria defined by Beaumanoir and Dravet[3] and by Kaminska et al.,[54] including a complete clinical and EEG picture with predominantly tonic seizures, episodes of nonconvulsive status, and runs of 10-Hz discharges, report the worst outcome. In such cases, the characteristic types of Lennox-Gastaut syndrome seizures continue into adolescence and early adulthood and the degree of mental

deficit is severe. In patients with less typical features and clear evidence of focal clinical and EEG manifestations, the characteristic seizures of Lennox-Gastaut syndrome are often replaced by other seizure types, usually focal.[3] In such cases the Lennox-Gastaut syndrome may be only a transient phase in the course of a focal or multifocal epilepsy.

The itellectual disability following Lennox-Gastaut syndrome is often severe (see above). Children in whom Lennox-Gastaut syndrome was preceded by infantile spasms have a particularly poor outcome with regard to seizure control. In contrast, the outlook is better for children in whom myoclonic or myo-atonic seizures are a prominent feature[5,6] or in whom myoclonic-astatic epilepsy precedes Lennox-Gastaut syndrome.[7]

The SSW pattern generally tends to persist.[3,13] Focal or multifocal spikes become superimposed in 75 per cent of cases and may replace the diffuse SSW pattern in some. When diffuse spike-waves are replaced by multiple independent spike foci, there is often associated clinical or imaging evidence of cortical damage and the prognosis tends to be worse.[46]

A symptomatic etiology, early age of onset (even in cryptogenic cases), high frequency of tonic seizures, the occurrence of repeated episodes of nonconvulsive status epilepticus and a constantly slow EEG background were reported by Roger[55] to be associated with a poor outcome. Patients with onset of seizures after 4 years, myoclonic seizures, normal neuroimaging, a precipitation of SSW with paroxysmal response to hyperventilation, or a relatively high proportion of fast (3-Hz) spike-waves do better.

DIAGNOSIS AND NOSOLOGIC ISSUES

The diagnosis of Lennox-Gastaut syndrome may be complicated because many patients exhibit most, but not all, of the characteristic features. Although tonic seizures and runs of fast rhythms are probably the most suggestive features, both of these are not present in every case. In addition, there are many causes of Lennox-Gastaut syndrome and the cause may have prognostic and even therapeutic significance.

Neuroimaging may help to demonstrate the etiology but is normal in the majority of cases. PET studies have given variable results.[56,57] Focal, multifocal or diffuse areas of hypometabolism were observed.

The etiological heterogeneity of Lennox-Gastaut syndrome probably contributes to the different clinical patterns. Beaumanoir[43] found that only 63 per cent of 103 patients presented with the typical picture of tonic seizures, 10-Hz EEG bursts and episodes of status, whereas 37 per cent of them exhibited only some of the classic features and also had other seizure types, such as focal seizures or, rarely, generalized tonic-clonic seizures, or even absence seizures suggestive of primary generalized epilepsy. Some investigators have suggested that some clinical patterns should be separated from typical Lennox-Gastaut syndrome. Gastaut and Zifkin[58] suggested that cases characterized by the predominance of atonic drop attacks, commonly observed in association with focal seizures and focal EEG anomalies, should be separated from Lennox-Gastaut syndrome. They considered that these patients had focal epileptogenic lesions and secondary bilateral synchrony that resembled the cases of 'partial epilepsy with a turn for the worse' reported by Pazzaglia et al.[52] As such, these cases differed from 'true' Lennox-Gastaut syndrome, which was classified as a generalized epilepsy. However, the rationale for excluding patients who fulfill the clinical and EEG criteria of Lennox-Gastaut syndrome on the basis of supposed pathophysiological mechanisms is not warranted in our present stage of knowledge. Thus, asymmetry of the EEG and focal neurologic signs, including hemiparesis, are well recognized in Lennox-Gastaut syndrome.[58] An 'intermediate petit mal' was proposed by Lugaresi et al.[59] to describe those patients who differ from Lennox-Gastaut syndrome by the presence of relatively typical absence seizures during the initial course and by the high proportion of fast (3-Hz) spike-waves in addition to the SSW of Lennox-Gastaut syndrome. Exclusion of such patients from Lennox-Gastaut syndrome on the basis of a single feature or a combination of features does not appear to be warranted. The 'myoclonic variant' of the Lennox-Gastaut syndrome describes patients with prominent myoclonic or myo-astatic seizures,[6,60] who frequently have episodes of absence status, often with marked erratic myoclonus. Tonic seizures were less frequent, usually of late onset, and almost exclusively nocturnal. The age of onset was later and the outcome more favorable. The EEG variably featured fast and slow spike-wave complexes. The duration and repetition of the episodes of absence status seemed to be causally related to the development of cognitive deterioration and tonic attacks.[7,54,61]

OTHER EPILEPSY SYNDROMES RESEMBLING LENNOX–GASTAUT SYNDROME

Severe myoclonic epilepsy of infancy or Dravet syndrome[6,62,63] (see Chapter 9E), also termed polymorphic epilepsy of infants,[64] also features brief seizures with falls and cognitive deterioration. However, the early history of affected children is quite different. The onset is virtually always in the first year of life and is characterized by repeated and often long-lasting convulsive seizures, commonly precipitated by mild fevers. The EEG never features SSW and tonic seizures, if they do occur, are rare and start much later. The less severe myoclonic epilepsies (including benign myoclonic epilepsy) and other imperfectly classified types do not feature tonic attacks or SSW, except in rare cases.[44,65,66]

Atypical partial benign epilepsy,[67] also termed **pseudo-Lennox syndrome**,[68,69] is associated with multiple falls and has diffuse slow spike-waves during sleep. It is characterized by rare, focal seizures that are often nocturnal, and by active periods, usually of a few weeks' duration, during which intense clinical and EEG epileptic activity is evident. During these periods, there are atonic seizures that can be focal or generalized and result in multiple daily falls. The EEG abnormalities include brief discharges of spike-waves associated with the falls and 'continuous spike-waves of slow sleep'. The intervals between active periods can last for several months and only a few (2–5) active periods occur before complete recovery.[39,70,71] The cognitive and behavioral outcome is usually favorable but deterioration may also occur, especially when bouts of seizures are multiple and prolonged. Atypical partial benign epilepsy probably represents an intermittent form of the syndrome of continuous spike-waves of slow sleep.

Patients with tonic seizures only do not meet the criteria of Lennox-Gastaut syndrome. However, some have a course quite similar to patients with Lennox-Gastaut syndrome and probably can be regarded as a variant of Lennox-Gastaut syndrome, whereas others may have different syndromes. Vigilance-dependent tonic seizures[72] and other sleep-related tonic seizures[73] probably represent focal seizures of frontal lobe origin and these conditions are rarely difficult to distinguish from Lennox-Gastaut syndrome.

TREATMENT

Lennox-Gastaut syndrome is notoriously resistant to therapy. Although complete seizure control is rare, drug treatment can decrease the frequency of seizures in a significant proportion of patients. The frequent resistance to drug treatment results often in the use of multiple drugs at high dosage. This, however, may depress the level of consciousness and result in a paradoxical increase in seizure frequency, particularly if drugs with sedative effects are used. Thus, patients are usually improved by a decrease in polypharmacy, even though complete control may not be achieved. Monotherapy is rarely effective, and drug combinations are often used. However, only a limited number of drugs have been tested adequately and most therapeutic recommendations are based on clinical experience only.

Valproic acid is commonly used and thought to be effective, especially in cryptogenic Lennox-Gastaut syndrome.[74]

The benzodiazepines, especially clobazam, are also first-line treatment. Benzodiazepines should be used with caution in nonconvulsive status as they may precipitate tonic status. The combination of valproic acid with a benzodiazepine, especially clobazam, seems often to be effective.[44]

Felbamate was the first drug shown in a randomized controlled trial (RCT) to be effective as adjunctive therapy in the treatment of Lennox-Gastaut syndrome.[75] Unfortunately, hematological and hepatic toxicity have limited the use of this agent. Repeated measurements of blood counts and transaminase activities are recommended. However, the frequency of severe toxicity is low in children in whom no case of aplastic anemia has been reported.[76] Lamotrigine has also been shown in an RCT to be safe and effective and is commonly used.[77] The drug may be particularly efficacious against atypical absences and falls. The combination of lamotrigine with a benzodiazepine has also been recommended.[78] Finally, topiramate has been proven to be effective in placebo-controlled studies.[79,80] There have been no studies comparing lamotrigine, topiramate or valproic acid. Currently, I prefer lamotrigine, which is better tolerated, but all three agents should be tried in the frequent cases of refractoriness or only partial response.

Carbamazepine may be active against tonic seizures but should be used with caution when myoclonic seizures are prominent.[81] Other drugs reported to be effective in open-label, uncontrolled studies include vigabatrin[82–85] and zonisamide[86] as adjunctive drugs. The risk-benefit ratio of these agents is not yet clearly defined. The retinal toxicity associated with vigabatrin limits its use in this condition.

Nonconventional agents have been used. Corticosteroids or ACTH may be indicated to tide the patient over a particularly difficult period,[44] but their prolonged use is fraught with undesirable side-effects. The value of immunoglobulins has not been properly assessed, although some favorable results have been reported.[87,88] Some authors have used amantadine[89] and thyroid-releasing hormone in small numbers of patients, but the trials appear to have been discontinued.

The ketogenic diet is clearly effective in a proportion of cases[90–92] and is used extensively in several centres.[10,93] There has been no controlled study of the ketogenic diet in Lennox-Gastaut syndrome and its use is considered by some to be controversial, but clinical opinion tends to be favorable.

Resective surgery has been used in a few cases in which a focal lesion, especially cortical dysplasia,[22] was thought to be responsible for the syndrome. In most case, the only surgical possibility is anterior or total callosotomy. This operation has proved useful in the treatment of drop attacks, which are the most incapacitating type of seizure.[94,95]

KEY POINTS

- Lennox-Gastaut syndrome is characterized by
  - **multiple seizure types**, including brief tonic, atonic, myoclonic and atypical absence seizures
  - interictal EEG pattern of diffuse, **slow (<2.5 Hz) spike-wave complexes**
- Some authors consider that two **additional criteria** are necessary for the diagnosis:
  - generalized tonic seizures
  - runs of fast (10 Hz) rhythms, especially during non-REM sleep
- **Intellectual disability** is very frequent but not a constant feature
- **Focal seizures, unilateral seizures, and generalized tonic-clonic seizures** may occur before and after the appearance of Lennox-Gastaut syndrome
- Lennox-Gastaut syndrome **can follow other epilepsy syndromes**, including West syndrome and myoclonic-astatic epilepsy
- The onset of the seizures is between 1 and 7 years of age with a peak age of onset between 3 and 5 years of age
- Lennox-Gastaut syndrome is associated with a variety of different causes: brain malformations are the most common abnormality demonstrated and genetic factors are generally less important
- 50–75 per cent of patients with Lennox-Gastaut syndrome have episodes of **nonconvulsive status**, which often last hours or days and may be difficult to recognize
- Prolonged episodes of nonconvulsive status affect **mental outcome**
- Few patients achieve complete seizure control but **AEDs can reduce the seizure frequency**
- A **poor outcome** is more common in those patients with a symptomatic etiology, early age of onset, high frequency of tonic seizures, the occurrence of repeated episodes of nonconvulsive status epilepticus, a consistently slow EEG background, and abnormal brain imaging

REFERENCES

1. Commission on Classification and Terminology of the International League Against Epilepsy. Proposal for revised classification of epilepsy and epileptic syndromes. *Epilepsia* 1989; **30**: 389–399.
2. Aicardi J, Levy Gomes A. The Lennox-Gastaut syndrome: clinical and electroencephalographic features. In: Niedermeyer E,

Degen R (eds) *The Lennox-Gastaut Syndrome*. New York: Alan Liss, 1988; 25–46.

3. Beaumanoir A, Dravet C. The Lennox-Gastaut syndrome. In: Roger J, Dravet C, Bureau M *et al.* (eds) *Epileptic Syndromes in Infancy, Childhood and Adolescence*. London: John Libbey, 1992; 115–132.

4. Roger J, Gobbi G, Bureau M, *et al.* Severe partial epilepsies in childhood. In: Fukuyama Y, Kamoshita S, Ohtsuka C, Suzuki Y (eds) *Modern Perspectives of Child Neurology*. Tokyo: Japanese Society of Child Neurology, 1991; 223–230.

5. Chevrie JJ, Aicardi J. Childhood epileptic encephalopathy with slow spike-wave: a statistical study of 80 cases. *Epilepsia* 1972; **13**: 259–271.

6. Dravet C, Roger J, Bureau M, Dalla Bernardina B. Myoclonic epilepsies in childhood. In: Akimoto A, Kazamatsuri A, Seino M, Ward A (eds) *Advances in Epileptology; XIIIth Epilepsy International Symposium* New York: Raven Press, 1982; 135–140.

7. Hoffmann-Riem M, Diener W, Beninger C, *et al.* Nonconvulsive status epilepticus: a possible cause of mental retardation in patients with Lennox-Gastaut syndrome. *Neuropediatrics* 2000; **31**: 169–174.

8. Gastaut H, Dravet C, Loubier D, *et al.* Evolution clinique et pronostic du syndrome de Lennox-Gastaut. In: Lugaresi E, Pazzaglia P, Tassinari CA (eds) *Evolution and Prognosis of Epilepsies*. Bologna: Aulo Gaggi, 1973; 133–154.

9. Luna D, Chiron C, Dulac O, Pajot N. Epidémiologie des épilepsies de l'enfant dans le département de l'Oise (France). In: Jallon P (ed.) *Epidémiologie des Epilepsies, Journées d'Étude de la Ligue Française contre l'Épilepsie*. London: John Libbey, 1988; 41–53.

10. Trevathan E. Infantile spasms and Lennox-Gastaut syndrome. *Journal of Child Neurology* 2002; **17**: 2S9–22.

11. Steffenburg U, Hagberg G, Viggedal G, Kyllerman M. Active epilepsy in mentally retarded children. I. Prevalence and additional neuroimpairments. *Acta Paediatrica* 1995; **84**: 1147–1152.

12. Mariani E, Ferini-Strambi L, Sala M, Erminio C, Smirne C. Epilepsy in institutionalized patients with encephalopathy: Clinical aspects and nosological considerations. *American Journal on Mental Retardation* 1993; **98**(Suppl): 27–33.

13. Roger J, Remy C, Bureau M, *et al.* Le syndrome de Lennox-Gastaut chez l'adulte. *Revue Neurologique* 1987; **143**: 401–405.

14. Ohtahara S. Lennox-Gastaut syndrome: considerations in its concept and categorization. *Japanese Journal of Psychiatry and Neurology* 1988; **42**: 535–542.

15. Boniver C, Dravet C, Bureau M, Roger J. Idiopathic Lennox-Gastaut syndrome. In: Wolf P, Dam M, Janz D, Dreifuss F (eds) *Advances in Epileptology, 16th Epilepsy International Symposium*. New York: Raven Press, 1987; 195–200.

16. Ohtahara S, Ohtsuka Y, Yoshinaga H, *et al.* Lennox-Gastaut syndrome: etiological considerations. In: Niedermeyer E, Degen R (eds) *The Lennox-Gastaut Syndrome*. New York: Alan Liss, 1988; 47–63.

17. Dravet C, Roger J. The Lennox-Gastaut syndrome: historical aspects from 1966 to 1987. In: Niedermeter E, Degen R (eds) *The Lennox-Gastaut Syndrome*. New York: Alan Liss, 1988; 9–23.

18. Guerrini R, Dravet C, Gobbi G, Ricci S, Dulac O. Idiopathic generalized epilepsies with myoclonus in infancy and childhood. In: Malafosse AZ *et al.* (eds) *Idiopathic Generalized Epilepsies; Clinical and Genetic Aspects*. London: John Libbey, 1994; 267–80.

19. Guerrini R, Dravet C, Raybaud C, *et al.* Epilepsy and gyral anomalies detected by MRI: electroclinicomorphological correlations and follow up. *Developmental Medicine and Child Neurology* 1992; **34**: 706–718.

20. Ricci B, Cusmai R, Fariello G, *et al.* Double cortex: a neuronal migration anomaly as a possible cause of Lennox-Gastaut syndrome. *Archives of Neurology* 1992; **48**: 61–65.

21. Kuzniecky R, *et al.* Congenital bilateral perisylvian syndrome. *Lancet* 1993; **341**: 608–612.

22. Palmini A, Andermann F, Tampieri D. Neuronal migration disorders: a contribution of modern neuroimaging to the etiologic diagnosis of epilepsy. *Canadian Journal of Neurological Sciences* 1991; **18**: 580–587.

23. Palmini A, Andermann F, Olivier A, *et al.* Focal neuronal migration disorders and intractable partial epilepsy; results of surgical treatment. *Annals of Neurology* 1991; **30**: 750–757.

24. Guerrini R, Andermann F, Canapicchi R, *et al.* (eds). *Dysplasias of Cerebral Cortex and Epilepsy*. Philadelphia: Lippincott-Raven, 1996.

25. Chevrie JJ, Specola N, Aicardi J. Secondary bilateral synchrony in unilateral pial angiomatosis: successful surgical treatment. *Journal of Neurology, Neurosurgery and Psychiatry* 1988; **51**: 663–670.

26. Roger J, Gambardelli-Dubois D. Neuropathological studies of the Lennox-Gastaut syndrome. In: Niedermeyer E, Degen R (eds) *The Lennox-Gastaut Syndrome*. New York: Alan Liss, 1988; 73–93.

27. Angelini L, Brogli G, Riva D, Solero CL. A case of Lennox-Gastaut syndrome successfully treated by removal of a parieto-temporal astrocytoma. *Epilepsia* 1979; **20**: 665–669.

28. Berkovic S, Andermann F, Melanson D, *et al.* Hypothalamic hamartoma and ictal laughter: evolution of a characteristic epileptic syndrome and diagnostic value of magnetic resonance imaging. *Annals of Neurology* 1988; **23**: 429–439.

29. Renier WO. Neuromorphological and biochemical analysis of a brain biopsy in a second case of idiopathic lennox-Gastaut syndrome. In: Niedermeyer E, Degen R (eds) *The Lennox-Gastaut Syndrome*. New York: Alan Liss, 1988; 427–432.

30. Renier WO, Gabreels FJM, Jaspar HHJ. Morphological and biochemical analysis of a brain biopsy in a case of idiopathic Lennox-Gastaut syndrome. *Epilepsia* 1988; **29**: 644–649.

31. Palm A, Brandt M, Korinthenberg R. West syndrome and Lennox-Gastaut syndrome in children with porencephalic cysts. In: Niedermeyer E, Degen R (eds) *The Lennox-Gastaut Syndrome*. New York: Alan Liss, 1988; 418–426.

32. Niedermeyer E. *The Generalized Epilepsies*. Springfield, IL: CC Thomas, 1972.

33. Donat JF, Wright FS. Seizures in series; similarities between seizures in the West and Lennox-Gastaut syndromes. *Epilepsia* 1991; **32**: 504–509.

34. Gastaut H, Zifkin B. Secondary bilateral synchrony and Lennox-Gastaut syndrome. In: Niedermeyer E, Degen R (eds) *The Lennox-Gastaut Syndrome*. New York: Alan Liss, 1988; 221–242.

35. Tassinari CA, Bureau M, Thomas P. Epilepsy with myoclonic absences. In: Roger J, *et al.* (eds) *Epileptic Syndromes in Infancy, Childhood and Adolescence*, 2nd edn. London: John Libbey, 1992; 151–160.

36. Egli M, Mothersill I, O'Kane M, O'Kane F. Axial spasm – the predominant type of drop-seizure in patients with secondary generalized epileptic encephalopathy (Lennox-Gastaut syndrome). *Epilepsia* 1985; **26**: 401–405.

37. Ikeno T, Shigematsu H, Miyakashi M, *et al.* An analytical study of epileptic falls. *Epilepsia* 1985; **26**: 612–621.

38. Oller Daurella L. A special type of attack observed in the Lennox-Gastaut syndrome in adults. *Electroencephalography and Clinical Neurophysiology* 1970; **29**: 529.

39. Aicardi J, Levy Gomes A. Clinical and EEG symptomatology of the 'genuine' Lennox-Gastaut syndrome and its differentiation from other forms of epilepsy in early childhood. In: Degen R (ed.) *The Benign Localized and Generalized Epilepsies of Early Childhood.* Amsterdam: Elsevier, 1992; 185–193.

40. Bonanni P, Parmeggiani L, Guerrini R. Different neurophysiologic patterns of myoclonus characterize Lennox-Gastaut syndrome and myoclonic astatic epilepsy. *Epilepsia* 2002; **43**(6): 609–615.

41. Dravet C, Natale O and Magaudda A, *et al.* Les états de mal dans le syndrome de Lennox-Gastaut. *Revue d'Electroencéphalographie et de Neurophysiologie Clinique* 1985; **15**: 361–368.

42. Beaumanoir A, Foletti G, Magistris M, Volanschi D. Status epilepticus in the Lennox-Gastaut syndrome. In: Niedermeyer E, Degen R (eds) *The Lennox-Gastaut Syndrome.* New York: Allan Liss, 1988; 283–299.

43. Beaumanoir A. The Lennox-Gastaut syndrome. In: Roger J *et al.* (eds) *Epileptic Syndromes in Infancy, Childhood and Adolescence.* London: John Libbey Eurotext, 1985; 89–99.

44. Aicardi J. *Epilepsy in children*, 2nd edn. New York: Raven Press, 1994.

45. Engel J. A proposed diagnostic scheme for people with epileptic seizures and with epilepsy: Report of the ILAE Task Force on Classification and Terminology. *Epilepsia* 2001; **42**(6): 796–803.

46. Ohtsuka Y, Amano R, Mizukawa M, Ohtahara S. Long-term prognosis of the Lennox-Gastaut syndrome. *Japanese Journal of Psychiatry and Neurology* 1990; **44**: 257–264.

47. Oller Daurella L. Evolution et pronostic du syndrome de Lennox-Gastaut. In: Lugaresi E, Pazzaglia P, Tassinari CA (eds) *Evolution and Prognosis of Epilepsies.* Bologna: Aulo Gaggi, 1973; 156–164.

48. Blume WT. The EEG features of the Lennox-Gastaut syndrome. In: Niedermeyer E, Degen R (eds) *The Lennox-Gastaut Syndrome.* New York: Allan Liss, 1988; 159–176.

49. Blume WT, David RB, Gomez MR. Generalized sharp and slow wave complexes-associated clinical features and long-term follow up. *Brain* 1973; **96**: 289–306.

50. Niedermeyer E. The Lennox-Gastaut syndrome. A severe type of childhood epilepsy. *Deutsche Zeitschrift für Nervenheilkunde* 1969; **195**: 263–282.

51. Baldy-Moulinier M, Touchon J, Billiard M, *et al.* Nocturnal sleep studies in the Lennox-Gastaut syndrome. In: Niedermeyer E, Degen R (eds) *The Lennox-Gastaut Syndrome.* New York: Allan Liss, 1988; 243–260.

52. Pazzaglia P, d'Alessandro R, Ambrosetto G, Lugaresi E. Drop attacks: an ominous change in the evolution of partial epilepsy. *Neurology* 1985; **33**: 1725–1730.

53. Degen R, Degen HE. Sleep and sleep deprivation in epileptology. In: Degen R, Niedermeyer E (eds) *Epilepsy, Sleep and Sleep Deprivation.* Amsterdam: Elsevier Science, 1984; 273–286.

54. Kaminska A, Ickowicz A, Plouin P, *et al.* Delineation of cryptogenic Lennox-Gastaut syndrome and myoclonic-astatic epilepsy using multiple correspondence analysis. *Epilepsy Research* 1999; **36**: 15–29.

55. Roger J. Introduction: partial epilepsies symposium. *Epilepsia* 1989; **30**: 797.

56. Chugani HT, Mazziota JC, Engel J Jr, Phelps ME. The Lennox Gastaut syndrome: metabolic subtypes determined by 2 fluoro-D-glucose positron emission tomography. *Annals of Neurology* 1987; **21**: 4–13.

57. Theodore WH, Rose D, Patronas W, *et al.* Cerebral glucose metabolism in the Lennox-Gastaut syndrome. *Annals of Neurology* 1987; **21**: 14–21.

58. Gastaut H, Zifkin BJ. Secondary bilateral synchrony and Lennox-Gastaut syndrome. In: Niedermeyer E, Degen R (eds) *The Lennox-Gastaut Syndrome.* New York: Alan Liss, 1988; 221–242.

59. Lugaresi E, Cirignotta P, Montagna P. Nocturnal paroxysmal dystonia. *Journal of Neurology, Neurosurgery and Psychiatry* 1986; **49**: 375–380.

60. Aicardi J, Chevrie JJ. Myoclonic epilepsies of childhood. *Neuropediatrie* 1971; **3**: 177–190.

61. Doose H, Völzke E. Petit mal status in early childhood and dementia. *Neuropediatrie* 1979; **10**: 10–14.

62. Dravet C, Bureau M, Guerrini R, *et al.* Severe myoclonic epilepsy of infants. In: Roger J *et al.* (eds) *Epileptic Syndromes in Infancy, Childhood and Adolescence.* London: John Libbey, 1992; 75–88.

63. Dalla Bernardina B, Capovilla G, Gattoni MB, *et al.* Epilepsie myoclonique grave de la première année. *Revue d'Electroencéphalographie et de Neurophysiolgie Clinique* 1982; **12**: 21–25.

64. Aicardi J. Myoclonic epilepsies in childhood. *International Pediatrics* 1991; **6**: 195–200.

65. Dravet C, Bureau M, Roger J. Benign myoclonic epilepsy in infants. In: Roger J *et al.* (eds) *Epileptic Syndromes in Infancy, Childhood and Adolescence.* London: John Libbey, 1992; 67–74.

66. Guerrini R, Dravet C, Gobbi G, Ricci S, Dulac O. Idiopathic generalized epilepsies with myoclonus in infancy and childhood. In: Malafosse AZ *et al.* (eds) *Idiopathic Generalized Epilepsies; Clinical and Genetic Aspects.* London: John Libbey, 1994; 267–280.

67. Aicardi J, Chevrie JJ. Atypical benign partial epilepsy of childhood. *Developmental Medicine and Child Neurology* 1982; **24**: 281–292.

68. Doose H, Baier WK. Benign partial epilepsies and related syndromes – multifactorial pathogenesis with hereditary impairment of brain maturation. *European Journal of Pediatrics* 1989; **149**: 152–158.

69. Hahn 2001, Pistohl J, Neubauer BA, Stephani U. Atypical 'benign' partial epilepsy or pseudo-Lennox syndrome. Part I: symptomatology and long-term prognosis. *Neuropediatrics* 2001; **32**: 1–8.

70. Aicardi J. *Epilepsy in children*, 2nd edn. New York: Raven Press, 1994.

71. Deonna T, Ziegler AL, Despland PA. Combined myoclonic-astatic and benign focal epilepsy of childhood ('atypical benign partial

epilepsy of childhood'). A separate syndrome. *Neuropediatrics* 1986; **17**: 144–151.

72. Rajna P, Kundra O, Halasz P. Vigilance level-dependent tonic seizures. Epilepsy or sleep disorder? *Epilepsia* 1983; **24**: 725–733.

73. Vigevano F, Fusco L. Hypnic tonic postural seizures in healthy children provide evidence for a partial epilepsy syndrome of frontal origin. *Epilepsia* 1993; **34**: 110–119.

74. Farrell K. Secondary generalized epilepsy and Lennox-Gastaut syndrome. In: Wyllie E (ed.) *The Treatment of Epilepsy: Principles and Practice*. Philadelphia: Lea and Febiger, 1993; 604–613.

75. Efficacy of felbamate in childhood epileptic encephalopathy (Lennox-Gastaut syndrome). The Felbamate Study Group in Lennox-Gastaut Syndrome. *New England Journal of Medicine* 1993; **328**: 29–33.

76. Pellock JM, Dodson WE, Bourgeois B (eds) *Pediatric Epilepsy: Diagnosis and Therapy*, 2nd edn. New York: Demos, 2000; 201–218.

77. Motte J, Trevathan E, Arvidson JF, *et al.* Lamotrigine for generalized seizures associated with the Lennox-Gastaut syndrome. *New England Journal of Medicine* 1997; **337**: 1807–1812.

78. Pisani F, Di Perri E, Perucca E, Richens A. Interaction of lamotrigine with sodium valproate. *Lancet* 1993; **341**: 1224.

79. Sachdeo RC, Glauser TA, Ritter F, *et al.* A double-blind randomized trial of topiramate in Lennox-Gastaut syndrome. *Neurology* 1999; **52**: 1282–1287.

80. Glauser TA, Morita DA. Encephalopathic epilepsy after infancy. In: Pellock JM, Dodson WE, Bourgeois B (eds) *Pediatric Epilepsy: Diagnosis and Therapy*, 2nd edn. New York: Demos, 2000; 201–218.

81. Guerrini R, Dravet C, Genton P, *et al.* Lamotrigine and seizure aggravation in severe myoclonic epilepsy. *Epilepsia* 1998; **39**(5): 508–512.

82. Dulac O, Chiron C, Luna D, *et al.* Vigabatrin in childhood epilepsy. *Journal of Child Neurology* 1991; **6**(Suppl. 2): 30–37.

83. Feucht M, Brantner-Inthaler S. Gamma-vinyl Gaba (vigabatrin) in the therapy of Lennox-Gastaut syndrome: an open study. *Epilepsia* 1994; **35**: 993–998.

84. Appleton RE. Vigabatrin in the management of generalized seizures in children. *Seizure* 1995; **4**: 45–48.

85. Maldonado C, Castello J, Fuentes E. Vigabatrin in the management of Lennox-Gastaut syndrome. *Epilepsia* 1995; **36**: 102.

86. Yamatogi Y, Ohtahara S. Current topics of treatment. In: Ohtahara S and Roger J (eds) *Proceedings of the International Symposium, New Trends in Pediatric Epileptology*. Okayama, Japan: University of Okayama, 1991; 136–148.

87. Rapin F, Astruc J, Echenne B. Utilisation pédiatrique des immunoglobulines intraveineues en immunomodulation; A propos de 34 observations. *Annales de Pédiatrie* 1988; **35**: 381–488.

88. Engelen BG Van, Renier WO, Weemaed CM, *et al.* High-dose intratravenous immunoglobulin treatment in cryptogenic West and Lennox-Gastaut syndromes: an add-on study. *European Journal of Pediatrics* 1994; **153**: 762–769.

89. Shields WD, Lake JL, Chugani HT. Amantadine in the treatment of refractory epilepsy: an open trial in 10 patients. *Neurology* 1985; **35**: 579–581.

90. O'Donohoe N. *Epilepsies of Childhood*, 2nd edn. London: Butterworths, 1985.

91. Schwartz RH, Eaton J, Ainsley-Green A, Bower BD. Ketogenic diet in the management of childhood epilepsy. In: Clifford-Rose F (ed.) *Research Progress in Epilepsy*. London: Pitman, 1983; 326–332.

92. Kinsman SL, Vining EPG, Quaskey SA, *et al.* Efficacy of the ketogenic diet for intractable seizure disorders. Review of 58 cases. *Epilepsia* 1992; **33**: 1132–1136.

93. Abram HS, Turk WR. Lennox-Gastaut syndrome. In: *Management of Epilepsy in Children: the Need for Consensus. Consensus in Child Neurology*. Hamilton, Ontario: Decker Periodicals, 1997; 10–15.

94. Oguni H, Fukuyama Y, Imaizumi Y, Uehara T. Video-EEG analysis of drop seizures in myoclonic epilepsy of early childhood (Doose syndrome). *Epilepsia* 1992; **33**: 805–813.

95. Pinard JM. Anterior and total callosotomy in epileptic children: prospective one-year follow-up study. *Epilepsia* 1991; **32**(Suppl. 3): 54.

Derby Hospitals NHS Foundation
Trust
Library and Knowledge Service

11

Epileptic syndromes with onset in middle childhood

Childhood absence epilepsy

ROBERTO MICHELUCCI AND CARLO ALBERTO TASSINARI

Childhood absence epilepsy (CAE), otherwise known as **petit mal**, **pyknolepsy** or **Friedmann syndrome**, is an age-dependent, idiopathic form of generalized epilepsy, characterized by the following features:[1–5]

- a strong family history of similar seizures
- onset before puberty in previously normal children
- female preponderance
- typical absence seizures as the initial and predominant seizure type
- multiple typical absence seizures each day
- ictal EEG pattern characterized by a bilateral, symmetric, and synchronous discharge of regular 3-Hz spike-waves on a normal background (Figure 11A.1)
- predisposition to development of generalized tonic-clonic seizures (GTCS) during adolescence
- good response to treatment and good prognosis.

CAE represents the paradigm of idiopathic generalized epilepsy. Typical absence seizures, however, are not exclusive of CAE and may be the symptom of a variety of other generalized epilepsies, including juvenile absence epilepsy, juvenile myoclonic epilepsy, myoclonic absence epilepsy and a number of conditions awaiting further studies and confirmation.

ETIOLOGY AND BIOLOGICAL BASIS

A positive family history of epilepsy is reported in 15–44 per cent[6,7] of children with typical absence seizures. In two large series, 17 per cent of patients with CAE had first-degree relatives with epilepsy manifesting with absence seizures, generalized tonic-clonic seizures or both.[4,8] The risk of epilepsy in the offspring of subjects having had CAE has been estimated to be 6–8 per cent.[9] There is a high concordance for the same epilepsy type in the relatives of children with CAE. In 24 families with a CAE proband, 33 per cent of first-degree relatives had CAE, whereas febrile seizures (47 per cent) and GTCS (30 per cent) were more common in distant relatives.[10] In a large twin study, the concordance for epilepsy was 75 per cent in monozygotic pairs with CAE, which was 16 times greater than in dyzigotic twins.[11] Overall, there is a great deal of evidence for a genetic component to etiology of CAE, but the mechanism of inheritance and the genes involved remain largely unknown. As concordance in monozygotic twins is not 100 per cent, nongenetic factors are also likely and CAE is regarded as a multifactorial condition, resulting from interactions between genetic and acquired factors.[12]

Recent advances in mapping and positional cloning of CAE have suggested the existence of two separate gene loci: chromosome 1 p for typical absence seizures evolving to juvenile myoclonic epilepsy, and chromosome 8q24 for CAE with grand mal seizures.[13] As to the candidate genes for CAE, available evidence suggests that mutations in genes encoding GABA receptors or brain-expressed voltage-gated calcium channels may underlie CAE. Indeed, genetic animal models of typical absence seizures have been found to harbor mutations of the P/Q-type voltage-gated calcium channel genes.[14] A patient with a phenotype combining typical AS (absence seizures) GTCS and episodic and progressive ataxia showed mutations of

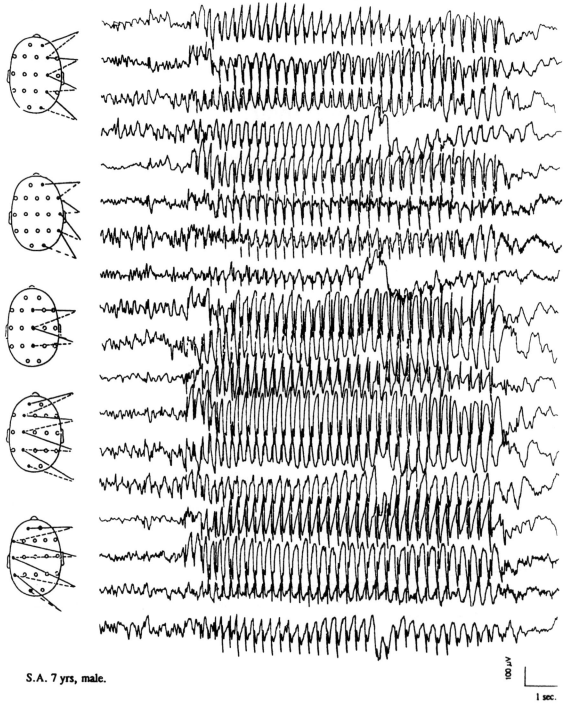

S.A. 7 yrs, male.

100 µV

1 sec.

Figure 11A.1 *Childhood absence epilepsy: a typical simple absence seizure. The generalized SWs have highest amplitude under the frontocentral leads. The frequency of the discharge is faster, about 4 Hz at the onset and slows to 2.5–3 Hz towards the end of the absence seizure.*

the P/Q-type voltage-gated calcium channel gene.[15] Recently two families exhibiting a phenotypic spectrum of CAE and febrile seizures have been reported showing mutations of the $GABA_A$ receptor γ2 subunit (GABRG2).[16–18] However, mutations of GABRG2 have not been found in a large number of patients with CAE.[17,18]

CLINICAL DATA

General

CAE accounts for 8 per cent of school-aged children with epilepsy.[19] In two recent prospective community-based studies, the prevalence of CAE in children less than 16 years of age with epilepsy was 10 per cent[8] and 12.3 per cent.[20] The annual incidence rate of CAE has been estimated to be 6.3/100 000[21] to 8.0/100 000[22] in children aged 0–15 years. There is a female preponderance, with 60–76 per cent of affected children being girls.

The onset of CAE is classically considered to be between 4 and 10 years of age, with a peak around 5–7 years. However, onset before 4 years has been described in an Italian series[23] and onset after the age of 10 has occasionally been described.[5]

Description of seizures

TYPICAL ABSENCES

These seizures are the hallmark of CAE. The essence of an absence seizure consists of a loss of awareness and responsiveness with cessation of ongoing activities. Different degrees of altered consciousness have been described, but a complete abolition of awareness, responsiveness and memory is usual in typical absence seizures.

Classic studies with intensive video-EEG monitoring[24–26] have demonstrated that loss of consciousness represents the only finding (simple absence) in less than 10 per cent of absence seizures. More frequently, there are associated clinical features such as clonic, tonic, and atonic activity, vegetative components or automatisms. Mild **clonic** components occur in approximately half of the cases and consist of eye blinking (at a rhythm of 3 Hz) or, less often, facial twitching. In some attacks there may be an increase in postural tone with **tonic** muscular contraction, usually limited to the eyes (which deviate upwards) or the head (which draws backwards). Decrease in postural tone may also occur, resulting in a gradual lowering of the head and/or arms. The **atonic** components rarely cause the patient to fall. **Automatisms** occur in 60 per cent of absence seizures and may be either perseverative, in which the patient persists in what he or she is doing, or *de novo,* with simple or complex movements. The frequency of automatisms increases with increasing seizure duration.[27] **Autonomic or vegetative** phenomena may also occur, including pupil dilatation, color change, piloerection, tachycardia, urinary incontinence and salivation. Several components may occur during a given absence seizure, and several types of absence seizure may be present in the same patient.

Absence seizures are characterized by a short duration (5–30 s in most cases) and abrupt onset and termination. In CAE, absence seizures occur frequently (10–100 per day), are often precipitated by emotional, intellectual or metabolic (e.g. hyperventilation) factors, and may occur at particular times of day. The true frequency of absence seizures is often difficult to estimate because of the short duration of the attacks, and prolonged EEG recordings

are sometimes necessary to assess seizure frequency and evaluate the efficacy of therapy.

Episodes of absence seizure status, sometimes called **spike-wave stupor** or **petit mal status**, are relatively rare in CAE and are reported in 10–16 per cent of patients.[28]

OTHER SEIZURE TYPES

GTCS as a presenting seizure type is not consistent with a diagnosis of CAE. Myoclonic jerks and GTCS do not occur at the same stage as the AS[4,5]. However, infrequent GTCS occur in 16–45 per cent of patients in adolescence or adult life [1,3–5].

NEUROPHYSIOLOGIC DATA

Interictal EEG

The interictal EEG background activity is usually normal. Interictal paroxysmal activity consists of single or brief discharges of generalized 3 Hz spike-waves, which occurs either spontaneously or during hyperventilation. These paroxysms are found in almost all children with active CAE. If repeated EEG recordings with hyperventilation fail to show generalized discharges or clinical absence seizures, the diagnosis of CAE must be questioned. The interictal spike-wave discharges are also numerous during non-REM sleep, when they are usually briefer, irregular and slower, around 1.5–2.5 Hz[29] (Figure 11A.2). Some children exhibit a particular posterior delta rhythm, characterized by long bursts of symmetric or asymmetric, high amplitude, sinusoidal 3-Hz activity, which is maximal in the occipitoparietal areas, is blocked by eye opening and enhanced by hyperventilation[30] (Figure 11A.3). The interictal paroxysmal abnormalities in CAE are 'generalized' by definition. However, there is a link between CAE and benign epilepsy of childhood with centrotemporal spikes,[31] and unilateral 'central' or 'midtemporal' spike-waves (Figure 11A.4) or persistent focal abnormalities may be observed.[32] In some patients, isolated interictal fast spike-waves either predominate over or occasionally involve one or both frontal regions; this occurs particularly during sleep.[33]

Paroxysmal response to intermittent photic stimulation is not usually found in CAE and has been proposed as an exclusion criterion by some[5,32] but not all authors.[34]

Ictal EEG

The ictal EEG consists of rhythmic 3-Hz, bilateral, synchronous and symmetric, spike-wave discharge with the highest amplitude in the frontocentral leads (Figures 11A.1, 11A.3). The onset of the discharge is abrupt, but

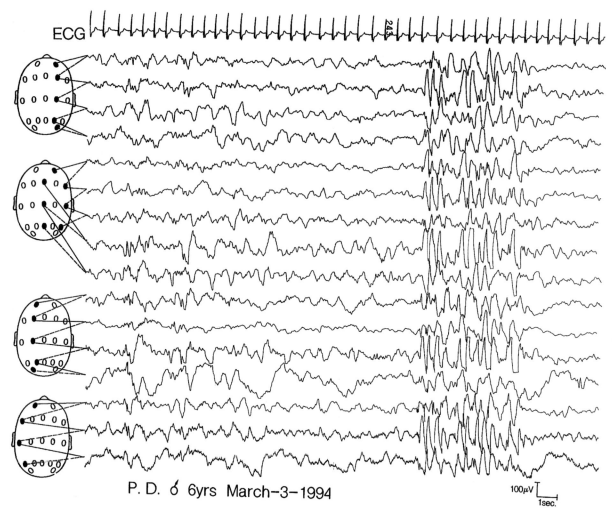

Figure 11A.2 *Childhood absence epilepsy: interictal paroxysmal abnormalities during slow sleep (phase III). The discharges are briefer, slower and more irregular when compared to wakefulness.*

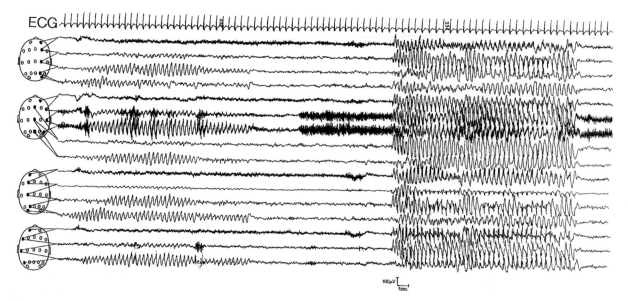

Figure 11A.3 *Same patient as in Figure 11A.2. On the left: long bursts of high sinusoidal activity at 3 Hz over both occipitoparietal areas. On the right: typical absence seizure.*

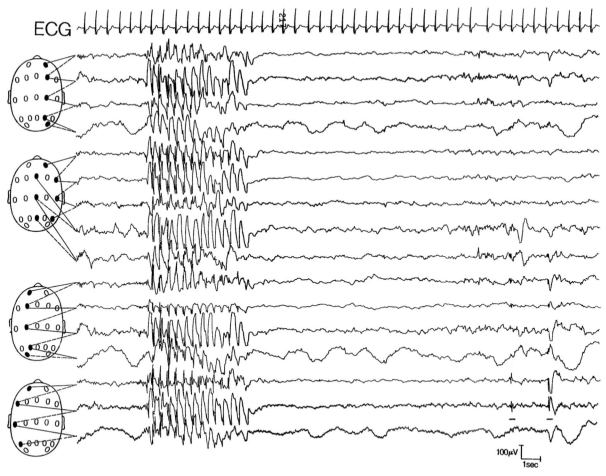

Figure 11A.4 *Same patient as in Figures 11A.2 and 11A.3. Slow sleep (phase II). On the left: an apparently subclinical discharge of spike-waves at 3 Hz. On the right: left focal temporal spikes and spike-waves.*

termination is less sudden. The frequency tends to be faster, about 4 Hz, at the onset and slows to 2.5–2 Hz towards the end of the discharge.

More irregular spike-wave discharges (polyspike-waves, changing rhythms within a discharge) are compatible with a diagnosis of CAE[35] but are more common in absences persisting to adult life.[36] EEG spike topography of absence seizures shows a maximum positivity as well as negativity of the individual spike-wave complexes over both frontal areas.[37]

In CAE, the distinction between 'ictal' and 'interictal' EEG paroxysms is sometimes difficult. Isolated spike-wave discharges are usually interictal and subclinical. However, they may also be ictal and manifest as a brief lapse of consciousness (**micro-absence** or **phantom absence**) or transient autonomic phenomena (pupillary hippus, an electrodermal response, etc.).[33] Sophisticated testing including continuous performance tasks and response testing has demonstrated impairment even with paroxysms less than 3 s in duration.[2]

EVOLUTION AND PROGNOSIS

Descriptions of the evolution and prognosis of CAE are rather inconclusive because of the heterogeneity in diagnostic criteria and insufficient follow-up periods of the different series. Nonetheless, CAE is generally considered a syndrome with an excellent prognosis. Typical absence seizures are controlled with appropriate therapy in about 80 per cent of patients.[35,38,39] The absence seizures may cease soon after the onset of therapy or persist for a time, so that a complete resolution of CAE may occur at varying ages and not just at puberty. Recent findings indicate that the absence seizures in patients with CAE, even if they persist for several years, finally disappear with age in more than 90 per cent of patients.[4] In a Swedish population-based study, a 91 per cent remission rate was found when patients with absence epilepsy had only absence seizures.[32] Gradual withdrawal of medication is recommended in children who are seizure-free for 1–2 years and have a normalized EEG. In a minority of patients (about 6 per cent), absence seizures are refractory to treatment and continue during adulthood, although at a lower frequency.[7]

Whatever the evolution of the absence seizures, GTCS develop in 16–44 per cent of patients with CAE.[4,7,35] GTCS usually begin between 8 and 15 years of age, occur infrequently and are easily controlled by treatment. Predisposing factors for the development of GTCS include onset of absence seizures after 8 years of age, male gender, a poor response to initial treatment, incorrect therapy, abnormal background activity and photosensitivity.[4]

Although CAE occurs usually in neurologically and intellectually normal children, some degree of cognitive dysfunction, mild cognitive decline or behavioral problems is observed in about one third of patients.[3–5] These problems can be due to a variety of causes including antiepileptic therapy, frequency of absence seizures and parents' attitude. However, they are most often the result of the ongoing ictal and interictal discharges.

DIAGNOSIS

A great deal of confusion and misunderstanding arose in the past from the fact that all epilepsies with absence seizures were called 'petit mal'. Only in the last two decades has progress been made in classifying the epileptic syndromes,[1] and a number of conditions featuring absence seizures as a prominent seizure type have been recognized as distinct clinical entities. CAE should be differentiated from the following disorders:

- **Juvenile absence epilepsy,** in which absence seizures begin during adolescence and occur at a lower frequency.
- **Epilepsy with myoclonic absences,** in which absence seizures are accompanied by rhythmic jerks of the proximal muscles of the upper limbs and may be resistant to treatment.
- **Juvenile myoclonic epilepsy,** in which absence seizures occur in 10–38 per cent of cases and usually begin 1–9 years before the onset of myoclonic jerks and GTCS. Absence seizures heralding juvenile myoclonic epilepsy are less frequent and briefer than in CAE and are probably accompanied by a different EEG pattern.
- **Other forms of idiopathic generalized epilepsy,** in which absence seizures show distinctive features, include eyelid myoclonia,[40] perioral myoclonia,[5] absence epilepsy of early childhood (with onset before the age of 5 and heterogeneous prognosis),[41] absence epilepsy of the first year of life[42] and absence epilepsy occurring after 'initial grand mal'.[43] The

ILAE commission has not currently accepted most of these conditions as autonomous or individual syndromes.[44]

CAE should also be differentiated from other entities whose ictal clinical manifestations are similar, yet definitely different from typical absence seizures; these include the following forms:

- **Symptomatic or probably symptomatic generalized epilepsies,** such as Lennox-Gastaut syndrome, in which absence seizures are 'atypical'. Atypical absence seizures are associated with 1.5–2.5 Hz, irregular or asymmetric spike-wave discharges and are characterized by a less abrupt onset and cessation, more pronounced changes in tone, and longer duration than the typical absence seizures seen in CAE.[45] Absence seizures have been also reported in progressive encephalopathies, such as lipidosis[46] and progressive myoclonus epilepsies.[47]
- **Partial epilepsies of frontal origin,** in which more or less regular bilateral spike-wave discharges may arise from frontal foci. Some frontal epilepsies give rise to seizures that closely resemble absence seizures. Focal motor components, asymmetrical ictal discharges and the occurrence of interictal frontal foci may help to differentiate these frontal lobe seizures. Head trauma and brain tumors have been reported to be possible causes of absence seizures of frontal origin.[48]

TREATMENT

Valproic acid is usually considered the drug of first choice. The main reason for preferring it is that, unlike ethosuximide, valproic acid is also effective against GTCS.

When valproic acid does not control absence seizures, ethosuximide alone is the drug of second choice. Sometimes a combination of valproic acid plus ethosuximide is needed to obtain seizure control. Lamotrigine is achieving an increasing place in the therapy of CAE, either added to valproic acid in refractory patients or as monotherapy in untreated patients.[49] Clonazepam and clobazam are also effective against absence seizures, but display frequent side-effects and tolerance develops in one-half of the cases. Acetazolamide may also be effective and should be considered in the few patients that do not respond to the above drugs. There is clinical and experimental evidence that carbamazepine, vigabatrin and tiagabine may exacerbate absence seizures and these drugs are contraindicated.[49] Benzodiazepines, given either intravenously or orally, are the first-line drugs for the treatment of 'absence status'.[50]

KEY POINTS

- 60–76 per cent of patients are **female**
- A **family history** of similar seizures is common
- **Absence seizures** start between 4 and 10 years of age
- Typical absence seizures are the initial and predominant seizure type; they occur many times per day and are precipitated by hyperventilation
- Ictal **EEG** pattern is characterized by bilateral, symmetric, 3-Hz regular spike-waves on a normal background.
- Absence seizures usually **respond to appropriate treatment and remit** in 90 per cent of patients.
- 16–44 per cent of patients develop **GTCS**, usually between 8 and 15 years of age

REFERENCES

1. Commission on Classification and Terminology of the International League Against Epilepsy. Proposal for revised classification of epilepsies and epileptic syndromes. *Epilepsia* 1989; **30**: 389–399.
2. Dreifuss FE. Absence epilepsies. In: Dam M, Gram L (eds) *Comprehensive Epileptology*. New York: Raven Press, 1990; 145–153.
3. Loiseau P. Childhood absence epilepsy. In: Roger J, Bureau M, Dravet C, *et al.* (eds) *Epileptic Syndromes in Infancy, Childhood and Adolescence,* 2nd edn. London: John Libbey,1992; 135–150.
4. Loiseau P, Duché B, Pedespan JM. Absence epilepsies. *Epilepsia* 1995; **36**: 1182–1186.
5. Loiseau P, Panayiotopoulos CP, Hirsch E. Childhood absence epilepsy and related syndromes. In: Roger J, Bureau M, Dravet C, *et al.* (eds) *Epileptic syndromes in Infancy, Childhood and Adolescence,* 3rd edn. London: John Libbey, 2002; 285–303.
6. Lugaresi E, Pazzaglia P, Franck L, *et al.* Evolution and prognosis of primary generalized epilepsy of the petit mal absence type. In: Lugaresi E, Pazzaglia P, Tassinari CA (eds) *Evolution and Prognosis of Epilepsy.* Bologna: Aulo Gaggi, 1973; 2–22.
7. Currier RD, Kooi KA, Saidman LJ. Prognosis of pure petit mal: a follow-up study. *Neurology* 1963; **13**: 959–967.
8. Callenbach PMC, Geerts AT, Arts WFM, *et al.* Familial occurrence of epilepsy in children with newly diagnosed multiple seizures: Dutch study of epilepsy in childhood. *Epilepsia* 1998; **39**: 331–336.
9. Beck-Mannagetta G, Janz D, Hoffmeister G, *et al.* Morbidity risk for seizures and epilepsy in offspring of patients with epilepsy. In: Beck-Mannagetta G, Anderson VE, Doose H, Janz D (eds) *Genetics of the Epilepsies.* Berlin: Springer-Verlag, 1989; 119–126.
10. Bianchi A, and the Italian LAE Collaborative Group. Study of concordance of symptoms in families with absence epilepsies. In: Duncan JS, Panayiotopoulos CP (eds) *Typical Absences and Related Epileptic Syndromes.* London: Churchill Communications Europe, 1995; 328–337.
11. Lennox WG, Lennox MA. *Epilepsy and Related Disorders.* Boston: Little, Brown, 1960; 546–574.
12. Berkovic SF, Howell RA, Hay DA, Hopper JL. Epilepsies in twins: genetics of the major epilepsy syndromes. *Annals of Neurology* 1998; **43**: 435–445.
13. Delgado-Escueta AV, Medina MT, Serratosa JM, *et al.* Mapping and positional cloning of common idiopathic generalized epilepsies: juvenile myoclonus epilepsy and childhood absence epilepsy. *Advances in Neurology* 1999; **79**: 351–374.
14. Fletcher CF, Frankel WN. Ataxic mouse mutants and molecular mechanisms of absence epilepsy. *Human Molecular Genetics* 1999; **8**: 1907–1912.
15. Jouvenceau A, Eunson LH, Spauschus A, *et al.* Human epilepsy associated with dysfunction of the brain P/Q-type calcium channel. *Lancet* 2001; **358**: 801–807.
16. Wallace RH, Marini C, Petrou S, *et al.* Mutant GABA-A gamma-2-subunit in childhood absence epilepsy and febrile seizures. *Nature Genetics* 2001; **28**: 49–52.
17. Kananura C, Haug K, Sander T, *et al.* A splice-site mutation in GABRG2 associated with childhood absence epilepsy and febrile convulsions. *Archives of Neurology* 2002; **59**: 1137–1141.
18. Marini C, Harkin LA, Wallace RH, *et al.* Childhood absence epilepsy and febrile seizures: a family with a GABA-A receptor mutation. *Brain* 2003; **126**: 230–240.
19. Cavazzuti GB. Epidemiology of different types of epilepsy in school-age children of Modena, Italy. *Epilepsia* 1980; **21**: 57–62.
20. Berg AT, Shinnar S, Levy SR, *et al.* How well can epilepsy syndromes be identified at diagnosis? A reassessment two years after initial diagnosis. *Epilepsia* 2000; **41**: 1267–1275.
21. Loiseau J, Loiseau P, Guyot M, *et al.* Survey of seizure disorders in the French Southwest. I: incidence of epileptic syndromes. *Epilepsia* 1990; **31**: 391–396.
22. Blom S, Heijbel J, Bergfors PG. Incidence of epilepsy in children: a follow-up study three years after the first seizure. *Epilepsia* 1978; **19**: 343–350.
23. Darra F, Fontana E, Scaramuzzi V, *et al.* Typical absence seizures in the first three years of life: electroclinical study of 31 cases. *Epilepsia* 1996; **37**(Suppl. 4): 95.
24. Penry JK, Porter RJ, Dreifuss FE. Simultaneous recording of absence seizures with video tape and electroencephalography. *Brain* 1975; **98**: 427–440.
25. Holmes GL, Mckeever M, Adamson M. Absence seizures in children: clinical and electroencephalographic features. *Annals of Neurology* 1987; **21**: 268–273.
26. Panayiotopoulos CP, Obeid T, Waheed G. Differentiation of typical absence seizures in epileptic syndromes: a video EEG study of 224 seizures in 20 patients. *Brain* 1989; **112**: 1039–1056.
27. Penry JK, Dreifuss FE. Automatisms associated with the absence petit mal epilepsy. *Archives of Neurology* 1969; **21**: 142–148.
28. Porter RJ, Penry JK. Petit mal status. In: Delgado-Escueta AV, Wasterlain CG, Treiman DM, Porter RJ. (eds) *Status Epilepticus: Mechanisms of Brain Damage and Treatment.* New York: Raven Press,1983; 61–67.
29. Sato S, Dreifuss FE, Penry JK. The effect of sleep on spike-wave discharges in absence seizures. *Neurology* 1973; **23**: 1335–1345.

30. Cobb WA, Gordon N, Matthews C, Nieman EA. The occipital delta rhythm in petit mal. *Electroencephalography and Clinical Neurophysiology* 1961; **13**: 142–143.

31. Beaumanoir A, Ballis T, Warfis G, Ansari K. Benign epilepsy of childhood with rolandic spikes. *Epilepsia* 1974; **15**: 301–315.

32. Hedstrom A, Olsson I. Epidemiology of absence epilepsy: EEG findings and their predictive value. *Pediatric Neurology* 1991; **7**: 100–104.

33. Gastaut H, Broughton R, Roger J, Tassinari CA. Generalized nonconvulsive seizures. In: Magnus O, Lorentz De Haas AM. (eds) *The Epilepsies, Handbook of Clinical Neurology.* Amsterdam: North-Holland, 1974; 130–144.

34. Wolf P, Goosses R. Relation of photosensitivity to epileptic syndromes. *Journal of Neurology, Neurosurgery and Psychiatry* 1986; **49**: 1386–1391.

35. Livingstone S, Torres I, Pauli LL, Rider RV. Petit mal epilepsy. Results of prolonged follow-up study of 117 patients. *JAMA* 1965; **194**: 113–118.

36. Michelucci R, Rubboli G, Passarelli D, *et al.* Electroclinical features of idiopathic generalized epilepsy with persisting absences in adult life. *Journal of Neurology, Neurosurgery and Psychiatry* 1996; **61**: 471–477.

37. Rodin E, Ancheta O. Cerebral electrical fields during petit mal absences. *Electroencephalography and Clinical Neurophysiology* 1987; **66**: 457–466.

38. Dalby MA. Epilepsy and 3 per second spike and wave rhythms. A clinical, electroencephalographic and prognostic analysis of 346 patients. *Acta Neurologica Scandinavica* 1969; **45**(Suppl.): 1–83.

39. Sato S, Dreifuss FE, Penry JK, *et al.* Long-term follow-up of absence seizures. *Neurology* 1983; **33**: 1590–1595.

40. Jeavons PM. Nosological problems of myoclonic epilepsies in childhood and adolescence. *Developmental Medicine and Child Neurology* 1977; **19**: 3–8.

41. Doose H. Absence epilepsy of early childhood. *European Journal of Pediatrics* 1994; **153**: 372–377.

42. Cavazzuti GB, Ferrari F, Galli V, Benatti A. Epilepsy with typical absence seizures with onset during the first year of life. *Epilepsia* 1989; **30**: 802–806.

43. Dieterich E, Doose H, Baier WK, Fichsel H. Long-term follow-up of childhood epilepsy with absences. II: absence-epilepsy with initial grand mal. *Neuropediatrics* 1985; **16**: 155–158.

44. Engel J. Jr. A proposed diagnostic scheme for people with epileptic seizures and with epilepsy: report of the ILAE task force on classification and terminology. *Epilepsia* 2001; **42**: 1–8.

45. Commission on Classification and Terminology of the International League Against Epilepsy. Proposal for revised clinical and electroencephalographic classification of epileptic seizures. *Epilepsia* 1981; **22**: 489–501.

46. Andermann F. Absence attacks and diffuse neuronal disease. *Neurology* 1967; **17**: 205–12.

47. Michelucci R, Serratosa JM, Genton P, Tassinari CA. Seizures, myoclonus and cerebellar dysfunction in progressive myoclonus epilepsies. In: Guerrini R, Aicardi J, Andermann F, Hallet M (eds) *Epilepsy and Movement Disorders.* Cambridge: Cambridge University Press, 2002; 227–249.

48. Loiseau P, Cohadon F. *Le petit mal et ses frontieres.* Paris: Masson, 1971.

49. Panayiotopoulos CP. Typical absence seizures and their treatment. *Archives of Disease in Childhood* 1999; **81**: 351–5.

50. Tassinari CA, Daniele O, Michelucci R, *et al.* Benzodiazepines: efficacy in status epilepticus. In: Delgado-Escueta AV, Wastenlain CC, Treiman DM, Porter RJ (eds) *Advances in Neurology: Status Epilepticus.* New York: Raven Press, 1983; 465–475.

11B

Epilepsy with myoclonic absences

CARLO ALBERTO TASSINARI, GUIDO RUBBOLI, ELENA GARDELLA AND ROBERTO MICHELUCCI

Epilepsy with myoclonic absences is characterized clinically by absence seizures accompanied by rhythmic, bilateral myoclonic jerks of severe intensity. On polygraphic recording (EEG-EMG of deltoid muscles), myoclonic absences correspond to a rhythmic, bilateral, synchronous, symmetric 3-Hz spike-wave discharge (similar to that in typical absences), associated with EMG myoclonic bursts at 3 Hz, superimposed on an increasing tonic contraction.

Since the early description of myoclonic absences,[1–3] it has been generally believed that an epileptic syndrome characterized by the presence of myoclonic absences (MAs) as the only or predominant seizure type could be differentiated from other forms of generalized epilepsy, such as childhood absence epilepsy. This view was accepted by the Commission on Classification and Terminology of the International League Against Epilepsy (ILAE), and **epilepsy with myoclonic absences** was recognized as a distinct syndrome.[4] In the 1989 classification, epilepsy with myoclonic absences was included in the group of cryptogenic or symptomatic generalized epilepsies, based largely on the very variable and sometimes quite poor prognosis. However, in the recent 'Proposed diagnostic scheme for people with epileptic seizures and with epilepsy' produced by the ILAE Task Force on Classification and Terminology, it has been tentatively placed among the idiopathic generalized epilepsies.[5] Indeed, in their recent review on this epileptic condition, Bureau and Tassinari[6] described the existence of at least two forms of epilepsy with myoclonic absences. One form is characterized by a more benign course, eventual disappearance of seizures, and the occurrence of myoclonic absences as the sole, or predominant, seizure type. In the second form, myoclonic absences are associated with other seizure types, particularly generalized tonic-clonic seizures, and this has a much poorer prognosis than the other idiopathic generalized epilepsies. Furthermore, there have been reports of 'atypical' cases characterized by the association of MAs with some degree of mental retardation, neurological abnormalities (e.g. congenital hemiparesis), and chromosomal disorders.[7,8]

CLINICAL DATA

General

Epilepsy with myoclonic absences is a rare condition, accounting for 0.5–1 per cent of the epilepsies observed in a selected population with epilepsy who attend the Centre Saint-Paul in Marseilles (France). There is a male preponderance (69 per cent), in contrast to the female preponderance in childhood absence epilepsy. Etiologic factors have been reported in about 35 per cent of cases and include prematurity, perinatal brain injury, consanguinity, congenital hemiparesis, and chromosomal disorders.[6] The recent description of associated chromosomal dysfunction in some cases has led to the hypothesis that abnormal expression of genes located in the affected chromosome segments may play a role in the pathogenesis of myoclonic absence epilepsy.[7,8] A genetic susceptibility, as demonstrated by a positive family history of epilepsy, has been observed in about 20 per cent of cases. The mean age of onset of myoclonic absences is 7 years, with a range between 11 months and 12.2 years. However, some reports have described cases with onset of myoclonic absences in the first year of life.[9–12]

MYOCLONIC ABSENCES

Myoclonic absences are characterized by:

- **impairment of consciousness**, which is quite variable in intensity, ranging from a mild disruption of contact to a complete loss of consciousness. Sometimes the patients are aware of the jerks and may recall the words pronounced by the examiner during the seizures.
- **motor manifestations**, which consist of bilateral myoclonic jerks, often associated with a discrete tonic contraction. The myoclonias mainly involve the muscles of shoulders, arms and legs. When facial myoclonias occur, they are more evident around the chin and the mouth, whereas eyelid twitching is typically absent or rare. Owing to concomitant tonic contraction, the jerking of the arms is accompanied by a progressive elevation of the upper extremities, giving rise to a quite constant and recognizable pattern. Head and body deviation can be a feature in some patients but rarely results in a fall.
- **autonomic manifestations**, which consist of an arrest of respiration and occasional loss of urine.

Myoclonic absences last for 10–60 s, and recur at a high frequency (many seizures per day), often being precipitated by hyperventilation or awakening. They may be also observed during the early stages of sleep. Episodes of myoclonic absences status are distinctly rare.

SEIZURES OTHER THAN MYOCLONIC ABSENCES

Myoclonic absences are the only seizure type in about one third of cases. In the remaining patients, generalized tonic-clonic seizures, absences, or epileptic falls occur either before the onset of myoclonic absences or in association with them.

NEUROLOGIC AND NEUROPSYCHOLOGIC EXAMINATION

Neurologic examination is normal, except in those cases with congenital hemiparesis. Intellectual disability is present in about 45 per cent of cases before the onset of myoclonic absences. During the course of myoclonic absences, intellectual disability may worsen or even appear in previously normal patients, particularly if there have been frequent tonic-clonic seizures associated with myoclonic absences. These cognitive features differ significantly from those observed in childhood absence epilepsy.

NEUROPHYSIOLOGIC DATA

Interictal EEG

The interictal EEG shows a normal background activity in all cases, with superimposed generalized spike-wave in one third of cases and, more rarely, focal or multifocal spike-wave. It is noteworthy that the sinusoidal posterior slow rhythm reported in childhood absence epilepsy has never been observed in epilepsy with myoclonic absences.

Ictal EEG

The ictal EEG consists of rhythmic spike-wave discharges at 3 Hz, which are bilateral, synchronous and symmetric, as observed in typical absences. The onset and the end of spike-wave discharges are abrupt. Polygraphic (EEG-EMG) recording discloses the appearance of bilateral myoclonias, at the same frequency as the spike-wave, which begin 1 s after the onset of EEG paroxysmal discharges and are followed by a tonic contraction, maximal in the shoulder and deltoid muscles (Figure 11B.1). Tassinari et al.[1,13] provided a detailed analysis of the relationships between the EEG spike-wave and motor events by means of high-speed oscilloscopic recording. There is a strict and constant relationship between the spike of the spike-wave discharge and the myoclonia. In the spike there is a positive transient[14] of high amplitude, which is followed on the EMG by a myoclonia with a latency of 15–40 ms for the more proximal muscles and of 50–70 ms for the more distal muscles (Figures 11B.2, 11B.3). This myoclonia is followed by a brief silent period (60–120 ms) which breaks the tonic contraction. Gardella et al.[15] demonstrated that the first myoclonic jerks are restricted to the facial musculature, and that subsequent jerks spread to involve the neck and upper limb muscles. Back-averaging of the EEG activity triggered from the onset of the first myoclonia has confirmed the correlation of the myoclonic phenomenon with the positive transient of the spike-wave complex.

Sleep EEG

Sleep organization is normal and physiologic patterns are symmetrically present. During sleep the evolution of the spike-wave discharges is similar, on the whole, to that

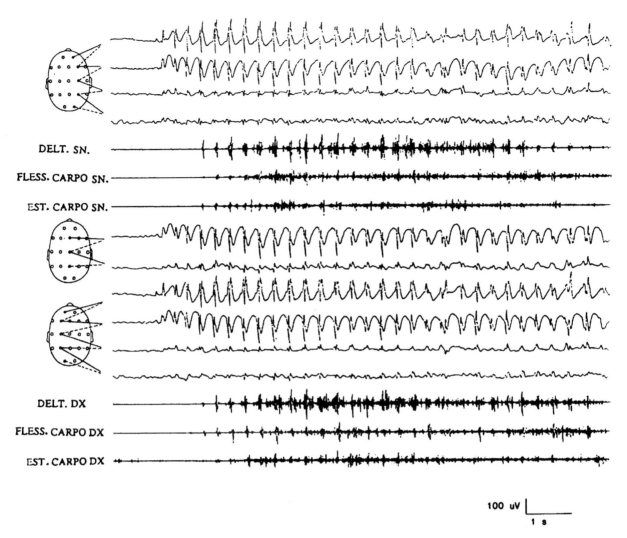

Figure 11B.1 *Spontaneous myoclonic absence. EEG: rhythmic spike-wave discharge at 3 Hz, bilateral, synchronous and symmetrical, as observed in typical absences. EMG: rhythmic myoclonias, at the same frequency of the spike-waves, which involve the upper extremities, begin 1 s after the onset of the EEG paroxysmal discharge and are progressively associated with a tonic contraction.*

observed in childhood absence epilepsy.[16] Myoclonic absences may occur during stage I of sleep, awakening the subject. During stage II, spike-wave discharges, of short or long duration, are also observed, sometimes associated with bursts of myoclonias.

EVOLUTION

The MAs are still present in about two thirds of the patients followed for a mean period of 10 years and disappear in the remaining patients after a mean period of 5.5 years from the onset.[3] Patients with 'refractory' myoclonic absences have a high incidence (80 per cent) of associated seizures, mainly generalized tonic-clonic and atonic seizures, whereas patients who remit have a lower incidence (40 per cent) of associated seizures, which

are mainly absence seizures. The duration of the myoclonic absences probably plays an important role in the appearance of intellectual disability, in that cognitive function is always preserved in children with rapid remission of myoclonic absences. Very rarely, the disappearance of myoclonic absences has been followed by the onset of other seizure types, namely absences with atypical spike-wave discharges, and clinical and subclinical tonic seizures, giving rise to a clinical picture similar to the Lennox-Gastaut syndrome.[9,17]

DIAGNOSIS

The diagnosis of myoclonic absences is based mainly on the demonstration of 3-Hz spike-wave discharges (as in typical absences) accompanied by rhythmic myoclonias.

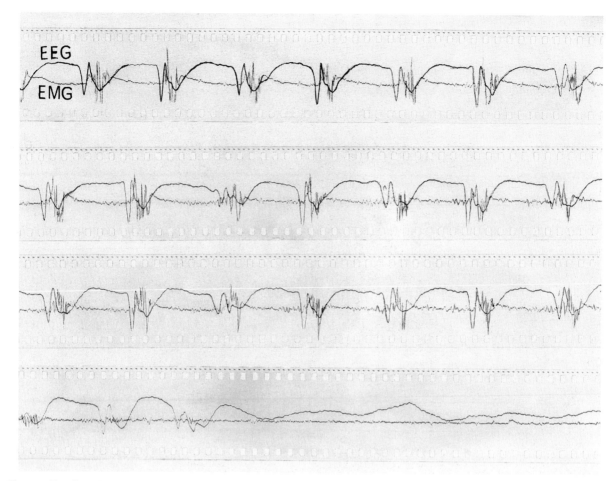

Figure 11B.2 *Superimposition of two oscilloscopic traces, recording EEG (Fz–Cz) and EMG (right deltoid) activities during a myoclonic absence seizure, showing the relationship between the positive transient of the spike-wave complex and the myoclonic potential. In the two lower strips, the progressive decrement of the positive transient is associated with the progressive disappearance of the myoclonic activity.*

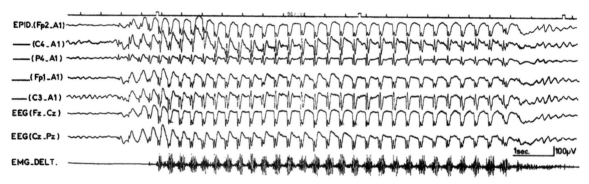

Figure 11B.3 *Epidural recording of right frontal (Fp2, C4, P4, ref. A1) and left frontal (Fp1, C3, ref. A1), approximately corresponding to the 10–20 International System; EEG recording from the vertex region; EMG: left deltoid. On the scalp EEG (Fz–Cz and Cz–Pz), there is a spike-wave discharge with evident positive transient, corresponding to a spike in the epidural recording. The positive transients, as the spikes in the epidural tracing, are consistently related to the myoclonic potentials in the EMG.*

Therefore, polygraphic recording should be performed when there is a clinical suspicion of myoclonic absences. The parent or patient's memory of the episodes can be misleading and asymmetric myoclonic absences may be misdiagnosed as partial motor seizures. Similarly, myoclonic absences with mild myoclonias may be misdiagnosed as typical petit mal absences. Consequently, it is our practice to perform polygraphic recording in patients with refractory absence, myoclonic or partial motor seizures.

Capovilla *et al.*[18] reported a group of patients with childhood absence epilepsy in whom the absence seizures were associated with mild myoclonic jerks, involving mainly facial and neck muscles (eyebrows, nostrils, perioral region, chin, sternocleidomastoideus). The electroclinical characteristics that differentiated this condition from epilepsy with myoclonic absences were (1) the mild myoclonia occurred without a background of tonic contraction, and (2) the benign course, characterized by an excellent response to treatment and possible remission of the epilepsy.

TREATMENT

The most effective therapy for myoclonic absences is the combined use of valproic acid and ethosuximide at high doses, with serum plasma levels ranging from 80 to 130 μg/mL (555–900 mol/L) and 70–110 μg/mL (495–780 mol/L) respectively. Good seizure control has also been achieved using the combination of phenobarbital, valproic acid and a benzodiazepine. More recently, lamotrigine, particularly in combination with valproate, and ethosuximide have been reported to be useful when other measures have failed.[11,19]

KEY POINTS

- Myoclonic absence seizures last for 10–60 s, occur many times per day, and are characterized by
  - a variable degree of **impairment of consciousness**
  - **bilateral myoclonic jerks**, which occur at the same frequency as the spike-wave, begin 1 s after the onset of EEG paroxysmal discharges, and are followed by a tonic contraction
  - **autonomic manifestations**, such as arrest of respiration or occasionally loss of urine
- The ictal **EEG** consists of rhythmic 3 Hz spike-wave discharges, which are bilateral, synchronous, and symmetric, similar to those observed in typical absences
- Epilepsy with myoclonic absence seizures **occurs more often in boys**, in contrast to the female preponderance in childhood absence epilepsy. The age of onset ranges from 11 months to 12 years, with a mean age of 7 years
- There is a positive **family history of epilepsy** in about 20 per cent of cases
- **Etiologic factors** have been reported in about 35 per cent of cases and include prematurity,

perinatal brain injury, consanguinity, congenital hemiparesis, and chromosomal disorders
- **Generalized tonic-clonic seizures, absences or epileptic falls** occur either before the onset of myoclonic absence seizures or in association with them in about two third of cases
- **Intellectual disability** is present in approximately 45 per cent of cases before the onset of myoclonic absence seizures. During the course of the seizures, intellectual disability may worsen or even appear in previously normal patients, particularly if there have been frequent tonic-clonic seizures
- Myoclonic absence seizures **remit** in approximately one third of the patients followed for 10 years. The mean time to remission is 5.5 years from the onset. Patients with 'refractory' myoclonic absence seizures have a high incidence of associated seizures, usually generalized tonic-clonic or atonic seizures

ACKNOWLEDGMENTS

We thank Professor G. Avanzini and Dr. S. Franceschetti from the Neurological Institute 'C. Besta' in Milan for providing the case illustrated in Figure 11B.1, and Mrs. C. Giardini for her help in the preparation of the manuscript.

REFERENCES

1. Tassinari CA, Lyagoubi S, Santos V, *et al.* Etude des décharges de pointes ondes chez l'homme. II. Les aspects cliniques et electroencephalographiques des absences myocloniques. *Revue Neurologique* 1969; **121**: 379–383.

2. Lugaresi E, Pazzaglia P, Franck L, *et al.* Evolution and prognosis of primary generalized epilepsy of the petit mal absence type. In E. Lugaresi E, Pazzaglia P, Tassinari CA (eds) *Evolution and Prognosis of Epilepsy*. Bologna: Aulo Gaggi, 1973; 2–22.

3. Tassinari CA, Bureau M. Epilepsy with myoclonic absences. In: Roger J, Dravet C, Bureau M, Dreifuss FE, Wolf P (eds) *Epileptic Syndromes in Infancy, Childhood and Adolescence*. London: John Libbey, 1985; 123–131.

4. Commission on Classification and Terminology of the International League Against Epilepsy. Proposal for revised classification of epilepsies and epileptic syndromes. *Epilepsia* 1989; **30**: 389–399.

5. Engel J, Jr. A proposed diagnostic scheme for people with epileptic seizures and with epilepsy: Report of the ILAE Task Force on Classification and Terminology. *Epilepsia* 2001; **42**: 796–803.

6. Bureau M, Tassinari CA. The syndrome of myoclonic absences. In: Roger J, *et al.* (eds) *Epileptic Syndromes in Infancy, Childhood and Adolescence*, 3rd edn. London: John Libbey: 2002; 305–312.

7. Elia M, Musumeci SA, Ferri R, Cammarata M. Trisomy 12p and epilepsy with myoclonic absences. *Brain Development* 1998; **20**: 127–130.

8. Elia M, Guerrini R, Musumeci SA, Bonanni P, Gambardella A, Aguglia U. Myoclonic absence-like seizures and chromosome abnormality syndrome. *Epilepsia* 1998; **39**: 660–663.

9. Tassinari CA, Bureau M, Thomas P. Epilepsy with myoclonic absences. In: Roger J, *et al.* (eds) *Epileptic Syndromes in Infancy, Childhood and Adolescence*, 2nd edn. London: John Libbey, 1992; 151–160.

10. Aicardi J. Typical absences in the first two years of life. In: Duncan JS, Panayiotopoulos CP (eds) *Typical Absences and Related Syndromes*. London: Churchill Livingstone, 1995; 284–288.

11. Manonmani V, Wallace S. Epilepsy with myoclonic absences. *Archives of Disease in Childhood* 1994; **70**: 288–290.

12. Verrotti A, Greco R, Chiarelli F, *et al.* Epilepsy with myoclonic absences with early onset: a follow-up study. *Journal of Child Neurology* 1999; **14**: 746–749.

13. Tassinari CA, Lyagoubi S, Gambarelli F, *et al.* (1971) Relationships between EEG discharge and neuromuscular phenomena. *Electroencephalography and Clinical Neurophysiology* 1971; **31**: 176.

14. Weir, B. (1965) The morphology of the spike-wave complex. *Electroencephalography and Clinical Neurophysiology* 1965; **19**: 284–290.

15. Gardella E, Rubboli G, Meletti S, Volpi L, Tassinari CA. Polygraphic study of muscular activation pattern in myoclonic absence seizures. *Epilepsia* 2002; **43**(Suppl. 8): 98–99.

16. Tassinari CA, Bureau-Paillas M, Dalla Bernardina B, *et al.* Generalized epilepsies and seizures during sleep: a polygraphic study. In: Van Praag HM, Meinardi H (eds) *Brain and Sleep*. Amsterdam: De Erven Bhon, 1974; 154–66.

17. Tassinari CA, Michelucci R, Rubboli G, *et al.* Myoclonic absence epilepsy. In: Duncan JS, Panayiotopoulos CP (eds), *Typical Absences and Related Syndromes*. London: Churchill Livingstone, 1995; 187–195.

18. Capovilla G, Rubboli G, Beccaria F, *et al.* A clinical spectrum of the myoclonic manifestations associated with typical absences in childhood absence epilepsy. A video-polygraphic study. *Epileptic Disorders* 2001; **3**: 57–61.

19. Wallace SJ. Myoclonus and epilepsy in childhood: a review of treatment with valproate, ethosuximide, lamotrigine and zonisamide. *Epilepsy Research* 1998; **29**: 147–154.

11C

Eyelid myoclonia with absences

COLIN D FERRIE

EYELID MYOCLONIA

Eyelid myoclonia is sudden involuntary jerks of the eyelids. They can be single or multiple; rhythmic or arrhythmic; violent or subtle; and are often accompanied by tonic components of the involved muscles, causing the eyelids and head to retract and the eyeballs to deviate upwards.[1] Eyelid myoclonus is the main seizure type in eyelid myoclonia with absences (EMWA), but it may also occur in other idiopathic generalized epilepsies and in symptomatic focal and generalized epilepsies.[1,2] The ILAE diagnostic scheme[3] recognizes two seizure types: eyelid myoclonia with and without absences.[1,4]

THE SYNDROME OF EYELID MYOCLONIA WITH ABSENCES (EMWA)

The first case was recognized in 1932.[1,5] Subsequently, Jeavons described EMWA in detail:[6]

> Eyelid myoclonia and absences show a marked jerking of the eyelids immediately after eye closure and there is an associated brief bilateral spike and wave activity. The eyelid movement is like rapid blinking and the eyes deviate upwards, in contrast to the very slight flicker of eyelids, which may be seen in a typical absence in which the eyes look straight ahead. Brief absences may occur spontaneously and are accompanied by 3 cycles per second spike and wave discharges. The spike and wave discharges seen immediately after eye closure do not occur in the dark. Their presence in the routine EEG is a very reliable warning that abnormality will be evoked by photic stimulation.

Many consider this report to justify the eponym **Jeavons syndrome**. Over 100 cases have now been described in all ages.[1,4,7–19]

Definition

EMWA usually starts in childhood, and persists well into adult life. Frequent brief seizures are characterized by fast eyelid myoclonia (4–6 Hz) with and without absences. All patients are highly photosensitive. Self-induction may precipitate seizures in an undetermined proportion of patients. Other ictal events include generalized tonic-clonic seizures, which are probably inevitable; occasional myoclonic jerks of the limbs; and possibly typical absences without eyelid myoclonia. The ictal EEG consists mainly of generalized discharges of polyspikes or polyspikes and slow waves at 3–6 Hz.

Epidemiology

The incidence and prevalence are not known for unselected populations. In specialized pediatric neurology services, 2 of 41 children with absence epilepsies (excluding myoclonic absence epilepsy and perioral myoclonia with absences), and 3 of 50 with 'drug-resistant absence-like attacks' had EMWA.[1] Other reported prevalences are:

- almost 3 per cent in patients aged over 16 years of age with all types of epilepsy
- 13 per cent amongst those with idiopathic generalized epilepsies with typical absences.[1]

There is a marked female preponderance.[1,4,14] In a study of adults, the mean age of onset was 7.8 ± 3.8 years (range 2–14 years).[4] The first manifestations can be around 2 years of age. In all cases the first seizures are eyelid myoclonia with or without absences. Generalized tonic clonic seizures inevitably appear at 12.2 ± 5.0 years (range 3–19 years).[4]

Genetics

There are several reports of familial cases,[1,10,14,19] but not all the families have typical features. The pattern of inheritance is not yet established. The strong female preponderance remains unexplained, though it parallels the disproportionate female tendency to photosensitivity. A high incidence of epilepsies other than EMWA is found in the families of probands.

Neurodevelopmental background

Subjects have normal intelligence and normal neurological examinations. No pregnancy- or birth-related antecedents are found. The EEG is the only abnormal investigation.

Clinical symptoms

Brief episodes of eyelid myoclonia with and without absences are very frequent: sometimes hundreds occur each day. They are particularly likely to present in bright sunlight and may come in clusters as the patient moves from indoors to outdoors. Other photic factors may also induce attacks. Rare generalized tonic-clonic seizures are not usually problematical in younger children; but, in older subjects, they may be precipitated both by photic factors and nonspecific activators, e.g. sleep deprivation, stress, alcohol. Infrequent myoclonic jerks of the limbs occur in many subjects. Typical absences, independent of eyelid myoclonia are uncommon, and do not occur in adults with EMWA.[4] They have not yet been confirmed by video-EEG. Nonconvulsive status epilepticus with eyelid myoclonia has been described.[15–17]

EEG, eye closure and photosensitivity

The background EEG is normal. However, in most subjects, especially if untreated, there are frequent epileptiform discharges that are increased by hyperventilation and, usually, also by sleep. The typical ictal discharges of generalized 3–6-Hz polyspike or polyspike and slow waves are illustrated in Figure 11C.1. These are readily precipitated by eye closure in an illuminated room, and

by intermittent photic stimulation. The electroclinical features are best demonstrated by video-EEG. Home video-recordings can also be very helpful.

The controversy over self-induction

Many subjects who are photosensitive induce seizures or apparently subclinical discharges.[20,21] One technique is a slow eye closure maneuver, which is accompanied by a more sustained upward deflection of the eye than is normal. A 6-Hz tremor of the eyelids may be superimposed. Oculographic features can help distinguish such self-induced seizures from involuntary ictal eyelid myoclonia.[1] Details of a patient in whom nonconvulsive status epilepticus with eyelid myoclonia developed in total darkness, after the myoclonia, precipitated by sunlight, had been eliminated and the interictal EEG was normal, contribute to continuing uncertainties.[17] Many children with EMWA experience compulsive or tic-like symptoms, including premonitory sensations; urges that are compulsive and difficult to resist; and a sense of relief associated with the absences.[16] Possibly, the initial tic-like symptoms cause absences and characteristic EEG discharges in subjects who are photosensitive. Currently the possible role of self-induction in eyelid myoclonia is unresolved.

Differential diagnosis

The ictal manifestations are often misdiagnosed as tics. EMWA is more a myoclonic than an absence epilepsy and is very different in both its clinical and EEG features from childhood and juvenile absence epilepsies (Chapters 11A, 12C).

Treatment and prognosis

There are no controlled therapeutic trials, and the eyelid myoclonia tend to be resistant to therapy. Anecdotal evidence[1] suggests valproic acid should be used alone as first-line therapy, followed by either ethosuximide monotherapy or a combination of valproic acid and ethosuximide, though the use of ethosuximide as monotherapy in subjects who are highly photosensitive may not be wise. Other suggestions are lamotrigine, either alone or combined with valproic acid and/or ethosuximide; or, for resistant cases, benzodiazepines. Carbamazepine, vigabatrin, gabapentin, tiagabine and phenytoin should be avoided. No information is available on topiramate and levetiracetam in EMWA, but the latter could be promising. Associated generalized tonic-clonic seizures respond to medication.

EEG discharges associated with eyelid myoclonia in patients with Jeavons syndrome

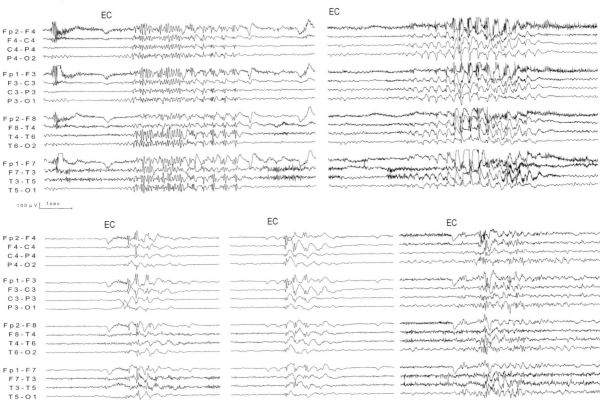

Figure 11C.1 *EEG discharges associated with eyelid myoclonia from four patients with Jeavons syndrome. All discharges were associated with eyelid myoclonia confirmed by simultaneous video recordings.* **Top left:** *Woman aged 35 years. Generalized discharges of mainly multiple spikes occur after eye-closure in the presence of light.* **Top right:** *Woman aged 33 years. Spontaneous generalized discharge of mainly spikes and slow waves.* **Bottom left and middle:** *Girl aged 10 years. Brief generalized discharges after eye closure and during photic stimulation.* **Bottom right:** *Girl aged 16 years. A brief generalized discharge during photic stimulation. (With thanks to Dr CP Panayiotopoulos.)*

KEY POINTS

- Eyelid myoclonia with and without absences are the **characteristic seizure types** of the syndrome of EMWA, which is an idiopathic generalized epilepsy, starting in childhood and persisting into adult life
- All subjects are highly **photosensitive**
- The **EEG features** are brief discharges of polyspikes or polyspike waves often precipitated by eye closure or intermittent photic stimulation
- The characteristic seizures are usually **very frequent**, occurring many times each day. In older children, adolescents and adults, rare generalized tonic-clonic seizures are usual
- Valproic acid, ethosuximide and lamotrigine are commonly used in treatment. However, the myoclonia are often **resistant**

REFERENCES

1. Panayiotopoulos CP (ed.) *Eyelid Myoclonia with Absences.* London: John Libbey; 1996; 17–26.
2. Scuderi C, Musumeci SA, Ferri R, *et al.* Eyelid myoclonia with absences in three subjects with mental retardation. *Neurological Sciences* 2000; **21**; 247–250.
3. Engel J Jr. A proposed diagnostic scheme for people with epileptic seizures and with epilepsy: report of the ILAE Task Force on Classification and Terminology. *Epilepsia* 2001; **42**: 796–803.
4. Giannakodimos S, Panayiotopoulos CP. Eyelid myoclonia with absences in adults: a clinical and video-EEG study. *Epilepsia* 1996; **37**: 36–44.
5. Radovici A, Misirliou V, Gluckman ML. Epilepsy reflexe provoquée par excitations optiques des rayons solaires. *Revue Neurologique* 1932; **1**: 1305–1307.
6. Jeavons PM. Nosological problems of myoclonic epilepsies in childhood and adolescence. *Developmental Medicine and Child Neurology* 1977; **19**: 3–8.

7. Gobbi G, Tinuper P, Tassinari CA, Dravet C, *et al.* Eyelid myoclonia absences. *Bollettino-Lega Italiania Contro L'Epielessia* 1985; **51/52**: 225–226.

8. Gobbi G, Bruno L, Mainetti S, *et al.* Eye closure seizures. In: Beaumanoir A (ed.) *Reflex Seizures and Reflex Epilepsies: International Symposium on Reflex Seizures and Reflex Epilepsies.* Geneva: Medicine & Hygiene; 1989; 181–191.

9. Dalla Bernadina B, Sgro V, Fontana E, *et al.* Eyelid myoclonia with absences. In: Beaumanoir A (ed.) *Reflex Seizures and Reflex Epilepsies: International Symposium on Reflex Seizures and Reflex Epilepsies.* Geneva: Medicine & Hygiene; 1989; 193–200.

10. DeMarco P. Eyelid myoclonia with absences (EMA) in two monovular twins. *Clinical Electroencephalography* 1989; **20**: 193–195.

11. Panayiotopoulos CP, Chroni E, Daskalopoulos C, *et al.* Typical absence seizures in adults: clinical, EEG, video-EEG findings and diagnostic/syndromic considerations. *Journal of Neurology, Neurosurgery and Psychiatry* 1992; **55**: 1002–1008.

12. Appleton RE, Panayiotopoulos CP, Acomb BA, Beirne M. Eyelid myoclonia with typical absences: an epilepsy syndrome. *Journal of Neurology, Neurosurgery and Psychiatry* 1993; **56**: 1312–1316.

13. Covanis A, Skiadas K, Loli N, *et al.* Eyelid myoclonia with absence. *Epilepsia* 1994; **35**(Suppl. 7): 13.

14. Panayiotopoulos CP (ed.) *Typical Absences and Related Epileptic Syndromes.* London: Churchill Communications, 1995.

15. Agathonikou A, Panayiotopoulos CP, Giannakodimos S, Koutroumanidis M. Typical absence status in adults: diagnostic and syndromic considerations. *Epilepsia* 1998; **39**: 265–276.

16. Kent L, Blake A, Whitehouse W. Eyelid myoclonia with absences: phenomenology in children. *Seizure* 1998; **7**: 193–199.

17. Wakamoto H, Nagao H, Manabe K, Kobayashi H, Hayashi M. Nonconvulsive status epilepticus in eyelid myoclonia with absences—evidence of provocation unrelated to photosensitivity. *Neuropediatrics* 1999; **30**: 149–150.

18. Baykan-Kurt B, Gokyigit A, Parman Y, *et al.* Eye closure related spike and wave discharges: clinical and syndromic associations. *Clinical Electroencephalography* 1999; **30**: 106–110.

19. Yagi S, Matsuzawa J, Hongou K, *et al.* [Two siblings with eyelid myoclonia with absences]. (in Japanese) *No To Hattatsu* 2001; **33**: 517–522.

20. Binnie CD, Darby CE, De Korte RA, Wilkins AJ. Self-induction of epileptic seizures by eye closure: incidence and recognition. *Journal of Neurology, Neurosurgery and Psychiatryy* 1980; **43**: 386–389.

21. Kasteleijn-Nolst Trenité DGA. Photosensitivity in epilepsy: electrophysiological and clinical correlates. *Acta Neurologica Scandinavica* 1989; Suppl. 125.

Benign partial epilepsies

KAZUYOSHI WATANABE

BENIGN CHILDHOOD EPILEPSY WITH CENTROTEMPORAL SPIKES (BENIGN ROLANDIC EPILEPSY)

Definition

Benign childhood epilepsy with centrotemporal spikes (BCECT) is a syndrome of brief, simple, partial, hemifacial motor seizures, frequently having associated somatosensory symptoms, which have a tendency to evolve into generalized tonic-clonic seizures.[1] Both seizure types occur more often in sleep, and the initial hemifacial seizures are often missed during nocturnal sleep in patients with nocturnal generalized convulsions. The EEG has blunt high-voltage centrotemporal spikes, often followed by slow waves that are activated by sleep and tend to spread or shift from side to side. Oropharyngeal symptoms and arrest of speech are also frequent[2] and should be incorporated into the definition, in addition to hemifacial seizures.

Clinical features

This syndrome represents 8–23 per cent of all epileptic seizures in children aged 0–15 years.[3] Heijbel et al.[4] reported an incidence of 21 in 100 000 among children aged 0–15 years in a region in Sweden, but more recent population-based studies describe an annual incidence ranging from 6.2 to 10.7 per 100 000 children.[5–7] The EEG abnormality is more common and only 9 per cent of children with benign focal sharp waves have clinical seizures.[8] The ratio of boys to girls is 6:4.

The age of onset ranges from 2 to 12 years, but is mostly between 4 and 10 years with a peak at 7–9 years.[8] As a rule, the patients have normal neurologic development and a normal neurologic examination. However, BCECT is very prevalent and the presence of development retardation or neurologic deficits does not preclude its diagnosis.[9,10]

Higher mental functions such as language may be affected by focal sharp waves even in these benign partial epileptic syndromes.[11] Transitory cognitive impairment occurs in association with rolandic spikes,[12,13] and in some patients interferes with scholastic performance[14] or with general psychosocial functioning.[15] More recent studies have also demonstrated minor auditory-verbal or visual spatial impairments, attention deficits, executive dysfunction, reading errors, learning disabilities and behavioral problems in this syndrome.[16–23] Staden et al.[21] reported a specific pattern of language impairment. The patients failed significantly more often in five language functions: reading, spelling, auditory verbal learning, auditory discrimination with background noise and expressive grammar. Deonna et al.,[18] however, did not observe a single pattern of dysfunction and postulated that the differences in cognitive profiles and abilities could be explained by the location and spread of paroxysmal activities, interindividual variability in cerebral organization, age at onset of the epilepsy, and/or its duration and severity. Baglietto et al.[24] correlated neuropsychological dysfunctions with activation of interictal epileptic discharges. At time of marked activation of interictal epilepic discharges during sleep, patients showed a mean Full-Scale IQ score within the normal range, but significantly below that of control participants; neuropsychological assessment revealed disorders in visuospatial short-term memory attention, and cognitive flexibility, picture naming, and fluency of visuoperceptual skill and visuomotor coordination. At the time of EEG remission, neuropsychological re-evaluation showed a notable increase in IQ score and a significant improvement in visuomotor coordination, nonverbal short-term memory, sustained attention and mental flexibility, picture naming and visual-perceptual performance. A prospective study has shown that 10 (28 per cent) of 35 patients with typical BCECT developed behavioral problems and cognitive dysfunctions.[25] These problems were correlated with impulsivity, learning difficulties, attention disorders, and minor (7/35 cases, 20 per cent) or serious (3/35 cases, 8 per cent) auditory-verbal or visual-spatial deficits. Worsening of behavior and cognitive dysfunction started 2–36 months after onset and persisted for 9–39 months. Occurrence of such atypical evolutions was significantly correlated with different combinations of three of six interictal EEG patterns: intermittent slow-wave focus, multiple asynchronous spike-wave foci, long spike-wave clusters, generalized 3-Hz 'absence-like' spike-wave discharges, conjunction of interictal paroxysms with negative or positive myoclonia, and abundance of interictal abnormalities during wakefulness and sleep. Saint-Martin et al.[26] classified the symptoms into three major categories: classical focal seizures; spike and wave related symptoms; and paraictal symptoms. **Spike and wave related symptoms** are brief neurological or neuropsychological phenomena having a relatively strict temporal relation with individual components of isolated focal or generalized spikes and waves. **Paraictal symptoms** consist of acquired progressive and fluctuating motor or cognitive deficits.

Recurrent headaches or migraine are reported frequently in patients with BCECT,[27–29] but may not be significantly more frequent than in control children.[30,31] In a long-term controlled study, Septien et al.[32] observed migraine in 63 per cent of patients with a history of BCECT and concluded that the association of the two conditions was not fortuitous. A recent study[33] that evaluated the long-term evolution of headache in patients with rolandic centrotemporal spikes found a good correlation between centrotemporal spikes and the number of headaches.

Genetics

There is a high incidence of a positive family history of epilepsy and of sharp waves on EEG,[8,9,34–38] suggesting that genetic factors are important in this disorder. This is also supported by the study of monozygotic twins.[39] Most authors postulate an autosomal dominant inheritance

with age-dependent penetrance. Eeg-Olofsson[40] also suggested dominant inheritance on the basis of his study on HLA (human lymphocyte antigens) antigens and haplotypes. Some 7–10 per cent of patients also have a past history of febrile seizures. This may indicate a genetic link between the two conditions, or a genetic predisposition to febrile seizures at a younger age in patients with BCECT. Some differences in the clinical manifestations of patients with a past history of febrile seizures suggest that these conditions may occur independently but with closely linked genes.[41] Several linkage studies have given negative results,[42–44] but a recent study reported evidence for linkage to a region on chromosome 15q14.[45] There seem to be common genetic mechanisms underlying the pathogenesis of idiopathic neonatal seizures and benign partial epilepsies.[46,47] BCECT has also been reported in a patient with chromosome 7q deletion[48] and a patient with velocardiofacial syndrome.[49] Guerrini et al.[50] reported a pedigree in which three members in the same generation were affected by rolandic epilepsy, paroxysmal exercise-induced dystonia and writer's cramp. Both the seizures and the paroxysmal dystonia had a strong age-related expression that peaked during childhood, whereas the writer's cramp also appeared in childhood but persisted into adult life. Linkage analysis identified a common homozygous haplotype on chromosome 16p12–11.2.

Seizure manifestations

The seizure manifestations are related to the somatosensory and motor area in the lower rolandic region just above the sylvian fissure. They consist of unilateral paresthesiae involving the tongue, lips, gums and inner cheeks, and unilateral motor phenomena involving the face, lips, tongue, pharyngeal and laryngeal muscles.[2,51] Difficulty with speech and vocalization is caused by a peripheral type of motor disturbance or dysarthria and is independent of the laterality of the epileptogenic focus. Sialorrhea, drooling, gurgling sounds from the throat and a feeling of suffocation are common, and should not be mistaken for oral automatisms. Speech and oromotor deficits may be the initial or only symptom of the disorder and may be observed in the absence of typical clinical seizures.[52–57] The oromotor deficits consist of hypersialorrhea, difficulties in chewing, swallowing, reduced speech fluency, and difficulties in pronunciation and articulation. Consciousness is usually preserved unless seizures become secondarily generalized. Failure to respond may be due to arrest of speech and should not be mistaken for impaired consciousness. Hemifacial seizures may spread to the upper arm but rarely to the lower limb. In diurnal seizures, somatosensory symptoms may be the only manifestation. Screaming may occur as a focal seizure component. Todd's paralysis has been reported to occur in 7 per cent.[58]

Secondary generalization of seizures is rare during wakefulness, but frequent during sleep. The initial focal manifestations of the nocturnal seizures are often not recognized and it is often not appreciated that the nocturnal tonic-clonic seizures are secondarily generalized. Three types of nocturnal seizures occur:[59]

- hemifacial seizures associated with speech arrest and drooling
- seizures similar to the above but with loss of consciousness, usually with gurgling or grunting noises
- generalized convulsions.

The presence or absence of consciousness is often difficult to determine in nocturnal seizures in children with speech arrest and uncertain memory. In one series, hemifacial seizures occurred more often in older children, whereas hemiconvulsive or generalized nocturnal seizures were more frequent in younger ones.[60] However, Ishikawa et al.[61] did not observe any difference in seizure type according to age. Haga et al.[41] reported that those who had a family and/or a past history of febrile seizures tended to have generalized seizures.

The duration of seizures is usually brief, lasting several seconds to a few minutes, although status epilepticus has been reported.[53,61–64] The status is characterized by unilateral motor seizures dominant on the face with persistent anarthria and sialorrhea, or prolonged status of anarthria and sialorrhea. Diurnal seizures, especially those showing somatosensory symptoms, are usually of short duration. Seizures occur only during sleep in 51–80 per cent of the patients, both during sleep and wakefulness in 13–40 per cent, and only during wakefulness in 0–32 per cent.[8]

The frequency of seizures is usually low.[65,66] Some 50–60 per cent of the patients have sporadic seizures infrequently at intervals of 2–12 months and 10–20 per cent experience only a single seizure. In 20 per cent, seizures occur frequently and usually in clusters.

EEG features

The background activity is generally considered normal, at least on visual analysis. Power spectral analyses have demonstrated slower occipital basic rhythms,[67] power reduction in alpha and beta ranges in 7–9-year-old patients, and power increase at delta and theta frequency ranges in 10–12-year-old patients.[68] Focal rhythmic slow waves often seen in the same region of the rolandic discharges are though to be a part of the morphology of rolandic discharges, since they were abolished with clonazepam.[69]

The interictal EEG shows characteristic focal spikes in the left or right central and/or midtemporal region (Figure 11D.1). However, when the field distribution of interictal spikes is evaluated using closely spaced electrodes arranged over the perisylvian cortex, none of the patients showed maximum negativity in the midtemporal regions (T3/T4).[70] Instead, maximum negativity was evident in the high central region (C3/C4) in 30 per cent of the patients and in the low central region (C5/C6) in 70 per cent. Hand involvement was significantly more frequent in the high central group, and drooling with oromotor involvement was a distinctive symptom in the low central group. These spikes are typically a negative sharp wave with a blunted peak, preceded by a small positive wave and followed by a prominent positive wave with an amplitude frequently up to 50 per cent that of the preceding negative sharp wave. This may be followed by an inconspicuous negative slow wave of lower amplitude than the preceding negative sharp wave.[8] Van der Meij et al.[71] reported that the morphology of rolandic spikes did not provide a clue to the presence or absence of an organic cerebral lesion. Frost et al.[72] analyzed spike morphology of different childhood partial epilepsies more precisely and found the spikes of this syndrome to be higher in amplitude, longer in duration and less sharp than those of patients with other syndromes. When effective drug treatment results in clinical seizure control, the amplitude and duration of spikes decreases, and the sharpness increases.[73] When these sharp waves occur unilaterally, they are always synchronous in the central and midtemporal regions;[74] and when bilateral they may be bilaterally asynchronous, and occur with different frequencies and amplitudes in the left and the right hemispheres. The spike focus is unilateral in about 60 per cent of patients and bilateral in 40 per cent. When bilateral, the spike foci tend to shift from side to side. They may be ipsi- or contralateral to the symptomatogenic side. During sleep, rolandic spikes occur maximally in slow wave sleep and minimally in REM sleep.[75]

Centrotemporal sharp waves have a typical field of distribution forming a dipole with a negative pole at the mid-temporal–central region and a positive pole at the superior frontal area.[8] This has been confirmed by topographic mapping analysis,[76–78] and further supported by more recent investigations using a dipole localization method, a dipole tracing method or a dipole source analysis. The dipoles of children with BCECT were found to be more concentrated in the rolandic region compared with those with features similar to BCECT but with signs of brain damage.[79–81] The presence of a dipole field usually indicates a better clinical course of epilepsy, and the occurrence of multiple foci does not imply a poor clinical course.[82]

Magnetoencephalographic (MEG) studies have also shown that the dipoles of prominent negative sharp waves of rolandic discharges appeared as tangential dipoles in the rolandic region, positive poles being situated anteriorly.[83,84] In contrast, MEG dipoles in symptomatic rolandic-sylvian epilepsy tend to be multiple and randomly oriented.[85] However, van der Meij et al.[86] did not find clear differences between various clinical groups in the localization

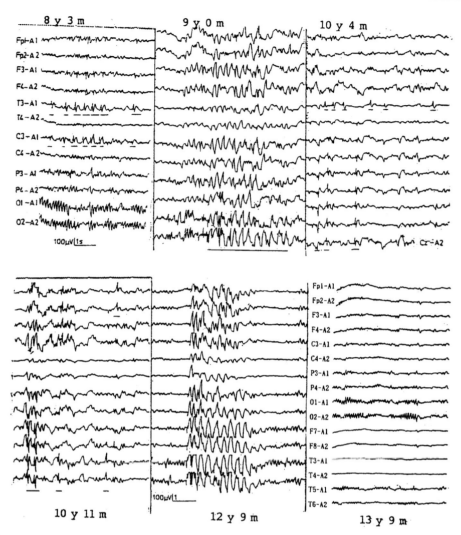

Figure 11D.1 *This neurologically and developmentally normal 15-year-old girl with a past history of febrile convulsions had typical nocturnal sylvian seizures at the age of 8 years. The EEG at 8 years 3 months disclosed typical sharp and slow wave discharges in the left midtemporal and central regions. The EEG at 9 years showed spike and wave complexes in both occipital regions on eye closure. The EEG at 10 years 4 months also displayed sporadic sharp waves in the left midtemporal area and spike and waves in the occipitoparietal regions independently. The EEG at 10 years 11 months demonstrated sporadic sharp waves independently in both frontal and occipital regions. She complained of blurred vision and headache occasionally. The EEG at 12 years 9 months revealed parieto-occipital dominant diffuse spike and wave bursts. EEG at 13 years 9 months and thereafter were normal. She has been seizure free without treatment.*

and the orientation of the dipole sources of the rolandic discharges. Neither the exact location nor dipolar distribution of rolandic spikes helps to differentiate between neurodevelopmentally normal patients with and without clinical seizures.[87] Sequential topographic mapping disclosed two types of potential field: stationary and nonstationary patterns.[88] The latter topographic pattern was statistically more frequently associated with an increased probability for clinical seizures.

The frequency of rolandic spikes was significantly lower during hyperventilation and the 2 min following hyperventilation than during normal wakefulness.[89] The voluntary maneuver of protrusion of the tongue induced inhibition of centrotemporal spikes,[90–92] and appeared to terminate the seizure.[92] The decrease in discharge rate during tongue movements was not significant in patients with cerebral lesion, but a significant reduction was evident in those without cerebral lesion.

Benign rolandic discharges occur in patients with symptomatic partial epilepsy. Three possible explanations have been postulated:[93]

- The organic lesion may lower the seizure threshold and result in expression of the genetically determined benign discharges.
- A lowering of the seizure threshold by benign partial epileptic discharges may have activated a symptomatic epilepsy.

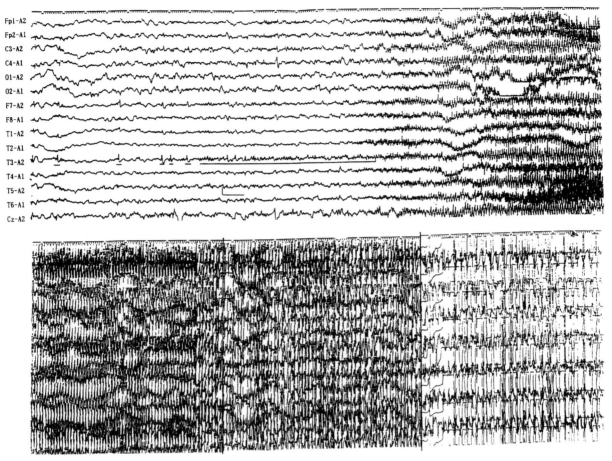

Figure 11D.2 *Ictal EEG of a 9-year-old girl with benign childhood epilepsy with centrotemporal spikes. During phase II sleep semirhythmic alpha activity appeared from the left midtemporal region which propagated to other areas with increasing and decreasing frequency. Seven seconds later, the right corner of her mouth was drawn downward to the right. Ten seconds later, she opened her eyes. Fifteen seconds later, her head rotated to the right, followed by generalized tonic-clonic convulsions.*

- The benign focal discharges may have occurred coincidentally with the symptomatic partial epilepsy.

Centrotemporal spikes can be present in nonepileptic children and adolescents. They disappear spontaneously and only a small percentage of subjects who have persistence of this pattern develops rolandic epilepsy.[92]

The centrotemporal regions are not exclusive locations of the sharp waves in BCECT. Drury and Beydoun[94] found a focus outside the centrotemporal area in one fifth of patients with histories and clinical courses completely compatible with BCECT. A number of authors have mentioned the coexistence of other foci, multiple independent sharp wave foci, shifting of the location of sharp waves from a posterior to a centrotemporal location, and vice versa[59,65,95–100] (Figure 12D.1). Generalized spike-waves are also observed in some patients.[59,65,95,99,101] Degen and Degen[35] observed generalized spike-wave complexes in 32 per cent of the siblings of patients with BCECT but focal discharges in various locations in only 6 per cent.

There have been a few documentations of ictal recordings.[36,102] They usually show frequent rhythmic spikes or low-voltage fast activity beginning in the centrotemporal region on one side (Figure 11D.2). The paroxysmal discharges increase in amplitude and decrease in frequency, spreading to the adjacent regions and then to the whole hemisphere, evolving to high-amplitude rhythmic spikes, and then to spike and waves when secondary generalization occurs. Lerman[74] recorded a diurnal seizure beginning with focal decremental activity followed by dense spikes in the centrotemporal area during the tonic phase and spike-waves in the clonic phase with no spread and no postictal slowing. One of our patients showed frequent discharges of sharp waves in the right midtemporal, central and left central areas during a diurnal simple partial seizure (Figure 11D.3). Guiterrez *et al.*[103] and Silva *et al.*[104] each recorded a subclinical seizure with paroxysmal discharges showing a dipole reversal relative to the interictal discharges. Gutierrez *et al.*[103] postulated the origin of the seizure discharge to be deep in the sylvian fissure in areas

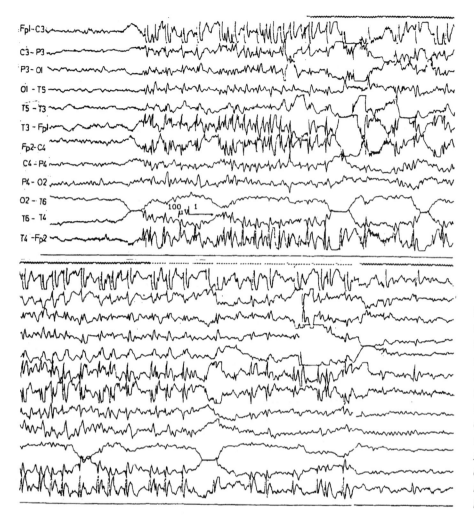

Figure 11D.3 *Ictal EEG of a diurnal simple partial seizure in a 9-year-old girl with benign childhood epilepsy with centrotemporal spikes. A burst of repetitive spikes was observed in the right and left midtemporal and central regions in association with an attack consisting of speech arrest and salivation. The dipole shows negativity in the midtemporal region and positivity in the frontal region.*

within cortical folds. The spike component of contralateral interictal rolandic spike-wave complexes may be associated with single and rhythmic facial myoclonia during active worsening phases of the disease, although the majority of interictal discharges are asymptomatic. The amplitudes of the positive and negative spikes and of the slow wave are significantly higher during symptomatic than during asymptomatic discharges.[56]

Pathophysiology

Both the seizure semiology and the location of EEG foci suggest that the epileptogenic focus is in the part of the lower rolandic cortex representing the face and the oropharynx. The bluntness of the spikes and the frequent association with slow waves both suggest a focus deep in the sylvian fissure.[51] This has been confirmed by the above-mentioned studies using topographic mapping, various kinds of dipole analyses and MEG.[71,81,83,84,105–107] A recent study with high-resolution EEG, MEG and fMRI has also confirmed that the epileptic focus resides in

the lower sensorimotor cortex, and high-resolution EEG revealed two distinct sourses, one in the post- and the other in the precentral cortex.[108]

Some children with BCECT demonstrate extremely high amplitude somatosensory evoked potentials. The evoked responses showed a morphology, dipole configuration and source localization similar to rolandic spikes, suggesting the same cortical generators for both.[109] Evoked spikes and spontaneous spikes are both sensitive to stimulus rate, suggesting that these generators can be influenced by afferent input, which provides important information regarding the functional mechanisms involved in modulating cortical excitability in benign rolandic epilepsy.[110] A fMRI study in a patient with this type of benign rolandic epilepsy demonstrated a highly focal activation of sensorimotor areas related to subclinical evoked spikes in benign rolandic epilepsy.[111] Giant somatosensory evoked potentials show a clear developmental change with age, and are not present in subjects older than 12 years of age.[112] This phenomenon mirrors the disappearance of rolandic discharges in most patients with BCECT after this age.[113] Kubota *et al.*[114] investigated patients with rolandic epilepsy associated with giant somatosensory responses to median nerve stimulation using MEG. The initial positive peak and large negative peak of rolandic discharges were considered identical to P30m and N70m. They suggest that the rolandic discharge generator mechanism in these patients could be closely related to developmental alteration of excitability in the primary somatosensory cortex, posterior parietal cortex and secondary somatosensory cortex, which decreased with age, and it could share a common neuronal pathway, at least in part, with the giant P30m–N70m (N90m) in the somatosensory evoked magnetic field through the sequential and parallel processing of somatosensory information. Manganotti and Zanette[115] investigated motor evoked potentials (MEP) in hand muscles by transcranial magnetic stimulation which were conditioned by electrical digital stimulation producing evoked spikes. Digital stimulation produced an increase in MEP amplitude, and this MEP facilitation showed a time course overlapping the ascending phase and peak of the evoked spike, whereas no significant MEP changes were found during the early positive peak and the descending phase of the spike, or during the following slow wave. The authors considered that the short-lasting M1 facilitation is related to the spread of an abnormal hypersynchronous discharge of the S1 neurons to functionally related motor areas via cortico-cortical connections.

Only a fraction of patients with typical rolandic sharp waves have clinical seizures. The factors that contribute to the expression of clinical epilepsy have not been elucidated. Heijbel et al.[116] postulated the existence of an inhibitory factor, capable of preventing seizures, which can be breached by external or internal factors. Lerman[74] suggested that a precipitating factor was needed to convert the inherited trait into the overt disease. The marked age dependency of symptoms and almost regular disappearance of seizures and EEG abnormalities at puberty has led Doose and Baier[117] to postulate an hereditary impairment of brain maturation.

The fact that patients with typical rolandic spikes may develop occipital spikes typical of benign occipital epilepsy (Figure 11D.1), while patients with typical occipital spikes may develop typical rolandic spikes and generalized spikewaves typical of idiopathic generalized epilepsy (Figure 11D.4), strongly suggests that there are close links between these disorders.[118] Manifestations during a rolandic seizure that are suggestive of occipital lobe involvement are extremely rare. Parmeggiani and Guerrini[119] reported a patient with idiopathic partial epilepsy who presented a seizure consisting of initial rolandic and late occipital involvement, suggesting susceptibility of cortical neurons of both areas to develop seizures at the age range of both benign rolandic epilepsy and early onset benign occipital epilepsy. Some children with idiopathic partial epilepsy may present occipital and rolandic seizures at different ages.

Although concomitance or sequential occurrence of BCECT and childhood absence epilepsy has been reported,[120,121] such a combination is extremely rare. Moreover, brief bursts of bilateral diffuse spike and wave discharges frequently seen in patients with BCECT occur mostly during sleepiness. BCECT does not evolve into idiopathic generalized epilepsy. Therefore, there is no neurobiological and genetic continuum between the two epileptic syndromes.[122]

Investigation

Neuroimaging procedures have been considered unnecessary in most patients with BCECT but may be indicated in those with atypical features such as persistent seizures and/or long duration of active epilepsy. Typical rolandic sharp waves may be seen in children with tumors and other organic lesions.[123–125] Sheth et al.[126] used dipole analysis to study a patient with BCECT and an underlying cortical dysplasia in the sylvian region and found that the discharges had the features of BCECT rather than those of a cortical dysplasia. Gelisse et al.[127] recently reported a patient with BCECT who displayed marked hippocampal atrophy and considered that this association seemed coincidental. However, Lundberg et al.[128] has described hippocampal asymmetries and white matter abnormalities in one third of children with BCECT examined with MRI. All of the hippocampal abnormalities were ipsilateral to the main EEG findings, and Lundberg commented that it was of interest to consider the function of an abnormal hippocampus in epileptogenesis especially in sylvian seizures.

Van Bogaert et al.[129] used FDG-PET to study the regional cerebral metabolism in children with centrotemporal spikes and did not find any metabolic changes associated with interictal spiking. They suggested that this technique could be helpful for the differentiation between idiopathic and symptomatic cases of partial epilepsy in children. de Saint-Martin et al.[56] found a bilateral increase of glucose metabolism in both opercular regions in a patient with BCECT during the worsening period when the patient presented interictal facial myoclonia and oromotor deficit. Laub et al.[130] found localized hypoperfusion in about 40 per cent of the patients using SPECT with technetium-99 m hexamethyl propylene amine oxime (HMPAO). The significance of their findings is unknown because of the absence of correlation between the localization of the EEG focus and the site of the hypoperfused area.

Visual and somatosensory evoked potentials have been reported to be of high amplitude with no changes in morphology and latency.[131,132] Overnight sleep recordings in children with BCECT do not show significant modifications in sleep organization.[133,134]

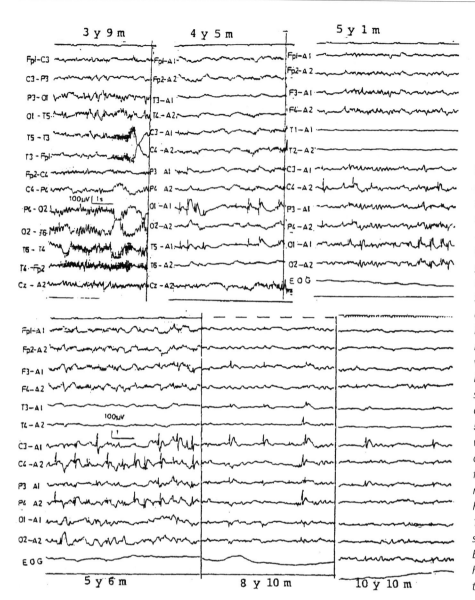

Figure 11D.4 *This neurologically and developmentally normal 14-year-old boy had had several febrile seizures up to 7 years 6 months, when he developed afebrile nocturnal generalized convulsions. The EEG was normal at 3 years of age. At 3 years 9 months small spikes and slow waves were seen in the left occipital region, becoming more definite and of high voltage at 4 years 5 months. The EEG at 5 years 1 months showed sporadic spikes in the right central area, in addition. At 5 years 6 months abundant spikes were seen in the left or right central and parietal areas, but fewer came from the occipital regions. Occipital spikes were hardly seen at 8 years and at 10 years 10 months only central spikes were demonstrable. The EEG normalized at 12 years and he has been seizure free without treatment for 3 years.*

Treatment

In view of the benign nature of the condition, intensive therapy is unnecessary. Peters *et al.*[136] reported that antiepileptic drugs significantly reduced generalized seizures but did not reduce partial seizures and that all patients eventually entered remission without medication or injury whether treated or not.

Ambrosetto *et al.*[66] advise withholding treatment even after the second seizure if it occurs more than 6 months after the first. The same authors reported no differences in seizure frequency, recurrence or duration of active epilepsy between untreated and treated patients with BCECT.[135]

If treatment is initiated, carbamazepine is considered the drug of first choice, although a possible worsening of seizures has rarely been reported with this medication.[137] Carbamazepine may exert its aggravating effect only during a period of spontaneous activation of epilepsy in a susceptible patient. It may induce epileptic negative myoclonus.[138] Carbamazepine treatment has been reported to cause memory difficulties in patients with benign rolandic epilepsy.[139] Phenobarbital, phenytoin, and valproic acid have been reported as equally effective, but have been associated with behavioral, cosmetic and hematologic side-effects respectively. A double-blind, randomized and placebo-controlled study reported the efficacy of gabapentin monotherapy (30 mg kg^{-1} day^{-1}).[140] Low-dose sulthiame monotherapy (5 mg kg^{-1} day^{-1} in three divided doses) has also been demonstrated in a randomized, double-blind, placebo-controlled study to be effective.[141] Sulthiame is well tolerated without serious side-effects, but may rarely be associated with poor concentration, depressed mood, lack of drive and listlessness even at low dose,[142] and with elevation of liver enzymes.[143]

Once-daily administration at bedtime may be sufficient in the case of nocturnal seizures. We have found once-daily administration of a low dose of clonazepam or clobazam highly effective in most cases. Although most patients respond to a low dose of a single drug, a few are highly drug-resistant. In such cases, monotherapy at a moderate dose with some persisting seizures may be better than high-dose polypharmacy with neurotoxic side-effects.[144]

Although some authors advocate anticonvulsant therapy until the age of 14–16 years,[144] anticonvulsants may be successfuly discontinued in patients with normal EEGs who have been seizure-free for more than 2 years. Some 80 per cent of patients followed by De Romanis et al.[145] became seizure-free, and remained so for at least 6–12 months when drug therapy was discontinued after 2 years of treatment. It is more important to give the parents a full explanation of the benign nature of the disorder, in order to avoid unnecessary psychologic reactions, than to prescribe drugs.[74]

Spike discharges typical of those seen in benign partial epilepsies of childhood can also be observed in patients with abdominal pain, cyclic vomiting, etc. Such children should not be treated with antiepileptic drugs.[58]

Prognosis

Seizures eventually disappear and EEGs normalize irrespective of treatment: 92 per cent are in remission by 12 years of age 99.8 per cent by 18 years.[113] The duration of active epilepsy is longer in patients with earlier ages of onset.[146] Seizures are more easily controlled in patients with secondarily generalized seizures than in those with only partial seizures.[41] In 1–2 per cent of patients, partial or generalized tonic-clonic seizures recur during adolescence or occasionally adulthood.[146–149] These tend to be isolated or infrequent and have been considered to represent another form of idiopathic epilepsy rather than a relapse of the same syndrome.[144] The absence of typical EEG sharp waves and seizures characteristic of this syndrome in adults also indicates that this syndrome improves before adulthood.

In patients followed up for long periods, temporal changes in the EEG often make allocation into discrete syndromes impossible (Figures 11D.1, 11D.4, 11D.5). The electroclinical patterns overlap and the determining factor for prognosis is not the location but the morphology of the sharp waves.[150] Morikawa et al.[151] conducted a longitudinal study of children with partial seizures and rolandic discharges and found that rolandic discharges disappeared in an age-related manner in idiopathic patients, but tended to persist in the symptomatic ones. They concluded that the presence of rolandic discharges was not a hallmark of a benign outcome, but that the presence of sylvian seizures indicated a favorable prognosis.

A small proportion of patients with typical features of BCECT show atypical evolution of their syndrome. Twenty-six (6.9 per cent) of 378 patients studied by Fejerman et al.[64] showed atypical evolution. Eleven of them developed atypical benign partial epilepsy of childhood (ABPEC), three Landau-Kleffner syndrome, seven status epilepticus, and five mixed features with or without continuous spikes and waves during slow sleep, mixed features (MF). Prognosis is generally favorable for ABPEC and status epilepticus, but Landau-Kleffner syndrome and MF may be associated with the risk of persistent language, cognitive and behavioral deterioration. In a long-term follow-up study, the patients with atypical rolandic epilepsy had a significantly higher percentage of learning and behavioral disabilities than children with the classical form of rolandic epilepsy.[152]

BENIGN CHILDHOOD EPILEPSY WITH OCCIPITAL PAROXYSMS

Definition

Benign childhood epilepsy with occipital paroxysms (BCEOP) is defined in the International Classification[1] as a syndrome generally similar to BCECT, but characterized by seizures which start with visual symptoms (amaurosis, phosphenes, illusions, or hallucinations) that are often followed by a hemiclonic seizure or automatisms. One quarter of the seizures are followed immediately by a migrainous headache. The EEG has paroxysms of high-amplitude spike-waves or sharp waves recurring rhythmically in the occipital and posterior temporal areas of one or both hemispheres, but only when the eyes are closed. During seizures, the occipital discharge may spread to the central or temporal regions.

The current definition is based largely on the description by Gastaut[153,154] and Gastaut and Zifkin.[155] Some authors have questioned the existence of BCEOP as a distinct clinical entity, and have questioned the benign nature of the condition.[156–161] Roger and Bureau[162] have alluded to the difficulty in diagnosing this syndrome with confidence. They have drawn attention to the nonspecific nature of the interictal EEG features, as described by Gastaut,[154] which can also be observed in symptomatic or cryptogenic partial epilepsies that often have unfavorable outcomes. The only selection criterion that they used was the presence of occipital spikes, occurring when the eyes were closed; thus they included patients with organic brain lesions or mental retardation. However, fixation-off sensitivity (FOS) is not specific to any clinical condition and cannot be used as a sole diagnostic criterion.[163] Moreover, in some of the previous cases, paroxysmal discharges are not increased in slow wave sleep and even disappear during

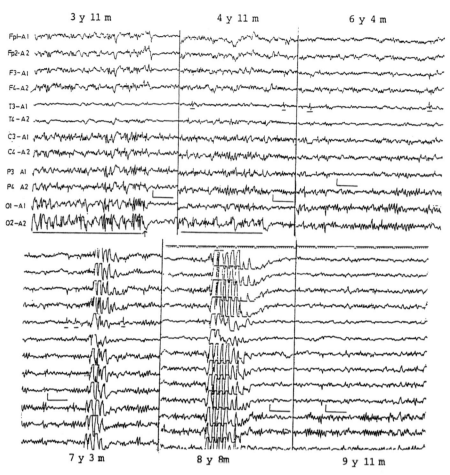

Figure 11D.5 *This neurologically and developmentally normal 12-year-old boy had several febrile seizures starting at 13 months. The EEG showed small spikes in the right occipital region at 3 years 5 months and spike and wave bursts attenuated on eye opening at 3 years and 11 months. Around this time, he developed seizures characterized by deviation of the eyes to the left. At 4 years 4 months, he had an attack consisting of deviation of the eyes to the left, vomiting and stiffening of the body. At 4 years 4 months and 4 years 11 months the EEG displayed focal spikes in the left midtemporal area, in addition to occipital spikes, but occipital spikes disappeared at 6 years 4 months and thereafter. At 7 years 3 months, there were short burst of generalized spikes and waves in addition to midtemporal spikes; these disappeared at 8 years 8 months. The EEG was normal at 9 years 11 months and thereafter. He has been seizure free without treatment for 3 years.*

slow wave sleep, which is unusual in BCEOP.[164–166] Only idiopathic patients with normal neurodevelopment status should be considered to have BCEOP.

The specificity of BCEOP is not as high as that of BCECT, in which the electroclinical picture is rarely seen in symptomatic or cryptogenic partial epilepsy. Thus, stricter criteria should be developed to define BCEOP.

Clinical features

The exact incidence of BCEOP is not well established, but Dalla Bernardina, Bondavalli and Colomaria[167] found that 19 (7 per cent) of 260 patients with various types of benign partial epilepsies had BCEOP in contrast to 162 (62 per cent) with BCECT. The age of onset ranges from 15 months to 17 years, with a peak age of onset between 5 and 7

years.[154,168] The clinical manifestations depend on the age of onset. Younger children more often present with nocturnal seizures, mainly consisting of motor seizures; whereas children above 8 years of age tend to have diurnal attacks characterized by visual seizures.[168] No convincing gender difference has been demonstrated.[168,169]

Gastaut[151] elicited a family history of epilepsy in 37 per cent and migraine in 16 per cent, but other authors did not find positive family histories.[168,170] Kuzniecky and Rosenblatt[171] postulated an autosomal dominant inheritance for the EEG abnormalities with age-dependent expression and variable penetrance for the seizures. Nagendran et al.[172] suggested autosomal dominant inheritance, reporting a familial case in which the mother and two children were affected.

The patients have normal psychomotor development and a neurologic examination. Headache and vomiting occur commonly in this syndrome.[154,161,173–175] Lerman and Kivity[174] observed that headache was the presenting symptom in 29 per cent, occurred simultaneously with the visual symptoms in 37 per cent and was postictal in 33 per cent of their patients. Although postictal migrainous headache occurs frequently in BCEOP, it is not exclusive to this syndrome. The relationship between epilepsy and migraine is complex,[176,177] and it has been suggested that the epileptic discharges trigger migrainous phenomena in patients with postictal headache.[176]

Seizure manifestations

The seizures are characterized mainly by visual symptomatology, often followed by hemiclonic seizures or automatisms and postictal headache. The visual seizures consist of transient partial or complete visual loss in the entire visual field, sometimes preceded by initial hemianopsia, elementary visual hallucinations (i.e. phosphenes or moving flashing spots occupying the half or the entire visual field), complex visual hallucinations, or visual illusions such as micropsia, metamorphosia or palinopsia.[154] Younger children may underreport these visual phenomena. Visual symptoms may be followed by several ictal phenomena: hemiclonic seizures; complex partial seizures with automatisms, indistinguishable from those typical of temporal lobe epilepsy; adversive seizures; and/or secondarily generalized tonic-clonic seizures. These are often followed by a postictal diffuse headache, which is only rarely hemicrania and which is sometimes associated with nausea and vomiting. This sequence of symptoms may create some difficulties in differentiating migraine and epilepsy.[176] The visual epileptic symptoms are predominantly multicolored and circular/spheric in contrast with the predominantly black and white linear pattern of migraine.[178] Seizures may be provoked by light extinction, by entering a dark room, or going from a dark area into a brighter one.[179,180,154]

EEG features

The interictal EEG shows characteristic occipital paroxysms on normal background activity.[154,168,178] The occipital paroxysms typically consist of high-voltage, repetitive spikes, sharp waves and slow wave complexes over the occipital and posterior temporal regions, which are often bilateral, asymmetric and attenuate on eye opening (Figure 11D.4). Individual complexes consist of a diphasic spike component in which a main negative peak in the occipital electrodes is followed by a relatively small positive peak and a negative slow wave.[168] The spike component is usually higher in amplitude than the negative slow wave, similar to centrotemporal spikes in benign rolandic epilepsy. The paroxysms are rarely isolated and usually

recur pseudorhythmically in bursts of from 1 to 3 Hz or in trains at irregular intervals.[154] They disappear promptly with opening of the eyes in 94 per cent of cases and reappear 1–20 s after eye closure. They are further attenuated by fixation and induced by elimination of central vision.[168] Darkness is not a prerequisite for inducing occipital paroxysms. Thus, the term fixation-off sensitivity is preferable to scotosensitive epilepsy.[178] They are also inhibited by monocular elimination of central vision and monocular fixation. Neither occipital paroxysms nor fixation-off sensitivity is diagnostic of benign occipital epilepsy with occipital paroxysms. Fixation-off sensitivity is not always demonstrable in this syndrome.[178] Polyspikes, small spikes intermixed with slow waves, scattered occipital spikes as seen in photosensitive patients, or slow waves which happen to attenuate with eyes open are not features of the occipital paroxysms in BCEOP.[178] In contrast to Panayiotopoulos,[178] Vigevano and Ricci[181] never observed the induction of occipital paroxysms in response to eye closure. Intermittent photic stimulation has an inhibitory effect particularly at high frequencies. Unlike Terasaki et al.[173] and Lerman and Kivity,[174] Gastaut[154] did not find that hyperventilation had an activating effect. No consistent effect of sleep has been observed, in contrast to BCECT where sleep almost always activates spikes. Lerman and Kivity[174] reported that non REM sleep activated or disclosed the occipital discharges, but Gastaut[154] found reinforcement by slow sleep in only 15 per cent of his cases. Gastaut and Zifkin[155] reported that drowsiness and sleep caused the disappearance of occipital paroxysms in 59 per cent of cases, but the discharges occurred more frequently during sleep in another study.[182] In some patients, the occipital paroxysms are associated with generalized bisynchronus spike and waves or focal spikes in other regions such as centrotemporal spikes in the same or subsequent records.[154,168] The location of spikes may change during the clinical course and shift from the occipital area to other areas, sometimes showing multifocality[183] (Figures 11D.4, 11D.5). Not all children with occipital paroxysms develop clinical seizures.[184,185]

The ictal EEG of a diurnal seizure recorded by Beaumanoir[186] disclosed focal rapid spikes, becoming progressively slower. The ictal EEG of nocturnal seizures showed disappearance of interictal occipital paroxysms followed by a tonic discharge of low-voltage spikes of progressively increasing amplitude in an occipital region, followed by spike and waves localized to one or more of the posterior areas.

Pathophysiology

The varying clinical seizure patterns seen in this syndrome can be explained by the propagation of the occipital ictal discharges to anterior regions.[154] Purely visual seizures are associated with focal occipital discharges limited to the occipital region. Visual auras followed by hemisensory and/or hemiconvulsive seizures are related to the spread of the occipital discharge to the central region. Visual auras followed by psychomotor automatisms are due to the spread of the occipital discharge to the temporal lobe and/or related structures. Seizures without visual phenomena result from the secondary spread of the occipital discharge in which visual symptoms are not reported, or from the discharge of an independent focus separate from the primary occipital focus.[154] Gastaut and Zifkin[155] suggested a subcortical mechanism for the electrogenesis of occipital paroxysms. They postulated that the postictal migrainous symptoms were due to the persistence, in the territory of the posterior cerebral and basilar arteries, of the initial vasodilatation accompanying the occipital ictal activity, and that they occurred in children with impaired or labile cerebrovascular autoregulation due to a predisposition to migraine.

Investigation

The occipital paroxysms are not specific to BCEOP and may be seen in patients with occipital lesions. Gobbi et al.[187] and Giroud et al.[28] reported patients, initially considered to have benign occipital epilepsy, who subsequently showed mental deterioration and worsening of seizures and were found to have occipital calcification. Therefore, neuroimaging is indicated patients with features of BCEOP.

Treatment

Carbamazepine has been the drug of choice, although almost all of the classic anticonvulsants, including phenobarbital, valproic acid and benzodiazepines, are effective.[154]

Prognosis

The prognosis is usually good, with complete seizure control achieved in 60 per cent of cases. No patients have typical seizures persisting past adolescence, but other types of seizures have been reported in 5 per cent in adulthood.[154] A longitudinal prospective study has shown that the prognosis is less favorable than in BCECT.[163]

PANAYIOTOPOULOS SYNDROME

Definition

The seizures are brief or prolonged, usually nocturnal, infrequent partial seizures consisting of deviation of the eyes and vomiting. The clinical manifestations of this syndrome were described initially in a study of children with occipital paroxysms. Therefore, the syndrome was initially considered to represent early-onset variant of BCEOP.[178,188] The syndrome was later called **early onset benign childhood occipital seizure syndrome** or Panayiotopoulos syndrome.[189] Numerous studies[190–195] have been published since the initial report by Panayiotopoulos[196] and a subsequent international collaborative study.[197] Panayiotopoulos described another syndrome characterized by the same symptomatology but with extraoccipital spikes, and named it **extraoccipital benign childhood partial seizures with ictal vomiting and excellent prognosis**.[198] Because of the frequent occurrence of concurrent or subsequent extraoccipital spikes and the infrequent occurrence of generalized discharges in early-onset childhood epilepsy with occipital spikes, he suggested that these syndromes be combined as Panayiotopoulos syndrome.[199] He emphasized that this was not exclusively an occipital epilepsy, but rather part of a childhood seizure susceptibility syndrome with age-related EEG and clinical manifestations.

Clinical features

The syndrome is common, comprising 28 per cent of all cases of benign childhood partial seizures, as opposed to 67 per cent of benign rolandic epilepsy.[200] The age of onset ranges from 1 to 14 years with a peak at 4–5 years. The children have normal physical and neuropsychological development. There is a high prevalence of febrile seizures[201] in family members but usually no family history of other benign childhood seizure disorders, other epilepsies or migraine.

Seizure manifestations

The seizures are characterized by nausea, vomiting, tonic eye deviation and often impairment of consciousness that can progress to hemi- or generalized convulsions. Seizures may last for a few minutes or persist for several hours constituting partial status epilepticus and giving rise to concerns about a serious cerebral insult.[202–204] Although dramatic and prolonged, seizures occur infrequently and may be solitary. Even after the most severe seizures and status, the patient returns to normal after a few hours' sleep without any residual neurological or mental abnormalities. They are usually nocturnal and are rarely diurnal.[178] Postictal headache, migraine and ictal visual symptoms are rare. The clinical seizure manifestations appear independent of the interictal EEG localization, although there may be slightly less autonomic and slightly more focal motor features at onset in children without occipital spikes.[199] About 10 per cent of patients with early-onset benign occipital seizures also had ictal visual symptoms, and were considered overlap cases.[205] Some children with this syndrome have concurrent symptoms of rolandic epilepsy, or may develop rolandic seizures after remission.[192]

EEG features

The EEG background is usually normal, but diffuse or localized slow-wave abnormalities may occur. The interictal EEG commonly reveals functional, mainly multifocal high amplitude sharp and slow wave complexes. All brain regions are involved though the posterior predominate. EEG abnormalities may appear only several months after the first seizure.[206] Two thirds of patients have at least one EEG with occipital spikes, which are often concurrent with extraoccipital spikes. The other third never show occipital spikes. These patients either have only extraoccipital spikes, a consistently normal EEG or only brief generalized discharges. Those with occipital sharp waves have a higher rate of frontal foci than those without.[207] Spikes are usually of high amplitude and morphologically similar to the centrotemporal (rolandic) spikes. However, small and even inconspicuous spikes may also be seen in children with giant spikes. Brief generalized discharges of slow waves intermixed with small spikes may occur either alone or more often with focal spikes. The occipital paroxysms are commonly activated by the elimination of central vision and fixation, whereas rolandic discharges may be elicited by somatosensory stimuli. Occipital photosensitivity is an exceptional finding. Functional spikes in whatever location are accentuated by sleep. EEG abnormalities, particularly functional spikes, may persist after clinical remission for many years until the mid-teens. Conversely, spikes may appear only once in one series of EEGs. Frequency, location and persistence of functional spikes do not determine clinical manifestations, duration, severity and frequency of seizures or prognosis.

Ictal EEG recordings have rarely been reported. The seizure discharge consists mainly of rhythmic theta or delta activity intermixed usually with small spikes.[208] Onset is unilateral, often posterior, but may also be anterior and not strictly localized to one electrode.

Pathophysiology

Clinical and EEG findings suggest that there is a diffuse cortical hyperexcitability, which is maturation-related. This diffuse epileptogenicity may be unequally distributed, predominating in one area, which is often posterior. The frequent emetic and autonomic symptoms may be due to epileptic discharges generated at various cortical locations influencing the emetic centers and the hypothalamus in vulnerable children.[199] Panayiotopoulos has suggested that febrile seizures, Panayiotopoulos syndrome and benign rolandic seizures may represent an age-related continuum of childhood seizure susceptibility.

Investigation

As in any idiopathic epilepsy, the neurological development, neurologic examination and MRI are normal. Approximately 10–20 per cent of children with similar seizures have brain abnormalities and an MRI is normally performed. Interictal SPECT revealed decreased cerebral blood flow in the occipital region corresponding to the EEG focus in a patient with this syndrome.[209]

Prognosis

Panayiotopoulos syndrome is a remarkably benign condition, despite the high incidence of partial status epilepticus. Twenty-seven per cent of patients have a single seizure only, 47 per cent have between 2 and 5 seizures and only 5 per cent have more than 10 seizures. Furthermore, the duration of the epilepsy is very brief with remission occurring within 1–2 years from onset. The outcome is favorable even in those with frequent seizures. The risk of developing epilepsy in adult life is probably no more than of the general population. However, 21 per cent may develop other seizure types, which tend to occur infrequently. Rolandic seizures (13 per cent) are the most common other seizure type and these occur during childhood and early teens, and remit before the age of 16 years. Atypical evolutions with absences, atonic seizures and continuous spike-waves during slow sleep like those occurring in rolandic epilepsy are exceptional.[210]

Treatment

Continuous anticonvulsant therapy is not recommended for children with single or brief seizures. Most clinicians use carbamazepine for recurrent seizures, but clobazam or clonazepam, administered once daily at bedtime, is fairly effective. Lengthy seizures are a medical emergency and rectal diazepam should be prescribed for home administration in patients with a previous episode of status epilepticus. Recurrent and lengthy seizures create anxiety in parents and patients, and appropriate education and emotional support should be provided.[199] Supportive family management includes education about Panayiotopoulos syndrome and specific instructions about emergency procedures for possible subsequent seizures.

BENIGN EPILEPSY OF CHILDHOOD WITH COMPLEX PARTIAL SEIZURES

This syndrome was identified in 26 of 145 children with benign partial epilepsies, and is characterized by seizures consisting of impaired consciousness, often accompanied by staring or eye deviation (66 per cent), nausea and/or vomiting (50 per cent) and focal motor symptoms (31 per cent). Automatisms are infrequent (8 per cent).[211,212] The seizures are usually brief, not frequent and respond well to the initial drug. During the clinical course, focal spikes, sharp waves or spike and waves are seen in varying regions except anterior temporal regions and do not have a fixed focus. Multifocal epileptiform discharges and shifting of the foci are common. Prognosis is excellent with disappearance of epileptiform discharges. Recognition of this syndrome is more difficult because the clinical features are not as homogeneous as in BCECT. Some of these patients may belong to Panayiotopoulos syndrome.

Among patients with complex partial seizures following febrile seizures, there is a subgroup with an extremely benign outcome.[213] The characteristic features are

- no history of remote neurologic injury, no underlying disorder, normal neurological examination, and normal cognitive function
- no past history of prolonged febrile convulsions
- EEG spike foci other than the anterior temporal type
- easily controlled CPS with full recovery.

We have termed this **disorder benign epilepsy of childhood with complex partial seizures after febrile convulsions**. It is important to distinguish these children from those with mesial temporal sclerosis following prolonged febrile convulsions because of the excellent prognosis.

BENIGN PARTIAL EPILEPSY WITH AFFECTIVE SYMPTOMATOLOGY

This syndrome was first described by Dalla Bernardina et al.[214,215] and is characterized by ictal affective symptoms, especially fear, as the predominant manifestation and a favorable outcome.

Clinical features

The age of onset in 26 patients reported by Dalla Bernardina et al.[215] ranged from 2 to 9 years with two peaks at 2–5 years and 6–9 years. The patients were neurologically normal with normal development. CT scans were normal in all cases. A family history of epilepsy was noted in 38 per cent and a past history of febrile convulsions of brief duration in 19 per cent.

Seizure manifestations

The predominant feature of the seizure in these 26 patients was sudden fright or terror manifesting itself as screaming, yelling or calling for the mother (46 per cent), clinging to somebody nearby (54 per cent) or trying to hide (12 per cent). The terrorized expression was sometimes associated with either chewing or swallowing movements (23 per cent); distressed laugh (15 per cent); arrest of speech with glottal noises, moans, and salivation (23 per cent); or autonomic symptoms such as pallor, sweating or abdominal pain (27 per cent). Consciousness seemed to be impaired to some extent. The mean duration of the attack was 1–2 min, maximally 10 min. The seizures took place during sleep and wakefulness and often became frequent soon after the onset, occurring several times a day in 50 per cent of cases. No postictal deficit was observed, although the patient might be sleepy or tired. A few brief nocturnal orofacial clonic seizures were observed at the same period in 15 per cent. No tonic, clonic, tonic-clonic or atonic seizures occurred during the clinical course in any child.

EEG features

The background activity was normal with normal organization of sleep, even during periods with frequent seizures. The commonest interictal paroxysmal abnormalities were sharp waves or sharp and slow waves, similar to the rolandic spikes of BCECT, occurring in the frontotemporal or parietotemporal regions of one or both hemispheres and activated by sleep, without changes in morphology. These occurred in 73 per cent of patients. Brief bursts of generalized spike and waves may be observed alone or in association with focal abnormalities. These generalized discharges might appear during drowsiness but never increased in slow wave sleep.

Ictal records usually showed localized discharges in the frontotemporal, centrotemporal or parietal regions, but more diffuse abnormalities occasionally made localization of the initial discharge difficult.

Pathophysiology

This syndrome has been considered to be a benign functional epilepsy because of its similarity to BCECT, i.e. occurrence in normal children, age of onset, high incidence of positive family history, brief seizures, response to treatment, morphology of spikes, sleep enhancement, and brief generalized spike and waves,[215] but its pathophysiology is unknown. Fright as a main seizure manifestation is of little value in localizing the seizure origin and may only be a nonspecific response of the child to subjective phenomena. The origin of ictal discharges in these children is not as specific as in BCECT.[215] Inconsistency of the origin of ictal discharges and the poor correlation between the focus and affective symptoms suggest that this syndrome may not be a disease entity. Indeed, Dalla Bernardina et al.[215] suggested that benign partial epilepsy with affective symptomatology (BPEA) might not constitute an independent form of idiopathic partial epilepsy but rather a relatively rare variant of BCECT.

We have also had several patients who showed frequent attacks of sudden fright which responded well to carbamazepine, but in whom the interictal EEG did not show spikes. Attempted withdrawal of the medication resulted in relapse of the subjective symptoms in some patients even after treatment for more than 5 years. We considered that these patients probably had frontal lobe epilepsy based on their ictal EEGs. In contrast, those patients who showed similar attacks of terror and interictal rolandic spike-like discharges in the centrotemporal region ultimately became free from seizures on no treatment after the intermittent use of once-daily large doses of diazepam. Thus, the symptoms in benign partial epilepsy with affective symptomatology may represent a nonspecific affective response of young children to somatosensory phenomena occurring in rolandic epilepsy or related conditions, and the affective symptoms may themselves not be epileptic manifestations.

Treatment

Carbamazepine or phenobarbital are the most effective drugs. When the seizure frequency is low, medication may not be necessary.

Prognosis

Most patients respond well to antiepileptic treatment. Three of the 26 patients followed by Dalla Bernardina et al.[214] were never treated and 21 were followed longitudinally. Sixteen of the 21 were eventually seizure-free and off treatment whereas 5 patients, all over 18 years of age, had persistent seizures despite treatment. At the time of frequent seizures, some patients exhibited behavioral and/or intellectual disturbances.

KEY POINTS

Benign childhood epilepsy with centrotemporal spikes (BCECT):

- BCECT is characterized by **brief, simple, partial, hemifacial motor seizures**, frequently having associated somatosensory symptoms, which may evolve into generalized tonic-clonic seizures. Oropharyngeal symptoms and arrest of speech occur frequently
- Seizures occur more often in **sleep**
- The **EEG** has blunt high-voltage centrotemporal spikes, often followed by slow waves that are activated by sleep and tend to shift from side to side

- Only 9 per cent of children with the typical centrotemporal spikes that are characteristic of BCECT have **clinical seizures**
- The **age of onset** is mostly between 4 and 10 years with a peak at 7–9 years
- **Transient behavioral problems and mild cognitive dysfunctions** may occur when the discharges are occurring most frequently but resolve as the epilepsy remits
- All patients eventually enter **remission** without medication whether treated or not

Benign childhood epilepsy with occipital paroxysms (BCEOP):

- The seizures start with **visual symptoms** (amaurosis, phosphenes, illusions, or hallucinations) that are often followed by a hemiclonic seizure or automatisms
- One quarter of the seizures are followed immediately by a **migrainous headache**
- The **EEG** has paroxysms of high-amplitude spike-waves or sharp waves recurring rhythmically in the occipital and posterior temporal areas of one or both hemispheres, but only when the eyes are closed
- Patients have **normal neurologic development, normal neurologic examination** and **normal neuroimaging**
- Complete **seizure control** is achieved in 60 per cent of cases. No patients have typical seizures persisting past adolescence, but other types of seizures have been reported in 5 per cent in adulthood

Panayiotopoulos syndrome:

- The seizures are brief or prolonged, usually nocturnal, **infrequent partial seizures** consisting of deviation of the eyes and vomiting
- The interictal **EEG** demonstrates multifocal high amplitude sharp and slow wave complexes that predominate posteriorly but can involve all brain regions
- The **age of onset** ranges from 1 to 14 years with a peak at 4–5 years
- The children have **normal neurologic development** and a **normal neurologic examination**
- There is often a **family history of febrile seizures**
- Approximately 10–20 per cent of children with similar seizures have brain pathology, and an **MRI** should be considered
- **Remission** occurs within 1 to 2 years from onset but 21 per cent of patients develop other seizure types, usually rolandic seizures, during later childhood and early teens

Benign epilepsy of childhood with complex partial seizures:

- The seizures consist of **impaired consciousness**, often accompanied by staring or eye deviation, nausea and/or vomiting, and focal motor symptoms. Automatisms are infrequent
- The seizures are usually brief, infrequent and **respond well to the initial drug**
- Focal spikes, sharp waves or spike and waves are seen in varying regions except the anterior temporal regions and **do not have a fixed focus**
- **Prognosis is excellent** with disappearance of epileptiform discharges

Benign partial epilepsy with affective symptomatology (BPEA):

- The seizures in these patients involve **sudden fear or terror** and occur both in wakefulness or sleep. There may be swallowing movements, arrest of speech, salivation or autonomic symptoms such as pallor, sweating or abdominal pain
- The episodes **usually last 1–2 min and always <10 min.** The seizures often become frequent soon after the onset and may occur several times a day
- The **age of onset** ranges from 2 to 9 years
- The patients are **neurologically normal with normal development**
- A **family history of epilepsy** was noted in 38 per cent and a past history of febrile convulsions of brief duration in 19 per cent
- The commonest **interictal abnormalities** are sharp waves or sharp and slow waves, similar to the rolandic spikes of BCECT
- Most patients **respond well to antiepileptic treatment** and three quarters are eventually seizure-free off treatment

REFERENCES

1. Proposal for revised classification of epilepsies and epileptic syndromes. Commission on Classification and Terminology of the International League Against Epilepsy. *Epilepsia* 1989; **30**: 389–399.
2. Loiseau P, Beaussart M. The seizures of benign childhood epilepsy with rolandic paroxysmal discharge. *Epilepsia* 1973; **14**: 381–389.
3. Panayiotopoulos CP. The benign occipital epilepsies of childhood: how many syndromes? *Epilepsia* 1999; **40**: 1320–1323.
4. Heijbel J, Blom S, Bergfors PG. Benign epilepsy of children with centro-temporal EEG foci. A study of incidence rate in outpatient care. *Epilepsia* 1975; **16**: 657–664.
5. Sidenvall R, Forsgren L, Blomquist HK, Heijbel J. A community-based prospective incidence study of epileptic seizures in children. *Acta Paediatrica* 1993; **82**: 60–65.
6. Braathen G, Theorell K. A general hospital population of childhood epilepsy. *Acta Paediatrica* 1995; **84**: 1143–1146.
7. Astradsson A, Olafsson E, Ludvigsson P, Bjorgvinsson H, Hauser WA. Rolandic epilepsy: an incidence study in Iceland. *Epilepsia* 1998; **39**: 884–886.
8. Luders H, Lesser RP, Dinner DS, Morris HH III. Benign focal epilepsy of childhood. In: Luders H, Lesser RP (eds) *Electroclinical Syndromes.* Berlin: Springer-Verlag, 1987: 303–346.
9. Blom S, Heijbel J, Bergfors PG. Benign epilepsy of children with centrotemporal EEG foci. Prevalence and follow-up study of 40 patients. *Epilepsia* 1972; **13**: 609–619.
10. Santanelli P, Bureau M, Magaudda A, *et al.* Benign partial epilepsy with centro-temporal (or rolandic) spikes and brain lesion. *Epilepsia* 1989; **30**: 182–188.
11. Piccirilli M, D'Alessandro P, Tiacci C, Ferroni A. Language lateralization in children with benign partial epilepsy. *Epilepsia* 1988; **29**: 19–25.
12. D'Alessandro P, Piccirilli M, Tiacci C, *et al.* Neuropsychological features of benign partial epilepsy in children. *Italian Journal of Neurological Sciences* 1990; **11**: 265–269.
13. Binnie CD, de Silva M, Hurst A. Rolandic spikes and cognitive function. In: Degen R, Dreifuss FE (eds) *Benign Localized and Generalized Epilepsies of Early Childhood (Epilepsy Research,* Suppl. 6). Amsterdam: Elsevier, 1992; 71–73.
14. Kasteleijn-Nolst Trenité DGA, Bakker DJ, *et al.* Psychological effects of subclinical epileptiform EEG discharges. I. Scholastic skills. *Epilepsy Research,* 1988; **2**: 111–116.
15. Aarts JHP, Binnie CD, Smit AM, Wilkins AJ. Selective cognitive impairment during focal and generalized epileptiform EEG activity. *Brain* 1984; **107**: 293–308.
16. Carlsson G, Igelbrink-Schulze N, Neubauer BA, Stephani U. Neuropsychological long-term outcome of rolandic EEG traits. *Epileptic Disorders* 2000; **2**: S63–S66.
17. Croona C, Kihlgren M, Lundberg S, Eeg-Olofsson O, Eeg-Olofsson KE. Neuropsychological findings in children with benign childhood epilepsy with centrotemporal spikes. *Developmental Medicine and Child Neurology,* 1999; **41**: 813–818.
18. Deonna T, Zesiger P, Davidoff V, Maeder M, Mayor C, Roulet E. Benign partial epilepsy of childhood: longitudinal neuropsychological and EEG study of cognitive function. *Developmental Medicine and Child Neurology,* 2000; **42**: 595–603.
19. Gunduz E, Demirbilek V, Korkmaz B. Benign rolandic epilepsy: neuropsychological findings. *Seizure* 1999; **8**: 246–249.
20. Piccirilli M, D'Alessandro P, Sciarma T, *et al.* Attention problems in epilepsy: possible significance of the epileptogenic focus. *Epilepsia* 1994; **35**: 1091–1096.
21. Staden U, Isaaca E, Boyd SG, Brandl U, Neville BG. Language dysfunction in children with Rolandic epilepsy. *Neuropediatrics* 1998; **29**: 242–248.
22. Yung AW, Park YD, Cohen MJ, Garrison TN. Cognitive and behavioral problems in children with centrotemporal spiles. *Pediatric Neurology* 2000; **23**: 391–395.
23. Weglage J, Demsky A, Pietsch M, Kurlemann G. Neuropsychological, intellectual, and behavioral findings in patients with centrotemporal spikes with and without seizures. *Developmental Medicine and Child Neurology* 1997; **39**: 646–651.

24. Baglietto MG, Battaglia FM, Nobili L, *et al.* Neuropsychological disorders related to interictal epileptic discharges during sleep in benign epilepsy of childhood with centrotemporal or Rolandic spikes. *Developmental Medicine and Child Neurology* 2001; **43**: 407–412.

25. Massa R, de Saint-Martin A, Carcangiu R, *et al.* EEG criteria predictive of complicated evolution in idiopathic rolandic epilepsy. *Neurology* 2001; **57**: 1071–1079.

26. Saint-Martin AD, Carcangiu R, Arzimanoglou A, *et al.* Semiology of typical and atypical Rolandic Epilepsy: a video-EEG analysis. *Epileptic Disorders* 2001; **3**: 173–182.

27. Bladin PF. The association of benign rolandic epilepsy with migraine. In: Andermann F, Lugaresi E (eds) *Migraine and Epilepsy.* London: Butterworths, 1987; 145–152.

28. Giroud M, Borsotti JP, Michiel SR, *et al.* Epilepsie et calcifications occipitales bi-laterales: 3 cas. *Revue Neurologique* 1990; **146**: 288–292.

29. Andermann F. Migraine and the benign partial epilepsies of childhood: evidence for an association. *Epileptic Disorders* 2000; **2**: S37–39.

30. Santucci M, Giovanardi Rossi P, Ambrosetto G, *et al.* Migraine and benign epilepsy with rolandic spikes in childhood: a case-control study. *Developmental Medicine and Child Neurology* 1985; **27**: 60–62.

31. Giovanardi Rossi P, Santucci M, Gobbi G, *et al.* Epidemiological study of migraine in epileptic patients. In: Andermann F, Lugaresi E (eds) *Migraine and Epilepsy.* London: Butterworths, 1987; 312–322.

32. Septien L, Pelletier JL, Brunotte F, *et al.* Migraine in patients with history of centro-temporal epilepsy in childhood: a Hm-PAO SPECT study. *Cephalalgia* 1991; **11**: 281–284.

33. Melchionda D, Verrotti A, Chiarelli F, *et al.* Headache in children with centrotemporal spikes. *Neurophysiologie Clinique* 1999; **29**: 90–100.

34. Blom S, Heijbel J. Benign epilepsy of children with centro-temporal EEG foci: discharge rate during sleep. *Epilepsia* 1975; **16**: 133–140.

35. Degen R, Degen HE. Some genetic aspects of rolandic epilepsy: waking and sleep EEGS in siblings. *Epilepsia* 1990; **31**: 795–801.

36. Roger J, Bureau M, Genton P, Dravet C. Idiopathic partial epilepsies. In: Dam M, Gram L (eds) *Comprehensive Epileptology.* New York: Raven Press, 1990; 155–170.

37. Degen R, Degen HE. Contribution to the genetics of rolandic epilepsy: waking and sleep EEGS in siblings. In: Degen R, Dreifuss FE (eds) *Benign Localized and Generalized Epilepsies of Early Childhood.* Amsterdam: Elsevier, 1992; 49–52.

38. Holmes GL. Benign focal epilepsies of childhood. *Epilepsia* 1993; **34**: S49–61.

39. Kajitani T, Nakamura M, Ueoka K, Koduchi S. Three pairs of monozygotic twins with rolandic discharges. In: Wada JA, Penny JK (eds) *Advances in Epileptology, The Tenth International Symposium.* New York: Raven Press, 1980: 171–175.

40. Eeg-Olofsson O. Further genetic aspects in benign localized epilepsies in early childhood. In: Degen R, Dreifuss FE (eds) *Benign Localized and Generalized Epilepsies of Early Childhood* (*Epilepsy Research,* Suppl. 6). Amsterdam: Elsevier, 1992: 117–119.

41. Haga Y, Watanabe K, Negoro T, *et al.* Children with centro-temporal EEG foci. *Journal of the Japanese Epileptic Society* 1992; **10**: 113–118.

42. Rees M, Diebold U, Parker K, Doose H, *et al.* Benign childhood epilepsy with centrotemporal spikes and the focal sharp wave trait is not linked to the fragile X region. *Neuropediatrics* 1993; **24**: 211–213.

43. Whitehouse W, Diebold U, Rees M, *et al.* Exclusion of linkage of genetic focal sharp waves to the HLA region on chromosome 6p in families with benign partial epilepsy with centrotemporal sharp waves. *Neuropediatrics* 1993; **24**: 208–210.

44. Neubauer BA, Moises HW, Lassker U, *et al.* Benign childhood epilepsy with centrotemporal spikes and electroencephalography trait are not linked to EBN1 and EBN2 of benign neonatal familial convulsions. *Epilepsia* 1997; **38**: 782–787.

45. Neubauer BA, Fiedler B, Himmelein B, *et al.* Centrotemporal spikes in families with rolandic epilepsy: linkage to chromosome 15q14. *Neurology* 1998; **51**: 1608–1612.

46. Maihara T, Tsuji M, Higuchi Y, Hattori H. Benign familial neonatal convulsions followed by benign epilepsy with centrotemporal spikes in two siblings. *Epilepsia* 1999; **40**: 110–113.

47. Doose H, Koudriavseva K, Neubauer BA. Multifactorial pathogenesis of neonatal seizures – relationships to the benign partial epilepsies. *Epileptic Disorders* 2000; **2**: 195–201.

48. Burke MS, Carroll JE, Burket RC. Benign rolandic epilepsy and chromosome 7q deletion. *Journal of Child Neurology* 1997; **12**: 148–149.

49. Coppola G, Sciscio N, Russo F, Caliendo G, Pascotto A. Benign idiopathic partial seizures in the velocardiofacial syndrome: Report of two cases. *American Journal of Medical Genetics* 2001; **103**: 172–175.

50. Guerrini R, Bonanni P, Nardocci N, *et al.* Autosomal recessive rolandic epilepsy with paroxysmal exercise-induced dystonia and writer's cramp: delineation of the syndrome and gene mapping to chromosome16p12–11.2. *Annals of Neurology* 1999; **45**: 344–352.

51. Lombroso CT. Sylvian seizures and mid temporal spike foci in children. *Archives of Neurology* 1967; **17**: 52–59.

52. Kellerman K. Recurrent aphasia with subclinical status epilepticus during sleep. *European Journal of Pediatrics* 1978; **128**: 207–212.

53. Roulet E, Deonna T, Despland P.A. Prolonged intermittent drooling and oromotor dyspraxia in benign childhood epilepsy with centro-temporal spikes. *Epilepsia* 1989; **30**: 564–568.

54. Boulloche J, Husson A, Le Luyer B, Le Roux P. Dysphagie, troubles du langage et pointes ondes centro-temporales. *Archives Françaises de Pediatrie,* 1990; **47**: 115–117.

55. Deonna TW, Roulet E, Fontan D, Marcoz J.-P. Speech and oromotor deficits of epileptic origin in benign partial epilepsy of childhood with rolandic spikes (BPERS). Relationship to the acquired aphasia-epilepsy syndrome. *Neuropediatrics* 1993; **24**: 83–87.

56. de Saint-Martin A, Petiau C, Massa R, *et al.* Idiopathic rolandic epilepsy with 'interictal' facial myoclonia and oromotor deficit: a longitudinal EEG and PET study. *Epilepsia* 1999; **40**: 614–620.

57. Kramer U, Ben-Zeev B, Harel S, Kivity S. Transient oromotor deficits in children with benign childhood epilepsy with central temporal spikes. *Epilepsia* 2001; **42**: 616–620.

58. Wirrell EC, Camfield PR, Gordon KE, Dooley JM, Camfield CS. Benign rolandic epilepsy: atypical features are very common. *Journal of Child Neurology* 1995; **10**: 455–458.

59. Lerman P, Kivity S. Focal epileptic EEG discharges in children not suffering from clinical epilepsy. In: Degen R,

Dreifuss FE (eds) *Benign Localized and Generalized Epilepsies of Early Childhood* (*Epilepsy Research*, Suppl. 6). Amsterdam: Elsevier, 1992; 99–103.

60. Beaussart M. Benign epilepsy of children with rolandic (centrotemporal) paroxysmal foci. A clinical entity. Study of 221 cases. *Epilepsia* 1972; **13**: 795–911.

61. Ishikawa T, Nakazato M, Awaya A, *et al.* Benign childhood epilepsy with centrotemporal spikes. Evolution of seizure types. *Acta Paediatrica Japonica* 1988; **30**: 73–77.

62. Fejerman N, Di Blasi AM. Status epilepticus of benign partial epilepsies in children: report of two cases. *Epilepsia* 1987; **28**: 351–355.

63. Colamaria V, Sgro V, Caraballo R. *et al.* Status epilepticus in benign rolandic epilepsy manifesting as anterior opercular syndrome. *Epilepsia* 1991; **32**: 329–334.

64. Fejerman N, Caraballo V, Korkmaz B, Dervent A, Townes BD. Neuropsychological function in idiopathic occipital lobe epilepsy. *Epilepsia* 2000; **41**: 405–411.

65. Lerman P, Kivity S. Benign focal epilepsy of childhood, A follow up of 100 recovered patients. *Archives of Neurology* 1975; **32**: 261–264.

66. Ambrosetto G, Giovanardi Rossi P, Tassinari CA. Predictive factors of seizure frequency and duration of antiepileptic treatment in rolandic epilepsy: a retrospective study. *Brain Development* 1987; **9**: 300–304.

67. Hongo K, Naganuma Y, Murakami M, *et al.* Development of EEG background activity in children with benign partial epilepsy. *Japanese Journal of Psychiatry and Neurology* 1990; **44**: 367–368.

68. Braga NI, Manzano GM, Nobrega JA. Quantitative analysis of EEG background activity in patients with rolandic spikes. *Clinical Neurophysiology* 2000; **111**: 1643–1645.

69. Mitsudome A, Ohu M, Yasumoto S, Ogawa A. Rhythmic slow activity in benign childhood epilepsy with centrotemporal spikes. *Clinical Electroencephalography* 1997; **28**: 44–48.

70. Legarda S, Jayakar P, Duchowny M, Alvarez L, Resnick T. Benign rolandic epilepsy: high central and low central subgroups. *Epilepsia* 1994; **35**: 1125–1129.

71. van der Meij W, Wieneke GH, van Huffelen AC, Schenk-Rootlieb AJ, Willemse J. Identical morphology of the rolandic spike-and-wave complex in different clinical entities. *Epilepsia* 1993; **34**: 540–550.

72. Frost JD Jr, Hrachovy RA, Glaze DG. Spike morphology in childhood focal epilepsy: relationship to syndromic classification. *Epilepsia* 1992; **33**: 531–536.

73. Kellaway P. The electroencephalographic features of benign centrotemporal (rolandic) epilepsy of childhood. *Epilepsia* 2000; **41**: 1053–1056.

74. Lerman, P. Benign partial epilepsy with centro-temporal spikes. In: Roger J, Bureau M, Dravet C *et al.* (eds) *Epileptic Syndromes in Infancy, Childhood and Adolescence*, 2nd edn. London: John Libbey, 1992; 189–200.

75. Clemens B, Majoros E. Sleep studies in benign epilepsy of childhood with rolandic spikes. II. Analysis of discharge frequency and its relation to sleep dynamics. *Epilepsia* 1987; **28**: 24–27.

76. Gregory DL, Wong PK. Topographical analysis of the centrotemporal discharges in benign rolandic epilepsy of childhood. *Epilepsia* 1984; **25**: 705–711.

77. Graf M, Lischka A, Gremel K. Benign rolandic epilepsy in children. Topographic EEG analysis. *Wiener Klinische Wochenschrift* 1990; **102**: 206–210.

78. Graf M, Lischka A. Topographic EEG analysis of rolandic spikes. *Clinical Electroencephalography* 1998; **29**: 132–137.

79. Wong PKH. Stability of source estimates in rolandic spikes. *Brain Topography* 1989; **2**: 31–36.

80. Weinberg H, Wong PKH, Crisp D. *et al.* Use of multiple dipole analysis for the classification of benign rolandic epilepsy. *Brain Topography* 1990; **3**: 183–190.

81. Yoshinaga H, Amano R, Oka E, Ohtahara S. Dipole tracing in childhood epilepsy with special reference to rolandic epilepsy. *Brain Topography* 1992; **4**: 193–199.

82. Tsai ML, Hung KL. Topographic mapping and clinical analysis of benign childhood epilepsy with centrotemporal spikes. *Brain Development* 1998; **20**: 27–32.

83. Minami T, Gondo K, Yamamoto T, Yanai S, Tasaki K, Ueda K. Magnetoencephalographic analysis of rolandic discharges in benign childhood epilepsy. *Annals of Neurology* 1996; **39**: 326–334.

84. Kamada K, Moller M, Kassubek J, *et al.* Localization analysis of neuronal activities in benign rolandic epilepsy using magnetoencephalography. *Journal of the Neurological Sciences* 1998; **154**: 164–172.

85. Otsubo H, Chitoku S, Ochi A, *et al.* Malignant rolandic-sylvian epilepsy in children: diagnosis, treatment, andoutcomes. *Neurology* 2001; **57**: 590–596.

86. Van der Meij W, Wieneke GH, van Huffelen AC. Dipole source analysis of rolandic spikes in benign rolandic epilepsy and other clinical syndromes. *Brain Topography* 1993; **5**: 203–213.

87. Legarda S, Jayakar P. Electroclinical significance of rolandic spikes and dipoles in neurodevelopmentally normal children. *Electroencephalography and Clinical Neurophysiology* 1995; **95**: 257–259.

88. Van der Meij W, Van Huffelen AC, Wieneke GH, Willemse J. Sequential EEG mapping may differentiate 'epileptic' from 'nonepileptic' rolandic spikes. *Electroencephalography and Clinical Neurophysiology* 1992; **82**: 408–414.

89. Nicholl JS, Willis JK, Rice J. The effect of hyperventilation on the frequency of rolandic spikes. *Clinical Electroencephalography* 1998; **29**: 181–182.

90. Colamaria V, Sgro V, Caraballo R, *et al.* Status epilepticus in benign rolandic epilepsy manifesting as anterior opercular syndrome. *Epilepsia* 1991; **32**: 329–334.

91. Fonseca LC, Tedrus GM, Bastos A, Bosco A, Laloni DT. Reactivity of rolandic spikes. *Clinical Electroencephalography* 1996; **27**: 116–120.

92. Veggiotti P, Beccaria F, Gatti A, *et al.* Can protrusion of the tongue stop seizures in rolandic epilepsy? *Epileptic Disorders* 1999; **1**: 217–220.

93. Degen R, Holthausen H, Pieper T, Txhorn I, Wolf P. Benign epileptic discharges in patients with lesional partial epilepsies. *Pediatric Neurology* 1999; **20**: 354–359.

94. Drury I, Beydoun A. Benign partial epilepsy of childhood with monomorphic sharp waves in centrotemporal and other locations. *Epilepsia* 1991; **32**: 662–667.

95. Dalla Bernardina B, Beghini G. Rolandic spikes in children with and without epilepsy (20 subjects polygraphically studied during sleep). *Epilepsia* 1976; **17**: 161–167.

96. Amit R. Benign focal epilepsy of childhood: Individual and intrafamilial multifocality of spikes. *Clinical Electroencephalography* 1987; **18**: 169–172.

97. Luders H, Lesser RP, Dinner DS, Morris HH III. Benign focal epilepsy of childhood. In: Luders H, Lesser RP (eds) *Electroclinical Syndromes*. Berlin: Springer-Verlag, 1987; 303–346.

98. Watanabe K. The localization related epilepsies: some problems with subclassification. *Japanese Journal of Psychiatry and Neurology* 1989; **43**: 471–475.

99. Beydoun A, Garofalo EA and Drury I.Generalized spike-waves, multiple loci, and clinical course in children with EEG features of benign epilepsy of childhood with centrotemporal spikes. *Epilepsia* 1992; **33**: 1091–1096.

100. Holmes GL. Rolandic epilepsy: clinical and electroencephalographic features. In: Degen R, Dreifuss FE (eds) *Benign Localized and Generalized Epilepsies of Early Childhood*. Amsterdam: Elsevier, 1992; 29–43.

101. Petersen J, Nielsen CJ, Gulmann NC. Atypical EEG abnormalities in children with benign partial (rolandic) epilepsy. *Acta Neurologica Scandinavica* 1983; **67**: 57–62.

102. Dalla Bernardina B, Tassinari CA. EEG of a nocturnal seizure in a patient with benign epilepsy of childhood with rolandic spikes. *Epilepsia* 1975; **16**: 497–501.

103. Gutierrez AR, Brick JF, Bodensteiner J. Dipole reversal: an ictal feature of benign partial epilepsy with centrotemporal spikes. *Epilepsia* 1990; **31**: 544–548.

104. Silva DF, Lima MM, Anghinah R, Zanoteli E, Lima JG. Dipole reversal: an ictal feature in a patient with benign partial epilepsy of childhood with centro-temporal spike. *Arquivos de Neuropsiquiatria*, 1995; **53**: 270–273.

105. Gregory DL, Wong PK. Topographical analysis of the centrotemporal discharges in benign rolandic epilepsy of childhood. *Epilepsia* 1984; **25**: 705–711.

106. Wong PK. Source modelling of the rolandic focus. *Brain Topography* 1991; **4**: 105–112.

107. Kubota M, Oka A, Kin S, Sakakihara Y. Generators of rolandic discharges identified by magnetoencephalography. *Electroencephalography and Clinical Neurophysiology* 1996; **47**: 393–401.

108. Van der Meij W, Huiskamp GJ, Rutlen GJ, et al. The existence of two sources in rolandic epilepsy: confirmation with high resolution EEG, MEG and fMRI. *Brain Topography* 2001; **13**: 275–282.

109. Manganotti P, Miniussi C, Santorum E, et al. Scalp topology and source analysis of interictal spontaneous spikes and evoked spikes by digital stimulation in benign rolandic epilepsy. *Electroencephalography and Clinical Neurophysiology* 1998; **107**: 18–26.

110. Manganotti P, Miniussi C, Santorum E, et al. Influence of somatosensory input on paroxysmal activity in benign rolandic epilepsy with 'extreme simatosensory evoked potentials'. *Brain* 1998; **121**: 647–658.

111. Manganotti P, Zanette G, Beltramello A, et al. Spike topography and functional magetic resonance imaging (FMRI) in benign rolandic epilepsy with spikes evoked by tapping stimulation. *Electroencephalography and Clinical Neurophysiology* 1998; **107**: 88–92.

112. Ferri R, Del Gracco S, Elia M, Musumeci SA. Age-related changes of cortical excitability in subjects with sleep enhanced centrotemporal spikes: a somatosensory evoked potential study. *Clinical Neurophysiology* 2000; **111**: 591–599.

113. Bouma PA, Bovenkerk AC, Westendorp RG, Brouwer OF. The course of benign partial epilepsy of childhood with centrotemporal spikes: a meta-analysis. *Neurology* 1997; **48**: 430–437.

114. Kubota M, Takeshita K, Sakakihara Y, Yanagisawa M. Magnetoencephalographic study of giant somatosensory evoked responses in patients with rolandic epilepsy. *Journal of Child Neurology* 2000; **15**: 370–379.

115. Manganotti P, Zanette G. Contribution of motor cortex in generation of evoked spiles in patients with benign rolandic epilepsy. *Clinical Neurophysiology* 2000; **111**: 964–974.

116. Heijbel J, Blom S, Rasmuson M. Benign epilepsy of children with centrotemporal EEG foci. A genetic study. *Epilepsia* 1975; **16**: 285–293.

117. Doose AH, Baier WK. Benign partial epilepsy and related conditions: multifactorial pathogenesis with hereditary impairment of brain maturation. *European Journal of Pediatrics* 1989; **149**: 152–158.

118. Panayiotopoulos CP. Benign childhood partial epilepsies: benign childhood seizure susceptibility syndrome. *Journal of Neurology Neurosurgery, and Psychiatry* 1993; **56**: 2–5.

119. Parmeggiani L, Guerrini R. Idiopathic partial epilepsy: electroclinical demonstration of a prolonged seizure with sequential rolantic and occipital involvement. Seizure spread due to regional susceptibility? *Epileptic Disorders* 1999; **1**: 35–40.

120. Ramelli GP, Donati F, Moser H, Vassella F. Concomitance of childhood absence and Rolandic epilepsy. *Clinical Electroencephalography* 1998; **29**: 177–180.

121. Gambardella A, Aguglia U, Guerrini R, et al. Sequential occurrence of benign partial epilepsy and childhood absence epilepsy in three patients. *Brain Development* 1996; **18**: 212–215.

122. Gelisse P, Genton P, Bureau M, et al. Are there generalised spike waves and typical absences in benign rolandic epilepsy? *Brain Development* 1999; **21**: 390–396.

123. Kraschnitz W, Scheer P, Korner K, et al. Rolandic spikes alselektroenzephalographische Manifestation eines Oligodendroglioma. *Pediatrie and Pedologie* 1988; **23**: 313–319.

124. Ambrosetto G. Unilateral opercular macrogyria and benign childhood epilepsy with centrotemporal (rolandic) spikes: report of a case. *Epilepsia* 1992; **33**: 499–503.

125. Shevell MI, Rosenblatt B, Watters GV, O'Gorman AM, Montes JL. 'Pseudo-BECRS': intracranial focal lesions suggestive of a primary partial epilepsy syndrome. *Pediatric Neurology* 1996; **14**: 31–35.

126. Sheth RD, Gutierrez AR, Rigga JE. Rolandic epilepsy and cortical dysplasia: MRI correlation of epileptiform discharges.*Pediatric Neurology* 1997; **17**: 177–179.

127. Gelisse P, Genton P,Raybaud C, Thiry A, Pincemaille O. Benign childhood epilepsy with centrotemporal spikes and hippocampal atrophy. *Epilepsia* 1999; **40**: 1312–1315.

128. Lundberg S, Eeg-Olfsson O, Raininko R, Eeg-Olfsson KE. Hippocampal asymmetries on MRI in benign childhood epilepsy with centrotemporal spikes. *Epilepsia* 1999; **40**: 1808–1815.

129. Van Bogaert P, Wikler D, Damhaut P, Szliwowski HB, Goldman S. Cerebral glucose metabolism and centrotemporal spikes. *Epilepsy Research* 1998; **29**: 123–127.

130. Laub MC, Funke R, Kirsch CM, Oberst U. BECT: comparison of cerebral flow imaging, neuropsychological testing and long-term EEG monitoring. In: Degen R, Dreifuss FE (eds) *Benign Localized and Generalized Epilepsies of Early Childhood* (*Epilepsy Research,* Suppl. 6). Amsterdam: Elsevier, 1992; 95–98.

131. Farnarier G, Bureau M, Mancini J. and Regis H. Etude des potentiels evoques multimodalitaires dans les epilepsies partielles de l'enfant. *Neurophysiologie Clinique* 1988; **18**: 243–254.

132. Plasmati R, Michelucci R, Forti A, *et al.* The neurophysiological features of benign partial epilepsy with rolandic spikes. In: Degen R, Dreifuss FE (eds) *Benign Localized and Generalized Epilepsies of Early Childhood* (*Epilepsy Research,* Suppl. 6). Amsterdam: Elsevier, 1992; 45–48.

133. Clemens B, Olah R. Sleep studies in benign epilepsy of childhood with rolandic spikes, I. Sleep pathology. *Epilepsia* 1987; **28**: 20–23.

134. Baldy-Moulinier M. Sleep organization in benign childhood partial epilepsies. In: Degen R, Dreifuss FE (eds) *Benign Localized and Generalized Epilepsies of Early Childhood* (*Epilepsy Research,* Suppl. 6). Amsterdam: Elsevier, 1992; 121–124.

135. Ambrosetto G, Tassinari CA. Antiepileptic drug treatment of benign childhood epilepsy with rolandic spikes: is it neccesary? *Epilepsia* 1990; **31**: 802–805.

136. Peters JM, Camfield CS, Camfield PR. Population study of benign rolandic epilepsy: is treatment needed? *Neurology* 2001; **57**: 537–539.

137. Corda D, Gelisse P, Genton P, Dravet C, Baldy-Moulinier M. Incidence of drug-induced aggravation in benign epilepsy with centrotemporal spikes. *Epilepsia* 2001; **42**: 754–759.

138. Nanba Y, Maegaki Y. Epileptic negative myoclonus by carbamazepin in a child with BECTS. Benign childhood epilepsy with centrotemporal spikes. *Pediatric Neurology* 1999; **21**: 664–667.

139. Seidel WT, Mitchell WG. Cognitive and behavioral effects of carbamazepine in children: data from benign rolandic epilepsy. *Journal of Child Neurology* 1999; **14**: 716–723.

140. Bourgeois BFD. Drug treatment of benign focal epilepsies of childhood. *Epilepsia* 2000; **41**: 1057–1058.

141. Rating D, Wolf C, Bast T. Sulthiame as monotherapy in children with benign childhood epilepsy with centrotemporal spikes: a 6-month randomized, double-blind, placebo-controlled study. Suithiame Study Group. *Epilepsia* 2000; **41**: 1284–1288.

142. Weglage J, Pietsch M, Sprinz A, *et al.* A previously unpublished side-effect of sulthiame in a patient with Rolandic epilepsy. *Neuropediatrics* 1999; **30**: 50.

143. Brockmann K, Hanefeld F. Progressive elevation of liver enzymes in a child treated with sulthiame. *Neuropediatrics* 2001; **32**: 165–166.

144. Loiseau P. Benign focal epilepsies of childhood. In: Wyllie E (ed.) *The Treatment of Epilepsy. Principle and Practice.* Philadelphia: Lea & Febiger, 1993; 503–512.

145. De Romanis F, Feliciani M, Ruggieri S. Rolandic paroxysmal epilepsy: a long term study in 150 children. *Italian Journal of the Neurological Sciences* 1986; **7**: 77–80.

146. Loiseau P, Duche B, Cordova S, *et al.* Prognosis of benign childhood epilepsy with centro-temporal spikes: a follow-up study of 168 patients. *Epilepsia* 1988; **29**: 229–235.

147. Blom S, Heijbel J. Benign epilepsy of children with centrotemporal EEG foci: a follow-up study in adulthood of patients initially studied as children. *Epilepsia* 1982; **23**: 629–632.

148. Ambrosetto G, Tinuper P, Baruzzi A. Relapse of benign partial epilepsy of children in adulthood: report of a case. *Journal of Neurology Neurosurgery and Psychiatry* 1985; **48**: 90.

149. Lerman P, Kivity S. The benign focal epilepsies of childhood. In: Pedley TA, Meldrum BS (eds) *Recent Advances in Epilepsy,* Vol. 11. Edinburgh: Churchill Livingstone, 1986; 137–156.

150. Loiseau P, Duche B, Cohadon S. Prognosis of benign localized epilepsy in early childhood. In: Degen R, Dreifuss FE (eds) *Benign Localized and Generalized Epilepsies of Early Childhood.* Amsterdam: Elsevier, 1992; 71–77.

151. Morikawa T, Seino M, Yagi K. Is rolandic discharge a hallmark of benign partial epilepsy of childhood? In: Degen R, Dreifuss FE (eds) *Benign Localized and Generalized Epilepsies of Early Childhood.* Amsterdam: Elsevier, 1992; 59–69.

152. Verrotti A, Latini G, Trotta D, *et al.* Typical and atypical rolandic epilepsy in childhood: a follow-up study. *Pediatric Neurology* 2002; **26**: 26–29.

153. Gastaut H. 'Benign' or 'functional' (versus 'organic') epilepsies in different stages of life: an analysis of the corresponding age-related variations in the predisposition to epilepsy. *Electroencephalography and Clinical Neurophysiology Supplement* 1982; 17–44.

154. Gastaut H. Benign epilepsy of childhood with occipital paroxysms. In: Roger J, Dravet C, Bureau M, Dreifuss FE, Wolf P (eds) *Epileptic Syndromes in Infancy, Childhood and Adolescence.* London: John Libbey Eurotext, 1985; 159–170.

155. Gastaut H, Zifkin BG. Benign epilepsy of childhood with occipital spike and wave complexes. In: Andermann F, Luagresi E (eds) *Migraine and Epilepsy.* London: Butterworths, 1987; 47–81.

156. Newton R, Aicardi J. Clinical findings in children with occipital spike wave complexes suppressed by eye opening. *Neurology* 1983; **33**: 1526–9152.

157. Aicardi J, Newton R. Clinical findings in children with occipital spike wave complexes suppressed by eye opening. In: Andermann F, Luagresi E (eds) *Migraine and Epilepsy.* London: Butterworths, 1987; 111–124.

158. Aso K, Watanabe K, Negoro T, *et al.* Visual seizures in children. *Epilepsy Research,* 1987; **1**: 246–253.

159. Aso K, Watanabe K, Negoro T, *et al.* Occipital epileptiform discharges in children. *Journal of the Japanese Epileptic Society* 1988; **6**: 103–110.

160. Cooper GW, Lee SI. Reactive occipital epileptiform activity: is it benign? *Epilepsia* 1991; **32**: 63–68.

161. Talwar D, Rask CA, Torres F. Clinical manifestations in children with occipital spike-wave paroxysms. *Epilepsia* 1992; **33**: 667–674.

162. Roger J, Bureau M. Benign epilepsy of childhood with occipital paroxysms. Update. In: Roger J, Bureau M, Dravet C *et al.* (eds) *Epileptic Syndromes in Infancy, Childhood and Adolescence.* London: John Libbey, 1992; 205–215.

163. Martinovic Z. Clinical correlations of electroencephalographic occipital epileptiform paroxysms in children. *Seizure* 2001; **10**: 379–381.

164. Dalla-Bernardina B, Chiamenti C, Capovilla, G. and Colomaria V. Benign partial epilepsies in childhood. In: Roger J, Bureau M, Dravet C et al. (eds) Epileptic Syndromes in Infancy, Childhood and Adolescence. London: John Libbey, 1985; 137–149.

165. Dalla Bernardina B, Sgro V, Fontana E, et al. Idiopathic partial epilepsies in children. In: Roger J, Bureau M, Dravet C et al. (eds) Epileptic Syndromes in Infancy, Childhood and Adolescence. London: John Libbey, 1992; 173–188.

166. Beaumanoir A, Thomas P. Benign epilepsy of childhood with occipital paroxysms. In: Degen R, Dreifuss FE (eds) Benign Localized and Generalized Epilepsies in Early Childhood. Amsterdam: Elsevier, 1992; 105–109.

167. Dalla-Bernardina B, Bondavalli S, Colomaria V. Benign epilepsy of childhood with rolandic spikes (BERS) during sleep. In: Sterman MB, Shouse MN, Passouant P (eds) Sleep and Epilepsy. London: Academic Press, 1985; 495–506.

168. Panayiotopoulos CP. Benign childhood epilepsy with occipital paroxysms. A 15 year prospective study. Annals of Neurology 1989; 26: 51–56.

169. Kivity S, Lermn P. Benign partial epilepsy of childhood with occipital discharges. In: Manelis J, Bental E, Loeber JN, Dreifuss FE (eds) The XVIIth Epilepsy International Symposium (Advances in Epileptology, vol. 17). New York: Raven Press, 1989; 371–373.

170. Fois A, Malandrini F, Tomaccini D. Clinical findings in children with occipital paroxysmal discharges. Epilepsia 1988; 29: 620–623.

171. Kuzniecky R, Rosenblatt B. Benign occipital epilepsy: a family study. Epilepsia 1987; 28: 346–350.

172. Nagendran K, Prior PF. Rossiter myoclonic absences. Benign occipital epilepsy of childhood: a family study. Journal of the Royal Society of Medicine 1989; 82: 684–685.

173. Terasaki T, Yamatogi Y, Ohtahara S. Electroclinical delineation of occipital lobe epilepsy in childhood. In: Andermann F, Lugaresi E (eds) Migraine and Epilepsy. London: Butterworth, 1987; 125–137.

174. Lerman P, Kivity S. The benign partial nonrolandic epilepsies. Journal of Clinical Neurophysiology 1991; 8: 275–287.

175. Andermann F, Zifkin B. The benign occipital epilepsies of childhood: an overview of the idiopathic syndromes and of the relationship to migraine. Epilepsia 1998; 39: S9–S23.

176. Panayiotopoulos CP. Difficulties in differentiating migraine and epilepsy based on clinical and electroencephalographic findings. In: Andermann F, Lugaresi E (eds) Migraine and Epilepsy. London: Butterworth, 1987; 31–46.

177. Terzano MG, Manzoni GC, Parrino, L. Benign epilepsy with occipital paroxysms and migraine: the question of intercalated attacks. In: Andermann F, Lugaresi E (eds) Migraine and Epilepsy. London: Butterworth, 1987; 83–96.

178. Panayiotopoulos CP. Benign childhood epilepsy with occipital paroxysms. In: Andermann F,. Beaumanoir A, Mira L, et al. (eds) Occipital Seizures and Epilepsies in Children. London: John Libbey, 1993; 151–164.

179. Panayiotopoulos CP, Inhibitory effect of central vision on occipital lobe seizure. Neurology 1981; 31: 1331–1333.

180. Lugaresi J, Cirignotta F, Montagna P. Occipital lobe epilepsy with scotosensitive seizures: the role of central vision. Epilepsia 1984; 25: 115–120.

181. Vivegano F, Ricci S. Benign occipital epilepsy of childhood with prolonged seizures and autonomic symptoms. In: Andermann F,

Beaumanoir A, Mira L, et al. (eds) Occipital Seizures and Epilepsies in Children. London: John Libbey, 1993; 133–140.

182. Fois A, Malandrini F, Tomaccini D. Clinical findings in children with occipital paroxysmal discharges. Epilepsia 1988; 29: 620–623.

183. Watanabe K. The localization related epilepsies: some problems with subclassification. Japanese Journal of Psychiatry and Neurology 1989; 43: 471–475.

184. Deonna T, Ziegler AL, Despland PA. Paroxysmal visual disturbances of epileptic origin and occipital epilepsy in children. Neuropediatrics 1984; 15: 131–135.

185. Herranz-Tanarro F, Saenz-Lope E, Cristobal-Sassot S. La pointe-onde occipitale avec et sans epilepsie benigne chez l'enfant. Revue d'Electroencephalographie et de Neurophysiologi Clinique 1984; 14: 1–7.

186. Beaumanoir A. Infantile epilepsy with occipital focus and good prognosis. European Neurology 1983; 22: 43–52.

187. Gobbi G, Sorrenti G, Santucci M, et al. Epilepsy with bilateral occipital calcifications: a benign onset with progressive severity. Neurology 1988; 38: 913–920.

188. Vivegano F, Ricci S. Benign occipital epilepsy of childhood with prolonged seizures and autonomic symptoms. In: Andermann F, Beaumanoir A, Mira L, et al. (eds) Occipital Seizures and Epilepsies in Children. London: John Libbey, 1993; 133–140.

189. Panayiotopoulos CP. Early-onset benign childhood occipital seizure susceptibility syndrome: a syndrome to recognize. Epilepsia 1999; 40: 621–630.

190. Yang S, Iwata Y, Negoro T, et al. [Benign childhood epilepsy with occipital paroxysms (early-onset variant)] (in Japanese). Shonika Rinsho 2000; 53: 197–202.

191. Verrotti A, Domizio S, Guerra M, et al. Childhood epilepsy with occipital paroxysms and benign nocturnal childhood occipital epilepsy. Journal of Child Neurology 2000; 15: 218–221.

192. Caraballo RH, Cersosimo R, Medina C, Fejerman N. Panayiotopoulos-type benign childhood occipital epilepsy: a prospective study. Neurology 2000; 55: 1096–1100.

193. Tsai ML, Lo HY, Chaou WT. Clinical and electroencephalographic findings in early and late onset benign childhood epilepsy with occipital paroxysms. Brain Development 2001; 23: 401–405.

194. Oguni H, Hayashi K, Imai K, et al. Study on the early-onset variant of benign childhood epilepsy with occipital paroxysms otherwise described as early-onset benign occipital seizure susceptibility syndrome. Epilepsia 1999; 40: 1020–1030.

195. Oguni H, Hayashi K, Funatsuka M, Osawa M. Study on early-onset benign occipital seizure susceptibility syndrome. Pediatric Neurology 2001; 25(4): 312–318.

196. Panayiotopoulos CP. Benign nocturnal childhood epilepsy: a new syndrome with nocturnal seizures, tonic deviation of the eyes, and vomiting. Journal of Child Neurology 1989; 4: 43–48.

197. Ferrie CD, Beaumanoir A, Guerrini R, et al. Early-onset benign occipital seizure susceptibility syndrome. Epilepsia 1997; 38: 285–293.

198. Panayiotopoulos CP. Extraoccipital benign childhood partial seizures with ictal vomiting and excellent prognosis. Journal of Neurology, Neurosurgery and Psychiatry 1999; 66: 82–85.

199. Panayiotopoulos CP. Panayiotopoulos Syndrome. A Common and Benign Childhood Epileptic Syndrome. London: John Libbey, 2002.

200. Panayiotopoulos CP. Benign childhood epileptic syndrome with occipital spikes: new classification proposed by the International League Against Epilepsy. *Journal of Child Neurology* 2000; **15**: 548–552.

201. Doose H, Petersen B, Neubauer BA. Occipital sharp waves in idiopathic partial epilepsies – clinical and genetic aspects. *Epilepsy Research* 2002; **48**: 121–130.

202. Panayiotopoulos CP, Igoe DM. Cerebral insult-like partial status epilepticus in the early-onset variant of benign childhood epilepsy with occipital paroxysms. *Seizure* 1992; **1**: 99–102.

203. Kivity S, Lerman P. Stormy onset with prolonged loss of consciousness in benign childhood epilepsy with occipital paroxysms. *Journal of Neurology, Neurosurgery and Psychiatry* 1992; **55**: 45–48.

204. Verrotti A, Domizio S, Melchionda D, *et al.* Stormy onset of benign childhood epilepsy with occipital paroxysmal discharges. *Child's Nervous System* 2000; **16**(1): 35–39.

205. Ferrie CD, Beaumanoir A, Guerrini R, *et al.* Early-onset benign occipital seizure susceptibility syndrome. *Epilepsia* 1997; **38**: 285–293.

206. Guerrini R, Bonanni P, Parmeggiani L, Belmonte A. Adolescent onset of idiopathic photosensitive occipital epilepsy after remission of benign rolandic epilepsy. *Epilepsia* 1997; **38**: 777–781.

207. Doose H, Petersen B, Neubauer BA. Occipital sharp waves in idiopathic partial epilepsies – clinical and genetic aspects. *Epilepsy Research* 2002; **48**: 121–130.

208. Vigevano F, Lispi ML, Ricci S. Early onset benign occipital susceptibility syndrome: video-EEG documentation of an illustrative case. *Clinical Neurophysiology* 2000; **111**(Suppl. 2): S81–86.

209. Sakagami M, Takahashi Y, Matsuoka H, *et al.* A case of early-onset benign occipital seizure susceptibility syndrome: decreased cerebral blood flow in the occipital region detected by interictal single photon emission computed tomography, corresponding to the epileptogenic focus. *Brain Development* 2001; **23**: 427–430.

210. Caraballo RH, Astorino F, Cersosimo R, Soprano AM, Fejerman N. Atypical evolution in childhood epilepsy with occipital paroxysms (Panayiotopoulos type). *Epileptic Disorders* 2001; **3**: 157–162.

211. Furune S, Nomura K, Matsumoto A, *et al.* Classification of epilepsies and epileptic syndromes in clinical practice. *Japanese Journal of Psychiatry and Neurology* 1994; **48**: 358–359.

212. Ishiguro Y, Okumura A, Nomura K, *et al.* A pilot study on benign partial epilepsy in children with complex partial seizures. *Seizure* 2001; **10**: 194–196.

213. Watanabe K, Takahashi I, Negoro T, Aso K, Miura K. Benign epilepsy of children with complex partial seizures following febrile convulsions. *Seizure* 1993; **2**: 57–61.

214. Dalla Bernardina B, Bureau M, Dravet C, *et al.* Epilepsie benigne de l'enfant avec crises à semiologie affective. *Revue d'Electroencephalographie et de Neurophysiologie Clinique* 1980; **10**: 8–18.

215. Dalla Bernardina B, Colamaria V, Chiamerti C, *et al.* Benign partial epilepsy with affective symptoms (benign psychomotor epilepsy). In: Roger J, Bureau M, Dravet C, *et al. Epileptic Syndromes in Infancy, Childhood and Adolescence.* London: John Libbey, 1992; 219–223.

Rasmussen syndrome

MARY B CONNOLLY AND KEVIN FARRELL

Rasmussen syndrome is a rare, progressive neurologic disorder, which begins in childhood and is characterized by seizures that are difficult to control, slowly progressive hemiparesis and progressive cognitive decline.[1,2] Unilateral, progressive hemispheric involvement is a characteristic feature and bilateral disease is rare. Epilepsia partialis continua (EPC) occurs in 50 per cent of patients and Rasmussen syndrome is the most common cause of EPC in childhood.

CLINICAL FEATURES

The illness begins typically between 14 months and 14 years of age, although onset in adulthood has been reported.[2] A viral or inflammatory illness occurred in the month before the onset of seizures in 40 per cent of patients in one retrospective series,[2] and an association with iritis has been reported.[3] Seizures are the commonest initial neurologic feature. Partial motor seizures are the most common seizure type and EPC, which is often difficult to control, occurs in half of the patients. Complex partial seizures, secondarily generalized tonic-clonic seizures and status epilepticus, also occur commonly. The seizures are usually difficult to control, and two thirds of the patients have daily seizures. There is a progressive hemiparesis in all patients, which usually evolves over months and years. Fine finger movement is eventually lost, but patients remain able to walk. Cognitive decline is characteristic and 85 per cent of patients become mentally retarded. Hemianopsia occurs in 50 per cent of patients and sensory deficits, dysarthria, dysphasia and psychiatric abnormalities are common.

DIFFERENTIAL DIAGNOSIS

Unilateral cortical dysplasia, mitochondrial disease, subacute measles in the immunocompromized patient and tick-borne Russian spring and summer encephalitis may also manifest with intractable seizures and progressive, unilateral hemispheric dysfunction.

INVESTIGATIONS

Electroencephalography

A persistent polymorphic delta activity, localized initially to one region, followed by slowing of the posterior dominant rhythm in the affected hemisphere, has been described early in the course of the disease.[4] Gradually the slow wave activity spreads to involve multiple lobes of the brain. When the disease is established, disturbance of background activity and focal delta activity occur in nearly all patients. These abnormalities may be bilateral, but there is a clear asymmetry in 90 per cent.[5] Multiple independent interictal epileptiform discharges are usually seen, occurring over the affected hemisphere in half of the patients and independently over both hemispheres in one third. Bilateral synchronous spike or sharp and slow wave complexes are observed in half of the patients, often with bifrontal predominance.

EPC may be associated with a contralateral spike wave focus involving the rolandic area,[5] but there is often no EEG correlate. Back-averaging of spikes may help to demonstrate an EEG correlate in some patients.[6] Seizures arising independently from both hemispheres have been reported rarely, usually later in the course of the disease.

Neuroimaging

CT and MRI demonstrate progressive cerebral atrophy that typically begins around the sylvian fissure and eventually may involve the entire affected hemisphere.[7] Atrophy of the contralateral hemisphere has been reported. PET and SPECT have demonstrated hypometabolism and hypoperfusion of the affected hemisphere.

Other investigations

Cerebrospinal fluid (CSF) is typically normal on examination, but lymphocytosis and oligoclonal bands have been observed.[8] Brain biopsy should be considered when hemispheric surgery or immunosuppressive therapy is contemplated, but may not be required when the clinical and neuroimaging evolution is classical. Brain biopsy is subject to sampling error, and a negative biopsy does not exclude the diagnosis.[8] Dual pathology with cortical dysplasia and neoplasms has been reported.[8]

PATHOLOGY

The characteristic pathologic features consist of perivascular lymphocytic cuffing with proliferation of microglial nodules. Neuronophagia may be seen, usually involving the medium-sized pyramidal cells of the external pyramidal layer.[8] The pathological process involves primarily the cerebral cortex; inflammation of deep white matter is rarely observed. Neuronal loss may be seen multifocally within the inflamed cortex and patchy distribution of abnormalities may result in a falsely negative brain biopsy. Involvement of the basal ganglia, cerebellum and inflammation of the meninges have been described in autopsy studies. Although neuropsychologic and EEG studies demonstrate bilateral abnormalities in many patients, seven of the ten brains studied at autopsy demonstrated no involvement of the contralateral hemisphere with only scattered perivascular cuffs in three.[9]

ETIOLOGY

The etiology of Rasmussen syndrome is unknown, but immune factors probably play a role. The genomes of various herpes viruses, including cytomegalovirus, herpes simplex virus types 1 and 6 and Epstein-Barr virus, have been identified in tissue resected from some but not all patients.[9] However, inclusion bodies and virus particles have never been described. In addition, the absence of a consistent CSF cellular response in patients with active cerebral inflammation differs from the findings in most patients with typical viral encephalitis.[10] There is no evidence of prion disease, and attempts to transmit the disease to animals have been unsuccessful.[10]

Several lines of evidence have suggested an autoimmune etiology. Iritis has been described in some patients.[3] IgM, IgG, IgA and C3 have been demonstrated in vessel walls.[11] Antibodies directed against glutamate receptors (GluR3) produced in animals an illness similar to Rasmussen encephalitis.[12] Antibodies to GluR3 have also been detected in the sera of humans with Rasmussen syndrome, although this test has not been established as a reliable investigation.[12,13] Finally, treatment with immunomodulating drugs has improved seizure control in some patients.

TREATMENT

Antiepileptic drugs are not effective in the long-term prevention of seizures. Focal resection has only limited benefit, and hemispheric disconnection is the surgical treatment of choice.[14] Surgery is typically performed when fine finger movement is lost,[14,15] but early hemispheric surgery has been advocated to limit the loss of motor function and prevent progressive cognitive decline.[15] Surgery in the dominant hemisphere requires careful evaluation of language function. Corticosteroids,[16,17] intravenous immunoglobulin[18] and plasmapheresis[19] may slow the course of the disease, particularly if used early, but have not been associated with long-term seizure control. The use of the antiviral agents ganciclovir and zidovudine has been reported, but with limited success.[20,21]

KEY POINTS

- Rasmussen syndrome begins in childhood and is characterized by **intractable seizures, slowly progressive hemiparesis and progressive cognitive decline**
- Unilateral, progressive hemispheric involvement is a characteristic feature and **bilateral disease is rare**
- **Partial motor seizures** are the most common seizure type. EPC occurs in 50 per cent of patients, and Rasmussen syndrome is the most common cause of EPC in childhood
- The seizures are usually difficult to control and **two thirds of the patients have daily seizures**

- **Cognitive decline** is characteristic and 85 per cent of patients become intellectually disabled
- **Hemianopsia** occurs in 50 per cent of patients and sensory deficits, dysarthria, dysphasia and psychiatric abnormalities are common
- CT and MRI demonstrate progressive **cerebral atrophy** that typically begins around the sylvian fissure
- The characteristic **pathologic features** consist of perivascular lymphocytic cuffing with proliferation of microglial nodules and neuronophagia
- The etiology of Rasmussen syndrome is unknown, but **immune factors** probably play a role
- **Antiepileptic drugs are not effective** in the long-term prevention of seizures
- Focal resection has only limited benefit and hemispheric disconnection is the **surgical treatment** of choice
- Treatment with **immunomodulating drugs** has improved seizure control in some patients

REFERENCES

1. Rasmussen T, Olsezewski J, Lloyd-Smith D. Focal seizures due to chronic localized encephalitis. *Neurology* 1958; **8**: 435–445.
2. Oguni H, Andermann F, Rasmussen TB. The natural history of the syndrome of chronic encephalitis and epilepsy: A study of the MNI series of 48 cases. In: Andermann F (ed.) *Chronic Encephalitis and Epilepsy. Rasmussen's Syndrome.* Boston: Butterworth-Heinemann; 1991; 7–35.
3. Harvey AS, Andermann F, Hopkins IJ, Kirkham TH, Berkovic SF. Chronic encephalitis (Rasmussen's syndrome) and ipsilateral uveitis. *Annals of Neurology* 1992; **32**: 826–829.
4. Capovilla G, Paladin F, Dallabernardina B. Rasmussen's syndrome: longitudinal EEG study from the first seizure to epilepsia partialis continua. *Epilepsia* 1997; **38**: 483–488.
5. So NK, Gloor P. Electroencephalographic and electrographic findings in chronic encephalitis of the Rasmussen type. In: Andermann F (ed.) *Chronic Encephalitis and Epilepsy. Rasmussen's Syndrome.* Boston: Butterworth-Heinemann; 1991; 37–45.
6. Shibasaki H, Yamashita Y, Kuroiwa Y. Electroencephalographic studies of myoclonus. Myoclonus related cortical spikes and high amplitude somatosensory evoked potentials. *Brain* 1978; **101**: 447–460.
7. Tampieri D, Melanson D, Ethier R. Imaging of chronic encephalitis. In: Andermann F (ed.) *Chronic Encephalitis and Epilepsy. Rasmussen's Syndrome.* Boston: Butterworth-Heinemann; 1991; 47–60.
8. Robitaille Y. Neuropathologic aspects of chronic encephalitis in chronic encephalitis and epilepsy. In: Andermann F (ed.) *Chronic Encephalitis and Epilepsy. Rasmussen's Syndrome.* Boston: Butterworth-Heinemann; 1991; 79–110.
9. So NK, Andermann F. Rasmussen's syndrome. In: Engel J Jr, Pedley TA (eds) *Epilepsy: A Comprehensive Textbook.* Philadelphia: Lippincott-Raven; 1997; 2379–2388.
10. Asher D, Gajdusek DC. Virologic studies in chronic encephalitis. In: Andermann F (ed.) *Chronic Encephalitis and Epilepsy. Rasmussen's Syndrome.* Boston: Butterworth-Heinemann; 1991; 147–158.
11. Andrews JM, Thompson JA, Pysher TJ, Walker ML, Hammond ME. Chronic encephalitis, epilepsy, and cerebrovascular immune complex deposits. *Annals of Neurology* 1990; **28**(1): 88–90.
12. Andrews PI, McNamara JO. Rasmussen's encephalitis: an autoimmune disorder? *Current Opinion in Neurology* 1996; **9**: 141–145.
13. Rogers SW, Andrews PI, Gahring LC *et al.* Auto-antibodies to glutamate receptor GluR3 in Rasmussen's encephalitis. *Science* 1994; **265**: 648–651.
14. Villemure JG, Andermann F, Rasmussen TB. Hemispherectomy for the treatment of epilepsy due to chronic encephalitis. In: Andermann F (ed.) *Chronic Encephalitis and Epilepsy. Rasmussen's Syndrome.* Boston: Butterworth-Heinemann; 1991; 235–241.
15. Vining EP, Freeman JM, Brandt J, Carson BS, Uematsu S. Progressive unilateral encephalopathy of childhood (Rasmussen's syndrome): a reappraisal. *Epilepsia* 1993; **34**: 639–650.
16. Dulac O, Robain O, Chiron C *et al.* High dose steroid treatment of Epilepsia partialis continua due to chronic focal epilepsy. In: Andermann F (ed.) *Chronic Encephalitis and Epilepsy. Rasmussen's Syndrome.* Boston: Butterworth-Heinemann; 1991; 193–199.
17. Hart YM, Cortez M, Andermann F *et al.* Medical treatment of Rasmussen's syndrome (chronic encephalitis and epilepsy): effect of high-dose steroids or immunoglobins in 19 patients. *Neurology* 1994; **44**: 1030–1036.
18. Walsh P. Treatment of Rasmussen's syndrome with intravenous gammaglobulin. In: Andermann F (ed.) *Chronic Encephalitis and Epilepsy. Rasmussen's Syndrome.* Boston: Butterworth-Heinemann; 1991; 201–204.
19. Andrews PI, Dichtor MA, Berkovic SF, Newton MR, McNamara JO. Plasmapheresis in Rasmussen's encephalitis. *Neurology* 1996; **46**: 242–246.
20. Machachlan RS, Levin S, Blume WT. Treatment of Rasmussen's syndrome with ganciclovir. *Neurology* 1996; **47**: 925–928.
21. De Toledo JC, Smith DB. Partially successful treatment of Rasmussen's encephalitis with zidovudine: systematic improvement followed by involvement of the contralateral hemisphere. *Epilepsia* 1994; **35**: 352–355.

12

Epileptic syndromes with onset in late childhood or adolescence

Idiopathic generalized epilepsy with generalized tonic-clonic seizures only

COLIN D FERRIE AND CP PANAYIOTOPOULOS

Idiopathic generalized epilepsies (IGEs) manifest clinically with the triad of **absences, myoclonic jerks** and **generalized tonic-clonic seizures** (GTCS), either alone or in combination. These, together with other symptoms, age at onset, prognosis and EEG findings define IGE syndromes.[1,2] Of the recognized syndromes of IGE, typical absences are the defining seizure type of childhood absence epilepsy, but GTCS may rarely occur in adolescence. In juvenile absence epilepsy, absences are the hallmark, but most of the patients also have GTCS, with random myoclonic jerks occurring less commonly. In juvenile myoclonic epilepsy, nearly all patients have GTCS in addition to myoclonic jerks; one third also have mild absences. Sleep deprivation, fatigue and excessive alcohol intake are the main precipitating factors in IGEs. Many patients also have photosensitivity of varying severity. In the IGEs, GTCS and myoclonic jerks mainly occur on awakening.

Therefore, GTCS are a common feature in IGEs. Overall GTCS are reported to occur on awakening in 17–53 per cent of patients, diffusely whilst awake in 23–36 per cent, during sleep in 27–44 per cent, or, randomly, in 13–26 per cent.[3] The proportion of these patients who also have other generalized seizures, characterized by jerks or absences, is undetermined.

CLASSIFICATION

'IGE with GTCS only' is considered a syndrome in the new ILAE diagnostic scheme,[2,4] and incorporates **epilepsy with GTCS on awakening** (EGTCSA), previously recognized as a separate syndrome.[1]

'IGE with GTCS only' has not been precisely defined by the ILAE.[2] Its name implies that it includes only those patients who have GTCS alone, i.e. without absences and/ or jerks, and that these may occur at any time. However, it is more likely that it constitutes a broader category, rather than a syndrome, of **'IGE with predominantly GTCS'**, which also includes patients with mild absences, myoclonic jerks or both. The GTCS is the most severe type of epileptic seizure; myoclonic jerks and absences may be mild and escape clinical detection.[5] A patient with a 'first GTCS' has often suffered from minor seizures, e.g. absences, myoclonic jerks or both, sometimes for many years, before the GTCS. Absences may be so mild that they are inconspicuous to the patient and imperceptible to observers: **phantom absences**.[5] The detection of myoclonic jerks and absences often requires meticulous history taking and/or video-EEG.

This chapter mainly deals with GTCS on awakening (EGTCSA) which has been most extensively studied by Janz.[6–8]

ILLUSTRATIVE CASES

GTCS on awakening

A 20-year-old man had, from the age of 16 years, six GTCS, which occurred within half an hour of awakening, when he was sleep deprived and drunk. An additional

GTCS had occurred late in the afternoon while he was relaxing after a successful job interview.

His EEG, which included recording during sleep and on awakening, showed some brief bursts of theta activity. Compliance with medication is poor. He is a heavy drinker who frequently stays out late. His maternal half-sister suffers from well-controlled idiopathic occipital lobe epilepsy. His father has frequent epileptic seizures.

GTCS on awakening with brief asymptomatic generalized discharges of 3–4-Hz spike-wave

A 19-year-old male student had two GTCS at age 14 and 18 years. Both occurred half an hour after awakening when

he was sleep deprived. He had had no absences or jerks. All his EEGs showed brief (up to 4 s) high-amplitude discharges of 3–4-Hz spikes/polyspikes and slow waves without clinical accompaniments (Figure 12A.1).

GTCS and phantom absences

A 24-year-old woman had a brief febrile convulsion at age 3 years. At 17 years of age she had a GTCS in the afternoon while talking to her teacher. There were no preceding symptoms or apparent precipitating factors. She was not aware of myoclonic jerks or absences. Video-EEGs documented phantom absences, that is brief generalized discharges of spike/multiple spike-wave associated with errors

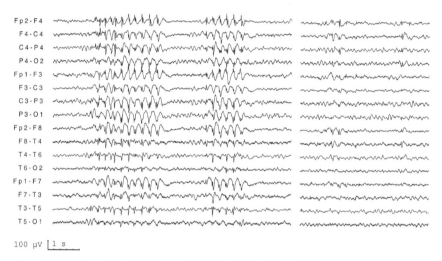

Figure 12A.1 *Asymptomatic brief generalized discharges of spike/multiple spike and slow waves in a 19-year-old man with two GTCS at ages 14 and 18 on awakening after sleep deprivation. There were no clinical manifestations during hyperventilation with breath counting. From Panayiotopoulos CP. A Clinical Guide to Epileptic Syndromes and Their Treatment.* Oxford: Bladon Medical Publishing, 2002 with the permission of the publisher.

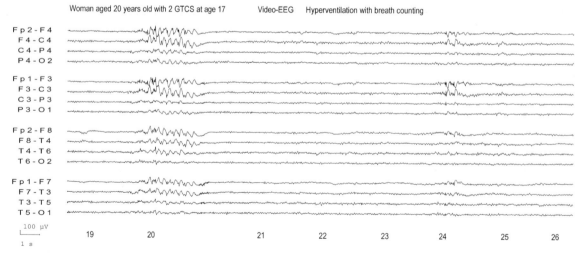

Figure 12A.2 *Brief generalized discharges of spike/multiple spike and slow wave are associated with significant delay during breath counting (annotated numbers) in a 20-year-old woman with two GTCS at age 17. From Panayiotopoulos CP. A Clinical Guide to Epileptic Syndromes and Their Treatment.* Oxford: Bladon Medical Publishing, 2002 with the permission of the publisher.

during breath counting (Figure 12A.2). Treatment with valproic acid 1000 mg daily was initiated. However, she had another GTCS, again in the afternoon, 5 days after stopping her medication. No further seizures occurred during the next 7 years, while she was on treatment with valproic acid.

PREVALENCE

The prevalence of 'IGE with GTCS only' is unknown. It is very rare if the criterion of GTCS only is strictly applied: of 1000 patients with one or more afebrile seizures we personally investigated during 10 years, 356 (35.6 per cent) had various syndromes of IGEs but only 9 (0.9 per cent) had GTCS only, though this was often the reason for referral.[5] The low yield of 'IGE with GTCS only' in this sample reflects that both patients and witnesses were methodically questioned with regard to the occurrence of minor seizures, and that long video-EEG recordings, including video-EEG during sleep and on awakening, were made. As a result of this approach, 14 patients mainly referred for late-onset GTCS, were found to have frequent 'phantom absences' consisting of mild ictal impairment of cognition associated with brief (3–4 s), generalized 3–4 Hz-spike/multiple spike- and slow-wave discharges (Figure 12A.2).[5]

The findings of other authors are different. In one group of 253 patients with IGEs, 30 (12 per cent) had EGTCSA and 39 (15 per cent) had 'a mild form of IGE characterized by infrequent GTCS and generalized interictal EEG discharges of spike-wave'.[9] The authors considered that this group probably had a mild form of IGE which they called 'non-syndromic grand mal'.[9] In a further series of 1033 patients with IGEs, 138 (13 per cent) had GTCS only, with onset from 3 to later than 18 years of age.[10] The reported prevalence of EGTCSA varies from 0 per cent[11] to as high as 17 per cent[8] of patients with epileptic seizures. Of 101 patients with IGE beginning in adolescence, only 10 had GTCS alone, but these occurred neither on awakening nor in the evening period of relaxation.[12] 'Pure' EGTCSA, i.e. GTCS only, was found in 10 per cent and 'mixed' EGTCSA, i.e. GTCS with absences and/or myoclonic jerks or other seizures, in 17 per cent of 4816 patients of Janz.[8]

Sex

The male/female ratio in 88 cases with pure EGTCSA was 1.8.[7] The male predominance is attributed to differences in alcohol exposure and sleep habits.

Genetics

There is a high incidence of epileptic disorders in families of patients with either the pure (4 per cent) or mixed (11–12.5 per cent) forms of EGTCSA.[3,7] Adolescent-onset

EGTCSA may be linked to the EJM-1 locus on chromosome 6 and may be genetically the same as juvenile myoclonic epilepsy.[13] Conversely, adolescent-onset idiopathic GTCS epilepsy with GTCS at any time whilst awake is not linked to the EJM-1 locus.[13]

Age

Age at onset of EGTCSA varies from 6 to 47 years and nearly 80 per cent of the cases have their first GTCS in the second decade of life, with a peak at 16–17 years.

CLINICAL MANIFESTATIONS, PRECIPITATING FACTORS AND DIFFERENTIAL DIAGNOSIS

By definition, in EGTCSA, patients suffer from GTCS, which occur within 1–2 h after awakening from either nocturnal or diurnal sleep. The seizure may occur while the patient is still in bed or having breakfast, or upon arriving at work. However, seizures may also occur in situations other than awakening and mainly during relaxation or leisure.[3,6,7] Sleep deprivation, fatigue and excessive alcohol consumption are the main seizure precipitants. Situations more relevant to adolescents than young children, such as shift work and other changes in sleep habits, particularly during holidays and celebrations, predispose to GTCS on awakening. With time, the interval between seizures becomes shorter and the attacks may become more random, occurring both diurnally and nocturnally, either as a result of the evolution of the disease or drug-induced modifications.[3,6,7] Thirteen per cent of patients are reported to show photosensitivity on EEG. The differential diagnosis is mainly from patients with other IGEs, which share with EGTCSA the same propensity to seizures after awakening and the same precipitating factors. Juvenile myoclonic epilepsy may cause diagnostic difficulties. Symptomatic partial epileptic seizures with secondary generalization may also occur, predominantly on awakening.

EEG

Generalized discharges of spike/multiple spike-slow waves are reported in approximately half of patients with pure EGTCSA (Figure 12A.1) and in 70 per cent of those with additional absences or myoclonic jerks preceding GTCS (Figure 12A.2). If the routine EEG is normal, this should prompt a request for a video-EEG performed on sleep and on awakening. Myoclonic jerks or, more frequently, brief absences will often be revealed. Focal EEG abnormalities, in the absence of generalized discharges, are rare. Photoparoxysmal responses are reported in 17 per cent of females and 9 per cent of males with EGTCSA.[3]

Personality characteristics and sleep patterns

Janz described patients with EGTCSA as unreliable, unstable and prone to neglect.[7,8] The sleep patterns of patients with EGTCSA are particularly unstable and modifiable by external factors, such as antiepileptic drugs, and the patients may suffer from chronic sleep deficit.[3,6,7]

PROGNOSIS

As in all other types of IGEs with onset in the mid-teens, EGTCSA is probably a life-long disease with a high (83 per cent) incidence of relapse on withdrawal of treatment.[7] Characteristically, the intervals between seizures become shorter with time, the precipitating factors less obvious, and GTCS may become more random and occur also during sleep.[7]

TREATMENT

Patients should be warned of the common seizure precipitants – sleep deprivation with early awaking and alcohol consumption – and, when possible, should avoid occupations involving night shifts. After adjusting their lifestyles, patients may become seizure-free. Drug treatment has not been properly evaluated, but retrospective open studies suggest that phenobarbital is more effective than phenytoin or carbamazepine.[3,8] Valproic acid and lamotrigine may be very effective. Bromide therapy has been 'rediscovered' to be useful in resistant cases of ECTCSA.[3]

KEY POINTS

- Idiopathic generalized epilepsies with generalized tonic-clonic seizures **only** is a **relatively rare** expression of IGE.
- The diagnosis can be confirmed only when **'phantom absences' and myoclonic jerks are excluded** by video-EEG, both in the normal waking state and after sleep deprivation.
- **Photosensitivity** is common.
- **Sleep deprivation** and **alcohol** should be avoided.
- Other family members commonly have IGE.

REFERENCES

1. Commission on Classification and Terminology of the International League Against Epilepsy. Proposal for revised classification of epilepsies and epileptic syndromes. *Epilepsia* 1989; **30**: 389–399.
2. Engel J, Jr. A proposed diagnostic scheme for people with epileptic seizures and with epilepsy: Report of the ILAE Task Force on Classification and Terminology. *Epilepsia* 2001; **42**: 796–803.
3. Wolf P. Epilepsy with grand mal on awakening. In: Roger J, Bureau M, Dravet C, *et al.* (eds) *Epileptic Syndromes in Infancy, Childhood and Adolescence.* London: John Libbey, 1992; 329–341.
4. Andermann F, Berkovic SF. Idiopathic generalized epilepsy with generalised and other seizures in adolescence. *Epilepsia* 2001; **42**: 317–320.
5. Panayiotopoulos CP, Koutroumanidis M, Giannakodimos S, Agathonikou A. Idiopathic generalised epilepsy in adults manifested by phantom absences, generalised tonic-clonic seizures, and frequent absence status. *Journal of Neurology, Neurosurgery and Psychiatry* 1997; **63**: 622–627.
6. Janz D. Epilepsy with grand mal on awakening and sleep-waking cycle. *Clinical Neurophysiology* 2000; **111**(Suppl. 2): S103–110.
7. Janz D. Pitfalls in the diagnosis of grand mal on awakening. In: Wolf P (ed.) *Epileptic Seizures and Syndromes.* London: John Libbey, 1994; 213–220.
8. Janz D. *Die Epilepsien: Spezielle Pathologie and Therapie.* Stuttgart: Georg Thieme, 1969.
9. Roger J, Bureau M, Oller Ferrer-Vidal L *et al.* Clinical and electroencephalographic characteristics of idiopathic generalised epilepsies. In Malafosse A, Genton P, Hirsch E, *et al.* (eds) *Idiopathic Generalised Epilepsies.* London: John Libbey, 1994; 7–18.
10. Oller-Daurella LFV, Oller L. *5000 epilepticos. Clinica y evolucion.* Barcelona: Ciba-Geigy, 1994.
11. Manford M, Hart YM, Sander JW, Shorvon SD. The National General Practice Study of Epilepsy. The syndromic classification of the International League Against Epilepsy applied to epilepsy in a general population. *Archives of Neurology* 1992; **49**: 801–808.
12. Reutens DC, Berkovic SF. Idiopathic generalized epilepsy of adolescence: are the syndromes clinically distinct? *Neurology* 1995; **45**: 1469–7146.
13. Greenberg DA, Durner M, Resor S, Rosenbaum D, Shinnar S. The genetics of idiopathic generalized epilepsies of adolescent onset: differences between juvenile myoclonic epilepsy and epilepsy with random grand mal and with awakening grand mal. *Neurology* 1995; **45**: 942–946.

Juvenile myoclonic epilepsy

RICHARD A GRÜNEWALD AND CP PANAYIOTOPOULOS

Juvenile myoclonic epilepsy (JME) is a genetically determined idiopathic generalized epilepsy (IGE), characterized by **myoclonic jerks on awakening, generalized tonic-clonic seizures** (GTCS) and, in around one third of patients, **typical absences** (Figure 12B.1).[1,2] Janz's contributions over the last 40 years in all aspects of JME fully justify the eponym **Janz syndrome**.[3-5]

CLINICAL MANIFESTATIONS

The following description, an extract from a patient's diary, epitomizes the clinical syndrome:[6]

> Lots of blanks and jerks; then I had a grand mal ... I usually have fits when rushing after getting up; usually does not happen later in the day.

Myoclonic jerks occurring after awakening are the most prominent and pathognomonic seizure type.[3,4,7-10] They are shock-like, irregular and arrhythmic, clonic movements of proximal and distal muscles, mainly of the upper extremities. They are often inconspicuous, restricted to the fingers, making the patient prone to drop things or look clumsy. They may be violent enough to cause falls. One fifth of the patients describe their jerks as unilateral, but video-EEG shows that the jerks affect both sides (Figure 12B.2).[4,11]

Some patients, less than 10 per cent, with mild forms of JME never develop GTCS.[10]

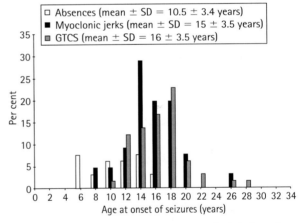

Figure 12B.1 *Age at onset of absences, myoclonic jerks and GTCS of 66 consecutive patients with JME. Modified from Panayiotopoulos et al. Juvenile myoclonic epilepsy: a 5-year prospective study. Epilepsia 1994; 35: 285–296 with the permission of Blackwell Publishing Ltd.[10]*

Typical absence seizures

One third of patients have typical absences, which are brief with subtle impairment of consciousness (Figure 12B.3). They are different from the absence seizures of childhood or juvenile absence epilepsy.[10,12,13] Those that appear before the age of 10 years may be more severe. They become less frequent and less severe with age.[10,12,13] One tenth of patients do not perceive absences, despite generalized spike-slow wave EEG discharges lasting more

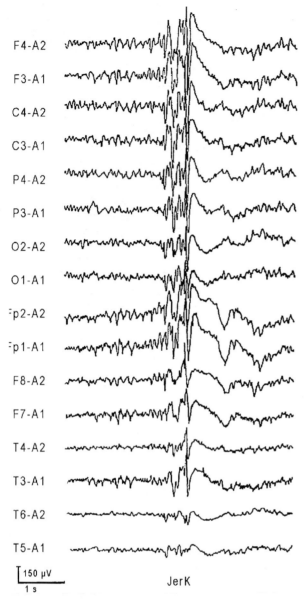

Figure 12B.2 *Typical EEG manifestations of myoclonic jerks in JME. From Panayiotopoulos et al. Juvenile myoclonic epilepsy: a 5-year prospective study. Epilepsia 1994; 35: 285–296 with the permission of Blackwell Publishing Ltd.[10]*

than 3 s.[10,12] However, on video-EEG with breath counting during hyperventilation, such EEG discharges often manifest with mild impairment of cognition, eyelid flickering or both.[14]

Generalized tonic–clonic seizures

GTCS usually follow the onset of myoclonic jerks.[3–5,7–10] Myoclonic jerks, usually in clusters and often with an accelerating frequency and severity, may precede GTCS, a so-called clonic-tonic-clonic generalized seizure.[4]

Status epilepticus

Myoclonic status epilepticus is probably more common than appreciated.[10] It almost invariably starts on awakening, associated with a precipitating factor such as sleep deprivation or missing medication. Consciousness may not be impaired, although some patients with myoclonic status epilepticus may also have absences interspersed with myoclonic jerks. Absence status epilepticus is exceptional,[15] and generalized tonic clonic status epilepticus infrequent.

Circadian distribution

Seizures, principally myoclonic jerks, occurring within 30–60 min of awakening are characteristic of JME.[3–5,7–10] Myoclonic jerks occur rarely at other times unless the patient is tired. GTCS occur mainly on awakening but may also be purely nocturnal or random. Absence seizures rarely show a circadian predilection.

Age at onset and sex

Absences, jerks, and GTCS show a characteristic age-related onset (Figure 12A.1). Absences, when a feature, begin between the ages of 5 and 16 years. Myoclonic jerks follow between 1 and 9, mean 4 years, later, usually around the age of 14–15 years. GTCS usually appear a few months later, occasionally earlier, than the myoclonic jerks. IGE with onset of myoclonic jerks in adulthood may be a variant of JME.[16] Men and women are equally affected.[3–5,7,8,10]

Seizure-precipitating factors

Sleep deprivation and fatigue, particularly after alcohol indulgence, are the most powerful precipitants of jerks and GTCS.[4,5,7,10] A brief sleep suddenly interrupted by early awakening in order to go to work or a trip, or an unscheduled early morning telephone call, may have disastrous effects. EEG photosensitivity occurs in one third of patients but probably less than one tenth experience seizures induced by photic stimulation. Other common precipitants are mental and psychological stress and arousal, failed expectations or frustration; all may interact.[10] Women may have premenstrual exacerbations.[10]

GENETIC ETIOLOGY

JME is genetically determined.[4,5,9,17] Inheritance is probably complex and polygenic.[18–20] Families with autosomal

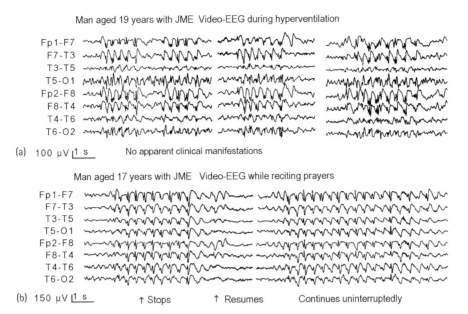

Man aged 19 years with JME Video-EEG during hyperventilation

Fp1-F7
F7-T3
T3-T5
T5-O1
Fp2-F8
F8-T4
T4-T6
T6-O2

(a)   100 µV ⌊1 s⌋   No apparent clinical manifestations

Man aged 17 years with JME Video-EEG while reciting prayers

Fp1-F7
F7-T3
T3-T5
T5-O1
Fp2-F8
F8-T4
T4-T6
T6-O2

(b)   150 µV ⌊1 s⌋   ↑ Stops   ↑ Resumes   Continues uninterruptedly

Figure 12B.3 *From video-EEG of 2 patients with JME: (a) 19-year-old man, video-EEG during hyperventilation. Generalized discharges of spike/multiple spike and slow waves are not associated with apparent clinical manifestations (but these may have been revealed if breath counting was performed during hyperventilation). (b) 17-year-old man, video-EEG while reading prayers. Generalized discharges of spike and slow waves are associated with mild impairment of cognition. Modified from Panayiotopoulos et al. Differentiation of typical absence seizures in epileptic syndromes. A video EEG study of 224 seizures in 20 patients.* Brain *1989;* 112: 1039–1056 with the permission of Oxford University Press.[13]

recessive[17] or dominant[17,18] inheritance have been described. Association studies favor a susceptibility locus for JME in chromosome 6p11–12 (EJM1) and 15q14 but these are still controversial.[20] A gene in the EJM1 region has been identified.[21] A reported association of JME with an HLA-DR allele[22,23] in patients with JME was not replicated.[24]

EPIDEMIOLOGY

The prevalence of JME has been reported as 2.7 per cent,[7] 5.7 per cent,[19] 8.7 per cent[25] and 10.2 per cent.[10]

EEG AND OTHER TESTS

The EEG is nearly always abnormal in untreated patients.[3–10,26] A normal EEG should prompt an EEG on sleep and awakening after partial sleep deprivation. The patients are asked to go to sleep 2 h later and wake 2 h earlier than usual. Video-EEG is recorded at mid-day during wakefulness, subsequent sleep and awakening. Paroxysmal abnormalities consist of generalized spike/ multiple spike-slow wave discharges (52 per cent) or brief generalized bursts of sharp theta activity with

interspersed small spikes (27 per cent) (Figures 12B.3, 12B.4).[10] Most of the discharges last for 1–3 s (range 1–20 s). Focal abnormalities are recorded in approximately one third of patients and are often misinterpreted as evidence of focal epilepsy (Figure 12B.4).[26] Hyperventilation accentuates the abnormalities in all patients. Photoparoxysmal discharges are evoked in 27 per cent of patients. The background EEG is usually normal. The typical EEG discharges of the myoclonic jerk (generalized bursts of multiple spikes of 0.5–2 s duration) and of the absences (generalized 3–5 Hz spike/poly-spikes and slow waves) are illustrated in Figures 12B.2 and 12B.3.

Brain imaging

Routine brain imaging is normal. However, using new MRI technologies, abnormalities involving mesiofrontal cortical structures have been reported in some patients with JME.[27]

DIAGNOSING JME

The rate of misdiagnosis of JME is as high as 90 per cent.[25,28] Factors responsible include lack of familiarity

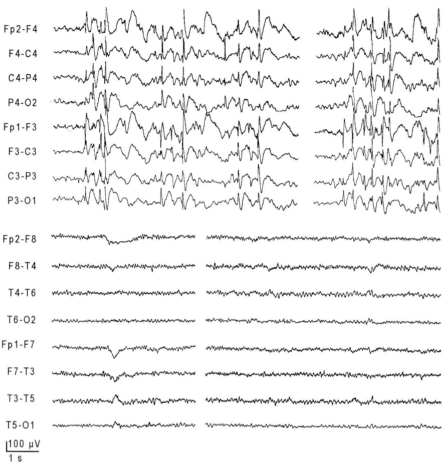

Figure 12B.4 *EEG recording of a 40 year old woman with JME (absences at 7 years, myoclonic jerks at 10 years and GTCS at 12 years). Initially diagnosed as suffering from complex partial and secondary generalized seizures, she had one or two GTCS per month and one to three absences per day while on carbamazepine and phenytoin. Absences and myoclonic jerks stopped after carbamazepine was replaced by valproic acid. She had five nocturnal GTCS in the last 2 years of follow-up. CT of the brain was normal. The EEG (upper trace) showed the typical JME pattern with Ws, discharge fragmentations, inconsistent spike and/or multiple spike-slow wave relation and intradischarge frequency variations. Focal spikes, independently right or more frequently left, were seen either at the onset or within the discharges. The resting EEG (lower trace) had also transients of slow waves localized either on the left or right midtemporal electrodes. From Panayiotopoulos et al. Typical absence seizures in adults: clinical, EEG, video-EEG findings and diagnostic syndromic considerations. Journal of Neurology Neurosurgery and Psychiatry 1992; 55: 1002–1008 with permission from the BMJ Publishing Group.*[37]

with JME, failure to elicit a history of myoclonic jerks, misinterpretation of absences as complex partial seizures, misinterpretation of jerks as partial motor seizures and high prevalence of focal EEG abnormalities.

Diagnosing myoclonic jerks in JME

It is often necessary to physically demonstrate mild myoclonic jerks. Questions like 'do you spill your morning tea?', 'do you drop things in the morning?', with simultaneous demonstration of how myoclonic jerks produce this effect, may elicit a positive response in those patients who denied myoclonic jerks on direct questioning.

Diagnosing absences in JME

Absences are difficult to reveal and diagnose in JME,[10,12,14] and often remain unrecognized for years or misdiagnosed as complex partial seizures.

Differential diagnosis

Juvenile absence epilepsy is characterized by severe absences. Myoclonic jerks, if they occur, are mild and random, often lacking the circadian predeliction of JME.

Diagnosis is difficult when JME presents with absences in childhood before the development of myoclonic jerks. Retrospective examination of EEG and clinical manifestations of these patients reveals absences distinct from childhood or juvenile absence epilepsy in that they are usually shorter, milder and associated with ictal EEG which often contain multiple spike-slow waves. It seems unlikely that true childhood absence epilepsy progresses to JME, as some authors have reported.[29]

PROGNOSIS

JME may vary in severity from mild myoclonic jerks to frequent GTCS with severe falls. Irrespective of severity, JME is generally associated with a lifelong predisposition to seizures.

Seizures are well controlled with appropriate medication in up to 90 per cent of patients.[4,6,9,10] A decline in seizure susceptibility after the fourth decade is possible.[10] Patients with all three types of seizure are more likely to be resistant to treatment.[30]

MANAGEMENT

Avoidance of precipitating factors and adherence to long-term medication is essential to avoid seizures. Some patients experience GTCS or myoclonic jerks only after encountering precipitating factors. Advice on the risks of alcohol and sleep deprivation is mandatory. Sleeping later the next morning may compensate for a late night, and patients should be advised to find what is right and wrong for them. Valproic acid is effective in treating absences, myoclonic jerks and GTCS.[14] The usual recommended dose is likely to be effective, but in resistant cases higher doses may be needed. Persistence of even mild myoclonic jerks imply a necessity to continue drug treatment. Valproic acid may be inappropriate in some women because of teratogenic effects, weight gain and polycystic ovarian syndrome,[31] although this is contentious.[32] Clonazepam controls myoclonic jerks but if used alone may precipitate GTCS.[10,33] Furthermore, clonazepam may deprive patients of the warning of an impending GTCS provided by the myoclonic jerks.[10,33] Phenobarbital is extensively used and effective in monotherapy.[5,7,9] Small doses of lamotrigine added to valproic acid are effective in resistant cases[14,34] possibly because of pharmacokinetic interactions.[14,35] Lamotrigine monotherapy is still controversial.[14,32] Worsening of seizure control has been reported.[36] Of the newest antiepileptic drugs, levitiracetam appears to be effective.[38] Contraindicated drugs include vigabatrin, tiagabine and carbamazepine. Lifelong anticonvulsant treatment is usually considered necessary in patients with JME. In mild forms of JME, it may be safe slowly to reduce the dose of medication, especially after the fourth decade of life. Persistence or recrudescence of myoclonic jerks necessitates continuation of medication.[30]

KEY POINTS

- As a result of failure to ask specific questions about early-morning myoclonic jerks and absences in adolescents who present with GTCS, JME is often **underdiagnosed**
- JME is associated with a **lifelong predisposition to seizures**
- Continued attention to **lifestyle measures**, avoidance of sleep-deprivation and moderation with regard to alcohol, are necessary
- **Lifelong antiepileptic drug medication** is usually needed
- Carbamazepine, vigabatrin and tiagabine are contraindicated

REFERENCES

1. Commission on Classification and Terminology of the International League Against Epilepsy. Proposal for revised classification of epilepsies and epileptic syndromes. *Epilepsia* 1989; **30**: 389–399.
2. Engel J, Jr. A proposed diagnostic scheme for people with epileptic seizures and with epilepsy: Report of the ILAE Task Force on Classification and Terminology. *Epilepsia* 2001; **42**: 796–803.
3. Schnitz B, Sander T (eds) *Juvenile Myoclonic Epilepsy: the Janz syndrome.* London: Wrightson Biomedical, 2000.
4. Delgado-Escueta AV, Enrile-Bacsal F. Juvenile myoclonic epilepsy of Janz. *Neurology* 1984; **34**: 285–294.
5. Canevini MP, Mai R, Di Marco C, *et al.* Juvenile myoclonic epilepsy of Janz: clinical observations in 60 patients. *Seizure* 1992; **1**: 291–298.
6. Grünewald RA, Panayiotopoulos CP. Juvenile myoclonic epilepsy. A review. *Archives of Neurology* 1993; **50**: 594–598.
7. Janz D, Christian W. Impulsiv-Petit mal. *Zeitschrift für Nervenheilkunde* 1957; **176**: 346–386. (English translatation by Genton P. In: Malafosse A, Genton P, Hirsch E, *et al.* (eds) *Idiopathic Generalised Epilepsies.* London: John Libbey, 1957; 229–251.
8. Panayiotopoulos CP. Juvenile myoclonic epilepsy: an uderdiagnosed syndrome. In: Wolf P (ed.) *Epileptic Seizures and Syndromes.* London: John Libbey, 1994; 221–230.
9. Janz D, Durner M. Juvenile myoclonic epilepsy. In: Engel JJ, Pedley TA (eds) *Epilepsy: A Comprehensive Textbook.* Philadelphia: Lippincott-Raven, 1997; 2389–2400.
10. Panayiotopoulos CP, Obeid T, Tahan AR. Juvenile myoclonic epilepsy: a 5-year prospective study. *Epilepsia* 1994; **35**: 285–296.
11. Oguni H, Mukahira K, Oguni M, *et al.* Video-polygraphic analysis of myoclonic seizures in juvenile myoclonic epilepsy. *Epilepsia* 1994; **35**: 307–316.
12. Panayiotopoulos CP, Obeid T, Waheed G. Absences in juvenile myoclonic epilepsy: a clinical and video-electroencephalographic study. *Annals of Neurology* 1989; **25**: 391–397.

13. Panayiotopoulos CP, Obeid T, Waheed G. Differentiation of typical absence seizures in epileptic syndromes. A video EEG study of 224 seizures in 20 patients. *Brain* 1989; **112**: 1039–1056.
14. Panayiotopoulos CP. Treatment of typical absence seizures and related epileptic syndromes. *Paediatric Drugs* 2001; **3**: 379–403.
15. Agathonikou A, Panayiotopoulos CP, Giannakodimos S, Koutroumanidis M. Typical absence status in adults: diagnostic and syndromic considerations. *Epilepsia* 1998; **39**: 1265–1276.
16. Gilliam F, Steinhoff BJ, Bittermann HJ, *et al*. Adult myoclonic epilepsy: a distinct syndrome of idiopathic generalized epilepsy. *Neurology* 2000; **55**: 1030–1033.
17. Panayiotopoulos CP, Obeid T. Juvenile myoclonic epilepsy: an autosomal recessive disease. *Annals of Neurology* 1989; **25**: 440–443.
18. Serratosa JM, Delgado-Escueta AV, Medina MT *et al*. Clinical and genetic analysis of a large pedigree with juvenile myoclonic epilepsy. *Annals of Neurology* 1996; **39**: 187–195.
19. Tsuboi T, Christian W. On the genetics of the primary generalised epilepsy with sporadic myoclonus of impulsive petit mal type. *Humangenetik* 1973; **19**: 155–182.
20. Delgado-Escueta AV, Medina MT, *et al*. Mapping and positional cloning of common idiopathic generalized epilepsies: juvenile myoclonus epilepsy and childhood absence epilepsy. *Advances in Neurology* 1999; **79**: 351–374.
21. Suzuki T, Ganesh S, Agarwala KL, *et al*. A novel gene in the chromosomal region for juvenile myoclonic epilepsy on 6p12 encodes a brain-specific lysosomal membrane protein. *Biochemistry and Biophysics Research Commununications* 2001; **288**: 626–636.
22. Greenberg DA, Durner M, Shinnar S, *et al*. Association of HLA class II alleles in patients with juvenile myoclonic epilepsy compared with patients with other forms of adolescent-onset generalized epilepsy. *Neurology* 1996; **47**: 750–755.
23. Obeid T, el Rab MO, Daif AK, *et al*. Is HLA-DRW13 (W6) associated with juvenile myoclonic epilepsy in Arab patients? *Epilepsia* 1994; **35**: 319–321.
24. Le Hellard S, Neidhart E, Thomas P, *et al*. Lack of association between juvenile myoclonic epilepsy and HLA- DR13. *Epilepsia* 1999; **40**: 117–119.
25. Grünewald RA, Chroni E, Panayiotopoulos CP. Delayed diagnosis of juvenile myoclonic epilepsy. *Journal of Neurology, Neurosurgery and Psychiatry* 1992; **55**: 497–499.
26. Aliberti V, Grünewald RA, Panayiotopoulos CP, Chroni E. Focal electroencephalographic abnormalities in juvenile myoclonic epilepsy. *Epilepsia* 1994; **35**: 297–301.
27. Woermann FG, Free SL, Koepp MJ, Sisodiya SM, Duncan JS. Abnormal cerebral structure in juvenile myoclonic epilepsy demonstrated with voxel-based analysis of MRI. *Brain* 1999; **122**: 2101–2108.
28. Panayiotopoulos CP, Tahan R, Obeid T. Juvenile myoclonic epilepsy: factors of error involved in the diagnosis and treatment. *Epilepsia* 1991; **32**: 672–676.
29. Wirrell EC, Camfield CS, Camfield PR, Gordon KE, Dooley JM. Long-term prognosis of typical childhood absence epilepsy: remission or progression to juvenile myoclonic epilepsy. *Neurology* 1996; **47**: 912–918.
30. Gelisse P, Genton P, Thomas P, *et al*. Clinical factors of drug resistance in juvenile myoclonic epilepsy. *Journal of Neurology, Neurosurgery and Psychiatry* 2001; **70**: 240–243.
31. Isojarvi JI, Tauboll E, Tapanainen JS, *et al*. On the association between valproate and polycystic ovary syndrome: A response and an alternative view. *Epilepsia* 2001; **42**: 305–310.
32. Genton P, Bauer J, Duncan S, *et al*. On the association between valproate and polycystic ovary syndrome. *Epilepsia* 2001; **42**: 295–304.
33. Obeid T, Panayiotopoulos CP. Clonazepam in juvenile myoclonic epilepsy. *Epilepsia* 1989; **30**: 603–606.
34. Buchanan N. The use of lamotrigine in juvenile myoclonic epilepsy. *Seizure* 1996; **5**: 149–151.
35. Ferrie CD, Robinson RO, Knott C, Panayiotopoulos CP. Lamotrigine as an add-on drug in typical absence seizures. *Acta Neurologica Scandinavica* 1995; **91**: 200–202.
36. Carrazana EJ, Wheeler SD. Exacerbation of juvenile myoclonic epilepsy with lamotrigine. *Neurology* 2001; **56**: 1424–1425.
37. Panayiotopoulos CP, Chroni E, Daskalopoulos C, *et al*. Typical absence seizures in adults: clinical, EEG, video-EEG findings and diagnostic/syndromic considerations. *Journal of Neurology, Neurosurgery and Psychiatry* 1992; **55**: 1002–1008.
38. Panayiotopolous CP. *A Clinical Guide to Epileptic Syndromes and Their Treatment.* Oxford: Bladon Medical Publishing, 2002, 139–145.

12C

Juvenile absence epilepsy

CP PANAYIOTOPOULOS

Juvenile absence epilepsy (JAE) is a syndrome of idiopathic generalized epilepsy (IGE)[1–3] mainly manifested with severe **absence seizures**. Nearly all patients (80 per cent) also suffer from **generalized tonic-clonic seizures (GTCS)** and one fifth from sporadic **myoclonic jerks**.

JAE is broadly defined by the ILAE by frequency of absences – less frequent than in childhood absence epilepsy (CAE) – and age at onset – around puberty.[1] These are insufficient criteria for the categorization of any syndrome.[3] Thus, epidemiology, genetics, age at onset, clinical manifestations, other type of seizures, long-term prognosis and treatment may not accurately reflect the syndrome of JAE. Recently, JAE has been redefined on a cluster of video-EEG-studied clinical and EEG manifestations.[3,4]

HISTORY

The first descriptions of JAE were probably by Janz and Christian in 1957[5] and Doose et al. in 1965.[6]

PREVALENCE

The exact prevalence of JAE is not known because of variable criteria. In patients older than 20 years, the prevalence of JAE may be around 2–3 per cent of all epilepsies and around 8–10 per cent of IGE.[7,8]

SEX AND AGE AT ONSET

Both sexes are equally affected.[9] The age at onset is from 9–13 years in 70 per cent of the patients, but the range is from 5 to 20 years.[3,10] Myoclonic jerks and GTCS usually begin 1–10 years after the onset of absences. Rarely, GTCS may precede the onset of absences.[3,9]

CLINICAL AND EEG MANIFESTATIONS

Frequent and severe typical absences are the characteristic and defining seizures of JAE (Figures 12C.1, 12C.2). The usual frequency of absences is approximately 1–10 per day, but this may be much higher for some patients.[3,9,10] The absences show the following features:[4]

- There is profound impairment of consciousness similar but not as severe as in CAE. Automatisms are frequent and proportional to the severity of the impairment of consciousness. Eyelid blinking or eyelid fluttering is a usual ictal motor manifestation of which the patient is rarely aware (Figure 12C.2).[7]
- The duration ranges from 4 to 30 s but on average the absences are usually long, around 16 s.
- The ictal EEG consists of 3–4-Hz generalized spike and/or multiple spike and slow wave discharge which is regular and continuous.
- The background interictal EEG is normal or with mild abnormalities only. However, focal epileptiform

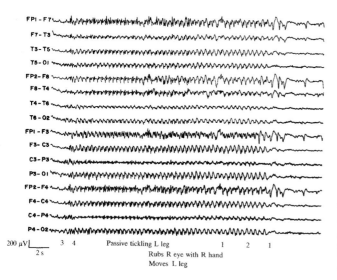

Figure 12C.1 *Video-EEG recording of a typical absence seizure from an 18-year-old patient who had severe and frequent absences daily from age 12 years. His monozygotic twin brother also had JAE. Both brothers also had infrequent GTCS. Breath-counting (annotated with numbers) stopped at the initial phase of the discharge but was resumed, in wrong sequence, 5 s before termination. Evoked automatisms from left leg and spontaneous from right foot occurred simultaneously. The EEG discharge is characterized by multiple spike and slow wave complexes without fragmentations. The regularity of the discharge is also apparent. Reproduced from Panayiotopoulos et al.[4] Differentiation of typical absence seizures in epileptic syndromes. A video EEG study of 224 seizures in 20 patients. Brain 1989; 112: 1039–1056 with the permission of Oxford University Press.*

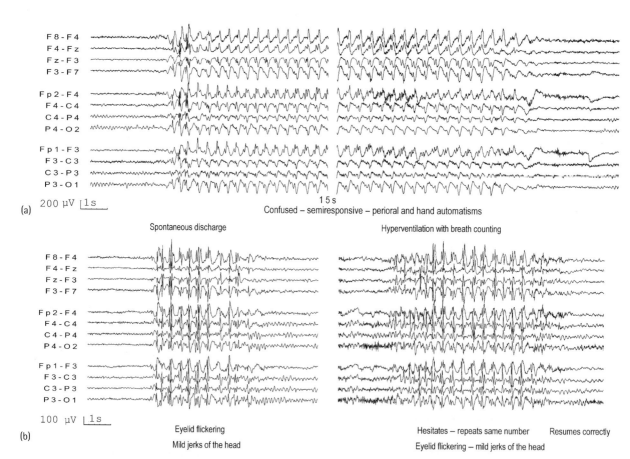

Figure 12C.2 *Video-EEG recorded absences of two adult patients with JAE: (a) A lengthy typical absence of a 31-year-old woman. She had onset of frequent and severe typical absences at age 10–11 years, but medical attendance was sought only after her first GTCS at age 15. Absences occur 5–10 times daily. They are usually long, lasting for half a minute, manifesting with severe impairment of consciousness and automatisms. GTCS, preceded by clusters of absences, occur every 3–4 months, mainly around her menstrual period. Occasionally, she also has random, infrequent and mild limb myoclonic jerks which started at the age of 20. Absences and GTCS were resistant to appropriate medication with high doses of valproic acid, also combined with lamotrigine or ethosuximide, clonazepam and acetazolamide. Absences disturb her daily life to the degree that she prefers to have GTCS instead of them. (b) Spontaneous and hyperventilation-induced absence seizures in a 48-year-old man with JAE. Irregular eyelid flickering associated with random mild jerks of the head to the left and mild impairment of consciousness were the stereotypical clinical features. Note the predominant polyspike*

abnormalities and abortive asymmetrical bursts of spike/multiple spike are common.

- One fifth of the patients with JAE develop absence status.[11,12]
- GTCS occur in 80 per cent of the patients, mainly after awakening, although nocturnal or diurnal GTCS may also be experienced.[3,6,7,9,10,13] GTCS are usually infrequent, but they may also become severe and intractable.
- Myoclonic jerks occurring in 15–25 per cent of the patients are infrequent, mild and of random distribution. They tend to occur in the afternoon hours, when the patient is tired, rather than in the morning after awakening.[3,12]

SEIZURE-PRECIPITATING FACTORS

Mental and psychological arousal are the main precipitating factors for typical absences. Conversely, sleep deprivation, fatigue, alcohol, excitement or lights (alone, or usually in combination) are the main precipitating factors for GTCS. Some authors have reported that 8 per cent of JAE patients suffer from photosensitivity clinically or on EEG.[9] However, clinical photosensitivity that is a consistent provocation for seizures, typical absences or GTCS may be incompatible with JAE. These patients may have other IGE syndromes.[3] EEG photosensitivity that consists of facilitation of absences by intermittent photic stimulation (IPS) may not be uncommon.

GENETICS AND ETIOLOGY

JAE is determined by genetic factors, but the mode of transmission and relation to other forms of IGE, and particularly CAE and juvenile myoclonic epilepsy (JME), has not yet been established; a single mendelian mode appears to be unlikely. There is an increased incidence of epileptic disorders in families of patients with JAE, including reports of monozygotic twins with JAE.[4,10,14]

A proband with JAE was found in 3 of 37 families selected because at least 3 members were affected by IGE in one or more generations.[15] However, only one sibling also had JAE; other members mainly had GTCS.[15] JAE still has to pass the test of genetic identification. It may be linked to chromosome 8,[16] 21,[17] 18[18] and probably 5.[18] Heterogeneity may be common, as indicated in animal models. Autopsy[19] and MRI studies[20] have found microdysgenesis and other cerebral structural changes in patients with JAE.

PROGNOSIS

JAE is a lifelong disorder, although seizures can be controlled in 70–80 per cent of the patients. There is a tendency for the absences to become less severe with age, in terms of impairment of cognition, duration and frequency, particularly after the fourth decade of life.[9,13] GTCS are usually infrequent, and are often precipitated by sleep deprivation, fatigue and alcohol consumption. Myoclonic jerks, if present, are not troublesome for the patient. However, one fifth of the patients may have frequent and sometimes intractable absences and GTCS (see caption of Figure 12C.2) and this proportion may be higher if appropriate treatment is not initiated at early stages of JAE.

MANAGEMENT

The treatment of IGE with absence seizures has been reviewed recently.[21] Currently, valproic acid, ethosuximide and lamotrigine alone or in combination are the primary drugs for the treatment of absence seizures. Of the newest drugs, levetiracetam and topiramate are promising. Vigabatrin, tiagabine, carbamazepine and phenytoin are strongly contraindicated. Patients should be warned with regard to precipitating factors of GTCS. Treatment may be lifelong: attempts to withdraw medication almost invariably lead to relapses, even after many years free of seizures. However, this has yet to be prospectively studied.

Figure 12C.2 *(Continued)*
component of the discharges. GTCS started at around the age of 10 years. They usually occurred within half an hour after awakening. They were very frequent, sometimes weekly, or every 1–3 months. They were preceded by brief absence seizures. Onset of absences could not be determined. These are frequent but not disturbing for him. He is aware of them because of 'eyelid flickering and becoming distant', 'observing rather than being there'. Numerous absences were recorded on video-EEG for many years, even after he was no longer aware of them. He also had myoclonic jerks that were mild and sporadic, occurring at any time of the day. They probably started at age 25 years. For many years he was inappropriately treated with phenytoin and phenobarbital. A dramatic improvement occurred at age 44 years with the appropriate introduction of valproic acid, later combined with ethosuximide. However, he continued to have infrequent GTCS. These stopped when lamotrigine was added. In the last 8 years he had only 4–5 GTCS, probably after missing his medication. From Panayiotopoulos CP. A clinical guide to epileptic syndromes and their treatment. Oxford: Bladon Medical Publishing, 2002 with the permission of the publisher.

DIFFERENTIAL DIAGNOSIS

In general and particularly in adults, absences are often misdiagnosed as complex partial seizures although it is easy to differentiate them.[3] The differentiation of JAE from other IGE with absences may be complex without appropriate video-EEG evaluation.[3,4,21] In children, it is often difficult to distinguish between CAE and JAE, because their features overlap and manifestations are similar. In JAE, absences often start later, usually they are less frequent and impairment of cognition is less severe.[4] Automatisms are equally prominent in both. Limb myoclonic jerks, at times other than during the absences, and/or GTCS in the presence of severe absences, indicate JAE. JAE is distinctly different from Jeavons syndrome of brief (3–6 s) absences with rapid eyelid myoclonia (Chapter 11C); from perioral myoclonia with absences accompanied by rhythmic perioral myoclonia during the absence; and from epilepsy with myoclonic absences where the absences are accompanied by rhythmic myoclonic jerks (Chapter 11B). In adolescents, the differential diagnosis between JAE and JME should not be difficult. Severe absences are the major problem in JAE, myoclonic jerks are the main seizure type in JME. Absences in JME are mild and often inconspicuous (Chapter 12B).

KEY POINTS

- JAE is an IGE syndrome
- Infrequent typical absences are **first seen round about the beginning of the second decade**
- **GTCS** occur in most patients
- Sporadic **myoclonic jerks** occur in about one fifth of patients
- The **precipitating factors** for the typical absences and the GTCS differ
- JAE is a **lifelong** epilepsy, which requires continued medication and attention to lifestyle

---

REFERENCES

1. Commission on Classification and Terminology of the International League Against Epilepsy. Proposal for revised classification of epilepsies and epileptic syndromes. *Epilepsia* 1989; **30**: 389–399.
2. Engel J Jr. A proposed diagnostic scheme for people with epileptic seizures and with epilepsy: Report of the ILAE Task Force on Classification and Terminology. *Epilepsia* 2001; **42**: 796–803.
3. Panayiotopoulos CP. Absence epilepsies. In: Engel JJ, Pedley TA (eds.) *Epilepsy: A Comprehensive Textbook*. Philadelphia: Lippincott-Raven, 1997: 2327–2346.
4. Panayiotopoulos CP, Obeid T, Waheed G. Differentiation of typical absence seizures in epileptic syndromes. A video EEG study of 224 seizures in 20 patients. *Brain* 1989; **112**: 1039–1056.
5. Janz D, Christian W. Impulsiv-Petit mal. *Zeitschrift für Nervenheilkunde* 1957; **176**: 346–386. (English translation by Genton P.) In: Malafosse A, Genton P, Hirsch E, *et al.* (eds) *Idiopathic Generalised Epilepsies*. London: John Libbey, 1957: 229–251.
6. Doose H, Volzke E, Scheffner D. Verlaufsformen kindlicher epilepsien mit spike wave-absencen. *Archiv für Psychiatrie und Nervenkrank* 1965; **207**: 394–415.
7. Panayiotopoulos CP, Giannakodimos S, Chroni E. Typical absences in adults. In: Duncan JS, Panayiotopoulos CP (eds) *Typical Absences and Related Epileptic Syndromes*. London: Churchill Communications Europe, 1995: 289–299.
8. ILAE classification of epilepsies: its applicability and practical value of different diagnostic categories. Osservatorio Regionale per L'Epilessia (OREp), Lombardy. *Epilepsia* 1996; **37**: 1051–1059.
9. Wolf P. Juvenile absence epilepsy. In Roger J, Bureau M, Dravet C *et al*, (eds) *Epileptic Syndromes in Infancy, Childhood and Adolescence*. London: John Libbey, 1992: 307–312.
10. Obeid T. Clinical and genetic aspects of juvenile absence epilepsy. *Journal of Neurology* 1994; **241**: 487–491.
11. Agathonikou A, Panayiotopoulos CP, Giannakodimos S, Koutroumanidis M. Typical absence status in adults: diagnostic and syndromic considerations. *Epilepsia* 1998; **39**: 1265–1276.
12. Panayiotopoulos CP. Absence status epilepticus. In: Gilman S (ed.) *Medlink Neurology*. San Diego, CA: Arbor Publishing, 2002.
13. Oller L. [Prospective study of the differences between the syndromes of infantile absence epilepsy and syndromes of juvenile absence epilepsy]. *Revue Neurologique* 1996; **24**: 930–936.
14. Berkovic SF, Howell RA, Hay DA, Hopper JL. Epilepsies in twins. In: Wolf P (ed.) *Epileptic Seizures and Syndromes*. London: John Libbey, 1994: 157–164.
15. Bianchi A, and the Italian LAE Collaborative Group. Study of concordance of symptoms in families with absence epilepsies. In: Duncan JS, Panayiotopoulos CP (eds) *Typical Absences and Related Epileptic Syndromes*. London: Churchill Communications Europe, 1995: 328–337.
16. Durner M, Zhou G, Fu D, *et al.* Evidence for linkage of adolescent-onset idiopathic generalized epilepsies to chromosome 8 and genetic heterogeneity. *American Journal of Human Genetics* 1999; **64**: 1411–1419.
17. Sander T, Hildmann T, Kretz R, *et al.* Allelic association of juvenile absence epilepsy with a GluR5 kainate receptor gene (GRIK1) polymorphism. *American Journal of Medical Genetics* 1997; **74**: 416–421.
18. Durner M, Keddache MA, Tomasini L, *et al.* Genome scan of idiopathic generalized epilepsy: evidence for major susceptibility gene and modifying genes influencing the seizure type. *Annals of Neurology* 2001; **49**: 328–335.
19. Meencke HJ, Janz D. The significance of microdysgenesia in primary generalized epilepsy: an answer to the considerations of Lyon and Gastaut. *Epilepsia* 1985; **26**: 368–371.
20. Woermann FG, Sisodiya SM, Free SL, Duncan JS. Quantitative MRI in patients with idiopathic generalized epilepsy. Evidence of widespread cerebral structural changes. *Brain* 1998; **121**: 1661–1667.
21. Panayiotopoulos CP. Treatment of typical absence seizures and related epileptic syndromes. *Paediatric Drugs* 2001; **3**: 379–403.

Benign partial seizures of adolescence

CP PANAYIOTOPOULOS

DEFINITION

Benign (isolated) partial seizures of adolescence constitute an idiopathic, short-duration and transient condition of the second decade of life with a peak at 13–15 years of age. This condition manifests with a single, or a cluster of 2–5 partial, mainly motor and sensory, seizures which, in half of the cases, progress to secondarily generalized tonic-clonic convulsions. There are no epileptic events before or after this limited seizure period which lasts for no more than 36 hours. The seizures are mainly diurnal and predominantly affect male teenagers. Physical and mental states, as well as EEG and brain imaging, are normal.

CASE HISTORIES

A typical case

A 14-year-old boy had a partial motor seizure consisting of tonic deviation of the head to the right, followed by forced circling movements before ending in a generalized tonic-clonic seizure. Postictally, he was confused for 15 minutes. MRI of the brain was normal. EEG showed mild, nonspecific, bitemporal theta activity. Treatment with carbamazepine was initiated, but the boy stopped medication after 2 weeks. Six years later, he remained well, with no seizures and a normal EEG.

A less typical case

An 18-year-old student rushed to catch the train back home after a hard day's work. He was hungry and thirsty. He looked at a small video display unit of travel information: after he looked away, the image of the screen persisted in the right upper corner of his vision and, nearly simultaneously, started flashing at a rate estimated at 3–5 Hz for 2 s. This was followed by the visual perception of the walls of the station and the other passengers closing in on him, ending in a generalized tonic-clonic seizure. Routine EEG, sleep deprivation EEG and MRI were all normal. No medication was prescribed. Two years later he remained well, with no further visual or other seizures.

HISTORY

The condition was described in 1978[1] as an 'unrecognized syndrome of benign focal epileptic seizures in teenagers'. This chapter is based on two later reviews of 108 patients from the original authors[2,3] and more recent reports of 55 cases.[4–7]

CLASSIFICATION

Although considered as a syndrome of 'isolated partial seizures of adolescence' by Loiseau and Jallon,[3] benign (isolated) partial seizures of adolescence is not recognized as a syndrome by the International League Against Epilepsy Task Force on Classification.[8] Its best position should be in the new category: 'Conditions with epileptic seizures that do not require a diagnosis of epilepsy'. This category includes '**single seizures or isolated clusters of seizures**, rarely repeated seizures (oligo-epilepsy)'.[8]

PREVALENCE, SEX, GENETICS, PRECIPITATING FACTORS AND CIRCADIAN DISTRIBUTION

According to the most extensive reviews,[2,3] one quarter of partial seizures with onset between 12 and 18 years of age have a benign course, i.e. they are single or occur in a cluster of up to five seizures during 36 hours, never to occur again. There is a 71 per cent male preponderance. A family or personal history of seizures is extremely rare. There are no apparent precipitating factors and the seizures are diurnal in 87 per cent. In a personal sample of 120 patients with onset of simple partial seizures in the second decade of life, nine cases satisfied the criteria of benign partial seizures of adolescence, as described in the two cases above. However, another study found 8 of 37 with partial epilepsy had benign partial seizures of adolescence.[7]

AGE

These isolated epileptic events occur between the ages of 10 and 20 years with a peak (one third of cases) at 13–15 years.

CLINICAL MANIFESTATIONS

Although the seizures are partial, the temporal lobes are rarely involved. Eighty-seven per cent of the seizures are diurnal. The teenager is fully aware and can give a reliable account of the onset of the clinical manifestations in 88 per cent of episodes. However, consciousness rarely remains intact throughout. Usually, there is evolution to impaired cognition, and/or to secondary generalized tonic-clonic convulsions, which occur in half of the cases. The commonest ictal clinical manifestations are motor, usually without Jacksonian marching, and somatosensory. Visual, vertiginous and autonomic symptoms are reported in one-fifth of the cases. Experiential phenomena practically never occur.

The physical and mental states of the patients are normal. Laboratory tests and brain imaging are also normal. The EEG may show some minor, nonspecific, abnormalities without spikes or focal slowing. In a recent report,[6]

about one quarter of 37 cases had functional spikes. This is incompatible with this syndrome, and a diagnosis of benign childhood partial seizures[9] seems more likely.

PROGNOSIS

Prognosis is excellent; in 80 per cent there is a single, isolated seizure event and in the remaining a cluster of 2–5 seizures, all occurring within 36 hours.

KEY POINTS

- This is an interesting seizure susceptibility in **otherwise normal** adolescents manifesting with one or a cluster of 2–5 partial seizures
- The seizures **should not be treated with drugs**
- **Diagnosis is difficult**, as there are no specific features at onset to differentiate these patients from others with similar clinical manifestations, but of different etiology
- All adolescents with onset of partial seizures should be investigated with **MRI and EEG**. If these are normal, the diagnosis of benign partial seizures of adolescence is more likely
- A definitive diagnosis cannot be made before **1–5 years of freedom from seizures**

REFERENCES

1. Loiseau P, Orgogozo JM. An unrecognized syndrome of benign focal epileptic seizures in teenagers? *Lancet* 1978; **2**: 1070–1071.
2. Loiseau P, Louiset P. In: Roger J, Bureau M, Dravet C, *et al.* (eds) *Epileptic Syndromes in Infancy, Childhood and Adolescence*. London: John Libbey, 1992; 343–345.
3. Loiseau P, Jallon P. In: Roger J, Bureau M, Dravet C, *et al.* (eds) *Epileptic Syndromes in Infancy, Childhood and Adolescence*, 3rd edn. London: John Libbey, 2002.
4. Mauri JA, Iniguez C, Jerico I, Morales F. Benign partial seizures of adolescence. *Epilepsia* 1996; **37**(Suppl. 4): 102.
5. Jallon P, Loiseau J, Loiseau P, *et al.* The risk of recurrence after a first unprovoked seizure in adolescence. *Epilepsia* 1999; **40**(Suppl. 7): 87–88.
6. Capovilla G, Gambardella A, Romeo A, *et al.* Benign partial epilepsies of adolescence: a report of 37 new cases. *Epilepsia* 2001; **42**: 1549–1552.
7. King MA, Newton MR, Berkovic SF. Benign partial seizures of adolescence. *Epilepsia* 1999; **40**: 1244–1247.
8. Engel J, Jr. A proposed diagnostic scheme for people with epileptic seizures and with epilepsy: Report of the ILAE Task Force on Classification and Terminology. *Epilepsia* 2001; **42**: 796–803.
9. Panayiotopoulos CP. *A Clinical Guide to Epileptic Syndromes and their Treatment.* Oxford: Bladon Medical Publishing, 2002; 89–113.

Reflex seizures and reflex epilepsies

MICHAEL KOUTROUMANIDIS AND CP PANAYIOTOPOULOS

The reflex epilepsies comprise a group of syndromes characterized by seizures that always or almost always occur in response to a specific stimulus (**reflex seizures**). The etiology may be idiopathic, symptomatic or probably symptomatic.

CLASSIFICATION AND NOMENCLATURE

According to the recently proposed ILAE glossary[1] and classification:[2]

- **Reflex seizures** are 'Objectively and consistently demonstrated to be evoked by a specific afferent stimulus or by activity of the patient. Afferent stimuli can be: elementary, i.e. unstructured: light flashes, startle, a monotone; or, elaborate i.e. structured. Activity may be elementary, e.g. motor, a movement; or elaborate, e.g. cognitive function, e.g. reading, chess playing, or both as in reading aloud.'
- **Reflex epilepsy syndrome** is 'A syndrome in which all epileptic seizures are precipitated by sensory stimuli. Reflex seizures that occur in focal and generalized epilepsy syndromes that are also associated with spontaneous seizures are listed as seizure types. Isolated reflex seizures can also occur in situations that do not necessarily require a diagnosis of epilepsy. Seizures precipitated by other special circumstances, such as fever or alcohol withdrawal, are not reflex seizures.'

Reflex epilepsies are determined by the specific precipitant, the stimulus, and the clinical-EEG response, the seizure. The type of the stimulus is used for descriptive purposes (Table 12E.1). Some principal forms of simple and complex reflex epilepsies are briefly reviewed here, and some basic references cited for the remainder.

STIMULUS

The stimulus, or trigger, is specific for a given patient and may be simple (i.e. flashes of light, tactile stimuli, etc.) or complex (eating, reading, etc.).

With complex stimuli (complex reflex epilepsies), the latency from the stimulus onset to the clinical or EEG response is typically longer than in simple reflex epilepsies.

RESPONSE

The response may consist of combined clinical and EEG manifestations, subclinical EEG activation only, or clinical changes without conspicuous surface EEG changes. Reflex seizures may be generalized, e.g. absences, myoclonic jerks and generalized tonic/tonic clonic seizures (GTCS), or focal such as visual, motor or sensory. GTCS may constitute the first clinical response, follow a cluster of absences or myoclonic jerks, or be secondary to a partial, simple or complex seizure. Myoclonic jerks are by far the commonest, manifested in the limbs and trunk, or regionally, as in the jaw muscles in reading epilepsy, or the eyelids, as in eyelid myoclonia with absences. The electroclinical events may reflect activation of the stimulus-related

Table 12E.1 *The main stimulus-sensitive (reflex) epilepsies and their responsible stimuli*

I Somatosensory stimuli
  1 Exteroceptive simple somatosensory stimuli
    a Tapping epilepsy (as in benign childhood epilepsy with somatosensory evoked spikes)[3]
    b Sensory (tactile) evoked idiopathic myoclonic seizures in infancy[4]
    c Tooth-brushing epilepsy[5]
    d Hot water epilepsy[6]
  2 Complex proprioceptive stimuli
    a Eating epilepsy[7]
    b Gait epilepsy[8]
    c Epileptic paroxysmal kinesiogenic choreoathetosis[9]

II Visual stimuli
    a Photosensitive epilepsies
    b Pattern-induced epilepsies
    c Fixation-off induced epilepsies
    d Scotogenic epilepsy
    e Self-induced photo- and pattern-sensitive epilepsy

III Auditory and olfactory stimuli
    a Seizures induced by pure sounds or words[10]
    b Music-induced seizures[11]
    c Eating-induced (multifactorial, triggered by sight, smell or taste)[7]
    d Startle epilepsy (sudden and unexpected stimuli, mainly auditory)[12]

IV High-level processes induced seizures (cognitive, emotional, decision-making tasks and other complex stimuli)
    a Thinking epilepsy (decision-making) epilepsy[46,47]
    b Noogenic (probably with prominent emotional element) epilepsies[13]

V Reading and language-induced epilepsies
    a Reading epilepsy
      With myoclonic seizures[14,51]
      With focal seizures (alexia)[14,49]
      With absences
    b Language-induced epilepsies[14]

brain region only, as in visually/photically-induced EEG occipital spikes; or become much wider, as in visually/photically-induced focal seizures that propagate in extra-occipital areas; and even generalized, as in the photoparoxysmal response that is associated with generalized seizures. Inter-individual responses to the same stimulus vary widely. For example, photic stimuli or reading may trigger both focal and generalized seizures.[14,15]

SIMPLE REFLEX EPILEPSIES

Visual-induced seizures and epilepsies

The commonest type of reflex seizure is the visual seizure, which is triggered by the physical characteristics of the visual stimulus and not by its cognitive effects. Photo- and pattern-sensitivity are the two main categories, but they frequently overlap. Both are genetically determined.[16] The interval between stimulus and response is very short, typically within seconds.

PHOTOSENSITIVITY, EPILEPSY SYNDROMES AND SEIZURES

Photosensitivity is the propensity to epileptic seizures in response to intermittent photic stimulation (IPS). Neurophysiological studies in humans have demonstrated that photic stimuli activate primarily the occipital cortex, from which the ictal discharge is generated.[17,18] Thus, despite the apparent paradox of photosensitivity being primarily associated with IGE,[19] photosensitive seizures are of regional, occipital lobe, origin. Although mainly encountered in IGE, photosensitivity features in various other forms of human epilepsy, including generalized and focal, idiopathic and symptomatic/probably symptomatic, and even situation-related seizures, and does not correspond to a particular epileptic syndrome. A list of the epilepsy syndromes that are associated with photosensitivity can be found elsewhere.[20] In pure photosensitive epilepsies seizures occur only in response to photic stimuli and not spontaneously.[21] According to the type of the provoked seizures, pure photosensitive epilepsy can be classified both amongst the IGE and the idiopathic focal, occipital lobe, epilepsies.[22] In the IGE-type photosensitive epilepsies, GTCS are considered the commonest type of seizures, but video-EEG recordings have documented that myoclonic jerks are much more common; absences may follow in prevalence. In half of these patients the resting EEG is normal but approximately 20 per cent of them show generalized discharges on eye-closure. The seizures are usually infrequent and the prognosis is often excellent. Avoidance of precipitating factors may be the only treatment. In the idiopathic photosensitive occipital lobe epilepsy, seizures have clear occipital symptomatology. Elementary visual hallucinations predominate and may progress to other manifestations from anterior spread and even evolve into GTCS. Spontaneous occipital or other types of generalized seizures may coexist in the less pure forms. This form should be differentiated from the rare cases of symptomatic photosensitive occipital epilepsy and in those patients with visual hallucinations only, from migraine.[23,24] The prognosis is usually good but a liability to seizures may persist.

PATTERN SENSITIVITY

Pattern-induced epilepsy refers to epileptic seizures induced by patterns.[21,25,26] All types of generalized seizures have been described, but absences are probably the commonest. Nearly all patients with clinical pattern sensitivity show photoparoxysmal responses on appropriate IPS testing.

Conversely, of clinically photosensitive patients, 30 per cent are also sensitive to stationary and 70 per cent to appropriately vibrating patterns of stripes. Thus, patterns alone appear to be less epileptogenic than photic stimuli, but enhance the effect of the latter under testing conditions and in real life.

PREVALENCE

Photosensitive seizures and epilepsies affect 1 in 4000 of the population, 5 per cent of patients with epileptic seizures. Two thirds are women. The peak age at onset is 12–13 years. Amongst the patients with photoparoxysmal responses and seizures, 42 per cent have only photically induced seizures, i.e. pure photosensitive epilepsy; 40 per cent also have spontaneous seizures, and the remainder have spontaneous seizures only.[21] In the UK the annual incidence of cases of epilepsy with photoparoxysmal responses on their first EEG is conservatively estimated to be 1.1 per 100 000, representing approximately 2 per cent of all new cases of epilepsy. In the age range 7–19 years, the annual incidence rises to 5.7 per 100 000, i.e. approximately 10 per cent of all new cases of epilepsy presenting in this age range.[27] EEG photosensitivity was found in 48 (0.35 per cent) of 13 625 healthy male Royal Air Force crew candidates, aged 17–25 years.[28]

Laboratory (EEG) and clinical photosensitivity

Many artificial or natural light sources can provoke epileptic seizures. Television, video-games, computer visual display units, night clubs and natural flickering light (in that order) are common triggers. Photosensitivity is demonstrated and quantified with EEG using appropriate IPS techniques.[29]

EEG PHENOMENA

The photoparoxysmal response to IPS is the EEG hallmark of photosensitivity (Figure 12E.1).[21,30,31] This consists of generalized spikes or multiple spike and slow-wave discharges, of higher amplitude in the anterior regions, but its onset, particularly if patterned IPS is employed, is often marked by occipital spikes.[17,32] The photoparoxysmal response is associated with up to 90 per cent likelihood of having clinical photosensitive seizures, particularly if it outlasts the stimulus train (Figure 12E.1, upper trace).[30] Milder abnormal responses to IPS consist of posterior abnormalities, which do not spread into the anterior regions. These mainly consist of occipital spikes (Figure 12E.1, bottom trace), which are often time-locked to the flicker, coinciding with the positive P100 of the visual evoked response.[17] Half of the subjects with posterior photoparoxysmal abnormalities suffer clinical seizures.[21]

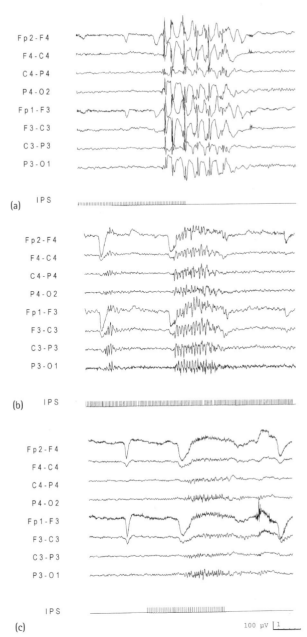

Figure 12E.1 *Various types of photoparoxysmal response: (a) Generalized photoparoxysmal response of spike and wave outlasting the stimulus train. These are often associated with clinical absences. (b) Generalized photoparoxysmal response of polyspikes limited within the stimulus train. These are often associated with jerks. (c) Posterior limited response consisting of occipital spikes. From Panayiotopoulos CP. A Clinical Guide to Epileptic Syndromes and their Treatment. Oxford: Bladon Medical Publishing, 2002 with the permission of the Publisher.*

CLINICAL ICTAL PHENOMENA

Complaints such as dizziness, eye fatigue or aches, headache and epigastric sensations, and simple visual hallucinations may reflect focal, occipital, ictal activity, and should be differentiated from normal phenomena or migraine.[24,33]

Such ictal activity may become self-sustained and give rise to focal seizures,[34] spreading to frontal or mesial temporal structures with varying semiology and propagation speed. Other photically induced seizure phenomena include regional (eyelids), bilateral, or generalized myoclonus, tonic unilateral version of head and eyes, absences and GTCS.

Seizures induced by video games

There is an increasing incidence of seizures induced by video games.[35–37] These can occur both with games using an interlaced video monitor (computer monitor or TV) and with small handheld liquid crystal displays and non-interlaced 70 Hz arcade games. Eighty-seven per cent of patients are aged 7–19 years: within this age group the annual incidence of first seizures triggered by playing electronic screen games is 1.5/100 000.[38] Photosensitivity is a major trigger (70 per cent) but these seizures may also occur in nonphotosensitive patients with IGE when sleep deprivation, fatigue, decision-making and praxis operate alone or in combination. Occipital lobe epilepsy with or without photosensitivity is the second most frequent type of epilepsy with seizures induced by video games.[35]

Self-induced seizures

Self-induction is a mode of seizure precipitation employed by mentally handicapped or normal photosensitive individuals. Its prevalence is debated.[21,39] Techniques include waving the outspread fingers in front of a bright light, viewing geometric patterns or slow eye-closure. Absences and myoclonic jerks are the commonest seizures in self-induction. Whether eyelid blinking or compulsive attraction to television or bright sun is mainly an attempt at self-induction or part of the seizure[40] is disputed, although both may be true.

Treatment

In patients with exclusive photosensitive seizures, avoidance of the provocative stimulus may be adequate. Patients should be advised to view TV in a well-lit room; to maintain a maximum comfortable viewing distance, typically more than 2.5 m for a 48-cm (19-inch) screen; to use the remote control; and, if approaching the screen, to cover one eye with their palm; and to avoid prolonged watching, particularly if sleep deprived and tired. Occlusion of one eye is also advised when photosensitive subjects are suddenly exposed to flickering lights e.g. in night clubs. Conditioning treatment[41] and wearing appropriate tinted glasses[42] have been recommended. Small doses of valproic acid may be needed in patients with possible spontaneous seizures or

coexistent spontaneous EEG discharges. Patients with distinct epileptic syndromes and photosensitivity are treated accordingly. Valproic acid controls all seizure types induced by light in more than 80 per cent of the patients, and clonazepam may control both absences and jerks. Levetiracetam has been shown to abolish photosensitivity.[43]

Fixation–off sensitive epilepsies (FOS)

The term denotes the form or forms of epilepsy and/or EEG abnormalities that are elicited by elimination of central vision and fixation.[44] Panayiotopoulos syndrome[45] and Gastaut-type childhood occipital epilepsy[33] are the model syndromes of FOS (Figure 12E.2). The term **scoto-sensitive** refers to patients with seizures and EEG abnormalities induced by the complete elimination of retinal light stimulation; most cases described as scotosensitive are probably FOS.[44]

COMPLEX REFLEX EPILEPSIES

Seizures induced by thinking, processing of spatial information and sequential decision-making

Thinking-induced seizures occur in response to high cognitive functions: effective triggers include mathematical calculations, drawing, playing cards, chess and other board games, and Rubik's cube. Decision-making and spatial tasks are essential elements in seizure provocation.[46] Thinking-induced seizures usually occur in the context of IGE.[47] They usually start during adolescence and are myoclonic, absences and GTCS; focal seizures are rare.[15] Neuropsychological analysis of the stimuli points to right parietal cortical dysfunction.

Reading– and language–induced seizures and epilepsies

Reading epilepsy is a distinct form of reflex epilepsy in which all or almost all seizures are precipitated by reading.[14,48] Regional, reading-induced myoclonic jerks appear typically in mid-teens, involve primarily the masticatory muscles and the tongue, and constitute the commonest seizure (Figure 12E.3, upper trace). Some patients have prolonged focal seizures manifested with alexia and possibly dysphasia (Figure 12E.3, lower trace),[14,49] but absences are exceptional. GTCS may ensue if reading continues. In the myoclonic variant, ictal EEG discharges are brief, bilateral synchronous or focal, often with a left hemisphere predominance, and ictal functional neuroimaging

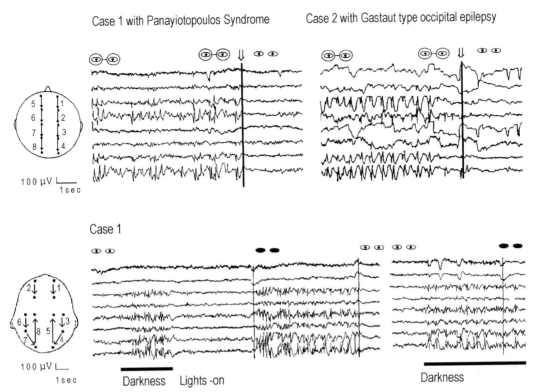

Case 1 with Panayiotopoulos Syndrome   Case 2 with Gastaut type occipital epilepsy

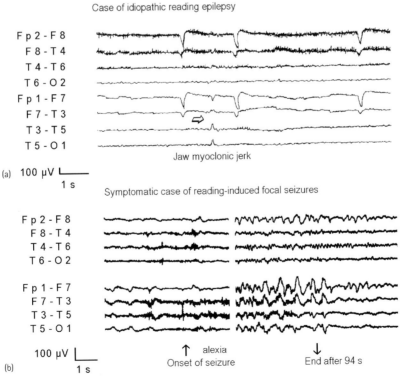

Figure 12E.2 *Fixation-off sensitivity. Case 1 had Panayiotopoulos syndrome, Case 2 Gastaut-type occipital epilepsy. Occipital paroxysms occur continuously only when fixation and central vision are eliminated. Eyes with glasses denote conditions of elimination of central vision and fixation. Modified from Panayiotopoulos CP, Inhibitory effect of central vision on occipital lobe seizures. Neurology 1981; 31: 1330–1333 with the permission of Lippincott, Williams & Wilkins.*

Case of idiopathic reading epilepsy

F p 2 - F 8
F 8 - T 4
T 4 - T 6
T 6 - O 2
F p 1 - F 7
F 7 - T 3
T 3 - T 5
T 5 - O 1

Jaw myoclonic jerk

(a) 100 µV ∟___
              1 s

Symptomatic case of reading-induced focal seizures

F p 2 - F 8
F 8 - T 4
T 4 - T 6
T 6 - O 2

F p 1 - F 7
F 7 - T 3
T 3 - T 5
T 5 - O 1

100 µV ∟___
          1 s

↑ alexia
Onset of seizure

↓
End after 94 s

(b)

Figure 12E.3 *Reading-induced seizures: (a) regional (jaw) myoclonic seizure; (b) prolonged partial seizure manifested with alexia. Modified from Koutroumanidis et al. The variants of reading epilepsy. A clinical and video-EEG study of 17 patients with reading-induced seizures. Brain 1998; 121: 1409–1427 with the permission of Oxford University Press.[14]*

studies have shown multiple cortical hyperexcitable areas, which are part of the neuronal network that subserves speech.[50] Seizures are usually well controlled with clonazepam or valproic acid. In many patients, clinically identical seizures can also be provoked by other linguistic activities, justifying the term **language-induced epilepsy**.[14] Whether reading or language-induced epilepsy should be classified amongst the generalized or the focal idiopathic epilepsies is still a matter of debate.[14,48,51]

KEY POINTS

- Reflex epilepsies are characterized by seizures that are evoked by **specific afferent stimuli**, or by activities of the patient
- The stimuli can be categorized as **simple**, e.g. flashes of light, or **complex**, e.g. eating or reading
- **Visual induced seizures** are the commonest
- Both photosensitivity and pattern-sensitivity are **genetically determined**
- Pure **photosensitivity** can be classified both amongst the IGE and the idiopathic, focal, occipital lobe epilepsies
- **Thinking-induced seizures** usually occur in the context of IGE
- **Reading epilepsy** is a distinct form: it is unclear whether this should be classified as a generalized or a focal epilepsy

---

REFERENCES

1. Blume WT, Luders HO, Mizrahi E, et al. Glossary of descriptive terminology for ictal semiology: report of the ILAE task force on classification and terminology. *Epilepsia* 2001; **42**(9): 1212–1218.
2. Engel J Jr. A proposed diagnostic scheme for people with epileptic seizures and with epilepsy: report of the ILAE Task Force on Classification and Terminology. *Epilepsia* 2001; **42**(6): 796–803.
3. De Marco P, Negrin P. Parietal focal spikes evoked by contralateral tactile somatotopic stimulation in four non-epileptic subjects. *Electroencephalography and Clinical Neurophysiology* 1973; **34**(3): 308–312.
4. Ricci S, Cusmai R, Fusco L, Vigevano F. Reflex myoclonic epilepsy in infancy: a new age-dependent idiopathic epileptic syndrome related to startle reaction. *Epilepsia* 1995; **36**(4): 342–348.
5. Koutroumanidis M, Pearce R, Sadoh DR, Panayiotopoulos CP. Tooth brushing-induced seizures: a case report. *Epilepsia* 2001; **42**(5): 686–688.
6. Bebek N, Gurses C, Gokyigit A, et al. Hot water epilepsy: clinical and electrophysiologic findings based on 21 cases. *Epilepsia* 2001; **42**(9): 1180–1184.
7. Remillard GM, Zifkin BG, Andermann F. Seizures induced by eating. *Advances in Neurology* 1998; **75**: 227–240.
8. Iriarte J, Sanchez-Carpintero R, Schlumberger E, et al. Gait epilepsy. A case report of gait-induced seizures. *Epilepsia* 2001; **42**(8): 1087–1090.
9. Perez-Borja C, Tassinari AC, Swanson AG. Paroxysmal choreoathetosis and seizures induced by movement (reflex epilepsy). *Epilepsia* 1967; **8**(4): 260–270.
10. Forster FM, Hansotia P, Cleeland CS, Ludwig A. A case of voice-induced epilepsy treated by conditioning. *Neurology* 1969; **19**(4): 325–331.
11. Wieser HG, Hungerbuhler H, Siegel AM, Buck A. Musicogenic epilepsy: review of the literature and case report with ictal single photon emission computed tomography. *Epilepsia* 1997; **38**(2): 200–207.
12. Saenz-Lope E, Herranz FJ, Masdeu JC. Startle epilepsy: a clinical study. *Annals of Neurology* 1984; **16**(1): 78–81.
13. Koutroumanidis M, Agathonikou A, Panayiotopoulos CP. Self induced noogenic seizures in a photosensitive patient [letter]. *Journal of Neurology, Neurosurgery and Psychiatry* 1998; **64**(1): 139–140.
14. Koutroumanidis M, Koepp MJ, Richardson MP, et al. The variants of reading epilepsy. A clinical and video-EEG study of 17 patients with reading-induced seizures. *Brain* 1998; **121**: 1409–1427.
15. Martinez O, Reisin R, Andermann F, Zifkin BG, Sevlever G. Evidence for reflex activation of experiential complex partial seizures. *Neurology* 2001; **56**(1): 121–123.
16. Doose H, Waltz S. Photosensitivity – genetics and clinical significance. *Neuropediatrics* 1993; **24**(5): 249–255.
17. Panayiotopoulos CP, Jeavons PM, Harding GF. Occipital spikes and their relation to visual responses in epilepsy, with particular reference to photosensitive epilepsy. *Electroencephalography and Clinical Neurophysiology* 1972; **32**(2): 179–190.
18. Wilkins AJ, Andermann F, Ives J. Stripes, complex cells and seizures. An attempt to determine the locus and nature of the trigger mechanism in pattern-sensitive epilepsy. *Brain* 1975; **98**(3): 365–380.
19. Commission on Classification and Terminology of the International League Against Epilepsy. Proposal for revised classification of epilepsies and epileptic syndromes. *Epilepsia* 1989; **30**: 389–399.
20. Kasteleijn-Nolst Trenité DG, Guerrini R, Binnie CD, Genton P. Visual sensitivity and epilepsy: a proposed terminology and classification for clinical and EEG phenomenology. *Epilepsia* 2001; **42**(5): 692–701.
21. Harding GFA, Jeavons PM. *Photosensitive Epilepsy*. London: MacKeith Press, 1994.
22. Guerrini R, Dravet C, Genton P, et al. Idiopathic photosensitive occipital lobe epilepsy. *Epilepsia* 1995; **36**(9):883–891.
23. Panayiotopoulos CP. Visual phenomena and headache in occipital epilepsy: a review, a systematic study and differentiation from migraine. *Epileptic Disorders* 1999; **1**(4): 205–216.
24. Panayiotopoulos CP. Elementary visual hallucinations in migraine and epilepsy. *Journal of Neurology, Neurosurgery and Psychiatry* 1994; **57**(11): 1371–1374.
25. Panayiotopoulos CP. Self-induced pattern-sensitive epilepsy. *Archives of Neurology* 1979; **36**(1): 48–50.

26. Wilkins AJ, Darby CE, Binnie CD. Neurophysiological aspects of pattern-sensitive epilepsy. *Brain* 1979; **102**(1): 1–25.

27. Quirk JA, Fish DR, Smith SJ, *et al*. Incidence of photosensitive epilepsy: a prospective national study. *Electroencephalography and Clinical Neurophysiology* 1995; **95**(4): 260–267.

28. Gregory RP, Oates T, Merry RTC. EEG epileptiform abnormalities in candidates for aircrew training. *Electroencephalography and Clinical Neurophysiology* 1993; **86**: 75–77.

29. Kasteleijn-Nolst Trenité DG, Binnie CD, Harding GF, Wilkins A. Photic stimulation: standardization of screening methods. *Epilepsia* 1999; **40**(Suppl. 4): 75–79.

30. Reilly EL, Peters JF. Relationship of some varieties of electroencephalographic photosensitivity to clinical convulsive disorders. *Neurology* 1973; **23**(10): 1050–1057.

31. Kasteleijn-Nolst Trenité DG. Photosensitivity in epilepsy: electrophysiological and clinical correlates. *Acta Neurologica Scandinavica* 1989; Suppl. **125**: 3–149.

32. Jeavons PM, Harding GFA, Panayiotopoulos CP, Drasdo N. The effect of geometric patterns combined with intermittent photic stimulation in photosensitive epilespy. *Electro-encephalography and Clinical Neurophysiology* 1972; **33**: 221–224.

33. Panayiotopoulos CP. *Benign Childhood Partial Seizures and Related Epileptic Syndromes.* London: John Libbey, 1999.

34. Hennessy MJ, Binnie CD. Photogenic partial seizures. *Epilepsia* 2000; **41**(1): 59–64.

35. Ferrie CD, De Marco P, Grunewald RA, Giannakodimos S, Panayiotopoulos CP. Video game induced seizures. *Journal of Neurology, Neurosurgery and Psychiatry* 1994; **57**(8): 925–931.

36. Graf WD, Chatrian GE, Glass ST, Knauss TA. Video game-related seizures: a report on 10 patients and a review of the literature. *Pediatrics* 1994; **93**(4): 551–556.

37. Kasteleijn-Nolst Trenite DG, da Silva AM, Ricci S, *et al*. Video-game epilepsy: a European study. *Epilepsia* 1999; **40**(Suppl. 4): 70–74.

38. Quirk JA, Fish DR, Smith SJ, *et al*. First seizures associated with playing electronic screen games: a community-based study in Great Britain. *Annals of Neurology* 1995; **37**(6): 733–737.

39. Tassinari CA, Rubboli G, Rizzi R, Gardella E, Michelucci R. Self-induction of visually-induced seizures. *Advances in Neurology* 1998; **75**: 179–192.

40. Panayiotopoulos CP, Giannakodimos S, Agathonikou A, Koutroumanidis M. Eyelid myoclonia is not a manoeuvre for self-induced seizures in eyelid myoclonia with absences. In: Duncan JS, Panayiotopoulos CP (eds) *Eyelid Myoclonia with Absences*. London: John Libbey, 1996; 93–106.

41. Forster FM. The classification and conditioning treatment of the reflex epilepsies. *International Journal of Neurology* 1972; **9**(1): 73–86.

42. Wilkins AJ, Baker A, Amin D, *et al*. Treatment of photosensitive epilepsy using coloured glasses. *Seizure* 1999; **8**(8): 444–449.

43. Kasteleijn-Nolst Trenité DG, Marescaux C, Stodieck S, Edelbroek PM, Oosting J. Photosensitive epilepsy: a model to study the effects of antiepileptic drugs. Evaluation of the piracetam analogue, levetiracetam. *Epilepsy Research* 1996; **25**(3): 225–230.

44. Panayiotopoulos CP. Fixation-off, scotosensitive, and other visual-related epilepsies. *Advances in Neurology* 1998; **75**: 139–157.

45. Panayiotopoulos CP. *Panayiotopoulos Syndrome: A Common and Benign Childhood Epileptic Syndrome.* London: John Libbey, 2002.

46. Wilkins AJ, Zifkin B, Andermann F, McGovern E. Seizures induced by thinking. *Annals of Neurology* 1982; **11**(6): 608–612.

47. Goossens LA, Andermann F, Andermann E, Remillard GM. Reflex seizures induced by calculation, card or board games, and spatial tasks: a review of 25 patients and delineation of the epileptic syndrome. *Neurology* 1990; **40**(8): 1171–1176.

48. Ramani V. Reading epilepsy. *Advances in Neurology* 1998; **75**: 241–262.

49. Gastaut H, Tassinari CA. Triggering mechanisms in epilepsy. The electroclinical point of view. *Epilepsia* 1966; **7**(2): 85–138.

50. Koepp MJ, Richardson MP, Brooks DJ, Duncan JS. Focal cortical release of endogenous opioids during reading-induced seizures. *Lancet* 1998; **352**(9132): 952–955.

51. Radhakrishnan K, Silbert PL, Klass DW. Reading epilepsy. An appraisal of 20 patients diagnosed at the Mayo Clinic, Rochester, Minnesota, between 1949 and 1989, and delineation of the epileptic syndrome. *Brain* 1995; **118**: 75–89.

13

Cognitive and behavioral manifestations of epilepsy in children

THIERRY DEONNA

The concept that epilepsy can be the only or main cause of acquired behavioral and cognitive problems in children is being increasingly accepted and tested. A chapter independent of those on the more classical and general 'psychosocial' or 'psychiatric' complications of epilepsy is thus particularly relevant. So many possible interrelated factors can account for cognitive or behavioral problems that most reviews contain indigestible and depressing lists, tacitly implying that these items cannot possibly be sorted out. Table 13.1 contrasts the general factors, always in the background, with the specific, direct effects of epileptic dysfunction in an individual. The precise aspects which could be the result of epilepsy[1] must also be considered in many forms of epilepsy other than those that present with cognitive and behavioral manifestations. In newly diagnosed 'typical' epilepsy, it is not exceptional to find rapid, unexpected and marked improvements in longstanding behavioral or cognitive problems when antiepileptic therapy is introduced. Since, at this point, neither psychological consequences of the diagnosis nor side-effects of treatment can be blamed, it is suggested that direct cognitive effects of epilepsy exist more often than is usually acknowledged.[2]

THE CONCEPT OF 'COGNITIVE' EPILEPSIES

In many forms of epilepsy, cognitive functions are altered during the seizure itself, the postictal state and sometimes during what is thought to be the normal interictal period. However, the cognitive dysfunction is only one among other epileptic manifestations and is not recognized or considered the main symptom.

Epilepsies with 'cognitive' symptomatology can be defined as those which manifest their effects mainly or exclusively in the cognitive sphere: the cognitive disturbance is itself the seizure, with no other visible manifestations beside the altered mental state. In reality, subtle signs, such as brief twitches, changes in posture or color, pupillary dilatation, etc. may occur, but these are not the main part of the seizure. Thus, it is somewhat arbitrary to draw firm boundaries in defining a 'cognitive' seizure and separate cognitive from behavioral manifestations. Indeed, behavioral disturbances can be the main or only symptom if the brain systems involved in social behavior and control of emotions are primarily involved by the epileptic process. However, this is a much more complex

Table 13.1 *Cognitive disorders and epilepsy in children: relationships*

General causes	Effects on brain function (cognition, behavior)	Comments
Brain lesion(s) causing epilepsy	Variable effects, possibly none	May be asymptomatic until becomes epileptogenic – physicians should not a priori blame pre-existing damage
Antiepileptic drugs	Specific antiepileptic effects, but also possible other effects (psychotropic) on cognition and mood	Final positive or negative clinical effect on cognition and mood depends on many factors (see text)
Psychological / emotional reactions (child, family)	Unspecific (chronic disease) and specific to epilepsy (unpredictable, loss of control)	Direct psychiatric manifestation of epilepsy and mental triggers of seizures (i.e. frontal, limbic) can be confounding factors
Epilepsy 'per se'[a] Ictal–postictal	Fluctuating deficit of variable duration (status epilepticus, postictal)	Repeated ictal–postictal states with no recovery of function between episodes may lead to prolonged chronic deficits
Brief unavailability of specific subsystem for cognitive function	Transient cognitive impairment related to EEG discharges	Possibly reduced cognitive efficiency
Prolonged cognitive epileptic deficits (paraictal[b])	Cognitive epilepsies: nature of deficit (selective or global) depends on cortical area(s) affected (i.e. language in Landau-Kleffner syndrome) and related networks	Usually sustained focal/diffuse epileptic EEG discharges and ±CSWS may occur without associated 'typical' seizures
Pathology induced by epilepsy	Epileptic 'damage' to developing networks	May apply only to early or special epilepsies. No generalization. Limits of animal models of epilepsy

[a] age at onset, location and spread of epileptic process, duration and type of epilepsy can be important additional factors not further discussed here.
[b] Paraictal: this term has been used for prolonged deficits observed in some partial epileptic syndromes not clearly attributable to a typical ictal or postictal state, but are also considered of functional epileptic origin.
CSWS: continuous spike waves during sleep.

and delicate dimension to evaluate.[3] In addition, any acquired disruption of cognitive function will have negative consequences on emotional or social behavior. The recognition that specific cognitive and/or behavioral disturbances can be epileptic manifestations requires a drastic conceptual change for the clinician. The typical rapid, paroxysmal change and recovery of function and clear-cut clinical-EEG correlations, usual in epileptic manifestations, are often not recognized. The episodic nature of symptoms, considered characteristic of epilepsy, is often not immediately apparent. The clinical disturbances must sometimes be measured over days or weeks; and, in special situations possibly, months or years. Gradual loss of cognitive functions, arrest or regression in development or new behavior disorders may thus be the presenting problems, with few or no hints of the epileptic origin.

Electroencephalographically, large parts of the brain which are important for behavior and cognition, such as the temporal and frontal lobes, are distant from the brain surface, so that scalp EEG may be normal, even during clinical seizures. Conversely, paroxysmal 'epileptic' EEG abnormalities can be found in normal children, or in different pathological situations without obvious correlations

with the clinical problem. Thus, some clinicians remain skeptical about the concept of 'cognitive' epilepsies and legitimately fear the risk of making an unprovable diagnosis with unwarranted practical implications. The present discussion emphasizes the need to acknowledge the problem and suggests some possible advances in this domain.

'COGNITIVE' EPILEPSIES IN THE CONTEXT OF MODERN EPILEPTOLOGY

Cognitive manifestations considered 'minimal' seizures are episodes of transient cognitive impairment documented during electroencephalographic epileptic discharges in children in whom no simultaneous sign of epileptic activity is clinically recognizable. A decrease in or loss of efficiency of performance occurs during the actual discharge.[4–6] Such immediate correlation is demonstrable only in older, cooperative children and only during simple-level cognitive processes (Chapter 23).

Temporary disturbances of cognitive function can be due either to focal epileptic seizures originating in brain areas which mediate particular cognitive functions or to generalized discharges which interfere with more global aspects of mental function (vigilance, execution). The observed deficit corresponds either to the ictal or to the postictal phase. Various forms of aphasia, apraxia, frontal lobe dysfunction, visuospatial disability or selective memory deficits have been reported, although precise details of these observations are rare in children.[7–12] More prolonged cognitive epileptic deficits are probably consequences of recurrent seizures with repeated postictal deficits and incomplete recovery of function between episodes. Logic suggests that frequent recurrent epileptic discharges in areas involved with complex developing mental functions can lead to more lasting consequences on cognition and behavior than those involving more elementary sensory and motor functions.

A specific cognitive status epilepticus (e.g. aphasic status epilepticus) can occur occasionally, but the commoner and best known of purely or mainly cognitive manifestations are those subsumed under the term **non-convulsive status epilepticus** (NCSE). This corresponds to a prolonged alteration of the mental state with continuous or sub-continuous generalized spikes or spike-wave discharges on the EEG. The prototype is **absence status** (**petit mal status**, **spike-wave stupor**, **minor epileptic status**),[13,14] where there is clouding of awareness but, presumably, no specific cognitive deficit. Apathy, drowsiness, slowness, inattention, perplexity, strange affect, amnesia, slow speech are the most obvious abnormal behaviors. It is not clear to what degree higher-level mental functions are truly preserved and what new memories can be formed during these episodes: detailed studies are rare.[15] These NCSE can be phases in primary generalized epilepsies, but may be manifestations of complex partial status epilepticus of temporal or frontal origin.[15] In temporal partial status epilepticus, only limited purposeful organized activity and responses to outside stimuli are possible and there is usually a total amnesia for the period. The epileptic nature is recognized by the presence, often subtle, of automatic motor behavior and vegetative phenomena.[16,17] A special form of frequent refractory nonconvulsive partial status epilepticus, associated with ring chromosome 20, is probably of frontal origin and, because it is so frequent, should allow exploration of the affected and preserved behaviors and memories during seizures.[18,19]

COGNITIVE DISTURBANCES IN IDIOPATHIC 'FUNCTIONAL' PARTIAL EPILEPSIES OF CHILDHOOD (BENIGN ROLANDIC EPILEPSIES AND VARIANTS)

Most children with benign partial epilepsy with rolandic spikes (BPERS) have no cognitive disturbances and benign

courses for the seizures. Nevertheless, prolonged reversible deficits of speech or oromotor function are sometimes encountered, despite an otherwise typically benign evolution.[20] Moderate and transient cognitive disturbances related to the active epilepsy phase can occasionally be of definite importance, are much more frequent than previously acknowledged, and have tended to be ignored or minimized.[21,22] Similar cognitive dysfunctions can be observed in children with only the EEG abnormalities, who have never had recognizable clinical seizures. The cognitive dysfunction seems closely related to the paroxysmal epileptic EEG activity, but may be due to special inhibitory mechanisms and not (or not only) corresponding to simple ictal and postictal phenomena.[23,24]

ACQUIRED EPILEPTIC APHASIA OR LANDAU–KLEFFNER SYNDROME

In acquired epileptic aphasia (AEA) or Landau-Kleffner syndrome, an insidious, or more rarely abrupt, onset of language deficit becomes apparent, most often between 3 and 7 years, usually with loss of verbal comprehension, due to auditory agnosia, followed by loss of oral expression. Generally few or sometimes no 'classical' seizures are noted: the 'visible' seizure disorder is usually 'benign' in conventional terms. No focal brain lesion is demonstrable and the diagnosis rests on the presence of severe, persistent, but fluctuant, focal paroxysmal bitemporal EEG abnormalities. The aphasia, of very variable severity and duration, may be protracted for years with remissions and recurrences and incomplete recovery.[25] The main physiopathological hypotheses are: abnormal electroencephalographic discharges are epiphenomena of an as-yet-unknown underlying encephalopathy; or, alternatively, secondary focal epilepsy with aphasic symptomatology is suggested, and apparently supported, by recent reports of AEA associated with various brain lesions in language areas. A prolonged aphasia can certainly result from a severe focal lesional epilepsy, such as a small focal dysplasia in a relevant brain area, but the physiopathology of the epilepsy in AEA is probably different.[26] There are many clinical and EEG similarities between BPERS and AEA,[22,27] so that AEA is increasingly considered to be the severest form of BPERS.

EPILEPSY WITH CONTINUOUS SPIKE-WAVES DURING SLEEP

Epilepsy with CSWS (continuous spike-waves during slow-wave sleep), or the syndrome of epilepsy with continuous spike-waves during sleep, refers to some cases of partial epilepsy in which marked increases of epileptic activity on the EEG during sleep (the so-called CSWS on the EEG) develop. It can last for months or years, and is accompanied by variable, minor or catastrophic, rapid or insidious stagnation or regression of one or several cognitive functions.[25,28–31] Correlative clinical and EEG data and evidence from electrophysiological studies and functional imaging[32] indicate that the nature and severity of the cognitive and/or behavioral dysfunction relates to the function played by the affected focal cortical area when the epileptic process becomes active, and possibly also to a disturbance of corticothalamic oscillatory mechanisms present during slow sleep, which seem to play a role in consolidation of material acquired during waking.[33,34] The **acquired epileptic frontal syndrome**[31,35] is one especially dramatic example of how partial epilepsy can lead to progressive dementia and/or massive behavioral regression.

CLINICAL EVALUATION OF CHILDREN WITH COGNITIVE EPILEPTIC MANIFESTATIONS

Ideally, children must be tested individually during and after episodes suspected of being cognitive ictal or postictal manifestations and direct correlations with EEG changes and treatment shown. This excludes the multiple variables in group studies which usually prevent evaluation of the direct role of epilepsy.[21,36,37] To ascertain which aspects of mental functions are affected during a suspected cognitive seizure (negative symptoms), interaction as well as observation is necessary, and it is difficult to plan systematic studies.[38] Positive symptoms such as hallucinations, memory recollections or acute emotional states – fear, ecstasy, etc. – certainly occur, but children are usually either unable or unwilling to express these experiences, and these events are, at best, underestimated. Sometimes the behavior of children who are 'concentrated' on, or afraid of, some bizarre sensations they experience may be interpreted as an absence or a panic reaction.

The practical and methodological problems of cognitive and behavioral assessment in children who are often said to be 'noncooperative' or 'untestable' and who need repeated EEGs are enormous. In order to document significant changes, children must be evaluated both at their best and at their worst. The emotional reaction of a child to the assessment may also limit collaboration. Such difficulties explain why convincing observations of 'cognitive' epilepsy are only exceptionally found in the literature. When epilepsy manifests itself with periods of fluctuating cognitive regression over long periods, for example in CSWS, specific circumstances are easier to plan and study.

HOW AND WHEN TO SUSPECT COGNITIVE MANIFESTATIONS OF EPILEPSY

It must be accepted that clear-cut paroxysmal clinical changes cannot always be documented; that subtle associated seizures, especially in very young children, are very difficult to diagnose; and that EEG changes are variable and often not conclusive. Cognitive seizures can be the causes of acquired learning or behavior disorders both in normally intelligent epileptic children without other previous problems, and in those with symptomatic epilepsy and known fixed cognitive deficits. Notable features in the history are: frequent mood changes; fluctuating attention; 'forgetfulness'; uneven memory skills; variable school results; uneven speed of performance; and transient failures in specific domains. Although none of these is specific, their combination and usually unexplained sudden occurrence and recurrence can be very suggestive that unrecognized 'cognitive' seizures are interfering with vigilance, attention, or with more specific functions, such as language or memory. Sometimes, the changes resemble those already seen in postictal states of previous more clear-cut episodes.

In schoolchildren, failure to encode, store and consolidate newly formed memories during or after seizures is probably an under-recognized cause of learning problems. Occult nocturnal episodes or seizures affecting limbic areas might have particular import. Transient memory impairment as the sole manifestation of complex partial seizures, known in adults as **epileptic amnesic attacks**[39] could easily go unrecognized in children. Misinterpretations of the causes for these fluctuations in behavior or performances are easy. Psychological explanations or antiepileptic therapy may be considered sufficient causes. Long delays, during which many psychological and other explanations may be proposed, can exist between the onset of cognitive or behavioral problems and the diagnosis of epilepsy. 'Cognitive' seizures must also be considered in brain-damaged children with epilepsy and chronic learning and behavioral disorders. Epilepsy can be responsible for, or aggravate, the chronic cognitive disturbances usually attributed to the basic focal lesion in congenital hemiplegia.[40] Although it is very difficult to show that fluctuating performances or regression in a domain which is already weak can be due to an additional direct effect of epilepsy, close attention should be paid to the possible negative role of epilepsy or paroxysmal EEG discharges on cognitive function in these situations.

PITFALLS AND PROBLEMS OF TREATMENT OF 'COGNITIVE' EPILEPSIES

Confirmation of cognitive seizures can come from the spectacular results of an antiepileptic drug trial which may, exceptionally, be justified before the diagnosis is certain. Apart from rare cases with immediate improvement, therapy in 'cognitive' epilepsies is fraught with as many difficulties as diagnosis. Improvement cannot always occur in a very short period and time has to be allowed to judge effects of treatment. A clear-cut chronological correlation between cognitive improvement and change of epileptic activity (as measured by EEG and drug effect) is rarely demonstrated. The lack of immediate improvement, or even worsening, of cognition or behavior is often taken as evidence that epilepsy is not the cause. This illogical reasoning has detracted clinicians from further drug trials and has probably delayed progress in the recognition of these epilepsies. The behavioral side-effects that occasionally present with any antiepileptic drug may be especially marked when the basic symptom specifically affects mental functions. Global cognitive and behavioral worsening could also correspond to increased numbers of seizures or to onset of new seizure types, as seen in other epilepsies when inappropriate drugs are used. Dissociations between cognitive and behavioral responses to treatment are sometimes seen, resulting in incorrect perceptions that are globally negative. In other words, the child becomes more difficult to handle, even though there is improvement in the cognitive domain.

Prolonged drug trials of uncertain benefit are sometimes necessary, carrying the risk of excessive focus on medical management, with poor attention to associated educational and psychological problems, which are obviously very important.

DEVELOPMENTAL DISORDERS: THE ROLE OF EPILEPSY

West syndrome (Chapter 9B), the most striking example of the cognitive and behavioral consequences of epilepsy starting very early, can be seen as a potentially reversible 'epileptic' dementia.[41] Behavioral changes usually occur before the motor manifestations and are sometimes the only signs of the epileptic disease. The recognition that some epilepsies with cognitive or language regression can start quite early raises the question whether epilepsy could be the main causal factor in children presenting with disorders such as developmental dysphasia or autistic behavior,[42,43] whether or not clinical seizures have occurred. Focal epileptic seizures or EEG discharges involving parts of the developing cerebral cortex which mediate particular cognitive functions at given ages, levels of experience and learning can be expected to produce nondevelopment, aberrant development, or loss of these functions, regardless of, or in addition to, the effects of the underlying brain pathology. Experimental data in animals show that focal discharges early in development can modify the structural development of the brain.

These data suggest possible roles of some early-onset epilepsies in cognitive development and have led to several studies which try to demonstrate direct relationships, and, particularly, positive effects, of antiepileptic drugs on development.[20,44–46] Currently, hard facts are limited, but it seems clear that in typical autism and specific language impairment, epilepsy is not a significant causal factor. Epilepsy is more directly involved in atypical cases with variable combinations of global retardation, language delay with autistic features, and where stagnation, regression or delayed recognition of developmental problems is reported.[43] Another important potential source of information on the role of early focal epilepsy in development will hopefully come from detailed prospective studies of those treated successfully with surgery, in whom the dynamics of development before and after surgery and the nature and evolution of deficits can be followed and correlated with specific epilepsy variables.

KEY POINTS

- A cognitive deficit or a behavioral disturbance can be the **main, the first and sometimes the unique manifestation of some forms of epilepsy** in children
- **Stagnation, regression or fluctuations in performance,** which are unlike the paroxysmal and transient events typically considered as epileptic can be observed in these situations
- These need to be recognized and distinguished from the **many other causes of cognitive and behavioral problems** frequently seen in children with epilepsy
- Epilepsy can occasionally be the main cause of some **developmental disturbances**

REFERENCES

1. Aicardi J. Epilepsy: The hidden part of the iceberg. *European Journal of Pediatric Neurology* 1999; **3**: 197–200.
2. Austin JK, Harezlak J, Dunn DW, *et al.* Behavior problems in children before first recognised seizure. *Pediatrics* 2001; **197**: 115–122.
3. Gillberg C, Schaumann H. Epilepsy presenting as infantile autism? Two case studies. *Neuropediatrics* 1983; **14**: 206–212.
4. Aarts HP, Binnie CD, Smit AM, Wilkins AJ. Selective cognitive impairment during focal and generalized epileptiform EEG activity. *Brain* 1984; **107**: 293–308.
5. Kasteleijn-Nolst Trénité DGA, Siebelink BM, Berends SGC, *et al.* Lateralized effects of subclinical epileptiform discharges on scholastic performance in children. *Epilepsia* 1990; **31**: 740–746.

6. Binnie CD, Marston D. Cognitive correlates of interictal discharges. *Epilepsia* 1992; **33**(Suppl. 6): S11–17.

7. Deonna T, Fletcher P, Voumard C. Temporary regression during language acquisition : A linguistic analysis of a 2½ year-old child with epileptic aphasia. *Developmental Medicine and Child Neurology* 1982; **24**: 156–163.

8. Deonna T, Chevrie C, Hornung E. Childhood epileptic speech disorder: prolonged isolated deficit of prosodic features. *Developmental Medicine and Child Neurology* 1987; **29**: 100–105.

9. Boone KB, Miller BL, Rosenberg I, *et al.* Neuropsychological and behavioral abnormalities in an adolescent with frontal lobe seizures. *Neurology* 1988; **38**: 583–586.

10. Jambaqué I, Dulac O. Syndrome frontal réversible et épilepsie chez un enfant de 8 ans. *Archives Françaises de Pediatrie* 1989; **46**: 525–529.

11. Deonna T. Annotation: Cognitive and behavioral correlates of epilepsy in children. *Journal of Child Psychology and Psychiatry* 1993; **34**: 611–620.

12. Deonna T, Davidoff V, Roulet E, Despland PA. Isolated disturbance of written language acquisition as an initial symptom of epileptic aphasia in a 7 year old girl. A 3-year follow-up study. *Aphasiology* 1993; **7**: 441–450.

13. Andermann F, Robb JP. Absence status: A reappraisal following review of 38 patients. *Epilepsia* 1972; **13**: 177–187.

14. Manning DJ, Rosenbloom L. Non-convulsive status epilepticus. *Archives of Diseases in Childhood* 1987; **62**: 37–40.

15. Thomas P, Zifkin B, Migneco O, *et al.* Nonconvulsive status epilepticus of frontal origin. *Neurology* 1999; **52**: 1174–1183.

16. McBride MC, Dooling EC, Oppenheimer EH. Complex partial status epilepticus in young children. *Annals of Neurology* 1981; **9**: 526–530.

17. Engel J, Lufwig BI, Fetell M. Prolonged partial complex status epilepticus: EEG and behavioral observations. *Neurology* 1986; **28**: 863–869.

18. Inoue Y, Fujiwara T, Matsuda K, *et al.* Ring chromosome 20 and nonconvulsive status epilepticus. A new epileptic syndrome. *Brain* 1997; **120**: 939–953.

19. Augustijn PB, Parra J, Wouters CH, *et al.* Ring chromosome 20 epilepsy syndrome in children: electroclinical features. *Neurology* 2001; **57**: 1108–1111.

20. Deonna T, Roulet E, Fontan D, Marcoz JP. Prolonged speech and oromotor deficits of epileptic origin in benign partial epilepsy with rolandic spikes: relationship to acquired epileptic aphasia. *Neuropediatrics* 1993; **24**: 83–87.

21. Deonna T. Rolandic epilepsy: Neuropsychology of the active epilepsy phase. *Epileptic Disorders* 2000; **2**(Suppl. 1): S59–61.

22. Deonna T. Acquired epileptic aphasia (AEA) or Landau-Kleffner syndrome: from childhood to adulthood. In: Bishop DVM, Leonard LB (eds) *Speech and Language Impairments in Children.* Hove: Psychology Press, 2000; 261–272.

23. Shewmon DA, Erwin RJ. Focal spike-induced cerebral dysfunction is related to the after-coming slow wave. *Annals of Neurology* 1988; **23**: 131–137.

24. De Saint-Martin A, Petiau C, Massa R, *et al.* Idiopathic rolandic epilepsy with 'interictal' facial myoclonia and oromotor deficit: A longitudinal EEG and PET study. *Epilepsia* 1999; **40**: 614–620.

25. Deonna T. Acquired epileptiform aphasia in children. (Landau-Kleffner syndrome) *Journal of Clinical Neurophysiology* 1991; **8**: 288–298.

26. Roulet Perez E, Seek M, Mayer E, *et al.* Childhood epilepsy with neuropsychological regression and continuous spike waves during sleep: epilepsy surgery in a young adult. *European Journal of Paediatric Neurology* 1998; **2**: 303–311.

27. Doose H, Baier WK. Benign partial epilepsy and related conditions: multifactorial pathogenesis with hereditary impairment of brain maturation. *European Journal of Paediatric Neurology* 1989; **149**: 152–158.

28. Deonna T, Davidoff V, Maeder-Ingvar M. *et al.* The spectrum of acquired cognitive disturbances in children with partial epilepsy and continuous spike-waves during sleep. A 4-year follow-up case study with prolonged reversible learning arrest and dysfluency. *European Journal of Paediatric Neurology* 1997; **1**: 19–29.

29. Boel M, Casaer P. Continuous spikes and waves during slow wave sleep: a 30 months follow-up study of neuropsychological recovery and EEG findings. *Neuropediatrics* 1989; **20**: 176–180.

30. Hirsch E, Marescaux C, Maquet P, *et al.* Landau-Kleffner syndrome: A clinical and EEG study of 5 cases. *Epilepsia* 1990; **31**: 768–777.

31. Roulet-Perez E, Davidoff V, Despland PA, Deonna T. Mental deterioration in children with epilepsy and continuous spike-waves during sleep: Acquired epileptic frontal syndrome. *Developmental Medicine and Child Neurology.* 1993; **33**: 495–511.

32. Maquet P, Hirsch E, Metz-Lutz MN, *et al.* Regional cerebral glucose metabolism in children with deterioration of one or more cognitive functions and continuous spike-and-wave discharges during sleep. *Brain* 1995; **118**: 1497–1520.

33. Sjenowski TJ, Destexhe A. Why do we sleep. *Brain Research* 2000; **866**: 208–223.

34. Monteiro JP, Roulet Perez E, Davidoff V, Deonna T. Primary neonatal thalamic haemorrhage and epilepsy with continuous spike-wave during sleep: a longitudinal follow-up of a possible significant relation. *European Journal of Paediatric Neurology* 2001; **5**: 41–47.

35. Deonna T, Ziegler AL, Roulet E. Acquired epileptic frontal syndrome in children. In: *Frontal Seizures and Epilepsies in Children.* Paris: John Libbey, 2002.

36. Bourgeois B, Prensky Y, Palkes HS, *et al.* Intelligence in epilepsy: A prospective in children. *Annals of Neurology* 1983; **14**: 438–444.

37. Besag FMC. Cognitive deterioration in children with epilepsy. In: Trimble M, Reynolds EH (eds) *Epilepsy, Behavior and Cognitive Function.* New York: John Wiley, 1987: 113–127.

38. Gloor P. Neurobiological substrates of ictal behavioral discharges. *Advances in Neurology* 1991; **55**: 1–34.

39. Galassi R, Morreale A, Di Sarro R, Lugaresi E. Epileptic amnesic syndrome. *Epilepsia* 1993; **33**(Suppl. 6): S21–25.

40. Varga-Khadem F, Isaacs E, Van Der Werf S, *et al.* Development of intelligence and memory in children with hemiplegic cerebral palsy. The deleterious consequences of early seizures. *Brain* 1992; **115**: 315–329.

41. Guzzetta F, Crisafulli A, Isaya Crine M. Cognitive assessment of infants with West syndrome. How useful in diagnosis and prognosis? *Developmental Medicine and Child Neurology.* 1993; **35**: 379–387.

42. Echenne B, Cheminal R, Rivier F, *et al.* Epileptic encephalopathic abnormalities and developmental dysphasias: a study of 32 patients. *Brain Development* 1992; **14**: 216–225.

43. Uldall P, Sahlholdt L, Alving J. Landau-Kleffner syndrome with onset at 18 months and an initial diagnosis of pervasive developmental disorder. *European Journal of Paediatric Neurology* 2000; **4**: 81–86.

44. Deonna T, Ziegler AL, Moura-Serra J, Innocenti G. Autistic regression in relation to limbic pathology and epilepsy: Report of 2 cases. *Developmental Medicine and Child Neurology* 1993; **35**: 166–176.

45. Deonna T, Ziegler AL, Maeder Ingvar M, Ansermet F, Roulet E. Reversible behavioural autistic-like regression: a manifestation of a special (new?) epileptic syndrome in a 28-month-old child. A 2-year longitudinal study. *Neurocase* 1995; **1**: 91–99.

46. Lewine JD, Andrews R, Chez M, *et al.* Magnetoencephalographic patterns of epileptiform activity in children with regressive autism spectrum disorders. *Pediatrics* 1999; **104**: 405–418.

14

Progressive myoclonus epilepsies

CHARLOTTE DRAVET AND ALAIN MALAFOSSE

The progressive myoclonus epilepsy (PME) syndrome is characterized by:

- a combination of fragmentary or segmental, arrhythmic, asynchronous symmetric or asymmetric myoclonus, and massive myoclonias
- other epileptic seizures, usually generalized tonic-clonic or clonic seizures
- abnormal neurologic signs, particularly cerebellar signs
- mental deterioration, which may culminate in dementia. This is a less constant component of the syndrome.[1]

PMEs in childhood and adolescence are rare and account only for about 1 per cent of patients in the population of the Centre Saint-Paul (Marseilles, France). The severity of the different clinical features varies with the etiology. Thus, the cognitive dysfunction in Unverrich-Lundborg disease progresses very slowly, if at all, whereas the cognitive dysfunction in Lafora disease evolves rapidly into dementia. There is also a wide range of neurologic abnormalities in the different PMEs, e.g. early blindness due to retinal impairment in juvenile ceroid lipofuscinosis, and deafness or optic atrophy in some mitochondrial encephalomyopathies. The rate of progression and severity of the neurological symptoms vary considerably both between diseases and also within each disease.

Classification of patients with PME can be difficult in spite of the advances in molecular genetics. In this chapter,

PMEs are listed by the usual age of presentation: infancy, early childhood, childhood and adolescence. The biochemical and metabolic aspects of PMEs are discussed in more detail in Chapter 4D. Table 14.1 summarizes the genetics, the anatomical and biological markers and the diagnostic procedures in the PMEs.

PROGRESSIVE MYOCLONUS EPILEPSIES IN INFANCY

Early infantile type of neuronal ceroid lipofuscinosis (Santavuori-Haltia-Hagberg disease)

This type of neuronal ceroid lipofuscinosis (NCL) presents between 3 and 18 months with myoclonias, hypotonia, arrest of psychomotor development evolving into mental deterioration and autistic features, acquired microcephaly, progressive loss of visual function and optic atrophy.[2] There is progressive flattening of the EEG activities, which has been described as **vanishing EEG**.[3,4] Skin, peripheral nerve or rectal biopsy confirms the diagnosis by showing characteristic inclusions (granular osmiophilic deposits). Death occurs around 10 years of age.

The transmission is autosomal recessive. The gene for the early infantile type of NCL (INCL; OMIM # 256730) has been localized to 1p35-p33.[5] Defects in the palmitoyl protein thioesterase (PPT) gene were identified in all of

Table 14.1 *Laboratory investigation of progressive myoclonic epilepsy*

Disease	Genetics	Biological/pathological marker	Procedure	Prenatal diagnosis
Ceroid lipofuscinosis	AR	Curvilinear granular inclusions, 'fingerprint' profiles, rectilinear profiles, osmiophilic granular profiles	Biopsy: skin, rectal mucosa	
1 Early infantile type	1p35–p33 defect in the palmitoyl protein thioesterase (PPT)			Possible 2 methods (see text)
2 Late infantile type	LINCL 11p15.5 pepstatin-insensitive lysosomal peptidase. Other variants: CLN5 13q21.1q32, CLN6 15q21–q23			Possible 2 methods (see text)
3. Juvenile type	Chromosome 16 near region 16q22			???
GM2 gangliosidosis	AR	Enzymatic defect (hexosaminidases)	Enzyme activity in serum, leucocytes, sometimes fibroblasts	Possible (amniotic cells, chorionic villi)
1 Tay-Sachs'	15q23–q24 beta-hexosaminidase A alpha subunit (HEX A)			
2 Sandhoff	5q13 HEX AB			
THB deficiencies	AR 1p15.1–16.1	Enzymatic defects → biopterin deficiency	Urine HVA, 5-HIA, biopterin levels; enzyme activity in liver and erythrocytes	Not easy (enzymatic dosages in amniocytes)
Alper's disease	Unknown	Brain atrophy (grey matter) and hepatic failure	None	Not possible
Huntington disease	AD paternal 4p16.3 – Huntingtin – expansion CAG triplets	none	Genetic study	Possible
Gaucher's (Type III)	AR 1q21	Beta-glucocerebrosidase deficit Beta-glucocerebroside storage	Gaucher's cells in bone marrow and reticuloendothelial tissue	Possible: enzymatic activity in trophoblasts
Sialidoses				
Type 1	AR 6p21.3	alpha-neuraminidase deficit	Urine oligosaccharide levels; enzyme activity in lymphocytes, fibroblasts	???
Type 2	20q13.1	alpha-neuraminidase deficit beta-galactosidase deficit	Urine oligosaccharide levels; enzyme activities in lymphocytes, fibroblasts	???
Lafora disease	AR 6q23–25 – Laforin	Lafora bodies (polyglucosans)	Skin biopsy (axilla)	Difficult
MERRF	Mitochondrial DNA maternal	Ragged-red fibers Respiratory metabolic chain deficit	Blood lactate; muscle biopsy: enzymatic histochemistry genetic study	Not possible
Unverricht–Lundborg disease	AR 21q – cystatin B	None	Genetic study	Not possible
DRPLA	AD paternal 12p – expansion triplets CAG	None	Genetic study	???

AD, autosomal dominant; AR, autosomal recessive; PPT, palmitoyl protein thioesterase.

the Finnish and non-Finnish patients in one study.[6] Direct DNA sequencing depends on knowledge of the responsible mutation. More recently, a new fluorometric assay has been described that is able to detect PPT activity in chorionic villi cells and cultured fetal skin fibroblasts.[7,8]

Tay-Sachs and Sandhoff diseases (GM2 gangliodosis, A and O variants)

Tay-Sachs and Sandhoff diseases have similar clinical phenotypes. Infants present with sudden, nonepileptic startles provoked by noise. Epileptic seizures occur later as spontaneous and induced myoclonic jerks and focal seizures, accompanied by a slowing of the EEG background and the appearance of multifocal abnormalities.[9] There is neurologic regression with the development of microcephaly and loss of vision, often associated with a macular, cherry red spot. Death occurs usually before 4 years of age.

The transmission is autosomal recessive. The Tay-Sachs disease (OMIM # 272800) locus has been mapped to 15q23-q24.[10] The gene responsible has been shown to be the β-hexosaminidase A α-subunit (HEXA) gene.[10] The frequency of the Tay-Sachs mutation is high in Ashkenazi Jews of eastern European origin. Non-Jewish individuals should also be screened if they are spouses of Jewish carriers or relatives of probands. The use of DNA testing alone seems to be the most cost-effective and efficient approach to carrier screening for Tay-Sachs disease in individuals of confirmed Ashkenazi Jewish ancestry.[11] Sandhoff's disease (OMIM # 268800) is due to the HEXB gene which was assigned to chromosome 5q13 in 1975.[12] There is no ethnic predominance.

Tetrahydrobiopterin deficiencies

Progressive neurological abnormalities appear between 2 and 12 months of age. Truncal hypotonia, peripheral hypertonia and oculogyric crises precede the onset of erratic myoclonias and myoclonic seizures.[13] There is hyperphenylalaninemia and decreased blood and urine levels of homovanillic acid (HVA) and 5-hydroxyindolacetic acid (5-HIAA). The concentration of specific urinary biopterins can suggest the particular enzyme deficiency. Strict control of plasma phenylalanine concentrations, treatment with L-dopa and 5-hydroxytryptophan, in conjunction with carbidopa, for the central deficiency of serotonin and the catecholamines, and treatment with folinic acid for the central folate deficiency that arises in some cases should be started as early as possible because of the rapid neurological regression.

The transmission is autosomal recessive. The gene maps to chromosome 4p15.1-16.1. Measurement of enzyme activity in the amniocytes allows a prenatal diagnosis.

Poliodystrophies (Alper's disease)

The poliodystrophies (Alpers disease) are a heterogeneous group of diseases characterized by different seizure types, including myoclonic jerks, and neurologic deterioration that present usually during infancy. Epilepsy is often the first symptom and is characterized by myoclonias and focal seizures. There are often repeated episodes of focal status evolving into epilepsia partialis continua. There is associated slowing in psychomotor development and progressive brain atrophy. One form with associated hepatic dysfunction has been described.[14] The hepatic involvement often appears later in the course of the disease and is sometimes falsely attributed to valproic acid. The EEG performed during status epilepticus may show a characteristic pattern of repetitive small spikes and polyspikes, which are often unilateral.[15] The genetic basis is unknown. Familial cases have been described, particularly in those with hepatic involvement.

PROGRESSIVE MYOCLONUS EPILEPSIES OF EARLY CHILDHOOD

Juvenile myoclonic form of Huntington disease

The childhood-onset form of Huntington disease is rare.[16,17] Onset is after age 3 years, with loss of acquired psychomotor skills, cerebellar impairment, rigidity, dystonic posturing but not chorea. Epilepsy appears approximately 2 years after the onset, as tonic-clonic seizures, atypical absences and massive myoclonias. Erratic, asymmetric, spontaneous or action myoclonus may occur and coincides usually with worsening of the epilepsy and may culminate in myoclonic or tonic-clonic status.[18] The EEG may show clinical photosensitivity even before the onset of seizures and is later characterized by spontaneous bursts of spike-waves and polyspike-waves. The prognosis is very poor, death occurring at an average of 4–6 years after the onset.

The transmission is autosomal dominant and is through the father in the myoclonic forms. Huntington disease has been mapped to 4p16.3.[19] The abnormality is an expansion of CAG (cytosine–adenine–guanosine) triplets. Both preclinical and prenatal diagnoses are possible, which raises serious ethical issues.

Late infantile neuronal ceroid lipofuscinosis (Jansky-Bielschowsky disease)

The late infantile form of NCL is an autosomal recessive disease that is found in various ethnic groups.[20–22] Onset is between 15 months and 3 years of age. Ataxia, speech regression, gait disturbance and loss of mental skills are the first symptoms. These are soon followed by tonic-clonic and myoclonic seizures. Visual impairment becomes apparent between 2 and 5 years of age. Progression is rapid and children are usually blind, tetraplegic and bedridden by 5 years of age. Death occurs between 3 and 10 years of age. Optic atrophy can be observed from the age of 3, and the electroretinogram (ERG) is low in amplitude and later extinguished.[23] The EEG shows slowing of background activity, irregular slow waves and polyspikes. Single flash photic stimulation provokes very large polyphasic spikes over the posterior regions (Figure 14.1). Large visual evoked potentials persist throughout the course of the disease.[24] Later in the course, somatosensory evoked potentials may also be enlarged. The diagnosis may be confirmed by skin, peripheral nerve or rectal biopsy. The ultrastructural study shows curvilinear profiles and granular inclusions. A form of NCL intermediate between the late infantile and the juvenile forms was described as early juvenile NCL by Lake and Cavanagh in 1978.[25]

The gene for the late infantile type of NCL (LINCL; OMIM # 204500) maps to 11p15.5[26] and codes for a pepstatin-insensitive lysosomal peptidase.[27] For prenatal diagnosis, the choice between mutation analysis and electronmicroscopic examination of uncultured amniocytes for typical curvilinear bodies must be discussed case by case with a geneticist. Several variant forms of *LINCL* have been described and mapped to 13q21.1-q32 (CLN5)[28] and 15q21-q23 (CLN6).[29,30]

PROGRESSIVE MYOCLONUS EPILEPSIES IN CHILDHOOD AND ADOLESCENCE

Juvenile neuronal ceroid lipofuscinosis (Spielmeyer–Vogt–Sjögren disease)

This form is the most widespread and common presentation of NCL.[20] Onset is between ages 4 and 15 years.[31] Most patients present with progressive visual loss due to

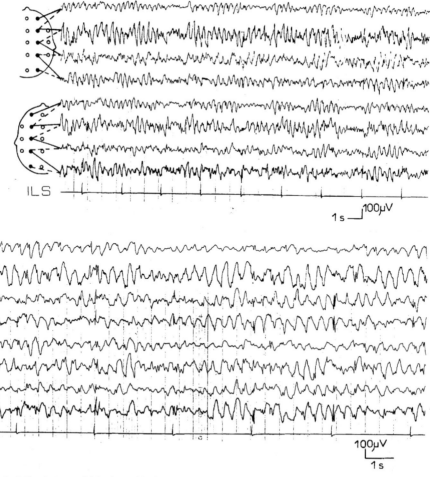

Figure 14.1 *Characteristic photosensitivity in a girl of 5 years 10 months, suffering from a late infantile NCL (Jansky-Bielschowsky). Abnormal potentials are evoked by each flash of stimulation at low frequency, in the posterior areas. Bottom: Sometimes more diffuse spikes can be seen more easily with a high recording speed.*

pigmentary degeneration of the retina. Intellectual impairment is less prominent at the onset and progresses slowly. Neurological signs begin 2–3 years after the onset. Absences, or more frequently tonic-clonic seizures, occur 1–4 years after the onset. Segmental and later massive myoclonus appears at the same time as the epileptic seizures. Myoclonias involving the face may be prominent and clonic status often occurs in the terminal stages. In some patients, the disease presents initially with seizures and myoclonus, and visual loss appears later.[32] The child adopts a typical stooping gait and dysarthria. Motor dyspraxia may become severe and confine the subjects to a wheelchair. Psychotic episodes may complicate the evolution. Death occurs generally around age 20. Treatment with antioxidant drugs has been reported to delay the progression of juvenile NCL,[33] but does not have the same effect in the other NCL types.

The EEG shows early slowing and disruption of the background activity, sharp waves and spike-waves that are activated by sleep. There is no photosensitivity. The amplitude of both ERG and visual evoked responses decreases over time. Somatosensory evoked potentials are enlarged. The diagnosis is confirmed by the presence of abnormal, vacuolized lymphocytes or by evidence of fingerprint membranous bodies or curvilinear and rectilinear bodies on skin biopsy.[34] According to Carpenter *et al.*, four types of inclusions can be found in the biopsy material of patients with NCL: curvilinear bodies (predominating in the late infantile form); fingerprint membranous profiles (in the juvenile form); rectilinear profiles (juvenile form); and granular osmiotic deposits (early infantile form). However, no type is absolutely specific for a particular clinical form.[34,35] The locus for Spielmeyer-Vogt disease has been mapped to 16q22, different from that of Santavuori disease (1p35-p33).[36] The gene encodes a novel 438-amino-acid protein of unknown function.[37] Antenatal diagnosis is possible either on cells obtained at amniocentesis[38] or by chorionic villus biopsy.[39]

Juvenile Gaucher disease (type III)

The juvenile form (type I) and the infantile neuropathic form (type II) of Gaucher disease do not present as PME. A heterogeneous group of patients, with proven histology and biochemistry of Gaucher disease, have been gathered as a type IIIb.[40] Age of onset varies between childhood and early adulthood. Presenting symptoms are generally myoclonus and saccadic horizontal eye movements. Splenomegaly may be present. Generalized or focal epileptic seizures, cerebellar impairment and some degree of dementia are usually present. In some families, a prominent, severe action myoclonus, touch myoclonus and photosensitivity may be found. Survival ranges between a decade and mid-adulthood.

The EEG shows normal or slow background activity and bursts of predominantly posterior, sometimes multifocal, 6–10-Hz polyspike-waves, which are enhanced by sleep.[41] Photic stimulation produces a myoclonic response. Visual evoked potentials are reported to be normal, but somatosensory evoked potentials may be enlarged in some patients.[42] The diagnosis is established by demonstration of storage of β-glucocerebroside in bone marrow (Gaucher cells), cultured fibroblasts, circulating lymphocytes, or other organs. Neuronal storage may be demonstrated also on rectal mucosal biopsy or in the appendix.

There is autosomal recessive transmission. The gene coding for β-glucocerebrosidase is located on the region q21 of chromosome 1. Many mutations have been demonstrated but no relationship has been established between a specific mutation and a particular phenotype.[43]

Sialidoses

Type I sialidosis is characterized by a deficiency in α-neuraminidase and has been termed the **cherry-red spot myoclonus syndrome**.[44–46] Age of onset is variable, the mean age being around 15 years. Onset is characterized by the occurrence of mild visual impairment, epileptic seizures, and neurologic signs without mental impairment.[47] The neurological signs may include 'burning feet' and cerebellar impairment. Myoclonus becomes increasingly evident and includes spontaneous, intermittent, irregular myoclonias of the face and mouth that are not stimulus-sensitive and persist during sleep. A macular cherry-red spot may be seen but can disappear during the course of the disease. The prognosis is poor and the myoclonus is difficult to control.

The EEG background is normal or shows fast, low voltage activity, which slows down when dementia occurs. There is no photosensitivity. Massive myoclonias are associated with generalized PSWs (polyspike waves). Facial myoclonias are not associated with EEG changes. Visual evoked potentials are usually decreased, but somatosensory evoked potentials are greatly enhanced.

There is an oligosacchariduria containing sialic acid. Foamy histiocytes may be seen in bone-marrow. α-neuraminidase activities can be measured in fibroblasts and chorionic villi. Prenatal diagnosis is possible. The transmission is autosomal recessive. The gene coding for α-neuraminidase is located on chromosome 6p21.3.

Type II sialidosis, or **galactosialidosis**, is characterized by a deficiency of α-neuraminidase and by a partial deficiency in β-galactosidase.[48] This form has been described mostly in Japanese patients. It presents usually in late childhood and adolescence with myoclonus, cerebellar ataxia and visual failure. A macular cherry-red spot can be seen. Onset of this disease may occur also in the neonate or in early infancy and is associated with visceromegaly, chondrodystrophy, and angiokeratoma. The gene is located on 20q13.

Lafora disease

Lafora disease is a well-defined entity with an autosomal recessive inheritance, characterized by the presence of Lafora bodies in brain tissue.[49–51] Deposits of polyglucosans can also be demonstrated in skin, mucosa, liver or muscle biopsy material.

The age of onset varies from 6 to 19 years.[52] The clinical features include both generalized and focal seizures. Focal seizures with visual phenomena and photosensitivity are characteristic features, but may not be present in Indian patients.[53,54] A severe and progressive myoclonic syndrome with erratic resting and action myoclonus is accompanied by a rapidly progressive dementia, with early and severe impairment of higher cortical functions

and marked depression.[52] The clinical course is marked by spontaneous episodes of rapid worsening, followed by periods of apparent stabilization. Death occurs within 2–10 years of the onset of disease.

Early EEGs show normal background activity, isolated bursts of spike-waves and polyspike-waves, with clinical photosensitivity. Erratic myoclonus is not associated with EEG changes. The presence of erratic myoclonus and the lack of activation of EEG abnormalities during sleep are features that distinguish Lafora disease from idiopathic generalized epilepsy. The EEG evolves to show slowing of the background activity, fast generalized polyspikes and PSWs, focal occipital or multifocal spikes, disappearance of physiologic sleep patterns and persisting erratic myoclonus (Figure 14.2). Photosensitivity may persist throughout the evolution. Brainstem evoked potentials may be delayed; enlarged somatosensory evoked potentials have also been found.

The characteristic clinical and EEG features can suggest the diagnosis early in the course of the disease.

Resting

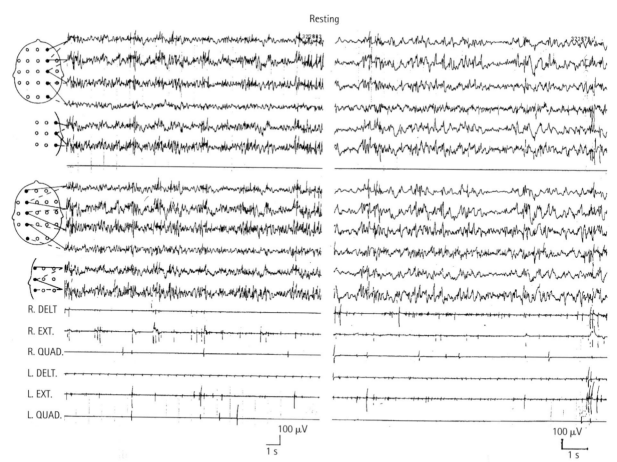

Figure 14.2 *Typical EEG and polygraphic recording in a girl of 17 years with Lafora disease. No recognizable normal posterior background. Succession of more or less diffuse spikes, spike-waves and polyspikes. Continuous erratic, fragmentary and segmental myoclonias recorded on different muscles.* **Right***: the high-speed recording shows the absence of constant relationship between the myoclonias and the spikes.*

Biopsy of axillary skin seems to be the most practical procedure for early diagnosis.[55,56] The deposits are particularly visible in eccrine sweat glands, but are also seen in muscle or liver biopsies.

The inheritance is autosomal recessive and the gene for Lafora disease (OMIM # 254780) has been mapped to chromosome 6q23-q25 (*EPM2A*).[57] Between 13 per cent[58] and 20 per cent[59] of the families with this condition are not linked to 6q23-q25. With the existence of several different mutations in the 6q-linked families, this nonallelic genetic heterogeneity makes the prenatal diagnosis difficult. A mutation in the *EPM2A* gene that encodes a protein called laforin has also been described.[60] This novel gene encoded a protein with consensus amino acid sequence indicative of a protein tyrosine phosphatase (PTP).

Myoclonus epilepsy with ragged-red fibers

Myoclonus is a prominent feature in a group of diseases that are maternally inherited disorders of mitochondrial metabolism.[61,62] The boundaries between the different syndromes are not well established, and precise relationships between the metabolic defects and the clinical expression have yet to be established. This is similar to the mitochondrial myopathies, in which there is nonconsistent phenotype, and symptoms and signs may be similar in patients with different biochemical defects.[63]

Myoclonus epilepsy with ragged-red fibers (MERRF) is associated with progressive myoclonus epilepsy. Age of onset varies widely between 5 and 42 years. Myoclonus and ataxia are the most constant features. Tonic-clonic seizures and dementia are less constant. A majority of patients present with prominent associated features such as short stature, deafness, optic atrophy, peripheral neuropathy, pes cavus and endocrine dysfunction.[64] Myopathic symptoms are often very slight and sometimes absent. The clinical presentation and prognosis vary considerably but the course of the disease is relatively slow but progressive in most patients. Some patients with MERRF have eventually also shown symptoms of **mitochondrial encephalomyopathy with lactic acidosis and stroke-like episodes** (MELAS).[65]

Skeletal muscle biopsy typically shows ragged-red fibers.[64] Swollen/abnormal mitochondria may be present in some tissue (skin) and absent on CNS biopsy material. The muscle biopsy may, however, be normal in MERRF, even in tissue in which the enzyme defect can be demonstrated. Conversely, asymptomatic family members and those with only limited clinical involvement (e.g. with isolated hearing loss) may show ragged-red fibers on muscle biopsy.[66] The biochemical deficit can be demonstrated by measurement of the mitochondrial respiratory chain enzyme activities.[67] Treatment with coenzyme Q_{10}, which

plays a pivotal role in electron transfer in the respiratory chain, has been reported to be of benefit, but high doses can worsen the symptoms.[68]

A heteroplasmic A/G mutation has been reported in position 8344 in mitochondrial DNA in patients affected by MERRF and in some of their relatives.[69]

Unverricht-Lundborg disease

This condition was described initially in two large groups of patients. The Marseilles school described these patients successively under the names of **Ramsay-Hunt syndrome**,[70] **dyssynergia cerebellaris myoclonica with epilepsy**[71] and **Mediterranean myoclonus**.[72] The other group was reported in Finland as **progressive myoclonus epilepsy with no Lafora bodies**[73] and as **Baltic myoclonus**.[74] Advances in molecular biology have demonstrated that these represent the same syndrome, and the Marseilles Consensus Group recommended the term **Unverricht-Lundborg disease**.[75]

The age of onset is 6–18 years. It begins either insidiously with action myoclonus, noticeable in the morning upon wakening, or more suddenly with nocturnal clonic or clonic-tonic-clonic seizures. The myoclonus gradually becomes incapacitating and myoclonias make some movements difficult to perform. Eating and drinking become difficult. Myoclonus attacks may be triggered by performing difficult movements and may develop into full-scale clonic or clonic–tonic–clonic seizures, often involving a partial loss of consciousness. Absence seizures have been observed much less frequently. A variable degree of ataxia is generally present but may be difficult to assess because of the jerks. Other neurologic signs are uncommon, but mild pes cavus and absent deep tendon reflexes have been described. In the Marseilles series, optic atrophy, sensory disorders, pyramidal or extrapyramidal impairments and amyotrophy have not been observed. Cognitive abilities are not severely affected but emotional disorders are common. Myoclonus and ataxia worsen slowly but steadily. The epilepsy can be controlled by medication and lessens with time. The patients' condition tends to fluctuate sharply between 'good periods', during which they are only slightly handicapped, and 'bad periods', when the myoclonus does not permit walking, sometimes ending in a series of seizures. The periods of remission tend to shorten progressively during the course of the disease and last from one day to several weeks. The disease tends to stabilize once the patient is over 40, and the debilitating effects of the myoclonus subside. We have not observed dementia in our patients.

The EEG shows normal background activity, with a few slow waves, in the early stages of the disease. There are short, generalized spike-waves, which may sometimes be associated with massive myoclonias. Action myoclonus is not accompanied by any changes in the EEG. Clinical and EEG sensitivity to photostimulation is observed in almost 90 per cent of cases. Normal physiologic sleep patterns are present. The paroxysmal abnormalities are not aggravated during slow wave sleep, whereas fast spike and polyspike discharge occur around the vertex during REM sleep.[76] The amplitude of the somatosensory evoked potentials is abnormally high.[77,78] The abnormalities tend to diminish with time. A moderate slowing of the background activity and a slight attenuation of the physiologic sleep patterns during stage 2 sleep are observed in patients followed for many years.

Antiepileptic drugs successfully control the seizures, but the myclonus responds only transiently to drug therapy. Alcohol can reduce its intensity, but its effects are short-lived and there is a risk of rapid habituation.[79] More interestingly, high doses of oral piracetam have been reported to be the most effective treatment.[80] Conversely, carbamazepine and phenytoin must be avoided because they tend to worsen the myoclonic syndrome. The more severe course and shortened life expectancy described initially in Finnish patients appears to have related to high doses of phenytoin.[74,81]

The diagnosis can be established relatively simply by molecular genetic tests but other laboratory tests are unremarkable. Muscle biopsy is normal[78] and mitochondrial DNA does not show the mutation found in families with MERRF.[82]

Unverrich-Lundborg disease is inherited by autosomal recessive transmission. The gene has been mapped to 21q22.3[83] and the locus (*EPM1*) subsequently shown to be linked to both the Baltic and the Mediterranean forms of the disease.[84] A significant allelic association between the disease mutation and 21q haplotypes has been demonstrated in the Mediterranean form, suggesting a founder effect in Mediterraneann myoclonus.[85,86] Using positional cloning strategy, a clone encoding a previously described protein, cystatin B (also known as stefin B), a cysteine protease inhibitor, has been described.[87] The most common type of mutation in Unverrich-Lundborg disease is an expansion of a dodecamer (CCCCGCCC-CGCG) in the 5'-untranslated region.[88] The only *EPM1*-related point mutation in the cystatin B gene found in homozygous state was the G4R amino acid substitution in a Moroccan patient.[89] All other point mutations identified in *EPM1* patients have been found as compound heterozygotes with the 12-bp repeat expansion allele. The repeat expansion allele was also homozygous in some patients, particularly in those of Mediterranean origin.[86,88] In contrast to other diseases with triplet expansions, such as the Huntington disease, no correlation has been found between the number of repeat expansions and the age at onset or the severity of the disease in Unverrich-Lundborg disease.[90] Due to the high frequency of the 12-bp repeat expansion, and the shortness of the cystatin B gene, the molecular diagnosis of Unverrich-Lundborg disease is relatively simple.[90]

Dentato-rubral-pallido-luysian atrophy (DRPLA)

This disease, with predominantly autosomal dominant transmission, involves degeneration of both the dentato-rubral and the pallido-luysian systems.[91,92] Although most reports have come from Japan, a number of cases with similar clinical findings have been reported from the UK, Denmark and North Carolina, USA, where it was called **Haw River syndrome**.[93] Diverse clinical pictures have been described and the onset occurs between 6 and 69 years of age. When the onset occurs between childhood and adulthood, nearly half of the patients present with a PME. There may be other neurologic manifestations, such as choreoathetosis, rapidly developing dementia and ataxia. The EEG shows slow bursts and generalized spike-waves, but no consistent pattern of photosensitivity has been observed.

The juvenile type of DRPLA, like Huntington disease, is most commonly inherited via paternal transmission of the gene. Recently, Koide *et al.* have identified an unstable expansion of a CAG in a gene on chromosome 12 in all the 22 DRPLA patients examined.[94]

KEY POINTS

- PMEs are rare diseases characterized by **progressive myoclonus associated with other epileptic seizures and abnormal neurological signs**
- **Mental deterioration** is observed in most patients
- **Metabolic studies, muscle biopsy, skin biopsy and molecular genetic testing** permit a definite diagnosis in many cases
- Treatment involves the judicious use of **antiepileptic drugs and psychological support**
- **Reversal** of the underlying disease is rarely possible
- **Molecular genetic studies** have identified the gene in a number of entities
- **Genetic counseling** is important and prenatal diagnosis is feasible in some diseases

REFERENCES

1. Roger J, Genton P, Bureau M, Dravet C. Progressive myoclonus epilepsy in childhood and adolescence. In: Roger J, Bureau M, Dravet C, *et al.* (eds) *Epileptic Syndromes in Infancy, Childhood and Adolescence*, 2nd edn. London: John Libbey; Paris: Eurotext, 1992; 381–400.

2. Santavuori P, Haltia M, Rapola J. Infantile type of so-called neuronal ceroid lipofuscinosis. *Developmental Medicine and Child Neurology* 1974; **16**: 644–653.

3. Santavuori P. EEG in the infantile type of so-called neuronal ceroid lipofuscinosis. *Neuropaediatrics* 1973; **4**: 375–387.

4. Pampiglione G, Harden A. An infantile form of neuronal 'storage' disease with characteristic evolution of neurophysiological features. *Brain* 1974; **97**: 355–360.

5. Järvela I, Schleutker J, Haataja L, *et al.* Infantile form of neuronal ceroid lipofuscinosis (CLN1) maps to the short arm of chromosome 1. *Genomics* 1991; **9**: 170–173.

6. Vesa J, Hellsten E, Verkruyse LA, *et al.* Mutations in the palmitoyl protein thioesterase gene causing infantile neuronal ceroid lipofuscinosis. *Nature* 1995; **376**: 584–588.

7. Voznyi YV, Keulemans JLM, Mancini GMS, *et al.* A new simple enzyme assay for pre- and postnatal diagnosis of infantile neuronal ceroid lipofuscinosis (INCL) and its variants. *Journal of Medical Genetics* 1999; **36**(6): 471–474.

8. de Vries BBA, Kleijer WJ, Keulemans JLM, *et al.* First-trimester diagnosis of infantile neuronal ceroid lipofuscinosis (INCL) using PPT enzyme assay and CLN1 mutation analysis. *Prenatal Diagnosis* 1999; **19**: 559–562.

9. Aicardi J. Epilepsy and inborn errors of metabolism. In: Roger J, Bureau M, Dravet C, *et al.* (eds) *Epileptic Syndromes in Infancy, Childhood and Adolescence*, 2nd edn. London: John Libbey; Paris: Eurotext, 1992; 97–102.

10. Takeda K, Nakai H, Hagiwara H, *et al.* Fine assignment of beta-hexosaminidase A alpha-subunit on 15q23-q24 by high resolution *in situ* hybridization. *Experimental Medicine* 1990; **160**: 203–211.

11. Bach G, Tomczak J, Risch N, Ekstein J. Tay-Sachs screening in the Jewish Ashkenazi population: DNA testing is the preferred procedure. *American Journal of Medical Genetics* 2001; **99**: 70–75.

12. Gilbert F, Kucherlapati RS, Creagan RP, *et al.* Tay-Sachs' and Sandhoff's diseases: the assignment of genes for hexosaminidase A and B to individual human chromosomes. *Proceedings of the National Academy of Sciences of the USA* 1975; **72**: 263–267.

13. Rey F, Harpey JP, Leeming RJ, *et al.* Les hyperphénylalaninémies avec activité normale de la phénylalanine-hydroxylase. *Archives Françaises de Pédiatrie* 1977; **34**: 109–120.

14. Harding BN, Egger J, Portmann B, Erdohazi M. Progressive neuronal degeneration of childhood with liver disease. *Brain* 1986; **109**: 181–206.

15. Boyd SG, Harden A, Egger J, Pampiglione G. Progressive neuronal degeneration of childhood with liver disease ('Alpers disease'): characteristic neurophysiological features. *Neuropaediatrics* 1986; **17**: 75–80.

16. Jervis GA. Huntington's chorea in childhood. *Archives of Neurology* 1963; **9**: 244–257.

17. Bruyn GW. Huntington's chorea: historical, clinical and laboratory synopsis. In: Vinken PS, Bruyn GW (eds) *Handbook of Clinical Neurology*, vol. 6. Amsterdam: Elsevier North-Holland, 1968; 298–378.

18. Garrel S, Joannard A, Feuerstein J, Serre F. Formes myocloniques de la chorée de Huntington. *Revue d'Electroencephalographie et de Neurophysiologie* 1978; **8**: 123–128.

19. Macdonald ME, Ambrose CM, Duyao MP, *et al.* Novel gene containing a trinucleotide repeat that is expanded and unstable on Huntington's disease chromosomes. *Cell* 1993; **72**: 971–983.

20. Zeman W, Donahue S, Dyken P, Green J. The neuronal ceroid-lipofuscinoses (Batten–Vogt syndrome). In: Vinken PS, Bruyn GW (eds) *Handbook of Clinical Neurology*, vol. 10. Amsterdam: Elsevier North-Holland, 1970; 588–679.

21. Aicardi J, Plouin P, Goutières F. Les céroïde-lipofuscinoses. *Revue d'Electroencephalographie et de Neurophysiologie* 1978; **8**: 149–160.

22. Warburg M. The natural history of Jansky–Bielschowsky's and Batten's diseases. In: Armstrong D, Koopand, Rider JA (eds) *Ceroid Lipofuscinosis (Batten's Disease)*. Amsterdam: Elsevier Biomedical Press, 1982; 35–44.

23. Harden A, Pampiglione G, Picton-Robinson N. Electro-retinogram and visual evoked response in a form of 'neuronal lipidosis' with diagnostic EEG features. *Journal of Neurology, Neurosurgery and Psychiatry* 1973; **36**: 61–67.

24. Pampiglione G, Harden A. Neurophysiological identification of a late infantile form of 'neuronal lipidosis'. *Journal of Neurology, Neurosurgery and Psychiatry* 1977; **36**: 323–330.

25. Lake BD, Cavanagh NPC. Early juvenile Batten's disease. A comparative subgroup distinct from other forms of Batten's disease. *Journal of the Neurological Sciences* 1978; **36**: 265–71.

26. Haines JL, Boustany RMN, Alroy J, *et al.* Chromosomal localization of two genes underlying late-infantile neuronal ceroid lipofuscinosis. *Neurogenetics* 1998; **1**: 217–222.

27. Sleat DE, Donnelly RJ, Lackland H, *et al.* Association of mutations in a lysosomal protein with classical late-infantile neuronal ceroid lipofuscinosis. *Science* 1997; **277**: 1802–1805.

28. Savukoski M, Kestila M, Williams R, *et al.* Defined chromosomal assignment of CLN5 demonstrates that at least four loci are involved in the pathogenenesis of human ceroid lipofuscinosis. *American Journal of Human Genetics* 1994; **55**: 695–701.

29. Sharp JD, Wheeler RB, Lake BD, *et al.* Loci for classical and variant late infantile neuronal ceroid lipofuscinosis map to chromosome 11p15 and 15q21-23. *Human Molecular Genetics* 1997; **6**: 591–595.

30. Gao H, Boustany RMN, Alroy J. Mutations in a novel CLN6 – encoded transmembrane protein cause variant neuronal ceroid lipofuscinosis in man and mouse. *American Journal of Human Genetics* 2002; **70**: 324–335.

31. Sorensen JB, Parnas P. A clinical study of 44 patients with juvenile amaurotic idiocy. *Acta Psychiatrica Scandinavica* 1979; **59**: 449–461.

32. Berkovic SF, Andermann F. The progressive myoclonus epilepsies. In: Pedley TA, Meldrum BS (eds) *Recent Advances in Epilepsy*, vol. 3 . Edinburgh: Churchill Livingston, 1986; 157–187.

33. Santavuori P, Heiskala H, Westermarck T, *et al.* Experience over 17 years with antioxidant treatment in Spielmeyer-Sjögren

disease. *American Journal of Medical Genetics, supplement* 1988; **5**: 265–274.

34. Bagh K, Hortling H. Blodfynd vid juvenil amaurotisk idioti. *Nordisk Medicin* 1948; **38**: 1072–1076.

35. Carpenter S, Karpati G, Andermann F, *et al.* The ultrastructural characteristics of the abnormal cytosomes in Batten-Kuf's disease. *Brain* 1977; **100**: 137–156.

36. Eiberg H, Gardiner RM, Mohr J. Batten disease (Spielmeyer-Sjögren disease) and haptoglobins (HP): indication of linkage and assignment to CH. 16. *Clinical Genetics* 1989; **36**: 217–218.

37. International Batten Disease Consortium. Isolation of a novel gene underlying Batten disease, CLN3. *Cell* 1995; **82**: 949–957.

38. McLeod PM, Nag S, Berry G. Ultrastructural studies as a method of prenatal diagnosis of neuronal ceroid lipofuscinosis. *American Journal of Medical Genetics* 1988; Suppl. 5: 93–97.

39. Conradi G, Uvebrant P, Hökegärd KH, *et al.* First trimester diagnosis of juvenile neuronal ceroid lipofuscinosis by demonstration of fingerprint inclusion in chorionic villi. *Prenatal Diagnosis* 1989; **9**: 283–287.

40. Winkelman MD, Banker BQ, Wictor M, Moser HW. Non-infantile neuronopathic Gaucher's disease: a clinicopathologic study. *Neurology* 1983; **33**: 994–1008.

41. Nishimura R, Omos-Lau N, Ajmone-Marsan C, Baranger JA. Electroencephalographic findings in Gaucher Disease. *Neurology* 1980; **30**: 152–159.

42. Halliday AM, Halliday E. (1980) Cerebro-somatosensory and visual evoked potentials in different clinical forms of myoclonus. In: Desmedt JE (ed.) *Clinical Uses of Cerebral, Brainstem and Spinal Somatosensory Potentials*, vol. 7. Basel: Karger, 1980; 292–310.

43. Mistry PK, Smith SJ, Ali M, *et al.* Genetic diagnosis of Gaucher's disease. *Lancet* 1992; **339**: 889–892.

44. Rapin I, Goldfisher S, Katzman R, Engel J, O'Brien JS. The cherry-red spot myoclonus syndrome. *Annals of Neurology* 1978; **3**: 234–342.

45. Thomas PK, Abrams JD, Swallow D, Stewart G. (1979) Sialidosis type I: cherry-red spot-myoclonus syndrome with sialidase deficiency and altered electrophoretic mobilities of some enzymes known to be glyocoproteins. 1 Clinical findings. *Journal of Neurology, Neurosurgery and Psychiatry* 1979; **42**: 873–880.

46. Federico A, Cecio A, Apponi Battini G, Michalski JC, Strecker G, Guazzi G. Macular cherry-red spot and myoclonus syndrome. Juvenile form of sialidosis. *Journal of the Neurological Sciences* 1980; **48**: 157–169.

47. Steinman L, Tharp BR, Dorfman LJ, *et al.* Peripheral neuropathy in the cherry-red spot myoclonus syndrome (sialidosis type 1). *Annals of Neurology* 1980; **7**: 450–456.

48. Sakuraba H, Suzuki Y, Akagi M, Sakai M, Amano N. β-Galactosidase-neuraminidase deficiency (galactosialidosis): clinical, pathological and enzymatic studies in a postmortem case. *Annals of Neurology* 1983; **13**: 497–503.

49. Lafora GR. Über das Vorkommen amyloider Körperchen im Innenrender Ganglienzellen. *Virchows Archiv für Pathologie und Anatomie* 1911; **205**: 295–303.

50. Van Heycop Ten Ham MW, De Jager H. Progressive myoclonus epilepsy with Lafora bodies. Clinical-pathological features. *Epilepsia* 1963; **4**: 95–119.

51. Roger J, Gastaut H, Boudouresques J, *et al.* Epilepsie myoclonique progressive avec corps de Lafora. Etude clinique et polygraphique. Contrôle anatomique ultrastructural. *Revue Neurologuque* 1967; **116**: 197–212.

52. Tassinari CA, Bureau-Paillas M, Dalla Bernardina B, *et al.* La maladie de Lafora. *Revue d'Electroencephalographie et de Neurophysiologie* 1978; **8**: 107–122.

53. Roger J, Pellissier JF, Bureau M, *et al.* Le diagnostic précoce de la maladie de Lafora. Importance des manifestations paroxystiques visuelles et intérêt de la biopsie cutanée. *Revue d'Electroencephalographie et de Neurophysiologie* 1983; **139**: 115–124.

54. Acharya NJ, Satishchandra P, Asha T, Shankar SK. Lafora disease in South India: a clinical, electrophysiological, and pathologic study. *Epilepsia* 1993; **34**: 476–487.

55. Carpenter S, Karpati G. Sweat gland duct cells in Lafora disease: diagnosis by skin biopsy. *Neurology* 1981; **31**: 1564–1568.

56. Tinuper P, Aguglia U, Pellissier JF, Gastaut H. Visual ictal phenomena in a case of Lafora disease proven by skin biopsy. *Epilepsia* 1983; **24**: 214–218.

57. Serratosa JM, Delgado-Escueta AV, Posada I. *et al.* The gene for progressive myoclonus epilepsy of the Lafora type maps to chromosome 6q. *Human Molecular Genetics* 1995; **9**: 1657–1663.

58. Gomez-Garre P, Sanz Y, Rodriguez de Cordoba SR, Serratosa JM. Mutational spectrum of the EPM2A gene in progressive myoclonus epilepsy of Lafora: high degree of allelic heterogeneity and prevalence of deletions. *European Journal of Human Genetics* 2000; **12**: 946–954.

59. Serratosa JM, Gardiner RM, Lehesjoki AE, Pennachio LA, Myers RM. The molecular genetic bases of the progressive myoclonus epilepsies. *Advances in Neurology* 1999; **79**: 383–398.

60. Minassian BA, Lee JR, Herbrick JA, *et al.* Mutations in a gene encoding a novel protein tyrosine phosphatase cause progressive myoclonus epilepsy. *Nature Genetics* 1998; **2**: 171–174.

61. Tsairis P, Engel WK, Kark F. Familial myoclonic epilepsy syndrome associated with skeletal muscle mitochondrial abnormalities. *Neurology* 1973; **23**: 408.

62. Fukuhara N, Tokiguchi S, Shirakawa K, Tsubaki T. Myoclonus epilepsy asociated with ragged-red fibers (mitochondrial abnormalities). Disease entity or a syndrome? *Journal of the Neurological Sciences* 1980; **47**: 117–133.

63. Di Mauro S, Bonilla E, Zeviani M, Nakagawa M, de Vivo DC. Mitochondrial myopathies. *Annals of Neurology* 1985; **17**: 521–538.

64. Roger J, Pellissier JF, Dravet C, *et al.* Dégénérescence spino-cérébelleuse. Atrophie optique. Epilepsie-myoclonies. Myopathie mitochondriale. *Revue Neurologique* 1982; **138**: 187–200.

65. Byrne E, Trounce I, Dennett X, *et al.* (1988): Progress from MERRF to MELAS phenotype in a patient with respiratory complex I and IV deficiency. *Journal of the Neurological Sciences* 1988; **88**: 327–337.

66. Rosing HS, Hopkins LC, Wallace DC, Epstein CM, Weidenheim K. Maternally inherited mitochondrial myopathy and myoclonic epilepsy. *Annals of Neurology* 1985; **17**: 228–237.

67. Bindoff LA, Desnuelle C, Birch-Machin MA, *et al.* Multiple defects of the mitochondrial respiratory chain in mitochondrial

encephalopathy (MERRF): a clinical, biochemical and molecular study. *Journal of the Neurological Sciences* 1991; **102**: 17–24.

68. Wallace DC, Shoffner JM, Lott MT, Hopkins LC. Myoclonic epilepsy and ragged-red fiber disease (MERRF): a mitochondrial tRNALys mutation responsive to coenzyme Q10 (CoQ) therapy. *Neurology* 1991; **41**(Suppl. 1): 586S; 280.

69. Schoffner JM, Lon MT, Lezza AMS, et al. Myoclonic epilepsy and ragged-red fiber disease (MERRF) is associated with a mitochondrial DNA tRNALys mutation. *Cell* 1990; **61**: 931–937.

70. Roger J, Soulayrol R, Hassoun J. La dyssynergie cérébelleuse myoclonique (syndrome de Ramsay-Hunt). *Revue Neurologique* 1968; **119**: 85–106.

71. Roger J, Genton P, Bureau M, Dravet C, Tassinari CA. Dyssynergia cerebellaris myoclonica (Ramsay-Hunt syndrome) associated with epilepsy. A study of 32 cases. *Neuropediatrics* 1987; **118**: 117.

72. Genton P, Michelucci R, Tassinari CA, Roger J. The Ramsay Hunt Syndrome revisited: Mediterranean Myoclonus versus mitochondrial encephalomyopathy with ragged red fibers and Baltic Myoclonus. *Acta Neurologica Scandinavica* 1990; **81**: 8–15.

73. Koskiniemi ML, Toivakka E, Donner M. Progressive myoclonus epilepsy. Electroencephalographic findings. *Acta Neurologica Scandinavica* 1974; **50**: 333–359.

74. Koskiniemi ML. Baltic myoclonus. In: Fahn S, Marsden CD, Van Woert M (eds) *Myoclonus. Advances in Neurology*, vol. 43. New York: Raven Press, 1986; 57–64.

75. Marseille Consensus Group. Classification of progressive myoclonus epilepsies and related disorders. *Annals of Neurology* 1990; **28**: 113–116.

76. Tassinari CA, Bureau-Paillas M, Dalla Bernardina B, Grasso E, Roger J. Etude electroencéphalographique de la dyssynergie cérébelleuse myoclonique avec épilepsie (syndrome de Ramsay-Hunt). *Revue d'Electroencephalographie et de Neurophysiologie* 1974; **4**: 407–428.

77. Mauguière F, Bard J, Courjon J. Les potentiels évoqués somesthésiques précoces dans la dyssynergie cérébelleuse myoclonique progressive. *Revue d'Electroencephalographie et de Neurophysiologie* 1981; **11**: 174–182.

78. Tassinari CA, Michelucci R, Genton P, Pellissier JF, Roger J. Dyssynergia cerebellaris myoclonica (Ramsay Hunt syndrome): an autonomous condition unrelated to mitochondrial encephalomyopathies. *Journal of Neurology, Neurosurgery and Psychiatry* 1989; **52**: 262–265.

79. Genton P. and Guerrini R. Antimyoclonic effects of alcohol in progressive myoclonus epilepsy. *Neurology* 1990; **40**: 1412–1416.

80. Remy C, Genton P. Effect of high doses of oral piracetam on myoclonus in progressive myoclonus epilepsy (Mediterranean myoclonus). *Epilepsia* 1991; **32**(Suppl. 3): 6 (abstract).

81. Elridge R, Ilvanainen M, Stern R, Koerber I, Wilder BJ. Baltic myoclonus epilepsy: hereditary disorder of childhood made worse by phenytoin. *Lancet* 1983 **ii**; 838–842.

82. Tassinari CA, Michelucci R, Forti A, et al. Ramsay-Hunt syndrome and MERRF: Two unrelated conditions as demonstrated by mitochondrial DNA study. *Neurology* 1991; **41**(Suppl. 1): 587S; 281.

83. Lehesjoki AE, Koskiniemi M, Sistonen P, et al. Localization of a gene for progressive myoclonus epilepsy to chromosome 21q22. *Proceedings of the National Academy of Sciences of the USA* 1991; **88**: 3606–3699.

84. Malafosse A, Lehesjoki AE, Genton P et al. Evidence in favour of a same genetic locus to Baltic and Mediterranean myoclonus. *Lancet* 1992; **39**: 1080–1081.

85. Labauge P, Ouazzani R, M'Rabet A, et al. Allele heterogeneity of Mediterranean myoclonus and the cystatin B gene. *An Neurol* 1997; **41**: 686–689.

86. Moulard B, Genton P, Grid D, et al. Haplotype study of West European and North African Unverricht-Lundborg chromosomes: evidence for a few founder mutations. *Human Genetics* 2002; **111**: 255–262.

87. Pennachio LA, Lehesjoki AE, Stone NE. Mutations in the gene encoding cystatin B in progressive myoclonus epilepsy (EPM1). *Science* 1996; **271**: 1731–1734.

88. Lalioti M, Scott HS, Buresi C, et al. Dodecamer repeat in *Cystatin B* in progressive myoclonus epilepsy (EPM1). *Nature* 1997; **386**: 847–851.

89. Lalioti M, Mirotsou M, Buresi C, et al. Identification of mutations in *Cystatin B*, the gene responsible for the Unverricht-Lundborg type of progressive myoclonus epilepsy (EPM1). *American Journal of Human Genetics* 1997; **60**: 342–352.

90. Lalioti M, Scott HS, Genton P, et al. A PCR amplification method reveals instability of the dodecamer repeat in progressive myoclonus epilepsy (EPM1) and no correlation between the size of the repeat and the age of onset. *American Journal of Human Genetics* 1998; **62**: 842–847.

91. Naito H, Oyanagi S. Familial myoclonus epilepsy and choreoathetosis: hereditary dentato rubral-pallido luysian atrophy. *Neurology* 1982; **32**: 798–807.

92. Iizuka R, Hirayama K, Maehara K. Dentato-rubro-pallido-luysian atrophy: a clinicopathological study. *Journal of Neurology, Neurosurgery and Psychiatry* 1984; **47**: 1288–1298.

93. Burke JR, Winfield MS, Lewis KE, et al. The Haw River syndrome: dentato rubro pallido luysian atrophy (DRPLA) in an African American family. *Nature Genetics* 1994; **7**: 521–524.

94. Koide R, Ikuchi T, Onodesa O, et al. Unstable expansion of CAG repeat in hereditary dentato rubral-pallidol uysian atrophy (DRPLA). *Nature Genetics* 1994; **6**: 9–12.

15

Epilepsies symptomatic of structural lesions

PAOLO CURATOLO

Symptomatic epilepsies and syndromes are considered to be consequences of known or strongly suspected disorders of the CNS.[1] They include both location-related epilepsies, in which seizure semiology or findings at investigation disclose a localized origin of the seizures, and generalized epilepsies, in which the first clinical changes indicate initial involvement of both hemispheres and the ictal EEG patterns are apparently bilateral. They are a heterogeneous group of epilepsies with different pathophysiologic mechanisms, causes, and clinical manifestations, including syndromes of great individual variability. Their diagnoses lie not only in the correct identification of seizure types and clinical and EEG features, but also in the anatomic localization of the structural causes and in their etiology, when known (Chapter 6). Nonetheless, epilepsies symptomatic of structural lesions share some common characteristics, including uncertain prognoses, frequent associations with neurologic and/or mental abnormalities, and, often, some degree of resistance to drug treatment. Factors associated with more favorable outcomes include absence of neurologic and mental abnormalities, a limited number of seizures, the presence of a single type of seizure; absence of tonic, atonic and secondarily generalized seizures and of episodes of status epilepticus; a relatively late onset of seizures (i.e. after the age of 3 years); and absence of secondary bilateral synchrony on EEG. The prognoses for children with epilepsies symptomatic of structural lesions are generally poor and depend mainly on the type, extension and topography of brain abnormalities. Therefore, prognostic studies should be performed on etiologically homogeneous cohorts of individuals. Epidemiologic studies examining the strength of the association between a probable cause of epilepsy and the time of onset of the condition could provide clues to the major and minor etiologic agents and their potential interaction. Systematic study of the etiologies of epilepsy is the key to prevention. Furthermore, epilepsy, intellectual disability and/or cerebral palsy are often associated in the same child, as a result of the same underlying brain abnormalities. Therefore, prognostic studies should stratify different homogeneous groups that present with only epilepsy, or, concurrent epilepsy and intellectual disability and/or cerebral palsy.

The etiology of some epilepsies can be strongly suspected from clinical and EEG features, but in most children, the identification of a structural cause requires the use of neuroimaging techniques, particularly since epilepsies sharing the same basic pathology may have different clinical expressions. An etiologic approach and a careful search for the underlying cause are mandatory in order to compare the natural history and the efficacy of treatment in homogeneous groups of children. Unfortunately, morphologic changes seen in symptomatic epilepsies may have no bearing on the genesis of seizures. Despite the progress in developmental neuropathology, a structural abnormality in neurons that could unquestionably act as a direct cause of seizures has yet to be identified. Therefore, the possible morphologic basis of epileptic seizures often remains unknown. Symptomatic epilepsies may be intractable because of a serious associated brain disease. Brain tumors are one possible cause, but any structural lesion of the brain in an epileptogenic area is likely to lead to difficulties in seizure control. Such patients are potential candidates for surgical treatment, as discussed in Chapters 19 and 22D.

GENERAL CONSIDERATIONS

Clinical features

It is important to try to localize the site of origin of a seizure, but this can be difficult. The first sign or symptom is often the most important indicator of the site of origin of the seizure discharge, whereas the subsequent sequence of ictal events can reflect its further propagation throughout the brain. The total sequence can help in localizing the site of origin. However, one of the major problems is that the initial discharges may start in clinically silent regions. In such situations, the first clinically recognizable events occur only after subsequent spread to sites that are more or less distant from the zones of the initial discharges. Another problem is that a subtle focal onset of a secondary generalized seizure may not be recognized and this seizure may be incorrectly defined as generalized. Many types of generalized seizures, including myoclonic, tonic and atonic seizures, may complicate different diseases, such as malformations or inborn errors of metabolism. Any type of partial seizure may be present in epilepsies symptomatic of structural lesions. The following tentative description of syndromes related to anatomic localization summarizes data which include findings from electrocorticographic recordings (see also Chapter 6).

FRONTAL LOBE EPILEPSIES

These are characterized by simple partial, complex partial or secondarily generalized seizures, or by various combinations of these types of seizures. Seizures often occur several times in a 24-h period, and are characterized by short duration and rapid secondary generalization. They frequently occur during sleep, with prominent motor manifestations that are often tonic or postural. Complex gestural automatisms are common at onset. There is minimal or no postictal confusion. Drop attacks responsible for multiple falls are common when the discharge is bilateral. Status epilepticus is a frequent complication. Supplementary motor seizures are characterized by focal tonic manifestations, with vocalization, speech arrest and fencing postures. Anterior frontopolar seizure patterns include loss of contact and adversive movements of the head and eyes with possible subsequent evolution, including axial clonic jerks and falls and autonomic signs. Opercular seizures include mastication, salivation, swallowing, speech arrest, epigastric aura, and autonomic phenomena. In frontal lobe seizures interictal EEG recordings may show frontal spikes, sharp waves or slow waves, either unilateral or frequently bilateral. Frontal lobe epilepsies are mainly characterized by a severe course that is frequently resistant to antiepileptic drugs and commonly associated with intellectual disability.

TEMPORAL LOBE EPILEPSIES

These are characterized by simple partial seizures, complex partial seizures and secondary generalized seizures, or combinations of these. A family history of seizures is common. The simple partial seizures are typically characterized by both autonomic and psychic symptoms and certain sensory phenomena, such as epigastric sensations or olfactory and auditory illusions. The complex partial seizures are characterized by motor arrest followed by oroalimentary automatisms. In lateral temporal seizures, when the focus is located in the dominant hemisphere a language disorder may occur. Postictal confusion and memory deficits are usual. Interictal EEG patterns include unilateral or bilateral temporal spikes, sharp waves and slow waves, often asynchronous. These events are not always confined to the temporal regions.

PARIETAL LOBE EPILEPSIES

These are usually characterized by simple partial and secondarily generalized seizures. Seizures are predominantly sensory. Positive phenomena include a feeling of electricity that is initially confined, subsequently spreading in a Jacksonian manner; facial and tongue sensations; and a desire to move a body part. Metamorphopsia with distortions and parietal lobe visual phenomena, such as hallucinations, may also occur. Negative phenomena include numbness and a loss of awareness of a part of the body. Disorientation in space and vertigo may be indicative of inferior parietal lobe seizures. Seizures in the dominant parietal lobe result in a variety of receptive or conductive language disturbances.

OCCIPITAL LOBE EPILEPSIES

These are usually characterized by simple partial and secondarily generalized seizures. Complex partial seizures may occur and may spread beyond the occipital lobe. The clinical manifestations usually include visual phenomena which are either positive, such as flashes and phosphenes, or (more rarely) negative, such as amaurosis, hemianopsia and scotomata. Disperceptive illusions, including a change in size, distance or shape may occur. Illusional and hallucinatory visual seizures involve epileptic discharges in the temporo-parieto-occipital junction. The initial signs may also include tonic or clonic deviation of the eyes and head. The discharge may spread to the temporal lobe, producing seizure manifestations of lateral temporal or amygdalo-hippocampal seizures.

EEG FINDINGS

EEG, especially video-EEG, can be very useful in localizing origins of seizures. Changes in background rhythms can be as useful as epileptic discharges, but neither is infallible. Video-EEG recording has greatly improved the ability to precisely classify seizures by accurately illustrating the chronologic relationship between seizures and ictal EEG abnormalities. The ictal EEG recording is of great importance. Certain features are generally considered to be indicative of symptomatic partial epilepsies: specifically, rhythmic slow waves or rapid, low-amplitude bilateral activity recorded in frontal epilepsies. However, the anatomic origin of certain epilepsies is sometimes difficult to assign to specific lobes. For example, perirolandic seizures may include both precentral and postcentral symptomatology. Interictal scalp EEG, may be misleading. The absence of interictal abnormalities does not eliminate the possibility of a lesional epilepsy. Furthermore, some focal abnormalities may temporarily disappear during antiepileptic treatment, even in cases of brain tumors. Certain nonparoxysmal abnormalities are of great value because they are generally related to etiology rather than to the epileptic phenomenon. They include abnormal basic rhythms, focal polymorphic or even monomorphic slow waves, localized depression of rhythms in one hemisphere, and asymmetry of rhythms during hyperventilation and sleep. Paroxysmal focal abnormalities may assume the morphology of unifocal spike-waves, multifocal spike-waves, and even bilateral synchronous or asynchronous spike and wave. Multifocal spike-waves recorded on the awake EEG are often asynchronous and blend into slow background activity. These may evolve from a hypsarrhythmic pattern and generally occur in the context of bilateral lesions in severe lesional epilepsies associated with encephalopathy. Difficulties in accurate topographic localization of epileptogenic foci by visual inspection of the tracings may arise due to the presence of apparently bilateral synchronous EEG abnormalities, associated with multifocal spike-waves, suggesting the possible existence of a secondary bilateral synchrony. This type of synchrony is defined by the occurrence of bilateral synchronous spike-wave or polyspike-wave complexes on EEG recordings, in which spike-wave bursts are immediately preceded by a sequence of focal spikes or sharp waves lasting at least 2 s.[2] Secondary bilateral synchrony is thought to originate from a limited area of abnormal cortex in one hemisphere and to spread rapidly to both sides. This phenomenon is particularly frequent in relation to discharges originating in the frontal regions. The bilateral nature of these abnormalities is probably linked to a number of factors: ease of propagation and bilateralization from a unilateral frontal focus, the existence of multiple foci and the existence of an epileptic predisposition.[2,3] The finding of bilateral synchronous paroxysmal EEG activity should not automatically exclude the possibility of surgical treatment of an epilepsy, at least in the presence of a detectable unilateral lesion. It is well known that in cases of unilateral brain damage, bilateral

paroxysmal abnormalities may be present, and they may be larger over the healthy hemisphere where even ictal onset may appear to be located.[4] Some children who have paroxysmal EEG manifestations similar to those who have clinical problems never have overt seizures: a situation which is difficult to explain.

LOCATION–RELATED SYMPTOMATIC EPILEPSIES WITH SPECIFIC ETIOLOGY

Epileptic seizures may complicate many disease states. Diseases in which seizures are a presenting or predominant feature are included under this heading.

Cerebral palsy

Cerebral palsy is a chronic disability of CNS origin, characterized by abnormal control of movement or posture, appearing early in life. It is not a single disease, but a group of disorders resulting from nonprogressive abnormalities in the developing brain, occurring prenatally or acquired peri- or postnatally. The risk of epilepsy is increased among children with cerebral palsy, particularly in those who are mentally retarded (see also Chapter 16). Cerebral palsy and epilepsy may have an intricate multifactorial relationship involving adverse prenatal or perinatal events. Neuropathologic states that occur in pre- or perinatal hypoxic-ischemic brain injury and that may account for both cerebral palsy and epilepsy include focal and multifocal ischemic brain injuries, selective neuronal necrosis and parasagittal cerebral injury, as discussed in Chapter 5. Epilepsy is estimated to occur in 10–40 per cent of children with cerebral palsy. The incidence of seizures is greatest in patients with hemiplegic or tetraplegic palsies.[5] However, the prevalence is generally lower when epilepsy is defined as recurrent afebrile seizures than when single seizures are included.[6]

Seizures are common in spastic cerebral palsy, especially in congenital hemiplegia, in which half of the patients have seizures. Athetoid, ataxic, and diplegic cerebral palsy are only rarely associated with seizures. Children with quadriplegic cerebral palsy almost always have multifocal or secondarily generalized seizures; those with hemipareses are more likely to show partial Jacksonian or generalized tonic-clonic seizures. Compared with children who are seizure-free, those who have epilepsy are more likely to be mentally retarded, especially if left-sided hemiparesis or tetraplegia coexist. The onset of seizures is most frequently in the first 2 years of life, but is sometimes much later, and is characterized by generalized seizures of focal or multifocal origin. However, almost any form of seizure may occur. Tonic-clonic, myoclonic and atonic seizures are relatively common among severely retarded children and may be intractable. Predictors of the long-term evolution of epilepsy associated with hemiparesis have been identified.[7] Those factors significantly associated with severe and drug-resistant epilepsy include cortical lesions identified by MRI, nonvascular etiology, and mixed and frequent seizures during the first 2 years of life. Patients with a prenatal anomaly may have a higher incidence of epilepsy and an earlier onset of seizures than those with perinatal injury.[8]

Among the epilepsies observed in children with cerebral palsy, startle epilepsy is a well-defined clinical entity related to early lesions of the motor cortex.[9] Complex partial seizures may be symptomatic of parieto-occipital lesions secondary to circulatory disorders occurring during the perinatal period. Genetic susceptibility may be a contributory factor: a familial predisposition to epilepsy is often found in children with cerebral palsy and symptomatic epilepsy, supporting the view that the manifestation of epileptic attacks results from the interaction of endogenous genetic factors and exogenous mechanisms of brain damage.[10] In a case-control study of risk factors for partial epilepsies with onset in the first 3 years in children with cerebral palsy and intellectual disability, a surprisingly high family history of epilepsy was found in first-degree relatives.[10] Other risk factors associated with partial epilepsy in children with cerebral palsy and intellectual disability are placental pathologies, low gestational age, low birthweight for gestational age, cardiopulmonary resuscitation and neonatal convulsions. However, only epidemiologic studies carried out on homogeneous populations, not only for the type of seizures but also for age at onset, can improve identification of risk factors for partial epilepsy associated with cerebral palsy and provide clues for their prevention. Prognoses both for seizures and for their control vary according to the type, extension and topography of the brain abnormalities underlying both cerebral palsy and epilepsy. Therefore, a detailed investigation of lesions is essential in all children. Seizures commonly occur following hypoxic-ischemic cerebral injury, especially in the full-term infant. Spasms associated with periventricular leukomalacia have a better prognosis than those associated with hypoxic-ischemic brain injury in the term infant. Perfusion failure and hypoxia during the second half of gestation are associated with both epilepsy and cerebral palsy. Unfortunately, a diagnosis of prenatal brain ischemia is sometimes difficult after the event, even with MRI. Some children show neuroradiologic findings of both cerebral malformations and hypoxic-ischemic insult.

Prenatal perfusion failures occurring after the end of neuronal migration and before the establishment of gyration may cause microgyria associated with the early onset of severe epilepsy and with poor prognosis.[11] However, the nature and pathogenesis of ischemic disturbances affecting prenatal development of the CNS remains largely unknown. Factors relevant to labor and delivery appear to contribute little to childhood seizure disorders. Given the high human and financial costs of care and treatment of affected individuals, further studies on the etiology and on the co-occurrence of these conditions are needed. Identification of antecedents may be helpful in the development of preventive measures. Given the strong and consistent association between cerebral palsy and epilepsy, prevention of cerebral palsy should reduce the incidence of epilepsy among children.

Head injury

Head trauma caused by accidents is becoming increasingly common during infancy, childhood and adolescence. However, epilepsy develops in only a small percentage of head-injured patients. Head trauma is a potentially preventable risk factor for epilepsy, and identification of patients with head trauma at risk for epilepsy is of practical importance. Seizures may occur acutely, or many years after a head injury. Approximately 5 per cent of children hospitalized for head injuries have a seizure within the first week. A family history of seizures is commoner amongst individuals who develop epilepsy compared with those who do not, suggesting that genetic susceptibility contributes to seizure occurrence. The seizures, which may occur predominantly in the first 24 h following trauma, are likely to be focal, and 75 per cent are partial motor in type. They may be followed by localizing signs and be associated with temporary alterations in consciousness. Status epilepticus following head trauma is common, occurring in 22 per cent of children less than 5 years old.[12] Nevertheless, approximately one third of affected patients have only one attack. Thus, the earliest seizures often remain isolated, and, consequently, should not be regarded as epilepsy. **Early post-traumatic epilepsy** does not indicate the presence of a neurosurgical complication, but is often a precursor of **late post-traumatic epilepsy**. All seizures that occur more than 1 week after head trauma are termed late post-traumatic epilepsy. Although this can develop at any time following trauma, the relative risk decreases after the first 2 years. Late seizures are more often complex partial or apparently generalized, mainly with frontal or frontotemporal lesions. An increased risk for early post-traumatic epilepsy exists in association with the following: penetrating cranial trauma, early posttraumatic seizures, acute intracranial hemorrhage, focal neurological signs, unconsciousness for more than 24 h, depressed fracture with dural laceration and fractures at the base of the skull.[13]

The EEG is only marginally useful in the prediction of a continuing liability to epilepsy. Nevertheless, persistence of focal abnormalities related to the site of the trauma is usually associated with late epilepsy. On the other hand, localized paroxysmal abnormalities can persist for up to 10 years or more without the development of seizures. Prophylactic treatment is based on the concept that antiepileptic drugs given early enough after trauma can prevent the development of an epileptic focus, but there is no proven basis for this concept. Decisions about treatment must take into account the likely benefit and risk of this strategy in terms of adverse behavioral effects.

The pathogenesis of post-traumatic epilepsy remains unknown, despite the standard explanations suggesting that meningocerebral scars and focal ischemic lesions may be factors. Early post-traumatic seizures have been linked with focal injury to the brain and with local ischemia and metabolic changes. Late epilepsy has been attributed to scarring and has been associated with tissue distortion, vascular involvement, and mechanical irritation of the brain. Iron deposition following hemorrhage is also considered a possible risk factor. Pathological considerations are examined in detail in Chapter 5.

Hydrocephalus

Risks of epilepsy relate to the etiology of the hydrocephalus. Hydrocephalus, per se, is not commonly recognized as a cause of seizures, but epilepsy is reported to be frequent in children with shunt-treated hydrocephalus. The mechanisms underlying an increased risk of epileptic seizures after shunt placement remain controversial. One study[14] found seizures were not related to the site of shunt insertion, number of shunt revisions, number of shunt infections or age at shunt insertion. However, the insult to the brain at the time of the ventricular catheter insertion, the presence of the shunt tube itself as a foreign body, the number of shunt revisions after malfunction and associated infection are thought by others to be related to the risk of epilepsy. In children less than 2 years old, age at the time of initial shunt placement also seems to be an important factor, since early shunting is a well known determinant of risk in shunt obstruction.[15]

Seizures are relatively common in children with congenital hydrocephalus, with a reported incidence of 48 per cent in children with congenital hydrocephalus alone, and up to 16 per cent in those with myelomeningocele and hydrocephalus.[16,17] When children with hydrocephalus are considered as a group, including those with posthemorrhagic and other pathologies, the incidence of seizures is approximately 50 per cent. Within this group, there are variable risks, related to the pathologic condition producing hydrocephalus: e.g. injury to the cortex as a result of shunt insertion; damage from shunt complications, such as infection or obstruction resulting in higher intracranial pressure; other intracerebral abnormalities, e.g. neuronal migration disorders; posthemorrhagic or periventricular ischemic lesions, etc. Some patients have seizures following

an episode of shunt dysfunction. The location of EEG foci has been found to correspond to the location of the ventricular catheter. However, the cause of hydrocephalus may also be responsible for the epilepsy, and a topographic correlation between EEG foci and the position of the catheter has not been confirmed by all authors. Intellectual disability, often in combination with cerebral malformation other than hydrocephalus, is associated with seizure occurrence and seizure persistence. Approximately one third of children with epilepsy in association with isolated hydrocephalus continue to have frequent seizures despite treatment. In contrast, in the vast majority of children with hydrocephalus and myelomeningocele there is an excellent prognosis for seizure control, and, in these, discontinuation of drug treatment after relatively brief seizure-free periods does not increase the risk of recurrent convulsions. In children with congenital hydrocephalus who are of normal intelligence, and, who, as a result of anticonvulsants, have been seizure-free for 3 years, it is safe to discontinue therapy.

Intracranial tumors

Brain tumors are uncommon causes of epilepsy in children. However, hemispheric tumors may present with epileptic seizures which may remain the only clinical symptom for prolonged periods, ranging from a few months to many years. Generally, such seizures are not immediately associated with other neurologic signs and symptoms, especially in patients with normal intellect.[18] Tumors located close to the brain surface have a greater propensity to cause seizures than deep subcortical tumors. Seizures are more commonly associated with slower growing tumors, than rapidly growing lesions. Since most tumors that give rise to seizures are benign, e.g. low-grade astrocytomas and oligodendrogliomas (Figure 15.1), early diagnosis is important because complete recovery may be possible following surgical treatment. Thus, identification of those few children whose attacks are likely to be caused by brain tumors is very important. In the past the mean interval between the first seizure and the diagnosis of a tumor has been 5.6 years[19] and intervals as long as 20 years have been reported.[20] The main factors considered to be responsible for these delays are: initial EEG normal or soon normalized after the onset of the treatment, misinterpretation of CT, and remission of seizures with or without antiepileptic drug treatment.[21] Epilepsies caused by hemispheric tumors are mainly characterized by simple or complex partial seizures; but, apparently generalized seizures and bilaterally synchronous interictal EEG abnormalities may also be present. Some seizures are described as generalized because the localizing symptoms are missed or they originate from a clinically silent zone of the brain. Suspicion should be

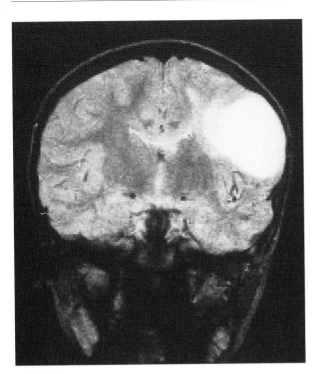

Figure 15.1 *MRI of a 2-year-old girl who had three partial motor seizures. Large area of hyperdensity of the left rolandic area was shown to be a low-grade astrocytoma. After surgical removal the seizures disappeared.*

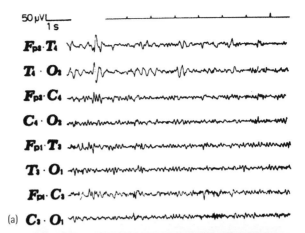

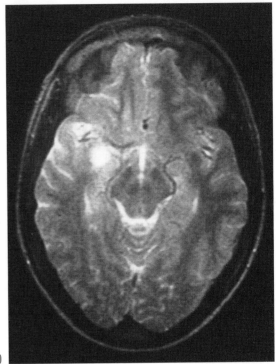

Figure 15.2 *Interictal EEG showing sporadic sharp waves over the right temporal region in a 12-year-old boy with seizures characterized by olfactory-gustatory aura, oral automatisms and loss of contact. Hyperdense signal of the right temporal region detected by MRI is an oligodendroglioma.*

heightened when seizures are partial and refractory, particularly if intelligence and physical examination are normal or if there is a progressive deterioration in behavior. Localized EEG foci of polymorphic slow waves or sharp waves on a slow disorganized EEG background are suggestive of a tumor (Figure 15.2a, b). In a series of 20 children with seizures who had histologically confirmed cerebral tumors mainly involving the temporal and the frontal lobes, 40 per cent were aged 15 months or younger at onset of the first partial seizure.[22] Initial misdiagnosis occurred in 25 per cent of these infants. Examination was normal in 75 per cent. EEG at onset revealed focal abnormalities in 62 per cent and generalized abnormalities in 25 per cent. CT scan findings were not diagnostic in 40 per cent: conversely, MRI confirmed the presence of tumors in all the children. Although MRI findings are not specific, such imaging has made the diagnosis of brain tumors easier and faster, allowing for an accurate evaluation of all regions.

Outcome with regard to seizures is generally considered favorable. Postoperative freedom from seizures is probable when complete or near-complete resection of epileptogenic cortex is achieved. A clear trend towards improvement of neuropsychologic and cognitive functions is also noted.[23] Tumors are further considered in Chapters 5 and 22D.

GELASTIC EPILEPSY

Seizures begin before 3 years of age, and often before 1 year of age. At the onset or during evolution the ictal manifestations are characterized by laughter, eventually followed by a more complex event characterized by head and eye deviation and automatisms. The seizures are brief, but very frequent. Neurologic examination is generally normal. Gelastic epilepsy should always arouse a strong suspicion of a tumor of the floor of the third ventricle, especially a hamartoma.[24] The onset of gelastic epilepsy and precocious puberty in childhood is potentially serious since,

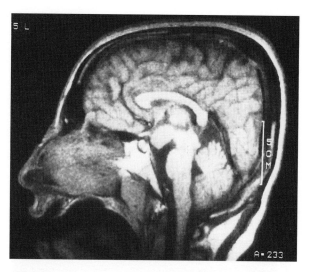

Figure 15.3 *Sagittal MRI showing hypothalamic hamartoma in a boy with precocious puberty and gelastic epilepsy from the age of 2 years.*

rarely, this combination has been reported to be associated with a low-grade astrocytoma. However, the most common association is with a posterior hypothalamic hamartoma, a tumor-like collection of normal tissue lodged in an abnormal location. The attacks of laughter can be confused with behavioral or emotional disorders, but their stereotyped recurrence, the absence of any precipitating factor, other manifestations of epilepsy (generalized, temporal-lobe and psychomotor seizures), and no other obvious cause for the pathologic laughter make the diagnosis of gelastic epilepsy highly probable. Ictal and interictal awake EEG show localized discharges of spikes, predominantly originating in the temporal or frontotemporal areas and generalized slow spike and wave discharges.[24] Investigation with MRI or CT may confirm the diagnosis by detecting a posterior hypothalamic tumour. MRI is superior to CT in showing the exact size and anatomic location of the hamartomata (Figure 15.3). These lesions are not expansive and are not readily accessible to surgery. The evolution is characterized by the presence of seizures, intellectual disability and behavioral problems.

DYSEMBRYOPLASTIC NEUROEPITHELIAL TUMORS

Dysembryoplastic neuroepithelial tumors (DNET) are newly described, pathologically benign, tumors originating in the supratentorial cortex which have an invariable association with intractable partial complex seizures. The age of onset of the partial seizures ranges from 2 to 19 years. MRI demonstrates a well-circumscribed focal cortical mass, located in the temporal lobe or more rarely in the occipital lobe. These lesions have an increased signal intensity on T2-weighted images and may simulate benign cysts or low-grade astrocytomata.[25]

NEUROCUTANEOUS SYNDROMES

Advances in neuroimaging and developmental neuropathology are providing new and exciting information on the structure of the brain in neurocutaneous syndromes. Previously unknown relationships with the neurologic complications of neurocutaneous syndromes, including seizures, are becoming apparent. A large number of neurocutaneous syndromes are associated with migrational disorders (Chapters 4A, 4C), accounting for the coexistence of brain and skin pigmentary pathology. Sometimes, seizures are the presenting symptoms or contribute significantly to the severity of the disease. The prognosis for seizure control and neurologic development is influenced particularly by the underlying cause. For example, in children with tuberous sclerosis, spasms have a very poor outcome, but spasms associated with neurofibromatosis have an excellent prognosis.

Tuberous sclerosis complex (TSC)

TSC is a congenital hamartomatosis with variable expression in seizures, intellectual disability, behavioral disturbance and pathology in multiple organs. It is transmitted by autosomal dominant inheritance. TSC shows genetic heterogeneity with linkage to chromosomes 9q34 and 16p13. Pathologically, TSC is a disorder of cellular migration, proliferation and differentiation. Cortical tubers constitute the hallmark of the disease and are pathognomonic tumors originating in the supratentorial regions in cerebral TSC. There is variability in the range and extent of the neurologic problems, of which seizures are the most common, occurring in 92 per cent of patients. The complex relationships between the TSC1 and TSC2 gene products are currently under investigation. Several lines of evidence support a direct interaction between hamartin and tuberin, suggesting that both these two proteins participate in some common cellular functions. Compared to patients with TSC2 mutations, sporadic patients with TSC1 mutations have, on average, milder disease, with lower frequencies of seizures and moderate/severe intellectual disability; fewer subependymal nodules and cortical tubers; less severe kidney involvement; no retinal hamartomas; and less severe facial angiofibroma.[26] In addition, TSC2 mutations are associated with a significantly earlier epilepsy presentation than TSC1 mutations, with the result that infantile spasms are frequent.[27] In TSC, epilepsy often begins in the first year of life, and, in most cases, in the very first months of life, when the commonest types of seizure are partial motor and infantile spasms (Chapter 9B). The high incidence of infantile spasms and hypsarrhythmia has long been emphasized, but the possibility that infants with TSC exhibit some specific clinical, and interictal and ictal EEG features, which distinguish them from those with classic infantile spasms and hypsarrhythmia, has not been clarified. In the same child partial seizures may precede, coexist or evolve into infantile spasms.

A vast number of subtle partial seizures such as unilateral tonic or clonic phenomena, mainly localized to the face or limbs, and other subtle lateralizing features, such as tonic eye deviation, head turning and unilateral grimacing, can be missed by the parents until the third or fourth month of life when infantile spasms occur.

At the onset, the awake EEG shows multifocal or focal spike discharges and irregular slow focal activity. Although EEG foci can be located in any region of the brain, the commonest locations for focal EEG discharges, at the age when infantile spasms occur, are the posterior temporal and occipital regions. During sleep, an increase in epileptiform activity is usually observed, and the multifocal abnormalities tend to generalize, giving a semblance of hypsarrhythmia.

Video-EEG monitoring and polygraphic recordings of the spasms have shown that the ictal phenomenon is a single seizure. Each spasm consists of a combination of both focal and bilateral manifestations. The ictal EEG starts with a focal discharge of spikes and polyspikes, often originating from the temporal, rolandic or occipital regions, and is followed by a generalized irregular slow transient and an abrupt flattening of the background activity in all regions.

The vast majority of patients who have infantile spasms at onset later manifest either partial motor or complex partial seizures or apparently generalized seizures. In the EEG of older patients, the pseudotype pattern of hypsarrhythmia tends to disappear, and tracings tend to exhibit bifocal or multifocal spikes or slowing. After 2 years of age, additional foci with a frontal localization become progressively evident. Cortical tubers detected by MRI represent the epileptogenic foci of TSC, and a topographic relationship exists between EEG abnormalities and the largest MRI high-signal lesions.[28] MRI lesions in the occipital lobes show the best correlation with the EEG foci, while the weakest correlation is in the frontal lobes.[29,30] The age of seizure onset and the age of occurrence of EEG foci may depend on the localization of cortical tubers, with an earlier expression for parietal and occipital lesions than for frontal ones. This may result from maturational phenomena. Since perfusion of the occipital lobes decreases with age and frontal areas reach complete maturation only in the second year of life, there is no paradox in the finding that cortical lesions which are associated with infantile spasms are not epileptogenic as the child gets older; and, that, in the same child, complex partial seizures originating from a more anterior tuber may become evident only some years later. Patients with multiple lesions may have a greater tendency to show hypsarrhythmia at an early age with subsequent development of bilateral synchronization. In the tubers, disarray

of the neuronal architecture is associated with malformed neurons and astrocytes and neural cells of indeterminate identity, suggesting a defect in neuronal and glial differentiation and migration (Chapter 4C) and providing a likely anatomic substrate for epilepsy.[31]

Immunohistochemical and molecular analysis have indicated that the neuronal populations of cortical tubers might have intrinsic epileptogenicity and actively participate in the generation of partial seizures, through the release of neurotransmitters or neuromodulators into the adjacent brain tissue. Giant cells in tubers express neurotransmitter-producing enzymes and neurotransmitter receptors, such as NMDA receptor subunit 1 and $GABA_A$ receptor subunits.[32] Furthermore, it has been suggested that changes in the properties of $GABA_A$ receptors, possibly related to plastic changes in subunit combinations, may result in an altered regulation of inhibitory function. On the basis of these findings a decrease in GABAergic inhibition in cortical tubers can be postulated. This could represent a fertile field for further investigation. The idea that epileptogenesis in TSC may be related to an impairment of GABAergic transmission is supported by the effectiveness of drugs with affinity with $GABA_A$-benzodiazepine receptor in the treatment of epilepsy. Elevated GABA levels have been reported in brain biopsies of subjects with intractable epilepsy and TSC, and not from other causes. Furthermore, several studies have indicated that vigabatrin, a specific and irreversible inhibitor of γ-aminobutyric acid aminotransferase, has a higher efficacy in infantile spasms and in partial seizures due to TSC than in those related to other etiologies. It is possible to suppose that epilepsy in TSC may result from 'aberrant plasticity' that may involve a subunit switch of $GABA_A$ receptors and changes in a regulatory system.

A consistent association between seizures and intellectual disability has been observed. Both the number and the localization of cortical tubers play important roles in mental outcome, suggesting that epilepsy and intellectual disability reflect the underlying brain dysfunction caused by cortical tubers.[33] Late-onset partial seizures or transient infantile spasms may be the only seizure types observed in nonretarded patients.[33] All patients with favorable evolutions of their epilepsy have normal psychomotor development before the onset of the first seizure and generally show only one seizure type. Children with normal intelligence have small isolated cortical tubers, mainly localized to the parietal and rolandic regions. In contrast, patients with intellectual disability suffer from frequent partial seizures, developing multifocal or secondary generalized epilepsy, and show multiple bilateral cortical tubers on MRI (Figure 15.4). Progressive mental deterioration, observed in children with intractable seizures, may be due to a particular epileptogenicity of parasagittal frontal tubers. Difficulties in accurate topographic localization of epileptogenic foci by visual inspection of the tracing may arise as a result of the presence of apparently bisynchronous EEG abnormalities. This phenomenon is particularly frequent for discharges originating in the frontal regions. Children with bilateral involvement, with three or more affected lobes demonstrated on MRI, are more likely to show bilateral synchronization on EEG, when, mainly during sleep, a multifocal frontally dominant pattern of

bursts of bilateral and more synchronous slow spike waves, tending to assume the appearance of a Lennox-Gastaut pattern, is characteristic.

In children with apparently bilateral synchronous spike-wave bursts on standard EEG, high-time-resolution topographic spike mapping enables the recognition of a focal frontal onset with propagation of the contralateral

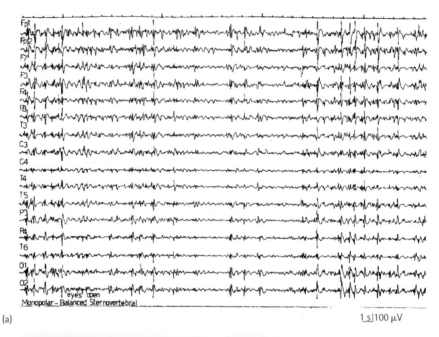

(a)   1 s | 100 μV

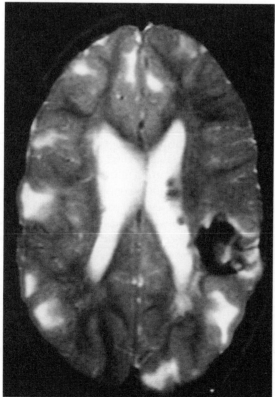

(b)

Figure 15.4 *Interictal EEG showing apparently generalized spike and wave discharges in a girl with tuberous sclerosis, intractable epilepsy and severe mental retardation. MRI reveals multiple tubers in both hemispheres.*

homologous region, in topographic concordance with the site of a prominent MRI lesion.[34] These findings support the concept that apparently generalized spike-wave discharges are of focal origin in most children, with a subsequent phenomenon of secondary bilateral synchrony. This has important implications not only in the clinical management, but also in the therapeutic approach, since the presence of multifocal and generalized interictal EEG abnormalities and/or multiple areas of cerebral involvement cannot be automatic bases for exclusion of consideration for surgical treatment.

Correlations between cortical tubers and epileptogenic areas are far from being definitive in TSC. The combined use of topographic mapping of EEG and dipole-localization methods may provide important clues to localization of epileptogenic areas even in cases with apparently synchronous spike wave bursts. Mapping the results on a three-dimensional MRI reconstruction can more accurately localize the zone of the cortical focal abnormalities and can help the surgeon to make tailored and conservative resections in children with intractable seizures. However, MRI is not yet able to detect all the cortical tubers that may be identified pathologically. Therefore, the disturbance of cerebral function may be more extensive than is indicated by morphologic imaging alone.[35] Evidence from multiple imaging modalities suggests that not all lesions in children with TSC are epileptogenic. Whenever possible, the identification of a single epileptogenic area is essential. Selective surgical removal can significantly improve the quality of life of patients with TSC.

Other neurocutaneous syndromes

NEUROFIBROMATOSIS

Neurofibromatosis 1 (NF1) (previously known as **von Recklinhausen's neurofibromatosis**) is an autosomal dominant disorder affecting about 1 in 3000 individuals. It is characterized by multiple hyperpigmented areas and peripheral neurofibromata. Anomalous migration and localization of neural crest cells occurs (Chapters 4A, 4C). The gene for NF1 has been mapped to chromosome 17. Brain findings include cortical architectural abnormalities, with random orientations of neurons and disarray of normal cortical lamination, heterotopic neurons within the cortical molecular layer in the subcortical or deep cerebral white matter, and gross cerebral malformations such as polymicrogyria, pachygyria and hemimegalencephaly.[36] In recent years MRI has improved the diagnosis of brain abnormalities in NF1, particularly in relation to dysembryoplastic lesions and heterotopic foci. The incidental discovery of high-signal MRI lesions localized in the basal ganglia, brainstem and cerebellum has been reported in as many as 60 per cent of these children. Since MRI abnormalities have been detected both in

children affected by early-onset partial seizures and in asymptomatic individuals, these findings do not seem to have any correlation with neurologic dysfunction.

Seizures are 10 times more frequent in NF1 than in the general population, but are rarely the presenting symptom. They are generally sporadic and respond rapidly to drug treatment.

Infantile spasms (Chapter 9B) with onset between 4 and 6 months and associated with an EEG pattern of hypsarrhythmia have been observed in children with NF1; they are usually associated with a favorable evolution and a normal developmental outcome. Older children may occasionally have localization related, generalized tonic-clonic seizures, or atypical absences. Discontinuation of anticonvulsants is possible in the vast majority of patients.

EPIDERMAL NEVUS SYNDROME

Epidermal nevus is a sporadic congenital skin lesion characterized by a slightly raised, yellow-brown plaque usually located in the midline of the forehead and nose, associated with congenital abnormalities of the brain and other systems. A subgroup with a recognizable neurologic variant has been described.[37] These patients have facial epidermal nevi, ipsilateral hemimegalencephaly, gyral malformation, contralateral hemiparesis, intellectual disability, seizures and often facial hemihypertrophy. Seizures may begin between birth and 6 months. Both partial seizures and infantile spasms are commonly reported. EEG abnormalities at the onset are usually ipsilateral to the major brain abnormality.

HYPOMELANOSIS OF ITO

Hypomelanosis of Ito is characterized by areas of skin hypopigmentation in the form of streaks or whorls. Neurologic abnormalities such as intellectual disability and seizures are present in more than half of the reported cases and can probably be explained by abnormal neuronal migration (Chapter 4C). A large spectrum of brain abnormalities, including pachygyria, multiple gray matter heterotopias and hemimegalencephaly has been reported in individuals with hypomelanosis of Ito, supporting the concept that the bases of the CNS lesions are probably neuronal migration disorders. Seizures (infantile spasms or partial seizures) usually become manifest during the first year of life and tend to be refractory to anticonvulsants. Abnormal rhythmic EEG activity and radiologic images of neuronal migration defects also seem to be correlated.[38]

INCONTINENTIA PIGMENTI

Incontinentia pigmenti is probably transmitted as an X-linked dominant trait, affecting females in 95 per cent of cases. The syndrome is characterized by various hyperpigmented skin lesions that are apparent at birth or during the first weeks of life as vesiculobullous lesions, becoming hyperpigmented gray-brown macular lesions during the first years of life. Most patients have symptoms and signs of neurologic abnormalities, manifested by developmental delay, spastic cerebral palsies and seizures. Seizures are observed in about 20 per cent of individuals. Partial seizures or infantile spasms may begin during the first months of life, and may persist with great frequency and severity during the first year. Intellectual disability, observed in a minority of individuals, is most frequent in association with early seizures and with structural changes in the brain.

INCONTINENTIA PIGMENTI ACHROMIANS

Incontinentia pigmenti achromians is characterized by bilateral, asymmetric, hypopigmented whorls associated with CNS abnormalities, including seizures, intellectual disability, and motor system dysfunction. Abnormalities of neuronal migration, such as micropolygyria, are also reported.

INTRACRANIAL VASCULAR DISORDERS

Seizures may develop throughout childhood as a result of vascular disorders. Focal seizures may occur in neonatal cerebral infarction and in children with cerebral embolism, dural sinus or cortical vein thrombosis. The diagnosis of cerebrovascular lesions can be difficult, especially in children with clinically atypical features. However, widespread use of modern diagnostic techniques, including magnetic resonance imaging and other studies, has improved the ability to confirm the presence of vascular lesions and often to identify their causes, even when the clinical presentation is subtle or atypical.

Sturge–Weber syndrome

Sturge-Weber syndrome is characterized by a nevus of the upper face, ipsilateral leptomeningeal angiomatosis, contralateral hemiparesis or hemianopia, contralateral partial or secondary generalized seizures and, frequently, intellectual disability. The association and localization of aberrant vasculature in the facial skin, eyes and meninges are compatible with a single early localized defect in vascular morphogenesis at a very early stage of development in the tissue from which the vasculature of these three regions eventually develops. The degree of CNS involvement is variable. Seizures most commonly begin between 2 and 7 months of age and are often the presenting symptom, usually preceding the motor deficit and intellectual disability. Partial motor and/or secondary generalized seizures occur in almost all patients; infantile spasms are rarely reported. The first seizure is often asymmetric or unilateral, long-lasting

and followed by a transient paralysis. The EEG is characterized by decreased amplitude and frequency of background electrocerebral activity over the affected hemisphere. Unilateral or diffuse multiple independent spike foci are commonly associated. As time goes on there is a notable increase in seizure frequency and severity, with progressive worsening of the hemiparesis, and dementia; generalized tonic, tonic-clonic or myoclonic seizures may become manifest and may be refractory to drug treatment. Despite the topographic localization of the intracranial angioma in the occipital region, visual seizures and complex partial seizures are rare. Seizures occur in about 75 per cent of individuals affected by Sturge-Weber syndrome. In a retrospective study of 102 patients, 88 individuals had one cerebral hemisphere affected, and 14 showed bilateral hemispheric involvement.[39] Sixty-three of the 88 patients with unilateral hemispheric disease had seizures, with a mean age of seizure onset of 24 months; whereas 13 of 14 individuals with bilateral hemispheric lesions had seizure disorders, with a mean age of seizure onset of 6 months. Intellectual disability was present in about half of the patients and was generally more severe in patients with bihemispheric lesions and persistence of seizures. In contrast, all 25 patients with unihemispheric leptomeningeal involvement, who did not have seizures, were of average intelligence. Therefore, seizures must play some role in determining intellectual disability and in causing deterioration of mental function.

Several new antiepileptic drugs have been released and complete seizure control may not be as difficult as previously. In one series of patients, reported in 1995, half achieved complete control, and an additional 39 per cent had partial control of their seizures.[40] Some patients experience long seizure free intervals, whereas other children have frequent and/or prolonged seizures despite high doses of multiple antiepileptic drugs. Usually more extensive intracranial lesions tend to cause seizures that are more difficult to control.

CT, MRI, SPECT and PET can be used to define the extent of the intracerebral angioma and to carefully select candidates for early focal resection. Serial PET scanning can be useful in documenting the progression of the disease (Chapter 19B). The delineation of hypoperfusion or hypometabolism in the region of the angioma can provide an accurate definition of the epileptogenic zone to be resected in children with early-onset intractable seizures.[41,42]

Hemispherectomy can sometimes improve seizure control and enhance intellectual development.[43,44]

Arteriovenous malformations

The presenting features of arteriovenous malformations include intracranial hemorrhage, seizures, and focal deficits. The mean age at onset of clinical manifestations is about 10 years.[45] The seizure focus is typically adjacent to the malformation, and the seizure type is often focal motor or complex partial. However, secondary generalization of the seizures may occur so rapidly that sometimes it is difficult to distinguish a focal onset on clinical findings alone. Seizures occur as the first clinical manifestation in about 20 per cent of patients.[46] Arteriovenous malformations which involve the temporal lobe cause seizures twice as often as lesions at other sites.

Acute headache, vomiting and alterations of consciousness are characteristic of hemorrhage. Sometimes episodic headache similar to migraine without signs of intracranial hemorrhage is the initial symptom of the vascular malformation. Arteriovenous malformations can be identified by MRI from the flow void determined by the rapidly moving blood within the lesion.

Cavernous malformations

A cavernous malformation is a vascular abnormality characterized by abnormally dilated vessels which are not separated by brain tissue and do not communicate directly with the arterial system. Cavernous malformations are typically identified because of epileptic seizures, acute focal motor deficits, or, more rarely, with intracranial hemorrhage. Patients diagnosed because of seizures tend to fare better than those who present with bleeding.[47] The commonest presentations of the cavernous malformation are seizures, which occur in two thirds of patients.[48] Seizures may appear at any age from infancy to adulthood, are partial in type and often difficult to control. Cavernous malformations have a significant familial incidence, with a dominant transmission and an almost complete penetrance. A gene mapping to chromosome 7q seems to be responsible.[49]

Autoimmune vascular disorders

Both systemic lupus erythematosis and Hashimoto's thyroiditis can present with status epilepticus (personal communication, SJ Wallace). Affected children show signs of involvement of other systems in addition to the CNS, e.g. poor growth, proteinuria, skin lesions and/or myopathic changes.

KEY POINTS

- Epilepsies symptomatic of structural lesions can manifest with either **localized or generalized seizures, or both**
- **Anatomical localization and etiology of** structural pathology are important for both treatment and prognosis
- **Localization can be difficult** despite careful observation of the seizure and detailed scrutiny of the EEG. Ictal video-EEG provides the best information
- **MRI** can identify lesions which are not seen on CT
- The presence of a lesion, identified on imaging, does not always mean that this is the **source** of the seizures
- Epilepsies secondary to structural lesions are commonly associated with **physical and mental disabilities**
- They are often **resistant to medical treatment**
- Epilepsy may be **associated** with cerebral palsy, hydrocephalus, tumors, neurocutaneous syndromes, intracranial vascular disorders, or follow head injuries

REFERENCES

1. Commission on Classification and Terminology of the International League Against Epilepsy. Proposal for revised classification of epilepsies and epileptic syndromes. *Epilepsia* 1989; **30**: 389–399.
2. Blume WT, Pillay N. Electrographic and clinical correlates of secondary bilateral synchrony. *Epilepsia* 1985; **26**: 636–641.
3. Gastaut H, Zifkin B, Magaudda A, Mariani E. Symptomatic partial epilepsies with secondary bilateral synchrony: differentiation from symptomatic generalized epilepsies of the Lennox-Gastaut type. In: Wieser HG, Elger CE (eds) *Presurgical Evaluation of Epilepsies*. Berlin: Springer Verlag, 1987; 308–316.
4. Sammaritano M, De Lobiniere A, Andermann F, *et al.* False lateralization by surface EEG of seizure onset in patients with temporal lobe epilepsy and gross focal cerebral lesions. *Annals of Neurology* 1987; **21**: 361–369.
5. Bruck I, Antoniuk SA, Spessatto A, *et al.* Epilepsy in children with cerebral palsy. *Arquivos de Neuro-Psiquiatria (Sao Paulo)* 2001; **59**: 35–39.
6. Nelson KB, Ellenberg JK. Antecedents of seizure disorders in early childhood. *American Journal of Diseases of Children* 1986; **140**: 1053–1061.
7. Gaggero R, Devescovi R, Zaccone A, Ravera G. Epilepsy associated with infantile hemiparesis: predictors of long-term evolution. *Brain Development* 2001; **23**: 12–17.
8. Okumura A, Hayakawa F, Kato T, *et al.* Epilepsy in patients with spastic cerebral palsy: correlation with MRI findings at 5 years of age. *Brain Development* 1999; **21**: 540–543.
9. Chauvel P, Vignal JP, Liegeois-Chauvel C, *et al.* Startle epilepsy with infantile brain damage: clinical and neurophysiological rationale for surgical therapy. In: Wieser HG, Elger CE (eds) *Presurgical Evaluation of Epilepsies*. Berlin: Springer Verlag, 1987; 306–307.
10. Curatolo P, Arpino C, Stazi MA, Medda E. Risk factors for early symptomatic localized epilesies. *Epilepsia* 1991; **32**: 22.

11. Curatolo P, Cusmai R, Pruna D, Feliciani M. Polymicrogyria: a case detected by MRI. *Brain Development,* 1989; **11**: 257–259.

12. Jennett B. Trauma as a cause of epilepsy in childhood. *Developmental Medicine and Child Neurology* 1973; **15**: 56–72.

13. Jacobi G. (1992) Post-traumatic epilepsy. *Monatsschrift Kinderheilkunde* 1992; **140**: 619–623.

14. Stellman GR, Bannister CM, Hillier V. The incidence of seizure disorder in children with acquired and congenital hydrocephalus. *Zeitschrift fur Kinderchiurgier* 1986; **41**: 38–41.

15. Sato O, Yamguchi T, Kittaka M, Toyama H. Hydrocephalus and epilepsy. *Child's Nervous System* 2001; **17**: 76–86.

16. Noetzel M, Blake JN. Prognosis for seizure control and remission in children with myelomeningocele. *Developmental Medicine and Child Neurology* 1991; **33**: 803–810.

17. Noetzel MJ, Blake JN. Seizures in children with congenital hydrocephalus: long term outcome. *Neurology* 1992; **42**: 1277–1281.

18. Blume WT, Girvin JP, Kaufmann JCE. Childhood brain tumors presenting as chronic uncontrolled focal seizure disorder. *Annals of Neurology* 1982; **12**: 538–541.

19. Aicardi J, Praud E, Bancaud J, *et al.* Epilepsies cliniquement primitives et tumeurs cerebrales chez l'enfant. *Archives Françaises de Pediatrie,* 1970; **27**: 1041–1055.

20. Spencer DD, Spencer SS, Mattson RH, Williamson PD. Intracerebral masses in patients with intractable partial epilepsy. *Neurology* 1984; **34**: 432–436.

21. Sjors K, Blennow G, Lantz G. Seizures as the presenting symptom of brain tumors in children. *Acta Pediatrica* 1993; **82**: 66–70.

22. Williams BA, Abbott KJ, Manson JI. Cerebral tumors in children presenting with epilepsy. *Journal of Child Neurology* 1992; **7**: 291–294.

23. Adelson PD, Peacock WJ, Chugani HT *et al.* Temporal and extended temporal resections for the treatment of intractable seizures in early childhood. *Pediatric Neurosurgery* 1992; **18**: 169–178.

24. Curatolo P, Cusmai R, Finocchi G, Boscherini B. Gelastic epilepsy and true precocious puberty due to hypothalamic hamartoma. *Developmental Medicine and Child Neurology* 1984; **26**: 509–514.

25. Koeller KK, Dillon WP. Dysembryoplastic neuroepithelial tumors: MRI appearance. *American Journal of Neuroradiology* 1992; **13**: 1319–1325.

26. Dabora SL, Jozwiak S, Franz DN *et al.* Mutational analysis in a cohort of 224 tuberous sclerosis patients indicates increased severity of TSC2, compared with TSC1, disease in multiple organs. *American Journal of Human Genetics* 2001; **68**: 64–80.

27. Jozwiak S, Kwiatkowski DJ, Kasprzyk-Obara J, *et al.* Epilepsy and especially infantile spasms are more frequent among patients with TSC2 mutations. *Journal of Child Neurology* 2001; **16**: 675.

28. Curatolo P, Cusmai R. MRI in Bourneville disease: relationship with EEG findings. *Neurophysiologie Clinique,* 1988; **18**: 149–157.

29. Cusmai R, Chiron C, Curatolo P, *et al.* Topographic comparative study of MRI and EEG in 34 children with tuberous sclerosis. *Epilepsia* 1990; **31**: 747–755.

30. Tamaki K, Okuno T, Ito M, *et al.* MRI in relation to EEG epileptic foci in tuberous sclerosis. *Brain Development* 1990; **12**: 316–320.

31. Huttenlocher PR, Wolman RL. Cellular neuropathology of tuberous sclerosis. *Annals of the New York Academy of Sciences* 1991; **615**: 140–148.

32. Crino PB, Henske EP. New development in neurobiology of tuberous sclerosis complex. *Neurology* 1999; **53**: 1384–1390.

33. Curatolo P, Cusmai R, Cortesi F, *et al.* Neuropsychiatric aspects of tuberous sclerosis. *Annals of the New York Academy of Science,* 1991; **615**: 8–16.

34. Curatolo P, Seri S, Cerquiglini A. Topographic spike mapping of EEG in tuberous sclerosis. *Neuropediatrics* 1993; **24**: 178.

35. Curatolo P, Verdecchia M, Bombardieri R. Tuberous sclerosis complex: a review of neurological aspects. *European Journal of Paediatric Neurology* 2002; **6**: 15–23.

36. Cusmai R, Curatolo P, Mangano S, *et al.* Hemimegalencephaly and neurofibromatosis. *Neuropediatrics* 1990; **21**: 179–182.

37. Pavone L, Curatolo P, Rizzo R, *et al.* Epidermal nevus syndrome: a neurologic variant with hemimegalencephaly, gyral malformation, mental retardation, seizures and facial hemihypertrophy. *Neurology* 1991; **4**: 266–271.

38. Esquival EE, Pitt MC, Boyd SG. EEG findings in hypomelanosis of Ito. *Neuropediatrics* 1991; **22**: 216–219.

39. Bebin EM, Gomez MR. Prognosis in Sturge-Weber disease: comparison of unihemispheric and bihemispheric involvement. *Journal of Child Neurology* 1988; **3**: 181–184.

40. Sujansky E, Conradi S. Sturge-Weber syndrome; age of onset of seizures and glaucoma and the prognosis for affected children. *Journal of Child Neurology* 1995; **10**: 49–58.

41. Chiron C, Raynaud C, Tzourio N, *et al.* Regional cerebral blood flow by SPECT imaging in Sturge-Weber disease: an aid for diagnosis. *Journal of Neurology, Neurosurgery and Psychiatry* 1989; **52**: 1402–1409.

42. Chugani HT, Mazziotta JC, Phelps ME. Sturge-Weber syndrome: a study of cerebral glucose utilization with PET. *Journal of Pediatrics* 1989; **114**: 244–253.

43. Carson BS, Javedan SP, Freman JM, *et al.* Hemispherectomy: a hemidecortication approach and review of 52 cases. *Journal of Neurosurgery* 1996; **84**: 903–911.

44. Peacock WJ, Wehby-Grant MC, Shields WD, *et al.* Hemispherectomy for intractable seizures in children: a report of 58 cases. *Child's Nervous System* 1996; **12**: 376–384.

45. Murphy MJ. Long-term follow-up seizures, associated with cerebral arteriovenous malformations. Results of therapy. *Archives of Neurology* 1985; **42**: 477–479.

46. Crawford PM, West CR, Chardwick DW, *et al.* Arteriovenous malformations of the brain: Natural history in unoperated patients. *Journal of Neurology, Neurosurgery and Psychiatry* 1986; **49**: 1–10.

47. Simard JM, Garcia-Bengochea F, Ballenger WE, *et al.* Cavernous angioma: A review of 126 collected and 12 new clinical cases. *Neurosurgery* 1986; **18**: 162–172.

48. Kattapong VJ, Hart BL, Davis LE. Familial cerebral cavernous angiomas: clinical and radiological studies. *Neurology* 1995; **45**: 492–497.

49. Dubovsky J, Zabramski JM, Kurth J, *et al.* A gene responsible for cavernous malformations of the brain maps to chromosome 7q. *Human Molecular Genetics* 1995; **4**: 453–458.

16

Epilepsy in people with intellectual disability

MATTI SILLANPÄÄ

Epilepsy and intellectual disability (mental retardation) are two of the commonest major neurodevelopmental disabilities. They often occur in combination. Intellectual disability is defined as a chronic or lifelong inability to care for oneself in a manner comparable to one's peers, resulting from a low intelligence level (IQ < 70) before the age of 18 years. When associated with intellectual disability, epilepsy tends to be difficult to treat or completely intractable. Therefore, epilepsy combined with intellectual disability constitutes both a serious medical challenge and an economic load on the health care system. Investments in prevention, early diagnosis and treatment and management of both intellectual disability and epilepsy may markedly diminish institutionalization and other costs of care, and help patients to become more independent.

EPIDEMIOLOGICAL ASPECTS

Reports on epilepsy associated with intellectual disability deal with the prevalence of epilepsy in selected, institutionalized subjects; or in patients seen in hospital;[1-3] or, in patients with intellectual disability from population studies of epilepsy.[4-6] However, data on epilepsy among people with intellectual disability[7-13] are most illustrative of the magnitude of the problem.

Epilepsy in inpatients with intellectual disability

The prevalence of epilepsy is higher in institutionalized than in unselected populations. In 816 consecutive hospital patients, epilepsy was found in 34 per cent overall, and in 38 per cent with cerebral palsy and 31 per cent without, respectively.[1] With severe intellectual disability, the prevalence rates were 54 per cent with and 47 per cent without cerebral palsy.[1] In a retrospective study of 338 of 1000 patients consecutively admitted to an institution for the mentally retarded during the years 1943 to 1966 and alive at the end of 1966, the lifetime prevalence of epilepsy was 62 per cent.[2] Seizures were focal in 22 per cent, generalized in 18 per cent and miscellaneous in 49 per cent. In the whole group of 1000, comprising survivors and those who had died before 1966, the lifetime prevalence was 44 per cent.[14] A more recent study of 1023 institutionalized patients with intellectual disability with an encephalopathy[3] found 32 per cent with epilepsy. Seizures were much more likely to be generalized than partial (65 per cent vs. 33 per cent).

Epilepsy in populations with intellectual disability

Studies relating to the occurrence of epilepsy in populations with intellectual disability (Table 16.1) are often

Table 16.1 *Prevalence of epilepsy (per cent) in populations with intellectual disability*

Age of patients (yrs)	N	IQ			Reference
		50–70	<50	≤70	
1–16	122			30	9
5–16	161		36		15
5–16	171	22			18
1–16	91	12			19
All ages	1479	11	23	20	11
22	221	10	35	15	12
6–16	1602			13	16
6–13	378	15	45	26	13
22	151	7	35	21	17

cross-sectional, yielding a point prevalence or period prevalence of an 'active' epilepsy.[7,9,11,15] In one report, at least one seizure occurred in 32 per cent of children with intellectual disability up to age 14 years, but the period prevalence for 1 year was only 19 per cent.[8] Unselected cohort studies are preferable and the only ones which give reliable data. Table 16.1 shows that the overall prevalence of epilepsy is approximately 15 per cent (range 7–22 per cent) in patients with mild intellectual disability (IQ 50–70)[11–13,16–19] and 30 per cent (range 23–45 per cent) in those with severe intellectual disability (IQ < 50).[11–13,17] The prevalence of intellectual disability in patients with epilepsy seems to be much the same as that of epilepsy in intellectual disability, ranging from 14–41 per cent.[4–6,20,21] In Finland, intellectual disability is reported to be severe in 15–33 per cent and mild in 6–7 per cent.[4,5] In the National Collaborative Perinatal Project (NCPP), intellectual disability was reported in 14 per cent of patients and 5 per cent of their siblings followed up to the age of 7.[6] In Sweden, 23–52 per cent of those with severe intellectual disability and 11–21 per cent with mild disability are reported with epilepsy.[11,15] In 1962, in three groups of British children, born in 1951–1955 and matched for city of residence, age and sex, epilepsy occurred in 27 per cent with severe intellectual disability, 11 per cent with borderline disability and 4 per cent with normal intelligence.[10] Epilepsy started at younger ages and persisted longer in those with severe intellectual disability.

A further prospective study found epilepsy in 15 per cent and one febrile or afebrile seizure in an additional 7 per cent by age 22 years.[12] The cumulative incidences of epilepsy were 9 per cent, 11 per cent, 13 per cent and 15 per cent at 5, 10, 15 and 22 years, respectively. With severe intellectual disability, epilepsy occurred in 35 per cent and one or more seizures in 44 per cent. Another comparable study gave similar results:[8] at least one seizure occurred in 32 per cent of patients with severe disability. Age at onset of epilepsy is as early as or earlier than in the general population.[10–12] Seizure frequency is usually high, with 60–70 per cent having annual seizures.[11]

TYPES OF EPILEPTIC SEIZURES AND SYNDROMES IN PEOPLE WITH INTELLECTUAL DISABILITY

Classification of seizures in people with intellectual disability presents several difficulties. Inadequate or defective verbal communication can result in underestimation of focal seizures. Most patients with intellectual disability have mixed seizure types. Generalized tonic-clonic seizures are easiest to identify and are reported to be the commonest (58–68 per cent) in population-based studies.[5,11,22,23] Those with focal seizures with or without secondary generalization may be more readily recognized in studies of institutionalized patients, making the distribution of seizure types less clear.[3,24] Focal epilepsies are associated with more severe handicaps and institutionalization. Since seizure types are age-related, they vary in distribution. As age increases, the proportions of generalized tonic-clonic and focal seizures increase, and seizures typical of early childhood decrease.[11] Convulsive status epilepticus occurs in about one fifth of patients.

The International Classification of Epilepsies and Epileptic Syndromes is not easily applicable in cases of intellectual disability, with only 28–34 per cent of patients' epilepsies classifiable.[3,25] Some epilepsies and epileptic syndromes are of importance in association with intellectual disability. Ohtahara syndrome, early infantile epileptic encephalopathy (see Chapter 1) presents with very early onset and drug-resistant tonic spasms and suppression-burst on the EEG, and is associated with early death or with frequent evolution to West syndrome[26–28] and further to Lennox-Gastaut syndrome. West syndrome[27] (see Chapter 9B) accounts for 7 per cent of the intellectually disabled population with onset of epilepsy during the first year of life.[11] Lennox-Gastaut syndrome[27] (see Chapter 10B) evolves from West syndrome in 23–54 per cent,[27,29,30] most commonly in those with focal etiologies.[27] Intellectual disability, severe personality disturbances and drug-resistance occur in addition to epilepsy with predominantly tonic seizures. In contrast to West syndrome, the prognosis for neurologic and mental outcome in patients with cryptogenic Lennox-Gastaut syndrome is no better than in those with a symptomatic etiology, and all patients with West syndrome and subsequent Lennox-Gastaut syndrome are more or less intellectually disabled.[27] Common etiologies in both symptomatic West syndrome and Lennox-Gastaut syndrome are cerebral malformations, such as Aicardi syndrome,[31] various forms of cerebral dysplasia,[32] neurocutaneous syndromes, e.g. tuberous sclerosis,[33] hypoxic-ischemic encephalopathy[34] and Down syndrome.[35]

EPILEPSY IN CERTAIN INTELLECTUAL DISABILITY SYNDROMES

Chromosomal abnormalities (see also Chapter 4B)

Down himself[36] and other earlier authors[1,37,38] did not associate Down syndrome with epilepsy. Later, the prevalence reported varied from 1 to 9 per cent,[39,40] probably as a result of small patient series, definitions of epilepsy, characteristics of source populations, difficulties in case identification and ages of the subjects. In a series of 1654 patients, the incidence of epilepsy showed a bimodal distribution of age at onset, with the first peak between 16 and 23, and the second between 35 and 54 years of age.[41] The higher age-related incidence is ascribed to the occurrence of Alzheimer-like alterations in the brain. Further information from this study showed the onset of epilepsy at 35 years or more was significantly associated with dementia, but the incidence was remarkably low between 30 and 49 years.[42] Patients with Down syndrome and Alzheimer-like dementia have a seven-fold increase in epilepsy compared with those with Alzheimer disease alone,[43,44] suggesting a specific epileptogenic factor in Down patients.[45]

In fragile X syndrome, recurrent partial and generalized convulsive seizures and infantile spasms may occur in 25 per cent. High prevalences of epilepsy also occur in other, less common chrosomosomal disorders, such as Angelman and Prader-Willi syndromes (epilepsy in 84–90 per cent),[46–48] and Wolf-Hirschhorn syndrome (70 per cent).[49]

Dysplastic conditions (see also Chapter 15)

Intellectual disability and epilepsy are almost invariably associated in tuberous sclerosis, where half of all patients have infantile spasms,[50] and in Sturge-Weber syndrome. Aicardi syndrome, megalencephaly and other cerebral malformations also present with West syndrome, Lennox-Gastaut syndrome or other epilepsy syndromes. In these conditions, 41–100 per cent suffer from epilepsy.[8]

Neurometabolic and degenerative abnormalities (see also Chapter 14)

Forty-one per cent of patients with metabolic diseases and intellectual disability have been reported with epilepsy.[8]

Myoclonic seizures are invariable in children with infantile and late infantile types of ceroid lipofuscinosis. Seizures also occur in 83 per cent of those with the juvenile form.[51] Seizures usually start at age 3–5 years in patients with Rett syndrome, but very early onset is possible: partial, or generalized seizures or atypical infantile spasms, which may be very therapy-resistant, occur in 70–80 per cent.[52,53] Phenylketonuria, maple syrup urine disease, metachromatic leukodystrophy and several organic acidemias are frequently complicated by epilepsy.

CONCOMITANT HANDICAPS

Although a firm relationship between the occurrence of epilepsy and degree of intellectual disability, neurological disability or electroencephalographic changes is not always found,[23] numerous cohort studies with long-term follow-up have found intellectual disability to be a significant independent risk factor in the occurrence or persistence of seizures. The prevalences of epilepsy associated with cerebral palsy and varying degrees of intellectual disability have been briefly considered above. Further data on 43 692 people, of whom 95 per cent had intellectual disability, found that epilepsy occurred in 23 per cent and cerebral palsy in 16 per cent of those less than 22 years of age.[54] In the mildly affected, intellectual disability combined with cerebral palsy raised the prevalence of epilepsy slightly from 19 to 22 per cent,[18] but in severe intellectual disability the coexistence of cerebral palsy had a less obvious effect (55 per cent vs. 46 per cent[15]). A retrospective study that included both children and adults[11] found 20 per cent of 1479 patients with intellectual disability alone, and 33 per cent with additional cerebral palsy, had epilepsy. Fourteen per cent of children with mild intellectual disability and cerebral palsy and 59 per cent of those with severe intellectual disability and cerebral palsy had epilepsy; the prevalence was highest in tetraplegic (100 per cent) and hemiplegic (83 per cent) cerebral palsy.[13] The etiology of intellectual disability can play a major role.[10,12] In a study where the incidence of epilepsy was unrelated to the severity of intellectual disability in the subgroup of intellectual disability only, it was about seven-fold (38 per cent vs. 5 per cent) in children with intellectual disability and cerebral palsy and 15-fold (75 per cent vs. 5 per cent) in children with intellectual disability and a postnatal injury. Thus, significantly increased incidences of epilepsy in severe compared with mild intellectual disability (35 per cent vs. 10 per

Derby Hospitals NHS Foundation Trust
Library and Knowledge Service

cent) may be ascribed to the occurrence of cerebral palsy, and even more so to a postnatal brain lesion. The cumulative incidence of febrile seizures was 9 per cent; one third of those affected developed epilepsy. If children develop expansive hydrocephalus at age less than 1 year, epilepsy is significantly more frequent in children with, than in those without, intellectual disability (74 per cent vs. 28 per cent).[55]

ADAPTIVE BEHAVIORAL PROBLEMS

Institutionalized adults who suffer from intellectual disability and epilepsy have poorer life skills than matched controls without epilepsy.[56] Behavioral problems are substantially more frequent and severe in epileptic patients with intellectual disability than in those with normal intelligence, but qualitatively there is no difference:[57] poor language skills and life circumstances probably contribute.[58] Aggressiveness, and emotional and self-injurious problems are more frequent and social competence is less in people with intellectual disability.[8,59] Behavioral disorder has been reported in 40 per cent, temper tantrums in 38 per cent, hyperkinesis in 30 per cent and childhood autism in 15 per cent.[8] Behavioral disturbances were severer with drug-resistant seizures.[56]

COMMON PROBLEMS OF IDENTIFICATION AND CLASSIFICATION OF SEIZURES

In intellectual disability, problems with expression of subjective symptoms and sensations, specifically in relation to auras and aspects of ictal consciousness, often lead to difficulties with diagnosis of seizure types and differentiation from nonepileptic seizures. Nonepileptic seizures are considered in detail in Chapter 2. Those seen most often with intellectual disability are classified on the basis of underlying principal mechanisms in Table 16.2. Keeping in mind the possibility of occurrence, most of them may be identified without difficulty. Emotionally triggered episodes, such as aggression and rage, unresponsiveness with staring, masturbation and nocturnal phenomena can lead to particular difficulties. A multifaceted psychopathology may be obscured by these disorders, including anxiety, dissociative, psychotic and factitious disorders, malingering and rarely rage attacks.[60] Patients with intellectual disability frequently suffer from sleep disturbances which precipitate the occurrence of seizures.[61,62] Particularly in patients with intellectual disability, nonepileptic attacks may be combined with epileptic seizures[63] and thus less easily detectable. Video-EEG recording is often necessary for a correct diagnosis. If raised, the serum prolactin level may contribute.[60]

Table 16.2 *Differential diagnosis of epileptic seizures in intellectual disability*

Cerebral hypoxic states
Reflex and mechanical syncope
Transient global cerebral ischemia
Cardiogenic
Migraine

Disturbed homeostasis
Hypoglycaemia
Electrolyte imbalance
Disturbed thermoregulation

Involuntary paroxysmal movements
Paroxysmal dystonia or choreoathetosis
Drug-related dyskinesias
Startle responses
Nystagmus and other oculomotor disorders
Tic
Stereotypic rocking and hand-waving

Sleep disorders
Night terrors
Pavor nocturnus
Head banging
REM sleep-related violence
Somnambulism
Benign nocturnal myoclonus
Sleep apnea

Diurnal psychogenic episodes
Episodic rage attacks
Hyperventilation syndrome
Masturbation
Self-injurious behaviour
Panic attacks
Breath-holding spells

Gastrointestinal disorders
Vomiting, regurgitation, and rumination
Gastro-oesophageal reflux
Urinary and stool incontinence

Other
Unresponsiveness or 'staring'
Tonic episodes due to brainstem compression
Self-induced seizures

Self-induced seizures are mostly a sign of photosensitive epilepsy. By waving a hand rhythmically across the eyes, flickering is elicited. Apparently, self-provoked seizures produce pleasure and the patient is often reluctant to discontinue seizure-provoking behavior.

ETIOLOGY OF EPILEPSY IN PEOPLE WITH INTELLECTUAL DISABILITY

The etiology of severe intellectual disability is reportedly prenatal in 55–72 per cent, perinatal in 8–15 per cent, postnatal in 1–12 per cent and unknown in 13–22 per cent.[13,15,64,65] The corresponding figures for mild intellectual disability are 23–43 per cent, 7–18 per cent, 4–5 per cent, and 43–55 per cent.[18,64] The etiology of epilepsy cannot be differentiated from that of intellectual disability. Epilepsy can result from any pre-, peri- or postnatal brain injury which is a presumed cause of intellectual disability. However, not every abnormal event in the pre-, peri- or postnatal history is necessarily of importance.

TREATMENT AND MANAGEMENT

Antiepileptic drugs with clear-cut sedative side-effects, such as phenobarbital and phenytoin,[66] should be avoided in patients with intellectual disability. These drugs may further weaken the patients' mental capacity even at acceptable blood levels. Discontinuation of phenobarbital does not necessarily worsen and can improve seizure control and behavior patterns.[67] Phenytoin-induced cerebellar atrophy has been reported in intellectual disability.[68] Multiply handicapped children with intellectual disability seem especially sensitive to phenytoin.[69] In intellectual disability, side-effects may be masked by pre-existing neurologic abnormalities and are therefore less easily detectable. Monotherapy should always be preferred. However, epilepsies that are difficult to treat and special epileptic syndromes, such as refractory atypical absences and epilepsy with multiple seizure types, may require two or more drugs. If seizures are resistant despite trials of several combinations, a reduction of polytherapy may not change the seizure frequency but may diminish side-effects. If the epilepsy is worsening, drug toxicity, poor compliance, and, rarely, the development of an intracranial tumor or raised intracranial pressure should be considered.

Broad-spectrum drugs with several modes of action are preferable for patients with intellectual disability. Valproic acid is effective and widely used in several seizure types, including infantile spasms,[70] and, with less effect, in Lennox-Gastaut syndrome. The risk of an idiosyncratic reaction is particularly high in intellectually disabled children aged up to 4 years.[71,72] Up to the end of 1991, 129 fatal valproate-treated cases had been reported. Dementia as a side-effect of valproic acid is also possible.[73] Lamotrigine, in addition to effects on focal and generalized seizures, can also be very useful for otherwise intractable seizures, particularly in Lennox-Gastaut syndrome.[74] In a retrospective review of 44 patients institutionalized for multiple handicaps who were treated with lamotrigine, 32 per cent experienced 75–100 per cent decrease in seizure frequency, 23 per cent experienced 50–74 per cent decrease and 25 per cent less than 50 per cent decrease.[75] Twenty per cent had more seizures, which were mostly myoclonic. Topiramate has also proved to be effective against refractory focal and generalized seizures. In Lennox-Gastaut syndrome, a significant decrease in drop attacks has been demonstrated,[76,77] and, with continued treatment, at least 50 per cent decreases in generalized, tonic-clonic, myoclonic and atypical absence seizures have been maintained by 60 per cent, 53 per cent and 53 per cent of the patients, respectively. Topiramate may also be used for treatment of infantile spasms.[78,79] Soon after its introduction, felbamate was proved to be effective against several types of refractory seizures. Unfortunately, dangerous adverse effects have greatly restricted its use.[80] Levetiracetam is a promising newcomer.[80] Formal trials in people with intellectual disability are so far lacking, but there are anecdotal data reporting favorable effects on photosensitive seizures, and in myoclonic seizures in progressive myoclonus epilepsy.[81] Zonisamide has comparable efficacy to carbamazepine and valproic acid, and is effective also for myoclonias and generalized seizures in progressive myoclonus epilepsy.[82] Carbamazepine is still widely used for focal and secondarily generalized tonic-clonic seizures in people with intellectual disability. It is well tolerated, with minimal cognitive, emotional and behavioral side-effects. However, in patients with pretreatment behavioral problems, side-effects of carbamazepine which might be similar can be difficult to detect. In people with intellectual disability, carbamazepine may also provoke atypical absence, atonic and myoclonic seizures.[83,84] Oxcarbazepine has an antiepileptic profile and efficacy equivalent to carbamazepine, but fewer serious and other adverse effects and interactions. Recently, vigabatrin has been shown to be an effective add-on therapy in patients with drug-resistant seizures.[24,85] The most favorable results have been in infantile spasms, particularly those associated with tuberous sclerosis.[86] Adverse effects include hyperactive agitation or aggression,[87] myoclonic jerks[88] and, most importantly, but especially difficult to assess in people with intellectual disability, restriction of visual fields.[89] Other GABAergic antiepileptics, including gabapentin, and tiagabine, have virtually similar antiepileptic efficacy to vigabatrin. With the exception of visual field defects, they also possess similar side-effects such as aggressiveness, other behavioral disturbances, increase in seizure frequency and ataxia or lethargy.[90–93]

Antiepileptic drugs are very important, but are not the only ways to care for epilepsy in people with intellectual disability. A multidisciplinary approach and team work are needed to train professionals of various categories and families in the observation of seizures, side-effects, and long-term neurologic and behavior changes, so that the adverse effects of drugs are minimized. Surgical intervention may be indicated in resistant epilepsy if there is unilateral spike-wave activity, which should be prevented from spreading to the other hemisphere. Here, corpus callosotomy or commissurotomy could be the preferred approach, but in some cases, cortical resection, lobectomy or hemispherectomy will be feasible.

In the management of patients with intellectual disability and epilepsy, several specific aspects must be considered. They may be associated with intellectual disability or seizures or both, and include risks of aspiration; drowning, for example in bath water; nutritional deficiencies due to swallowing difficulties; and gastrointestinal disorders arising from constipation or other dysfunctions. Fatal and nonfatal, seizure-related and other injuries should be prevented by avoidance of identified risk factors, enhanced staff supervision, minimization of risks in the structural environment, and development of reasonable activities for patients so that boredom and restlessness are avoided.

PROGNOSIS

The association of intellectual disability with epilepsy has generally been regarded as unfavorable in relation to seizure prognosis,[94–95] but some authors have not found any difference in outcome related to the severity of intellectual disability in patients on or off medication.[96,97] Even though intellectual disability will affect the seizure prognosis it is important to recognize that patients with intellectual disability may also become seizure free. In a personal, prospective, 35-year follow-up study of 150 epilepsy patients with incidence cases (unpublished data), 74 per cent of mentally normal patients, 61 per cent with mild intellectual disability and 28 per cent with severe intellectual disability achieved a 5-year terminal remission on or off medication. In a comparison of 44 institutionalized subnormal patients with at least 50 convulsive seizures during the first 9 months of the year 1976 and 29 matched controls who had had no seizures during the same period of time, the seizure outcome after 20–22 years of follow-up was predictable with an 80 per cent probability on the basis of admission EEG characteristics and clinical findings.[98] In the group with a poor outcome, early-onset seizures with high initial frequency, multiple seizure types and severe intellectual disability predominated, and was combined with absence of posterior dominant rhythmic activity, generalized delta activity and frequent generalized paroxysmal discharges on the EEG. Freedom from seizures for 5 years on or off medication has been reported in 39 per cent of patients with intellectual disability by age 22.[12] The etiology of intellectual disability was clearly related to the prognosis. The remission rate was 56 per cent in the subgroup of intellectual disability only, 47 per cent in the group with intellectual disability and cerebral palsy and 11 per cent in patients with intellectual disability resulting from a perinatal brain injury. It has been shown that medically fragile patients with severe intellectual disability and complex epilepsy could be successfully transferred from an institution into the community by early initiation of seizure therapy, reducing polypharmacy and improving staff education.[99]

KEY POINTS

- Epilepsy occurs in about **one third** of those with severe intellectual disability and in about **one sixth** of those with mild intellectual disability
- The **coexistence of cerebral palsy** increases the likelihood of epilepsy, particularly if there is a postnatal etiology
- The same **pathology** is responsible for both epilepsy and intellectual disability
- **Classification of seizures and epilepsy syndromes** can present particular difficulties in intellectual disability
- Care is needed in the **choice of drug therapy**. It is easy to overlook or misinterpret **adverse events**, particularly sedation and behavioral changes
- Aspects of **care**, other than drug therapy, are important
- Some patients with intellectual disability can have **remission** of their epilepsy

REFERENCES

1. Illingworth RS. Convulsions in mentally retarded children with or without cerebral palsy. *Journal of Mental Deficiency Research* 1959; **3**: 88–93.
2. Iivanainen M. *A Study of Origins of Mental Retardation.* Clinics in Developmental Medicine No. 51. London: William Heinemann Medical Books for Spastics International Publications, 1974.
3. Mariani E, Ferini-Strambi L, Sala M, Erminio C, Smirne C. Epilepsy in institutionalized patients with encephalopathy: Clinical aspects and nosological considerations. *American Journal on Mental Retardation* 1993; **98**(Suppl.): 27–33.
4. Sillanpää M. Social functioning and seizure status of young adults with onset of epilepsy in childhood. An epidemiologic 20 year follow-up study. *Acta Neurologica Scandinavica* 1983; **68**(Suppl.): 96: 1–77.
5. von Wendt L, Rantakallio P, Saukkonen AL, Mäkinen H. Epilepsy and associated handicaps in a 1 year birth cohort in Northern Finland. *European Journal of Paediatrics* 1985; **144**: 149–151.
6. Ellenberg JH, Hirtz DG, Nelson KB. Do seizures cause intellectual deterioration? *New England Journal of Medicine* 1986; **314**: 1085–1088.
7. Drillien CM, Jameson S, Wilkinson EM. Studies in mental handicap. Part I: Prevalence and distribution by clinical type and severity of defect. *Archives of Disease in Childhood* 1966; **41**: 528–538.

8. Corbett JA, Harris R, Robinson R. Epilepsy. In: Wortis J (ed.) *Mental Retardation and Developmental Disabilities*, vol. VII. New York: Raven Press, 1975: 79–111.

9. Gustavson KH, Hagberg B, Hagberg K, Sars K. Severe mental retardation in a Swedish county. I. Epidemiology, gestational age, birthweight and associated CNS handicaps in children born 1959-70. *Acta Paediatrica Scandinavica* 1977; **66**: 373–379.

10. Richardson SA, Koller H, Katz M. McLaren J. Seizures and epilepsy in a mentally retarded population over the first 22 years of life. *Applied Research in Mental retardation* 1980; **1**: 123–138.

11. Forsgren L, Edvinsson SO, Blomquist HK, Heijbel J, Sidenvall R. Epilepsy in a population of mentally retarded children and adults. *Epilepsy Research* 1990; **6**: 234–248.

12. Goulden KJ, Shinnar S, Koller H, Katz M, Richardson SA. Epilepsy in children with mental retardation: a cohort study. *Epilepsia* 1991; **32**: 690–697.

13. Steffenburg U, Hagberg G, Viggedal G, Kyllerman M. Active epilepsy in mentally retarded children. I. Prevalence and additional neuroimpairments. *Acta Paediatrica* 1995; **84**: 1147–1152.

14. Iivanainen M. *Brain Developmental Disorders Leading to Mental Retardation. Modern Principles of Diagnosis.* Springfield: CC Thomas, 1990.

15. Gustavson KH, Holmgren G, Jonsell R, Blomquist HK. Severe mental retardation in children in a Northern Swedish county. *Journal of Mental Deficiency Research* 1977; **21**: 161–180.

16. Wellesley D, Hockey A, Stanley F. The aetiology of intellectual disability in Western Australia: a community-based study. *Developmental Medicine and Child Neurology* 1991; **33**: 963–973.

17. Airaksinen EM, Matilainen R, Mononen T, *et al*. A population-based study on epilepsy in mentally retarded children. *Epilepsia* 2000; **41**: 1214–1220.

18. Blomquist HK, Gustavson KH, Holmgren G. Mild mental retardation in children in a Northern Swedish county. *Journal of Mental Deficiency Research* 1981; **25**: 92–109.

19. Hagberg B, Hagberg G, Lewerth A, Lindberg U. Mild mental retardation in Swedish school children. II. Etiologic and pathogenetic aspects. *Acta Paediatrica Scandinavica* 1981; **70**: 445–452.

20. Ross EM, Peckham CS, West PB, Butler NR. Epilepsy in childhood: findings from the National Child Development Study. *BMJ* 1980; **280**: 207–210.

21. Sidenvall R, Forsgren L, Heijbel J. Prevalence and characteristics of epilepsy in children in northern Sweden. *Seizure* 1996; **6**: 21–26.

22. Baldev KS, Towle PO. Antiepileptic drug status in adult outpatients with mental retardation. *American Journal on Mental Retardation* 1993; **98**(Suppl.): 41–46.

23. Marcus JC. Control of epilepsy in a mentally retarded population: lack of correlation with IQ, neurological status, and electroencephalogram. *American Journal on Mental Retardation* 1993; **98**(Suppl.): 47–51.

24. Matilainen R, Pitkänen A, Ruutiainen T, *et al*. Effect of vigabatrin on epilepsy in mentally retarded patients: A 7-month follow-up study. *Neurology* 1988; **38**: 743–747.

25. Manford M, Hart YM, Sander JW, Shorvon SD. The national general practice study of epilepsy: The syndromic classification of the International League Against Epilepsy in a general population. *Archives of Neurology* 1992; **49**: 801–808.

26. Lombroso CT. Early myoclonic encephalopathy, early infantile epileptic encephalopathy, and benign and severe infantile myoclonic epilepsies: a critical review and personal contributions. *Journal of Clinical Neurophysiology* 1990; **7**: 380–408.

27. Rantala H, Putkonen T. Occurrence, outcome and prognostic factors of infantile spasms and Lennox-Gastaut syndrome. *Epilepsia* 1999; **40**: 286–289.

28. Sillanpää M. Medico-social prognosis of children with epilepsy. Epidemiological study and analysis of 245 cases. *Acta Paediatrica Scandinavica* 1973; **62**(Suppl. 237): 1–104.

29. Lombroso CT. A prospective study of infantile spasms: clinical and therapeutic correlations. *Epilepsia* 1983; **24**: 135–158.

30. Ohtahara S, Yamatogi Y, Ohtsuka Y, Oka E, Ishida T. Prognosis of West syndrome with special reference to Lennox syndrome: a developmental study. In: Wada JA, Penry JK (eds). *Advances in Epileptology: The Xth Epilepsy International Symposium.* New York: Raven Press 1980, 149–154.

31. Bour F, Chiron C, Dulac O, *et al*. Caratères électrocliniques des crises dans le syndrome d'Aicardi. *Revue d'Electroencéphalographie et de Neurophysiogie Clinique* 1986; **16**: 341–353.

32. Dulac O, Plouin P, Perulli L, *et al*. L'épilepsie dans l'agyrie-pachygyrie classique. *Revue d'Electroencéphalographie et de Neurophysiogie Clinique* 1983; **13**: 232–239.

33. Jeavons PM, Bower BD. Infantile spasms. In: Vinken PJ, Bruyn GW (eds). *Handbook of Clinical Neurology*, vol 15. *The Epilepsies.* Amsterdam: Elsevier-North Holland, 1974: 219–34.

34. Watanabe K, Takeuchi T, Hakamada S, Hayakawa F. Neurophysiological features preceding infantile spasms. *Brain Review* 1987; **9**: 391–398.

35. Stafstrom CE, Konkol RJ. Infantile spasms in Down syndrome. *Developmental Medicine and Child Neurology* 1994; **36**: 576–585.

36. Down JLH. Observations on an ethnic classification of idiots. *London Hospital Clinical Lectures and Reports* 1866; **3**: 259–262.

37. Shuttleworth GE. Mongolian imbecility. *British Medical Journal* 1909; **2**: 661–665.

38. Wilmarth AW. Report on the examination of one hundred brains of feeble-minded children. *Alienist and Neurologist* 1890; **11**: 520–533.

39. Engler M. *Mongolism.* Bristol: J Wright, 1949.

40. Kirman BH. Epilepsy in mongolism. *Archives of Disease in Childhood* 1951; **26**: 501–503.

41. Veall RM. The prevalence of epilepsy among mongols related to age. *Journal of Mental Deficiency Research* 1974; **18**: 99–106.

42. Collacott A. Epilepsy, dementia and adaptive behaviour in Down's syndrome. *Journal of Intellectual Disability Research* 1993; **37**: 153–160.

43. Hauser WA, Morris ML, Heston LL, Anderson VE. Seizures and myoclonus in patients with Alzheimer's disease. *Neurology* 1986; **36**: 1226–1230.

44. Lai F, Williams RS. A prospective study of Alzheimer disease in Down syndrome. *Archives of Neurology* 1989; **46**: 849–853.

45. Stafstrom CE. Epilepsy in Down syndrome: clinical aspects and possible mechanisms. *American Journal on Mental Retardation* 1993; **98**: 12–26.

46. Viani F, Romeo A, Viri M, Mastrangelo M, *et al.* Seizure and EEG patterns in Angelman syndrome. *Journal of Child Neurology* 1995; **10**: 467–471.

47. Zori RTY, Henrickson J, Woolven S, *et al.* Angelman syndrome: clinical profile. *Journal of Child Neurology* 1992; **7**: 270–280.

48. Cassidy SB, Schwartz S. *Reviews in Molecular Medicine: Prader-Willi and Angelman Syndromes, Disorders of Genomic Imprinting.* Baltimore: Williams & Wilkins 1998: 140–151.

49. Jennings MT, Bird TD. Genetic influences in the epilepsies. *American Journal of Diseases in Children* 1981; **135**: 450–457.

50. Jeavons PM, Bower BD. *Infantile Spasms: a Review of the Literature and a Study of 112 Cases.* London: Heinemann Medical, 1964.

51. Aberg LE, Backman M, Kirveskari E, Santavuori P. Epilepsy and antiepileptic drug therapy in juvenile neuronal ceroid lipofuscinosis. *Epilepsia* 2000; **41**: 1296–1302.

52. Perry A. Rett syndrome: a comprehensive review of the literature. *American Journal on Mental Retardation* 1991; **3**: 275–290.

53. Hagberg B. Rett syndrome: clinical peculiarities and biological mysteries. *Acta Paediatrica* 1996; **84**: 971–976.

54. Jacobson JW, Janicki MP. Observed prevalence in multiple mental disabilities. *Mental Retardation* 1983; **21**: 87–94.

55. Voutilainen A. Lapsuusiän hydrokefalian esiintyvyys, etiologia ja ennuste aikuisikään saakka]Incidence, etiology and outcome up to adulthood of infantile hydrocephalus]. PhD Thesis. Helsinki **1992**: 1–143. (In Finnish, with English summary).

56. Espie CA, Pashley AS, Bonham KG, Sourindhrin I, O'Donovan M. The mentally handicapped person with epilepsy: a comparative study investigating psychosocial functioning. *Journal of Mental Deficiency Research* 1989; **33**: 123–135.

57. Reber M. Mental retardation. *Psychiatric Clinics of North America* 1992; **15**: 511–522.

58. Szymanski L, King LH. Practice parameters for the assessment and treatment of children, adolescents and adults with mental retardation and comorbid mental disorders. American Academy of Child and Adolescent Psychiatry working group on quality issues. *Journal of American Academy of Child and Adolescent Psychiatry* 1999; **38**(Suppl.): 5–31.

59. Hermann BP. Neuropsychological functioning and psychopathology in children with epilepsy. *Epilepsia* 1982; **23**: 545–554.

60. Kloster R. Pseudo-epileptics V. epileptic seizures: a comparison. In: Gram L, Johannessen SI, Osterman PO, Sillanpää M (eds) *Pseudo-epileptic Seizures.* Petersfield: Wrightson Medical Publishing, 1993: 3–16.

61. Aird RB. The importance of seizure-inducing factors in the control of refractory forms of epilepsy. *Epilepsia* 1983; **24**: 567–583.

62. Papini M, Pasquinelli A, Armellini M, Orlandi D. Alertness and incidence of seizures in patients with Gastaut-Lennox syndrome. *Epilepsia* 1984; **25**: 161–167.

63. Metrick ME, Ritter FJ, Gates JR, Jacobs MP *et al.* Nonepileptic events in childhood. *Epilepsia* 1991; **32**: 322–328.

64. Hagberg B, Kyllerman M. Epidemiology of mental retardation – a Swedish survey. *Brain and Development* 1983; **5**: 441–449.

65. Linna SL. Prevalence, aetiology, associated handicaps and self care ability in 5–19-old severely mentally retarded. Doctoral thesis, University of Oulu, 1985: 1–166.

66. Corbett JA, Trimble MR, Nichol T. Behavioral and cognitive impairment in children with epilepsy: the long-term effects of anticonvulsant therapy. *Journal of the American Academy of Child Psychiatry* 1985; **23**: 17–23.

67. Pointdexter AR, Berglund JA, Kolstoe PD. Changes in antiepileptic drug prescribing patterns in large institutions: preliminary results of a five-year experience. *American Journal on Mental Retardation* 1993; **98**: 34–40.

68. Iivanainen M, Viukari. M, Helle, EP. Cerebellar atrophy in phenytoin-treated mentally retarded epileptics. *Epilepsia* 1977; **18**: 375–385.

69. Zielinski JJ. Childhood epilepsy and mental retardation. In: Hermann BP, Seidenberg M (eds). *Childhood Epilepsies: Neuropsychological, Psychosocial and Intervention Aspects.* Chichester: John Wiley, 1989: 221–245.

70. Friis ML. Valproate in the treatment of epilepsy in people with intellectual disability. *Journal of Intellectual Disability Research* 1998; **42**(Suppl. 1): 32–35.

71. Scheffner D, König, St, Rauterberg-Ruland I, *et al.* Fatal liver failure in 16 children on valproate therapy. *Epilepsia* 1988; **29**: 530–541.

72. Dreifuss FE, Langer EH, Moline KA, Maxwell JE. Valproic acid fatalities. II. US experience since 1984. *Neurology* 1989; **39**: 201–207.

73. Zaret BS, Cohen RA. Reversible valproic acid dementia: a case report. *Epilepsia* 1986; **27**: 234–240.

74. Motte J, Trevathan E, Barrera MN, Mullens EL, Manasco P. Lamotrigine for generalized seizures associated with Lennox-Gastaut syndrome. *New England Journal of Medicine* 1997; **337**: 1807–1812.

75. Gidal BE, Walker JK, Lott RS, *et al.* Efficacy of lamotrigine in institutionalized, developmentally disabled patients with epilepsy: a retrospective evaluation. *Seizure* 2000; **9**: 131–136.

76. Sachdeo RC, Reife RA, Lim P, Pledger G. A double-blind randomized trial of topiramate in Lennox-Gastaut syndrome. Topiramate YL Study Group. *Neurology* 1999; **52**: 1882–1887.

77. Glauser TA, Levisohn PM, Ritter F, Sachdeo RC, and the Topiramate YL Study Group. Topiramate in Lennox-Gastaut syndrome: open-label treatment of patients completing a randomized controlled trial. *Epilepsia* 2000; **41**(Suppl. 1): 86–90.

78. Glauser TA, Clark PO, Strawburg R. A pilot study of topiramate in the treatment of infantile spasms. *Epilepsia* 1998; **39**: 1324–1328.

79. Glauser TA, Clark PO, McGee K. Long-term response to topiramate in patients with West syndrome. *Epilepsia* 2000; **41**(Suppl. 1): 91–94.

80. Shorvon SD, Lowenthal A, Janz D, Bielen E, Loiseau P. Multicenter, double-blind randomized, placebo-controlled trial of levetiracetam as add-on therapy in patients with refractory seizures. European Levetiracetam Study Group. *Epilepsia* 2000; **41**: 1179–1186.

81. Shorvon SD. *Handbook of Epilepsy Treatment.* Oxford: Blackwell Science, 2000: 113–116.

82. Kyllerman M, Ben-Menachem E. Zonisamide for progressive myoclonus epilepsy: long-term observations in seven patients. *Epilepsy Research* 1998; **29**: 109–114.

83. Genton P, MacMenamin J. Aggravation of seizures by antiepileptic drugs: what to do in clinical practice. *Epilepsia* 1998; **39**(Suppl. 3): 26–29.

84. Guerrini R, Belmonte A, Genton P. Antiepileptic drug-induced worsening of seizures in children. *Epilepsia* 1998; **39**(Suppl. 3): 2–10.

85. Pitkänen A, Ylinen A, Matilainen R, *et al.* Long-term antepileptic efficacy of vigabatrin in drug-refractory epilepsy in mentally retarded patients. A five-year follow-up study. *Archives of Neurology* 1993; **50**: 24–29.

86. Chiron C, Dulac O, Beaumont D, *et al.* Therapeutic trial of vigabatrin in refractory infantile spasms. *Journal of Child Neurology* 1991; **6**: 52–59.

87. Dulac O, Chiron C, Luna D, *et al.* Vigabatrin in childhood epilepsy. *Journal of Child Neurology* 1991; **6**(Suppl. 2): 30–37.

88. Dean C, Mosier M, Penry K. Dose-response study of vigabatrin as add-on therapy in patients with uncontrolled complex partial seizures. *Epilepsia* 1999; **40**: 74–82.

89. Kälviäinen R, Nousiainen I. Visual field defects with vigabatrin: epidemiology and therapeutic implications. *CNS Drugs* 2001; **15**: 217–230.

90. Mikati ME, Choueri R, Khurana DS, *et al.* Gabapentin in the treatment of refractory partial epilepsy in children with mental disability. *Journal of Intellectual Disability Research* 1998; **42**(Suppl. 1): 57–62.

91. Tallian KB, Nahata MC, Lo W, Tsao CY. Gabapentin associated with aggressive behavior in pediatric patients with seizures. *Epilepsia* 1996; **37**: 501–502.

92. Zupanc ML, Shroeder VM. Behavioral changes in children with gabapentin. *Epilepsia* 1995; **36**(Suppl. 4): 73.

93. So EL, Fessler AJ, Cascino GD, Britton JW. Tiagabine-associated encephalopathy. *Epilepsia* 2001; **42**(Suppl. 7): 261.

94. Brorson LO, Wranne L. Long-term prognosis of childhood epilepsy: survival and seizure prognosis. *Epilepsia* 1987; **28**: 324–330.

95. Sillanpää M. Children with epilepsy as adults: Outcome after 30 years of follow-up. *Acta Paediatrica Scandinavica* 1990; **79**(Suppl. 368): 1–78.

96. Theodore WH, Schulman EA, Porter RJ. Intractable seizures: long-term follow-up after prolonged inpatient treatment in an epilepsy unit. *Epilepsia* 1983; **24**: 336–343.

97. Shinnar SS, Vining EPG, Mellits E, *et al.* Discontinuing antiepileptic medication in children with epilepsy after two years without seizures. *New England Journal of Medicine* 1985; **313**: 976–980.

98. Rowan AJ, Overveg J, Sadikoglu S, *et al.* Seizure prognosis in long-stay mentally subnormal epileptic patients: interrater EEG and clinical studies. *Epilepsia* 1980; **21**: 219–26.

99. Lizinger MJ, Duvall B, Little P. Movement of individuals with complex epilepsy from an institution into the community: seizure control and functional outcomes. *American Journal on Mental Retardation* 1993; **98**: 52–57.

Status epilepticus

JOHN H LIVINGSTON

Status epilepticus (SE) is common in pediatric practice, particularly in infants: 40 per cent of all SE occurs in children under 2 years.[1–4] In a prospective study of patients with newly diagnosed epilepsy, 9 per cent of 613 children had had one or more episodes of SE by the time of diagnosis.[5] In a long-term follow-up study of a population-based cohort of 150 children with epilepsy, 27 per cent had at least one episode of SE, usually within 2 years of onset.[6]

DEFINITIONS

Gastaut[7] defined SE as

> a condition in which epileptic seizures are sufficiently prolonged or repeated at such frequent intervals as to produce an enduring epileptic condition.

More recently, the ILAE TaskForce on Classification and Terminology[8] proposed that SE be defined as

> A seizure that shows no clinical signs of arresting after a duration encompassing the great majority of seizures of that type in most patients *or* recurrent seizures without interictal resumption of baseline central nervous system function.

Both definitions are of limited value in a clinical context. For many years the accepted operational definition of SE was

> recurrent epileptic seizures continuing for more than 30 min without full recovery of consciousness before the

next seizure begins, or continuous clinical and/or electrical seizure activity lasting for more than 30 min whether or not consciousness is impaired.[9]

However, video-EEG studies have demonstrated that most generalized (including secondary generalized) tonic-clonic seizures have a duration of less than 2 min and that seizures continuing for more than 5 min are more likely to continue.[10,11] An important study by DeLorenzo et al.,[12] which included 91 children, compared the outcome of seizures lasting 10–29 min with that of traditionally defined SE. Almost half of the 10–29-min group stopped spontaneously and this group had no mortality. The patients in the 10–29-min group that required treatment had a mortality of 4.4 per cent compared with 19 per cent for the SE group.

It has been proposed that the duration of seizure that is defined as SE should be lowered to 10 min.[11–13] Although there is general agreement that seizures continuing for longer than 5 min should usually be treated, there is nevertheless a concern that overaggressive treatment may lead to avoidable morbidity.[14] There is no consensus on this change of definition in children, and further research is required to address this question.[15]

CLASSIFICATION

SE can be classified in the same way as epileptic seizures. In the classification of epileptic seizures put forward in 2001 by the ILAE Task Force on Classification and

Table 17.1 *Classification of status epilepticus*

Convulsive status epilepticus		Nonconvulsive status epilepticus	
Generalized	Tonic Tonic-clonic Clonic Myoclonic	Absence	Typical Atypical
Focal (partial)	Focal motor Focal motor with secondary generalization	Focal SE	With sensory symptomatology With affective symptomatology
	Epilepsia partialis continua		Complex partial SE[a]
Other			Continuous spike and wave during slow sleep

[a] No wholly satisfactory term for complex partial SE is proposed in the new ILAE classification.

Terminology,[16] a list of 'continuous seizure types', which are either generalized or focal, is proposed. It also proposes to omit the words 'convulsion' or 'convulsive' from the classification. However, there needs to be some readily understandable term to distinguish SE in which there is a major motor component from SE with only minor or no motor features. The previous empirical classification into convulsive and nonconvulsive status epilepticus (NCSE) is easy to apply and is used in this chapter (Table 17.1).

Electrical SE, which refers to continuous seizure activity on the EEG in a context where no obvious clinical features of a seizure are present, represents a heterogeneous group of disorders. It may occur in the syndromes of continuous spike and wave of slow sleep and the Landau-Kleffner syndrome (see Chapter 13). However, electrical status[17] may also occur in comatose or pharmacologically sedated or paralyzed patients where the pathophysiologic significance is clearly quite different. In addition, it has been suggested that epileptic encephalopathies with hypsarrythmia or other severely abnormal and long lasting EEG patterns can be considered to be a form of NCSE.[18,19] There is no question that these disorders are 'enduring epileptic conditions', but the pathophysiological basis for these disorders may be quite different from other forms of SE.

ETIOLOGY

Status epilepticus can be classified etiologically into four approximately equal groups: febrile, idiopathic, remote symptomatic and acute symptomatic. Two large series, although separated by two decades, show remarkably similar proportions when examined by etiology.[2,3] However, the etiology may also be influenced by the geographical region. In a recent very large series of SE from Senegal,[4] infection was the cause in 67 per cent of patients.

- **Febrile SE** occurs in febrile children with no previous history of afebrile seizures and no evidence of CNS infection or other acute CNS process. This is the commonest group between 1 and 3 years of age.

Table 17.2 *Aetiology of status epilepticus (see refs 2, 3, 20, 23)*

	Percentage
Febrile	20–29
Idiopathic	16–39
Chronic static CNS disorder	
Remote symptomatic	14–23
Acute symptomatic:	23–40
CNS infection	
CNS trauma	
hypoxic-ischaemic damage	
cerebrovascular	
metabolic/electrolyte disturbance	
intoxication	
drugs, e.g. theophylline derivatives,	
tricyclic antidepressants, insulin,	
amphetamines	
tumor	
acute AED withdrawal	
Progressive encephalopathy	2–6

- **Idiopathic SE** occurs in the absence of any acute CNS or systemic insult in neurologically normal children, and includes SE occurring in idiopathic epilepsy.
- **Remote symptomatic SE** occurs in children with a known prior neurological insult with or without a prior history of epilepsy. Most of these children will have cerebral palsy and/or mental retardation or other neurological abnormalities.
- **Acute symptomatic SE** occurs during the course of an acute illness affecting the CNS, accounts for 25–50 per cent of cases in most series, and is particularly common in infants[2,3,20,21] (see Table 17.2). Most of the mortality associated with SE occurs in this group, which accounts also for most seizures lasting longer than 1 h. Intravenous benzodiazepines may precipitate tonic SE in children with epileptic encephalopathies,[22,23] and tiagabine has recently been reported as precipitating NCSE in patients with refractory focal epilepsy.[24–26]

SYSTEMIC AND METABOLIC EFFECTS

Convulsive SE is associated initially with an increase in sympathetic output resulting in tachycardia and hypertension, increased intracranial pressure, hyperglycemia and hyperpyrexia. Metabolic acidosis may develop secondary to a release of lactic acid. Decompensation eventually occurs and may manifest with hypotension, cardiac arrhythmias, hypoglycemia, pulmonary edema, hypoxia and hypoventilation.[27] Rhabdomyolysis and myoglobinuria with renal failure may occur. Leukocytosis and CSF pleocytosis may be seen.[28] The onset of decompensation is variable but generally occurs 30–60 min after the seizure onset.

There is a 3–4 fold increase in cerebral blood flow with a comparable increase in metabolic rate.[29] ATP levels and energy reserves fall during a prolonged seizure, and neuronal damage eventually occurs in selectively vulnerable areas. Factors contributing to neuronal damage include mismatch between blood flow and metabolism, self-sustaining seizure activity, and calcium-mediated excitotoxicity.[27] These effects are also seen, albeit to a lesser degree, in well-oxygenated, ventilated and paralyzed animals[30,31] and are influenced by the age at which the status occurs.[32]

Diffusion-weighted brain MRI studies in both experimental animals and humans have demonstrated abnormalities that have been interpreted as seizure induced cytotoxic edema, which in some cases is followed by neuronal necrosis.[33–36]

CLINICAL FEATURES

Convulsive status epilepticus

Convulsive SE comprises either a series of partial-onset or generalized-onset tonic-clonic seizures or a more or less continuous clonic seizure.[37] When tonic-clonic seizures are repetitive, each seizure usually lasts 1–3 min and the patient is in a coma interictally. The tonic phase may become less conspicuous as the status continues and the seizure evolves into continuous clonic SE. The motor features often shift from side to side, wax and wane in intensity and involve different segments of the body at different times.[37–39] The motor features may become less dramatic and the seizure evolve into a 'subtle generalized convulsive status epilepticus'.[39] This **electroclinical dissociation** usually indicates that the normal compensatory mechanisms have been exhausted.

Tonic status epilepticus

Tonic SE is relatively uncommon and occurs almost exclusively in children with previous epilepsy, particularly the Lennox-Gastaut syndrome. Hypoventilation, salivation and cyanosis are often marked. The motor features may become less prominent, and tonic SE may last up to several days. Tonic SE can be precipitated by intravenous benzodiazepines.[22,23]

Myoclonic status epilepticus

Myoclonic SE is characterized by repeated massive myoclonic jerks. It may occur in a child with a previous history of myoclonic or generalized epilepsy, as part of a progressive myoclonic epilepsy syndrome, or following an acute brain injury e.g. severe hypoxic-ischemic brain injury.

Focal convulsive status epilepticus

One part of the body is involved in focal convulsive SE. In contrast, the whole of one side of the body is involved in unilateral SE, which often occurs during an attack of generalized SE.[37] Focal SE often becomes secondarily generalized. Focal motor status is usually diagnosed quite easily, but more subtle forms of focal SE may involve only eye deviation, eye jerking or unusual movements such as trunk rotation.

Epilepsia partialis continua (EPC) is a form of continuous motor status. It is a prominent feature of Rasmussen's syndrome (see Chapter 11E). A non-progressive form of EPC may occur at any age and may be due to a neoplasm, vascular lesion, infection, or developmental brain abnormality.

DIFFERENTIAL DIAGNOSIS OF CONVULSIVE STATUS EPILEPTICUS

A number of non-epileptic paroxysmal disorders may be mistaken for epileptic seizures and may be mistaken for SE when they are repeated frequently, are continuous or occur in a comatose child (see Table 17.3). Repetitive tonic extensor spasms in a child with reduced level of consciousness are usually due to acute brainstem dysfunction, secondary to transtentorial herniation, ischemia, severe metabolic disturbance or a combination of these factors. Aggressive treatment with antiepileptic drugs (AEDs) in these patients may cause hypoventilation and hypotension, which can further exacerbate an already critical state. Acute dystonic reactions to drugs may produce florid motor features, usually without alteration of consciousness. Chorea, hemiballismus or a paroxysmal dyskinesia may develop during an acute encephalopathic illness or following trauma. In such cases it may be difficult to exclude SE without EEG verification. Fictitious epilepsy may occasionally take the form

Table 17.3 *Differential diagnosis of convulsive status epilepticus*

Tonic extensor spasms:
   tentorial herniation
   acute brainstem dysfunction
Rigors
Acute dystonic reaction (particularly phenothiazines or
   butyrophcnones)
Chorea/ballismus
Paroxysmal dyskinesia
Psychogenic status epilepticus

Table 17.4 *Management of status epilepticus*

Immediate stabilization and resuscitation
Check airway
Suction
Nasogastric tube
100 per cent oxygen
Monitor oxygen saturation
Assess ventilation
Establish IV access
Blood tests
   glucose
   urea and electrolytes
   calcium
   magnesium
   AED level
Start IV infusion 5 per cent dextrose/0.45 per cent saline

Confirmation of diagnosis of SE
Observation of ictal behaviour
Documentation of duration
If in doubt, further observation and EEG

Initial evaluation
History (including history of recent trauma, infection,
   ingestion, drug history and history of seizures)
Examination (including temperature, cardiorespiratory status,
   neurologic examination, signs of trauma, rashes or
   neurocutaneous stigmata)

Investigation
All patients: Glucose, urea and electrolytes, calcium,
   magnesium, blood gases and AED levels (where appropriate)
Selected patients: Plasma ammonia, lactate, and amino acids;
   and urine organic acids and toxicology

Treatment (see Tables 17.5 and 17.6)

of prolonged **pseudo-status epilepticus**.[40,41] Prolonged nocturnal episodes with prominent motor features suggestive of sexual behavior have been described in young women following sexual abuse,[40] but similar movements may occur in frontal lobe seizures.

MANAGEMENT OF CONVULSIVE STATUS EPILEPTICUS

SE has a significant morbidity and mortality. A well-designed protocol, familiar to staff in the emergency department, wards and intensive care unit (ICU), is more important than the choice of AED. Improvement in quality of management of SE has been demonstrated after the introduction of a treatment algorithm combined with staff education.[42] The aims of treatment are to control seizures rapidly and to treat any reversible causes. Most protocols recommend proceeding to general anesthesia within 60 min but this requires the support of pediatric anesthetic staff and adequate monitoring facilities (see Table 17.4).

Initial stabilization

It is essential to document the time at which treatment commences. The first priority is protection of the airway and circulation. A nasogastric tube should be passed to decompress the stomach. Oxygen at 100 per cent should be administered to all patients. If there is inadequate ventilation, the child should be intubated. It is difficult to assess the depth of coma in a child during SE, but the level of consciousness should be documented once the status has been controlled. If there are signs of hypovolemia or hypotension, these should be treated. Early vascular access is important for optimal administration of AEDs and for continued resuscitation and treatment. If peripheral cannulation is not possible, a central line should be inserted. Intraosseous infusion has been used with success in children under 6 years of age when vascular access cannot be found.[43,44]

Confirmation of diagnosis

During the initial assessment, it is important that the clinician determine whether the episode is consistent with SE. If the child is having repetitive seizures, it is worthwhile observing at least two cycles of seizures.[45] If the behavior is not typical of SE, an emergency EEG may be helpful.

Initial evaluation

It is important to take a history, carry out a brief clinical examination, and carry out some basic investigations (see Table 17.4). If the cause of the SE is unknown, blood and urine collected on presentation should be sent for toxicological screen and, in infants and young children, a metabolic screen. An urgent CT head scan should be performed in all patients in whom the SE is unexplained or associated with new, focal neurological signs. Meningitis is an important cause of SE, especially in infants. Children who present with SE and fever should receive appropriate

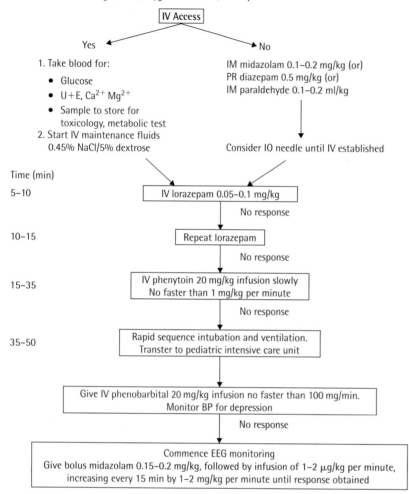

Initial stabilization

1. Confirm diagnosis
2. Check airway, administer oxygen, give suction
3. Monitor vital signs, ECG, oxygen saturation, blood pressure

IV Access

Yes → No

1. Take blood for:
   - Glucose
   - U+E, Ca²⁺ Mg²⁺
   - Sample to store for toxicology, metabolic test
2. Start IV maintenance fluids 0.45% NaCl/5% dextrose

IM midazolam 0.1–0.2 mg/kg (or)
PR diazepam 0.5 mg/kg (or)
IM paraldehyde 0.1–0.2 ml/kg

Consider IO needle until IV established

Time (min)

5–10   IV lorazepam 0.05–0.1 mg/kg
No response

10–15   Repeat lorazepam
No response

15–35   IV phenytoin 20 mg/kg infusion slowly
No faster than 1 mg/kg per minute
No response

35–50   Rapid sequence intubation and ventilation.
Transter to pediatric intensive care unit
No response

Give IV phenobarbital 20 mg/kg infusion no faster than 100 mg/min.
Monitor BP for depression
No response

Commence EEG monitoring
Give bolus midazolam 0.15–0.2 mg/kg, followed by infusion of 1–2 μg/kg per minute,
increasing every 15 min by 1–2 mg/kg per minute until response obtained

Figure 17.1 *A protocol for the management of status epilepticus.*

antibiotics at antimeningitic doses and aciclovir until CNS infection has been excluded. Lumbar puncture should not be performed until the SE has been controlled and the level of consciousness improves or until brain swelling and a mass lesion have been excluded.

First-line treatment of status epilepticus

The ideal pharmacokinetic features of a drug used to treat SE include rapid brain entry; long distribution half-life; short elimination half-life; and absence of cardiac or respiratory side-effects or sedation.[45] The first-line drugs used in the treatment of SE include benzodiazepines (lorazepam, diazepam); phenytoin and fosphenytoin; and phenobarbital. A suggested treatment protocol is shown in Figure 17.1. If there are problems with intravenous access, rectal diazepam or intramuscular midazolam may be given. The intraosseous route may be used to administer phenytoin and benzodiazepines.

Refractory status epilepticus

SE is regarded as refractory if seizures continue in spite of optimal treatment with lorazepam/diazepam, phenytoin and phenobarbital. General anesthesia is generally recommended for seizures continuing for longer than 40–60 min. More recently, intravenous midazolam infusion has been shown to be effective. Children should be managed in a unit that is skilled in pediatric and neurointensive care.

General anesthesia has used barbiturates, including thiopentone, pentobarbitone and phenobarbital, and the inhalational agent isofluorane (see Table 17.6). These carry significant risks of cardiac depression, ventilation problems and the risk of pharmacological paralysis. If the child is anesthetized, EEG monitoring is essential and continuous monitoring is preferable. No entirely adequate system is available and feasible for most ICUs, but cerebral function monitors do allow detection of most seizures and assessment of the depth of anesthesia.[46] The dose commonly used is that required to control the seizures and achieve a burst suppression pattern on the EEG. The importance of achieving burst suppression has not been established.

When **midazolam** is used in the treatment of for refractory SE, a bolus dose is administered and thereafter the rate of infusion is increased gradually to achieve seizure control.[47–51] A preliminary comparative study has demonstrated that midazolam is as effective as thiopentone and has fewer complications.[52] A recent meta-analysis of the treatment of refractory convulsive SE in children suggested that mortality was lower in those treated with midazolam than with barbiturates, diazepam or isoflurane.[53]

A trial of intravenous **pyridoxine** 100 mg should be given to all infants who have unexplained SE that is resistant to AED treatment or recurs (see Chapter 4E).

Intravenous lignocaine (lidocaine), chlormethiazole, valproic acid and propofol have been used in SE but cannot be regarded as first-line drugs. These should only be used in refractory SE and therefore not outside the intensive care setting. None has been subject to controlled studies.

Out-of-hospital treatment

Seizure clusters may evolve into SE,[54] and there is general agreement that seizure clusters should be treated. Benzodiazepines administered by paramedics out of hospital have been demonstrated to be effective in terminating prolonged seizures and seizure clusters.[55,56] In addition, a comparison between intravenous diazepam and rectal diazepam in children[55] demonstrated no difference with regard to seizure duration, need for intubation or recurrent seizures in hospital. This supports the initiation of treatment of prolonged seizures or seizure clusters with rectal diazepam, buccal/nasal midazolam or sublingual lorazepam by the guardian or caregiver.

DRUGS USED FOR STATUS EPILEPTICUS

The pediatric doses, time to peak effect, duration of action and common adverse effects are described in Tables 17.5 and 17.6.

Diazepam

The onset of action following intravenous administration is within 1–3 min and 80 per cent of patients are controlled within 5 min.[57] Rapid distribution to other tissues results in a very short duration of action and seizures often recur after 15–20 min. Therefore, diazepam should be used with a longer-acting AED, such as phenytoin.

Diazepam is rapidly absorbed from the rectum and peak levels are reached within 4–10 min. The usual dose is 0.5mg/kg, maximum 10 mg. Rectal diazepam is mainly of value when intravenous access in an infant is proving difficult, or for the parent of a young child to start treatment before admission to hospital.

Lorazepam

Intravenous lorazepam has a rapid onset of action. It is less lipophilic and has a smaller volume of distribution than diazepam resulting in a longer duration of action, which lasts for several hours and up to 48 h.[57,58] Lorazepam has been shown to be at least as effective as other benzodiazepines and as phenytoin,[57–60] and is superior to phenytoin alone.[61] Thus, many treatment protocols now recommend lorazepam as the first-line agent of choice.

Midazolam

This extremely potent, short-acting benzodiazepine is water soluble and, unlike diazepam and lorazepam, is rapidly absorbed and nonirritant following intramuscular injection.[62,63] Its short duration of action requires that it be given by frequent boluses or continuous infusion. It is increasingly used for refractory SE and has also been used as first-line treatment of SE.[64]

Midazolam is rapidly absorbed from both the nasal and the buccal mucosa.[65–67] Buccal midazolam has been demonstrated to be as safe and effective as rectal diazepam in the treatment of prolonged seizures in children.[68] Several noncomparative studies of nasal midazolam have demonstrated its safety and efficacy.[67,69–71] The main disadvantage of nasal or buccal midazolam, at present, is the need to use the intravenous preparation. The usual dose is 0.2 mg/kg.

Phenytoin

Intravenous phenytoin controls SE in 70–80 per cent of patients.[72,73] The main advantage of phenytoin is its lack of sedative side-effects. The loading dose of 20 mg/kg must be given intravenously over 20 min and peak activity in the brain does not occur for 10–30 min. Thus, the maximal clinical effect may not be seen for 50 min. Consequently, phenytoin should be given with a benzodiazepine. Hypotension, bradycardia and arrhythmias may be precipitated if the infusion rate exceeds 1 mg/kg per minute. Phenytoin is highly alkaline and poorly soluble in water and should be diluted in normal saline.[43] When patients on phenytoin present with SE, it is usually safe to give a full loading dose.[74] The maintenance dose

Table 17.5 *First-line drugs for the treatment of status epilepticus*

Drug	Route	Dosage and administration	Time to peak effect	Duration of action	Adverse effect
Diazepam	IV	0.2–0.3 mg/kg	1.5 min	15–20 min	Respiratory depression Sedation
Lorazepam	IV	0.05–0.1 mg/kg	1–5 min	12–48 h	Respiratory depression Sedation
Midazolam[a]	IV/IM	0.1–0.2 mg/kg, max dose 5 mg	1–5 min	1–5 h	Respiratory depression Sedation
Phenytoin	IV	20 mg/kg slow infusion, no faster than $1\,mg\,kg^{-1}min^{-1}$	10–30 min	12–24 h	Cardiac effect if infused too rapidly
Phenobarbital	IV	20–25 mg/kg infused no faster than $100\,mg\,min^{-1}$	10–20 min	24–72 h	Cardiorespiratory depression if infused too rapidly Sedation

[a] Midazolam is not currently recommended as first-line drug, but if there is no IV access it can be given IM (intramuscularly). However, see refs 62 and 63.

Table 17.6 *Drugs for the treatment of refractory status epilepticus*

Drug	Loading dose	Maintenance	Comment	References
Midazolam	0.15–0.2 mg/kg	$1–2\,\mu g\,kg^{-1}\,min^{-1}$ Increased every 15 min until control achieved		49–53
Thiopentone	5–30 mg/kg	$2–10\,mg\,kg^{-1}\,h^{-1}$	Hypotension frequent Inotrope support often, but not on lower dose regime	130, 131
Phenobarbital	10–20 mg/kg Repeated boluses every 30–60 min until control			132
Isoflurane	0.5–3.0 per cent inhalational anesthetic		Circulatory support necessary in all patients reported by Kofke *et al.*	133, 134

required is variable and the serum level should be maintained between 40–80 μmol/L (10–20 mg/L). Recent studies have attempted to produce dosage recommendations based on early blood level monitoring.[75,76]

Fosphenytoin

Fosphenytoin is a phenytoin pro-drug, which does not require an organic solvent and high alkaline pH for solubility and does not precipitate with commonly used intravenous diluents. The dose is expressed as phenytoin equivalent (PE): 1.5 mg of fosphenytoin is equivalent to 1 mg of phenytoin. It can be given by intramuscular injection or infused rapidly, and does not cause tissue necrosis or discomfort on intravenous administration.[77] Fosphenytoin can be infused at three times the rate of phenytoin (3 mg/kg per minute of PE) and conversion rates to phenytoin are similar across all age groups (mean conversion time 8.3 min).[77,78] It therefore offers several advantages over phenytoin, particularly for infants and neonates.

Phenobarbital

Phenobarbital is a very effective agent for the treatment of SE and is relatively nontoxic.[79,80] Its prolonged half-life results in a long duration of action after a single dose. The main disadvantages of phenobarbital are depression of conscious level, respiration and blood pressure, which are more likely to occur if the patient has received a benzodiazepine.

Rectal paraldehyde

In children who are resistant to benzodiazepines, rectal paraldehyde offers an alternative approach. It is given in a dose of 1 mL per year of age (or 0.1 0.2 mL/kg) diluted in a 1:1 solution of olive/mineral oil. The slow and erratic absorption is a disadvantage.[81]

Lignocaine (lidocaine)

This is given as an initial intravenous bolus of 1–2 mg/kg followed by infusion of 6 mg/kg per hour.[81,82] The effects are rapid but short lived; seizures may be induced if the dose is too high, and arrhythmias and cardiac depression may occur.

Chlormethiazole

This may be effective in focal and generalized SE.[81,83,84] Slow infusion is necessary because of the risk of apnea if it is administered by rapid bolus. The suggested rate of infusion is 5–10 mg/kg per hour. Adverse effects include fever, sedation, hypotension, apnea, thrombophlebitis, hiccups and severe headaches, and limit its usefulness.[84]

Intravenous valproic acid

This has been used in refractory status in children using a loading dose of 20–40 mg/kg followed by a continuous infusion of 5 mg/kg per hour.[85] Most studies have suggested that it is safe and well tolerated, but severe hypotension was reported in an 11 year old after treatment with 30 mg/kg intravenous valproic acid.[86]

Propofol

This has been reported to be effective in the treatment of refractory status,[47,87] but a number of deaths have been associated with propofol infusion in children.[88]

OUTCOME OF CONVULSIVE STATUS EPILEPTICUS

The morbidity and mortality associated with convulsive SE are determined primarily by the cause and are highest following acute symptomatic SE. The poor outcome of SE in infants parallels the higher proportion of acute symptomatic cases in this age group.[89,90]

Mortality

A mortality rate of 11 per cent was described in 1970,[2] but more recent studies have described mortality rates between 3.6 and 7 per cent.[3,20,89] A meta-analysis of **refractory** GCSE described a mortality rate of 16 per cent.[53] Death occurs primarily in those with acute symptomatic SE or progressive encephalopathy. In the series of Maytal et al.[3] no deaths were associated with either febrile

or unprovoked SE. On the other hand, Philips and Shanahan[89] described one child who died following febrile SE.

Morbidity

The morbidity associated with convulsive SE also appears to be declining. In 1970 neurologic sequelae were reported in 20 per cent and mental retardation in 33 per cent of survivors of SE,[2] but recent morbidity rates have ranged from 9 to 28 per cent.[3,20,89] Morbidity is very low following febrile or idiopathic SE. No neurologic abnormalities were documented in 67 children who had idiopathic, remote symptomatic or febrile SE.[3]

The development of epilepsy after SE is strongly influenced by the etiology. In children presenting with idiopathic SE as their first seizure, the risk of seizure recurrence does not differ from that following an initial short seizure.[91,92] Although epilepsy developed later in 4 per cent of children following febrile SE,[93] a higher rate than those who experience brief febrile seizures,[94] this may relate to the higher rate of prior neurological abnormality, neonatal seizures and family history of epilepsy in those with febrile SE. The risk of a subsequent unprovoked seizure following acute symptomatic SE was reported to be 41 per cent, compared with a risk of 13 per cent for those with an acute symptomatic seizure without SE.[95] Whether the increased rate is a marker of the severity of the injury, damage due to the SE itself, or an indication of an underlying susceptibility to SE and seizures, remains unclear. Patients with a preceding chronic neurologic disorder who present with SE as a first seizure have a very high risk of subsequent epilepsy and recurrent SE.[90,96]

Recurrent status epilepticus

The risk of a further episode of SE is between 11 and 25 per cent,[90,97] and is primarily related to the presence of neurologic abnormalities predating the original SE. In the remote symptomatic or progressive encephalopathies group, the risk of recurrent SE is 50 per cent.

Prophylactic AED treatment is recommended for patients with preceding chronic neurologic abnormalities because of the high risk of recurrent SE.[90] The risk of subsequent epilepsy is low in the other three groups and long-term AED therapy is not always recommended after SE.[98] There is no evidence that long-term AED treatment reduces the subsequent likelihood of developing epilepsy in the acute symptomatic group.

NONCONVULSIVE STATUS EPILEPTICUS

When evaluating a patient in coma, it is important to consider the possibility of both subtle GCSE and other forms

Table 17.7 *Differential diagnosis of nonconvulsive status epilepticus*

Chronic intoxication
Prolonged postictal state
Progressive ataxia (when associated with depressed conscious level)
   intoxication
   hydrocephalus
   tumors
   metabolic disease
Dementia
   neurodegenerative disease
   metabolic disease
Psychiatric disease

of NCSE,[17] and an EEG should be performed if the cause of the coma is not apparent. For the reasons already discussed, subtle GCSE will not be included in this section on NCSE. The differential diagnosis of NCSE is listed in Table 17.7.

Complex partial status epilepticus

Complex partial status epilepticus (CPSE) is characterized by fluctuating impairment of consciousness, lack of interaction with familiar people, staring, speech arrest and automatisms.[45,99,100] Focal motor activity may occur. CPSE may manifest as repeated complex partial seizures without complete return to normal between attacks, or as continuous long-lasting confusion and altered behaviour.[45] CPSE may occasionally be the first manifestation of epilepsy.[100] The EEG characteristically shows the features of individual complex partial seizures. Low-voltage activity followed by a build up of higher amplitude slow wave activity may be seen and spike and slow wave activity in the temporal or occipital regions, which may wax and wane, can occur. The diagnosis is easily overlooked and CPSE should be considered in any situation where there is an unexplained prolonged change in a child's behavior.[100–102]

Other forms of nonconvulsive partial status epilepticus

Prolonged simple partial seizures may occur with sensory or affective symptomatology, and include such symptoms as isolated fear, simple auditory sensations, cognitive symptoms and true dysphasia.[103–108] Recurrent episodes of generalized NCSE associated with nocturnal frontal lobe seizures have recently been identified as one of the characteristic features of the ring chromosome 20 epilepsy syndrome.[109,110]

Absence status epilepticus

Absence SE has been defined as a prolonged period of diminished awareness associated with generalized spike-wave discharges.[111] Other terms that have been used are **petit mal status**, **spike-wave stupor** and **prolonged epileptic twilight state**.[112–114] Typical absence SE is associated with generalized (synchronous/symmetric) 3-Hz spike-wave discharges and occurs only rarely in children with idiopathic generalized epilepsy, including childhood absence epilepsy. Atypical absence SE, on the other hand, occurs much more frequently and largely in children with Lennox-Gastaut syndrome, myoclonic astatic epilepsy, severe myoclonic epilepsy of infancy, or following West syndrome. The child appears to lose contact with the external environment, responses are very delayed, speech may be lost, drooling and feeding difficulties are very common, and the gait may deteriorate (**pseudo-ataxia**). There may be frequent motor manifestations such as brief head nods, jerks of the face, limbs and trunk, and eyelid myoclonias. The clinical features may be very subtle and difficult to distinguish from preexisting cognitive problems. Thus, the diagnosis is often delayed. Video-EEG monitoring with cognitive testing may be necessary to identify ictal events.[115] The associated EEG changes are variable. There is often continuous generalized slow spike-wave activity, which may be synchronous and rhythmic, but is more often very irregular with asynchronous spike and wave bursts, sometimes approaching a hypsarrhythmic pattern. There may be poor correlation between the clinical and EEG changes. The adverse effects of AEDs, particularly polytherapy, can also produce a very similar picture.

Treatment of nonconvulsive status epilepticus

NCSE is not life threatening but is associated with neurologic morbidity. Consequently, it should be treated aggressively. EEG monitoring is usually required to determine when the status has ceased. The adverse effects of AED treatment may be difficult to distinguish from the NCSE itself and there is a real risk of over-treatment.[116] Whether general anesthesia should ever be recommended for NCSE is a matter of some debate.

COMPLEX PARTIAL STATUS EPILEPTICUS

In most patients, CPSE will respond rapidly to intravenous phenytoin or benzodiazepines.[100,117]

ABSENCE STATUS EPILEPTICUS

Typical absence status responds rapidly and completely to intravenous benzodiazepines. Valproic acid may be equally effective.[114,118]

ATYPICAL ABSENCE STATUS EPILEPTICUS

This is often very resistant to treatment. Benzodiazepines are much less effective in this type of SE than in all other types.[119,120] Furthermore, benzodiazepines may precipitate tonic SE in children with the Lennox-Gastaut syndrome. Sodium valproic acid or lamotrigine may be effective. The risk of provoking a serious drug rash by adding lamotrigine at a high dose limits its usefulness in the acute management of NCSE. Nevertheless rapid oral loading with lamotrigine has been reported in a 17 year old with tonic SE and was not associated with adverse effects.[121] Steroids or ACTH may be effective but there is a risk of relapse on discontinuation of treatment and severe side-effects may occur. Intravenous propofol infusion was recently been reported to be effective in terminating NCS in a child with Lennox-Gastaut syndrome.[122]

Outcome of nonconvulsive status epilepticus

COMPLEX PARTIAL STATUS EPILEPTICUS

There are case reports of long-term neurologic and behavioral problems, particularly memory deficits, following CPSE.[123]

ABSENCE STATUS EPILEPTICUS

Typical absence SE is generally considered to have a good prognosis. Children who have atypical absence SE have a high incidence of severe epilepsy on follow-up and many demonstrate cognitive deterioration.[115,124,125] However, it is difficult to determine the extent to which the NCSE contributed to these problems. Beaumanoir et al.[126] did not observe cognitive deterioration in their patients with Lennox-Gastaut syndrome who developed NCSE. There is experimental evidence that NCSE is detrimental.[127,128] However, the models used may not be valid for NCSE in humans. A new animal model for NCSE has recently been reported.[129]

KEY POINTS

- Status epilepticus is common in childhood with the **highest incidence in the first 2 years of life**
- There is no consensus on the **duration of seizure** required for the diagnosis of status epilepticus Many commentators have proposed that a seizure longer than 10 min should be regarded as SE
- **Nonepileptic conditions** may mimic status epilepticus
- The **management** of SE is directed towards stopping the seizure and diagnosing and treating the underlying cause

- The use of a suitably designed **treatment algorithm** improves the management of SE. This requires education of all hospital staff involved in the treatment
- There are no randomized controlled trials to show that one drug is superior to another in SE. Most protocols recommend **lorazepam** as the first-line agent, followed by phenytoin if unsuccessful
- For refractory SE, **continuous infusion of midazolam** appears to be as effective as other agents, and has fewer complications than thiopentone
- The **outcome** of SE is primarily related to the cause. Mortality and morbidity is greatest in acute symptomatic SE whereas febrile SE has a low morbidity. Febrile SE, however, is associated with a greater risk of recurrent afebrile or febrile seizures, and of recurrent SE than a brief febrile seizure

REFERENCES

1. Shinnar S, Pellock JL, Moshe SL, et al. In whom does status epilepticus occur: age related differences in children. Epilepsia 1997; **38**: 907–914.
2. Aicardi J, Chevrie JJ. Convulsive status epilepticus in infants and children: a study of 239 cases. Epilepsia 1970; **11**: 187–197.
3. Maytal J, Shinnar S, Moshe SL, Alvarez LA. Low morbidity and mortality of status epilepticus in children. Pediatrics 1989; **83**: 323–331.
4. Mbodj I, Ndiaye M, Sene F, et al. Treatment of status epilepticus in a developing country. Neurophysiologie Clinique 2000; **30**: 165–169.
5. Berg AT, Shinnar S, Levy SR, Testa FM. Status epilepticus in children with newly diagnosed epilepsy. Annals of Neurology 1999; **45**: 618–623.
6. Silanpaa M, Shinnar S. Status epilepticus in a population-based cohort with childhood-onset epilepsy in Finland. Annals of Neurology 2002; **52**: 303–310.
7. Gastaut H. Dictionary of Epilepsy. Part 1. Geneva: World Health Organisation, 1973.
8. Blume WT, Luders HO, Mizrahi E, et al. Glossary of descriptive terminology for ictal semiology: report of the ILAE Task Force on Classification and Terminology. Epilepsia 2001; **42**: 1212–1218.
9. Treiman DM. Generalised convulsive status epilepticus in adults. Epilepsia 1993; **34**(Suppl. 1): S2–11.
10. Lowenstein DH, Bleck T, Macdonald RL. It's time to revise the definition of status epilepticus. Epilepsia 1999; **40**: 120–122.
11. Fountain NB. Status epilepticus: risk factors and complications. Epilepsia 2000; **41**(Suppl. 2): S23–30.
12. DeLorenzo RJ, Garnett LK, Towne AR, et al. Comparison of status epilepticus with prolonged seizure episodes lasting from 10 to 29 minutes. Epilepsia 1999; **40**: 164–169.
13. Meldrum BS. The revised operational definition of generalized tonic-clonic (TC) status epilepticus in adults. Epilepsia 1999; **40**: 123–124.

14. Tasker RC. Emergency treatment of acute seizures and status epilepticus. *Archives of Disease in Childhood* 1998; **79**: 78–83.

15. Mitchell WG. Status epilepticus and acute serial seizures in children. *Journal of Child Neurology* 2002; **17**: S36–43.

16. Engel J Jr. A proposed diagnostic scheme for people with epileptic seizures and with epilepsy: Report of the ILAE Task Force on classification and terminology. *Epilepsia* 2001; **42**: 1–8.

17. Towne AR, Waterhouse EJ, Boggs JG, *et al.* Prevalence of nonconvulsive status epilepticus in comatose patients. *Neurology* 2000; **54**(2): 340–345.

18. Doose H. Nonconvulsive status epilepticus in childhood: clinical aspects and classification. In: Delgado-Escueta AV, Wasterlain CG, Treiman DM, Porter RJ. (eds) *Status Epilepticus: Mechanisms of Brain Damage and Treatment.* New York: Raven Press, 1983: 83–92.

19. Livingston JH, Brown JK. Diagnosis and management of nonconvulsive status epilepticus. *Pediatric Review Communications* 1988; **2**: 283–315.

20. Dunn DW. Status epilepticus in children: etiology, clinical features and outcome. *Journal of Child Neurology* 1988; **3**: 167–173.

21. Dulac O, Aubourg P, Chercoury A, *et al.* Infantile status epilepticus, etiological and prognostic aspects. *Revue d'Electroencephalographique et de Neurophysiologie* 1985; **14**: 255–262.

22. Tassinari CA, Dravet C, Roger J, *et al.* Tonic status epilepticus precipitated by intravenous benzodiazepines in five patients with Lennox-Gastaut syndrome. *Epilepsia* 1972; **13**: 421–435.

23. Prior PF, McLaine GN, Scott DF, Laurance BM. Tonic status epilepticus precipitated by intravenous diazepam in a child with petit mal status. *Epilepsia* 1972; **13**: 467–472.

24. Ettinger AB, Bernal OG, Andriola MR, *et al.* Two cases of nonconvulsive status epilepticus in association with tiagabine therapy. *Epilepsia* 1999; **40**: 1159–1162.

25. Piccinelli P, Borgatti R, Perucca E, *et al.* Frontal nonconvulsive status epilepticus associated with high-dose tiagabine therapy in a child with familial bilateral perisylvian polymicrogyria. *Epilepsia* 2000; **41**: 1485–1488.

26. Balslev T, Uldall P, Buchholt J. Provocation of non-convulsive status epilepticus by tiagabine in three adolescent patients. *European Journal of Paediatric Neurology* 2000; **4**: 169–170.

27. Wasterlain CG, Fujikawa DG, Penix L, Sankar R. Pathophysiological mechanisms of brain damage from status epilepticus. *Epilepsia* 1993; **34**:(Suppl. 1) S37–53.

28. Aminoff MJ, Simon RP. Status epilepticus. Causes, clinical features and consequences in 98 patients. *American Journal of Medicine* 1980; **69**: 657–666.

29. Chapman AG, Meldrum BS, Siesjo BK. Cerebral metabolic changes during prolonged epileptic seizures in rats. *Journal of Neurochemistry* 1977; **28**: 1025–1035.

30. Meldrum BS, Vigouroux RA, Brierley JB. Systemic factors and epileptic brain damage. Prolonged seizures in paralysed artificially ventilated baboons. *Archives of Neurology* 1973; **29**: 82–87.

31. Nevander G, Ingvar M, Auer R, Siesjo BK. Status epilepticus in well oxygenated rats causes neuronal necrosis. *Annals of Neurology* 1984; **18**: 281–290.

32. Sankar R, Shin D, Mazarati AM, *et al.* Epileptogenesis after status epilepticus reflects age- and model-dependent plasticity. *Annals of Neurology* 2000; **48**: 580–589.

33. Wall CJ, Kendall EJ, Obenaus A. Rapid alterations in diffusion-weighted images with anatomic correlates in a rodent model of status epilepticus. *AJNR* 2000; **21**: 1782–1783.

34. Hisano T, Ohno M, Egawa T, *et al.* Changes in diffusion-weighted MRI after status epilepticus. *Pediatric Neurology* 2000; **22**: 327–329.

35. Chu K, Kang DW, Kim JY, *et al.* Diffusion-weighted magnetic resonance imaging in nonconvulsive status epilepticus. *Archives of Neurology* 2001; **58**: 993–998.

36. Kim JA, Chung JI, Yoon PH, *et al.* Transient MR signal changes in patients with generalized tonicoclonic seizures or status epilepticus: pericital diffusion-weighted imaging. *AJNR* 2001; **22**: 1149–1160.

37. Aicardi J. Status epilepticus. In: *Epilepsy in Children.* New York: Raven Press, 1986: 240–259.

38. Roger J, Lob H, Tassinari CA. Status epilepticus. In: Vinken PJ, Bruyn GW. (eds) *Handbook of Neurology,* vol. 15, *The Epilepsies.* Amsterdam: North Holland, 1974: 145–188.

39. Treiman DM. Electroclinical features of status epilepticus. *Journal of Clinical Neurophysiology* 1995; **12**: 343–362.

40. Betts T, Boden S. Diagnosis, management and prognosis of a group of 128 patients with non epileptic attack disorder. *Seizure* 1992; **1**: 19–32.

41. Pakalnis A, Paolicchi J, Gilles E. Psychogenic status epilepticus in children: psychiatric and other risk factors. *Neurology* 2000; **54**: 969–970.

42. Gilbert KL. Evaluation of an algorithm for treatment of status epilepticus in adult patients undergoing video/EEG monitoring. *Journal of Neuroscience Nursing* 2000; **32**: 101–107.

43. Tunik MG, Young GM. Status epilepticus in children: the acute management. *Pediatric Clinics of North America* 1992; **39**: 1007–1030.

44. Lathers CM, Jim KF, Spivey WH. A comparison of intraosseous and intravenous routes of administration for antiseizure agents. *Epilepsia* 1989; **30**: 472–479.

45. Delgado-Escueta AV, Swartz B, Abad-Herrera P. Status epilepticus. In: Dam M, Gram L. (eds) *Comprehensive Epileptology.* New York: Raven Press, 1990: 251–270.

46. Murdoch-Eaton D, Darowski M, Livingston J. Cerebral function monitoring in paediatric intensive care: useful features for predicting outcome. *Developmental Medicine and Child Neurology* 2001; **43**: 91–96.

47. Claassen J, Hirsch LJ, Emerson RG, Mayer SA. Treatment of refractory status epilepticus with pentobarbital, propofol, or midazolam: a systematic review. *Epilepsia* 2002; **43**: 146–153.

48. Fountain NB, Adams RE. Midazolam treatment of acute and refractory status epilepticus. *Clinical Neuropharmacology* 1999; **22**: 261–267.

49. Igartua J, Silver P, Maytal J, Sagy M. Midazolam coma for refractory status epilepticus in children. *Critical Care Medicine* 1999; **27**: 1982–1985.

50. Holmes GL, Riviello JJ Jr. Midazolam and pentothal for refractory status epilepticus. *Pediatric Neurology* 1999; **20**: 259–264.

51. Pellock JM. Use of midazolam for refractory status epilepticus in pediatric patients. *Journal of Child Neurology* 1998; **13**: 581–587.

52. Lohr A Jr, Werneck LC. Comparative non-randomized study with midazolam versus thiopental in children with refractory status epilepticus. *Arquivos de Neuro-Psiquiatria* 2000; **58**: 282–287.

53. Gilbert DL, Gartside PS, Glauser TA. Efficacy and mortality in treatment of refractory generalized convulsive status epilepticus in children: A meta-analysis. *Journal of Child Neurology* 1999; **14**: 602–609.

54. Haut SR, Shinnar S, Moshe SL, *et al.* The association between seizure clustering and convulsive status epilepticus in patients with intractable complex partial seizures. *Epilepsia* 1999; **40**: 1832–1834.

55. Alldredge BK, Wall DB, Ferriero DM. Effect of prehospital treatment on the outcome of status epilepticus in children. *Pediatric Neurology* 1995: **12**: 213–216.

56. Alldredge BK, Gelb AM, Isaacs SM, *et al.* A comparison of lorazepam, diazepam, and placebo for the treatment of out-of-hospital status epilepticus. *New England Journal of Medicine* 2001; **345**: 631–637.

57. Treiman DM. The role of benzodiazepines in the management of status epilepticus. *Neurology* 1990; **4**(Suppl. 2): 32–42.

58. Crawford TO, Mitchell WG, Snodgrass SR. Lorazepam in childhood status epilepticus and serial seizures: effectiveness and tachyphylaxis. *Neurology* 1987; **37**: 190–195.

59. Giang DW, McBride MC. Lorazepam versus diazepam for the treatment of status epilepticus. *Pediatric Neurology* 1988; **4**: 358–361.

60. Lacey DJ, Singer WD, Horwitz SJ, *et al.* Lorazepam therapy of status epilepticus in children and adolescents. *Journal of Pediatrics* 1986; **108**: 771–774.

61. Treiman DM, Meyers PD, Walton NY, *et al.* A comparison of four treatments for generalized convulsive status epilepticus. *New England Journal of Medicine* 1998; **339**: 792–798.

62. Chamberlain JM, Altieri MA, Futterman C, *et al.* A prospective, randomized study comparing intramuscular midazolam with intravenous diazepam for the treatment of seizures in children. *Pediatric Emergency Care* 1997; **13**: 92–94.

63. Towne AR, DeLorenzo RJ. Use of intramuscular midazolam for status epilepticus. *Journal of Emergency Medicine* 1999; **17**: 323–328.

64. Yoshikawa H, Yamazaki S, Abe T, Oda Y. Midazolam as a first-line agent for status epilepticus in children. *Brain and Development* 2000; **22**: 239–242.

65. Scott RC, Besag FM, Boyd SG, *et al.* Buccal absorption of midazolam: Pharmacokinetics and EEG pharmacodynamics. *Epilepsia* 1998; **39**: 290–294.

66. Rey E, Delaunay L, Pons G, *et al.* Pharmacokinetics of midazolam in children: Comparative study of intranasal and intravenous administration. *European Journal of Clinical Pharmacology* 1991; **41**: 355–357.

67. Lahat E, Goldman M, Barr J, *et al.* Intranasal midazolam for childhood seizures. *Lancet* 1998; **352**: 620.

68. Scott RC, Besag FM, Neville BG. Buccal midazolam and rectal diazepam for treatment of prolonged seizures in childhood and adolescence: A randomized trial. *Lancet* 1999; **353**: 623–626.

69. O, Regan ME, Brown JK, Clarke M. Nasal rather than rectal benzodiazepines in the management of acute childhood seizures? *Developmental Medicine and Child Neurology* 1996; **38**: 1037–1045.

70. Chattopadhyay A, Morris, Blackburn L, *et al.* Buccal midazolam and rectal diazepam for epilepsy (letter). *Lancet* 1999; **353**: 1798.

71. Jeannet PY, Roulet E, Maeder-Ingvar M, *et al.* Home and hospital treatment of acute seizures in children with nasal midazolam. *European Journal of Paediatric Neurology* 1999; **3**: 73–77.

72. Wilder BJ, Ramsay RE, Willmore LJ, *et al.* Efficacy of intravenous phenytoin in the treatment of status epilepticus: kinetics of central nervous system penetration. *Annals of Neurology* 1977; **1**: 511–518.

73. Cranford RE, Leppik IE, Patrick B, *et al.* Intravenous phenytoin in acute management of seizures. *Neurology* 1979; **29**: 1474–1479.

74. Simon RP. Management of status epilepticus. In: Pedley TA, Meldrum BS. (eds) *Recent Advances in Epilepsy 2.* Edinburgh: Churchill Livingstone, 1985: 137–160.

75. Riviello JJ. Jr, Roe EJ. Jr, Sapin JJ, Grover WD. Timing of maintenance phenytoin therapy after intravenous loading dose. *Pediatric Neurology* 1991; **7**: 262–265.

76. Richard MO, Chiron C, d'Athis P, *et al.* Phenytoin monitoring in status epilepticus. *Epilepsia* 1993; **34**: 144–150.

77. Morton LD. Clinical experience with fosphenytoin in children. *Journal of Child Neurology* 1998; **13**: (Suppl. 1), S19–22.

78. Pellock JM. Fosphenytoin use in children. *Neurology* 1996; **46**: (Suppl. 1), S14–16.

79. Shaner DM, McCurdy SA, Herring MO, *et al.* Treatment of status epilepticus: a prospective comparison of diazepam and phenytoin versus phenobarbital and optional phenytoin. *Neurology* 1988; **38**: 202–207.

80. Dunn DW. Status epilepticus in infancy and childhood. *Neurologic Clinics* 1990; **8**: 647–657.

81. Browne TR. Paraldehyde, chlormethiazole and lidocaine for treatment of status epilepticus. In: Delgado-Escueta AV, Wasterlain CG, Treiman DM, Porter RJ. (eds) *Status Epilepticus: Mechanisms of Brain Damage and Treatment.* New York: Raven Press, 1983: 509–517.

82. Pascual J, Sedano MJ, Polo JM, *et al.* Intravenous lidocaine for status epilepticus. *Epilepsia* 1988; **29**: 584–589.

83. Harvey PK, Higenbottom TM, Loh L. Chlormethiazole in the treatment of status epilepticus. *BMJ* 1975; **2**: 603–605.

84. Lingam S, Bertwhistle H, Ellison HM, Wilson J. Problems with intravenous chlormethiazole (heminevrin) in status epilepticus. *BMJ* 1980; **280**: 155–156.

85. Uberall MA, Trollman R, Wunsiedler U, *et al.* Intravenous valproate in pediatric epilepsy patients with refractory status epilepticus. *Neurology* 2000; **54**: 2188–2189.

86. White JR, Santos CS. Intravenous valproate associated with significant hypotension in the treatment of status epilepticus. *Journal of Child Neurology* 1999; **14**: 822–823.

87. Mackenzie SJ, Kapadia F, Grant IS. Propofol infusion for control of status epilepticus. *Anaesthesia* 1990; **45**: 1043–1045.

88. Parke JJ, Stevens JE, Rice ASC, *et al.* Metabolic acidosis and fatal myocardial failure after propofol infusion in children: five case reports. *BMJ* 1992; **305**: 613–616.

89. Philips SA, Shanahan RJ. Etiology and mortality of status epilepticus in children: a recent update. *Archives of Neurology* 1989; **46**: 74–76.

90. Gross-Tsur V, Shinnar S. Convulsive status epilepticus in children. *Epilepsia* 1993; **34**(Suppl. 1): S12–20.

91. Shinnar S, Berg AT, Moshe SL, *et al.* The risk of seizure recurrence following a first unprovoked seizure in childhood, a prospective study. *Pediatrics* 1990; **85**: 1076–1085.

92. Hauser WA, Rich SS, Annegers JF, Anderson VE. Seizure recurrence following a first unprovoked seizure: an extended follow up. *Neurology* 1990; **40**: 1163–1170.

93. Maytal J, Shinnar S. Febrile status epilepticus. *Pediatrics* 1990; **86**: 611–616.

94. Shinnar S, Pellock JM, Berg AT, *et al.* Short-term outcomes of children with febrile status epilepticus. *Epilepsia* 2001; **42**: 47–53.

95. Hesdorffer DC, Logroscino G, Cascino G, *et al.* Risk of unprovoked seizures after acute symptomatic seizure: effect of status epilepticus. *Annals of Neurology* 1998; **44**: 908–912.

96. Berg AT, Shinnar S. The risk of recurrence following a first unprovoked seizure: a meta-analysis. *Pediatrics* 1991; **41**: 965–972.

97. Shinnar S, Maytal J, Krasnoff L, Moshe SL. Recurrent status epilepticus in children. *Annals of Neurology* 1992; **31**: 598–604.

98. Freeman JM. Status epilepticus: it's not what we've thought or taught. *Pediatrics* 1989; **83**: 444–445.

99. McBride MC, Dooling EC, Oppenheimer EY. Complex partial status epilepticus in young children. *Annals of Neurology* 1981; **9**: 526–530.

100. Mayeux R, Lueders H. Complex partial epilepticus, case report and proposal for diagnostic criteria. *Neurology* 1978; **28**: 957–961.

101. Ballenger CE, King DW, Gallagher BB. Partial complex status epilepticus. *Neurology* 1983; **33**: 1545–1552.

102. Shalev RS, Amir N. Complex partial status epilepticus. *Archives of Neurology* 1983; **40**: 90–92.

103. De Pasquet E, Gaudin E, Bianchi A, De Zmendilaharsu S. Prolonged and monosymptomatic dysphasic status epilepticus. *Neurology* 1976; **25**: 244–247.

104. McLachlan RS, Blume WT. Isolated fear in complex partial status epilepticus. *Annals of Neurology* 1980; **8**: 639–641.

105. Dinner DS, Lueders H, Lederman R, Gretter TE. Aphasic status epilepticus; a case report. *Neurology* 1981; **31**: 888–891.

106. Nakada T, Lee H, Kwee IL, Lerner AM. Epileptic Kluver-Bucy syndrome: case report. *Journal of Psychiatry* 1984; **45**: 87–88.

107. Wieser HG, Kailemariam S, Regard M, Landis T. Unilateral limbic epileptic status activity: stereo EEG, behavioural and cognitive data. *Epilepsia* 1985; **26**: 19–29.

108. DeToledo JC, Minagar A, Lowe MR. Persisting aphasia as the sole manifestation of partial status epilepticus. *Clinical Neurology and Neurosurgery* 2000; **102**: 144–148.

109. Augustijn PB, Parra J, Wouters CH, *et al.* Ring chromosome 20 epilepsy syndrome in children: electroclinical features. *Neurology* 2001; **57**: 1108–1111.

110. Inoue Y, Fijiwara T, Matsuda K, *et al.* Ring chromosome 20 and nonconvulsive status epilepticus. A new epileptic syndrome. *Brain* 1997; **120**: 939–953.

111. Gastaut H. Clinical and electroencephalographical classification of epileptic seizures. *Epilepsia* 1970; **11**: 102–113.

112. Zappoli R. Prolonged epileptic twilight state with almost continuous 'wave-spikes'. *Electroencephalography and Clinical Neurophysiology* 1955; **3**: 421–423.

113. Niedermeyer E, Kalifeh R. Petit mal status ('spike wave stupor'). An electro clinical appraisal. *Epilepsia* 1965; **6**: 250–262.

114. Porter RJ, Penry JK. Petit mal status. In: Delgado-Escueta AV, Wasterlain CG, Treiman DM, Porter RJ. (eds) *Status Epilepticus: Mechanisms of Brain Damage and Treatment.* New York: Raven Press, 1983: 61–68.

115. Stores G. Non convulsive status epilepticus in children. In: Pedley TA, Meldrum BS. (eds) *Recent Advances in Epilepsy 3.* Edinburgh: Churchill Livingstone, 1986: 295–310.

116. Kaplan PW. No, some types of nonconvulsive status epilepticus cause little permanent sequelae (or: 'the cure may be worse than the disease'). *Neurophysiologie Clinique* 2000; **30**: 377–382.

117. Treiman DM, Delgado-Escueta AV. Complex partial status epilepticus. In: Delgado-Escueta AV, Wasterlain CG, Treiman DM, Porter RJ. (eds) *Status Epilepticus: Mechanisms of Brain Damage and Treatment.* New York: Raven Press, 1983: 69–82.

118. Shields WD. Status epilepticus. *Pediatric Clinics of North America* 1989; **36**: 383–393.

119. Tassinari CA, Daniele O, Michelucci R, *et al.* Benzodiazepines: efficacy in status epilepticus. In: Delgado-Escueta AV, Wasterlain CG, Treiman DM, Porter RJ. (eds) *Status Epilepticus: Mechanisms of Brain Damage and Treatment.* New York: Raven Press, 1983: 465–476.

120. Livingston JH, Brown JK. Non convulsive status epilepticus resistant to benzodiazepines. *Archives of Disease in Childhood* 1987; **62**: 41–44.

121. Pisani F, Gallitto G, Di Perri R. Could lamotrigine be useful in status epilepticus? A case report. *Journal of Neurology, Neurosurgery and Psychiatry* 1991; **54**: 845–846.

122. Crouteau D, Shevell M, Rosenblatt B, *et al.* Treatment of absence status in the Lennox-Gastaut syndrome with propofol. *Neurology* 1998; **51**: 315–316.

123. Treiman DM, Delgado-Escueta AV, Clark MA. Impairment of memory following prolonged complex partial status epilepticus. *Neurology* 1981; **31**: 109.

124. Brett E. Minor epileptic status. *Journal of the Neurological Sciences* 1966; **3**: 52–75.

125. Doose H, Volzke E. Petit mal status and early childhood dementia. *Neuropadiatrie* 1979; **10**: 10–14.

126. Beaumanoir A, Foletti G, Magistris M, *et al.* Status epilepticus in the Lennox-Gastaut syndrome. In: Niedermeyer E, Degen R. (eds) *The Lennox-Gastaut Syndrome.* New York: Alan R. Liss, 1988: 283–99.

127. Meldrum B. Metabolic factors during prolonged seizures and their relation to nerve cell death. In: Delgado-Escueta AV, Wasterlain CG, Treiman DM, Porter RJ. (eds) *Status Epilepticus: Mechanisms of Brain Damage and Treatment.* New York: Raven Press, 1983: 261–277.

128. Wasterlain CG. Inhibition of cerebral protein synthesis by epileptic seizures without motor manifestation. *Neurology(Minn)* 1976; **24**: 175–180.

129. Krsek P, Mikulecka A, Druga R, *et al.* An animal model of nonconvulsive status epilepticus: a contribution to clinical controversies. *Epilepsia* 2001; **42**: 171–180.

130. Tasker RC, Boyd SG, Harden A, Matthew DJ. EEG monitoring of prolonged thiopentone administration for intractable seizures and status epilepticus in infants and children. *Neuropediatrics* 1989; **20**: 147–153.

131. Amit R, Goitein KJ, Mathot I, Yatziu S. Prolonged electrocerebral silent barbiturate coma in intractable seizure disorders. *Epilepsia* 1988; **29**: 63–66.

132. Crawford TO, Mitchell WG, Fishman LS, *et al.* Very high dose phenobarbital for refractory status epilepticus in children. *Neurology* 1988; **38**: 1035–1040.

133. Kofke WA, Young RSK, Davis P, *et al.* Isoflurane for refractory status epilepticus: a clinical series. *Anesthesiology* 1989; **71**: 653–659.

134. Meeke RI, Soifer BE, Gelb AW. Isoflurane for management of status epilepticus. *Drug Intelligence and Clinical Pharmacy* 1989; **23**: 579–581.

18

Neurophysiological investigations

MARY B CONNOLLY AND PETER KH WONG

Neurophysiological techniques have an important role in the diagnosis and management of epilepsy. EEG is the most informative laboratory test in patients with epileptic seizures. It can play an important role in the diagnosis of epilepsy, classification of the epileptic seizure type and epilepsy syndrome, localization of the epileptogenic zone, assessment of the response to treatment, and estimation of the risk of seizure recurrence after discontinuation of antiepileptic medication.

The diagnosis of epilepsy is usually based on the history. Because of the paroxysmal nature of epileptic seizures, the EEG is typically recorded between seizures and conclusions are based on the interictal findings. The number and length of recordings, use of additional electrodes, activation methods used and epilepsy type influence the detection of interictal epileptiform abnormalities. If the epileptogenic area is deep in the brain, such as in the mesial frontal or temporal lobes, the interictal EEG may be normal. Indeed, even repeated EEGs may be normal in some patients with epilepsy. In contrast, epileptiform EEG patterns occur in approximately 1–2 per cent of patients with no history of epileptic seizures.[1] Similarly, relatives of patients with absence epilepsy may have 3-Hz spike-wave discharges and not have clinically detectable seizures.[2] In addition, patients with structural cortical lesions, such as infarction or tumor, may have sharp waves or spikes without having clinical seizures.

- **Video-EEG** monitoring allows simultaneous recording of the EEG and video data and is very useful in the evaluation of patients for epilepsy surgery and in the differentiation of epileptic from nonepileptic clinical events. Children have more frequent seizures than adults and we have performed video-EEG during routine EEG recordings carried out in our laboratory over the past 10 years. Seizures have been recorded in approximately 10 per cent of 23 000 EEGs performed, and review of the video recording has often resulted in a change in classification of the seizure type or epilepsy classification.

- **Ambulatory EEG** allows continuous EEG monitoring during normal activities and can be helpful in the assessment of seizure frequency and determination of the nature of clinical behaviors.

- **High-resolution EEG** involves application of 100–200 scalp electrodes. The precise role of this new technique has not been established, but it may provide more accurate localization of the epileptic zone in presurgical assessment.

- **Invasive EEG** using subdural and depth electrodes is used in patients undergoing epilepsy surgery where the epileptogenic zone cannot be sufficiently defined with noninvasive monitoring and where mapping of eloquent brain function (language and motor) is required.

- **Evoked potentials** have a more limited role in the evaluation of patients with epilepsy but may yield useful information in specific conditions, such as progressive myoclonic epilepsies, neurodegenerative diseases or epilepsia partialis continua.

- **Magnetoencephalography** (MEG), which measures the weak magnetic fields generated by ionic currents within the brain, is being evaluated as a noninvasive method of localization of the epileptogenic zone.

TECHNICAL ASPECTS OF EEG

The EEG measures the difference in electrical potential between two points on the head, i.e. it is a tracing of voltage fluctuations (in microvolts, μV) over time recorded from electrodes placed over the scalp in a specific array. This represents fluctuating dendritic membrane potentials from superficial cortical layers. The EEG is attenuated by 50–90 per cent by the skull, scalp and CSF. The EEG measured at the scalp is extremely weak (10–200 μV) and is smaller than many sources of biological signals (noise). Thus, the EEG must be amplified to permit recording from the scalp.

Technical aspects influence the quality of the EEG recording markedly. It is beyond the scope of this chapter to address all technical aspects of EEG recording.[3] It is imperative that there are accurate measurements for electrode position and that the electrodes be applied according to the 10–20 system.[4] This international system of electrode placement was established in 1958; electrodes are spaced at 10–20 per cent of distances between specific anatomical landmarks. The basic number of electrodes recommended is 19 plus reference electrodes, but the addition of other electrodes can increase spatial resolution, permit recording from specific areas, and allow monitoring of other activity, such as electrooculogram and electrocardiogram (ECG).[5] Surface sphenoidal electrodes yield as much information in temporal lobe epilepsy as

sphenoidal electrodes and are not invasive.[6,7] With mesial frontal, central or parietal foci, additional electrodes may be applied in order to detect epileptiform activity close to the midline.

The reference electrodes should be chosen carefully to minimize contamination. Theoretically, a reference electrode should be electrically silent, but this is impossible and a reference that is not contaminated by the activity in question is optimal. An ear reference is associated with less contamination from EMG and ECG but is prone to contamination if there are temporal abnormalities (Figure 18.1). A cheek reference may be contaminated by eye movement and frontal polar abnormalities, and linked cheek reference reduces ECG contamination. The central midline electrode (CZ) can be used as a reference in the waking state, but may be confusing in drowsiness and sleep. The average reference is useful for detection of focal abnormalities but it is important to remove abnormal electrodes and frontal polar electrodes (due to eye movement) from the average reference.

A large number of montages may be used but the recording should include at least referential, longitudinal and coronal bipolar montages. Bipolar montages have the advantages of localization by phase reversal, less contamination and less movement artifact, but pose difficulty when the EEG abnormalities are at the end of a chain (occipital or frontal polar) or when there are dipolar fields recorded. A coronal bipolar montage is useful in

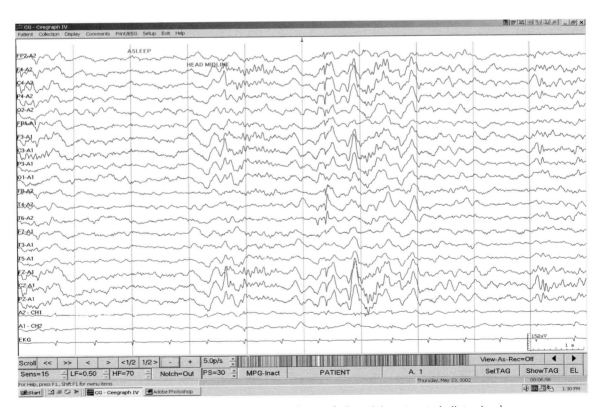

Figure 18.1 *Right temporal spike contaminating the right ear reference (referential montage to ipsilateral ear).*

the interpretation of activity close to the midline and for seeing sleep potentials. A posterior halo (Figure 18.2) provides good coverage of the occipital areas.

Since the original report of the EEG in humans by Hans Berger,[8] collection and management of large amounts of data have been influenced dramatically by computerization.[9] This has culminated in the development of digital EEG, which has the major advantage of being able to alter montages after collection of the EEG data.[10,11] Thus, montages may be created that enhance the abnormal activity.

Response testing is important during episodes of alteration of awareness or 3-Hz spike-wave discharges. We give the child a word or words to remember and, if the discharge lasts long enough, have the child do age-appropriate mathematics or point to an object. If the episodes are frequent enough, the child can sit up or perform a task such as clapping while hyperventilating. This may demonstrate any loss of tone or coordination during the event.

Activation procedures

Various methods of activation are used to enhance paroxysmal activity on the EEG or epileptic seizures. Eye opening and closing enhance assessment of the posterior dominant rhythm, and eye closure may demonstrate abnormal activity in certain forms of epilepsy, e.g. benign occipital epilepsy. Sleep is an important part of the EEG recording,

in that the epileptiform activity may be limited to light sleep in many individuals with epilepsy. Thus, an EEG without sleep is an incomplete recording. The mechanism by which sleep activates epileptiform patterns is poorly understood, but it has been suggested that it is the fatigue rather than sleep per se that is the main trigger.[12,13] Sleep deprivation is an important activator of focal epileptiform abnormalities. It is also a potent activator of epileptic seizures, particularly in individuals who have a history of seizures associated with sleep deprivation. Consequently, one should be prepared to manage an epileptic seizure in the laboratory.

Hyperventilation is an activation procedure that influences particularly absence seizures and the generalized 3-Hz spike-wave discharge. The precise duration of hyperventilation required to activate 3-Hz spike-wave is unclear. We typically have patients hyperventilate for 3 min, except children with a history suggestive of absence seizures, where hyperventilation is performed for 4 min twice during the EEG. Children under 4 years or older children with impaired cognition are often unable to cooperate to perform hyperventilation. Focal slowing induced by hyperventilation may be seen in children with structural or vascular lesions. Hyperventilation results in hypocarbia and vasoconstriction and typical clinical events may be precipitated by hyperventilation in moya–moya disease. For this reason, it should be performed with caution in

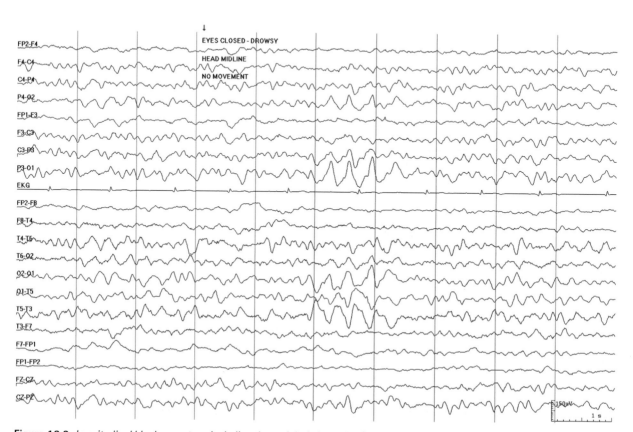

Figure 18.2 *Longitudinal bipolar montage including the occipital electrodes (posterior halo) to demonstrate occipital delta activity.*

individuals with known or suspected moya–moya disease, vascular disorders, completed stroke and transient ischemic attacks. It is contraindicated in patients with significant cardiac disease (recent cardiac arrest or cardiac abnormalities), severe respiratory problems and sickle cell anemia. High-amplitude rhythmic slowing may occur during hyperventilation and clinically mimic an absence seizure. The EEG change may occur with or without clinical change and is not considered to be an ictal pattern.[14,15]

Intermittent photic stimulation is primarily an activator of generalized spike-wave or polyspike-wave in individuals with idiopathic generalized and myoclonic epilepsies. Generalized spike-wave induced by intermittent photic stimulation is a genetic pattern and may be seen in individuals with no history of epileptic seizures. Thus, photosensitivity should be interpreted appropriately and not result in inappropriate treatment with antiepileptic medications (AEDs). A spike-wave discharge that outlasts the duration of the photic stimulation or is associated with clinical signs, such as a myoclonic or an absence seizure, is a photoconvulsive response and is clearly an abnormal pattern.

In the evaluation of patients for epilepsy surgery, it may be necessary to gradually reduce or withdraw AEDs in order to precipitate infrequent seizures. There is a risk that atypical seizures may be induced or that status epilepticus may occur, particularly if there is a history of prolonged seizures. However, no effect on spike localization or seizure symptomatology was noted with acute withdrawal of antiepileptic medication in one study.[16] The withdrawal of AEDs should be individualized for each patient. The rapid withdrawal of benzodiazepines and barbiturates is not recommended. In patients who have seizures several times each week, it is usually not necessary to alter the dose of AEDs. It is often possible to start reducing medications gradually before hospital admission in those with less frequent seizures. Proconvulsant medications such as methohexital may be used in certain circumstances to activate temporal lobe spikes.[17]

NORMAL PATTERNS

Maturation of the EEG

In his first report on EEG in humans, Berger studied 17 children between 8 days and 5 years of age and recognized age-dependent changes.[8] It is important to appreciate the normal evolution and maturation of the EEG from the premature brain to adulthood and to recognize normal variants and patterns, which have a low association with epileptic seizures.[18–20] Table 18.1 summarizes the main features of the neonatal EEG at specific conceptual ages.[21] Up to the age of 4 months, attention to the background voltage, symmetry, synchrony and continuity are more important than the presence of sharp transients, which are seen in many neonates without a history of seizures and correlate poorly with epileptic seizures or outcome.[22]

A posterior dominant rhythm first appears at the age of 3 months, and is 3 Hz in the alert state. Table 18.2 describes the evolution of the posterior dominant rhythm. By 3 years of age, the posterior dominant rhythm reaches alpha frequency. Alpha rhythm is an 8–12-Hz rhythm occurring during wakefulness over the posterior head region, with higher voltage over the occipital area. It is best seen with the eyes closed and in a relaxed state. It is blocked by attention, e.g. eye opening or mental effort. Prominent bursts of rhythmic slowing, maximal in the parasagittal area, are a normal finding in the drowsy state in the first few years of life and are known as **hypnagogic hypersynchrony** (Figure 18.3). These changes are abnormal if they occur in an older child or adult. Sleep potentials occur in stage II sleep and are 12–15 Hz, sharply contoured, waveforms located in the central parietal area. They are seen from 2 months onwards and may be asynchronous until 18 months of age. Asynchronous sleep potentials beyond 18 months may be seen with abnormalities of the corpus callosum. Stage III, IV and rapid eye movement (REM)

Table 18.1 *Neonatal EEG: characteristic findings and gestation*

Active sleep	Irregular respirations, rapid eye movements, continuous EMG and variations in heart rate, restless movements of distal limbs, grimacing and smiling
Quiet sleep	Regular respirations, slow eye movements, intermittent EMG, proximal limb movements
Transitional sleep	Irregular and regular respirations, eye movements and both types of limb movements
28 weeks	*Trace discontinue*, flats less than 5 μV lasting up to 3 min, asynchrony, 4–5 Hz theta in temporal areas, sharp transients maximal frontally
28–32 weeks	Active and quiet periods, *trace discontinue*, temporal theta, synchronous bioccipital delta, delta brushes
32–36 weeks	Flat periods increase in voltage, bursts synchronous, delta brushes most prominent until 35 weeks in active sleep and 35 weeks in quiet sleep
36–40 weeks	80% synchrony, *trace alernant* 50–50 bursts/flats at 37 weeks, attenuation on stimulation, frontal sharp transients, anterior dysrhythmia, delta brushes rare but may be seen in quiet sleep
40–44 weeks	Active and quiet sleep, increase in quiet sleep, *trace alternant* with increasing delta in bursts and increasing voltage of flats, reduction in frontal sharp transients, no delta brushes
44 weeks	80% quiet sleep, continuous except slight bursting in quiet sleep, attenuation on stimulation, high voltage slow waves, rare sharp waves in rolandic regions, rudimentary spindles

sleep are rarely seen in a routine sleep recording but are seen in an overnight EEG recording. The frequent delta activity normally seen in these states should be interpreted appropriately. Prominent occipital delta is a normal observation in stage I and II sleep in the first 18 months of life.

Normal variants

Mu rhythm, described first by Gastaut and also referred to as '*rhythme rolandique en arceau*',[23] is a 7–11-Hz rhythm seen in the central area (Figure 18.4). Mu rhythm is observed in 15 per cent of recordings, may be unilateral or bilateral, and may shift from side to side. It is attenuated by touch, movement, or even thought of movement, of the contralateral hand.

Lambda is low-amplitude ($<20\,\mu$V), sharp, transient activity seen over the occipital region in the waking state during visual exploration and attenuated by closing the eyes or darkening the room (Figure 18.5). This waveform

Table 18.2 *Waking posterior dominant rhythm (PDR) and age*

Age	PDR (Hz)
4 months	4
12 months	6
3 years	8
10 years	10–12

lasts 200–300 ms and is bi- or triphasic with the most prominent phase being surface positive.

Positive occipital sharp transients of sleep (POSTS) occur in all stages of non-REM sleep, particularly drowsiness and stage I. They are occipital in location, 4–6 Hz, and with a sharp lambdoid appearance (Figure 18.6). They may be asymmetric or unilateral, may occur in short runs and can be difficult to differentiate from occipital sharp waves in a patient with epilepsy.

Posterior slow waves are 1–4-Hz slow waves that interrupt the posterior dominant rhythm and extend from the occipital area to the posterior temporal and, less frequently, to the parietal area. They may be lateralized to one hemisphere or bilateral (Figure 18.7). They are more prominent in the first decade and diminish in adolescence.

Ctenoids, or **14 and 6 cycle positive spikes**, are a surface-positive comb-shaped rhythm at 14 or 6 Hz frequency (Figure 18.8). This rhythm is seen maximally in the posterior head region with spread to the temporal area. It is seen primarily in drowsiness and light sleep and may persist into stage II sleep. It is unilateral or bilateral, synchronous or independent, and typically lasts 0.5–1 s. It is seen most frequently between 5 and 15 years of age.

6-Hertz spike-wave is a common variant that is often misinterpreted as epileptiform spike-wave activity (Figure 18.9). It consists of bisynchronous low amplitude 5–7-Hz spike-wave rhythm and is most prevalent in drowsiness and light sleep. It is usually well-organized, bilateral,

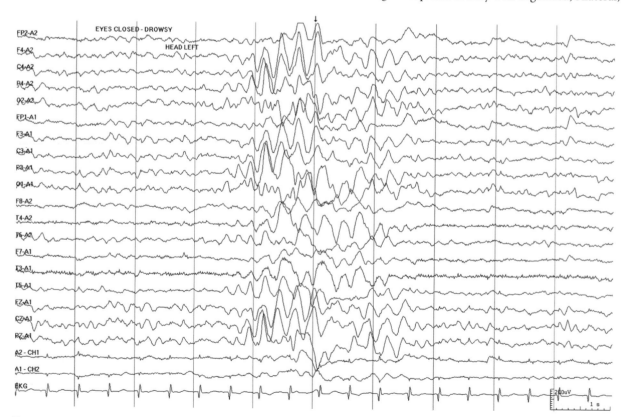

Figure 18.3 *A hypnagogic hypersynchrony burst seen at sensitivity of 20 µV/mm on a referential montage.*

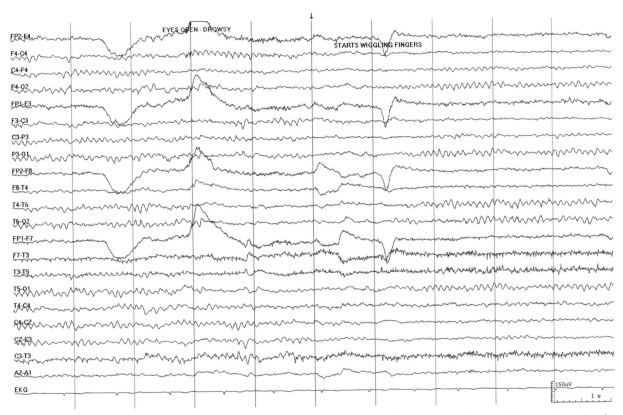

Figure 18.4 *Central mu rhythm viewed on a longitudinal bipolar montage attenuated by wiggling the fingers of the contralateral hand.*

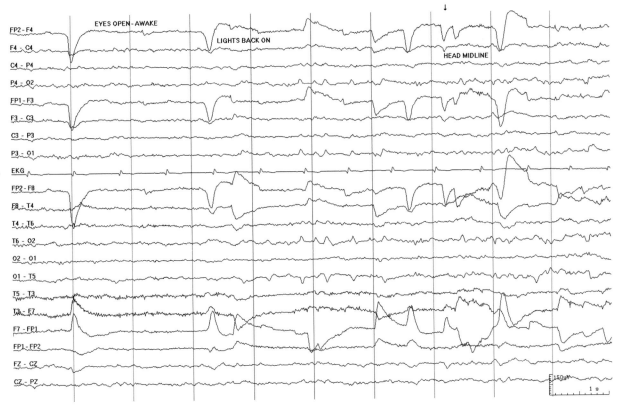

Figure 18.5 *Lambda rhythm viewed on a longitudinal bipolar montage with the lights on in the room.*

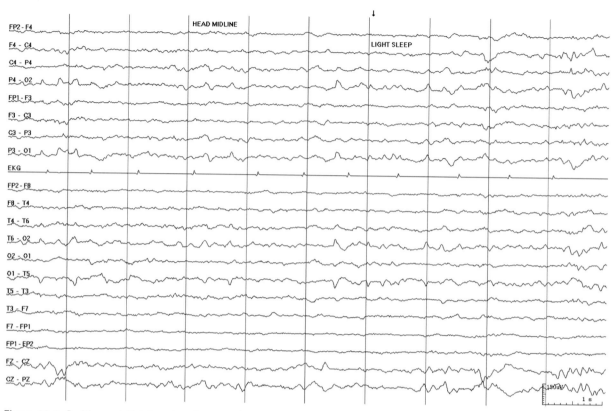

Figure 18.6 *Positive occipital sharp transients on a longitudinal bipolar montage in light sleep.*

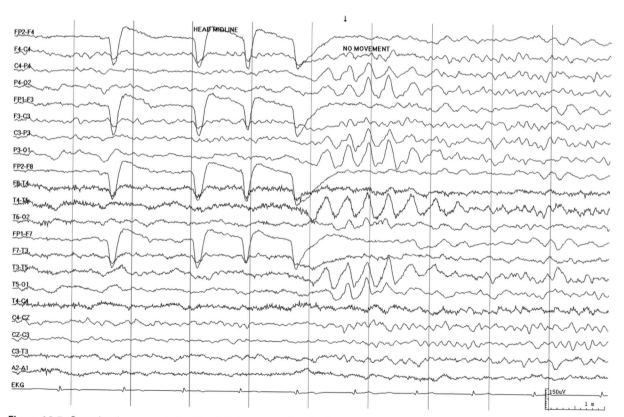

Figure 18.7 *Posterior slow waves in the bioccipital areas on a longitudinal bipolar montage.*

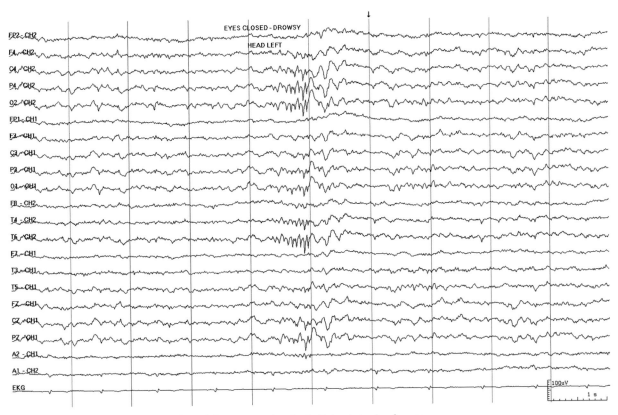

Figure 18.8 *Ctenoids viewed on a referential montage using the ipsilateral cheek reference.*

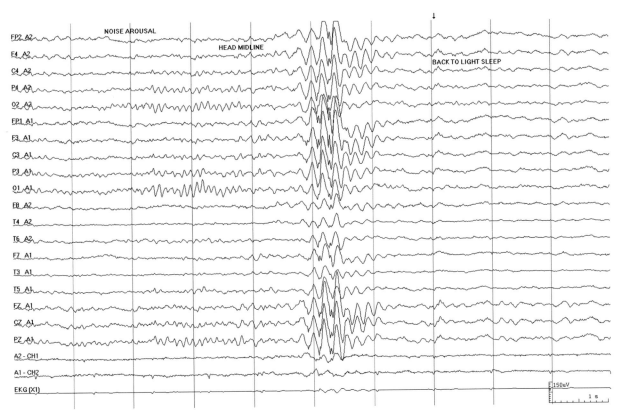

Figure 18.9 *6-Hz spike-wave viewed on referential montage to the ipsilateral ear.*

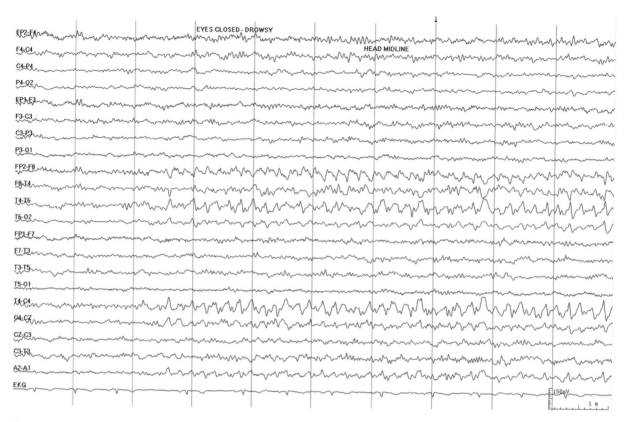

Figure 18.10 *Rhythmic midtemporal theta on the right side viewed on a longitudinal bipolar montage.*

gradual onset/offset (crescendo/decrescendo) and maximal at midcentral or midparietal electrodes. It occurs in both adolescents and adults with a peak incidence between 11 and 15 years.

Rhythmic mid temporal theta (previously called **psychomotor variant**) is a theta rhythm at 5–7 Hz, which is seen in the temporal region and may be unilateral or bilateral. It is often misinterpreted as an ictal pattern but, in contrast to an ictal rhythm, does not evolve (Figure 18.10). It occurs in relaxed wakefulness and drowsiness, is attenuated by alerting the patient, and disappears in stage II sleep. It typically lasts 5–10 s but may last 30–60 s. It is more common in adolescents.

Small sharp spikes are monophasic or biphasic, low-to-medium amplitude spikes ($<135\,\mu V$) that are of short duration (35–90 ms) (Figure 18.11). They are best seen in the anterior and midtemporal areas and have a diffuse field. They are common in drowsiness and light sleep. They have a low association with epileptogenicity.

Frontal arousal rhythm (FAR) consists of bursts of rhythmic notched theta (6–8 Hz) with a beta component of 16–20 Hz in some patients (Figure 18.12). It occurs in the midfrontal regions and after arousal from sleep. It is seen between 2 and 14 years, lasts up to 20 s, and may wax and wane if the child remains drowsy. It may resemble an ictal pattern but there is no evolution in rhythm and amplitude.

ABNORMAL PATTERNS

Abnormalities of the EEG background

Changes in EEG background activity are important to recognize and may be subtle. Amplitude asymmetries of less than 50 per cent may be normal. Technical factors such as interelectrode distance, electrolyte salt bridge, subcutaneous edema, abnormal filter setting and impedance of the electrodes should always be considered if there is background asymmetry. Amplitude may be increased or decreased over the side of a lesion. Asymmetry of voltage of EEG activity in one hemisphere such as lower amplitude posterior dominant rhythm, generalized lower amplitude EEG activity, and lower amplitude vertex waves or sleep potentials are seen with extrinsic lesions such as large extradural or subdural hematomata, Sturge-Weber syndrome or intrinsic lesions such as cerebral infarction or progressive atrophy associated with CNS infection or Rasmussen encephalitis. Asymmetry of photic-induced driving may also be seen with focal lesions and the photic driving response may be more or less pronounced over the affected hemisphere. However, asymmetries up to 75 per cent in the photic driving response may be normal.

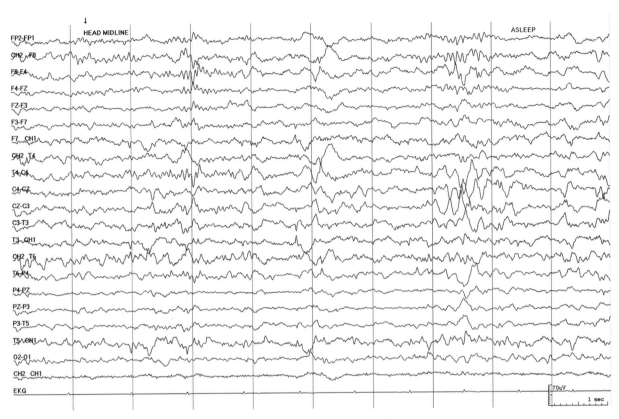

Figure 18.11 *Small sharp spikes in the left temporal area viewed on a coronal bipolar montage.*

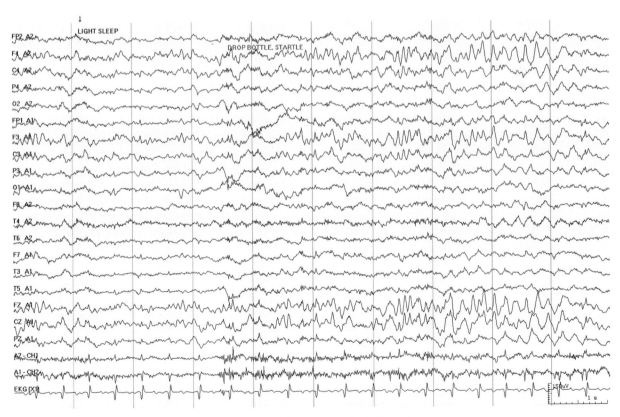

Figure 18.12 *Frontal arousal rhythm viewed on a referential montage to the ipsilateral ear.*

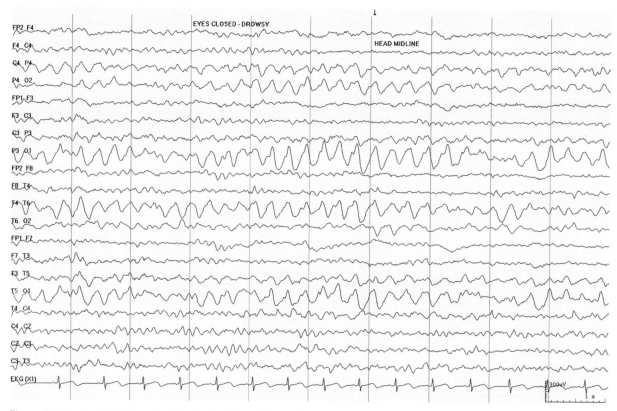

Figure 18.13 *Occipital intermittent rhythmic delta activity in drowsiness viewed on a longitudinal bipolar montage.*

Persistent changes in the EEG background are highly suggestive of a structural lesion. Lower-amplitude background without slowing may be seen with grey matter dysfunction, whereas slowing is more indicative of white matter dysfunction. Focal lesions located predominantly in the white matter are often associated with **polymorphic delta**. This is an arrhythmic waveform, varying in duration and amplitude, which may be continuous, intermittent, focal or generalized. It is generally unreactive to different physiologic states, showing little change on eye opening, and persisting into sleep. It may be accentuated by hyperventilation. Continuous focal polymorphic delta is often associated with focal structural lesions, particularly involving the white-gray matter interface, but may also occur transiently after a focal seizure or complex migraine episode. Such postictal slowing usually disappears by 24 h but may persist for several days. Generalized continuous polymorphic delta activity indicates more diffuse alteration in cerebral function such as toxic/metabolic, postictal effects or progressive white matter disorders.

Intermittent rhythmic delta activity (IRDA) consists of paroxysmal bursts of 2.5–4-Hz high-amplitude sinusoidal delta waves lasting 1–4 s. They are usually bilateral but may be unilateral, are accentuated by hyperventilation and drowsiness, attenuated by eye opening and alerting, and disappear in stage II–IV sleep. The anatomic and pathologic basis of IRDA is poorly understood, but

suggests abnormal thalamocortical interactions. The location is maximal in the occipital area in children less than 10 years (**occipital intermittent rhythmic delta activity**, OIRDA) (Figure 18.13) and maximal in the frontal regions in individuals over 10 years of age (**frontal intermittent rhythmic delta activity**, FIRDA) (Figure 18.14).

Posterior bilateral delta activity (PBDA) is rhythmic high-amplitude paroxysmal bursts of 3-Hz delta intermixed with low-voltage spike activity and is also seen in the bilateral posterior head regions, maximal occipitally (Figure 18.15). Unlike OIRDA, it is enhanced by hyperventilation, attenuated by eye opening and disappears in stage II sleep. It may evolve to 3-Hz spike-wave activity. It is seen in individuals with primary generalized epilepsy, particularly childhood absence epilepsy (40–60 per cent of patients with absence epilepsy have PBDA). **Temporal intermittent rhythmic delta activity** (TIRDA) may be seen in temporal lobe epilepsy.

Beta activity is increased with barbiturates, benzodiazepines and chloral hydrate, and is usually maximal frontally although may be seen in a generalized distribution. If there is a skull defect, beta activity may be more prominent and higher in amplitude in this area (**breach rhythm**). Asymmetry of beta voltage may indicate a brain lesion and the voltage may be increased or decreased over the affected hemisphere.

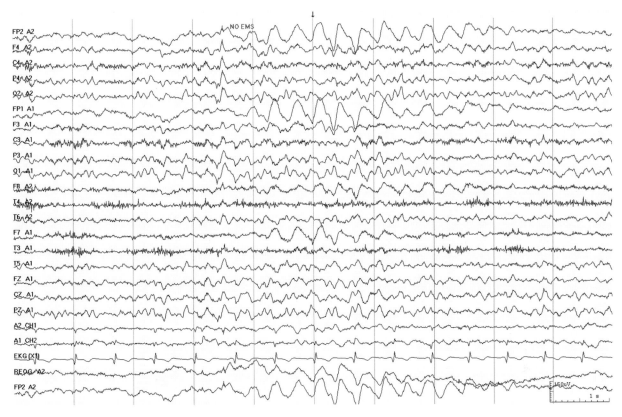

Figure 18.14 *Frontal intermittent rhythmic delta activity viewed on a referential montage.*

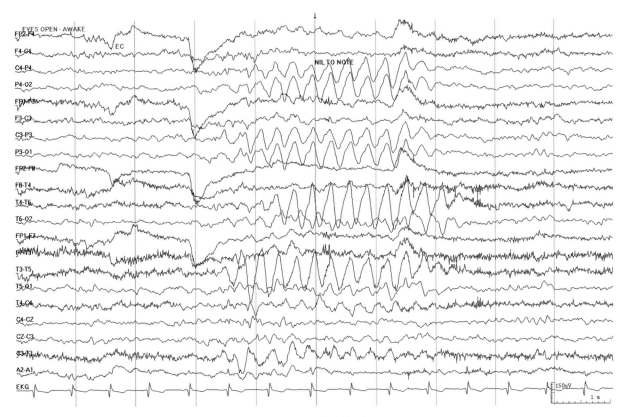

Figure 18.15 *Posterior bilateral delta activity viewed on a longitudinal bipolar montage.*

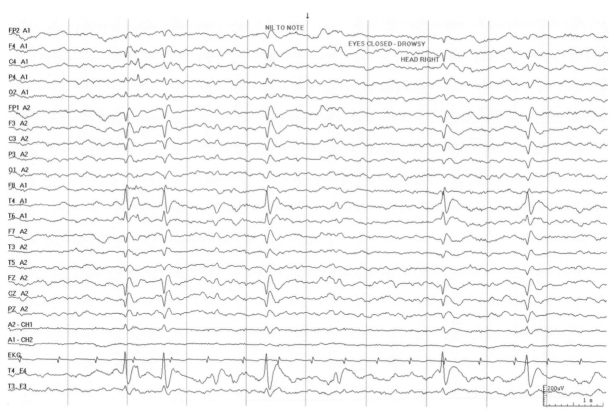

Figure 18.16 *Right midtemporal spike dipole with maximum negativity at the mid temporal electrode and positivity in the bifrontal areas (referential montage).*

Interictal epileptiform abnormalities

Interictal spikes and sharp waves are defined as transient waveforms, which are easily differentiated from the background EEG activity. **Spikes** are 20–70 ms in duration, diphasic or triphasic, usually surface negative and often followed by a slow wave; **sharp waves** are 70–200 ms in duration. The voltage of spikes and sharp waves may vary. They are typically surface negative in polarity, but spikes with a positive polarity may also occur. With certain types of epileptiform discharge, one may appreciate both the positive and negative ends of the dipole depending on the orientation of the spike generator. This is seen classically in the central temporal discharges characteristic of benign partial epilepsy with central temporal spikes (BCECTS), where the generator orientation is horizontal (Figure 18.16). The maximum amplitude or voltage determines the location of the spike or sharp wave. This is best appreciated on a referential montage, but phase reversal on a bipolar montage may assist in localization. When a spike or sharp wave occurs at the end of a chain, such as in the occipital or frontopolar region, phase reversal will not be seen unless one uses a montage that includes the occipital or frontalpolar electrodes within the chain.

Interictal epileptiform patterns in idiopathic partial epilepsies

A **central temporal spike with a dipole configuration** (rolandic spike dipole) is one of the most common interictal epileptiform patterns seen in children.[24,25] These are high-voltage diphasic spikes or sharp waves, with maximum negativity seen in the midtemporal area and simultaneous positivity in the frontal area. They are seen independently in both rolandic areas in 30 per cent of children. This pattern is more common in drowsiness and sleep and spikes or sharp waves may occur rhythmically in sleep. This abnormality is seen between 3 and 15 years. Epileptic seizures occur in 70 per cent of children with this EEG pattern, most commonly in BCECTS. This EEG pattern occurs on a genetic basis and may be observed in individuals without epilepsy. Horizontal spike dipoles are not specific for BCECTS and may occur in other types of epilepsy. However, if they occur in developmentally normal children with the characteristic clinical seizure pattern, a specific diagnosis may be made.

Central spikes without a dipole configuration are seen in many children and are a nonspecific finding. They are more frequent in drowsiness and sleep and not influenced by hyperventilation or photic stimulation. Fifty to seventy

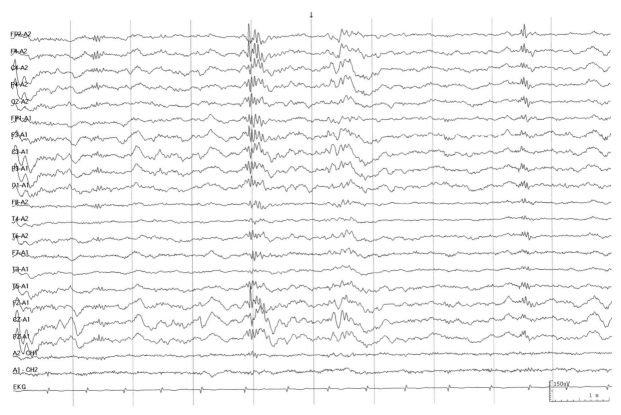

Figure 18.17 *Generalized polyspikes viewed on a referential montage.*

Table 18.3 *Ictal EEG patterns*

Seizure type	EEG pattern
Absence	3-Hz spike-wave
Atypical absence	Slow spike-wave
Myoclonic	Polyspike-wave
Tonic	Electrodecremental pattern
Atonic	Attenuation, generalized atypical spike-wave or rhythmic spikes
Tonic-clonic	Rhythmic spikes evolving
Infantile spasm	Generalized attenuation/ electrodecremental pattern
Focal seizure	Recruiting pattern

per cent of patients have seizures, which may be focal or generalized. Central spikes with low amplitude only evoked by tapping the hands or feet have a low association with epileptic seizures.[26] They are seen maximally in sleep and the spikes occur 18–20 ms after tapping the feet.

Occipital spikes or spike-wave enhanced by eye-closure is characteristic of benign occipital epilepsy (Figure 18.17). Differentiation from low-amplitude spikes with a very sharp morphology is important, as the latter morphology spikes may be seen in individuals with visual impairment. Diagnosis of benign occipital epilepsy requires characteristic clinical seizures with visual aura or migraine features and the characteristic EEG pattern.

Fifty to sixty per cent of patients with occipital spikes have epileptic seizures, which may be focal with or without secondary generalization. They may also occur in individuals with visual impairment on an ocular or occipital basis. In some patients the cause of occipital spikes is unclear.

Autosomal dominant nocturnal frontal lobe epilepsy may begin in childhood.[27] The seizures are typically nocturnal and may be misdiagnosed as a sleep disturbance. There is no pathognomonic interictal EEG pattern. No interictal epileptiform activity was seen in 31 of 37 patients.[27] Bilateral sharp and slow wave was seen in the bilateral frontal lobes in 3 patients and bifrontotemporal or unilateral frontotemporal in 3. Ictal video-EEG monitoring was performed in 10 of the 34 patients. Six of the 10 showed no clear ictal change, 3 had bilateral frontal dominant, sharp and slow wave activity, and there was an arousal response followed by diffuse 9-Hz rhythm in one patient.

Interictal EEG patterns in cryptogenic and symptomatic partial epilepsies

There are no interictal patterns that are pathognomonic of the cryptogenic or symptomatic epilepsies, but certain patterns are commonly seen. If the source of the seizures is deep within the brain in the mesial frontal, temporal, or parietal regions, or in the orbitofrontal area, the surface

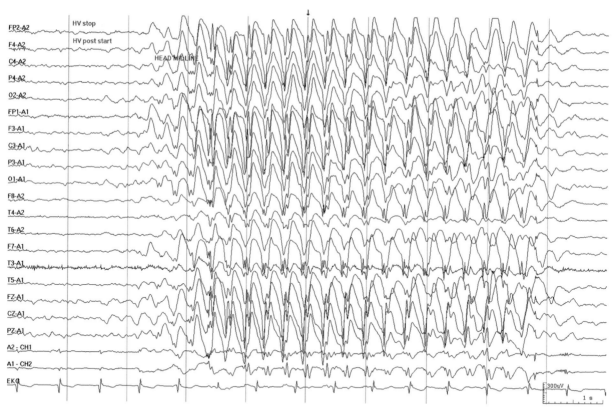

Figure 18.18 *3-Hz spike-wave viewed on a referential montage.*

EEG may demonstrate no abnormality. In that situation, the application of additional electrodes may permit identification of interictal spikes or sharp waves. In frontal lobe epilepsy, epileptiform discharges may be seen in the frontal polar area or in the frontal or central area. With orbitofrontal epilepsy, the interictal discharges may be seen over the F8 or F7 electrodes. In mesial temporal lobe epilepsy, the interictal spikes or sharp waves may only be appreciated using surface sphenoidal or T1 and T2 electrodes. However, anterior, mid or posterior temporal epileptiform discharges are more likely to be seen if the epileptogenic focus is neocortical rather than mesial. Parietal or occipital spikes may be appreciated more readily than frontal or temporal abnormalities.

Interictal and ictal epileptiform patterns in idiopathic generalized epilepsies

The characteristic pattern of idiopathic generalized epilepsies is **generalized spike-wave**, which is often 3 Hz in frequency (Figure 18.18). Generalized 3-Hz spike-wave may start at a faster frequency and decrease to 3 Hz and to 2.5 Hz. It occurs between 18 months and 25 years and is maximally seen in the frontal area. It has an abrupt onset and offset and is associated with a normal EEG background and often with PBDA (Figure 18.15). Hyperventilation is a potent activator for generalized 3-Hz

Table 18.4 *Epilepsy syndromes and characteristic EEG patterns*

Syndrome	EEG pattern
Ohtahara syndrome	Burst suppression
West syndrome	Hypsarrhythmia
Benign myoclonic epilepsy	Photosensitivity
Severe myoclonic epilepsy of infancy	Photosensitivity
Childhood absence epilepsy	3-Hz spike-wave
Juvenile absence epilepsy	3-Hz spike-wave
BCECTS	Rolandic spike dipoles
Benign occipital epilepsy	Occipital spike or sharp and slow wave
Juvenile myoclonic epilepsy	Generalized polyspike-wave
Lennox-Gastaut syndrome	Slow background, 1–2.5-Hz spike or sharp and slow wave and generalized fast spikes

spike-wave activity. It is seen maximally in hyperventilation, drowsiness and sleep. Fragments of spike-wave may be seen in sleep and may be difficult to differentiate from a focal epileptic abnormality. Generalized spike wave results from volleys from the thalamus, which normally produce sleep potentials, which in the presence of cortical hyperexcitability and reduced inhibition by the brain stem result in 3-Hz spike-wave. Seizures occur in 90 per cent of patients with generalized spike-wave discharges.

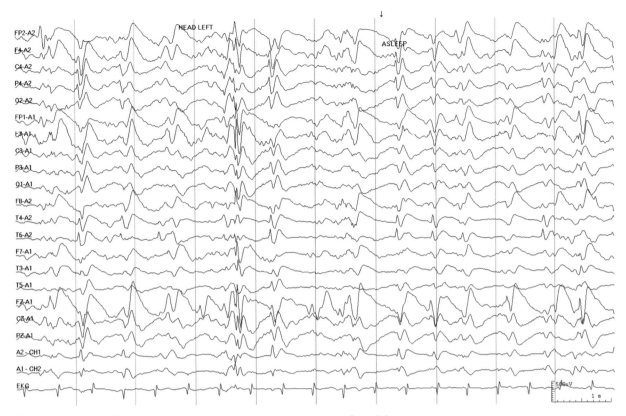

Figure 18.19 *Generalized sharp and slow wave complexes viewed on a referential montage.*

Polyspikes are complex paroxysmal patterns consisting of five or more polyphasic spike components that occur rhythmically in bursts of variable duration (0.2–1.5 s) (Figure 18.18). They usually occur as bilateral generalized synchronous discharges, maximal frontally, and can be an interictal or an ictal pattern. Activation by photic stimulation and sleep is common. Polyspikes are seen as a photoparoxysmal response, which is usually genetic. Polyspikes are associated with photosensitive epilepsies, myoclonic seizures, generalized tonic-clonic seizures and myoclonic astatic epilepsy. They may also be associated with diffuse or progressive encephalopathies, such as in patients with progressive myoclonic epilepsy. The prognosis in children with polyspikes depends on the underlying etiology and seizure type.

Interictal and ictal epileptiform patterns in Lennox–Gastaut syndrome and other symptomatic generalized epilepsies

The Lennox-Gastaut syndrome is an electroclinical syndrome characterized by mixed seizures, tonic, atypical absence, atonic and generalized tonic-clonic seizures and a characteristic EEG pattern. The latter is characterized by slowing of the background of the EEG, 1–2.5-Hz spike or sharp and slow wave activity (Figure 18.19) and bursts of fast rhythmic 10–25-Hz spikes or beta rhythm

(Figure 18.20).[28] The spike or sharp and slow wave activity is diffusely distributed but may be more anterior or posterior. It is usually bilaterally synchronous and symmetrical but transient shifting asymmetries may be seen. It is more prominent in drowsiness and sleep and attenuated by alerting. It is not affected by hyperventilation or photic stimulation. Normal sleep potentials may be absent in individuals with slow spike or sharp and slow wave activity.

There are other symptomatic generalized epilepsies which have quite similar EEG features, but tonic seizures and bursts of rhythmic spikes are usually not observed except in the Lennox-Gastaut syndrome. Slow spike-wave complexes may be seen in children with diffuse brain dysfunction following previous hypoxic-ischemic brain injury, meningitis or severe head injury and in patients with a prior history of infantile spasms.

An **electrodecremental event** (EDE) is an EEG pattern characterized by a suppression of EEG activity, which may be generalized or focal (Figure 18.21). It may be preceded by a 10–20-Hz rhythm, following which there is a sudden cessation of activity for a few seconds. It is usually an ictal pattern associated with a tonic seizure. The clinical features may be extremely subtle with upward eye deviation (*sursum vergens*). The duration of EDEs is typically 5–20 s and is seen more commonly in drowsiness and on arousal. Ninety-eight per cent of patients have epileptic seizures, tonic, atonic or infantile spasms. Atypical

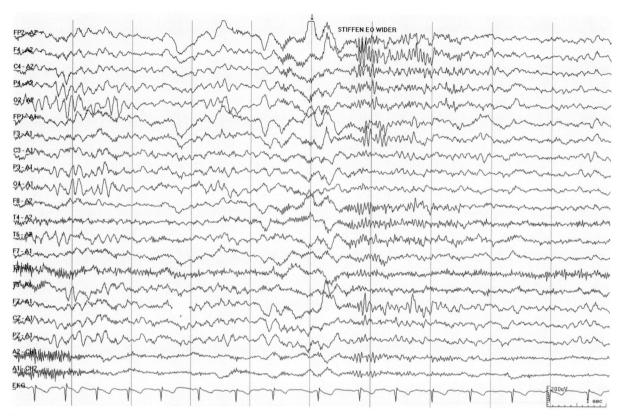

Figure 18.20 *Burst of rhythmic spikes associated with a tonic seizure (referential montage).*

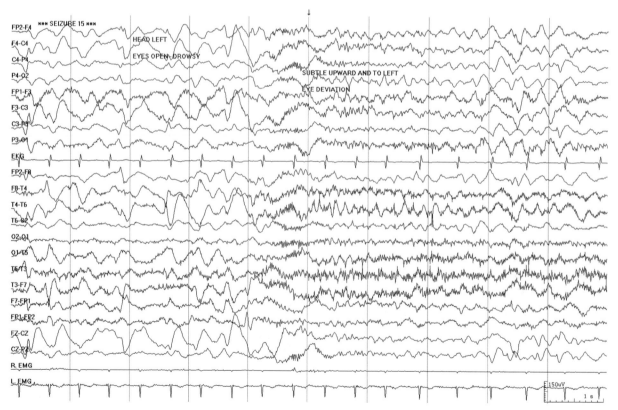

Figure 18.21 *Electrodecremental pattern associated with an infantile spasm (longitudinal bipolar montage).*

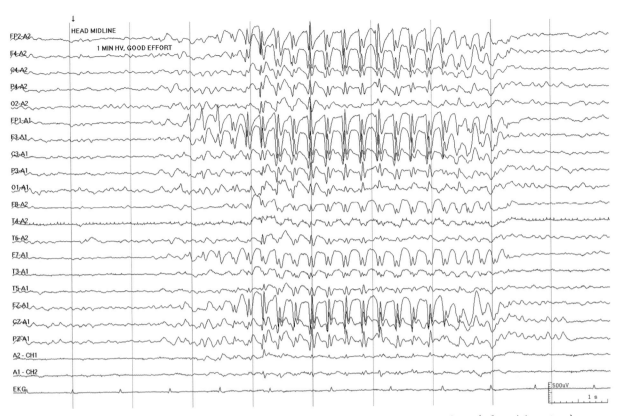

Figure 18.22 *Secondary bilateral synchrony with onset of spike-wave in the left frontal temporal area (referential montage).*

absence seizures are associated with diffuse slow spike-wave discharges at approximately 2–2.5 Hz and may be difficult to differentiate from the interictal pattern. Atonic seizures and myoclonic seizures may be associated with a variety of EEG abnormalities including slow spike-wave, polyspike wave or diffuse rapid rhythms.[28]

Hypsarrhythmia

Gibbs and Gibbs defined hypsarrhythmia as an EEG pattern characterized by:

> ... random high voltage slow waves and spikes. These spikes vary from moment to moment, both in location and durations. At times they appear to be focal and a few seconds later appear to originate from multiple foci. Occasionally, the spike discharge becomes generalized but it never appears as a rhythmically repetitive and highly organized pattern that could be confused with a discharge of the petit mal variant. The abnormality is almost continuous ...[29]

The key ingredients are: chaotic background, multifocal spike or sharp waves and electrodecremental events.

Secondary bilateral synchrony

Secondary bilateral synchrony involves unilateral, focal spikes or sharp waves that consistently precede a generalized

epileptiform discharge by 100–200 ms (Figure 18.22). There may be also a unilateral offset to the burst. It is seen in multifocal or focal cortical disease. Approximately half of the patients are mentally handicapped and one third have focal neurologic signs. The origin is in the frontal lobe in 50 per cent of patients and approximately one third have more than one seizure type.[30] Approximately half of the patients have cognitive dysfunction and one third have focal neurological findings on examination.[30]

Multiple independent spike foci

Spikes or sharp waves arising from three or more non-contiguous electrodes with at least one focus in each hemisphere characterize this pattern. It indicates multiple areas of cerebral irritability. It is usually associated with diffuse brain disease such as in hypoxic ischemic brain injury, traumatic, infectious or degenerative diseases.

Periodic lateralized epileptiform discharges

Periodic lateralized epileptiform discharges (PLEDS) are lateralized, high-amplitude 50–150 μV discharges occurring every 0.3–5 s, and often associated with disturbance of the background (Figure 18.23). They may also be seen bilaterally and are then referred to as bilateral independent periodic lateralized epileptiform discharges (BIPLEDs).

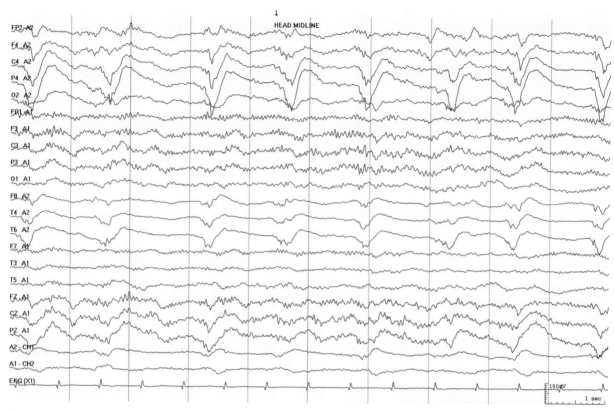

Figure 18.23 *Periodic lateralized epileptiform discharges in the right hemisphere viewed on a referential montage.*

They are not affected by state or activation procedures such as hyperventilation or sleep. They are associated with cerebral infarction, mass lesions such as tumors, CNS infection or inflammation, and seizures occur in 90 per cent of patients. The seizures are most commonly focal motor, epilepsia partialis continua and complex partial seizures.

Burst suppression

This pattern is characterized by high-voltage slow waves with intermixed sharp transients or spikes with a suppressed EEG background <5 μV (Figure 18.24). It is invariant and unreactive to stimulation and may be periodic. It is indicative of severe CNS depression, which may be drug-induced such as pentobarbital coma to control seizures. It may be seen in the rare infantile epileptic encephalopathy of Ohtahara syndrome or infantile encephalopathy with suppression bursts. It is often associated with coma. Myoclonus may be seen with or without EEG changes.

Triphasic waves

This pattern is usually seen synchronously and symmetrically in trains over both hemispheres maximal in the anterior head region (see Figure 18.27). They may only be seen in waking and disappear in sleep. They are associated with liver disease, renal failure, metabolic disturbance, and hypoxic encephalopathy.

SPECIAL TECHNIQUES

Video–EEG monitoring

Video-EEG monitoring, the simultaneous recording of EEG and video data, is useful for differentiation of epileptic from nonepileptic behaviors, characterization of epileptic seizures and measurement of seizure frequency. It is expensive, labor intensive, and requires admission to hospital. In most centers, EEG technologists or nurses are not available to assess individuals continuously during video-EEG monitoring. It is our practice to have a parent, caregiver or other family member present for the duration of the monitoring in order to assess the level of awareness, language and motor function of the child during and after a seizure. In infants and very young children, only limited response testing may be possible, e.g. following a toy. It is important to instruct the observers not to obstruct the camera view, as the video data may be useless in this situation. It is important

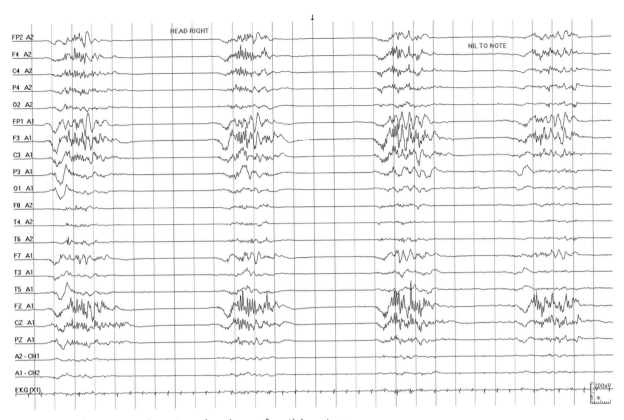

Figure 18.24 *Burst suppression pattern viewed on a referential montage.*

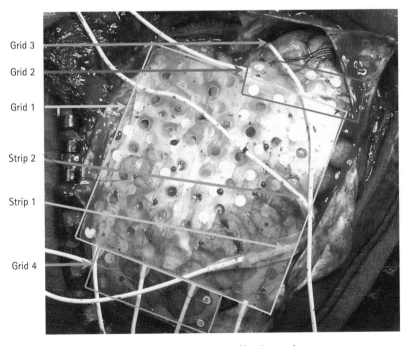

Figure 18.25 *Subdural electrodes covering the frontal parietal area. (See Plate 4.)*

to prepare the child and family for this procedure and we use a teaching video to explain the procedures involved. To optimize the information acquired, careful attention to ambient lighting, other sources of noise and technical interference is recommended.

Invasive EEG

Invasive EEG monitoring may be required in some patients to accurately define the ictal onset zone. This occurs particularly in nonlesional extratemporal lobe epilepsy or

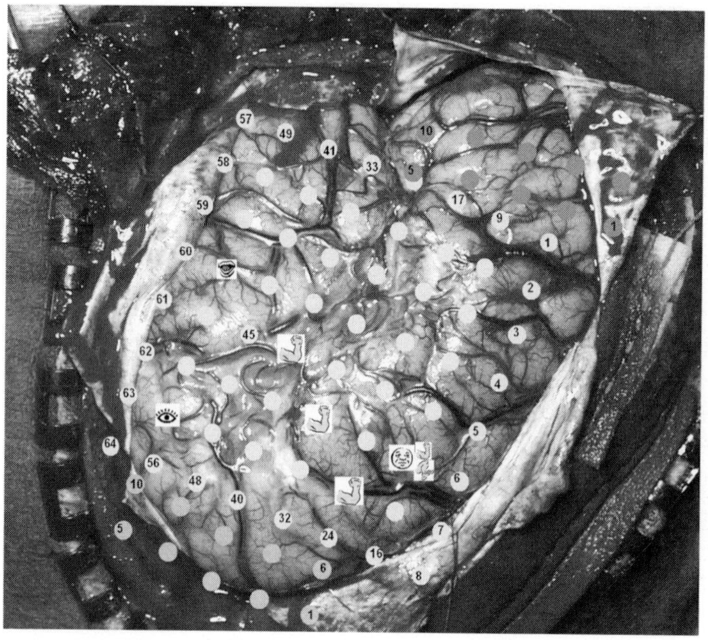

Figure 18.26 *Mapping of eloquent brain function using cortical stimulation. (See Plate 5.)*

when the zone is close to eloquent brain function, such as language and the motor area for the hand. The advances in high-resolution MRI, fMRI, and ictal single photon CT, subtraction ictal SPECT co-registered with MRI, and interictal PET reduce the need for invasive EEG or allow a more precise planning of invasive EEG monitoring.

Invasive EEG involves placing subdural strip and grid electrodes directly on the brain surface and/or the use of depth electrodes, which are placed directly within the substance of the brain (Figure 18.25). There are limitations to the amount of brain tissue that can be sampled with either method, which is a major limitation of invasive EEG. The cortex sampled must include the entire ictal generator. Hence, it is important to acquire as much data as possible noninvasively before determining the area to be studied with intracranial electrodes. Invasive EEG requires a craniotomy in the case of subdural grid electrodes and burr holes for depth or strip electrodes. The venous anatomy may interfere with the planned placement of subdural electrodes and the risk of hemorrhage may prevent adequate coverage of the brain region of interest. Other potential complications include infection, anesthesia risks and incorrect localization of the epileptogenic zone. The potential benefits of invasive EEG monitoring are precise localization of the ictal onset zone, and mapping of eloquent brain function using direct cortical stimulation (Figure 18.26) and somatosensory evoked responses (Figure 18.27). This reduces the risk of loss of function following cortical resection and indicates when multiple subpial transections may be a safer approach.

Ambulatory EEG monitoring

Ambulatory EEG involves continuous recording of EEG activity, during which time the patient may continue normal activities. It is important that the clinician clearly define the specific question that the ambulatory EEG is expected to answer. It is often useful in the differentiation of epileptic from nonepileptic behaviors, when these occur frequently. Ambulatory EEG usually does not answer the specific question raised if events do not occur at least several times each week. Ambulatory EEG may also be used with simultaneous neuropsychological assessment, which can permit subtle clinical events to be recognized. Finally, it can also be used to assess epileptiform activity occurring in sleep. This may be important in children with regression in language function, or with nocturnal episodes of uncertain nature. It is important to recognize that some types of partial epilepsy may not be associated with a surface ictal EEG abnormality and absence of an EEG abnormality does not preclude a diagnosis of epilepsy. This is particularly important when attempting to distinguish between frontal lobe epilepsy and a parasomnia (see section above on autosomal dominant nocturnal frontal lobe epilepsy). In this situation, video-EEG monitoring permits the clinical event to be studied in addition to the EEG and may be more useful.

Ambulatory EEG monitoring is less expensive than video-EEG monitoring and can be performed on an outpatient basis. However, setting up the patient, instruction on how to use the system, and analysis of the data are labor

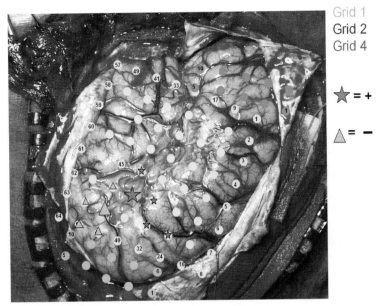

Grid 1
Grid 2
Grid 4

★ = +

△ = −

Figure 18.27 *Median nerve somatosensory evoked potential demonstrating area of maximum positivity and negativity on the cortical grid electrodes. Stars indicate positive areas, triangles negative. (See Plate 6.)*

intensive. Ambulatory systems are battery operated and most require recharging after 24 h. Thus, the patient must return to the laboratory if monitoring needs to be performed for longer than 24 h. The system may be programmed to save a sample of interictal EEG each hour and to record events where the event marker is pressed. Several minutes of EEG are usually saved before the event marker is pressed, in addition to the recording of the event. The system may also be programmed to record continuously in sleep. Technical problems such as artifacts from poor electrode contact and touching the electrodes affect the quality of the EEG information. Finally, ambulatory systems are expensive and fragile, and may be damaged when they are used for patients with major behavioral problems.

High-resolution EEG

The usual number of scalp electrodes used in clinical EEG is 19, in addition to the reference electrodes. Such a number of electrodes spread over the entire scalp represents a fairly low density electrode array. This has been the clinical standard for some 20 years. Under normal circumstances, such an electrode array may have difficulty differentiating signals arising from either hemisphere. Using electrodes arrays up to 128 channels, Gevins et al.[31] demonstrated the superiority in localization of higher density arrays. In clinical practice it is difficult to contemplate application of 128 channels on a routine basis. Under certain circumstances, this may be completely justified and necessary.

The EEG recorded with high density arrays affords a much improved view of the topography around regions of interests. With 128 electrodes, the interelectrode distance is approximately 2–2.5 cm in children, which approximates the minimum practical distance to physically apply electrodes of ~5 mm diameter. This yields higher spatial definition of focal signals, allowing more accurate pinpointing of spike locations. It can be demonstrated that recording the same event with 19 scalp channels may produce localization errors of up to several centimeters.[32] Although this may not be of critical importance in the identification or diagnosis of epilepsy, it is best avoided during preoperative investigations. The placement of subcortical grid electrode arrays must completely cover the cortical region responsible for generating ictal events. The placement is guided by the scalp localization of recorded seizures. Should the latter be mislocalized, then the grid electrode placement would be subject to unacceptably large errors, not conducive to good surgical outcome.

EEG recorded from scalp electrodes is subject to dispersion from volume conduction, attenuation through poorly conducting bone, regional variation of bone thickness, different degradation of different frequency components, etc., so that the final result is a poor version of the real cortical signal. High-resolution EEG allows the calculation of the negative effects of scalp, skull and soft tissue, and further allows a rigorous mathematical approach to remove these confounding effects. Such a procedure is essentially a computed approximation to the recording of the same signals directly from cortical

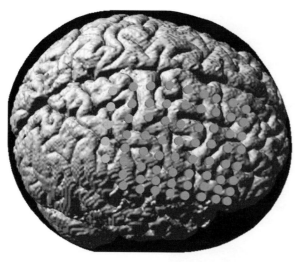

Figure 18.28 *Segmentation result of the patient's brain after removal of extracranial tissue. Dots denote the superimposed subdural grid electrode positions. (See Plate 7.)*

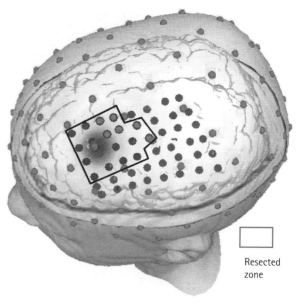

Resected zone

Figure 18.29 *Same patient, with scalp/skull tissues rendered semi-transparent. Scalp and subdural grid electrodes are displayed. The resection zone is indicated by the black line. (See Plate 8.)*

surface (e.g. subdural grid recording). Gevins *et al.*[33] described their approach using a 'deblurring' technique, comparing the results with direct cortical recordings in human somatosensory evoked potentials. They demonstrated an acceptably high degree of accuracy. A side benefit is the availability of the exact cortical location underneath each scalp electrode position. This is done with computer software graphical manipulation of high-resolution MRI scan of the same patient's head, a process called **segmentation**, where all tissues down to the cortical surface are removed, resulting in an accurate rendering of the patient's brain surface, upon which the electrode positions can be superimposed (Figure 18.28). From this point on, one can then describe EEG signals as coming from a specific point on the cortical surface, rather than from a nominal position (e.g. T4) not exactly defined.

High-resolution EEG requires the co-registration of all the scalp electrodes referenced to known anatomic landmarks – usually nasion, inion and preauricular points. This is usually done by either a 3D measuring arm (electromagnetic measuring device) or digital calipers. This procedure calculates the exact position of each electrode within the framework of the skull, and allows the placement of each electrode on to the MRI of the patient's head (Figure 18.29). The latter can be any other radiological dataset (e.g. brain scan, PET, SPECT, fMRI etc.). Co-registration is required whenever we wish to superimpose datasets with each other. This permits viewing of one kind of data against the background of the patient's own brain anatomy, an obvious advantage over brain surgery carried out on the basis of intraoperative pencil drawings superimposed on to textbook figures of a brain.

The documentation of cortical surface features can best be done with good-quality digital photographs

taken just before and after the placement of grid electrodes. This provides unambiguous knowledge of the relationship of each of the grid electrodes to cortical surface landmarks. Once it has been decided which of the grid electrodes are active in seizure generation – the **seizure generator zone** – these can be marked on the digital photograph, then the electrode arrays can be removed while leaving these marks in place to denote the area of cortex to be resected. A third photograph should be taken before closure of the craniotomy in order to document the exact cortical area resected. Needless to say, all three photographs must be taken from the same vantage point with the same camera angle in order to be comparable (Figure 18.30).

Seizures recorded from ECoG electrode grid arrays can be visually analyzed in order to determine the cortical regions responsible for the events. Computer analysis using statistical techniques can also play a role in facilitating this process, although this type of analysis is still in the developmental stage and has not yet reached clinical application.

Using the above techniques, it is now routinely possible to view the estimated seizure generator zone superimposed on to a picture of the patient's cortical surface. With advanced computer techniques, one can anticipate even further improvement in accuracy, an obvious advantage for presurgical investigation. However, this comes at a price. Whereas the application of 19 scalp electrodes with low impedances will require some 20 min, the application of an electrode cap device with 128 channels in a cooperative child may require 2 h with practice. This will provide a set of stable electrodes with low impedance that can be maintained for several hours

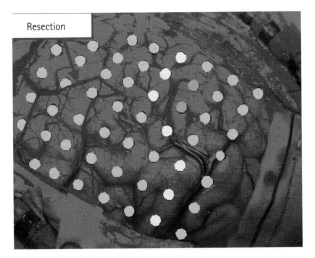

Figure 18.30 *Digital photograph of exposed craniotomy site, showing cortical features with resection zone marked. Dots denote subdural grid electrodes. (See Plate 9.)*

Resection

before deterioration. Only in patients with very frequent seizures can such a situation result in the harvesting of representative seizures of good technical quality. Future developments in high-density scalp electrode systems need to include the production of stable recording characteristics for several days.

Magnetoencephalography (MEG)

MEG is the measurement of very weak magnetic fields generated by ionic currents within the brain. Like EEG, MEG is recorded extracranially at multiple locations on the scalp. Despite differences in instrumentation and amplifier systems, the final output may be produced in its basic analog form and may be indistinguishable from EEG. The neural structures responsible for generation of extracranial magnetic field are similar to those producing scalp potentials recorded by EEG.[34] The differences between EEG and MEG are:

- MEG measures postsynaptic intracellular currents within similarly aligned apical dendrites of pyramidal cells tangential to the skull, i.e. in the cortical sulci, whereas EEG measures extracellular postsynaptic currents of pyramidal apical dendrites positioned both tangentially and radially, i.e. on gyri and in the sulci.
- MEG is a true monopolar measure of the magnetic field strength at a chosen extracranial site with no reference required while EEG signals are influenced by the reference.
- The conductive properties of the skull produce less distortion of MEG than of EEG.
- MEG shows increased spatial resolution over time.

Since the introduction of SQUID (superconducting quantum interference device) magnetometers in the 1970s, MEG has become somewhat more practical. SQUID can be regarded as a superconducting current amplifier. One of the major clinical applications of MEG has been in human seizure disorders as a noninvasive adjunct to the EEG both for detecting interictal and ictal phenomena and for localization of the epileptogenic zone in patients evaluated for epilepsy surgery and to locate normally functioning cerebral cortex prior to surgery. MEG is recorded from a matrix of closely spaced points centered on the anticipated region of the epileptic focus. Although there are many centers studying MEG, its role in the diagnosis and management of epilepsy and in the presurgical evaluation of patients remains undefined.

KEY POINTS

- The EEG can play an important role in:
  - the **diagnosis** of epilepsy
  - **classification** of the epileptic seizure type and epilepsy syndrome
  - **localization** of the epileptogenic zone
  - the **assessment** of the response to treatment
  - estimation of the risk of **seizure recurrence** after discontinuation of antiepileptic medication
- Recordings should include at least referential, longitudinal and coronal bipolar **montages**. Bipolar montages have the advantages of localization by phase reversal, less contamination and less movement artifact but pose difficulty when the EEG abnormalities are at the end of a chain.
- Epileptiform activity may be limited to light sleep in many individuals with epilepsy and **an EEG without sleep is an incomplete recording**.
- It is important to appreciate the normal **maturation patterns** of the EEG and to recognize **normal variants**, which have a low association with epileptic seizures.

REFERENCES

1. Zivkin L, Ajmone-Marsan C. Incidence and prognostic significance of 'epileptiform' activity in the EEG of non-epileptic subjects. *Brain* 1968; **91**: 751–778.
2. Metrakos K, Metrakos JD. Genetics of convulsive disorders. II. Genetic and electroencephalographic studies in centrencephalic epilepsy. *Neurology* 1961; **11**: 474–483.
3. American Electroencephalographic Society Guidelines in Electroencephalography, Evoked Potentials, and Polysomnography. *Journal of Clinical Neurophysiology* 1994; **11**(1): 1–147.

4. Jasper HH. The ten-twenty electrode system of the International Federation. *Electroencephalography and Clinical Neurophysiology* 1958; **10**: 371–375.

5. Risinger MW, Engel J, Van Ness PC, Henry TR, Crandal PH. Ictal localization of temporal lobe seizures with scalp/sphenoidal recordings. *Neurology* 1989; **39**: 1288–1293.

6. Sadler RM, Goodwin J. Multiple electrodes for detecting spikes in partial complex seizures. *Canadian Journal of Neurological Science* 1989; **16**: 326–329.

7. Sperling MR, Mendius JR, Engel J Jr. Mesial temporal epilepsy: a simultaneous comparison of sphenoidal, nasopharyngeal and ear electrodes. *Epilepsia*, 1986; **27**: 81–86.

8. Berger H. Uber das Elektroenzephalogramm des Menschen. *Archiv fur Psychiatrie und Nervenkrank* 1929; 87: 527–570 (for English translation see ref. 9).

9. Gloor P. *Hans Berger: On the Electroencephalogram of Man.* Amsterdam: Elsevier, 1969; 157–160.

10. Wong PKH. *Digital EEG in Clinical Practice.* Philadelphia: Lippincott-Raven, 1996.

11. Nuwer MR, Comi G, Emerson R, *et al.* IFCN Standards for digital recording of clinical EEG. *Electroencephalography and Clinical Neurophysiology* 1998; **106**: 259–261.

12. Binnie CD, Veldhuizen R, Beintema DJ. Evaluation of recording after sleep deprivation in the diagnostic EEG assessment of epilepsy. *Electroencephalography and Clinical Neurophysiology* 1982; **54**: 21–22.

13. Degen R, Degen HE. Sleep and sleep deprivation in epileptology. In: Degen R, Niedermeyer E (eds) *Epilepsy, Sleep and Sleep Deprivation.* Amsterdam: Elsevier, 1984; 273–286.

14. Epstein MA, Duchowny M, Jayakar P, Resnick TJ, Alvarez LA. Altered responsiveness during hyperventilation-induced EEG slowing: a non-epileptic phenomenon in normal children. *Epilepsia* 1994; **35**(6): 1204–1207.

15. Lum L, Connolly MB, Farrell K, Wong PKH. Hyperventilation induced high amplitude rhythmic slowing with altered awareness: a video-EEG comparison with absence seizures. *Epilepsia* 2002; **43**(11): 1372–1378.

16. Marks DA, Katz A, Scheyer R, Spencer SS. Clinical and electrographic effects of acute anticonvulsant withdrawal in epileptic patients. *Neurology* 1991; **41**: 508–512.

17. Wilder BJ. Activation of epileptic foci in psychomotor epilepsy. *Epilepsia* 1969; **10**: 418 (abstract).

18. Eeg-Olofsson O. The development of the EEG in normal children from age 1 to 15 years. The 14 and 6 positive spike phenomenon. *Neuropaediatrie* 1971; **4**: 405–427.

19. Eeg-Oloffson O, Pedersen I, Sellden U. The development of the electroencephalogram in normal children from the age of 1 through 15 years. Paroxysmal activity. *Neuropaeditrie* 1971; **2**: 375–404.

20. Eeg-Olofsson O. The development of the electroencephalogram in normal adolescents from the age of 16 through 21 years. *Neuropaediatrie* 1971; **3**: 11–45.

21. Lombroso CT. Neonatal EEG polygraphy in normal and abnormal newborns. In: Niedermeyer E, Lopes da Silva F (eds) *Electroencephalography: Basic Principles, Clinical Applications and Related Fields*, 3rd edn. Baltimore: Williams and Wilkins, 1993; 803–876.

22. Rose A, Lombroso CTL. Neonatal seizure states. *Pediatrics* 1970; **45**: 404–425.

23. Gastaut H. Etude electroencephalographique de la reativite des rhythmes rolandiques. *Revue Neurologique (Paris)* 1952; **87**: 176–182.

24. Gregory DL, Wong PK. Topographical analysis of the centrotemporal discharges in benign Rolandic epilepsy of childhood. *Epilepsia* 1984; **25**: 705–711.

25. Gregory DL, Wong PKH. Clinical relevance of a dipole field in Rolandic spikes. *Epilepsia* 1992; **33**: 36–44.

26. Langill L, Wong PKH. Tactile-evoked rolandic discharges – a benign finding? *Epilepsia* 2003; **2**: 221–227.

27. Scheffer IE, Bhatia KP, Lopes-Cendes I, *et al.* Autosomal dominant nocturnal frontal lobe epilepsy. *Brain* 1995; **118**: 61–73.

28. Roger J, Dravet C, Bureau M. The Lennox-Gastaut syndrome. *Cleveland Clinic Journal of Medicine* 1989; **56**: S172–180.

29. Gibbs FA, Gibbs EL. *Atlas of Electroencephalography: Epilepsy.* Cambridge, MA: Addison-Wesley, 1952; 2.

30. Blume WT, Pillay N. Electrographic and clinical correlates of secondary bilateral synchrony. *Epilepsia* 1985; **26**: 636–641.

31. Gevins A, Le J, Martin N, Brickett P, Desmond J, Reutter B. High resolution EEG: 124 channel recording, spatial deblurring and MRI integration methods. *Electroencephalography and Clinical Neurophysiology* 1994; **90**(5): 337–358.

32. Wong PKH, Bjornson B, Connolly M, *et al.* High resolution EEG and seizure localization. Proceedings of Human Brain Mapping Conference, Dusseldorf, Germany. *NeuroImage* 1999; **9**(6) Part II: S601.

33. Gevins A, Le J, Smith S. Deblurring. *Journal of Clinical Neurophysiology* 1999; **16**(3): 204–213.

34. Barth DS, Di S. The electrophysiological basis of epileptiform magnetic fields in neocortex. *Brain Research* 1990; **550**: 35–39.

19

Imaging

Anatomical imaging

RUBEN I KUZNIECKY

The impact of modern neuroimaging in the investigation and diagnosis of patients with neurologic diseases has been enormous. The impact in the management of patients with seizures and epilepsy can not be overemphasized, considering the high sensitivity and exquisite degree of anatomical resolution and metabolic information now available with different imaging techniques.[1–5] The most compelling example of this impact has been in the diagnosis of mesial temporal sclerosis. This entity was exclusively a pathologic diagnosis until a decade ago. Now, with MRI, this entity can be demonstrated *in vivo*.[6] The impact of this and other techniques extends beyond the simple detection of epileptic lesions by contributing to the proper classification of epileptic disorders and by delineating the genetics underlying some epileptic conditions. Lastly, modern neuroimaging techniques have directly and indirectly advanced our understanding of the basic pathophysiologic processes associated with the epilepsies.

This chapter compares the different anatomical imaging modalities and their specific role in children with seizures and epilepsy. It also discusses some of the special technical requirements and problems encountered when imaging the pediatric brain. The use of specific imaging modalities in neonates is briefly discussed.

TECHNICAL CONSIDERATIONS

Sedation

Appropriate and safe sedation is of paramount importance in the imaging of children.[7] Our experience suggests that is better not to initiate an examination without appropriate sedation because it is likely that motion artifact will render the examination invalid. This is particularly the case with MRI studies, which are highly sensitive to motion artifact. There are a number of sedation protocols using different drugs and routes of administration. Oral chloral hydrate is widely popular (50–100 mg/kg) but intravenous sodium pentobarbital is used in many centers. Proper physiologic monitoring with MR-compatible equipment is now available and should include heart and respiratory rate, blood pressure and oxygen and carbon dioxide concentrations following accepted sedation guidelines. In many medical centers, properly certified sedation teams have been successful by being cost effective and by providing optimal safety for imaging studies.

Scanning techniques

Although the techniques for scanning children are almost similar to those used for adults, there are a few technical aspects to be considered. CT studies should be done with thin slices (at least 5 mm) in all children. In view of the high water content of a newborn brain, appropriate windowing should be performed.

MRI studies should include a T1 weighted sagittal sequence to examine the midline structures. Axial images are done using the sagittal scout. It is important to obtain T1 and T2 information because of the maturational changes occurring during the first 18 months of life.[8] This is discussed further in the MRI section. In general, T1 images provide optimal anatomical delineation and T2 images provide the best sensitivity for water and iron containing lesions. The use of gradient echo images (for calcifications) and gadolinium diethylenetriamine pentaacetic acid

(Gd-DTPA) contrast agents is in general more limited and should be guided by the possible pathology.

To complete the study, we routinely acquire a 3D sequence yielding 1–1.5 mm images without gaps. This sequence is extremely useful to study the hippocampal structures and to detect small areas of focal cortical dysplasia. These images can be reconstructed in any plane with multiple angulations in a relatively short time. Over the past years, we have elected to routinely obtain inversion recovery sequences (IR) because they provide improved T1-weighted contrast and FLAIR (fluid attenuated inversion recovery) sequences in view of their excellent T2 contrast without CSF distortion. FLAIR sequences provide similar image quality in older children and adults. A host of new MR sequences are available as technology advances with improvement in speed and tissue contrast. Thus, it is difficult to provide protocols and image sequences since they are likely to be outdated in the very near future.

Contrast agents

CT contrast should not be given routinely in children with epilepsy. It should only be used if an abnormality is suspected in the initial uncontrasted scan. CT contrast agents doses should be 3 mL/kg up to a total dose of 120 mL. Similarly, MR contrast is in general of little use unless the pathology indicates a need for contrast or the initial images suggest an abnormality. Diagnostic information may be enhanced by MRI contrast use in patients with epilepsy and underlying expanding structural lesions, vascular malformations and Sturge-Weber syndrome.

IMAGING MODALITIES

Skull radiography

Skull radiography has a very limited role in the neuroimaging of children with epilepsy. In head trauma, skull radiographs may reveal linear fractures but CT provides both excellent bone and intracranial imaging information. Skull radiography is more helpful in operative planning such as the assessment of bone flaps, and to visualize the position of grids, strips and depth electrodes after electrode implantation. Its complementary role to MRI in patients with intracranial calcifications is marginal. Skull radiographs are useful for screening patients suspected of having non-compatible cranial MR material prior to MRI. Because of its limited diagnostic role in epilepsy, skull radiography will not be discussed further.

Cranial ultrasonography

Ultrasonography is a noninvasive, inexpensive, portable, real-time and multiplanar imaging modality well suited for the study of infants during the perinatal period. Except for special circumstances, ultrasonography is the imaging modality of choice to study premature infants.[9] It can provide an accurate delineation of the main brain structures, permit an accurate diagnosis of various lesions and may aid in the identification of etiologic and pathogenic factors associated with seizures. Ultrasonography can be used routinely in preterm infants through the anterior and posterior fontanels, and the examination can be performed in the neonatal unit with monitoring and adequate temperature control.

Ultrasound signals represent variations in acoustic reflections of tissues and tissue interfaces so that echogenic structures and sonolucent structures may be separated from one another and from the more uniform brain substance. Ultrasonography is operator-dependent and requires a window for adequate imaging. Cranial ultrasonography is most effective for viewing echogenic structures, intraventricular, periventricular, and intracerebral lesions (hemorrhage) as well as sonolucent structures such as CSF and other fluid-containing lesions, such as hydrocephalus.[10]

Ultrasonography is useful in its application to preterm infants with seizures. It is useful in the diagnosis of neonatal hypoxic-ischemic encephalopathy, suspected developmental malformations, infections, microcephaly and hemorrhagic manifestations of anoxic-ischemic injury.[10] It can also effectively image the evolution of ischemic injury, as well as the progression or resolution of hemorrhages or its consequences.[11]

Ultrasonography has also been used in the study of developmental anomalies of the ventricular system, including hydrocephalus, anomalies of the corpus callosum and other malformations. Although useful, it is not considered the procedure of choice for the delineation of developmental abnormalities of the CNS: MRI is preferred for the study of these malformations. In infants with macrocephaly and seizures, ultrasonography can provide an assessment of ventricular size for hydrocephalus or other pathologic entities associated with enlarged head size, but CT or MRI provides important additional information in such cases.

Although ultrasonography is extremely useful, MRI is often necessary for a definitive diagnosis. Because ultrasonography is limited to a well-defined population of infants, it will not be discussed further.

CT

CT uses ionizing radiation and can generate excellent hard-tissue imaging contrast with moderately good soft tissue resolution. The strengths of CT are its low cost, ready accessibility and easy use, which provides a relatively reliable imaging modality for unstable patients. Modern CT scanners can generate images of the brain in seconds.

The role of CT in the study of patients with epilepsy has been profoundly altered by the development of MRI. However, CT is still the technique of choice in the investigations of patients with seizures and epilepsy under certain conditions. In the neonate and young infant, CT is often of secondary or adjunctive importance, but it serves as a significant backup role to ultrasonography. This is particularly true if the ultrasound window is lost with age. A CT scan can accurately detect hemorrhage, infarctions, gross malformations, ventricular system pathologies and lesions with underlying calcification.[12–14]

The sensitivity of CT in patients with epilepsy has been reported to be approximately 30 per cent.[15–18] However, most studies are difficult to compare because of divergent patient selection criteria or technical differences. Nevertheless, CT has high sensitivity for the detection of hemispheric pathology such as tuberous sclerosis, Sturge-Weber syndrome or cerebral infarction. Unfortunately, CT has a low sensitivity overall because of poor resolution in the temporal fossa. Thus it is not surprising that CT is unable to detect mesial temporal sclerosis, the most common pathology in temporal lobe epilepsy.[19]

CT scan is the diagnostic imaging of choice in children with epilepsy if MRI is not available. It must be pointed out, however, that studies have shown that CT may fail to detect abnormalities in up to 40 per cent of patients with epileptogenic structural lesions such as small tumors and vascular malformations.[20] Contrast CT studies may provide useful information if the plain CT suggest an abnormality. In addition, CT may add information about bony involvement. CT is the technique of choice in the perioperative stage because it can rapidly detect recent hemorrhage, hydrocephalus and major structural changes.[4] Although highly diagnostic, the role of CT in the diagnosis of tuberous sclerosis, Sturge-Weber sydrome or other conditions with intracranial calcifications is complementary since MRI provides more information (noncalcified tubers).[21,22]

MRI

MRI is the imaging procedure of choice in the investigation of children with epilepsy.[23–25] The advantages of MRI include the use of nonionizing radiation, high sensitivity and higher specificity than CT scan, multiplanar imaging capability, improved contrast of soft tissue and high anatomical resolution.

Before we discuss the role of MRI in epilepsy, we should consider the important issue of brain maturation and myelination. It is important to recognize that interpretation of MRI in the infant must consider the normal development and maturational changes observed through

the first 2 years of life. In the neonate, the sylvian and posterior interhemispheric fissures are prominent and the cisterna magna and basilar cisterns are large. These normal findings should not be misinterpreted as atrophy. In addition, maturational changes are extremely important and can be studied with MRI.[8] Briefly, from birth to 6 months, the white matter is hyperintense relative to the gray matter on T2 weighted images. Between 6 and 18 months of age, the white matter slowly becomes hypointense (like the adult brain) in the same sequence. This means that during the first 6 months of life, T2 weighted images are necessary to detect cortical abnormalities and T1 contrast images are necessary to study brain maturation. After 6 months, the role of each sequence in assessing maturation and structure is reversed, with T2 weighted images necessary for maturational assessment. Failure to acquire both sequences and to understand the normal maturational process may result in improper image interpretation or underdetection of pathology.[26] Furthermore, the process of myelination takes place in an organized pattern and deviations of this pattern should be recognized. Myelination follows an anterior to posterior and midline to lateral pattern, with the frontal lobes and midline structures first to myelinate.

The sensitivity of MRI in detecting abnormalities in infants and children is dictated by the pathologies underlying childhood epilepsies (Table 19A.1) and by the MRI techniques and experience of the interpreting physician. Developmental malformations constitute the most common underlying pathology in infants and young children with epilepsy.[23,27] Of all new cases of infantile spasms presenting to our institution over a 12-month period, developmental malformations accounted for 40 per cent of cases. In the past, reports suggested that MRI was relatively insensitive to the detection of developmental pathology in infants with West syndrome.[28] However, studies indicate that this could be related to the lack of use of both T1 and T2 weighted sequences, critical for proper diagnosis during the maturational process as described above.[26] Because of the difficulties described above, it is recommended that children with persistent seizures and a normal MRI (done before age 2 years) should have a

Table 19A.1 *Pathologic substrates of childhood epilepsy*

Developmental malformations
Tumors
Hippocampal sclerosis
Prenatal and perinatal destructive injury
Neurocutaneous disorders
Infammatory
Infectious
Metabolic disorders
Vascular malformations
Degenerative disorders

repeated MRI study before age 5. Repeated MRIs are also indicated when there is a change in seizure semiology or new neurologic findings.

MRI is the imaging technique of choice in the investigation of patients with developmental disorders or malformations of cortical development. MRI can accurately define most of these malformations *in vivo*. The range and complexity of cortical developmental malformations is great, and appropriate classification is of utmost importance.[29] The following section describes important features of the most common developmental malformations.

Focal cortical dysplasia (FCD)

FCD is one of the most common forms of localized developmental disorder diagnosed in patients with intractable focal epilepsy.[28–31] The characteristic pathological abnormalities of these lesions consist of disruption of cortical lamination with poorly differentiated glial elements and balloon cells. Since its original description by Taylor *et al.*,[32] FCD has been recognized to encompass a spectrum of changes. These range from mild cortical disruption without apparent giant neurons to the most severe forms in which cortical dyslamination, large bizarre cells and astrocytosis are present.[33] It is the presence of so-called **balloon cells** that differentiates FCD type I (without balloon cells) from type II (with balloon cells). FCD with balloon cells has been reported in patients with tuberous sclerosis and in patients without skin anomalies.[32] The balloon cells are probably the result of proliferation of abnormal cells in the ventricular germinal zone. It is unclear whether they are of glial or neuronal lineage.

The clinical features of patients with FCD are variable.[24,29,34–36] Seizures begin in the first decade of life, usually after age 2 or 3 years but sometimes shortly after birth. The seizures may be simple partial motor, complex partial, or secondarily generalized. The majority of patients have extratemporal cortical dysplasia. Visualization of these lesions is best achieved with MRI. CT can detect a large FCD but with low specificity. The MRI features often consist of an abnormal cortex (cortical mantle) with abnormal gray-white matter architecture. T2 weighting and FLAIR are particularly useful in the detection of FCD. The presence of T2-weighted abnormalities in the underlying white matter correlates with balloon cells typical of type II cortical dysplasia.[31] Since some of these lesions are relatively small, the MRI examination should be targeted to the clinically suspected regions using both 3D volume techniques and IR sequences. Surface coils may help in the detection of these lesions since they improve the signal-to-noise ratio. A number of studies have reported improved detection rates with surface coils. However, placement of a surface coil demands either suspicion of a lesion or a well-defined electroclinical syndrome to guide placement. For unknown reasons the

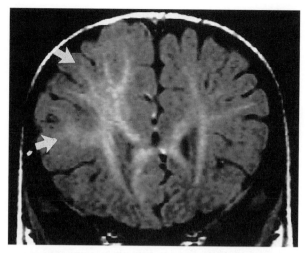

Figure 19A.1 *T1 weighted coronal image in a 6-month-old child with intractable seizures. Note abnormal frontal lobe (arrows). Size and gray-white matter pattern is abnormal. FCD found on pathology.*

frontal lobes and, in particular, the pre- and postcentral gyri are preferentially involved.[31,35,37] (Figure 19A.1).

FCD of the temporal lobe can also occur.[27,30] Involvement of both mesial and lateral neocortical structures can occur. Some patients have evidence of both mesial temporal sclerosis and neocortical cortical dysplasia (**dual pathology**). MRI shows cortical thickening of temporal convolutions associated with poor differentiation of the anterior temporal lobe gray-white junction. Bilateral amygdalo-hippocampal atrophy has been reported more commonly in these patients.[38] The pathology often shows type I cortical dysplasia. FLAIR and T2 weighted images often show these changes in the form of an abnormal gray-white matter junction.

Focal transmantle dysplasia

Focal transmantle dysplasia consists of a streak or column of abnormal cells, which extends from the ependyma to the pial surface, and the pathological appearance is similar to focal cortical dysplasia with balloon cells. Only a few patients with this entity have been described well in the literature, but experience suggests that this is not a rare condition. Diagnosis is based on the imaging features which consist of cortical thickening associated with a streak from the pial surface to the ventricular wall, well visualized on T2 weighted or FLAIR sequences.[39] In some patients, the column of abnormal cells is thick and can be visualized on T1 weighted images. The clinical and EEG features are similar to those of patients with FCD.

Cortical dysplasia with neoplastic changes

Several low-grade neoplasms have been associated with cortical dysplasia.[23] These include dysembryoplastic

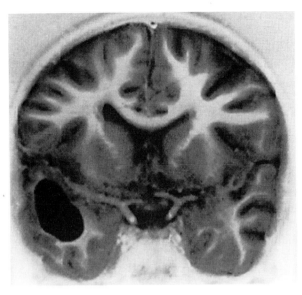

Figure 19A.2 *T1 weighted coronal MRI using IR. There is a large homogenous lesion involving the right temporal lobe. Note cystic component. DNET found on pathology.*

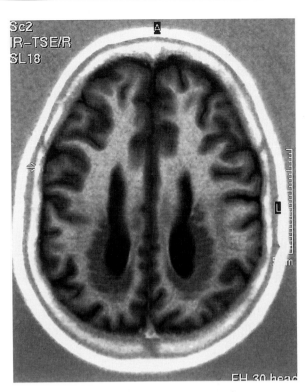

Figure 19A.3 *Laminar subcortical heterotopia. Gray matter surrounds the ventricles posteriorly. The underlying cortex appears to be normal. T1 weighted axial images.*

neuroepithelial tumor (DNET), ganglioglioma and gangliocytoma (Figure 19A.2). There is continuing controversy regarding the proper classification of these tumors. The frequency of these lesions in epilepsy surgical series is approximately 5–8 per cent, and they are seen most often in children or young adults. The tumors are most often located in the temporal lobes, where heterotopic neurons in the white matter are also common, but they can also be seen elsewhere.[13,40–42] The MRI appearance is characteristic, with moderately large cystic lesions without enhancement. T1 weighted images demonstrate hypointensity changes, with the opposite on T2 weighted images. Mass compression is often observed, but there is little perilesional edema. Ipsilateral hippocampal damage may be observed in some patients and may influence the surgical approach.

Heterotopia

Heterotopia are single or multiple nodules of gray matter which may be found in either a subcortical or subependymal location.[43] It is difficult to establish the true incidence of subependymal or subcortical heterotopia. Most patients with these conditions may present with developmental delay or mild pyramidal signs. Focal seizures associated with mild cognitive problems are frequent. Epilepsy may be the first symptom that brings medical attention or an imaging study.

Two major entities have been recognized by MRI: periventricular nodular heterotopia (PNH) and focal subcortical heterotopia. In typical periventricular subependymal heterotopia MRI is the diagnostic tool of choice since CT is unable to resolve these malformations because of its poor white/gray matter contrast. The heterotopic lesions consist of gray matter nodules in the subependymal region, most often in the trigone or in temporal or frontal white matter without underlying compression of the ventricles.[44,45] PNH are more frequent than single heterotopic lesions. At times the heterotopia has a laminar pattern (Figure 19A.3). In the familial form, a gene defect in the X chromosome has been found: the gene, Filamin 1, is crucial for neuronal migration along the radioglial fibers.[46]

In contrast to typical periventricular heterotopia, patients with subcortical heterotopia present with neurologic deficits since lesions are often localized in the pericentral region. Focal seizures are common and can be intractable. Subcortical heterotopia have no lobar predisposition, though the occipital lobes are less often involved. Identical twins discordant for subcortial heterotopia have been reported, suggesting that this entity is probably acquired rather than genetic.[47] The MRI often shows gray matter masses in the white matter of the temporal or frontal lobes. The lesions can range from small to large without mass effect (Figure 19A.4). If close to the ventricles, they may produce alterations in the regional anatomy. No abnormalities of the underlying vasculature are usually observed but large veins can be seen at times through the lesions.

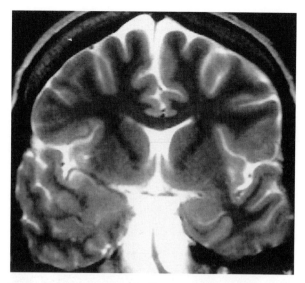

Figure 19A.4 *Focal subcortical heterotopia. Coronal T2 weighted image through temporal lobe showing abnormal cluster of gray matter in the right temporal lobe. The size of the temporal lobe is abnormal.*

Polymicrogyria/schizencephaly

Polymicrogyria is characterized by many small microgyri separated by shallow sulci, slightly thick cortex, neuronal heterotopia and often enlarged ventricles.[48] It often consists of areas of apparent pachygyria, which represent areas of fused gyri rather than true pachygyria. The best-known cause is intrauterine cytomegalovirus (CMV) infection, which is usually associated with diffuse or patchy white matter changes and often diffuse or multifocal periventricular calcifications.

The cortical abnormality is usually bilateral but may be either symmetrical or asymmetrical. Diffuse polymicrogyria may be truly diffuse, but often seems to spare the medial occipital region. Partial forms typically involve the frontal, perisylvian, parieto-occipital or mesial occipital regions or can be unilateral and involve one hemisphere. The CT appearance often suggests pachygyria, but high-resolution MRI or brain biopsy at the time of epilepsy surgery shows polymicrogyria rather than classical pachygyria.

Several families with bilateral perisylvian polymicrogyria appear to have X-linked dominant or autosomal recessive inheritance. Thus, the patterns of inheritance are unknown, although all are suspected to be genetic.

The clinical presentation in these conditions is variable except in the **congenital bilateral perisylvian syndrome** (CBPS) or **Kuzniecky syndrome**.[24,49–51] Patients with the congenital bilateral perisylvian syndrome have prominent pseudobulbar paresis, variable dysarthria and trouble swallowing. Motor involvement is dependent on the extent of the malformations. Seizures are reported in approximately 85 per cent of patients.

The diagnosis of CBPS can be made on the basis of the clinical features and can be confirmed by cranial MRI which is the imaging modality of choice. CT with thin cuts may show the perisylvian anomalies but MRI is more sensitive. The MRI demonstrates polymicrogyria in the perisylvian regions. Although the appearance of thick cortex may raise the suspicion of focal dysplasia or other malformation, the anatomical distribution is typical. The use of thin T1 weighted images is helpful in detecting the underlying small gyri or irregular inner and outer cortical surface typical of this condition. Further diagnostic improvement can be achieved by using surface coils or thin partition reconstruction. FLAIR or T2 weighted images do not show abnormal signal from the underlying cortex. The lesions may extend into the frontal or parietal areas, and may be symmetric though more often they are asymmetric. Calcifications are not observed and if present should raise doubts about the diagnosis.[24,49–51] The pathology in confirmed cases has been layered polymicrogyria.[52]

Focal unilateral polymicrogyria has typical clinical features with contralateral focal neurologic signs (pyramidal) and focal seizures. Outcome and features are not characteristics of any particular entity. However, a syndrome consisting of unilateral pericentral polymicrogyria and transient non-convulsive status epilepticus has been reported.[28] Patients present with epilepsy amenable to medical treatment until puberty when seizures become intractable and drop attacks develop. MRI shows typical changes in one opercular or perisylvian region with features consistent with polymicrogyria. It is important to examine the contralateral perisylvian region for subtle structural changes since polymicrogyria may be present. Other patient groups with bi-occipital, bifrontal or diffuse polymicrogyria have been reported. The imaging features are often similar to the ones described above for polymicrogyria.

Schizencephaly is included in the same category as polymicrogyria because the cortex around the lips of the cleft is polymicrogyric. Schizencephaly represents an extreme case of polymicrogyria.[53] Schizencephaly is morphologically classified according to the type of cleft, being either closed-lip (type I) or open-lip (type II).[53] Clinical manifestations are related to the type of defect, with type II clefts often associated with severe contralateral pyramidal signs and developmental delay. Callosal agenesis is also a marker for poor outcome. Seizures are usually focal but not necessarily intractable, with clinical variability observed.

MRI is the diagnostic modality of choice for accurate identification. The cleft extends from the ventricular wall to the pial surface. The cleft may be open, to the extreme of occupying an entire lobe or large part of an hemisphere. In those cases, semantic classification may question the difference between this entity and porencephaly.

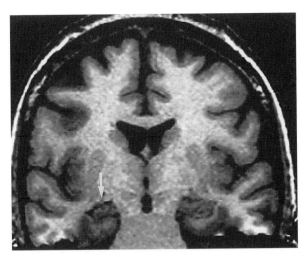

Figure 19A.5 *Mesial temporal sclerosis. T1 weighted images through hippocampal body showing atrophic hippocampus (arrow). In most patients the atrophy is in the body and varies from patient to patient.*

However, in schizencephaly, clusters of abnormal neurons are in the base and sides of the cleft while polymicrogyria borders the adjacent cortex. That is not found in porencephaly. Ventricles are usually normal unless compromised by the clefts.

Mesial temporal sclerosis (MTS)

MTS is the second major pathologic entity encountered in children with intractable epilepsy. This is pathologically characterized by the presence of a firm, atrophic hippocampus and the presence on histology of neuronal loss and gliosis in some of the hippocampal subfields. Until the advent of MRI, this entity was not diagnosed preoperatively. However, MRI is capable of detecting it with high sensitivity and specificity when hippocampal neuronal loss is at least 50 per cent. The typical MRI features of hippocampal sclerosis include:

* hippocampal atrophy (Figure 19A.5)
* increased signal on T2 weighted images or FLAIR
* decreased signal on IR sequence.

FLAIR has the advantage over regular T2 weighted sequences since it can resolve the hippocampus without the adjacent temporal horn CSF artifact. To best detect these abnormalities, the MRI study should be carried out with optimized imaging techniques. These include FLAIR and inversion recovery sequences which provide signal information. In addition, T1 weighted images provide the anatomical information needed. Although in the past it was desirable to obtain images using angulated coronal sections perpendicular to the long axis of the hippocampus, present software permits reconstruction of the images in any desirable plane and angle. Multiple images can be

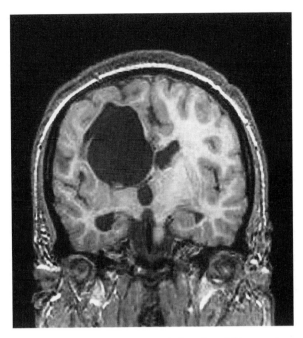

Figure 19A.6 *Congenital porencephaly and mesial temporal sclerosis. T1 weighted images through hippocampal body showing hippocampal atrophy (arrow) and ipsilateral porencephaly.*

obtained with thin slices without gap. Hippocampal volumetry is sensitive for lateralization of hippocampal atrophy. Multiple studies have reported similar findings with sensitivities ranging from 80 to 97 per cent. However, it is now clear that volumetry is not necessary in the majority of cases since qualitative assessment by trained observers can identify MTS in most patients.[54,55] A recent study from our laboratory indicates that a combination of techniques (anatomical resolution and signal alteration) is highly sensitive, with an overall 97 per cent detection rate when combined with volumetry.[6] Without volumetry, sensitivity was between 90 and 93 per cent. Mesial temporal sclerosis can also be detected in conjunction with other pathologies (dual pathology) as with cortical developmental malformations.

Ischemic injury

Early destructive or ischemic injuries constitute another major group of pathologies underlying diffuse or focal injury in children with epilepsy. The MRI appearance is dependent on the type and time of injury to the brain. Early injuries (first 6 months of gestation) will result in **porencephaly**. Late gestational, perinatal or postnatal injuries will result in **encephalomalacia** or **ulegyria**.[56] MRI can distinguish these conditions on the basis of imaging features.[7] Of importance however, is the fact that porencephaly can be associated with ipsilateral MTS (dual pathology), and MRI is of importance in the definition of the epileptic syndrome in these children (Figure 19A.6).

Encephalomalacias can be diffuse, as in anoxic injuries, or can be localized to the distribution of a cerebral artery branch. Ulegyria, which is less common, is typically localized to the posterior head regions (occipital lobe) with primary involvement of the sulci depth. Although porencephaly is common in children with epilepsy, it is not necessarily the cause of seizures.[57] Recent data suggest in fact, that most patients with porencephaly and seizures have temporal lobe seizures and associated MTS that can be detected with optimized techniques.[58]

NEW MR TECHNIQUES

New MR techniques are being applied to the study of patients with epilepsy. These techniques include magnetic resonance spectroscopy (MRS), magnetic resonance relaxometry (MRR) and functional magnetic resonance imaging (fMRI). It should be noted however, that limited data are available in children with epilepsy.

MRS can provide noninvasive biochemical measurements of specific brain metabolites.[59–62] In epilepsy, two major techniques have been applied ^{31}P (phosphorous) spectroscopy is designed to measure phospholipid metabolism and high-energy phosphate compounds. Studies in our laboratory[63] and others[62] have demonstrated a consistent abnormality in the epileptogenic region characterized by abnormal phosphocreatine/inorganic phosphate ratios. The pH, although at first thought to be alkaline in the epileptogenic focus, is normal as demonstrated by high-resolution MRS studies.[64]

^{1}H (proton) spectroscopy has demonstrated abnormalities of N-acetylaspartate (NAA), a mitochondrial neuronal compound, creatine and choline in patients with epilepsy. A consistent abnormality in NAA/creatine ratios has been found by several groups in correspondence with the epileptogenic focus in temporal and extratemporal lobe epilepsy[60,65,66] and in children.[67] The abnormal ratios may represent a drop in NAA due to neuronal dysfunction rather than pure neuronal loss and associated increases in creatine due to gliosis. The sensitivity of MRS appears higher than MRI.[68] Proton spectroscopy has also demonstrated bitemporal abnormalities in up to 40 per cent of patients, but the significance of these findings remains unclear. In other studies, Ng et al.[69] demonstrated a raise in lactate concentrations in the postictal state in the epileptogenic temporal lobe.

MRR for the evaluation of abnormal T1 and T2 signal has been applied to epilepsy. In hippocampal sclerosis, visually assessed hippocampal T2 weighted signal hyperintensity has typically been reported in 50–65 per cent of cases, with a range from 8 to 70 per cent.[70] Increased sensitivity for the detection of hippocampal pathology has been reported using T2 relaxation time as a quantitative measurement of tissue pathology in the hippocampal gray matter. In patients with temporal lobe epilepsy, approximately 80 per cent have abnormal ipsilateral T2 relaxation time with up to 30 per cent having abnormal contralateral hippocampal T2 values in addition to the ipsilateral abnormality; this may represent the bilateral hippocampal abnormalities described in pathology studies of hippocampal sclerosis.[71] The use of T2 relaxometry in other cortical regions is beginning to be explored.

fMRI has also been preliminarily applied to the study of seizure disorders. It utilizes very rapid scanning techniques that theoretically can demonstrate alterations in blood oxygenation. This technique has been applied to map functional areas before cranial surgery.[72] Since blood flow changes occur during seizures, it is theoretically possible to use this technique to demonstrate these abnormalities. Jackson et al.[73] demonstrated focal blood flow changes in a child with partial seizures using fMRI techniques. Detection of alterations in oxygenation in the epileptic focus may be possible using similar MR principles. fMRI has been applied to lateralized speech for surgery and motor function, with the advantage of being noninvasive. However, the technique is difficult in children because of motion. Recent experience suggests that with simple paradigms and training, children down to age 5–7 years are able to perform reliable tasks for fMRI. More recently, using bold techniques several investigators have been able to show blood flow changes linked to interictal discharges by using concurrent EEG/fMRI triggering techniques.

NEUROIMAGING IN PEDIATRIC EPILEPSY PRACTICE

Not all patients with epilepsy need neuroimaging studies. Such studies may not be necessary in patients with well-defined idiopathic generalized epilepsies such as childhood absence epilepsy (pyknolepsy). In addition, patients with typical idiopathic benign partial epilepsy with centrotemporal spikes may not require an imaging study. However, reports of patients with apparent generalized epilepsies or benign partial seizures in which structural abnormalities are seen on MRI have surfaced.[56] In general, the clinical course and the atypical features of such patients will identify those who require imaging studies. Similarly, patients with uncomplicated febrile convulsions and a normal neurological exam do not require imaging studies.

Conversely, all patients with symptomatic generalized or focal seizures should have a structural neuroimaging study. Since MRI is far superior to CT scan in the detection of structural lesions, it is suggested that MRI should be the imaging procedure of choice when evaluating children with seizures, especially if focal features are present on neurologic exam or EEG. In addition, MRI is indicated if seizures persist in the presence of a previously normal CT scan or when there are progressive neurological changes.

KEY POINTS

- **Cranial ultrasound** is the imaging modality of choice in premature infants. It can accurately delineate the main brain structures and may aid in identification of the etiology of the seizures. It is of limited value in detecting developmental abnormalities of the brain
- **CT head scan** can accurately detect hemorrhage, infarctions, gross malformations, ventricular system pathologies and lesions with underlying calcification
- CT is unable to detect **mesial temporal sclerosis**, the most common pathology in temporal lobe epilepsy, and may fail to detect abnormalities in up to 40 per cent of patients with epileptogenic structural lesions such as small tumors and vascular malformations
- **MRI is the imaging procedure of choice** in the investigation of children with epilepsy
- Major changes in MRI signal occur in the normal brain during the **first 2 years of life**. Children with persistent seizures and a normal MRI before 2 years of age should have a repeated MRI study before 5 years of age
- In general, **T1 images** provide optimal anatomical delineation while **T2 images** provide the best sensitivity for water- and iron-containing lesions. **Inversion recovery sequences** provide improved T1 weighted contrast and **FLAIR sequences** provide excellent T2 contrast without CSF distortion
- **Developmental brain malformations** are the most common underlying pathology in infants and young children with epilepsy and are delineated optimally using MRI
- **Mesial temporal sclerosis**, exclusively a pathologic diagnosis until a decade ago, can be detected by MRI in 90–97 per cent of cases
- Most patients with **porencephaly** and seizures have temporal lobe seizures and associated mesial temporal sclerosis that can be detected by MRI using optimized techniques

---

REFERENCES

1. Jackson G. New techniques in MR. *Epilepsia* 1994; **35**(6): S2–13.
2. Jackson GD, Connelly A, Duncan JS, Gadian DG, Grunewald RA. MRI detection of hippocampal pathology in intractable partial epilepsy: increased sensitivity with quantitative magnetic resonance T2 relaxometry. *Neurology* 1993; **43**: 1793–1799.
3. Cascino GD, Jack CR Jr, Parisi JE, *et al.*, Magnetic resonance imaging in intractable frontal lobe epilepsy: pathologic correlation and prognostic importance. *Epilepsy Research* 1992; **11**: 51–59.
4. Kuzniecky R, Jackson G. Neuroimaging in epilepsy. In: *Magnetic Resonance in Epilepsy.* New York: Raven Press, 1995: 27–48.
5. Kuzniecky R, Cascino GD, Palmini A, *et al.* Structural imaging. In: Engel JJ (ed) *Surgical Treatment of the Epilepsies*, 2nd edn. New York: Raven Press, 1993: 197–200.
6. Kuzniecky RI, Bilir E, Gilliam F, *et al.* Multimodality MRI in mesial temporal sclerosis: relative sensitivity and specificity. *Neurology*, 1997; **49**: 774–778.
7. Barkovich AJ. *Pediatric Neuroimaging*, 2nd edn New York: Raven Press, 1995: 668.
8. Barkovich A, Kjos BO, Jackson DE, Norman D. Normal maturation of the neonatal and infant brain: MR imaging at 1.5 T. *Radiology* 1988; **166**: 173–180.
9. Dubowitz LMS, Bydder GM, Mushin J. Developmental sequence of periventricular leukomalacia. Correlation of ultrasound, clinical, and nuclear magnetic resonance functions. *Archives of Disease in Childhood* 1985; **60**: 349–355.
10. Baarsma R, Laurini R, Baerts W, Okken A. Reliability of sonography in non-hemorrhagic periventricular leukomalacia. *Pediatric Radiology* 1987; **17**: 189–191.
11. Carson S, *et al.* Value of sonography in the diagnosis of intracranial hemorrhage and periventricular leukomalacia: a postmortem study of 35 cases. *AJNR* 1990; **11**: 677–684.
12. El Gammal T, Adams RJ, King DW, So EL, Gallagher BB. Modified CT techniques in the evaluation of temporal lobe epilepsy prior to lobectomy. *AJNR* 1987 **8**(1): 131–134.
13. Kishikawa H, Ohmoto T, Nishimoto A. Brain tumor with seizures in children. *Brain Development (Tokyo)* 1980; **12**(1): 19–26.
14. Kotagal P, Luders H. Recent advances in childhood epilepsy. *Brain and Development* 1994; **16**: 1–15.
15. Gastaut H, Gastaut JL. Computerized transverse axial tomography in epilepsy. *Epilepsia* 1976; **17**: 325–336.
16. Gastaut HL. Conclusions: computerized transverse axial tomography in epilepsy. *Epilepsia*, 1976; **17**: 337–338.
17. Heinz ER, Heinz TR, Radtke R, *et al.* Efficacy of MRI vs CT in epilepsy. *AJNR* 1988; **9**: 1123–1128.
18. Duncan R, Patterson J, Hadley DM, *et al.* CT, MR and SPECT imaging in temporal lobe epilepsy. *Journal of Neurology, Neurosurgery and Psychiatry* 1990; **53**(1): 11–15.
19. Babb TL, Pretorius JK. Pathological substrates of epilepsy. In: Wylie E (ed.) *The Treatment of Epilepsy: Principles and Practice.* Philadelphia: Lea & Febiger, 1993: 55–70.
20. Kuzniecky R, de la Sayette V, Ethier R, Melanson D, Andermann F. Magnetic resonance imaging in temporal lobe epilepsy: pathological correlations. *Annals of Neurology* 1987; **22**(3): 341–347.
21. Curatolo P, Cusmai R. Magnetic resonance imaging in the Bourneville syndrome: relations with EEG. *Neurophysiologie Clinique* 1988; **18**(5): 459–467.
22. Curatolo P, Cusmai R. The value of MRI in tuberous sclerosis. *Neuropediatrics* 1987; **18**(3): 184.
23. Kuzniecky R, Murro A, King D. Magnetic resonance imaging in childhood intractable partial epilepsies: Pathologic correlations. *Neurology* 1993; **43**: 681–687.

24. Guerrini R, Dravet C, Raybaud C, *et al.* Epilepsy and focal gyral anomalies detected by MRI: electroclinico-morphological correlations and follow-up. *Developmental Medicine and Child Neurology* 1992; **34**(8): 706–718.

25. Gulati P, Jena A, Tripathi RP, Gupta AK. Magnetic resonance imaging in childhood epilepsy. *Indian Pediatrics* 1991; **28**(7): 761–765.

26. Sankar R, Curran JG, Kevill JW, *et al.* Microscopic cortical dysplasia in infantile spasms: evolution of white matter abnormalities. *AJNR* 1995; **16**: 1265–1272.

27. Kuzniecky R, Ho SS, Martin R, *et al.* Temporal lobe developmental malformations and hippocampal sclerosis: epilepsy surgical outcome. *Neurology* 1999; **52**: 479–484.

28. Palmini A, Andermann F, Olivier A, *et al.* Neuronal migration disorders: a contribution to modern neuroimaging to the etiologic diagnosis of epilepsy. *Canadian Journal of the Neurological Sciences* 1991; **18**(4): 580–587.

29. Barkovich AJ, Kuzniecky RI, Jackson GD, Guerrini R, Dobyns WB. Classification system for malformations of cortical development: Update 2001. *Neurology* 2001; **57**: 2168–2178.

30. Kuzniecky R, Garcia JH, Faught E, Morawetz RB. Cortical dysplasia in TLE: MRI correlations. *Annals of Neurology* 1991; **29**: 293–298.

31. Kuzniecky R. Magnetic resonance imaging in developmental disorders of the cerebral cortex. *Epilepsia* 1994; **35**(6): S44–56.

32. Taylor DC, Falconer MA, Bruton CJ, Corsellis JAN. Focal dysplasia of the cerebral cortex in epilepsy. *Journal of Neurology, Neurosurgery and Psychiatry* 1971; **34**: 369–387.

33. Prayson RA, Estes M, Morris HH. Coexistence of neoplasia and cortical dysplasia in patients presenting with seizures. *Epilepsia* 1993; **34**: 609–615.

34. Barkovich A, Kuzniecky R. Neuroimaging of focal malformations of cortical development. *Journal of Clinical Neurophysiology* 1996; **13**:(6): 481–494.

35. Kuzniecky R, Berkovic S, Andermann F, *et al.* Focal cortical myoclonus and rolandic cortical dysphasia: clarification by MRI. *Annals of Neurology* 1988; **23**: 317–325.

36. Palmini A, Andermann F, Olivier A, Tampieri D, Robitaille Y. Focal neuronal migration disorders and intractable partial epilepsy: a study of 30 patients. *Annals of Neurology* 1991; **30**(6): 741–749.

37. Kuzniecky R, Powers R. Epilepsia partialis continua due to cortical dysplasia. *Journal of Child Neurology* 1993; **8**(4): 93–96.

38. Ho SS, Kuzniecky RI, Gilliam F, Faught E, Morawetz R. Temporal lobe developmental malformations and epilepsy: dual pathology and bilateral hippocampal abnormalities. *Neurology* 1998; **50**: 748–754.

39. Barkovich AJ, Kuzniecky RI, Bollen AW, Grant PE. Focal transmantle dysplasia: a specific malformation of cortical development. *Neurology* 1997; **49**: 1148–1152.

40. Koeller KK, Dillon WP. Dysembryoplastic neuroepithelial tumors: MR appearance. *AJNR* 1992; **13**: 1319–1325.

41. Peretti-Viton P, Perez-Castillo AM, Raybaud C, *et al.* Magnetic resonance imaging in gangliogliomas and gangliocytomas of the nervous system. *Journal of Neuroradiology* 1991; **18**(2): 189–199.

42. Daumas-Duport C. Dysembryoplastic neuroepithelial tumours. *Brain Pathology* 1993; **3**: 283–295.

43. Raymond AA, Fish DR, Sisodya SM, *et al.*, Abnormalities of gyration, heterotopias, tuberous sclerosis, focal cortical dysplasia, microdysgenesis, dysembryoplastic neuroepithelial tumor and dysgenesis of the archicortex in epilepsy. Clinical, EEG and neuroimaging features in 100 adult patients. *Brain* 1995; **118**(3): 629–660.

44. Harding B. Gray matter heterotopia. In: Guerrini R, Andermann F, Canapicchi R *et al* (eds) *Dysplasias of Cerebral Cortex and Epilepsy.* Lippincott-Raven: Philadelphia, 1995: 81–87.

45. Barkovich J, Kjos B. Nonlissencephalic cortical dysplasia: correlation of imaging findings with clinical deficits. *AJNR* 1992; **13**: 95–103.

46. Dobyns W, Andermann E, Andermann F. X-linked malformations of neuronal migration. *Neurology* 1996; **47**: 331–339.

47. Kuzniecky R, Gilliam F, Faught E. Discordant occurrence of cerebral unilateral heterotopia and epilepsy in monozygotic twins. *Epilepsia* 1995; **36**(11): 1155–1157.

48. Evrard P, Gaddisseux J, Lyon G. Les malformations du systeme nerveux. In: Royer P (ed.) *Naissance du cerveau.* Paris: Lafayette, 1982: 49–74.

49. Kuzniecky R, Andermann F, Tampieri D, *et al.*, Bilateral central macrogyria: epilepsy, pseudobulbar palsy and mental retardation: a recognizable neuronal migration disorder. *Annals of Neurology* 1989: **25**: 547–554.

50. Kuzniecky R, Andermann F, Guerrini R. Congenital bilateral perisylvian syndrome: study of 31 patients. *Lancet* 1993; **341**: 608–612.

51. Kuzniecky R, Andermann F. Congenital bilateral perisylvian syndrome: imaging findings in a multicenter study. *AJNR* 1994. **15**: 139–144.

52. Becker S, Dixon A, Troncoso J. Bilateral opercular polymicrogyria. *Annals of Neurology* 1989; **25**: 90–92.

53. Yakovlev P, Wadsworth R. Schizencephalies: a study of the congenital clefts in the cerebral mantle. I. clefts with fused lips. *Journal of Neuropathology and Experimental Neurology* 1946; **5**: 116–130.

54. Jack CR Jr, Sharbrough FW, Twomey CK, *et al.* Temporal lobe seizures: lateralization with MR volume measurements of the hippocampal formation. *Radiology* 1990; **175**(2): 423–429.

55. Jackson GD, Kuzniecky RI, Cascino GD. Hippocampal sclerosis without detectable hippocampal atrophy. *Neurology* 1994; **44**: 42–46.

56. Aicardi J. *Diseases of the Nervous System in Childhood.* London: MacKeith Press,1992.

57. Ho SS, Kuzniecky RI, Gilliam F, *et al.* Congenital porencephaly and hippocampal sclerosis. Clinical correlates. *Neurology* 1997; **49**: 1382–1388.

58. Ho SS, Kuzniecky RI, Gilliam F, *et al.* Congenital porencephaly: MR features and relationship to hippocampal sclerosis. *AJNR* 1998; **19**: 135–141.

59. Hetherington HP, Pan JW, Mason GF, *et al.* 2D 1H SI of the human brain at 4.1 T. *Magnetic Resonance in Medicine* 1994; **32**: 530–534.

60. Hetherington H, Kuzniecky R, Pan J, *et al.* Proton MRS in human temporal lobe epilepsy at 4.1 T. *Annals of Neurology* 1995; **38**(3): 396–404.

61. Gadian DG, Connelly A, Duncan JS. ^{1}H magnetic resonance spectroscopy in the investigation of intractable epilepsy. *Acta Neurologica Scandinavica* 1993; **152**: 116–122.

62. Laxer KD, Hubesch B, Sappey-Marinier D, Weiner MW. Increased pH and inorganic phosphate in temporal seizure foci, demonstrated by (31P) MRS. *Epilepsia* 1992; **33**: 618–623.

63. Kuzniecky R, Elgavish GA, Hetherington HP, Evanochko WT, Pohost GM. In vivo 31P nuclear magnetic resonance spectroscopy of human temporal lobe epilepsy. *Neurology* 1992; **42**(8): 1586–1590.

64. Chu WJ, Hetherington HP, Kuzniecky RJ, *et al.* Is the intracellular pH different from normal in the epileptic focus of patients with temporal lobe epilepsy? a 31 P NMR study. *Neurology* 1996; **47**: 756–760.

65. Connelly A, *et al.* Proton spectroscopy in the investigation of intractable temporal lobe epilepsy. In: *Book of Abstracts, Society of Magnetic Resonance in Medicine.* Berlin, 1992.

66. Cendes F, Caramanos Z, Andermann F, Dubeau F, Arnold DL. Proton MRSI and MRI volumetry in the lateralization of temporal lobe epilepsy: A series of 100 patients. *Annals of Neurology,* 1997; **42**: 737–746.

67. Cross H, Connelly A, Jackson GD, *et al.* Proton MRS in children with temporal lobe epilepsy. *Annals of Neurology* 1995; **39**: 107–113.

68. Kuzniecky R, Hugg JW, Hetherington H, *et al.* Relative utility of proton MRS and volumetry in the lateralization of mesial temporal sclerosis. *Neurology* 1998; **51**(1): 66–71.

69. Ng TC, Comair YG, Xue M, *et al.* Temporal lobe epilepsy: presurgical localization with proton chemical shift imaging. *Radiology* 1994; **193**: 465–472.

70. Jackson GD, Connelly A, Godian DG, *et al.* 1H MRS and T2 relaxometry of the contralateral temporal lobe after epilepsy surgery. *Epilepsia* 1993; **34**(Suppl. 6): 144.

71. Van Paesschen W, Sisodiya S, Connelly A, *et al.* Quantitative hippocampal MRI and intractable temporal lobe epilepsy. *Neurology* 1995; **45**: 2233–2240.

72. Detre JA, Sirven JI, Alsop DC, O'Connor MJ, French JA. Localization of subclinical ictal activity by functional magnetic resonance imaging: correlation with invasive monitoring. *Annals of Neurology* 1995; **38**: 618–624.

73. Jackson GD, Connelly A, Cross JH, Gordon I, Gadian DG. Functional magnetic resonance imaging of focal seizures. *Neurology* 1994: **44**: 1411–1417.

19B

Functional imaging

CSABA JUHÁSZ AND HARRY T CHUGANI

The advent of various types of high-resolution tomographic neuroimaging in recent years has had a significant impact on the diagnosis and management of epilepsy in children. Since epilepsy is primarily a **functional** disturbance of the brain, **functional neuroimaging** modalities, such as PET, SPECT and MRS are sensitive in detecting generalized and focal abnormalities in epilepsy. In general, the most common purpose in applying functional imaging to children with epilepsy is to localize the epileptogenic zone for surgical intervention. In some cases, abnormalities on FDG-PET and ictal SPECT can provide adequate localization so as to avoid the need for invasive intracranial EEG monitoring. However, when MRI findings are ambiguous or normal, or discordant with those of scalp EEG, localizing information from functional neuroimaging is used to guide the placement of intracranial electrodes for further localization of epileptogenic cortex. Functional imaging techniques using activation paradigms are also being used preoperatively to determine noninvasively **eloquent** (e.g. language, motor) cortex that should be preserved during resective epilepsy surgery.

MRI STUDIES OF BRAIN FUNCTION

fMRI

fMRI is a noninvasive technique to map activity of neural networks that underlie cognitive functions and epileptiform activity in both adults and children. The most commonly used technique is the blood oxygen level-dependent (BOLD) fMRI, which is based on a delayed (2–4 s after stimulus onset) change in oxy/deoxyhemoglobin ratio following regional brain activation. Application of fMRI in mapping brain activation in response to various tasks in children is particularly advantageous since it does not involve radiation exposure.

CLINICAL APPLICATIONS

There is no universally accepted clinical indication for fMRI.[1] In presurgical evaluation of children with intractable epilepsy, the two major goals of fMRI are:

- to localize eloquent cortex, and, ultimately, to replace invasive methods, such as the carotid amytal (Wada) test or direct cortical stimulation
- to aid in preoperative localization of the epileptic focus.

Cognitive functions investigated by fMRI in children have included working memory, spatial memory, verbal fluency, reading visual recognition, motor and sensory tasks.[2] fMRI was reported to be comparable in accuracy to the carotid amytal test for cerebral lateralization of language functions,[3] and may also provide clinically useful localizing information for sensory and motor function. In patients with intractable epilepsy, fMRI alone or combined with transcranial magnetic stimulation can demonstrate reorganization of motor function preoperatively,[4] thus predicting motor outcome following resection. The use of fMRI to identify the epileptic focus is feasible only in patients with very frequent seizures. Further, in patients with motor seizures or impaired cooperation during seizures, movement artifacts preclude meaningful data acquisition. There have been some promising attempts to localize interictal epileptiform activity using EEG-triggered fMRI,[5] and this potentially could become an additional noninvasive tool in presurgical evaluation.

INTERPRETATION

In children there are important physiologic and anatomic differences that may affect the acquisition, analysis and interpretation of pediatric fMRI data.[2] However, there appear to be some general similarities in the activation patterns observed between adults and 5–8-year-old children for various cognitive processes. Activation maps are fundamentally the same in normal children older than 8 years and adults. An obvious disadvantage of this technique is its sensitivity to motion artifacts. Patient cooperation, both in performing tasks and limiting motion, is often poor in young children, especially in those with cognitive impairment. Conditioning and personal interactions can improve compliance, and motion reduction techniques can successfully diminish artifacts due to head motion. In summary, fMRI holds the promise of being a safe, powerful clinical tool for noninvasive mapping of various brain functions in children with intractable epilepsy.

MRS

The MRS technique uses MRI equipment and the same radiofrequency coils, but is different from MRI in that it produces spectra that describe measurements of cellular energetics and metabolites. Proton (^{1}H) spectroscopy allows relative determinations of brain lactate, *N*-acetyl compounds (such as *N*-acetylaspartate (NAA)), various lipids, and can also be used to measure cerebral neurotransmitters, particularly γ-aminobutyric acid (GABA), glutamate and glutamine. Phosphorus (^{31}P) MRS is useful in the study of local high-energy phosphate levels *in vivo*.

CLINICAL APPLICATIONS

The sensitivity of MRS in lateralization of **temporal lobe epilepsy** (TLE) is about 90 per cent, similar to that of FDG-PET. Proton magnetic resonance spectroscopy (^{1}H-MRS) can provide evidence of temporal lobe abnormalities in TLE patients who show no abnormality on structural MRI. Phosphorus magnetic resonance spectroscopy (^{31}P-MRS) shows a decreased phosphocreatine/inorganic phosphate ratio in the epileptic temporal lobe compared both to controls and to the con-tralateral temporal lobe. Lateralization of the epileptic temporal lobe improves when a high-magnetic-field (4.1 Tesla) MR scanner is used to obtain ^{31}P-MRS data. In patients requiring intracranial EEG monitoring, a 78 per cent correspondence in lateralization was reported when using ^{31}P-MRS in contrast to a 33 per cent correspondence with MRI and 56 per cent correspondence with scalp EEG.[6]

^{1}H-MRS imaging (MRSI) can be useful in **extratemporal epilepsy**, showing widespread abnormalities greatest in the region of seizure focus. These abnormalities, however, do not appear to be specific for the epileptogenic region,[7] and the present limitation of sufficient spatial coverage limits clinical utility of MRSI in epilepsies of neocortical origin.

^{1}H-MRS has also been applied in the study of chronic **focal encephalitis** (Rasmussen syndrome). During epilepsia partialis continua, the lactate signal is usually increased in the area of seizure focus.[8] ^{1}H-MRS spectra acquired during focal status epilepticus in patients with cortical dysgenesis also show increased lactate, which recovers in the interictal state.[9]

Serial ^{1}H-MRS studies in children with **infantile spasms** who underwent ACTH therapy showed a reversible decrease of brain NAA concentration during the treatment period.[10] These findings may result from catabolic effects of ACTH on brain tissue, leading to cell loss, decrease in NAA synthesis in mitochondria, and/or leakage of NAA from cell membrane.

In vivo measurement of brain GABA levels by MRS is best achieved using high-magnetic-field MRI scanners that are currently not available in most epilepsy centers. The demonstration that brain GABA levels increase with vigabatrin therapy illustrates the ability of MRS to monitor effects of therapeutic interventions.[11] *In vivo* measurement of glutamate/glutamine concentration by MRS during prolonged seizures may contribute to a better understanding of the pathophysiology of seizure-related brain damage.[12]

INTERPRETATION

Decreased NAA on ^{1}H-MRS is considered to be a marker of neuronal loss and/or impaired neuronal function, although this concept has been challenged recently.[13] In TLE, bilateral temporal abnormalities commonly occur (in 35–45 per cent of cases) even in patients with unilateral seizure foci. Postsurgical increase of NAA levels in the nonresected contralateral temporal lobe following successful temporal lobectomy suggests that NAA abnormalities in patients with TLE are dynamic markers of both local and remote physiologic dysfunction associated with seizures.[14] Increased lactate concentration is a marker of impaired aerobic energy metabolism due to seizures or impaired mitochondrial function. Thus, ^{1}H-MRS can be used to document disturbances in oxidative metabolism in neurometabolic disorders, and occurrence of characteristic patterns of metabolite abnormalities may facilitate diagnosis of respiratory chain disorders.[15] Alterations of brain neurotransmitter concentrations measured by MRS in the ictal and interictal state may provide potentially valuable information on the pathomechanism of various types of epilepsy.

PET

PET is a noninvasive imaging method that can be used to measure local chemical functions in various body organs. The application of PET in the evaluation of children with epilepsy has had a significant impact on management, particularly when surgical intervention is being considered.

Basic concepts of PET methology

The PET technique employs a camera consisting of multiple pairs of oppositely-situated detectors which are used to record the paired high-energy (511 keV) photons traveling in opposite directions as a result of positron decay. Tracer kinetic models which mathematically describe physiological or biochemical reaction sequences of compounds labeled with positron-emitting isotopes permit a characterization of the kinetics and the mathematical expression for calculating actual rates of the biological process being studied. In the brain, PET has been applied in the study of local glucose (using the tracer 2-deoxy-2[^{18}F]fluoro-D-glucose [FDG]) and oxygen utilization, blood flow, protein synthesis, and neurotransmitter uptake and binding. Among several proposed PET tracers targeting various brain neurotransmitter systems, [^{11}C]flumazenil, (FMZ) has been quite extensively used in the past decade in several centers worldwide for measuring GABA$_A$ receptor binding. Others, such as [^{11}C]carfentanil for μ-opiate receptors, [^{11}C]doxepin for histamine H1 receptors, and (S)-[N-methyl-^{11}C]ketamine for NMDA receptors are potentially useful in detecting epileptic cortex, but have not been applied on a sufficient number of patients to determine whether they provide additional useful information. α-[^{11}C]methyl-L-tryptophan (AMT; an analog of the serotonin precursor tryptophan) is a promising new tracer that is being tested for its clinical utility to delineate epileptogenic brain regions.

FDG–PET studies

TEMPORAL LOBE EPILEPSY (TLE)

In adults and children with TLE, interictal studies performed with FDG-PET have identified areas of decreased glucose utilization, which correspond anatomically with pathologic and depth electrode EEG localization of epileptogenic lesions. PET can show relative temporal hypometabolism in more than 50 per cent of patients with nonlateralized surface ictal EEG findings.[16] Although ictal PET studies often reveal complex patterns of increased glucose metabolism, focal hypermetabolism may sometimes be seen on interictal PET scans in the presence of an active focal epileptiform discharge on the EEG.[17]

Therefore, continuous EEG monitoring during the FDG uptake period is essential.

The application of FDG-PET in the presurgical evaluation of TLE patients has led to a significant reduction in the need for intracranial EEG monitoring.[16] However, recent advances in analysis techniques of MRI (reviewed in the previous chapter) have eliminated the need for functional imaging or invasive EEG monitoring in the majority of patients with TLE. FDG-PET rarely provides additional clinical information when hippocampal atrophy is present and is increasingly reserved for those cases in which the MRI fails to provide the necessary localization.

An important finding has been that memory impairment, as determined by the intracarotid amobarbital procedure, was never present contralateral to the side of hypometabolism, but was found ipsilateral to hypometabolism in as many as 65 per cent of patients.[18] Similarly, a recent study confirmed that FDG-PET findings are strongly predictive of impaired memory on the intracarotid amobarbital test in patients with TLE.[19] **Bilateral temporal hypometabolism** may indicate bilateral TLE, and is often associated with severe behavioral abnormalities. For example, children with epilepsy and interictal aggression show a characteristic pattern of bilateral temporal neocortical and medial prefrontal hypometabolism[20] (Figure 19B.1). Interestingly, activity in the medial temporal structures is relatively preserved in these children, suggesting that their aggressive behavior is related to a widespread dysfunction of neocortical regions normally exerting an inhibitory effect on subcortical aggressive impulses. This metabolic pattern is different from that found in children with infantile spasms and autistic features, who often show severe bitemporal hypometabolism affecting both lateral and medial temporal structures.[21]

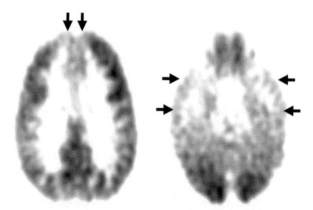

Figure 19B.1 *Bilateral temporal and prefrontal glucose hypometabolism (arrows) in a child with epilepsy and severe interictal aggressive episodes. Note the relative preservation of metabolism in the medial temporal structures.*

EXTRATEMPORAL LOBE EPILEPSY

Using high-resolution PET scanning, da Silva et al.[22] found unilateral frontal lobe hypometabolism in 85 per cent of epileptic children with a frontal lobe focus and normal CT and MRI scan. The location of frontal lobe PET abnormality corresponded to the area of seizure onset in 80 per cent of the patients. When onset of frontal lobe seizures is in the neonatal period or in infancy, an underlying structural lesion is often present even when the MRI is normal. Under these circumstances, FDG-PET can be quite useful in defining an area of hypometabolism which correlates with the extent of microdysgenesis. However, although FDG-PET can detect abnormal cortical areas in patients with normal structural neuroimaging, and can correctly identify the general region of the epileptogenic cortex, it has a limited specificity for the precise area of seizure onset.[23] Thus, the extent of glucose hypometabolism ipsilateral to the seizure focus does not correlate with the epileptogenic tissue to be resected as determined by intracranial EEG.[24] Nevertheless, findings from FDG-PET can be used to guide the placement of subdural electrodes which, otherwise, must rely only on seizure semiology and scalp electrode findings. Clearly, more specific PET ligands which are capable of identifying precisely the epileptogenic cortex to be resected would be desirable (see 'PET of neurotransmitter function', p. 346).

INFANTILE SPASMS

PET studies of cerebral glucose utilization have revolutionized the management of infants with intractable spasms and altered our concepts of the pathophysiology of infantile spasms. Most infants diagnosed with 'cryptogenic' spasms have, in fact, focal or multifocal cortical regions of decreased or increased glucose utilization on PET (Figure 19B.2). Focal ictal and/or interictal EEG abnormalities, which can occur before or after the development of hypsarrhythmia, correspond to the PET focus in most cases. When a single region of abnormal glucose utilization on PET corresponds to the EEG focus and the seizures are intractable, surgical removal of the PET focus can result not only in seizure control, but also in complete or partial reversal of the associated developmental delay. Neuropathological examination of the resected tissue reveals that the epileptogenic zone is typically a previously unsuspected area of cortical dysplasia.[25] Most patients with bilateral multifocal areas of hypometabolism are not surgical candidates, although resective surgery may improve seizure control and cognitive status if all the seizures arise from one area. When the pattern of glucose hypometabolism is symmetric, a lesional etiology is less likely and neurometabolic or neurogenetic disorders should be considered.

Infantile spasms have been considered to be generalized seizures resulting from complex cortico-subcortical

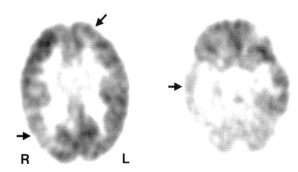

Figure 19B.2 *Multifocal hypometabolism in a 1.5-year-old girl with intractable infantile spasms starting at 3.5 months of age. The right temporal lobe showed the most severe abnormality on FDG-PET, and the seizures appeared to be originating from the right temporal region. This pattern of hypometabolism is often seen in multifocal cortical dysplasia (see also Figure 19B.7).*

interactions. PET studies have not only shown that cortical metabolic lesions are common in infants with spasms, but also that the lenticular nuclei and brainstem are often metabolically prominent. This constellation of findings suggests that spasms result from focal or diffuse cortical abnormalities interacting with subcortical structures.[26]

OTHER CHILDHOOD EPILEPSY SYNDROMES

PET scanning of cerebral glucose utilization has been applied in the study of a number of childhood epilepsy syndromes other than infantile spasms. In children with **Lennox-Gastaut syndrome**, four metabolic subtypes have been identified: unilateral focal, unilateral diffuse and bilateral diffuse hypometabolism, and normal patterns.[27] Patients with the unilateral focal and unilateral diffuse patterns may be considered for cortical resection provided that there is concordance between PET and ictal EEG findings.

In children and adults with advanced **Sturge-Weber syndrome**, PET typically reveals widespread unilateral hypometabolism ipsilateral to the facial nevus in a distribution that extends beyond the abnormalities depicted on CT or MRI scans. In contrast, infants under 1 year of age with Sturge-Weber syndrome may show a paradoxical pattern of **increased** glucose utilization in the cerebral cortex of the anatomically affected hemisphere on **interictal** PET.[28] PET has been useful both in guiding the extent of focal cortical resection (i.e. correlating better with intraoperative electrocorticography than CT or MRI) and in assessing candidacy for early hemispherectomy in patients with Sturge-Weber syndrome, providing not only a sensitive measure of the extent of early cerebral involvement, but also a means of monitoring disease progression. Children with mild but extensive glucose hypometabolism often have more frequent seizures and worse cognitive outcome than children with early and severe unilateral hypometabolism;[29] this suggests that early and rapid demise of the affected hemisphere may be beneficial in allowing unaffected areas to take over lost functions. In contrast, when the affected areas are slow to deteriorate, seizures tend to persist and plasticity mechanisms may not be called into play; these are perhaps the best candidates for resective surgery in our efforts to prevent cognitive decline.

Cortical tubers in **tuberous sclerosis** appear as multiple hypometabolic areas interictally on PET scanning, presumably due to the simplified dendritic arborization within tubers. Some hypometabolic regions on PET do not correspond to abnormalities on CT and MRI scans, and may represent either small tubers or areas of cortical dysplasia. A recently developed PET tracer (AMT) is able to differentiate, for the first time, between epileptogenic and nonepileptogenic tubers in the interictal state (see section, 'Increased uptake of AMT in epileptic foci', p. 347).

Hemimegalencephaly is a rare developmental brain malformation characterized by congenital hypertrophy of one cerebral hemisphere and ipsilateral ventriculomegaly. When the epilepsy is medically uncontrolled, cerebral hemispherectomy is recommended. However, irrespective of seizure control postoperatively, hemimegalencephalic children as a group have a worse cognitive outcome than children who have undergone hemispherectomy for other conditions, such as congenital hemiplegic cerebral palsy, Sturge-Weber syndrome or Rasmussen encephalitis. Glucose metabolism PET studies in children with hemimegalencephaly often also show less pronounced abnormalities in the opposite hemisphere that may account for the suboptimal cognitive outcome even with complete seizure control[30] (Figure 19B.3).

FDG-PET studies during sleep in children with **acquired epileptic aphasia (Landau-Kleffner syndrome)** have demonstrated right-sided, left-sided, or bilateral hypermetabolism or hypometabolism in the temporal lobes, confirming the general notion that this condition is heterogeneous. Abnormal glucose metabolism in the temporal lobes was a common feature in a study of 17 children, supporting the notion that temporal lobe dysfunction is central to the pathophysiology of this disorder.[31] The presence of variable additional cortical abnormalities in many of these children indicates that extensive brain functional disturbances may also exist in Landau-Kleffner syndrome.

In the early stages of **Rasmussen syndrome** (<1 year after onset of symptoms), when the MRI is normal, FDG-PET scanning shows areas of abnormal metabolism restricted mostly to the frontal and temporal regions, whereas the posterior cortex is usually preserved[32] (Figure 19B.4). Pathologic changes seen in the resected cortex are more pronounced in cortical areas of abnormal metabolism than in regions showing normal metabolism.

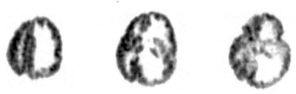

Figure 19B.3 *FDG-PET scan of a 1-year-old girl with hemimegalencephaly involving the left hemisphere (right side on the pictures). Preserved glucose metabolism in the contralateral hemisphere predicts favorable prognosis after hemispherectomy.*

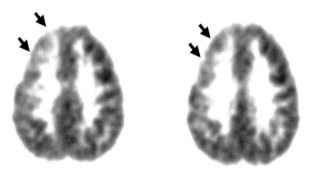

Figure 19B.4 *FDG-PET in early Rasmussen syndrome. The PET scan of this 7-year-old girl was performed after a normal MRI, and showed focal glucose hypometabolism in the right frontal region (arrows). Histology verified the diagnosis, and the patient underwent right hemispherectomy.*

Thus, FDG-PET performed early during the course of disease can facilitate the correct diagnosis and may also guide the site of brain biopsy when indicated.

PET of neurotransmitter function

PET technology allows the study of much more than glucose metabolism, and there has been considerable enthusiasm in further developing and applying PET to examine a number of neurotransmitter systems believed to be important in epileptic mechanisms.

IMAGING GABA$_A$ RECEPTORS BY FMZ-PET

Flumazenil is a benzodiazepine antagonist that binds to the α subunit of the GABA$_A$ receptor, and the PET tracer FMZ can be used to provide quantitative images of binding to these receptors. Initial studies using PET with FMZ showed significantly reduced binding in the epileptic focus of patients with partial epilepsy. FMZ-PET is more accurate in delineating the seizure focus than FDG-PET in some patients.[33] In children with **intractable epilepsy of extratemporal origin**, FMZ-PET was more sensitive than FDG-PET in delineating cortex with

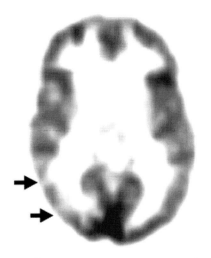

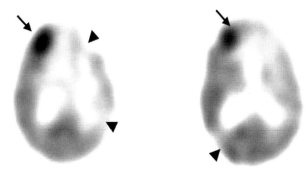

Figure 19B.6 *In children with tuberous sclerosis and intractable epilepsy, AMT-PET can select the epileptogenic tuber that shows increased tracer uptake (arrow) even in interictal state, whereas non-epileptogenic lesions show decreased AMT uptake (arrowheads).*

Figure 19B.5 *[¹¹C]Flumazenil PET can delineate epileptic neocortex. In this 13-year-old boy MRI was normal, and FDG-PET showed bilateral temporal and parietal hypometabolism. FMZ-PET indicated a focal area of decreased FMZ binding in the right superior temporal region (arrows). Video-EEG monitoring suggested that the seizures (brief body jerks) originated from the right frontotemporal region.*

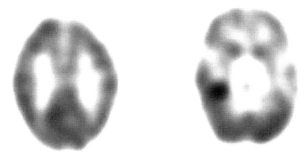

Figure 19B.7 *AMT-PET of a 1.5-year-old girl with infantile spasms. FDG-PET showed bilateral, multifocal abnormalities (see Figure 19B.2). AMT-PET revealed a single area with increased uptake in the right inferior temporal region, and this was consistent with the location of seizure onset shown by video-EEG monitoring.*

seizure onset and frequent interictal spiking as defined by intracranial EEG monitoring.[23] In patients with bilateral glucose hypometabolism associated with epileptic and nonepileptic abnormalities, FMZ-PET can be used to identify more specifically the epileptogenic cortex (Figure 19B.5). In children with **infantile spasms** associated with cortical dysplasia, FMZ-PET may indicate regions of decreased (or occasionally increased) FMZ binding consistent with subtle cortical abnormalities (dysplasia) not detected by MRI.[34] Recent studies have found abnormal FMZ binding in normal-appearing cortex adjacent to cortical developmental malformations, suggesting that abnormalities of GABA$_A$ receptors may extend well beyond MRI-detectable structural changes.[35] Because FMZ-PET is very sensitive in identifying hippocampal sclerosis, it is very useful in characterizing epileptogenic regions in patients with **dual pathology**.[36] This can have a major impact on the surgical strategy since resection of both the cortical lesion and the sclerotic hippocampus is required to achieve optimal surgical results.

INCREASED UPTAKE OF AMT IN EPILEPTIC FOCI

In vitro observations of increased serotonin content and immunoreactivity in human epileptic tissue led to the development of the PET tracer AMT. AMT is converted in the brain to α-[¹¹C]-methyl-serotonin, which accumulates in serotonergic terminals. AMT-PET has proven to be a powerful tool in the evaluation of children with tuberous

sclerosis and intractable epilepsy being considered for resective surgery[37] (Figure 19B.6). Indeed, AMT-PET is capable of differentiating between epileptogenic and nonepileptogenic lesions in children with tuberous sclerosis and in children with multifocal cortical dysplasia, by showing increased uptake of AMT in the epileptogenic regions and not in the nonepileptogenic areas. Interestingly, studies on the surgically resected tissues from these patients have shown that, at least in some cases, increased *in vivo* uptake of AMT may be due to an increased synthesis of quinolinic acid, which has a strong convulsant effect through its action as an agonist at NMDA receptors, and may play a key role in intractable seizures in these children. Recent studies have shown focally increased AMT uptake in proven epileptogenic cortical regions even when the FDG-PET scan is nonlocalizing or normal, with a sensitivity of approximately 50 per cent[38] (Figure 19B.7). In contrast, AMT-PET usually does not show increased tracer uptake in the sclerotic hippocampus.

SPECT

SPECT is a noninvasive functional imaging technique that uses simpler and less expensive equipment than PET. It provides tomographic imaging through the use of either a single, rapidly rotating gamma camera or multiple cameras to detect and reconstruct gamma-ray emissions. Because of the longer half-life of SPECT isotopes compared to those used in PET, and the readily available equipment, SPECT is suited for even the smallest hospitals and clinics. The isotopes can be obtained commercially and can be stored on site. However, the spatial resolution of SPECT images is about half of that achieved with PET, which is particularly relevant in pediatric studies. Furthermore, unlike PET, SPECT techniques are semi-quantitative at best.

In brain studies, SPECT has been used primarily to provide an index of cerebral blood flow using the iodoamines, xenon, technetium-99 m hexamethyl propylene amine oxime (^{99m}Tc-HMPAO) and the technetium-99m-ethyl cysteinate dimer (ECD). When ictal and postictal localization of seizure foci are desired, SPECT studies are particularly useful for several reasons. For example, the iodoamine N,N,N′-trimethyl-N′2-Hydroxy-3-Methyl-5-iodobenzyl-1,3-propanediamine iodine-131 (HIPDM) reaches 75 per cent of its peak brain concentration at 2 min after injection. Scanning of the brain can be initiated at leisure after the brain uptake phase because the trapped agent remains relatively stable for at least 1 h, and the isotopes used in SPECT have a rather long half-life (e.g. ^{123}I has a half-life of 13 h). In contrast, because of the short half-life of PET isotopes (e.g. 108 min for ^{18}F and 20 min for ^{11}C), it is extremely difficult to achieve planned ictal and postictal PET studies, although they have been done in a few cases with very frequent extratemporal seizures.[39] Furthermore, ictal FDG-PET studies typically include a prolonged postictal phase and are therefore often difficult to interpret.

Partial epilepsy

Interictal studies are generally less sensitive than ictal SPECT studies, but have some clinical utility in children with epilepsy. In a ^{99m}Tc-HMPAO-SPECT study of 14 children with frequent seizures, the typical finding in 11 patients with partial secondary generalized seizures was a single hypoperfused area. The 3 children with Lennox-Gastaut syndrome had multiple areas of hypoperfusion and a worse clinical outcome.[40] Similar sensitivity of interictal SPECT was found in another study of 14 children with intractable temporal lobe epilepsy.[41] This latter study

also demonstrated that a lack of perfusion asymmetry in the temporal lobes of some children may be attributed to bilateral temporal lobe damage, as determined by bilateral abnormalities on ^{1}H-MRS.

Ictal SPECT appears to be more sensitive in detecting the epileptic focus than interictal studies in both temporal and extratemporal epilepsy. Marks *et al.*[42] found ictal ^{99m}Tc-HMPAO-SPECT to be a valuable tool in the localization of extratemporal epileptic foci. A circumscribed area of increased perfusion was the most common finding, and was particularly useful in patients with nonlocalizing ictal EEG. In 65 children being considered for epilepsy surgery, ictal SPECT provided no additional prognostic information in those with a localized MRI lesion but gave additional localization data that could be used as a guide for the implantation of intracranial electrodes in patients without lesions.[43]

Sensitivity and spatial accuracy of ictal SPECT findings can be enhanced by using **subtraction ictal SPECT co-registered to MRI** (SISCOM).[44] In 40 children with epilepsy, SISCOM showed localized hyperperfusion in agreement with the seizure onset zone in 95 per cent of the cases. Importantly, a previously not appreciated MRI abnormality (subtle cortical dysplasia) was identified in 6 patients after coregistration of SPECT images.[45]

When seizures are brief, true ictal SPECT studies are very difficult to achieve. However, *postictal* SPECT studies have been reported to be superior to interictal SPECT by some investigators.[46] Increased uptake mainly in the anteromesial temporal region was seen in 83 per cent of patients with temporal lobe seizures during the first several minutes following the seizure. In most studies, this was accompanied by hypoperfusion in the lateral temporal and other areas of the ipsilateral cortex, which could last up to 20 min. Postictal SPECT permitted the unilateral seizure focus to be localized correctly in 31 of 45 patients.[47] Recent studies have demonstrated that postictal SPECT localization of epileptic foci can also be improved by subtraction studies coregistered with MRI.[48]

Epilepsy syndromes in infancy and childhood

Interictal areas of decreased perfusion usually correspond topographically to the CT scan abnormality in children with **Sturge-Weber syndrome** but may precede the appearance of defects on CT and MRI[49] suggesting that progressive structural abnormalities in Sturge-Weber syndrome are the consequence of progressive chronic ischemia and/or seizure-related neuronal damage. In young infants with Sturge-Weber syndrome, increased glucose metabolism can be associated with simultaneous hypo- and hyperperfusion.[50] These age-dependent phenomena are likely related to the pathophsysiology of Sturge-Weber syndrome, but are still poorly understood at present. In patients with more advanced disease, SPECT may reveal ischemic areas that often extend beyond the MRI-visualized lesions.

Focal areas of cortical hypoperfusion have been detected with ^{133}Xe-SPECT (Xenon-133 single photon emission computed tomography) in patients with **West syndrome**.[51] It was also shown that mean cerebral blood flow decreased just after steroid treatment. In a recent study of 40 children with West syndrome, localized cortical perfusion abnormalities were seen in 24 patients (60 per cent), confirming that focal cortical lesions play an important role in the development of West syndrome.[52] However, the existence of cortical dysfunction as defined by SPECT does not seem to predict seizure prognosis or developmental outcome. In longitudinal studies, areas of hypoperfusion appeared to be static as had been shown with FDG-PET, whereas frontal regions of increased perfusion tended to diminish as the spasms became controlled. Focal hyperperfusion has been observed in infants with **cortical dysgenesis** in several studies.[52,53] This pattern seems to be specific to young infants and is not observed in older patients.

Focal SPECT hypoperfusion in the parieto-occipital region is often associated with visual inattention at the time when the infants present with West syndrome, and with long-term cognitive compromise.[54] Both visual inattention and cognitive compromise have been reversed with successful focal cortical resection.[25]

The data reviewed above demonstrate that the clinical value of PET and SPECT studies (using various tracers) greatly varies according to the epilepsy syndrome as well as the clinical question being asked (see Table 19B.1). The clinician has to make a rational choice among several available imaging modalities in order to optimize the clinical effectiveness of these studies.

MULTIMODALITY IMAGING IN PRESURGICAL EVALUATION

Co-registration of various imaging modalities allows direct comparisons between structural and functional brain abnormalities, and enhances spatial accuracy of localization of epileptogenic regions during presurgical evaluation in children. For example, co-registered three-dimensional surface-rendered MRI and PET images can be displayed together with the subdural electrodes. This permits a comprehensive overview of the relative localization of ictal and interictal epileptiform activity, as well as results of motor, sensory and language mapping studies for direct comparison with the functional abnormalities obtained from FDG and/or neuroreceptor PET studies. This display provides an aid to the surgeon in performing a precise tailoring of the cortical resection, i.e. to maximize the excision of the epileptogenic zone while minimizing the

Table 19B.1 *Overview of clinical utility of interictal PET with different tracers, and ictal SPECT in childhood epilepsies*

	FDG-PET	FMZ-PET	AMT-PET	Ictal SPECT
Temporal lobe epilepsy	Very sensitive ($\geq$90%); often shows extratemporal hypometabolism	Very sensitive and specific for the epileptogenic hippocampus; sensitive for dual pathology	Not sensitive for medial temporal foci	Very sensitive ($\geq$90%), pattern depends on timing of injection
Extratemporal epilepsy	Sensitive (70–85%), but not specific for seizure onset	Sensitive for seizure onset in nonlesional cases; detects perilesional epileptic cortex	Very specific, up to 50% sensitive (even if MRI and/or FDG-PET is non-localizing)	Sensitive (70–90%) but less useful in brief seizures; provides additional localization in $\geq$50% of MRI-negative cases
Infantile spasms	Differentiates lesional vs. metabolic/genetic etiology; Reveals single focus in up to 20% of cryptogenic cases	Not evaluated systematically; may detect cortical dysplasia	Not evaluated systematically; may select epileptogenic lesion(s) in multifocal cortical dysplasia	Not feasible because seizures are short
Other childhood epilepsy syndromes	Hemimegalencephaly: assessment of functional integrity of the contralateral hemisphere; Rasmussen syndrome: early focal hypermetabolism may guide biopsy; Lennox-Gastaut syndrome: 4 metabolic subtypes; may help planning surgery	Not evaluated systematically	Tuberous sclerosis: differentiates epileptogenic from nonepileptogenic lesions	Sturge-Weber syndrome: occasionally helpful, detects ischemic areas and seizure focus

FDG, 2-deoxy-2[^{18}F]fluoro-D-glucose; FMZ, [^{11}C]flumazenil; AMT, α[^{11}C]methyl-L-tryptophan.

intrusion into vital areas. The advantage of multimodality imaging has been demonstrated clearly in children with tuberous sclerosis, where tracer uptake measured on AMT-PET (see above) in tubers delineated on coregistered FLAIR MRI and/or FDG-PET images was able to differentiate objectively between epileptogenic and nonepileptogenic tubers with a 91 per cent specificity.[55] Combination of functional mapping techniques (e.g. fMRI, magnetoencephalography and transcranial magnetic stimulation) to delineate eloquent cortex can aid precise noninvasive localization of such areas.[56]

KEY POINTS

- **fMRI** may be used to identify eloquent cortex and potentially the epileptic focus
- **FDG-PET** is a noninvasive investigation that has improved the selection of potential surgical candidates in children with temporal and extratemporal lobe epilepsy, infantile spasms and other epilepsy syndromes
- **FMZ-PET** can delineate the seizure focus more occurately than FDG-PET in some patients, particularly in those with extratemporal lobe epilepsy and in those with dual pathology
- **AMT-PET** may help to distinguish epileptogenic from nonepileptogenic abnormalities in children with tuberous sclerosis and multifocal cortical dysplasia.
- **Ictal SPECT** studies of cerebral blood flow can identify the epileptic focus, particularly when subtraction techniques are used
- **Multimodality imaging** in presurgical evaluation of children with intractable epilepsy is a powerful approach to display the epileptogenic zone for surgical resection

---

REFERENCES

1. ILAE Commission Report. Commission on diagnostic strategies. Recommendations for functional neuroimaging of persons with epilepsy. *Epilepsia* 2000; **41**: 1350–1356.
2. Gaillard WD, Grandin CB, Xu B. Developmental aspects of pediatric fMRI: considerations for image acquisition, analysis, and interpretation. *Neuroimage* 2001; **13**: 239–249.
3. Yetkin FZ, Swanson S, Fischer M, *et al.* Functional MR of frontal lobe activation: comparison with Wada language results. *AJNR 1998*; **19**: 1095–1098.
4. Macdonell RA, Jackson GD, Curatolo JM, *et al.* Motor cortex localization using functional MRI and transcranial magnetic stimulation. *Neurology* 1999; **53**: 1462–1467.
5. Krakow K, Woermann FG, Symms MR, *et al.* EEG-triggered functional MRI of interictal epileptiform activity in patients with partial seizures. *Brain* 1999; **122**: 1679–1688.
6. Chu WJ, Hetherington HP, Kuzniecky RI, *et al.* Lateralization of human temporal lobe epilepsy by ^{31}P NMR spectroscopic imaging at 4.1 T. *Neurology* 1998; **51**: 472–479.
7. Li LM, Cendes F, Andermann F, Dubeau F, Arnold DL. Spatial extent of neuronal metabolic dysfunction measured by proton MR spectroscopic imaging in patients with localization-related epilepsy. *Epilepsia* 2000; **41**: 666–674.
8. Park YD, Allison JD, Weiss KL, *et al.* Proton magnetic resonance spectroscopic observations of epilepsia partialis continua in children. *Journal of Child Neurology* 2000; **15**: 729–733.
9. Mueller SG, Kollias SS, Trabesinger AH, *et al.* Proton magnetic resonance spectroscopy characteristics of a focal cortical dysgenesis during status epilepticus and in the interictal state. *Seizure* 2001; **10**: 518–524.
10. Maeda H, Furune S, Nomura K, *et al.* Decrease of N-acetylaspartate after ACTH therapy in patients with infantile spasms. *Neuropediatrics* 1997; **28**: 262–267.
11. Novotny EJ Jr, Hyder F, Shevell M, Rothman DL. GABA changes with vigabatrin in the developing human brain. *Epilepsia* 1999; **40**: 462–466.
12. Sherwin AL. Neuroactive amino acids in focally epileptic human brain: a review. *Neurochemical Research* 1999; **24**: 1387–1395.
13. Martin E, Capone A, Schneider J, Hennig J, Thiel T. Absence of N-acetylaspartate in the human brain: impact on neurospectroscopy? *Annals of Neurology* 2001; **49**: 518–521.
14. Cendes F, Andermann F, Dubeau F, Matthews PM, Arnold DL. Normalization of neuronal metabolic dysfunction after surgery for temporal lobe epilepsy. Evidence from proton MR spectroscopic imaging. *Neurology* 1997; **49**: 1525–1533.
15. Duncan DB, Herholz K, Kugel H, *et al.* Positron emission tomography and magnetic resonance spectroscopy of cerebral glycolysis in children with congenital lactic acidosis. *Annals of Neurology* 1995; **37**: 351–358.
16. Theodore WH, Sato S, Kufta CV, Gaillard WD, Kelley K. FDG-positron emission tomography and invasive EEG: seizure focus detection and surgical outcome. Epilepsia 1997; **38**: 81–86.
17. Chugani HT, Shewmon DA, Khanna S, *et al.* Interictal and postictal focal hypermetabolism on positron emission tomography. *Pediatric Neurology* 1993; **9**: 10–15.
18. Salanova V, Morris HH, Rehm P, *et al.* Comparison of the intracarotid amobarbital procedure and interictal cerebral 18-fluorodeoxyglucose positron emission tomography scans in refractory temporal lobe epilepsy. *Epilepsia* 1992; **33**: 635–638.
19. Salanova V, Markand O, Worth R. Focal functional deficits in temporal lobe epilepsy on PET scans and the intracarotid amobarbital procedure: comparison of patients with unitemporal epilepsy with those requiring intracranial recordings. *Epilepsia* 2001; **42**: 198–203.
20. Juhász C, Behen ME, Muzik O, Chugani DC, Chugani HT. Bilateral medial prefrontal and temporal neocortical hypometabolism in children with epilepsy and aggression. *Epilepsia* 2001; **42**: 991–1001.
21. Chugani HT, Da Silva E, Chugani DC. Infantile spasms: III. Prognostic implications of bitemporal hypometabolism on positron emission tomography. *Annals of Neurology* 1996; **39**: 643–649.

22. da Silva EA, Chugani DC, Muzik O, Chugani HT. Identification of frontal lobe epileptic foci in children using positron emission tomography. *Epilepsia* 1997; **38**: 1198–1208.

23. Muzik O, da Silva E, Juhász C, *et al.* Intracranial EEG vs. flumazenil and glucose PET in children with extratemporal lobe epilepsy. *Neurology* 2000; **54**: 171–179.

24. Juhász C, Chugani DC, Muzik O, *et al.* Relationship of flumazenil and glucose PET abnormalities to neocortical epilepsy surgery outcome. *Neurology* 2001; **56**: 1650–1658.

25. Chugani HT, Shewmon DA, Shields WD, *et al.* Surgery for intractable infantile spasms: neuroimaging perspectives. *Epilepsia* 1993; **34**: 764–771.

26. Chugani HT, Chugani DC. Basic mechanisms of childhood epilepsies: studies with positron emission tomography. *Advances in Neurology* 1999; **79**: 883–891.

27. Chugani HT, Mazziotta JC, Engel J Jr, Phelps ME. The Lennox-Gastaut syndrome: metabolic subtypes determined by 2-deoxy-2[^{18}F]fluoro-D-glucose positron emission tomography. *Annals of Neurology* 1987; **21**: 4–13.

28. Chugani HT, Mazziotta JC, Phelps ME. Sturge-Weber syndrome: a study of cerebral glucose utilization with positron emission tomography. *Journal of Pediatrics* 1989; **114**: 244–253.

29. Lee JS, Asano E, Muzik O, *et al.* Sturge-Weber syndrome: correlation between clinical course and FDG PET findings. *Neurology* 2001; **57**: 189–195.

30. Rintahaka PJ, Chugani HT, Messa C, *et al.* Hemimegalencephaly: evaluation with positron emission tomography. *Pediatric Neurology* 1993; **9**: 21–28.

31. da Silva EA, Chugani DC, Muzik O, Chugani HT. Landau-Kleffner syndrome: metabolic abnormalities in temporal lobe are a common feature. *Journal of Child Neurology* 1997; **12**: 489–495.

32. Lee JS, Juhász C, Kaddurah AK, Chugani HT. Patterns of cerebral glucose metabolism in early and late stages of Rasmussen's syndrome. *Journal of Child Neurology* 2001; **16**: 798–805.

33. Ryvlin P, Bouvard S, Le Bars D, *et al.* Clinical utility of flumazenil-PET versus [^{18}F]fluorodeoxyglucose-PET and MRI in refractory partial epilepsy. A prospective study in 100 patients. *Brain* 1998; **121**: 2067–2081.

34. Juhász C, Chugani HT, Muzik O, Chugani DC. Neuroradiological assessment of brain structure and function and its implication in the pathogenesis of West syndrome. *Brain and Development* 2001; **23**: 488–495.

35. Hammers A, Koepp MJ, Richardson MP, *et al.* Central benzodiazepine receptors in malformations of cortical development: A quantitative study. *Brain* 2001; **124**: 1555–1565.

36. Juhász C, Nagy F, Muzik O, Watson C, Shah J, Chugani HT. [^{11}C]Flumazenil PET in patients with epilepsy with dual pathology. *Epilepsia* 1999; **40**: 566–574.

37. Chugani DC, Chugani HT, Muzik O, *et al.* Imaging epileptogenic tubers in children with tuberous sclerosis complex using alpha-[^{11}C]methyl-L-tryptophan positron emission tomography. *Annals of Neurology* 1998; **44**: 858–866.

38. Fedi M, Reutens D, Okazawa H, *et al.* Localizing value of alpha-methyl-L-tryptophan PET in intractable epilepsy of neocortical origin. *Neurology* 2001; **57**: 1629–1636.

39. Meltzer CC, Adelson PD, Brenner RP, *et al.* Planned ictal FDG PET imaging for localization of extratemporal epileptic foci. *Epilepsia* 2000; **41**: 193–200.

40. Heiskala H, Launes J, Pihko H, *et al.* Brain perfusion SPECT in children with frequent fits. *Brain and Development* 1993; **15**: 214–218.

41. Cross JH, Gordon I, Connelly A, *et al.* Interictal 99Tc(m) HMPAO SPECT and ^{1}H MRS in children with temporal lobe epilepsy. *Epilepsia* 1997; **38**: 338–345.

42. Marks DA, Katz A, Hoffer P, Spencer SS. Localization of extratemporal epileptic foci during ictal single photon emission computed tomography. *Annals of Neurology* 1992; **31**: 250–255.

43. Lawson JA, O'Brien TJ, Bleasel AF, *et al.* Evaluation of SPECT in the assessment and treatment of intractable childhood epilepsy. *Neurology* 2000; **55**: 1391–1393.

44. Vera P, Kaminska A, Cieuta C, *et al.* Use of subtraction ictal SPECT co-registered to MRI for optimizing the localization of seizure foci in children. *J Nucl Med* 1999; **40**: 786–792.

45. Chiron C, Vera P, Kaminska A, *et al.* Single-photon emission computed tomography: ictal perfusion in childhood epilepsies. *Brain and Development* 1999; **21**: 444–446.

46. Rowe CC, Berkovic SF, Sia STB, *et al.* Localization of epileptic foci with postictal single photon emission computed tomography. *Annals of Neurology* 1989; **26**: 660–668.

47. Rowe CC, Berkovic SF, Austin MC, *et al.* Patterns of postictal blood flow in temporal lobe epilepsy: qualitative and quantitative analysis. *Neurology* 1991; **41**: 1096–1103.

48. O'Brien TJ, So EL, Mullan BP, *et al.* Subtraction SPECT co-registered to MRI improves postictal SPECT localization of seizure foci. *Neurology* 1999; **52**: 137–146.

49. Reid DE, Maria BL, Drane WE, Quisling RG, Hoang KB. Central nervous system perfusion and metabolism abnormalities in Sturge-Weber syndrome. *Journal of Child Neurology* 1997; **12**: 218–222.

50. Pinton F, Chiron C, Enjolras O, Motte J, Syrota A, Dulac O. Early single photon emission computed tomography in Sturge-Weber syndrome. *Journal of Neurology, Neurosurgery and Psychiatry* 1997; **63**: 616–621.

51. Dulac O, Chiron C, Jambaque I, *et al.* Infantile spasms. *Progress in Clinical Neurosciences* 1987; **2**: 97–109.

52. Haginoya K, Kon K, Yokoyama H. The perfusion defect seen with SPECT in West syndrome is not correlated with seizure prognosis or developmental outcome. *Brain and Development* 2000; **22**: 16–23.

53. Hwang PA, Otsubo H, Koo BK, *et al.* Infantile spasms: cerebral blood flow abnormalities correlate with EEG, neuroimaging, and pathologic findings. *Pediatric Neurology* 1996; **14**: 220–225.

54. Jambaque I, Chiron C, Dulac O, *et al.* Visual inattention in West syndrome: a neuropsychological and neurofunctional imaging study. *Epilepsia* 1993; **34**: 692–700.

55. Asano E, Chugani DC, Muzik O, *et al.* Multimodality imaging for improved detection of epileptogenic foci in tuberous sclerosis complex. *Neurology* 2000; **54**: 1976–1984.

56. Morioka T, Mizushima A, Yamamoto T, *et al.* Functional mapping of the sensorimotor cortex: combined use of magneto-encephalography, functional MRI, and motor evoked potentials. *Neuroradiology* 1995; **37**: 526–530.

20

Investigation of the child with epilepsy

KATHERINE WAMBERA AND KEVIN FARRELL

Investigations are performed in children with epilepsy for four main reasons:

- to determine the underlying cause of the seizures
- to demonstrate the effect of repeated or prolonged seizures
- to detect adverse effects of treatment
- to measure the blood levels of antiepileptic drugs.

UNDERLYING CAUSE OF SEIZURES

Acute symptomatic seizures

Seizures may be a symptom of an acute illness that requires timely and specific treatment. The possibility of acute symptomatic seizures should be considered in any child presenting with a first seizure, particularly if the child is febrile or has other evidence of a systemic disturbance. Table 20.1 lists diseases that may manifest with acute symptomatic seizures.

Most children under 5 years of age who have a seizure with fever have benign febrile convulsions. However, the possibility that a seizure associated with fever is due to a CNS infection must always be considered. The clinical signs and symptoms of meningitis may be absent in infants younger than 12 months and may be subtle in infants between 12 and 18 months of age and in those who have received prior antibiotic treatment. Consequently, a lumbar puncture should be strongly considered when a first seizure with fever occurs in such children.[1] In children under 3 years of age with fever more than 39°C and no obvious cause, a complete blood count, blood culture and urinalysis should be performed unless the child looks well and can be monitored carefully. Routine blood studies, EEG and neuroimaging have not been demonstrated to be helpful in the assessment of a neurologically healthy child with a first simple febrile convulsion.[1]

Unprovoked epileptic seizures

Epileptic seizures are a common neurological symptom in children and are due to a variety of causes (see Table 20.2). In some children, several factors may contribute to the occurrence of seizures. Determination of the cause of the epilepsy can permit a more definitive prognosis and can have important implications regarding treatment. There may also be implications for genetic counseling.

Electroencephalogram

The EEG is the single most useful investigation in the child with an afebrile seizure (see Chapter 18). Thus, the EEG can be helpful in the diagnosis of seizure type, identification of a specific epileptic syndrome, and consequently, prediction of long-term outcome.[2] EEG recordings should include both sleep and waking states and should use hyperventilation and photic stimulation to maximize the chance of recording abnormalities.[3] In children with a first unprovoked seizure, EEG abnormalities occur at a substantially higher rate after 3 years of age.[4] A recent study of adults and children has suggested that the EEG may be more useful when performed within 24 h of a first seizure.[5] Approximately 60 per cent of children younger than 18 years of age with epilepsy have idiopathic epilepsy in which genetic factors play a prominent role.[6]

Table 20.1 *Causes of acute symptomatic seizures in children*

Infections
    Bacterial or viral meningitis
    Viral encephalitis
    Mycoplasma
    Brain abscess
Parainfectious encephalopathies
    Hemorrhagic shock
    Reye syndrome
    Acute disseminated encephalomyelopathy
Metabolic
    Hypoglycemia
    Hyponatremia
    Hypernatremia
    Hypocalcemia and hypomagnesemia
    Inborn error of metabolism
Acute hypoxic-ischemic brain injury
Acute organ dysfunction
    Renal: Acute glomerulonephritis
        Haemolytic uremic syndrome
        Renal failure
        Dialysis
    Hypertensive encephalopathy
    Hepatic encephalopathy
    Diabetic ketoacidosis
Drugs and toxins
    Cocaine, amphetamine, heroin, phencyclidine, ecstasy,
        γ-hydroxybutyrate
Head trauma
    Early epileptic seizure
    Intracranial hematoma
Vasculitic
    Henoch-Schonlein purpura
    Systemic lupus erythematosis
    Polyarteritis nodosa
    Kawasaki disease
Cerebrovascular/hematologic
    Intracranial hemorrhage: vascular malformation
    Bleeding disorder e.g. idiopathic thrombocytopenia
    Arterial thrombosis
    Venous thrombosis
    Leukemia

Table 20.2 *Causes of epileptic seizures in children*

Idiopathic
    Related to genetic factors and not
        associated with brain lesions. These
        can occur at all ages
Lesional
Prenatal
    Developmental brain abnormalities
    Phakomatoses
    Vascular malformation (e.g. cavernoma)
    Intrauterine infections
    Intrauterine hypoxic-ischemic injury or hemorrhage
    Some metabolic disorders (e.g. maternal phenylketonuria)
Perinatal
    Hypoxic-ischemic brain injury
    Intracranial hemorrhage
    Stroke
    Intracranial infection
    Metabolic (e.g. hypoglycemia)
Postnatal
    Trauma
    Hypoxic-ischemic brain injury
    Stroke (ischemic or hemorrhagic)
    Intracranial infections (bacterial meningitis, brain abscess,
        viral encephalitis, parasitic infection)
    Metabolic (inborn error of metabolism or hypoglycemia)

demonstrate clinically significant abnormalities that influence management.[2] In many of these patients, the clinical features and/or EEG abnormalities are strongly suggestive of a structural lesion. Emergent neuroimaging should be considered in any child with a prolonged post-ictal focal deficit or who does not recover within several hours of a seizure.[2] Nonurgent neuroimaging should be considered following an afebrile seizure in all children less than 1 year of age, in those with partial or generalized tonic-clonic, tonic or myoclonic seizures, and in those with an abnormal neurologic examination.[2] Children with the clinical and EEG features of idiopathic epilepsy do not require neuroimaging.

MRI is the most sensitive anatomical neuroimaging investigation for the detection of lesional causes of epilepsy (see Chapter 19A). Whether to obtain a CT or MRI will depend to some extent on the availability of these techniques, the age of the child and the need for sedation to perform the study.

Specific genetic testing

In a variety of diseases that manifest with epilepsy, the diagnosis can be confirmed best by genetic testing (Table 20.3). Most of these conditions are associated with a particular clinical and/or radiologic phenotype and the genetic investigations should only be performed where

These types of epilepsy tend to occur in individuals who are otherwise neurologically normal and in whom there is often a family history of epilepsy. These epilepsies are characterized by particular ictal and interictal EEG abnormalities. Thus, the EEG is normally the only investigation necessary in patients with benign childhood epilepsy with centrotemporal spikes, childhood or juvenile absence epilepsy, and juvenile myoclonic epilepsy.

Neuroimaging

Neuroimaging abnormalities occur in up to one third of children with a first seizure. However, only 2 per cent

Table 20.3 *Causes of epilepsy diagnosed by genetic testing*

Disease	Epilepsy/seizure type	Investigation	Chapter
Angelman	Myoclonic, atonic, atypical absence	Karyotype; FISH 15q11–13; = 15q11–13 methylation studies; UBE3A mutation analysis	2E
Miller-Dieker	Spasms, myoclonic, tonic	Karyotype; FISH 17p13.3	2E
Down syndrome	Spasms and reflex epilepsy	Karyotype	2E
1p36 deletion syndrome	Spasms, partial, tonic-clonic and myoclonic	Karyotype; FISH 1p36	2E
Wolf-Hirschorn syndrome	Partial, tonic-clonic, tonic, atypical absence, myoclonic	Karyotype; FISH 4p	2E
Ring chromosome 14	Partial, myoclonic, tonic-clonic	Karyotype	2E
Ring chromosome 20	Frequent episodes of nonconvulsive status. Onset between infancy and 14 years. No dysmorphic features and often of normal intelligence	Karyotype	2E
Fragile X	Partial seizures	Karyotype; *FMR1* antibody analysis; sizing of CGG expansion	2E
Rett syndrome	Partial seizures	*MECP2* mutation in 50% of patients	
Unverricht-Lundborg	Progressive myoclonic	21q dodecamer repeat expansion	14
Myoclonic epilepsy associated with ragged-redfibers (MERRF)	Progressive myoclonic	Missense mutation of mtDNA	
Lafora disease	Progressive myoclonic	6q24 *EPM2A* mutation	14
Dentato-rubro-pallido-luysian atrophy (DRPLA)	Progressive myoclonic	12p CAG repeat expansion	14

there is a clinical indication. Certain other disorders, such as ring chromosome 20 and Unverricht-Lundborg disease, are not associated with dysmorphic features and can occur in patients with normal intelligence. Investigations of these disorders should be considered in those with the appropriate clinical and EEG features[7] (see Chapters 2E and 4B).

Specific gene defects have been identified in patients with benign familial neonatal convulsions (KCNQ2, KCNQ3), benign familial infantile seizures (SCN2A), generalized epilepsy with febrile seizures plus (SCN1A, SCN1B, SCN2A, GABRG2), autosomal dominant juvenile myoclonic epilepsy (GABRA1), autosomal dominant nocturnal frontal lobe epilepsy (CHRNA4, CHRNB2) and autosomal dominant partial epilepsy with dominant features (LGI1) (see Chapter 4A). However, these investigations are not routinely available. Furthermore, there is often marked genetic heterogeneity even in syndromes that are clinically homogeneous.

Metabolic testing

Inherited disorders of metabolism are an uncommon cause of epilepsy in children. However, early diagnosis is important because of genetic counseling implications and because some require specific treatment. Table 20.4 outlines the more common metabolic disorders that may manifest with seizures. The clinical features and appropriate diagnostic tests are described in Chapters 4D and 14.

EFFECTS OF SEIZURES

Brief seizures are not generally associated with hematologic or biochemical changes. However, leukocytosis, thrombocytopenia and disseminated intravascular coagulation may complicate prolonged status epilepticus. Patients with prolonged status epilepticus may also develop hypoglycemia, hyponatremia, hypo- and hyperkalemia, metabolic and respiratory acidosis, hepatic and renal dysfunction, pancreatitis, rhabdomyolysis and myoglobinuria.[8]

MONITORING FOR THE ADVERSE EFFECTS OF ANTIEPILEPTIC DRUGS

The adverse effects of antiepileptic drugs (AEDs) are described in Chapters 21 and 22A. Dose-dependent, reversible side-effects are common. Abnormal laboratory tests are also common, and in most cases are significant only when there are clinical symptoms. Mildly elevated liver enzymes occur in 1–15 per cent of children receiving phenobarbital, phenytoin, carbamazepine or valproic acid.[9] Similarly, mild hyperammonemia commonly occurs in patients receiving valproic acid. These laboratory abnormalities are rarely associated with symptoms and are not predictive of serious toxicity. Consequently, routine laboratory investigations are not indicated in

Table 20.4 *Inherited disorders of metabolism associated with seizures*

Disorder	Neonates	Infants	Older children
	Time of seizure onset		
Nonketotic hyperglycinemia	•		
GABA transaminase deficiency	•		
Sulfite oxidase deficiency and molybdenum cofactor deficiency	•		
Vitamin B_6 dependency	•	•	
Folinic acid responsive seizures	•	•	
Urea cycle disorers (hyperammonemia)	•	•	
Peroxisomal disorders	•	•	
Phenylketonuria		•	
Tetrahydrobiopterin disorders		•	
Tay-Sachs and Sandhoff diseases		•	•
Mitochondrial disorders	•	•	•
Neuronal ceroid lipofuscinosis		•	•
Glutaric aciduria type 1		•	•
Biotiniase deficiency		•	•
Various organic acidurias		•	•
Serine deficiency disorders		•	•
Disorders of pyrimidine metabolism		•	•
Glucose transporter deficiency		•	
Fucosidosis		•	•
Schindler's disease		•	•
Sialidosis and galactosialidosis		•	•
Niemann-Pick type C			•
Gaucher disease type III			•

For details of investigations and references, see Chapters 4D and 14.

children with epilepsy and these tests are normally done only in patients with symptoms.[10]

Hyponatremia occurs in approximately 3 per cent of patients receiving oxcarbazepine and electrolytes should be measured in patients who become symptomatic. Acetazolamide and topiramate may be associated with urolithiasis. Urinalysis should be performed in patients who develop abdominal pain and should also be done periodically in severely handicapped children receiving either of these drugs. Blood amylase should be performed in patients receiving valproic acid who develop unexplained abdominal pain or vomiting. Finally, patients receiving valproic acid should have a platelet count measured if they develop bruising or petechiae and should have a more detailed coagulation assessment prior to any major surgery.

Certain AEDs have been associated with rare, life-threatening adverse reactions, including aplastic anaemia, agranulocytosis, pancytopenia, hepatic failure and pancreatitis. Although recommendations have been produced by manufacturers for the routine laboratory monitoring of these adverse affects in patients receiving AEDs, there is no convincing evidence that laboratory monitoring alters the outcome for patients who develop these side-effects.[11]

A more helpful approach is for parents and patients to be educated about the clinical signs and symptoms of possible serious adverse effects and what they should do if these occur. Ideally, the patient and parent should be provided with written information in addition to the oral instructions. When a patient has clinical symptoms consistent with a serious adverse event, laboratory investigations should be performed urgently in order to confirm or rule out the diagnosis.

THERAPEUTIC DRUG MONITORING

Antiepileptic drug levels can be useful in the management of epilepsy but are unfortunately often measured inappropriately. In particular, the use of blood levels to adjust dosage so that numbers fall within the 'therapeutic range' is not only ineffective but may even be dangerous if effective and well-tolerated therapy is changed because levels are not in the published ranges.[12] The 'therapeutic range' holds true for the population as a whole but is not necessarily appropriate for the individual child being treated. Many children achieve seizure control at anticonvulsant blood levels that are below the 'therapeutic range,' whereas other patients achieve seizure control only at levels above the 'therapeutic range.' Similarly, some patients develop side-effects when the blood level is within the 'therapeutic range' whereas

Table 20.5 *Reasons for measurement of antiepileptic drug levels*

To determine:
- if a patient started on a new drug has achieved a blood level that is likely to be effective
- if poor seizure control might be due to an inadequate blood level
- if a low blood level is likely to be due to noncompliance
- if the clinical symptoms are likely to be due to drug toxicity
- if side-effects are likely to occur if the dose is increased

other patients have no side-effects at concentrations above the 'therapeutic range.' Consequently, as a general rule, changes in drug dosage should be based on clinical indications rather than drug levels. Measurement of drug levels is likely to be most helpful when there is a particular indication (see Table 20.5) and when the pretest probability is likely to be influenced by the result. 'Routine' measurement of drug levels should usually not be performed except in moderately or severely retarded children in whom the clinical manifestations of side-effects may be difficult to detect.

The value of measurement of drug levels has been demonstrated most convincingly in patients receiving phenytoin, which has complex pharmacokinetic properties. Indeed, phenytoin levels should probably be measured after any dosage change or when there is a change in the dose of a drug known to alter phenytoin metabolism or protein binding. Drug levels have also been used commonly in patients receiving phenobarbital, carbamazepine, ethosuximide and valproic acid. The value of measuring levels of the more recently introduced antiepileptic drugs is less well established.

Correct timing of the sample collection is essential. Thus, it is important to wait until the drug level has reached steady state, which may vary from 2 to 14 days (see Chapters 21 and 22A). In addition, the time of day at which the sampling occurs depends on the reason for measurement of the level. Levels performed because of poor seizure control are optimally performed before the first dose of the day, to capture to lowest level. In contrast, when toxicity is a concern, the level should be performed at the time of the symptoms or 3–4 h following the dose, when the peak concentration is estimated to occur. When levels are used to assess compliance, it is important to compare levels taken at the same time of day.

KEY POINTS

- The possibility of an acute symptomatic seizure should be considered in any child presenting with a first seizure, particularly if the child is febrile or has other evidence of a systemic disturbance
- Determination of the cause of the epilepsy can permit a more definitive prognosis, can have

important treatment implications, and may also have implications for genetic counseling
- The EEG is the single most useful investigation in the child with an afebrile seizure and is usually the only investigation necessary for the diagnosis of an idiopathic epilepsy
- MRI is the most sensitive anatomical neuroimaging investigation for children with epilepsy
- Routine laboratory investigations are not indicated in children on antiepileptic drugs
- Antiepileptic drug levels can be useful in the management of epilepsy but are often measured inappropriately
- Measurement of drug levels is particularly useful in patients receiving phenytoin, because of the pharmacokinetics involved, and in mentally handicapped patients in whom the clinical manifestations of side-effects may be difficult to detect

REFERENCES

1. American Academy of Pediatrics Policy Statement. Practice Parameter: the neurodiagnostic evaluation of the child with a first simple febrile seizure. *Pediatrics* 1996; **97**(5): 769–772.
2. Hirtz D, Ashwal S, Berg A *et al.* Practice parameter: Evaluating a first nonfebrile seizure in children. *Neurology* 2000; **55**: 616–623.
3. Guideline one: minimal technical requirements for performing clinical electroencephalography. *Journal of Clinical Neurophysiology* 1994; **11**: 2–5.
4. Shinnar S, Kang H, Berg AT, *et al.* EEG abnormalities in children with a first unprovoked seizure. *Epilepsia* 1994; **35**(3): 471–476.
5. King MA, Newton MR, Jackson GD, *et al.* Epileptology of the first-seizure presentation: a clinical, electroencephalographic, and magnetic resonance imaging study of 300 consecutive patients. *Lancet* 1998; **352**(9133): 1007–1011.
6. Hauser WA, Hesdorffer DC. *Epilepsy: Frequency, Causes and Consequences.* New York: Demos, 1990: 28–37.
7. Singh R, Gardner RJM, Crossland KM, Scheffer IE, Berkovic S. Chromosomal abnormalities and epilepsy: a review for clinicians and gene hunters. *Epilepsia* 2002; **43**: 127–140.
8. Shorvon S. *Status Epilepticus: Its Clinical Features and Treatment in Children and Adults.* Cambridge: Cambridge University Press, 1994; 175–182.
9. Camfield C, Camfield P, Smith E. Tibbles JA. Asymptomatic children with epilepsy: little benefit from screening for

anticonvulsant-induced liver, blood, or renal damage. *Neurology* 1986; **36**(6): 838–841.

10. Camfield P, Camfield C, Dooley J, *et al.* Routine screening of blood and urine for severe reactions to anticonvulsant drugs in asymptomatic patients is of doubtful value. *Canadian Medical Association Journal;* 1989; **140**(11): 1303–1305.

11. Pellock JM, Willmore J. A rational guide to routine blood monitoring in patients receiving antiepileptic drugs. *Neurology* 1991; **41**: 961–964.

12. Commission on Antiepileptic Drugs, International League Against Epilepsy. Guidelines for therapeutic monitoring on antiepileptic drugs. *Epilepsia* 1993; **34**(4): 585–587.

21

Pharmacology of antiepileptic drugs

ANDREW FISHER AND PHILIP N PATSALOS

Approximately 1 per cent of children are affected by epilepsy and in most instances the onset of symptoms occurs in infancy or early childhood. The immature brain may be susceptible to particular types of irreversible seizure-induced damage. Thus, it may be important, at least in some patients, to begin antiepileptic drug (AED) therapy as soon as possible after seizure presentation. Although we have a good understanding of the advantages and disadvantages of the long-established AEDs in children, novel AED treatments are evaluated initially only in adult patients. Our incomplete understanding of the pharmacokinetic, pharmacodynamic and safety profiles of these new medications in children limits their usefulness. A further issue particular to childhood epilepsy concerns the formulation of the drugs. Most adolescents are capable of swallowing capsules or tablets, but younger children may find liquid preparations or drug formulations that are liquid-soluble easier to take.

Therapeutic success depends not only on choosing the correct AED and formulation, but also identifying the optimal dose. In children, dose requirements may vary with time because of increasing body weight. In addition, children metabolize drugs much faster than adults because metabolic rate is inversely proportional to body surface area. Thus, an understanding of AED pharmacokinetics in children is essential.

This chapter reviews the pharmacology of AEDs, which are divided into two groups: those that are long-established and those new AEDs where limited data are available in relation to use in children. The mechanism of action, pharmacokinetic characteristics, interaction profile, safety profile and the role of therapeutic drug monitoring will be reviewed for each drug.

PHARMACOKINETICS IN CHILDREN

Absorption

GASTROINTESTINAL ABSORPTION

Gastrointestinal absorption in neonates is slow and unpredictable, particularly for relatively insoluble drugs such as carbamazepine and phenytoin, which exhibit poor bioavailability in the neonate. The gastric pH is neutral during the first 10–15 days of life, falling to adult levels at about 2 years of age. In addition, gastric emptying is slow and erratic for the first 6–8 months of life. Thus, oral bioavailability is not optimal in very young children. The different gastrointestinal flora in the neonate and infant may also influence bioavailability. Absorption processes rapidly become efficient during infancy, and oral bioavailability of AEDs in children is comparable to that of adults.[1,2]

Absorption rate is also dependent on formulation. Solutions, suspensions, chewable formulations and formulations that can be sprinkled on food will be absorbed faster than tablets or capsules. Enteric-coated tablets and other extended-release formulations are specifically designed to delay absorption.

Additional determinants of oral drug bioavailability include the activity of cytochrome P-450 (CYP) 3A4 and the expression of P-glycoprotein in the villus enterocytes of the small intestine.[3] Low P-glycoprotein activity in the gut wall results in shorter gut wall transit time, resulting in decreased gut wall CYP3A metabolism and increased drug bioavailability.

RECTAL ABSORPTION

When oral administration is not possible, the rectal route may provide a useful alternative. Rectal absorption can be rapid and efficient, particularly for lipid-soluble drugs such as diazepam. Indeed, rectal instillation of diazepam solution produces therapeutic plasma concentrations within a few minutes.[4] Rectal absorption of diazepam from suppositories is as fast as, but less efficient than, liquid formulations.

INTRAMUSCULAR ABSORPTION

Although intramuscular absorption of drugs is generally slow, new drug formulations have somewhat circumvented this therapeutic barrier. Drugs such as fosphenytoin, a phenytoin pro-drug, and midazolam are rapidly absorbed after intramuscular administration, allowing their use in an emergency situation such as status epilepticus.[5–7]

BUCCAL ABSORPTION

The surface area and pH of the mouth are similar to that of the rectum. They both have a rich blood supply and absorption occurs directly into the systemic circulation, which avoids high first-pass metabolism.[8] Indeed, midazolam has been shown to be rapidly absorbed after buccal administration and to have a rapid effect on the brain as determined electroencephalographically.[9] Furthermore, buccal midazolam appears at least as effective as rectal diazepam in the acute treatment of seizures.[10] This therapeutic approach has potential application, particularly for the treatment of acute seizures, since it is more socially acceptable and convenient.

Distribution

PLASMA PROTEIN BINDING

Many AEDs are protein bound in blood, primarily to albumin. It is the nonprotein-bound drug component that is available to cross the blood-brain barrier and exert its anticonvulsant effect. Thus, variability in plasma protein binding is clinically important. The plasma protein binding of AEDs such as phenytoin, phenobarbital and valproic acid is significantly reduced in the neonate, particularly if the baby is premature. This is a consequence of the persistence of fetal albumin (which is less able to bind drugs), hypoalbuminemia, and the displacement of drug by high levels of endogenous bilirubin and by free fatty acids. This results in an increased free fraction (free/total concentration ratio) but a decrease in the total plasma concentration. Correct interpretation of therapeutic drug monitoring data in the neonate needs an understanding of this phenomenon. Although monitoring free plasma concentrations would eliminate the effect of plasma protein binding, the larger sample volumes needed (200 μL of plasma) limit this approach in neonates.

TISSUE AND BRAIN DISTRIBUTION

The liver and the brain make up a larger proportion of body weight in the newborn, which is composed of less body fat and more water. Thus, drug distribution is reduced in the neonate and young infant, compared to older children and adults. Animal studies also suggest that a greater proportion of a protein-bound AED will cross the blood-brain barrier to reach the newborn brain, which may reflect changes in cerebral blood flow and capillary transit time during development.[11] The clinical significance of this is unknown, but it may enhance the neurotoxicity of AEDs in the newborn.

VOLUME OF DISTRIBUTION

The plasma concentration that results from a loading dose of a drug is inversely proportional to its volume of distribution (V_d). Age-related changes in V_d will alter loading dose requirements. The change in direction of the V_d is dependent on the characteristics described earlier (body water to body fat ratio, protein binding and tissue binding) and also on the physiochemical characteristics of the drug. Thus, the V_d of phenobarbital and phenytoin is larger in neonates than in older infants and children, whereas the V_d of diazepam and lorazepam is approximately the same.[12] Consequently, neonates will need larger loading doses (mg/kg) of phenytoin and phenobarbital to attain similar therapeutic concentrations as an adult.

Elimination

METABOLIC ELIMINATION

Most of the long-established AEDs are cleared almost exclusively by hepatic metabolism involving CYP and uridine diphosphate glucuronosyltransferase (UGT) enzymes. Among the new AEDs the exceptions to this are gabapentin, levetiracetam and vigabatrin. Five primary CYP isoenzymes (CYP1A2, CYP2C9, CYP2C19, CYP2D6 and CYP3A4) are involved in the hepatic metabolism of most AEDs. UGTs are involved in glucuronidation and there are two families, UGT1 and UGT2. The isoenzymes UGT1A and UGT1A4 are responsible for the glucuronidation of lamotrigine and the UGT2 family is responsible for the glucuronidation of valproic acid. In neonates, particularly those born prematurely, hepatic enzyme activity (CYP) is not fully developed ($\approx$50–70 per cent of adult levels), and consequently AEDs that require metabolism before removal from the body are eliminated very slowly. However, those neonates who may have been exposed transplacentally to hepatic enzyme-inducing

AEDs (carbamazepine, phenytoin, phenobarbital or primidone) will have more mature hepatic enzymes due to enzyme induction.

During postnatal development, hepatic enzyme activities increase rapidly and peak at 2–6-fold higher than adult activities by 6 months of age. The rate of hepatic metabolism decreases gradually to approximately 2 × adult activities by 6 years of age and reaches the adult rate around puberty. Thus, children who are receiving AED therapy should be monitored carefully for evidence of toxicity around this time. For example, phenytoin concentrations may rise during puberty without any change in drug dosage and result in drug toxicity. Metabolic processes that involve glucuronidation do not reach maturity until the age of 3–4 years, which has implications for those AEDs that are eliminated in this manner (e.g. lamotrigine and valproic acid).

RENAL ELIMINATION

None of the long-established AEDs are eliminated exclusively by renal excretion, although significant proportions of phenobarbital and primidone are excreted unchanged in urine. Interestingly, two of the seven new AEDs (gabapentin and vigabatrin) are eliminated exclusively by renal excretion in unchanged form, and the other five are in part excreted renally.[13] Premature newborns have decreased renal excretion, and AEDs excreted renally can be expected to have an increased half-life at this age.

THERAPEUTIC DRUG MONITORING IN CHILDREN

Therapeutic drug monitoring can be defined as 'the measurement and the clinical use of serum/plasma drug concentrations (levels) to adjust each patient's individual drug dosage and schedule to each patient's individual therapeutic requirement'. In practice, it is the patient that is treated and not the drug concentration. Thus, the drug concentration should be used as a guide to optimize its efficacy, identify toxicity and detect poor compliance. The criteria for monitoring AEDs in children are exactly the same as those for adults, but several additional factors need to be considered.[14,15] Neonates, infants and children undergo major and rapid age-related physiologic and biochemical changes, especially during the first year of life, which results not only in different clinical pharmacokinetic characteristics but also in different drug pharmacodynamics than adults. In addition, many children are unable to communicate whether or not they are experiencing drug-related adverse effects. Thus, therapeutic drug monitoring is a valuable tool in optimizing AED therapy in children.

Therapeutic drug monitoring is likely to be most helpful with AEDs that have a narrow therapeutic index (i.e. therapeutic doses are close to toxic doses). The pharmacological characteristics of some AEDs make them more suitable candidates for monitoring than others. The saturable pharmacokinetics of phenytoin makes it very difficult, if not impossible, to prescribe the optimum dose without measuring blood concentrations. There is a poor correlation between dosage and plasma concentrations of carbamazepine.[16–18] For carbamazepine and valproic acid, the interpretation of therapeutic drug monitoring is complicated by the presence of active metabolites, substantial diurnal variation in plasma concentrations and large interindividual variations in drug concentrations.

The concept of the target (therapeutic) range

Target ranges are widely quoted for AEDs (Table 21.1). It must be remembered that the target or therapeutic range is a population-derived statistical concept, which implies that within the range of drug concentrations, most patients receiving the drug will derive benefit from it with minimal side-effects. However, seizure control is often achieved at concentrations below the target range. In addition, seizure control may only be achieved in some patients at concentrations above the target range. Similarly, some patients experience toxicity at concentrations within the target range whereas others may have no side-effects at concentrations above the target range.[19,20] The target range must therefore be regarded as a guide and plasma drug concentrations must be considered in the context of a patient's symptoms and signs. In addition, there is evidence to suggest that different target ranges may apply for different seizure types[19,21,22] and that target or therapeutic ranges for children may be higher than those reported for adults.

For new AEDs the possible relationship between AED plasma drug concentrations, efficacy and side-effects is not usually systematically investigated during their clinical evaluation. Nevertheless, target ranges can be inferred from the clinical trial data and these ranges form the basis for the monitoring of new AEDs upon their license for general clinical use. These ranges can be expected to be refined as clinical experience accumulates.[15]

Altered plasma protein binding

Altered plasma protein binding can substantially effect the interpretation of drug concentration measurements. In most clinical settings the relationship between bound and unbound drug is constant and measurement of total

Table 21.1 *Guidelines for therapeutic drug monitoring of AEDs*

AED[a]	Time to steady state (days)	Putative target range[b]	
		μmol/L	mg/L
Established AEDs			
Carbamazepine	5[c]	12–50	3–12
Carbamazepine-epoxide		up to 9	up to 2
Clobazam	10	200–670[d,e]	60–200[f]
Clonazepam	17	80–270[d]	25–85[f]
Ethosuximide	12	300–700	40–100
Phenobarbital	20	40–170	10–40
Phenytoin	14–28	40–80 (adults)	10–20
		20–80 (children)	5–20
Primidone[g]	20	20–60	4–13
Valproic acid	3	350–700	50–100
New AEDs			
Felbamate	6	210–460	50–110
Gabapentin	2	12–120	2–20
Lamotrigine	13	4–60	1–15
Levetiracetam	2	35–118	6–20
Oxcarbazepine	2	50–110[e]	13–28
Tiagabine	1	200–1100[d]	80–450[f]
Topiramate	5	6–74	2–25
Vigabatrin	2	6–278	1–36
Zonisamide	12	50–190	10–40

[a] Carbamazepine, gabapentin, levetiracetam, tiagabine valproic acid and vigabatrin exhibit significant diurnal variation. Ideal sampling time is immediately before an oral dose. During suspected toxicity, sampling should be undertaken at time when adverse events are presenting.
[b] Target ranges as practiced in the author's laboratory. See text for further details.
[c] Because carbamazepine exhibits substantial autoinduction, 20 days need to elapse if the drug has been introduced for the first time.
[d] Drug values are in nmol/L.
[e] Refers to the pharmacologically active metabolite of clobazam (N-desmethyl clobazam) and oxcarbazepine (10-OH-carbazepine).
[f] drug values are in μg/L.
[g] During therapy with primidone, monitoring of only the active metabolite phenobarbital is recommended.

blood concentrations will suffice. However, when plasma protein binding is changed by disease (e.g. hepatic or renal disease), physiological change (e.g. pregnancy, aging) or iatrogenic procedures (e.g. surgery), the relationship between total drug concentration and the free concentration is substantialy changed. Plasma protein binding may also be altered during polytherapy with highly protein-bound drugs. For example, phenytoin is displaced from its protein binding sites by salicylates and valproic acid. In these circumstances, measurement of free drug concentrations may provide a better guide. However, free concentration monitoring should be restricted to highly protein bound (>90 per cent) drugs such as phenytoin and, possibly, valproic acid and tiagabine.

Monitoring of AEDs in saliva

Saliva can be used as an alternative to blood for the monitoring of AEDs.[23] The advantages of measuring salivary concentrations include:

- collection of saliva is simple and noninvasive and is achieved with minimal discomfort
- the procedure does not require venesection expertise and acquiring the sample may be cheaper
- the procedure is associated with less stress, fear and discomfort and avoids complications of infection and thrombosis
- measured concentrations reflect the free (pharmacologically relevant) concentration in blood.

Although saliva sampling is impracticable in neonates and infants, it can be readily achieved in older children.

There are substantial data suggesting useful correlation between saliva concentrations and free unbound drug in plasma for carbamazepine, phenytoin, primidone and ethosuximide.[24,25] This is not the case for valproic acid, and there is some controversy for phenobarbital.[25,26] The new AEDs are detectable in saliva, but the relationship between saliva and blood concentrations has not been established for these AEDs.

Patient sampling

A recommended method for monitoring is illustrated in Table 21.1. The timing of the blood sample is important. It is essential to ensure that sampling occurs at steady-state. This occurs at 4–6 half-lives after starting treatment or a dose change. If blood sampling is undertaken before steady-state, plasma concentration for a given dose will be underestimated and dosage increase may result in unnecessary toxicity for the patient.

It is also essential to select the sampling time in relation to dose. When there are concerns regarding efficacy or poor compliance, the ideal blood sampling time for all AEDs is immediately before the next oral dose (trough). If this is not possible, it is important to note the sampling time and the time medication was last ingested and to interpret the data with these in mind. If there is concern regarding toxicity, sampling should occur ideally around the time of the symptoms or, at least, when the peak concentration is expected to occur.

ESTABLISHED AEDs

Benzodiazepines

Clobazam, clonazepam, nitrazepam and diazepam are the most commonly used benzodiazepine compounds currently marketed as AEDs.

Table 21.2 *Mechanism of action of AEDs*

	↓ Na⁺ channels	↓ Ca²⁺ channels	↑ K⁺ channels	↑ Inhibitory transmission	↓ Excitatory transmission
Established AEDs					
Benzodiazepines				①	
Carbamazepine	①	③			
Ethosuximide		①			
Phenobarbital		③		①	③
Phenytoin	①	②			
Primidone		③		①	③
Valproic acid	③	③		②	③
New AEDs					
Felbamate	②	②		②	②
Gabapentin	③	③		②	
Lamotrigine	①	③			
Levetiracetam		③		③	③
Oxcarbazepine	①	③	③		
Tiagabine				①	
Topiramate	②	②		②	②
Vigabatrin				①	
Zonisamide	②	②			

① – primary action; ② – probable action; ③ – possible action.
Na⁺ – sodium; Ca²⁺ – calcium; K⁺ – potassium

MECHANISM OF ACTION

The benzodiazepine drugs exhibit similar effects to the barbiturate class of anticonvulsant on GABA$_A$ receptors (Table 21.2). The facilitation of chloride ion influx is mediated via an increase in channel opening frequency without affecting mean open duration or ion conductance.[27] This is in contrast to the barbiturates, which specifically increase mean channel open duration. Other mechanisms of action of the benzodiazepines include the inhibition of voltage-dependent sodium[28] and calcium channels.[29] However, these effects are only apparent at doses far exceeding normal therapeutic concentrations and are unlikely to have any clinical relevance except perhaps in the treatment of status epilepticus, where high doses of benzodiazepines are often used.

PHARMACOKINETICS

Benzodiazepines are generally rapidly and completely absorbed following oral administration, with peak plasma concentrations usually occurring within 1–4 h (Table 21.3). The rate of absorption can be reduced when the drugs are co-ingested with food. Clobazam, clonazepam and diazepam are highly protein bound (85–97 per cent) and therefore factors that alter protein binding may result in fluctuations in the total drug concentration. Benzodiazepines undergo hepatic metabolism and diazepam and clobazam are metabolized to desmethyldiazepam and desmethylclobazam respectively, which

are pharmacologically active. The elimination half-life of the benzodiazepines in children typically ranges from 10 to 50 h in young children but can be longer in neonates.

Diazepam is rapidly absorbed rectally, with peak plasma concentrations occurring within 10–20 min. Intravenous administration results in rapid brain penetration and an anticonvulsant effect can be seen within 1–2 min. However, it subsequently redistributes rapidly from the brain to muscle and fat, which markedly limits the duration of the anticonvulsant effect. Infused diazepam accumulates and its elimination is slow.[30] Consequently the neurotoxic effects wear off more slowly.

DRUG INTERACTIONS

Benzodiazepines have little if any effect on the metabolism of other AEDs, although patients receiving high doses of phenytoin have been observed to develop phenytoin toxicity when used in combination with clobazam (Table 21.4). Enzyme-inducing AEDs (phenobarbital, primidone, carbamazepine and phenytoin) enhance the metabolism of both clobazam and clonazepam and patients may require higher doses of these drugs in order to maintain adequate seizure control. For diazepam, the metabolism of the active metabolite is also enhanced. Valproic acid displaces diazepam from its plasma protein binding sites and also inhibits its metabolism, thus increasing the free concentration of diazepam.[31]

Table 21.3 *Pharmacokinetic characteristics of AEDs*

	Bioavailability (%)	T_{max} (h)	V_d (L/kg)	Protein binding (%)	$t^{1/2}$ (h)[a] Neonates	Infants	Children	Adults	Major route of elimination[b]
Established AEDs									
Carbamazepine	75–85	2–12[c]	0.8–2	75	8–35	3–15	3–15	5–25	HM
Clobazam	>90	1–4	–	85[d]				10–50	HM
Clonazepam	>90	1–4	2.0	85	20–45	20–30	20–30	25–40	HM
Diazepam	100		2.4	97	10–100	8–30	8–30	20–70	HM
Ethosuximide	>90	1–4	0.7	0	35–60		20–50	40–70	HM
Phenobarbital	>90	1–6	0.55	45	60–400	40–80	40–80	60–140	HM/RE
Phenytoin	>90	2–12	0.75	90	17–60[e]		12–22[e]	18–30[e]	HM
Primidone	>90	4–6	0.75	25	10–35		4–15	5–20	HM/RE
Valproic acid	100	1–8[c]	0.16	92	10–70		6–15	5–18	HM
New AEDs									
Felbamate	>90	2–6	0.75	25				14–23	HM/RE
Gabapentin	35–60	2–3	0.85	0				5–7	RE
Lamotrigine	>90	1–3	1.2	55				5–9	HM
Levetiracetam	100	0.6–1.3	0.5–0.7	0			5–7	6–8	NHM/RE
Oxcarbazepine[f]	>90	3–5	0.75	40				8–10	HM/RE
Tiagabine	90	1–2	1.4	96				5–8	HM
Topiramate	>80	1–4	0.65	15				19–25	HM/RE
Vigabatrin	80	0.5–2	0.8	0			4–7	5–8	RE
Zonisamide	95	2–6	1.5	55				27–70	HM/RE

[a] For drugs that undergo hepatic metabolism, half-life values will vary depending on whether or not concomitant enzyme inhibitors or inducers are co-prescribed.
[b] HM, hepatic metabolism; NHM, nonhepatic metabolism; RE, renal excretion; T_{max}, time to maximum plasma concentration after oral ingestion of drug; $t^{1/2}$ = elimination half-life, V_d, volume of distribution.
[c] Includes absorption of control release formulations.
[d] Refers to the pharmacologically active (N-desmethyl clobazam) metabolite of clobazam.
[e] Exhibits saturable kinetics. Half-life therefore dependent on plasma concentration.
[f] Refers to the pharmacologically active (10-hydroxy-carbazepine) metabolite of oxcarbazepine.

ADVERSE EFFECTS

Typical dose-related side-effects associated with benzodiazepines include ataxia, sedation, ocular disturbances, depression and the development of tolerance. Behavioral changes such as hyperactivity and aggression may also occur in some children.

THERAPEUTIC DRUG MONITORING

Therapeutic drug monitoring of benzodiazepines has not been demonstrated to be clinically useful.[32,33]

Carbamazepine

Carbamazepine is an iminodibenzyl derivative that is structurally related to the tricyclic antidepressants.

MECHANISM OF ACTION

Carbamazepine inhibits sustained, repetitive high-frequency neuronal firing via the blockade of voltage-gated sodium channels in a manner dependent on use and frequency (Table 21.2).[34,35] Moreover, carbamazepine was

reported to inhibit L-type calcium channels in cultured rat hippocampal neurons stimulated with glutamate receptor antagonists.[36] There are also reports that carbamazepine may modulate glutaminergic,[37] serotonergic,[38] dopaminergic[39] and purinergic[40,41] neurotransmission, although the significance of these actions on carbamazepine's clinical effectiveness is not clear at this time.

PHARMACOKINETICS

Carbamazepine is extremely water insoluble and is slowly and erratically absorbed after oral administration. The rate of absorption is greater in children than in adults. Malnourished children exhibit reduced absorption and bioavailability.[42] The different carbamazepine formulations have varying rates of absorption and bioavailability. Syrup formulations require a shorter time to reach maximum plasma concentration (T_{max}), but chewable formulations are similar to plain tablets in this respect.[43,44] The slow-release formulation is associated with a prolonged absorption phase. Diurnal variation in plasma concentrations is greater in children than in adults, which can result in intermittent side-effects. This effect can be minimized

Table 21.4 *Expected changes in plasma concentrations when an antiepileptic drug (AED) is added to an existing AED regimen*

AED added	Existing AED PB	PHT	PRM	ETS	CBZ	DZP	CZP	VPA	CLB	VGB	LTG	GBP	TPM	TGB	OXC	LEV	FBM	ZNS
PB	AI	PHT⇑⇓	NCCP	ETS⇓	CBZ⇓	DZP↓	CZP↓	VPA⇓	CLB↓ NDMC↑	NA	LTG⇓	NA	TPM⇓	TGB⇓	H-OXC↓	NA	FBM⇓	ZNS⇓
PHT	PB↑	AI	PRM↓ PB↑	ETS⇓	CBZ⇓	DZP↓	CZP↓	VPA⇓	CLB↓ NDMC↑	NA	LTG⇓	NA	TPM⇓	TGB⇓	H-OXC↓	NA	FBM⇓	ZNS⇓
PRM	NCCP	PHT⇑⇓	AI	ETS⇓	CBZ⇓	DZP↓	CZP↓	VPA⇓	NDMC↑	NA	LTG⇓	NA	TPM⇓	TGB⇓	?	NA	FBM⇓	ZNS⇓
ETS	NA	PHT↑	NA	—	NA	NA	NA	VPA↓	NA	NA	NA	NA	NA	NA	NA	NA	NA	NA
CBZ	NA	PHT↑*	PRM↓ PB↑	ETS⇓	AI	DZP↓	CZP↓	VPA⇓	NDMC↑	NA	LTG⇓	NA	TPM⇓	TGB⇓	H-OXC↓	NA	FBM⇓	ZNS⇓
DZP	NA	PHT↑⇓	NA	NA	NA	—	NA	NA	NA	NA	NA	NA	NA	NA	NA	NA	NA	NA
CZP	NA	PHT↑⇓	NA	NA	CBZ↓	NA	—	NA	NA	NA	NA	NA	NA	NA	NA	NA	?	NA
VPA	PB⇑	PHT↑*	PRM↑ PB⇑	ETS↑↓	CBZ↓ CBZ-E⇑	DZP↑*	NA	—	NA	NA	LTG⇑	NA	TPM↓	TPM↓	NA	NA	FBM⇑	NA
CLB	PB↑	PHT↑↓	PRM↑ PB↑	NA	CBZ↓	NA	CZP⇓	VPA↑	—	NA	NA	NA	NA	NA	NA	NA	NA	NA
VGB	PB↓	PHT⇓	PRM↓ PB↓	NA	CBZ↑	NA	NA	NA	NA	—	NA	NA	?	NA	?	NA	?	?
LTG	NA	NA	NA	NA	NA	NA	NA	NA	NA	NA	—	NA	NA	NA	NA	NA	NA	NA
GBP	NA	NA	NA	NA	NA	NA	NA	NA	NA	NA	—	—	NA	NA	—	NA	NA	NA
TPM	NA	PHT↑	NA	NA	NA	NA	NA	VPA↓	NA	NA	?	NA	—	?	?	NA	?	?
TGB	NA	NA	NA	NA	NA	NA	NA	VPA↓	NA	NA	NA	NA	—	—	NA	—	NA	NA
OXC	PB↑	PHT↑	?	?	CBZ⇓ CBZ-E↑	?	?	NA	?	NA	LTG↓	NA	TPM↓	?	—	NA	?	?
LEV	NA	NA	NA	NA	NA	NA	NA	NA	NA	NA	NA	NA	NA	NA	NA	—	NA	NA
FBM	PB⇑	PHT⇑	?	?	CBZ⇓ CBZ-E⇑	?	?	VPA⇓	?	NA	LTG↓	NA	?	?	NA	NA	—	?
ZNS	NA	PHT↑	NA	NA	CBZ↑	?	?	NA	?	NA	NA	NA	NA	NA	?	NA	?	—

CBZ, carbamazepine; CBZ-E, carbamazepine epoxide; CLB, clobazam; CZP, clonazepam; DZP, diazepam; ESM, ethosuximide; FBM, felbamate; GBP, gabapentin; H-OXC, 10-hydroxy-carbazepine; LTG, lamotrigine; NDMC, N-desmethylclobazam; OXC, oxcarbazepine; PB, phenobarbital; PHT, phenytoin; PRM, primidone; TGB, tiagabine; TPM, topiramate; VPA, valproic acid; VGB, vigabatrin; ZNS, zonisamide; NA, none anticipated; *, free pharmacologically active concentration; AI, autoinduction; NCCP, not commonly co-prescribed; ?, not known. ↓, an infrequently observed decrease in serum concentration; ⇓, a frequently observed decrease in serum concentration; ↑, an infrequently observed increase in serum concentration; ⇑, a frequently observed increase in serum concentration.

by more frequent dosing or by use of a slow release formulation, which has been reported to reduce the diurnal variation by 35–42 per cent.[45]

Carbamazepine is rapidly and extensively distributed to all body tissues with 75 per cent of drug bound to plasma proteins (Table 21.3). Carbamazepine is metabolized by the liver to carbamazepine-10,11-epoxide, which is hydrolyzed to carbamazepine-10,11-*trans*dihydrodiol. Carbamazepine-epoxide, a pharmacologically active metabolite, is 57 per cent protein bound. Infants metabolize carbamazepine more rapidly than adults, which results in carbamazepine-epoxide concentrations approaching those of the parent drug. Thus, carbamazepine-epoxide has a greater contribution to the pharmacologic effects (both beneficial and toxic) of carbamazepine in infants and children. Carbamazepine induces its own metabolism (autoinduction) with a resultant increase in clearance and reduction in plasma half-life during the first 4 weeks of administration.

DRUG INTERACTIONS

Carbamazepine metabolism is highly inducible by certain AEDs (Table 21.4). Thus co-medication with primidone, phenobarbital and phenytoin is commonly associated with significant reductions in carbamazepine plasma concentrations. Moreover, the diurnal variation in plasma carbamazepine concentrations, which may amount to 23–45 per cent on monotherapy, can be doubled when enzyme-inducing AEDs are added, which increases the risk of transient side-effects.

There is increasing evidence that the epoxide may contribute not only to the efficacy of carbamazepine but also to the toxicity. In recent years, interactions involving the selective inhibition of the metabolism of carbamazepine to its epoxide metabolite or the subsequent metabolism of the epoxide have been described.[46] These interactions may result in neurological toxicity at total carbamazepine concentrations that are unchanged. In this regard, the elevation of carbamazepine-epoxide concentrations by drugs such as valproic acid may be clinically significant in children.

Carbamazepine increases the metabolism of a wide variety of concurrently administered drugs including AEDs. Drugs whose clinical effects may be significantly affected include oral anticoagulants, beta-blockers, haloperidol, felodipine and theophylline.[47] The clinical significance of these interactions is variable and dosage adjustments may be necessary in some patients.

Macrolide antibiotics, including erythromycin, josamycin, triacetyloleandomycin, ponsinomycin and clarithromycin, inhibit carbamazepine metabolism and have been associated with carbamazepine toxicity.[47,48] Toxicity is observed shortly after starting erythromycin therapy, is rapidly reversed upon withdrawal of the antibiotic but can be severe if not recognized early. Plasma carbamazepine concentrations should be monitored if treatment with macrolide antibiotics is necessary.

ADVERSE EFFECTS

Carbamazepine is generally well tolerated although initial therapy can result in the appearance of hypersensitive rashes at doses that are comfortably tolerated later in the course of treatment.[49] Other dose-related side-effects include sedation, headache, nausea and cognitive and emotive disturbances. These effects are primarily reversible and can be prevented by slow and careful upward titration following initiation of treatment. Serious systemic toxicity is rare following treatment although there have been reported instances of aplastic anemia[50] and cardiac conduction disturbances[51] which may require discontinuation of therapy. Hyponatremia has also been reported.[52]

THERAPEUTIC DRUG MONITORING

The dose of carbamazepine is a poor guide to plasma concentrations. Carbamazepine exhibits autoinduction. Thus, after initiation of therapy, steady-state blood concentrations are only achieved after 20 days. As there is substantial variation in blood concentrations, sampling should be ideally undertaken just before the next scheduled dose (Table 21.1).

Ethosuximide

Ethosuximide is a succinimide used in the treatment of absence seizures.

MECHANISM OF ACTION

Ethosuximide blocks T-type calcium ion currents in thalamocortical[53] and in dorsal root ganglion neurons.[54] Low threshold T-type calcium channels play an integral role in the relationship between normal sleep pattern EEG and the 3 Hz spike and wave activity seen in absence epilepsy. By blocking these channels, ethosuximide prevents abnormal thalamocortical neuronal firing without affecting normal thalamic cell activity.[53]

PHARMACOKINETICS

Ethosuximide displays rapid absorption and has a bioavailability approaching 100 per cent after oral administration (Table 21.3). Peak plasma ethosuximide concentrations are reached within 3–7 h during chronic therapy. It is not protein bound and its V_d is 0.7 L/kg. Extensive hepatic metabolism by oxidation and then conjugation forms metabolites that are pharmacologically inert. Approximately 20 per cent of ethosuximide is excreted as unchanged drug in urine. The long elimination half-life is dose-dependent and allows once or twice daily dosing. Ethosuximide does not induce hepatic enzyme activity.

DRUG INTERACTIONS

Interactions with ethosuximide are rare and usually minor (Table 21.4). Enzyme-inducing AEDs enhance ethosuximide metabolism and reduce plasma concentrations.[55] Isoniazid and valproic acid may increase plasma ethosuximide concentrations in some patients by inhibition of metabolism.

ADVERSE EFFECTS

The most common dose-dependent side-effects are gastrointestinal disturbances, anorexia, lethargy, headache and behavioral disturbances. Nausea, which usually occurs shortly after initiation of treatment, can be alleviated by dose reduction. Anxiety, drowsiness, depression and sleep disturbances are seen occasionally in patients receiving ethosuximide and respond usually to drug withdrawal.

THERAPEUTIC DRUG MONITORING

In most patients routine monitoring of ethosuximide is generally unnecessary since ethosuximide plasma concentrations correlate well with dose and the dosage can be adjusted empirically on the basis of response (Table 21.1).

Phenobarbital

Phenobarbital is a substituted barbituric acid.

MECHANISM OF ACTION

Phenobarbital acts at the $GABA_A$ receptor and facilitates chloride ion influx by increasing the duration but not frequency of ion channel opening (Table 21.2).[56] Enhanced permeability of chloride ions generates hyperpolarization in the postsynaptic cell membrane and consequently hinders the conduction of epileptic activity. In addition, phenobarbital has been reported to inhibit voltage-dependent neurotransmitter release via inhibition of presynaptic calcium uptake.[57]

PHARMACOKINETICS

Phenobarbital exhibits good bioavailability following oral (>90 per cent) or intramuscular (80 per cent) administration in older infants and children. Oral bioavailability in neonates is typically lower because of poor absorption. Peak plasma concentrations are attained within 1–6 h (Table 21.3). In neonates the time to peak plasma concentrations is longer (9 h) than in infants and young children (3 h). After intramuscular injection of phenobarbital, the mean T_{max} varies from 7 to 40 h in premature infants, from 30 min to 27 h in fullterm neonates and from 45 min to 6 h in children. Phenobarbital is 45 percent protein bound. However, protein binding is 25–50 per cent lower in neonates than in older children and is even lower if there is hyperbilirubinemia.[58] The higher plasma concentrations of free drug during the first few days of life would suggest that the neonatal brain is exposed to higher concentrations of phenobarbital relative to plasma concentrations.[59] Phenobarbital is metabolized in the liver to numerous hydroxylated and conjugated metabolites, the primary metabolite being parahydroxy-phenobarbital, which is pharmacologically inactive. Elimination is age dependent and highly variable. Elimination in the neonate is slower and particularly variable.

DRUG INTERACTIONS

Perhaps the most predictable and clinically important interaction affecting phenobarbital is the elevation of plasma phenobarbital concentrations by valproic acid (Table 21.4). This inhibition of phenobarbital metabolism occurs in most patients and can lead to toxicity if the phenobarbital dosage is not reduced.[60] The degree of inhibition varies markedly and depends partly upon the phenobarbital baseline concentration.

As phenobarbital is a potent hepatic enzyme inducer, it enhances the metabolism of many AEDs (e.g. phenytoin, carbamazepine, valproic acid, lamotrigine and topiramate) and also drugs such as digitoxin, theophylline and warfarin. Higher doses of these drugs may be necessary to achieve therapeutic plasma concentrations.

ADVERSE EFFECTS

Behavioral and cognitive deficits commonly occur.[61] Sedation, ataxia and nystagmus are almost always encountered with higher doses whereas paradoxal drug-induced hyperactivity, aggression, irritability and insomnia have been reported in children treated with phenobarbital.[62] One of the main drawbacks in phenobarbital therapy is the risk of drug dependence. In most cases, abrupt withdrawal of phenobarbital has pronounced rebound effects manifested in the form of tremors, exacerbation of seizures or anxiogenesis.

THERAPEUTIC DRUG MONITORING

Monitoring of phenobarbital can be useful in improving compliance, for confirming the clinical diagnosis of toxicity and for minimizing the effects of drug interactions.

Phenytoin

Phenytoin is a hydantoin derivative.

MECHANISM OF ACTION

Phenytoin exerts many cellular effects but the main anticonvulsant properties relate to inhibition of voltage-dependent sodium channels (Table 21.2).[63] Phenytoin binds to the sodium channel use-dependently in its inactivated state and causes a reduction in the frequency of ictal excitability without affecting action potential amplitude or duration.[64] Thus, phenytoin will selectively act on sodium channels in neurons that are firing at high frequency following tonic activation, while exhibiting lower efficacy in neurons engaged in slow-rate neuronal firing.[65] Phenytoin has also been reported to reduce cortical excitability through a mechanism that involves the blockade of persistent sodium currents.[66] Blocking these persistent currents delays the time taken for the membrane potential to reach firing level during repeated stimulation culminating in prolonged interspike intervals and reduced neuronal firing.

Phenytoin inhibits calcium channels resulting in decreased intracellular calcium and reduction in calcium-calmodulin-regulated protein phosphorylation.[67–70] This has wide reaching consequences in many cellular processes and is thought to account for phenytoin's broad anticonvulsant profile.

PHARMACOKINETICS

Phenytoin is extremely insoluble at gastric pH and relies on the high pH of the small intestine for absorption. Food co-ingestion increases phenytoin absorption by as much as 40 per cent in the first year of life, during which time phenytoin is usually absorbed slowly and erratically. Food co-ingestion has a smaller effect in older children (+26 per cent between 1 and 6 years and +13 per cent between 7 and 18 years). In contrast, enteral feeding can markedly reduce the absorption of phenytoin suspension. The bioavailability of phenytoin is ≈95 per cent, but different formulations have dissimilar bioavailabilities. These differences can be clinically significant and thus different formulations should not be used interchangeably.

After oral ingestion peak plasma concentrations are typically achieved within 2–12 h (Table 21.3). Phenytoin is highly protein bound (90 per cent) with lower and more variable binding values seen in neonates. Hyperbilirubinemia further decreases phenytoin binding in neonates.[71] Furthermore, in patients receiving concomitant valproic acid therapy, the free phenytoin fraction is higher and indeed more variable than when phenytoin is administered as monotherapy.

Phenytoin is extensively metabolized in the liver by parahydroxylation of a phenyl ring followed by glucuronidation giving rise to a series of pharmacologically inert metabolites that are renally excreted. The metabolism of phenytoin is saturable at plasma concentrations within the target range. In addition, the concentration that is associated with saturation varies considerably from patient to patient. Consequently, the clearance of phenytoin is highly variable and an exponential increase in phenytoin plasma concentration can occur as a consequence of a small increment in phenytoin dose. Neonates eliminate phenytoin more slowly and children more rapidly than adults.

DRUG INTERACTIONS

Interactions with phenytoin are the most commonly observed interactions in epilepsy practice and this can be attributed to its rather unique pharmacokinetic characteristics (extensively bound to plasma proteins and also very loosely bound to hepatic CYP enzymes), which make it particularly susceptible to competitive displacement and inhibitory metabolic interactions (Table 21.4).[47] Additionally, phenytoin is also a potent inducer of hepatic enzyme activities and its metabolism is saturable at therapeutic concentrations. Thus, inhibition of metabolism may produce a disproportionate increase in circulating drug concentration and enhance the risk of toxicity. Induction of phenytoin metabolism is often not clinically significant. Plasma phenytoin concentrations should be monitored regularly when co-medication is introduced or withdrawn.

An important interaction of phenytoin is that seen with valproic acid. Valproic acid both displaces phenytoin from its binding sites and is also a weak inhibitor of phenytoin metabolism. This results in unpredictable changes in plasma phenytoin concentrations and complicates their interpretation. Phenytoin is a potent enzyme inducer and can be associated with as much as a 50 per cent reduction in the plasma concentrations of some other drugs. Thus, appropriate dosage adjustments need to be made if phenytoin is added or withdrawn.

ADVERSE EFFECTS

An allergic skin rash may occur with phenytoin treatment in children, especially when large loading doses of drug are administered. It occurs usually within 1–2 weeks after initiation of treatment. Dose-related side-effects include blurred vision, dizziness, unsteadiness, impaired cognitive function, headache, choreoathetosis and drowsiness. Nausea and constipation can be avoided by ingesting phenytoin with food.

THERAPEUTIC DRUG MONITORING

Phenytoin is a highly protein-bound drug and undergoes saturable hepatic metabolism. Therefore, small changes in dose or the introduction of a drug that displaces phenytoin from its protein binding sites or inhibits its metabolism can result in a disproportionate increase in phenytoin blood concentrations. Furthermore, there is considerable interpatient variability in the phenytoin concentration at which saturation of hepatic enzymes occurs. As a result, phenytoin treatment is very difficult without monitoring (Table 21.1). Because of the low elimination rate at high concentrations, phenytoin may take up to 4 weeks to achieve steady-state.

Primidone

Primidone is a desoxybarbiturate that was introduced into clinical practice in 1952. Although classified as a barbiturate, in fact it has few structural similarities to the barbiturate family of AEDs.

MECHANISM OF ACTION

Primidone is metabolized to two pharmacologically active metabolites, phenobarbital and phenylethylmalonamide (PEMA). Although primidone and PEMA have anticonvulsant activity, they are not considered to contribute significantly to the clinical efficacy of primidone, which is considered to be due to phenobarbital.

PHARMACOKINETICS

Primidone is rapidly absorbed after oral ingestion with peak plasma concentrations occurring within 4–6 h in children (Table 21.3).[72] Bioavailability is >90 per cent and binding to plasma proteins is low (25 per cent). As previously noted, primidone is rapidly metabolized to phenobarbital, which is then metabolized to the inactive metabolite para-hydroxyphenobarbital, and to PEMA. There is very high variability in the metabolism of primidone to phenobarbital and age-dependent changes in this metabolism are well documented.[72] Indeed, neonates and infants are unable to convert primidone to phenobarbital until 3–4 months of age and children have plasma phenobarbital/primidone ratios that are significantly lower than adolescents and adults.[73,74] These differences are reflected in the elimination half-life values of the drug.

DRUG INTERACTIONS

The interpretation of interactions between primidone and other drugs is complicated by the presence of its two pharmacologically active metabolites phenobarbital and PEMA. Thus, all the known interactions of phenobarbital (see above) may also be expected to occur in patients taking primidone. The most clinically significant interaction of primidone is the secondary inhibition of phenobarbital metabolism by valproic acid (Table 21.4). Furthermore, the phenobarbital metabolite induces the metabolism of a variety of drugs requiring dosage adjustment of concomitant drugs.

ADVERSE EFFECTS

Primidone has a similar toxicity profile to phenobarbital but nausea, dizziness, ataxia and sedation can be seen at low doses and can occur before phenobarbital is detected in the blood. This suggests that these effects are due to primidone itself and not to its metabolite. Tolerance to these effects occurs with chronic treatment, and patients can often subsequently cope with much higher doses of the drug.

THERAPEUTIC DRUG MONITORING

Primidone is metabolized to two pharmacologically active metabolites, phenobarbital and PEMA. If monitoring is indicated, measurement of phenobarbital only is recommended (Table 21.1).

Valproic acid

Valproic acid is a simple short-chain fatty acid.

MECHANISM OF ACTION

The precise mechanism of action of valproic acid is currently uncertain. It has been reported to exert an inhibitory action on voltage-sensitive sodium channels,[75] but differs from drugs such as phenytoin in that it does not appear to bind to these channels in its inactivated state.[76] Instead, valproic acid decreases the frequency potentiation in voltage-sensitive sodium channels and prolongs the afterdischarge generated by antidromic stimulation, possibly via a mechanism involving calcium-dependent potassium ion conductance.[77] Elevations in brain γ-aminobutyric acid (GABA) concentrations have been reported to be due to inhibition of GABA-transaminase, the enzyme responsible for GABA metabolism,[78] enhancement of the GABA synthesizing enzyme, glutamic acid decarboxylase,[78,79] increased GABA release[80] and decreased GABA uptake.[81] An increase in GABA neurotransmission may play a role in the anticonvulsant action of valproic acid, but high concentrations are required to elicit many of the effects described above. This suggests that there are probably additional, unidentified mechanisms responsible for the clinical efficacy of valproic acid.

PHARMACOKINETICS

Valproic acid, when formulated as its sodium salt, displays complete absorption and almost 100 per cent bioavailability within 1 h of ingestion (Table 21.3). Peak plasma concentrations of the drug are typically reached within 1–2 h in children except when slow release formulations are used. Absorption is relatively slower in neonates (mean T_{max} 4 h) and infants (2–3 h). Approximately 90 per cent of valproic acid is bound to plasma proteins, but this binding is saturable. Thus, the concentration of unbound drug increases from 7–9 per cent when plasma concentrations are below 520 μmol/L to 30 per cent when concentrations approach 1040 μmol/L.[82] This concentration-dependent alteration in free plasma concentrations of valproic acid influences the elimination kinetics of the drug and contributes to the interpatient variability in plasma concentrations. The interpatient variability may also be influenced by inter-individual differences in the concentration of binding proteins (mostly albumin) and endogenous binding modulators, particularly free fatty acids.[83] Hepatic elimination accounts for almost 100 per cent of valproic acid metabolism, with only 4 per cent of the compound excreted as unchanged drug. Metabolism results in numerous metabolites, which are pharmacologically active and may contribute to both its efficacy and toxicity. The elimination half-life is longer in neonates (10–70 h) than in children (6–15 h). The decline in the elimination half-life with age is thought to be attributable to a decrease in extravascular distribution volume and developmental-related enhancement of drug metabolism. These values are decreased by 30–50 per cent in patients co-prescribed hepatic enzyme-inducing AEDs.

DRUG INTERACTIONS

Valproic acid is a potent inhibitor both of oxidative pathways and of glucuronide conjugation pathways. Consequently it inhibits the metabolism of many AEDs (e.g. phenobarbital, phenytoin, ethosuximide, carbamazepine and lamotrigine). The inhibition of the metabolism of nimodipine may be particularly clinically significant.[84] Conversely, felbamate inhibits the metabolism of valproic acid, resulting in its clearance being decreased by as much as 50 per cent.[85] Thus, a reduction in the dose of valproic acid is necessary when felbamate is co-administered.

Because valproic acid is extensively metabolized in the liver, enzyme-inducing AEDs stimulate its metabolism resulting in the need to administer higher doses of valproic acid during co-medication with these AEDs.

ADVERSE EFFECTS

Valproic acid can result in serious hepatic toxicity in very young infants, particularly when used as polytherapy.[86] It also has a teratogenic effect and spina bifida occurs in 1 per cent of children born to mothers receiving valproic acid during pregnancy. In children, the most common dose-dependent side-effects include hyperammonemia,[87] tremor[88] and weight gain.[89]

THERAPEUTIC DRUG MONITORING

Valproic acid monitoring is probably unnecessary for most patients on monotherapy but may have a role when patients are on drugs that are known to interact with valproic acid and when noncompliance is suspected.

NEW AEDs

Felbamate

Felbamate is a carbamate derived from 1,3-propanediol.

MECHANISM OF ACTION

Felbamate has been shown to exert a direct antagonistic action on the N-methyl D-aspartate (NMDA) subtype of glutamate receptor. It reduces NMDA-mediated intracellular calcium ion passage,[90] reduces inward currents evoked by localized NMDA application on to striatal neurons[91] and impedes NMDA receptor-mediated excitatory postsynaptic potentials.[92] In addition, felbamate enhances the anticonvulsant actions of diazepam in animal seizure models, thereby suggesting a possible mode of action at the GABA receptor-ionophore complex.[93] However, ligand-binding studies failed to demonstrate any affinity of felbamate at the GABA, benzodiazepine or picrotoxin binding sites on the GABA receptor. It has been suggested that felbamate may enhance $GABA_A$ receptor-mediated neurotransmission,[94] although the exact location whereby felbamate binds to the $GABA_A$ receptor remains to be found.

PHARMACOKINETICS

After oral administration, felbamate displays complete absorption with peak plasma concentrations occurring by 2–6 h and a V_d of 0.75 L/kg (Table 21.3). Its bioavailability is >90 per cent and is unaffected by food.[95] Felbamate is minimally bound to plasma proteins (25 per cent) and is eliminated largely (50 per cent) unchanged in the urine. The remainder of the drug is either metabolized via an oxidative pathway mediated by CYP enzymes, or via a hydrolytic route that leads to the formation of mono-carbonate felbamate.[96] Formation of an intermediate metabolite, atropaldehyde, has been implicated in the pathogenesis of felbamate-related adverse idiosyncratic reactions.[96,97]

Felbamate displays linear kinetics with a half-life of 14–23 h in healthy volunteers, which is shortened to approximately 14–15 h in patients receiving enzyme-inducing AEDs.[98] Impaired renal function is associated with higher plasma felbamate concentrations and longer half-life values (27–34 h).[99]

DRUG INTERACTIONS

Clearance of felbamate is enhanced by carbamazepine and phenytoin (Table 21.4).[100] In contrast, valproic acid inhibits the metabolism of felbamate, increasing plasma felbamate concentrations. In children, carbamazepine and phenytoin increase the clearance of felbamate by 49 and 40 per cent respectively whereas valproic acid decreases it by 21 per cent.[101]

Plasma concentrations of phenytoin, phenobarbital, valproic acid, carbamazepine-epoxide and N-desmethyl-clobazam increase when felbamate is added to the treatment regimen.[100–104]

ADVERSE EFFECTS

Felbamate is associated with a high incidence of aplastic anemia and hepatotoxicity. Women over 17 years of age who have a prior history of an idiosyncratic drug reaction to other AEDs seem to be at most risk of developing aplastic anemia, whereas young children seem to be more predisposed to hepatotoxicity. An intermediate metabolite of felbamate, atropaldehyde, has been implicated in this toxicity. It has been suggested that measurement of the activity of the enzyme responsible for its production might identify patients predisposed to a felbamate-associated idiosyncratic reaction before treatment.[97,105,106]

THERAPEUTIC DRUG MONITORING

Optimal seizure control appears to be achieved at trough concentrations ranging from 210 to 460 μmol/L. Plasma concentrations are not easily predicted from the dosages. In addition, felbamate appears to have a narrow therapeutic window and a high propensity to interact with concomitant AEDs. Thus, therapeutic drug monitoring may be useful.

Fosphenytoin

Fosphenytoin is a phosphate ester pro-drug of phenytoin that was developed in an attempt to overcome complications associated with intravenous phenytoin. Phenytoin is insoluble in aqueous solutions and is typically supplied in a solution containing propylene glycol and ethanol adjusted to pH 12. This is irritating to tissue; soft tissue inflammation commonly occurs at the injection site and can lead to tissue necrosis. In contrast, fosphenytoin is readily soluble in aqueous solution and reduces this risk.

MECHANISM OF ACTION

As fosphenytoin is a phenytoin pro-drug, its mechanism of action is exactly that of phenytoin.

PHARMACOKINETICS

Fosphenytoin administered either intramuscularly or intravenously is 100 per cent bioavailable and its conversion half-life to phenytoin is 8–15 min. Thus, therapeutic plasma concentrations of phenytoin are usually attained within 10 min of intravenous infusion and 20 min after intramuscular administration.[107] Peak plasma concentrations after intramuscular administration are reached within 90 min.

DRUG INTERACTIONS

The interaction profile of fosphenytoin is similar to that of phenytoin (see phenytoin section pp. 366–7).

ADVERSE EFFECTS

Adverse effects associated with fosphenytoin treatment include dizziness, headache, tinnitus and somnolence. Cardiovascular complications have also been reported but are uncommon. Fosphenytoin is contraindicated in patients who display idiosyncratic reactions to phenytoin or other hydantoins, and in patients with a history of cardiovascular disease.

THERAPEUTIC DRUG MONITORING

The strategy for monitoring fosphenytoin is exactly that described for phenytoin (see phenytoin section pp. 366–7).

Gabapentin

Gabapentin is a structural analogue of GABA.

MECHANISM OF ACTION

Despite being designed as a GABA-mimetic, gabapentin failed to show affinity at any site on GABA receptors (Table 21.2).[108] Ligands that bind to the polyamine regulatory site of the NMDA receptor partially ($\approx$60 per cent) inhibit gabapentin binding.[109] In addition, several endogenous L-amino acids (leucine, isoleucine, phenylalanine and valine) all potently displace radiolabeled gabapentin binding.[110] Finally, gabapentin requires the L-amino acid transporter for transportation across cell membranes. These suggest that gabapentin may bind to the recognition site of a neuronal L-amino acid-like transporter.[110]

There is evidence that gabapentin may increase the synthesis[111] and nonvesicular release of GABA,[112] and may prevent its metabolism.[113] Gabapentin has been shown to augment GABA concentrations in the occipital cortex of epileptic patients.[114] Gabapentin binds to the $\alpha 2\delta$ subtype of voltage-gated calcium ion channels (VGCC), resulting in inhibition of calcium ion influx through presynaptic P/Q-type VGCCs[115] and culminates in a reduction in glutamate/aspartate release which in turn reduces the activation of α-amino-3-hydroxy-5-methyl-4-isoxazole propionic acid (AMPA) heteroreceptors on noradrenergic nerve terminals.[115] The extent to which each of these effects contributes to the mechanism of action of gabapentin has not been clarified.

PHARMACOKINETICS

After oral ingestion, gabapentin is rapidly absorbed, has a bioavailability of ≈60 per cent and is unaffected by food intake (Table 21.3).[116] Its absorption from the gut is mediated via a saturable L-amino acid transporter.[110,117] Consequently, absorption kinetics may be dose-dependent, such that increasing the dosage may decrease the percentage of gabapentin absorbed. Despite this phenomenon, there is a good correlation between dose and plasma concentration over the target dose range.[118] Gabapentin is not metabolized, is not protein bound and typically displays a half-life of 5–7 h. Gabapentin is excreted renally and its elimination is related to creatinine clearance. Therefore, clearance rates may be decreased in individuals with impaired cardiac function, renal impairment and in elderly patients.[119]

DRUG INTERACTIONS

Gabapentin is not protein bound, nor metabolized, and does not appear to induce liver enzymes. Thus, few drug interactions would be anticipated (Table 21.4). However, a reduction in renal clearance of gabapentin can occur with cimetidine, and antacids containing aluminium or magnesium can reduce gabapentin absorption by up to 20 per cent.[120]

ADVERSE EFFECTS

Gabapentin is generally well tolerated in pediatric patients and displays few significant side-effects. Behavioral symptoms associated with gabapentin include aggression, hyperexcitability and tantrums. However, these effects have only been observed in <10 per cent of children treated and appear to be most prevalent in individuals with a previous history of behavioral difficulties.[121]

THERAPEUTIC DRUG MONITORING

In clinical practice a good therapeutic outcome is typically seen when gabapentin plasma concentrations are in the range 12–120 μmol/L.[120]

Lamotrigine

Lamotrigine is a triazine derivative.

MECHANISM OF ACTION

Lamotrigine acts mainly through inhibition of use-dependent voltage-sensitive sodium channels and possibly VGCC (Table 21.2).[122] This results in stabilization of the presynaptic membrane by prevention of sustained repetitive firing of action potentials and reduction in excitatory neurotransmission.[123] Lamotrigine, unlike other sodium channel blockers such as phenytoin and carbamazepine, has a broad clinical spectrum of anticonvulsant activity suggesting that its interaction with these ion channels differs from typical sodium channel antagonists. Indeed, lamotrigine, unlike phenytoin, binds to the slow inactivated state of the sodium channel[124] and has been reported to display preferential binding to sodium channels on excitatory neurons.[125] However, these mechanisms alone are insufficient to explain the efficacy of lamotrigine in patients with absence epilepsy[121] and do not account for the reported efficacy of lamotrigine in the treatment of bipolar depression.[126] It would appear that there are undefined mechanism(s) of actions of lamotrigine that contribute to its clinical efficacy.

PHARMACOKINETICS

After oral ingestion, lamotrigine is rapidly absorbed with maximum plasma concentrations after 1–3 h (Table 21.3).[120] Absorption is unaffected by food intake. Lamotrigine has a bioavailability of ≈98 per cent and a V_d of 1.2 L/kg. It is ≈55 per cent protein bound and plasma concentrations increase linearly with dose. Lamotrigine undergoes extensive (≈90 per cent) metabolism by glucuronic acid conjugation in the liver, with the remaining 10 per cent of unmetabolized drug being excreted renally.

DRUG INTERACTIONS

The elimination half-life of lamotrigine (15–35 h) is markedly reduced (8–20 h) by the co-administration of hepatic enzyme-inducing AEDs, which enhance the metabolism of lamotrigine and decrease plasma concentrations by up to 50 per cent. It appears that phenytoin induces lamotrigine metabolism to a greater degree than phenobarbital or carbamazepine.[120] Co-administration of valproic acid reduces the rate of clearance and may more than double lamotrigine's half-life to about 60 h. Patients taking a combination of an enzyme-inducing AED with valproic acid will exhibit intermediate half-life values (≈28 h).

These interactions have important implications in children because the risk of developing a rash is greater when the initial lamotrigine concentration is higher and when the dosage escalation is rapid. Thus, it is necessary to employ smaller doses of lamotrigine when co-administered with valproic acid and to increase the dose very slowly. Sertraline has also been reported to increase lamotrigine concentrations, possibly by inhibition of lamotrigine glucuronidation.[127] Finally, acetaminophen and rifampacin have been reported to induce the metabolism of lamotrigine.[128,129]

Although lamotrigine does not generally affect the metabolism of other AEDs, it has been reported to elevate plasma concentrations of the primary metabolite of carbamazepine, carbamazepine-epoxide, in patients who are already taking maximum tolerated doses of carbamazepine.[130]

The report that low-dose lamotrigine in combination with valproic acid appears to have a synergistic effect on the prevention of typical absence seizures may imply a pharmacodynamic interaction.[131]

ADVERSE EFFECTS

Nausea, vomiting and rash, which appears usually within 2–8 weeks of dose initiation, are the most common side-effects. Children are at particular risk for the development of Stevens-Johnson syndrome or toxic epidermal necrolysis. They occur more often if the initial dose is high, the dosage escalation is rapid and valproic acid co-medication is used.[132] Although the risk was initially estimated to be approximately 1/50 in children and 1/1000 in adults,[133] a population-based study in which all affected patients were examined by a dermatologist has estimated the risk of developing Stevens-Johnson syndrome or toxic epidermal necrolysis in children to be approximately 3/10 000.[134]

THERAPEUTIC DRUG MONITORING

No clear-cut relationship exists between clinical response and serum lamotrigine concentrations.[134,135] However, the incidence of toxicity has been reported to rise markedly at concentrations above 60 μmol/L.[133,136] A target range of 4–60 μmol/L has been proposed.[120]

Levetiracetam

Levetiracetam is an *S*-enantiomer pyrrolidone derivative closely related to piracetam.

MECHANISM OF ACTION

Levetiracetam displays potent anticonvulsant effects in the audiogenic seizure-prone mouse model[137] and in other animal models of partial and generalized epilepsy.[138–140] Traditionally, compounds that are thought to possess anticonvulsant activity display an effect in either the maximal electroshock or pentylenetetrazol animal models. However, levetiracetam displayed no effect in either of these models despite effectively attenuating fully kindled seizures and the development of kindling. The possibility that levetiracetam can act prophylactically to prevent seizure progression has important implications in the treatment of children with epilepsy.[140] Most seizure disorders begin early in maturation, and it is desirable that the progression of seizures is halted as early in development as possible.

The mechanism of action of levetiracetam is unknown. Levetiracetam binds to a specific site in synaptic membranes of the rat brain in a reversible, saturable and stereoselective manner.[141] Levetiracetam does not have affinity for sodium, calcium or potassium ion channels, nor the GABA and glutamate neurotransmitter systems.[141,142] Levetiracetam has been reported to evoke changes in postsynaptic GABA function but appears to have no effect on whole-brain GABA synthesis, metabolism or concentration.[143] A recent study suggested that levetiracetam may act indirectly at $GABA_A$ receptors to modulate GABA-gated currents[144] and may also act on calcium-gated currents (Table 21.2).

PHARMACOKINETICS

After oral administration, levetiracetam is rapidly and almost completely absorbed. Absorption rates are unaffected by food intake and peak plasma concentrations are reached ≈ 1 h after drug administration (Table 21.3).[145] The elimination half-life of the drug is 5–7 h in children.[145] Levetiracetam is not protein bound and is not metabolized by the liver. It is transformed by enzymatic hydrolysis in the blood to an inactive metabolite and 93 per cent of the administered dose of drug is renally excreted within 24 h.[145]

DRUG INTERACTIONS

Because levetiracetam is not protein bound and does not undergo hepatic metabolism, it has a low propensity to interact pharmacokinetically with other drugs.[145,146] Levetiracetam does not appear to interfere with the metabolism of other AEDs, nor do other AEDs seem to exert any influence on its metabolism and excretion (Table 21.4). Furthermore, levetiracetam has been shown not to interact with oral contraceptives, digoxin, probenacid or warfarin.[145,147] A pharmacodynamic interaction with carbamazepine has been reported, in which symptoms compatible with carbamazepine toxicity occurred during combination therapy.[148]

ADVERSE EFFECTS

Levetiracetam has a very wide therapeutic index, unlike many AEDs.[138,139] Treatment-emergent side-effects in adult populations include asthenia, dizziness, headache and somnolence, with symptom manifestation typically occurring in early levetiracetam treatment. Recent studies have indicated a higher prevalence of neuropsychiatric symptoms such as hostility, irritability and hallucinations than previously reported.[149,150] Nonetheless, levetiracetam appears to be well tolerated.

THERAPEUTIC DRUG MONITORING

The relationship between levetiracetam plasma concentrations and clinical effect has not been ascertained and the value of plasma concentration measurements has not been established. There may be a role for drug monitoring of levetiracetam if noncompliance is suspected.

Oxcarbazepine

Oxcarbazepine is a 10-keto analogue of carbamazepine, which has a more favorable tolerability profile than carbamazepine.[151]

MECHANISM OF ACTION

Oxcarbazepine's anticonvulsant properties appear to be mediated, in part, through the blockade of voltage-dependent sodium channels (Table 21.2).[152] Oxcarbazepine has also been reported to inhibit the veratrine-induced release of glutamate, aspartate, GABA and dopamine in rodent striatal slices.[153] Oxcarbazepine is almost immediately converted to its active metabolite, a 10-monohydroxy derivative (MHD). In addition to sharing oxcarbazepine's propensity to block voltage-sensitive sodium channels, MHD also reversibly blocks high voltage-activated calcium ion currents.[154] Furthermore, MHD has been shown to reduce the frequency of penicillin-induced seizures. This action is believed to involve an enhancement of potassium ion conductance.[155]

PHARMACOKINETICS

Oxcarbazepine is considered a pro-drug since in humans it is rapidly metabolized to the pharmacologically active metabolite MHD (Table 21.3).[156] After oral ingestion, oxcarbazepine is rapidly and completely absorbed and food has no effect on the rate or extent of absorption. Peak plasma concentrations of oxcarbazepine occur within 1–2 h but MHD plasma concentrations peak somewhat later at 4–6 h.[157] The protein binding of MHD is 40 per cent.[158] The elimination half-life of oxcarbazepine is 1–3 h and that of MHD is 8–10 h. These appear to be stable during chronic therapy, even in patients receiving concomitant treatment with enzyme-inducing AEDs.[159,160] MHD is glucuronidated by UDP-glucuronosyltransferase and renally excreted. Indeed, the kidneys expel more than 96 per cent of administered oxcarbazepine; 83 per cent as MHD or its glucuronide conjugate, <1 per cent as unmetabolized oxcarbazepine and the remainder as inactive dihydroxide derivatives of MHD.[156] Hepatic abnormalities generally do not affect the pharmacokinetic characteristics of oxcarbazepine or MHD. However, patients with a creatine clearance <30 mL/min may experience significantly elevated levels of MHD.[161]

DRUG INTERACTIONS

As the biotransformation of oxcarbazepine to MHD is not CYP-mediated, the potential for interactions with other AEDs that interfere with CYPs is reduced. This, coupled with MHD's low affinity for plasma binding, suggests that oxcarbazepine would be unlikely to significantly interact with other medication. Nevertheless, oxcarbazepine is a weak hepatic enzyme inducer[158] and enzyme-inducing AEDs do enhance the metabolism of oxcarbazepine (Table 21.4). Furthermore, oxcarbazepine enhances the metabolism of lamotrigine resulting in lower lamotrigine concentrations.[162,163] Oxcarbazepine also enhances the metabolism of oral contraceptives.[164] At high doses (>1200 mg/day) oxcarbazepine increases phenytoin plasma concentrations by up to 40 per cent.[162]

ADVERSE EFFECTS

The most common adverse events associated with oxcarbazepine in adults and children are somnolence, headache, dizziness, nausea, fatigue and rash. Oxcarbazepine appears not to have an affect on pubertal development or growth.[165] Compared with carbamazepine, oxcarbazepine less frequently evokes allergic skin reactions although patients that are sensitized to carbamazepine may cross react with oxcarbazepine.[166] Oxcarbazepine is associated with hyponatremia, but this is usually asymptomatic.[167]

THERAPEUTIC DRUG MONITORING

A study of 19 seizure-free adult patients treated with oxcarbazepine in combination with other AEDs reported mean MHD serum concentrations of 64 µmol/L (range 12–128 µmol/L). The current target range for MHD is 50–110 µmol/L.

Tiagabine

Tiagabine is a nipecotic acid derivative that was specifically designed to increase GABA longevity in the synaptic cleft by preventing GABA reuptake into synaptosomal membranes, neurons and glia.

MECHANISM OF ACTION

Tiagabine has been shown to display selective affinity for the blockade of the GAT-1 subtype of GABA transporter, with little or no effect on GAT-2 or GAT-3 subtypes (Table 21.2).[168] The GAT-1 transporter is associated with the reuptake of GABA into the nerve terminals of inhibitory interneurons, but is also located in hippocampal glia cells.[169] Impeding the action of this transporter causes a prolongation of inhibitory postsynaptic potentials.[170] Tiagabine displays efficacy against bicuculline and picrotoxin-induced seizures in rodents.[171,172] and reduces the intensity and duration of epileptiform activity in amygdala-kindled rats.[172]

PHARMACOKINETICS

Tiagabine is rapidly and almost completely absorbed after oral administration (Table 21.3). The drug has a bioavailability of 90 per cent and reaches peak plasma concentrations within 2 h. Food intake reduces the rate of absorption, although the overall magnitude of absorption remains unaffected.[173] Tiagabine is highly protein bound (96 per cent) with a V_d of 1.4 L/kg. It is hepatically oxidized before being conjugated to inactive metabolites that are renally eliminated.[174] Medication that induces liver enzymes can increase the elimination rate of tiagabine and decrease the half-life of the drug from 5–8 h to 2–3 h.[171] The metabolism of tiagabine is reduced in patients with hepatic dysfunction, the half-life being 12–16 h.[175] Pediatric patients eliminate tiagabine more rapidly than adult patients.[176]

DRUG INTERACTIONS

Although tiagabine is neither an enzyme inducer nor an inhibitor itself, its metabolism can be induced or inhibited by other drugs (Table 21.4).[173,177–179] The enzyme-inducing AEDs carbamazepine, phenobarbital, phenytoin and primidone significantly shorten the half-life of tiagabine (to 2–3 h) and lower its plasma concentrations. Valproic acid displaces tiagabine from its protein binding sites, but the significance of this interaction is unknown.[177,178,180] This protein-binding displacement interaction is also observed with other highly protein-bound drugs such as naproxen and salicylates.[177]

ADVERSE EFFECTS

The most common adverse effects associated with tiagabine are asthenia, somnolence, depression, tremor, cognitive impairment and dizziness. Tiagabine at high doses (>40 mg/day) may be associated with the development of nonconvulsive status epilepticus.[179,181] Thus, caution is recommended in the use of tiagabine in any patient with previous evidence of generalized spike-wave discharges on EEG.

THERAPEUTIC DRUG MONITORING

There are few data available on the relationship between tiagabine plasma concentrations and therapeutic effect, and the usefulness of drug monitoring has yet to be established.[182]

Topiramate

Topiramate is a sulfamate-substituted monosaccharide derived from D-fructose.

MECHANISM OF ACTION

Topiramate is a compound with several mechanisms of action, all of which could contribute to its clinical efficacy (Table 21.2).[120] In vitro studies have demonstrated the effectiveness of topiramate in blocking voltage-dependent sodium channels[183] and N and L-type calcium ion electrogenesis,[184] although the importance of the latter mechanism in the anticonvulsant profile of topiramate remains to be elucidated. Topiramate is also thought to act via a novel mechanism at GABA receptors, culminating in a potentiation of GABA's inhibitory effects.[185] Moreover, topiramate may act directly at the GABA$_A$ receptor-ionophore complex, possibly via an interaction at a novel binding site.[186] A role of topiramate in the selective blockade of the AMPA/kainate subtype of glutamate receptor is also suggested.[187] In patients with epilepsy, topiramate has been associated with significant elevations in occipital cortex GABA as measured by nuclear magnetic resonance (NMR) spectroscopy.[188]

PHARMACOKINETICS

Topiramate is rapidly absorbed from the gastrointestinal tract with an estimated bioavailability of 80–95 per cent and a plasma elimination half-life of 19–25 h following monotherapy (Table 21.3). Peak plasma concentrations are reached within 1–4 h after oral administration.[189] Co-ingestion with food delays the absorption of topiramate, although the maximum plasma concentrations attained for any given dose remain unaffected.[190] Single-dose studies (100–1200 mg/day) show that topiramate exhibits dose-proportional and linear absorption kinetics, but only at the lower end of the dose range (100–400 mg/day).[191] Saturable binding of topiramate to erythrocytes has been implicated in the lack of dose-proportionality at higher doses.[191] Chronic studies have shown that dose-related linear absorption kinetics can be attained with doses of 50–200 mg/day given over a period of 2–3 weeks.[192] The V_d of topiramate is 0.65 L/kg, which is consistent with a distribution into total body water.[193] Topiramate is minimally protein bound (15 per cent) but because of the saturation of erythrocytes at higher doses, the blood/plasma concentration ratio decreases with increasing drug dosage. Consequently, differences arise between pharmacokinetic parameters calculated from whole blood and those from plasma.[190] Topiramate undergoes minimal metabolism and is renally eliminated. In adults, the mean elimination half-life for topiramate in plasma and urine are 21.5 and 18.5 h respectively and are independent of dose.[191] However, topiramate clearance in children appears to be 50 per cent greater than that in adults, resulting in plasma concentrations that are approximately 30 per cent lower in pediatric patients.[194,195]

DRUG INTERACTIONS

Hepatic enzyme-inducing AEDs enhance topiramate metabolism so that plasma concentrations of topiramate can be expected to be reduced by $\approx$50 per cent with an elimination half-life of 9–12 h (Table 21.4).[120,196] Oxcarbazepine also appears to enhance the metabolism of topiramate.[195] Conversely, topiramate exhibits a small inhibitory effect on phenytoin metabolism, which would be expected to be of minimal clinical significance in most patients. However, for individuals whose phenytoin metabolism is at, or near, saturation, this interaction may become clinically important.[120] Furthermore, valproic acid concentrations are decreased with increasing topiramate dose[197] and valproic acid is reportedly displaced from its plasma protein binding sites by topiramate.[198] The clinical implication of these findings remains to be determined. Finally, the oral clearance of digoxin was increased by 13 per cent following topiramate ingestion without an accompanying alteration in renal clearance.[199] This suggests that larger digoxin doses would be required in patients with topiramate co-therapy.

ADVERSE EFFECTS

The most commonly reported side-effects associated with topiramate therapy include impaired cognition, dizziness, headaches, ataxia, somnolence and anorexia. There is also a risk of nephrolithiasis, due to the inhibition of carbonic anhydrase. Children appear to be more susceptible to neuropsychiatric abnormalities and weight loss following topiramate treatment. The latter effect is thought to particularly affect children with pre-existing nutritional problems.

THERAPEUTIC DRUG MONITORING

Patients who responded to topiramate treatment in the initial clinical trials showed plasma topiramate concentrations ranging from 6–74 µmol/L. This range is considered to be the current putative target range for topiramate (Table 21.1).[15]

Vigabatrin

Vigabatrin, γ-vinyl GABA, is a structural homologue of GABA and was designed to mimic the natural inhibitory actions of the neurotransmitter. The drug is composed of a racemic mixture of R-($-$)- and S-($+$)-isomers in equal proportion, with the pharmacological profile of the drug solely attributable to the S-($+$)-enantiomer.

MECHANISM OF ACTION

Vigabatrin acts by irreversibly and covalently binding to GABA transaminase, the degradative enzyme of GABA.[200] Consequently, widespread increases in brain GABA levels occur, with a lengthening in effect of the actions of the inhibitory neurotransmitter on its receptors (Table 21.2).

PHARMACOKINETICS

After oral ingestion, vigabatrin is rapidly absorbed from the gastrointestinal tract with peak plasma concentrations occurring within 1 h (Table 21.3). The bioavailability is $\approx$80 per cent. Vigabatrin is not protein bound and has a V_d of 0.8 L/kg. Co-ingestion with food affects neither the rate nor the amount absorbed.[120] Vigabatrin is not metabolized and $\approx$70 per cent of the drug is excreted unchanged in the urine. The plasma half-life of the drug is relatively short (6–8 h), but because the drug irreversibly inhibits GABA transaminase the anticonvulsant effect can last several days until *de novo* synthesis of the enzyme occurs.

DRUG INTERACTIONS

Because vigabatrin is not metabolized and is not protein bound, it displays minimal pharmacokinetic interactions with co-administered medication. However, a decrease in phenytoin plasma concentrations has been reported in individuals concurrently prescribed vigabatrin as add-on therapy at approximately 1 month following initiation of treatment. The mechanism of action behind this interaction is presently unknown.[201] In addition, small decreases in plasma phenobarbital and primidone concentrations have been associated with adjunctive vigabatrin treatment. However, these decreases are considered clinically insignificant in most patients.[201]

ADVERSE EFFECTS

In adults the most prominent side-effects associated with vigabatrin treatment are drowsiness, fatigue, depression, psychosis, weight gain and visual field defects. In children, excitation and aggressive agitation may also be a feature.[202] The risk of visual defects is a major factor limiting its use.[203,204,205] The incidence of visual disturbances in children may be up to 50 per cent, a figure similar to that for adult patients.[206] Recently, chronic vigabatrin treatment has been shown to reduce $GABA_A$ receptor binding in epileptic children.[207] As the GABA ergic system has important implications in developmental plasticity, very careful consideration should be given before this drug is used in very young patients.

THERAPEUTIC DRUG MONITORING

Vigabatrin acts by irreversible inhibition of GABA-transaminase and there is a clear dissociation between its plasma concentration and the pharmacological effect. Thus therapeutic drug monitoring is not indicated, except possibly when noncompliance is an issue.

Zonisamide

Zonisamide is a liposoluble benzisoxazole compound.

MECHANISM OF ACTION

In animal models zonisamide prevents the tonic extensor component of maximal electroshock seizures, attenuates the fully kindled seizures and abolishes pentylenetetrazol-induced seizures.[208] Zonisamide is thought to act by impeding the sustained repetitive firing of voltage-sensitive sodium channels[209] and by retarding the current through voltage dependent T-type calcium channels (Table 21.2).[210]

PHARMACOKINETICS

Zonisamide is rapidly absorbed, with maximal plasma concentrations attained between 2–6 h after ingestion (Table 21.3). Its bioavailability is 95 per cent. The water solubility of zonisamide is pH dependent. Values below pH 8 are sparingly soluble in water (0.8 mg/ml), which makes production of formulations for oral use in small children difficult. It is 55 per cent bound to plasma proteins and has an elimination half-life ranging between 27 and 70 h. As zonisamide is partially metabolized in the liver, the half-life of the drug is dependent on whether or not the patient is concurrently taking hepatic enzyme-inducing AEDs. Approximately 48–60 per cent of an administered dose of zonisamide is excreted unchanged in the urine.[211]

DRUG INTERACTIONS

Hepatic enzyme-inducing AEDs accelerate the metabolism of zonisamide and reduce its half-life (Table 21.4). When added to existing carbamazepine treatment, zonisamide significantly increases the plasma concentration of carbamazepine-epoxide.[212]

ADVERSE EFFECTS

Common adverse effects associated with zonisamide therapy include fatigue, cognitive abnormalities, nephrolithiasis, somnolence and ataxia.[211] Zonisamide at steady-state plasma concentrations of more than 140 μmol/L is reported to adversely affect specific cognitive function in young children.[213] A study examining the concentration of this drug in plasma and breast milk of pregnant women taking zonisamide (400 mg/day) found that at this dose the transfer rates were 92 per cent via the placenta and 41–57 per cent through the breast milk.[214]

THERAPEUTIC DRUG MONITORING

No clear relationship between zonisamide plasma concentrations and clinical response has been found.[215]

KEY POINTS

- **Gastrointestinal absorption** in neonates and young infants is slow and unpredictable, and oral bioavailability is not optimal
- Most of the long-established AEDs are cleared almost exclusively by **hepatic metabolism**, which involves cytochrome P-450 and/or uridine diphosphate glucuronosyltransferase (UGT) enzymes
- **Cytochrome P-450** activities increase rapidly and peak at 2–6-fold higher than adult activities by 6 months of age. Metabolic processes that involve glucuronidation do not reach maturity until the age of 3–4 years. The rate of hepatic metabolism decreases gradually to reach the adult rate around puberty
- None of the long-established AEDs are eliminated exclusively by **renal excretion**, although significant proportions of phenobarbital and primidone are excreted unchanged in urine. In contrast, two of the seven new AEDs (gabapentin and vigabatrin) are eliminated unchanged exclusively by renal excretion and renal excretion is partially involved in the elimination of the other five
- **Drug concentrations** should be used as a guide to optimize efficacy, identify problematic drug interactions, to ascertain drug related toxicity, and to detect poor compliance
- The **target or therapeutic range** is a population-derived statistical concept, which implies that seizure control without side-effects is most often achieved within that range. However, seizure control is often achieved at concentrations below the target range and seizure control may only be achieved in some patients at concentrations above the target range. Similarly, some patients experience toxicity at concentrations within the target range whereas others may have no side-effects at concentrations above the target range
- It is essential to ensure that **sampling occurs at steady state**
- When there are concerns regarding efficacy or poor compliance, the ideal **blood sampling time** is immediately before the next oral dose (trough). If there is concern regarding toxicity, sampling should occur ideally around the time of the symptoms or alternatively when the peak concentration is expected to occur

- **Pharmacokinetic interactions** are common amongst AEDs and phenytoin has the greatest propensity to interact. The newer AEDs are associated with fewer interactions. Only two AEDs, gabapentin and levetiracetam, are truly noninteracting and thus can be prescribed without due regard to concomitant medication

REFERENCES

1. Cavell B. Gastric emptying in preterm infants. *Acta Paediatrica Scandinavica* 1979; **68**: 725–730.
2. Jalling B. Plasma and CSF concentrations of phenobarbitone in infants given single doses. *Developmental Medicine and Child Neurology* 1976; **16**: 781–793.
3. Benet LZ, Izumi T, Zhang Y, *et al.* Intestinal MDR transport proteins and P-450 enzymes as barriers to oral drug delivery. *Journal of Control Release* 1999; **62**: 25–31.
4. Knudsen FU. Plasma diazepam in infants after rectal administration in solution and by suppository. *Acta Paediatrica Scandinavica* 1977; **66**: 563–567.
5. Wilder BJ, Campbell K, Ramsey RE, *et al.* Safety and tolerance of multiple doses of intramuscular fosphenytoin substituted for oral phenytoin in epilepsy or neurosurgery. *Archives of Neurology* 1996; **53**: 764–768.
6. Bell DM, Richards G, Dhillon S, *et al.* A comparative pharmacokinetic study of intravenous and intramuscular midazolam in patients with epilepsy. *Epilepsy Research* 1991; **10**: 183–190.
7. Wroblewski BA, Joseph AB. The use of intramuscular midazolam for acute seizure cessation or behavioural emergencies in patients with traumatic brain injury. *Clinical Neuropharmacology* 1992; **15**: 44–49.
8. De Boer AG, De Leede LG, Breimer DD. Drug absorption by sublingual and rectal routes. *British Journal of Anaesthesia* 1984; **56**: 69–82.
9. Scott RC, Besag FMC, Boyd SG, Berry D, Neville BGR. Buccal absorption of midazolam: pharmacokinetics and EEG pharmacodynamics. *Epilepsia* 1998; **39**: 290–294.
10. Scott RC, Besag FMC, Neville BGR. Buccal midazolam and rectal diazepam for treatment of prolonged seizures in childhood and adolescence: a randomised trial. *Lancet* 1999; **353**: 623–626.
11. Cornford EM, Partridge WM, Braun LD, *et al.* Increased blood-brain barrier transport of protein bound anticonvulsant drugs in the newborn. *Journal of Cerebral Blood Flow and Metabolism* 1983; **3**: 280–286.
12. Painter MJ, Pippenger C, MacDonald H, *et al.* Phenobarbitone and diphenylhydantoin levels in neonates with seizures. *Journal of Pediatrics* 1978; **92**: 315–319.
13. Patsalos PN, Froscher W, Pisani F, van Rijn CN. The importance of drug interactions in epilepsy therapy. *Epilepsia* 2002; **43**: 365–385.
14. Loebstein R, Koren G. Clinical pharmacology and therapeutic drug monitoring in neonates and children. *Pediatric Review* 1998; **19**: 423–428.
15. Johannessen SI, Bettino D, Berry DJ, *et al.* Therapeutic drug monitoring of the new antiepileptic drugs. *Therapeutic Drug Monitoring* 2003; **25**(3): 347–363.
16. Callaghan N, O'Callaghan, Duggen B, Feely M. Carbamazepine as a single drug in the treatment of epilepsy. *Journal of Neurology, Neurosurgery and Psychiatry* 1978; **41**: 907–912.
17. Cereghino JJ, Brock JT, van Meter JC, *et al.* Carbamazepine for epilepsy: a controlled prospective evaluation. *Neurology* 1974; **24**: 401–410.
18. Bruni J, Wilder BJ, Willmore LJ, Perchalski RJ, Villareal HJ. Steady-state kinetics of valproic acid in epileptic patients. *Clinical Pharmacology and Therapeutics* 1978; **24**: 324–332.
19. Gannaway DJ, Mawer GE. Serum phenytoin concentration and clinical response in patients with epilepsy. *British Journal of Clinical Pharmacology* 1981; **2**: 833–839.
20. Woo E, Chan YM, Yu YL, Chan YW, Huang CY. If a well stabilized epileptic patient has a subtherapeutic antiepileptic drug level, should the dose be increased? A randomized prospective study. *Epilepsia* 1988; **29**: 129–139.
21. Callaghan N, Kenny RA, O'Neill B, Crowley M, Goggin TA. Prospective study between carbamazepine, phenytoin and sodium valproate as monotherapy in previously untreated and recently diagnosed patients with epilepsy. *Journal of Neurology, Neurosurgery and Psychiatry* 1985; **48**: 639–644.
22. Schmidt D, Einicke I, Haenel F. The influence of seizure type on the efficacy of plasma concentration of phenytoin, phenobarbitone and carbamazepine. *Archives of Neurology* 1986; **43**: 263–265.
23. Liu H, Delgado MR. Therapeutic drug concentration monitoring using saliva samples. Focus on anticonvulsants. *Clinical Pharmacokinetics* 1999; **36**: 453–470.
24. Drobitch RK, Svensson CK. Therapeutic drug monitoring in saliva: an update. *Clinical Pharmacokinetics* 1992; **23**: 365–379.
25. Gorodischer R, Burtin P, Verjee Z, Hwang P, Koren G. Is saliva suitable for therapeutic monitoring of anticonvulsants in children: an evaluation in the routine clinical setting. *Therapeutic Drug Monitoring* 1997; **19**: 637–642.
26. Luoma PV, Heikkinen JE, Ylostalo PR. Phenobarbitone pharmacokinetics and saliva and serum concentrations in pregnancy. *Therapeutic Drug Monitoring* 1982; **4**: 65–68.
27. Twyman RE, Rogers CJ, Macdonald RL. Differential regulation of gamma-aminobutyric acid receptor channels by diazepam and phenobarbitone. *Annals of Neurology* 1989; **25**: 213–220.
28. Macdonald RL, McLean MJ. Anticonvulsant drugs: mechanisms of action. *Advances in Neurology* 1986; **44**: 713–736.
29. Johansen J, Taft WC, Yang J, Kleinhaus AL, DeLorenzo RJ. Inhibition of Ca^{2+} conductance in identified leech neurons by benzodiazepines. *Proceedings of the National Academy of Sciences of the USA* 1985; **82**: 3935–3939.
30. Walker MC, Tong X, Brown S, Shorvon SD, Patsalos PN. Comparison of single- and repeated-dose pharmacokinetics of diazepam. *Epilepsia* 1998; **39**: 283–289.
31. Dhillon S, Richens A. Valproic acid and diazepam interaction in vivo. *British Journal of Clinical Pharmacology* 1982; **13**: 553–560.
32. Dreiffus FE, Penry JK, Rose SW, *et al.* Serum clonazepam concentrations in children with absence seizures. *Neurology* 1975; **25**: 255–259.
33. Naito H, Wachi M, Nishida M. Clinical effects and plasma concentrations of long-term clonazepam in monotherapy in

previously untreated epileptics. *Acta Neurologica Scandinavica* 1987; **76**: 58–63.

34. Courtney KR, Etter EF. Modulated anticonvulsant block of sodium channels in nerve and muscle. *European Journal of Pharmacology* 1983; **88**: 1–9.

35. Kuo CC, Chen RS, Lu L, Chen RC. Carbamazepine inhibition of neuronal Na^+ currents: quantitative distinction from phenytoin and possible therapeutic implications. *Molecular Pharmacology* 1997; **51**: 1077–1083.

36. Ambrósio AF, Silva AP, Malva JO, Soares-da-Silva P, Carvalho CM. Carbamazepine inhibits L-type Ca^{2+} channels in cultured rat hippocampal neurons stimulated with glutamate receptor antagonists. *Neuropharmacology* 1999; **38**: 1349–1359.

37. Ambrósio AF, Silva AP, Malva JO, Soares-da-Silva P, Carvalho CM. Inhibition of glutamate release by BIA 2-093 and BIA 2-024, two novel derivatives of carbamazepine, due to blockade of sodium but not calcium channels. *Biochemical Pharmacology* 2001; **406**: 191–201.

38. Dailey JW, Reith ME, Yan QS, Li MY, Jobe PC. Anticonvulsant doses of carbamazepine increase hippocampal extracellular serotonin in genetically epilepsy-prone rats: dose response relationships. *Neuroscience Letters* 1997; **227**: 13–16.

39. Ichikawa J, Meltzer HY. Valproate and carbamazepine: increase prefrontal dopamine release by 5 HT1A receptor activiation. *European Journal of Pharmacology* 1999; **380**: R1–3.

40. Skerritt JH, Davies LP, Johnston GA. Interactions of the anticonvulsant carbamazepine with adenosine receptors 1. Neurochemical studies. *Epilepsia* 1983; **24**: 634–642.

41. Skerritt JH, Johnston GA, Chow SC. Interactions of the anticonvulsant carbamazepine with adenosine receptors 2. Pharmacological studies. *Epilepsia* 1983; **24**: 643–650.

42. Bano G, Raina RK, Sharma DB. Pharmacokinetics of carbamazepine in protein energy malnutrition. *Pharmacology* 1986; **32**: 232–236.

43. Cornaggia C, Gianetti S, Battino D, *et al.* Comparative pharmacokinetic study of chewable and conventional carbamazepine in children. *Epilepsia* 1993; **34**: 158–160.

44. Miles MV, Lawless ST, Tennison MB, *et al.* Rapid loading of critical ill patients with carbamazepine suspension. *Pediatrics* 1990; **86**: 263–266.

45. Eeg-Olofsson O, Nilsson HL, Tonnby B, *et al.* Diurnal variation of carbamazepine and carbamazepine 10, 11-epoxide in plasma and saliva in children with epilepsy: a comparison between conventional and slow-release formulations. *Journal of Child Neurology* 1990; **5**: 159–165.

46. Patsalos PN. Phenobarbitone to gabapentin: a guide to 82 years of anti-epileptic drug pharmacokinetic interactions. *Seizure* 1994; **3**: 163–170.

47. Patsalos PN, Duncan JS. Antiepileptic drugs. A review of clinically significant interactions. *Drug Safety* 1993; **9**: 156–184.

48. Couet W, Istin B, Ingrand I, Girault J, Fourtillan JB. Effect of ponsinomycin on single-dose kinetics and metabolism of carbamazepine. *Therapeutic Drug Monitoring* 1990; **12**: 144–149.

49. Chadwick D, Shaw MD, Foy P, Rawlins MD, Turnbull DM. Serum anticonvulsant concentrations and the risk of drug induced skin eruptions. *Journal of Neurology Neurosurgery and Psychiatry* 1984; **47**: 642–644.

50. Seetharam MN, Pellock JM. Risk-benefit assessment of carbamazepine in children. *Drug Safety* 1991; **6**: 148–158.

51. Kenneback G, Bergfeldt L, Vallin H, Tomson T, Eldhag O. Electrophysiologic effects and clinical hazards of carbamazepine treatment for neurologic disorders in patients with abnormalities of the cardiac conduction system. *American Heart Journal* 1991; **121**: 1421–1429.

52. Perucca E, Garratt A, Hebdige S, Richens A. Water intoxication in epileptic patients receiving carbamazepine. *Journal of Neurology, Neurosurgery and Psychiatry* 1978; **41**; 713–718.

53. Coulter DA, Huguenard JR, Prince DA. Characterization of ethosuximide reduction of low threshold calcium current in thalamic neurons. *Annals of Neurology* 1989; **25**: 582–593.

54. Kostyuk PG, Molokanova EA, Pronchuk NF, Savchenko AN, Verkhratsky AN. Different action of ethosuximide on low- and high-threshold calcium currents in rat sensory neurons. *Neuroscience* 1992; **51**: 755–758.

55. Pisani F, Narbone MC, Trunfio C, *et al.* Valproic acid-ethosuximide interaction: a pharmacokinetic study. *Epilepsia* 1984; **25**: 229–233.

56. Macdonald RL, Rogers CJ, Twyman RE. Barbiturate regulation of kinetic properties of the $GABA_A$ receptor channel of mice spinal neurones in culture. *Journal of Physiology* 1989; **417**: 483–500.

57. Heyer EJ, Macdonald RL. Barbiturate reduction of calcium-dependent action potentials: correlation with anesthetic action. *Brain Research* 1982; **236**: 157–171.

58. Taburet AM, Chamouard C, Aymard P, *et al.* Phenobarbitone protein binding in neonates. *Developmental Pharmacology and Therapeutics* 1982; **4**(Suppl. 1): 129–134.

59. Aymard P, Taburet AM, Bauden JJ, *et al.* Kinetics and metabolism of phenobarbitone in the neonate. In: Johannesen SI, Morselli PL, Pippenger CE, *et al.* (eds) *Antiepileptic Therapy: Advances in Drug Monitoring.* New York: Raven Press, 1980; 1–8.

60. Yukawa E, Higuchi S, Aoyama T. The effect of concurrent administration of sodium valproate on serum concentrations of primidone and its metabolite phenobarbitone. *Journal of Clinical Pharmacy and Therapeutics* 1989; **14**: 387–392.

61. Calandre EP, Dominguez-Granados R, Gomez-Rubio M, Molina-Font JA. Cognitive effects of long-term treatment with phenobarbitone and valproic acid in school children. *Acta Neurologica Scandinavica* 1990; **81**: 504–506.

62. Burd L, Kerbeshian J, Fisher W. Does the use of phenobarbitone as an anticonvulsant permanently exacerbate hyperactivity? *Canadian Journal of Psychiatry* 1987; **32**: 10–13.

63. Tunnicliff G. Basis of the antiseizure action of phenytoin. *General Pharmacology* 1996; **27**: 1091–1097.

64. Schwarz JR, Grigat G. Phenytoin and carbamazepine: potential- and frequency-dependent block of Na currents in mammalian myelinated nerve fibers. *Epilepsia* 1989; **30**: 286–294.

65. Macdonald RL, Kelly KM. Antiepileptic drug mechanisms of action. *Epilepsia* 1995; **36**(Suppl. 2): S2–12.

66. Lampl I, Schwindt P, Crill W. Reduction of cortical pyramidal neuron excitability by the action of phenytoin on persistent Na^+ current. *Journal of Pharmacology and Experimental Therapeutics* 1998;1 **284**: 228–237.

67. Rivet M, Bois P, Cognard C, Raymond G. Phenytoin preferentially inhibits L-type calcium currents in whole-cell patch-clamped cardiac and skeletal muscle cells. *Cell Calcium* 1990; **11**: 581–588.

68. Schumacher TB, Beck H, Steinhauser C, Schramm J, Elger CE. Effects of phenytoin, carbamazepine and gabapentin on calcium channels in hippocampal granule cells from patients with temporal lobe epilepsy. *Epilepsia* 1998; **39**: 355–363.

69. Ferrendelli JA. Pharmacology of antiepileptic drugs. *Epilepsia* 1987; **28**(Suppl. 3): S14–16.

70. DeLorenzo RJ. Calmodulin systems in neuronal excitability: a molecular approach to epilepsy. *Annals of Neurology* 1984; **16**(Suppl. 1): S104–114.

71. Rane A, Lunde KM, Jalling B, *et al*. Plasma protein binding of diphenylhydantoin in normal and hyperbilirubinemic infants. *Journal of Pediatrics* 1971; **78**: 877–882.

72. Kauffman RE, Habersang R, Lansky L. Kinetics of primidone metabolism and excretion in children. *Clinical Pharmacology and Therapeutics* 1977; **22**: 200–205.

73. Powell C, Painter M, Pippenger CE. Primidone therapy in refractory neonatal seizures. *Journal of Pediatrics* 1984; **105**: 651–654.

74. Battino D, Avanzini G, Bossi L, *et al*. Plasma levels of primidone and its metabolite phenobarbitone: effect of age and associated treatment. *Therapeutic Drug Monitoring* 1983; **5**: 73–79.

75. McLean MJ, Macdonald RL. Sodium valproate, but not ethosuximide, produces use- and voltage-dependent limitation of high frequency repetitive firing of action potentials of mouse central neurons in cell culture. *Journal of Pharmacology and Experimental Therapeutics* 1986; **237**: 1001–1011.

76. Albus H, Williamson R. Electrophysiologic analysis of the actions of valproate on pyramidal neurons in the rat hippocampal slice. *Epilepsia* 1998; **39**: 124–139.

77. Franceschetti S, Hamon B, Heinemann U. The action of valproate on spontaneous epileptiform activity in the absence of synaptic transmission and on evoked changes in $[Ca^{2+}]$ and $[K^+]$ in the hippocampal slice. *Brain Research* 1986; **386**: 1–11.

78. Löscher W. Valproate: a reappraisal of its pharmacodynamic properties and mechanisms of action. *Progress in Neurobiology* 1999; **58**: 31–59.

79. Phillips NI, Fowler LJ. The effects of sodium valproate on gamma-aminobutyrate metabolism and behaviour in naive and ethanolamine-*O*-sulphate pretreated rats and mice. *Biochemical Pharmacology* 1982; **31**: 2257–2261.

80. Rowley HL, Marsden CA, Martin KF. Differential effects of phenytoin and sodium valproate on seizure-induced changes in gamma-aminobutyric acid and glutamate release in vivo. *European Journal of Pharmacology* 1995; **294**: 541–546.

81. Sills GJ, Leach JP, Butler E, *et al*. Antiepileptic drug action in primary cultures of rat cortical astrocytes. *Epilepsia* 1996; **37**(Suppl. 4): S116.

82. Cramer JA, Mattson RH, Bennett DM, Swick CT. Variable free and total valproic acid concentrations in sole- and multi-drug therapy. *Therapeutic Drug Monitoring* 1986; **8**: 411–415.

83. Riva R, Albani F, Franzoni E, *et al*. Valproic acid free fraction in epileptic children under chronic monotherapy. *Therapeutic Drug Monitoring* 1983; **5**: 197–200.

84. Tartara CA, Galimberti CA, Manni R, *et al*. Differential effects of valproic acid and enzyme-inducing antiepileptic drugs on nimodipine pharmacokinetics in epileptic patients. *British Journal of Clinical Pharmacology* 1991; **32**: 335–340.

85. Wagner ML, Graves NM, Leppik IE, *et al*. The effect of felbamate on valproic acid disposition. *Clinical Pharmacology and Therapeutics* 1994; **56**: 494–502.

86. Dreifuss FE. Fatal liver failure in children on valproate. *Lancet* 1987; **i**(8523): 47–48.

87. Thom H, Carter PE, Cole GF, Stevenson KL. Ammonia and carnitine concentrations in children treated with sodium valproate compared with other anticonvulsant drugs. *Developmental Medicine and Child Neurology* 1991; **33**: 795–802.

88. Wallace SJ. A comparative review of the adverse effects of anticonvulsants in children with epilepsy. *Drug Safety* 1996; **15**: 378–393.

89. Jallon P, Picard F. Bodyweight gain and anticonvulsants: a comparative review. *Drug Safety* 2001; **24**: 969–978.

90. Taylor LA, McQuade RD, Tice MA. Felbamate, a novel antiepileptic drug, reverses *N*-methyl-D-aspartate/glycine-stimulated increases in intracellular Ca^{2+} concentration. *European Journal of Pharmacology* 1995; **289**: 229–233.

91. Pisani A, Stefani A, Siniscalchi A, *et al*. Electrophysiological actions of felbamate on rat striatal neurones. *British Journal of Pharmacology* 1995; **16**: 2053–2061.

92. Pugliese AM, Corradetti R. Effects of the antiepileptic drug felbamate on long-term potentiation in the CA1 region of the rat hippocampal slices. *Neuroscience Letters* 1996; **215**: 21–24.

93. Gordon R, Gels M, Diamantis W, Sofia RD. Interaction of felbamate and diazepam against maximal electroshock seizures and chemoconvulsants in mice. *Pharmacology Biochemical Behaviour* 1991; **40**: 109–113.

94. Rho JM, Donevan SD, Rogawski MA. Mechanism of action of the anticonvulsant felbamate: opposing effects on the *N*-methyl-D-aspartate and γ-aminobutyric acid A receptors. *Annals of Neurology* 1994; **35**: 229–234.

95. Palmer KJ, McTavish D. Felbamate. A review of its pharmacodynamic and pharmacokinetic properties, and therapeutic efficacy in epilepsy. *Drugs* 1993; **45**: 1041–1065.

96. Thompson CD, Gulden PH, Macdonald TL. Identification of modified atropaldehyde mercapturic acids in rat and human urine after felbamate administration. *Chemical Research and Toxicology* 1997; **10**: 457–462.

97. Kapetanovic IM, Torchin CD, Thompson CD, *et al*. Potentially reactive cyclic carbamate metabolite of the antiepileptic drug felbamate produced by human liver tissue in vitro. *Drug Metabolism and Disposition* 1998; **26**: 1089–1095.

98. Wagner ML, Graves NM, Marienau K, *et al*. Discontinuation of phenytoin and carbamazepine in patients receiving felbamate. *Epilepsia* 1991; **32**: 398–406.

99. Glue P, Sulowicz W, Colucci R, *et al*. Single-dose pharmacokinetics of felbamate in patients with renal dysfunction. *British Journal of Clinical Pharmacology* 1997; **44**: 91–93.

100. Graves NM, Holmes GB, Fuerst RH, Leppik IE. Effect of felbamate on phenytoin and carbamazepine serum concentrations. *Epilepsia* 1989; **30**: 225–229.

101. Kelley MT, Walson PD, Cox S, Dusci LJ. Population pharmacokinetics of felbamate in children. *Therapeutic Drug Monitoring* 1997; **19**: 29–36.

102. Reidenberg P, Glue P, Banfield CR, *et al*. Effects of felbamate on the pharmacokinetics of phenobarbitone. *Clinical Pharmacology and Therapeutics* 1995; **58**: 279–287.

Derby Hospitals NHS Foundation
Trust
Library and Knowledge

103. Wagner ML, Graves NM, Leppik IE, *et al.* The effect of felbamate on valproic acid disposition. *Clinical Pharmacology and Therapeutics* 1994; **56**: 494–502.

104. Contin M, Riva R, Albani F, Baruzzi A. Effect of felbamate on clobazam and its metabolite kinetics in patients with epilepsy. *Therapeutic Drug Monitoring* 1999; **21**: 604–608.

105. Thompson CD, Kinter MT, Macdonald TL. Synthesis and in vitro reactivity of 3-carbamoyl-2-phenylpropionaldehyde and 2-phenylpropenal: putative reactive metabolites of felbamate. *Chemical Research and Toxicology* 1996; **9**: 1225–1229.

106. French J, Smith M, Faught E, Brown L. Practice advisory: The use of felbamate in the treatment of patients with intractable epilepsy. *Neurology* 1999; **52**: 1540–1545.

107. Pryor FM, Gidal B, Ramsay RE, DeToledo J, Morgan RO. Fosphenytoin: pharmacokinetics and tolerance of intramuscular loading doses. *Epilepsia* 2001; **42**: 245–250.

108. Suman-Chauhan N, Webdale L, Hill DR, Woodruff GN. Characteristics of 3H gabapentin binding to a novel site in rat brain: homogenate binding studies. *European Journal of Pharmacology* 1993; **244**: 293–301.

109. Brown JP, Boden P, Singh L, Gee NS. Mechanisms of action of gabapentin. *Reviews in Contemporary Pharmacotherapy* 1996; **7**: 203–214.

110. Thurlow RP, Brown JP, Gee NS, Hill DR, Woodruff GN. [3H]-Gabapentin may label a system-L-like neutral amino acid carrier in brain. *European Journal of Pharmacology* 1993; **247**: 341–345.

111. Taylor CP, Vartanian MG, Andruszkiewicz R, Silverman RB. 3-Alkyl GABA and 3-alkylglutamic acid analogues: two new classes of anticonvulsant agents. *Epilepsy Research* 1992; **11**: 103–110.

112. Gotz E, Feuerstein TJ, Meyer DK. Effects of gabapentin on release of γ-aminobutyric acid from slices of rat neostriatum. *Drug Research* 1993; **43**: 636–638.

113. Leach JP, Sills GJ, Butler E, *et al.* Neurochemical actions of gabapentin in mouse brain. *Epilepsy Research* 1997; **27**: 175–180.

114. Petroff OAC, Rothman DL, Behar KL, Lamoureux D, Mattson RH. The effect of gabapentin on brain γ-aminobutyric acid in patients with epilepsy. *Annals of Neurology* 1996; **39**: 95–99.

115. Fink K, Dooley DJ, Meder WP, Suman-Chauhan N, Duffy S, Clusmann H, Göthert M. Inhibition of neuronal Ca^{2+} influx by gabapentin and pregabalin in the human neocortex. *Neuropharmacology* 2002; **42**: 229–236.

116. Besag FMC. Gabapentin use with paediatric patients. *Reviews in Contemporary Pharmacotherapy* 1996; **7**: 233–238.

117. McLean MJ. Gabapentin. *Epilepsia* 1995; **36**(Suppl. 2): S57–86.

118. Wilson EA, Sills GJ, Forrest G, Brodie MJ. High dose gabapentin in refractory partial epilepsy: clinical observations in 50 patients. *Epilepsy Research* 1998; **29**: 161–166.

119. Dichter MA, Brodie MJ. New antiepileptic drugs. *New England Journal of Medicine* 1996; **334**: 1583–1590.

120. Patsalos PN. New antiepileptic drugs. *Annals of Clinical Biochemistry* 1999; **36**; 10–19.

121. Frank LM, Enlow T, Holmes GL, *et al.* Lamictal (lamotrigine) monotherapy for typical absence seizures in children. *Epilepsia* 1999; **40**: 973–979.

122. Stefani A, Spadoni F, Siniscalchi A, Bernadi G. Voltage-activated calcium channels: targets of antiepileptic drug therapy? *Epilepsia* 1997; **38**: 959–965.

123. Ramsey RE. Advances in the pharmacotherapy of epilepsy. *Epilepsia* 1993; **34**(Suppl. 5): S9–15.

124. Kuo CC, Lu L. Characterization of lamotrigine inhibition of Na$^+$ channels in rat hippocampal neurones. *British Journal of Pharmacology* 1997; **121**: 1231–1238.

125. Leach MJ, Marden CM, Miller AA. Pharmacological studies on lamotrigine, a novel potential antiepileptic drug: II. Neurochemical studies on the mechanism of action. *Epilepsia* 1986; **27**: 490–497.

126. Calabrese JR, Bowden CL, Sachs GS, *et al.* A double-blind placebo-controlled study of lamotrigine monotherapy in outpatients with bipolar I depression. *Journal of Clinical Psychiatry* 1999; **60**: 79–88.

127. Kaufman KR, Gerner R. Lamotrigine toxicity secondary to sertraline. *Seizure* 1998; **7**: 163–165.

128. Depot M, Powell JR, Messenheimer JA, Cloutier G, Dalton MJ. Kinetic effects of multiple oral doses of acetaminophen on a single oral dose of lamotrigine. *Clinical Pharmacology and Therapeutics* 1990; **48**: 346–355.

129. Ebert U, Thong NQ, Oertal R, Kirch W. Effects of rifampicin and cimetidine on pharmacokinetics and pharmacodynamics of lamotrigine in healthy subjects. *European Journal of Clinical Pharmacology* 2000; **56**: 299–304.

130. Warner T, Patsalos PN, Prevett M, Elyas AA, Duncan JS. Lamotrigine-induced carbamazepine toxicity: an interaction with carbamazepine-10, 11-epoxide. *Epilepsy Research* 1992; **11**: 147–150.

131. Ferrie CD, Robinson RO, Panayiotopoulos CP. Lamotrigine as add-on drug in typical absence seizures. *Acta Neurologica Scandinavica* 1995; **91**: 200–202.

132. Messenheimer J. Efficacy and safety of lamotrigine in pediatric patients. *Journal of Child Neurology* 2002; **17**(Suppl. 2): S34–42.

133. Besag FM, Berry DJ, Pool F, *et al.* Carbamazepine toxicity with lamotrigine: pharmacokinetic or pharmacodynamic interaction? *Epilepsia* 1998; **39**: 183–187.

134. Messenheimer J. Efficacy and safety of lamotrigine in pediatric patients. *Journal of Child Neurology* 2002; **17**: 2S34–42.

135. Bartoli A, Guerrini R, Belmonte A, *et al.* The influence of dosage, age, and comedication on steady state plasma lamotrigine concentrations in epileptic children: A prospective study with preliminary assessment of correlations with clinical response. *Therapeutic Drug Monitoring* 1997; **19**: 252–260.

136. Morris RG, Black AB, Harris AL, Batty AB, Sallustio BC. Lamotrigine and therapeutic drug monitoring: retrospective survey following the introduction of a routine service. *British Journal of Clinical Pharmacology* 1998; **46**: 547–551.

137. Gower AJ, Noyer M, Verloes R, Gobert J, Wülfert E. ucb L059, a novel anti-convulsant drug: pharmacological profile in animals. *European Journal of Pharmacology* 1992; **222**: 193–203.

138. Klitgaard H, Matagne A, Gobert J, Wülfert E. Evidence for a unique profile of levetiracetam in rodent models of seizure and epilepsy *European Journal of Pharmacology* 1998; **353**: 191–206.

139. Löscher W, Hönack D. Profile of ucb L059, a novel anticonvulsant drug, in models of partial and generalized epilepsy in mice and rats. *European Journal of Pharmacology* 1993; **232**: 147–158.

140. Löscher W, Hönack D, Rundfeldt C. Antiepileptogenic effects of the novel anticonvulsant levetiracetam (ucb L059) in the kindling model of temporal lobe epilepsy. *Journal of Pharmacology and Experimental Therapeutics* 1998; **284**: 474–479.

141. Noyer M, Gillard M, Matagne A, Henichart JP, Wülfert E. The novel antiepileptic drug levetiracetam (ucb L059) appears to act via a specific binding site in CNS membranes. *European Journal of Pharmacology* 1995; **286**: 137–146.

142. Zona C, Niespodziany I, Merchetti C, *et al.* Levetiracetam does not modulate neuronal voltage-gated Na^+ and T-type Ca^{2+} currents. *Seizure* 2001; **10**: 279–286.

143. Sills GJ, Leach JP, Kilpatrick WS, *et al.* Neurochemical studies with the novel anticonvulsant levetiracetam in mouse brain. *European Journal of Pharmacology* 1997; **325**: 35–40.

144. Poulain P, Margineanu DG. Levetiracetam opposes the action of $GABA_A$ antagonists in hypothalamic neurones. *Neuropharmacology* 2002; **42**: 346–352.

145. Patsalos PN. Pharmacokinetic profile of levetiracetam: toward ideal characteristics. *Pharmacology and Therapeutics* 2000; **85**: 77–85.

146. Nicolas JM, Collart P, Gerin B, *et al. In vitro* evaluation of potential drug interactions with levetiracetam, a new antiepileptic agent. *Drug Metabolism and Disposition* 1999; **27**: 250–254.

147. Levy RH, Ragueneau-Majlessi I, Baltes E. Repeated administration of the novel antiepileptic agent levetiracetam does not alter digoxin pharmacokinetics and pharmacodynamics in healthy volunteers. *Epilepsy Research* 2001; **46**: 93–99.

148. Sisodiya SM, Sander JWAS, Patsalos PN. Carbamazepine toxicity during combination therapy with levetiracetam: a pharmacodynamic interaction. *Epilepsy Research* 2002; **48**: 217–219.

149. Shorvon SD, Löwenthal A, Janz D, Bielen E, Loiseau P. Multicenter double-blind, randomized, placebo-controlled trial of levetiracetam as add-on therapy in patients with refractory epilepsy. *Epilepsy Research* 2000; **42**: 89–95.

150. Kossoff EH, Bergey GK, Freeman JM, Vining EPG. Levetiracetam psychosis in children with epilepsy. *Epilepsia* 2001; **42**: 1611–1613.

151. White HS. Comparative anticonvulsant and mechanistic profile of established and newer antiepileptic drugs. *Epilepsia* 1999; **40**(Suppl. 5): S2–10.

152. Schmutz M, Brugger F, Gentsch C, McLean MJ, Olpe HR. Oxcarbazepine: preclinical anticonvulsant profile and putative mechanisms of action. *Epilepsia* 1994; **35**(Suppl. 5): S47–50.

153. Parada A, Soares-da-Silva P. The novel anticonvulsant BIA 2-093 inhibits transmitter release during opening of voltage-gated sodium channels: a comparison with carbamazepine and oxcarbazepine. *Neurochemistry International* 2002; **40**: 435–440.

154. Stefani A, Pisani A, De Murtas M, *et al.* Action of GP 47779, the active metabolite of oxcarbazepine, on the corticostriatal system II. Modulation of high-voltage-activated calcium currents. *Epilepsia* 1995; **36**: 997–1002.

155. McLean MJ, Schmutz M, Wamil AW, *et al.* Oxcarbazepine: mechanisms of action. *Epilepsia* 1994; **35**: 5–9.

156. Tecoma ES. Oxcarbazepine. *Epilepsia* 1999; **40**(Suppl. 5): S37–46.

157. Theisohn M, Hamann G. Disposition of the antiepileptic drug oxcarbazepine and its metabolites in healthy volunteers. *European Journal of Pharmacology* 1982; **22**: 545–551.

158. Patsalos PN, Elyas AA, Zakrzewska JM. Protein binding of oxcarbazepine and its primary active metabolite, 10-hydroxycarbazepine, in patients with trigeminal neuralgia. *European Journal of Pharmacology* 1990; **39**: 413–415.

159. Dickinson RG, Hooper WD, Dunstan PR, Eadie MJ. First dose and steady-state pharmacokinetics of oxcarbazepine and its 10-hydroxy metabolite. *European Journal of Pharmacology* 1989; **37**: 69–74.

160. Lloyd P, Flesch G, Dieterle W. Clinical pharmacology and pharmacokinetics of oxcarbazepine. *Epilepsia* 1994; **35**(Suppl. 3): S10–13.

161. Rouan MC, Lecaillon LB, Godbillion J, *et al.* The effect of renal impairment on the pharmacokinetics of oxcarbazepine and its metabolites *European Journal of Clinical Pharmacology* 1994; **47**: 161–167.

162. Hossain M, Sallas W, Gaspparini M, *et al.* Drug-drug interaction profile of oxcarbazepine in children and adults. *Neurology* 1999; **52**(Suppl. 2): A525.

163. May TW, Rambeck B, Jürgens U. Influence of oxcarbazepine and methosuximide on lamotrigine concentrations in epileptic patients with and without valproic acid comedication: results of a retrospective study. *Therapeutic Drug Monitoring* 1999; **21**: 175–181.

164. Fattore C, Cipolla G, Gatti G, *et al.* Induction of ethinylestradiol and levonorgestrel metabolism by oxcarbazepine in healthy women. *Epilepsia* 1999; **40**: 783–787.

165. Rättyä J, Vainionpää L, Knip M, *et al.* The effects of valproate, carbamazepine and oxcarbazepine on growth and sexual maturation in girls with epilepsy. *Pediatrics* 1999; **103**: 588–593.

166. Beran RG. Cross-reactive skin eruption with both carbamazepine and oxcarbazepine. *Epilepsia* 1993; **34**: 163–165.

167. Van Amelsvoort T, Bakshi R, Devaux CB, *et al.* Hyponatremia associated with carbamazepine and oxcarbazepine therapy: a review. *Epilepsia* 1994; **35**: 181–188.

168. Borden LA, Dhar TGM, Smith KE, *et al.* Tiagabine, SK&F 89976-A, CI-966 and NNC-711 are selective for the cloned GABA transporter GAT-1. *European Journal of Pharmacology* 1994; **269**: 219–224.

169. Ribak CE, Tong WM, Brecha C. GABA plasma membrane transporters, GAT-1 and GAT-3, display different distributions in rat hippocampus. *Journal of Comparative Neurology* 1996; **367**: 595–606.

170. Thompson SM, Gähwiler BH. Effects of the GABA uptake inhibitor tiagabine on inhibitory synaptic potential in rat hippocampal slice cultures. *Journal of Neurophysiology* 1992; **67**: 1698–1701.

171. Nielsen EB, Suzdak PD, Andersen KE, *et al.* Characterization of tiagabine (NO-328), a new potent and selective GABA uptake inhibitor. *European Journal of Pharmacology* 1991; **196**: 257–266.

172. Suzdak PD, Jansen JA. A review of the preclinical pharmacology of tiagabine: a potent and selective anticonvulsant GABA uptake inhibitor. *Epilepsia* 1995; **36**: 612–626.

173. Wang X, Patsalos PN. The pharmacokinetic profile of tiagabine. *Reviews in Contemporary Pharmacotherapy* 2002; **12**: 225–233.

174. Adkins JC, Noble S. Tiagabine. A review of its pharmaco-dynamic and pharmacokinetic properties and therapeutic potential in the management of epilepsy. *Drugs* 1998; **55**: 437–460.

175. Lau AH, Gustavson LE, Sperelakis R, *et al.* Pharmacokinetics and safety of tiagabine in subjects with various degrees of hepatic function. *Epilepsia* 1997; **38**: 445–451.

176. Gustavson LE, Boellner SW, Granneman GR, *et al.* A single dose study to define tiagabine pharmacokinetics in paediatric patients with complex partial seizures. *Neurology* 1997; **48**: 1032–1037.

177. So EL, Wolff D, Graves NM, *et al.* Pharmacokinetics of tiagabine as add-on therapy in patients taking enzyme-inducing antiepilepsy drugs. *Epilepsy Research* 1995; **22**: 221–226.

178. Brodie MJ. Tiagabine pharmacology in profile. *Epilepsia* 1995; **36**(Suppl. 6): S7–9.

179. Piccinelli P, Borgatti R, Perucca E, *et al.* Frontal non-convulsive status epilepticus associated with high-dose tiagabine therapy in a child with familial bilateral perisylvian polymicrogyria. *Epilepsia* 2000; **41**: 1485–1488.

180. Patsalos PN, Elyas AA, Ratnaraj N, Iley J. Concentration-dependent displacement of tiagabine by valproic acid. *Epilepsia* 2002; **43**(Suppl. 8): 143.

181. Buttery PC, Sisodiya SM. The safety, tolerability and adverse events profile of tiagabine. *Reviews in Contemporary Pharmacotherapy* 2002; **12**: 251–264.

182. Schmidt D, Gram L, Brodie MJ, *et al.* Tiagabine in the treatment of epilepsy – a clinical review with a guide for the prescribing physician. *Epilepsy Research* 2000; **41**: 245–251.

183. DeLorenzo RJ, Sombati S, Coulter DA. Effects of topiramate on sustained repetitive firing and spontaneous recurrent seizure discharges in cultured hippocampal neurons. *Epilepsia* 2000; **41**(Suppl. 1): S40–44.

184. Zhang X, Velumian AA, Jones OT, Carlen PL. Topiramate reduces high-voltage activated Ca^{2+} currents in CA1 pyramidal neurons in vitro. *Epilepsia* 1998; **39**(Suppl. 6): 44.

185. White HS, Brown SD, Skeen GA, Wolf HH, Twymann RE. The anticonvulsant topiramate displays a unique ability to potentiate GABA-evoked chloride currents. *Epilepsia* 1995; **36**(Suppl. 3): S39–40.

186. White HS, Brown SD, Woodhead JH, Skeen GA, Wolf HH. Topiramate enhances GABA-mediated chloride flux and GABA-evoked chloride currents in murine brain neurons and increases seizure threshold. *Epilepsy Research* 1997; **28**: 167–179.

187. Severt L, Coulter DA, Sombati S, DeLorenzo RJ. Topiramate selectively blocks kainate currents in cultured hippocampal neurons. *Epilepsia* 1995; **36**(Suppl. 4): 38.

188. Petroff OAC, Hyder F, Mattson RH, Rothman DL. Topiramate increases brain GABA, homocarnosine, and pyrrolidinone in patients with epilepsy. *Neurology* 1999; **52**: 473–478.

189. Nayak RK, Gisclon LG, Curtin CA, Benet LZ. Estimation of the absolute bioavailability of topiramate in humans without intravenous data. *Journal of Clinical Pharmacology* 1994; **34**: 1029.

190. Patsalos PN. The pharmacokinetic profile of topiramate. *Reviews in Contemporary Pharmacotherapy* 1999; **10**: 155–162.

191. Doose DR, Walker SA, Gisclon LG, Nayak RK. Single dose pharmacokinetics and effect of food on the bioavailability of topiramate, a novel antiepileptic drug. *Journal of Clinical Pharmacology* 1996; **36**: 884–891.

192. Doose DR, Scott VV, Margul BL, Marriot TB, Nayak RK. Multiple-dose pharmacokinetics of topiramate in healthy male subjects. *Epilepsia* 1988; **29**(Suppl. 5): 662.

193. Easterling DE, Zakszewski T, Moyer MD, *et al.* Plasma pharmacokinetics of topiramate, a new anticonvulsant in humans. *Epilepsia* 1988; **29**: 662.

194. Sachdeo RC, Sachdeo SK, Walker SA, *et al.* Steady-state pharmacokinetics of topiramate and carbamazepine in patients with epilepsy during monotherapy and concomitant therapy. *Epilepsia* 1996; **37**: 774–780.

195. May TW, Rambeck B, Jurgens U. Serum concentrations of topiramate in patients with epilepsy: influence of dose, age, and comedication. *Therapeutic Drug Monitoring* 2002; **24**: 366–374.

196. Contin M, Riva R, Albani F, Avoni P, Baruzzi A. Topiramate therapeutic monitoring in patients with epilepsy: effect of concomitant antiepileptic drugs. *Therapeutic Drug Monitoring* 2002; **24**: 332–337.

197. Rosenfeld WE, Liao S, Kramer LD, *et al.* Comparison of the steady-state pharmacokinetics of topiramate and valproate in patients with epilepsy during monotherapy and concomitant therapy. *Epilepsia* 1997; **38**: 324–333.

198. Yerby M. Topiramate displacement of valproic acid binding sites. *Epilepsia* 1997; **38**(Suppl. 3): 67–68.

199. Liao S, Palmer M. Digoxin and topiramate drug interaction in male volunteers. *Pharmaceutical Research* 1993; **10**: S405.

200. Lippert B, Metcalf B, Jung MJ, Casara P. 4-Amino-hex-5-enoic acid, a selective catalytic inhibitor of 4-aminobutyric acid transferase in mammalian brain. *European Journal of Biochemistry* 1977; **74**: 441–445.

201. Patsalos PN, Duncan JS. The pharmacology and pharmacokinetics of vigabatrin. *Reviews in Contemporary Pharmacotherapy* 1995; **6**: 447–456.

202. Sheth RD, Buckley D, Penney S, Hobbs GR. Vigabatrin in childhood epilepsy: comparable efficacy for generalized and partial seizures. *Clinical Neuropharmacology* 1996; **19**: 297–304.

203. Kälviänen R, Nousiainen I, Mäntyjärvi M, *et al.* Vigabatrin, a gabaergic antiepileptic drug, causes concentric visual field defects. *Neurology* 1999; **53**: 922–932.

204. Lawden MC, Eke T, Degg C, Harding GFA, Wild JM. Visual field defects associated with vigabatrin therapy. *Journal of Neurology, Neurosurgery and Psychiatry* 1999; **67**: 716–722.

205. Wild JM, Martinez C, Reinshagen G, Harding GFA. Characteristics of a unique visual field defect attributed to vigabatrin. *Epilepsia* 1999; **40**: 1784–1794.

206. Cross-Tsur V, Banin E, Shahar E, Shalev RS, Lahat E. Visual impairment in children with epilepsy treated with vigabatrin. *Annals of Neurology* 2000; **48**: 60–64.

207. Juhász C, Muzik O, Chugani DC, *et al.* Prolonged vigabatrin treatment modifies developmental changes of GABA$_A$-receptor binding in young children with epilepsy. *Epilepsia* 2002; **42**: 1310–1326.

208. Peters DH, Sorkin EM. Zonisamide. A review of its pharmacodynamic properties and therapeutic potential in epilepsy. *Drugs* 1993; **45**; 760–787.

209. Rock DM, Macdonald RL, Taylor CP. Blockade of sustained repetitive action potentials in cultured spinal cord neurons by zonisamide (AD 810, CI 912) a novel anticonvulsant. *Epilepsy Research* 1989; **3**: 138–143.

210. Suzuki S, Kawakami K, Nishimura S, *et al.* Zonisamide blocks T-type calcium channel in cultured neurons of rat cerebral cortex. *Epilepsy Research* 1992; **12**: 21–27.

211. Leppik IE. Zonisamide. *Epilepsia* 1999; **40**(Suppl. 5): S23–29.

212. Shinoda M, Akita M, Hasegawa M, Hasegawa T, Nabeshima T. The necessity of adjusting the dosage of zonisamide when coadministered with other anti-epileptic drugs. *Biological Pharmacy Bulletin* 1996; **19**: 1090–1092.

213. Berent S, Sackellares JC, Giordani B, *et al.* Zonisamide (CI-912) and cognition: results from preliminary study. *Epilepsia* 1987; **28**: 61–67.

214. Kawada K, Itoh S, Kusaka T, Isobe K, Ishii M. Pharmacokinetics of zonisamide in perinatal period. *Brain and Development* 2002; **24**: 95–97.

215. Mimaki T. Clinical pharmacology and therapeutic drug monitoring of zonisamide. *Therapeutic Drug Monitoring* 1998; **20**: 593–597.

22

Treatment of epilepsy

Antiepileptic drugs (AEDs)

BLAISE FD BOURGEOIS

REVIEW OF INDIVIDUAL DRUGS

Phenobarbital and primidone

EFFICACY

Despite its known sedative and behavioral side-effects, phenobarbital is still commonly used in the pediatric age range, because of its convenient pharmacokinetics and relative safety. Indications for phenobarbital include generalized tonic-clonic seizures, simple and complex partial seizures, generalized convulsive and simple or complex partial status epilepticus, juvenile myoclonic epilepsy, neonatal seizures and the prophylaxis of febrile seizures.

In the treatment of partial seizures, phenobarbital was found to be as effective as carbamazepine in children[1] and in adults.[2] It can also be effective in the treatment of juvenile myoclonic epilepsy, but it is not the preferred drug for this form of epilepsy. In the treatment of convulsive status epilepticus, phenobarbital is usually administered after a benzodiazepine and phenytoin, and it is as effective as diazepam and phenytoin.[3] The initial intravenous loading dose of phenobarbital in the treatment of status is 15–20 mg/kg. Very high doses of phenobarbital have been used in the treatment of refractory status epilepticus in children, with levels of 70–344 mg/L (302–1483 μmol/L).[4]

Phenobarbital remains a drug of first choice in neonates with seizures. The initial loading dose is 15–20 mg/kg, or even of up to 40 mg/kg,[5] and the maintenance dose is 3–4 mg/kg per day. When neonates with seizures were randomly assigned to receive either phenobarbital or phenytoin, both drugs were equally effective.[6] Efficacy of phenobarbital in preventing recurrence of febrile seizures could be demonstrated at levels above 15 μmg/L (65 μmol/L).[7] However, chronic prophylactic treatment of febrile seizures is now more the exception than the rule, and there are reservations about the possible detrimental effect on IQ.[8]

SIDE-EFFECTS

Phenobarbital and primidone share most of their long-term side-effects. The most common is sedation and drowsiness in adults, whereas children may also become hyperactive, aggressive, and irritable. Allergic rashes and hypersensitivity reactions can occur, but they are relatively rare. Organ toxicity from phenobarbital or primidone is exceedingly rare. In neonates of mothers treated with phenobarbital, vitamin K-deficient hemorrhagic disease can be prevented by administration of vitamin K to the mother before delivery.

PHARMACOKINETICS, INTERACTIONS, DOSAGE

The elimination half-life of phenobarbital is relatively long and it is age dependent, above 100 h in neonates,[9] 148 h in asphyxiated neonates,[10] 60 h during the first year of life, followed by a gradual prolongation until adult values of 80–100 h are reached.[11] Pharmacokinetic interactions involving phenobarbital reflect enzyme-inducing properties, which result in higher clearance and lower relative levels of several other AEDs, including carbamazepine, ethosuximide, felbamate, lamotrigine, oxcarbazepine metabolite, tiagabine, topiramate, valproic acid and zonisamide, and other drugs, including theophylline, warfarin, steroids and oral contraceptives. The most significant interaction affecting phenobarbital is the inhibition of its metabolism by valproic acid, resulting in a 50–100 per cent increase in phenobarbital levels.

The daily maintenance dose of phenobarbital in children varies between 2 and 8 mg/kg, and is inversely related to the child's age. The full maintenance dose can be given on the first day. Discontinuation should always be gradual over several weeks, because of the risk of withdrawal seizures upon rapid discontinuation.

Primidone

There has never been a clear demonstration that treatment with primidone truly differs from treatment with phenobarbital in clinical practice. Primidone is converted to phenobarbital. Independent seizure protection by primidone has been demonstrated in animals, but the actual contribution of primidone to the therapeutic effect during chronic therapy in humans is difficult to ascertain. It is unlikely that the other active metabolite of primidone, phenylethylmalonamide (PEMA), contributes to the clinical effect.[12,13]

Indications for primidone are similar to those for phenobarbital, but it is not available for parenteral administration and is not used in the acute treatment of status epilepticus. In clinical studies, primidone and phenobarbital were found to be equally effective.[14] In one crossover study, primidone was found to be slightly more effective against generalized tonic-clonic seizures than phenobarbital in the presence of similar phenobarbital levels.[15] In a controlled study in patients with partial and secondarily generalized seizures, primidone, phenytoin, carbamazepine and phenobarbital were equally effective, but failures occurred more often with primidone because of side-effects during the early phases of treatment.[2] Primidone is also effective in juvenile myoclonic epilepsy, but is not a drug of choice. Primidone has been evaluated as adjunctive therapy in neonates with seizures and found to be effective.[16,17] It appears that neonates cannot convert primidone to phenobarbital.

It is more rational to prescribe primidone as a monotherapy or in combination with a noninducing drug. The phenobarbital:primidone concentration ratio is increased by inducing drugs, and this obliterates any difference between prescribing primidone and prescribing phenobarbital. Primidone must be introduced slowly. The initial doses may cause transient dizziness, drowsiness, and nausea, and may have to be as low as 62.5–125 mg in adults (1–2 mg/kg in children), with dosage increases at intervals of 3 days. The final dose is about 10–20 mg/kg per day. Primidone appears to be tolerated better in children than in adults.[18] It causes the same pharmacokinetic interactions as phenobarbital.

Phenytoin

EFFICACY

Phenytoin can be useful in the treatment of generalized tonic-clonic seizures, simple and complex partial seizures, generalized convulsive status epilepticus, simple or complex partial status epilepticus, and neonatal seizures. It can be administered intravenously and has been used in every age group. In the treatment of status epilepticus, after administration of a benzodiazepine, phenytoin is the drug of choice for subsequent protection against recurrences. The dose for intravenous phenytoin in the treatment of status is 15–20 mg/kg. Additional doses can be given if needed, up to 30 mg/kg. In order to avoid bradyarrhythmia and hypotension, phenytoin needs to be administered slowly. The recommended rate is <50 mg/min in adolescents and adults. In children, the maximal rate is 1 mg/kg per minute. Because of its very high pH, the parenteral phenytoin preparation can cause significant irritation to the veins, as well as serious skin lesions when it infiltrates. Because of this, fosphenytoin is now preferred for intravenous administration. This water-soluble pro-drug that is rapidly converted to phenytoin in the blood is not irritating, but bradyarrhythmia and hypotension can still occur. The recommended infusion rate for fosphenytoin in children is 3 mg/kg per minute. The doses are indicated in 'phenytoin equivalents' and are the same as for phenytoin.

Phenytoin is a useful drug during the neonatal period. Usually, it is administered after phenobarbital has failed.[19] The initial intravenous loading dose of phenytoin in neonates is 15–20 mg/kg. When neonates with seizures were randomly assigned to receive either phenobarbital or phenytoin, both drugs were equally effective.[6]

SIDE-EFFECTS

The main side-effects of phenytoin consist of cosmetic changes, such as gingival hyperplasia and hypertrichosis or hirsutism, as well as of allergic reactions, including a hypersensitivity syndrome. Pseudolymphoma is rare and a polyneuropathy may be seen only after prolonged exposure. At high levels, first nystagmus then ataxia will appear.

PHARMACOKINETICS, INTERACTIONS, DOSAGE

Phenytoin has strong enzyme-inducing properties. This results in lower relative levels of several other drugs, including carbamazepine, ethosuximide, felbamate, lamotrigine, oxcarbazepine metabolite, tiagabine, topiramate, valproic acid and zonisamide, as well as theophylline, warfarin, steroids and oral contraceptives. Phenytoin distinguishes itself from all other AEDs by its nonlinear elimination kinetics, resulting in a disproportionate increase in steady-state serum levels as the maintenance dose is increased. The nonlinear kinetics of phenytoin initially described in adults were also demonstrated in children of any age,[20] including neonates.[21] In certain individuals, this can lead to very labile levels in the therapeutic range, dosage increases of 10–20 per cent being associated with increases in steady-state levels of 50–100 per cent.

The chronic maintenance dose of phenytoin is quite variable and age-dependent. It is advisable to adjust the dose in small increments. The initial dose should be about 5 mg/kg per day in older children and 8 mg/kg per day in young infants. Serum levels should be determined 2–3 weeks after any dosage adjustment. In neonates, the elimination of phenytoin is initially slow, but there is a rapid acceleration during the first month of life.[21] Subsequently, the elimination kinetics of phenytoin in infants less than 1 year old are faster than at any other age.[22] Accordingly, in older neonates and young infants, daily maintenance doses of phenytoin as high as 20 mg/kg may be required to maintain good therapeutic levels.

Carbamazepine and oxcarbazepine

EFFICACY

The role of carbamazepine is in the treatment of simple and complex partial seizures and of primarily or secondarily generalized tonic-clonic seizures. It is not available for parenteral administration. In adults, carbamazepine was found to be as effective as phenytoin, phenobarbital, primidone and valproic acid.[2,23] Carbamazepine was possibly more effective than any of the four other drugs against partial seizures without secondary generalization. Carbamazepine and phenobarbital in children with partial seizures did not differ in their efficacy.[1] Carbamazepine and valproic acid, compared in children with partial seizures, or primarily and secondarily generalized tonic-clonic seizures, were equally effective.[24] In children with the Lennox-Gastaut syndrome, carbamazepine can exacerbate certain seizures such as myoclonic and drop attacks.[25]

SIDE-EFFECTS

Carbamazepine seems to be well tolerated in children. In a comparative study of monotherapy with phenobarbital, primidone, phenytoin, carbamazepine and valproic acid,[18] serious side-effects requiring discontinuation of the drug were least common with carbamazepine. The main side-effects of carbamazepine are an allergic rash and leukopenia. Mild to moderate hyponatremia may develop, but this does not require routine monitoring. At high levels, carbamazepine can cause dizziness, diplopia, ataxia, and vomiting.

PHARMACOKINETICS, INTERACTIONS, DOSAGE

Co-medication with phenytoin or phenobarbital accelerates the elimination of carbamazepine. Inversely, carbamazepine is an enzyme inducer like phenobarbital, primidone and phenytoin. The initial maintenance dose of carbamazepine is 5–10 mg/kg per day. Carbamazepine accelerates its own elimination rate through hepatic enzyme induction, a phenomenon called **autoinduction**. The maintenance dose can be increased by 5–10 mg/kg per day at weekly intervals, and the final maintenance doses of 30 mg/kg per day or more are not unusual in children, especially in combination therapy.

Oxcarbazepine

This is closely related to carbamazepine, from which it differs structurally only by one oxo group on the central ring. Oxcarbazepine is rapidly converted to the mono-hydroxy derivative, which accumulates to a much larger extent and is responsible for the pharmacological effect. Only levels of the monohydroxy derivative are measured for the purpose of therapeutic monitoring. The spectrum of efficacy of oxcarbazepine does not differ from that of carbamazepine. Its efficacy in children with focal-onset seizures has been demonstrated in a placebo-controlled double-blind trial.[26] The side-effect profile of oxcarbazepine is also similar to that of carbamazepine, but there are minor differences. Leukopenia is less common and monitoring of the blood count is not necessary. However, hyponatremia may be more common than with carbamazepine.[27] Oxcarbazepine can cause allergic rashes like carbamazepine, but there seems to be only 25 per cent cross-reactivity.

Unlike carbamazepine, the metabolism of oxcarbazepine and of its active metabolite is not subject to autoinduction, and the drug causes less enzymatic induction than carbamazepine. Levels of the monohydroxy derivative are lowered by inducing drugs. In children, the recommended initial dose is 5–10 mg/kg per day. This dose can be increased weekly by increments of 5–10 mg/kg per day, up to 20–30 mg/kg per day.

Valproic acid

EFFICACY

Valproic acid is effective against a wide range of generalized seizures as well as against partial seizures. The administration of valproic acid reduces the frequency and duration of spike-and-wave discharges in patients with typical and atypical absences.[28] Against absence seizures, valproic acid and ethosuximide were found to be equally effective.[29,30] Valproic acid is also effective in generalized convulsive seizures.[31] It is currently one of the most effective drugs for myoclonic seizures, particularly those seen with primary or idiopathic generalized epilepsies. The role of valproic acid as the drug of choice in the treatment of juvenile myoclonic epilepsy is well established. Successful treatment with valproic acid in combination with clonazepam has been reported for tonic-clonic and myoclonic seizures in patients with severe progressive myoclonic epilepsy.[32] Valproic acid is widely used in the treatment of the Lennox-Gastaut syndrome and related forms of epilepsy. In 22 children with newly diagnosed infantile spasms, initial treatment with valproic acid controlled the spasms in 11 children after 4 weeks, and in 16 children after 3 months.[33]

In a multicenter trial in children with complex partial and primarily or secondarily generalized tonic-clonic seizures,[24] carbamazepine and valproic acid were equally effective. A comparative study of valproic acid, carbamazepine, phenytoin and phenobarbital was carried out in children.[34] Equal efficacy was found for all drugs against generalized and partial seizures. Valproic acid has been shown to be clearly effective in preventing the recurrence of febrile seizures.[35] However, based on risk versus benefit considerations, valproic acid cannot be recommended for this indication. Neonates with seizures have also been successfully treated with valproic acid.[36]

SIDE-EFFECTS

Neurological side-effects of valproic acid include a dose-related tremor, as well as occasional drowsiness and lethargy. A rare but rather specific side-effect is characterized by acute and reversible mental changes that can progress to stupor or coma.[37] Gastrointestinal adverse effects include nausea, vomiting and anorexia, as well as increased appetite and excessive weight gain.[38] Valproic acid can cause potentially fatal hepatotoxicity, mostly related to young age and polytherapy.[39] It is best identified on the basis of clinical symptoms that may include nausea, vomiting, anorexia, lethargy, as well as loss of seizure control, jaundice and edema. The occurrence of vomiting and abdominal pain should also raise the suspicion of hemorrhagic pancreatitis.[40] Thrombocytopenia is often seen at higher levels.[41] Hyperammonemia is common and mostly asymptomatic.[42]

Increased hair loss may be seen early during treatment with valproic acid and, although the hair tends to grow back, it may become different in texture or color. Facial or limb edema can occur in the absence of valproic acid-induced hepatic injury.[43] Children may develop nocturnal enuresis.[44]

In women, valproic acid can cause menstrual irregularities and hormonal changes.[45] A recent concern has been the possibility that it may cause polycystic ovaries, as well as endocrine and metabolic changes.[46,47] Treatment with valproic acid during the first trimester of pregnancy has been found to be associated with an estimated 1–2 per cent risk of neural tube defect in the newborn.[48,49] Folate supplementation appears to reduce the risk,[50] and a daily dose of at least 1 mg should be considered in all female patients of childbearing age who are taking valproic acid.

PHARMACOKINETICS, INTERACTIONS, DOSAGE

The elimination half-life of valproic acid is 13–16 h in adults not taking enzyme-inducing drugs,[51] and about 9 hours in the presence of inducing drugs.[52] Corresponding values in children are shorter, 11.6 and 7 h respectively.[53] Inducing drugs invariably lower valproic acid levels. Valproic acid itself markedly inhibits the elimination and raises the relative level of phenobarbital, ethosuximide and lamotrigine. Oral contraceptives are not affected by valproic acid.

Valproic acid therapy is usually initiated at a daily dose of 10–15 mg/kg. The dose can be increased at weekly intervals by 5–10 mg/kg per day. With valproic acid monotherapy, levels within the recommended therapeutic range and a satisfactory clinical response are usually achieved with doses between 10 and 20 mg/kg per day. Combination therapy with inducing drugs increases the dosage requirements to 30 mg/kg per day and above. If therapeutic levels of valproic acid are to be achieved rapidly, or in patients unable to take it orally, valproic acid can be administered intravenously.[54] This route has also been suggested for the treatment of status epilepticus, with an initial dose of 15 mg/kg followed by 1 mg/kg per hour.[55] A faster infusion rate of up to 6 mg/kg per minute has been tolerated.[56]

Ethosuximide

EFFICACY

Ethosuximide is still a drug of first choice in patients who have absence seizures only. It is highly effective against the typical absences seen in primary generalized epilepsies such as childhood absence epilepsy. Complete seizure control is achieved in approximately 80 per cent of the patients. With seizure control, a concomitant disappearance of spike-and-wave paroxysms in the EEG is the rule. It is a common observation that absence seizures that occur as the sole seizure type in a patient are more likely to be fully controlled by medication than if they occur in conjunction with another seizure type.[57] The therapeutic results with ethosuximide are also better against typical than against atypical absences.

The efficacy of ethosuximide in the control of absence seizures is similar to that of valproic acid.[29,30] Valproic acid and ethosuximide may have a beneficial synergistic interaction. A group of patients with absence seizures that had not been controlled by adequate trials of ethosuximide alone, or valproic acid alone, became free of seizures on a combination of ethosuximide and valproic acid.[58] Although there is no clear evidence that ethosuximide alone is effective against any other seizure type besides absences, as adjunctive therapy it may be effective against myoclonic seizures and against astatic seizures.[59,60]

SIDE-EFFECTS

Although its gastrointestinal side-effects may be bothersome (upset stomach, hiccups), ethosuximide is practically free of serious side-effects.

DOSAGE

Therapy with ethosuximide in children can be initiated at a dose of about 10 mg/kg per day. The dose can be titrated up at intervals of 5–7 days as necessary and as tolerated, up to a dose of approximately 30–40 mg/kg per day, preferably with or after meals in three divided doses, in order to minimize the occurrence of gastrointestinal side-effects.

Benzodiazepines

CLONAZEPAM

Clonazepam typifies the advantages and disadvantages of benzodiazepines. They have a rapid onset of action; can be administered orally, rectally, intramuscularly and intravenously; have a wide spectrum of efficacy; have some protective effect against every type of seizure; and have virtually no systemic or serious side-effects. Benzodiazepines have two major disadvantages: sedative and behavioral side-effects, and loss of efficacy in a high percentage of patients. Benzodiazepines are particularly useful for the acute and intermittent treatment of epilepsy, status epilepticus, intermittent prophylaxis of febrile seizures, periodic seizure clusters and catamenial epilepsy.

In children, clonazepam is most likely to be used as an adjunct in the treatment of various generalized epilepsies, including absence seizures. It is also used as a secondary drug against infantile spasms and myoclonic seizures. Clonazepam can be useful in combination with valproic acid, against absences, as well as against complex partial seizures.[61]

In the Lennox-Gastaut syndrome, the atypical absences, myoclonic seizures and falling spells can be reduced by clonazepam.[62] The combination of valproic acid and clonazepam can be of additional benefit.[61] Against infantile spasms, a favorable response has been documented.[62] Clonazepam has also been used successfully in the treatment of epilepsies with myoclonus as the predominant seizure type. Patients with severe myoclonus epilepsy can improve with the combination of clonazepam and valproic acid.[32] Clonazepam is also effective in controlling

the myoclonic seizures occurring in patients with juvenile myoclonic epilepsy, but it seems to be less effective against the generalized tonic-clonic seizures.[63]

Clonazepam has been used successfully in the treatment of status epilepticus in children.[64] Parenteral doses in children are usually 1–2 mg, up to a total of 4 mg. In patients with the Lennox-Gastaut syndrome, clonazepam can induce a generalized tonic state.[65] In neonates with frequent seizures refractory to phenobarbital,[66] excellent results were achieved with intravenous clonazepam at 0.1 mg/kg. Results were less encouraging at 0.2 mg/kg, suggesting an optimal response at the lower dose.

It is important to initiate therapy with clonazepam slowly, using initial doses of 0.01–0.03 mg/kg per day. Dosage increases should be carried out at intervals of 1 week or more, titrating the dose as necessary and as tolerated up to approximately 0.1–0.3 mg/kg per day, divided into two to three daily doses. In an attempt to avoid the development of tolerance with chronic use, administration of clonazepam on alternate days has been tried with some success.[67]

NITRAZEPAM

This is used mainly for infantile spasms with hypsarrhythmia and in children with the Lennox-Gastaut and related syndromes. Tolerance occurs, as with other benzodiazepines. Nitrazepam was compared with ACTH against infantile spasms in a randomized controlled study.[68] A 75–100 per cent seizure reduction could be achieved in 57 per cent of the patients treated with ACTH and in 53 per cent of the patients treated with nitrazepam.

Side-effects are similar to those of other benzodiazepines, but nitrazepam seems to more specifically cause drooling and aspiration, which may result in pneumonia and possible death.[69,70] The risk of death seems to be highest in children less than 3.4 years.[71] The maintenance dose of nitrazepam varies between 0.25 and 2.5 mg/kg per day but, because of the risk of death, it is recommended to maintain the dose below 1 mg/kg per day, especially in young children.

CLOBAZAM

This drug is a 1,5-benzodiazepine, as opposed to a 1,4-benzodiazepine (i.e. one nitrogen is in a different position). With the possible exception of milder side-effects, clobazam appears to have a similar spectrum of efficacy and to be associated with the same incidence of tolerance as other benzodiazepines. In countries where it is marketed, clobazam is now one of the favorite benzodiazepines in the treatment of epilepsy, particularly as adjunctive therapy of partial seizures.[72] In a placebo-controlled crossover study in institutionalized patients with refractory epilepsy, clobazam was associated with a highly significant decrease in seizure frequency,[73] but 77 per cent of the responders developed tolerance to the antiepileptic effect after a median interval of 3.5 months.[74] Good initial results with clobazam were obtained in monotherapy in children with various types of seizures.[75] The authors considered clobazam particularly effective in benign partial epilepsy. In a double-blind placebo-controlled study of clobazam in children with generalized and partial seizures, 52 per cent of the patients on clobazam had a greater than 50 per cent reduction in their seizure frequency.[76] Intermittent clobazam can be successful in the treatment of catamenial epilepsy.[77]

The maintenance dose is usually between 0.5 and 1 mg/kg per day. Side-effects are more likely at total daily doses of more than 30 mg/day, without clear evidence of improved effectiveness. Clobazam is not available for parenteral use but can be administered rectally in semiacute situations at doses of 20–30 mg.

Lamotrigine

EFFICACY

Lamotrigine has established itself as a major broad-spectrum drug in the treatment of pediatric epilepsy. A large body of evidence in adults supports the role of lamotrigine as an effective drug against seizures with focal onset.[78–80] No difference in efficacy could be found between lamotrigine and carbamazepine[81] or phenytoin.[82] The experience with lamotrigine in children with focal-onset seizures is derived from open studies in children with a broad spectrum of seizure types.[83,84]

The efficacy of lamotrigine in the treatment of patients with Lennox-Gastaut syndrome has been demonstrated in a double-blind study.[85] Lamotrigine was also found in open and in controlled studies to be effective against absence seizures,[86,87] as well as against generalized tonic-clonic seizures,[86] infantile spasms,[88] and juvenile myoclonic epilepsy.[89]

SIDE-EFFECTS

A rash that may evolve into Stevens-Johnson syndrome or toxic epidermal necrolysis is the only significant concern with lamotrigine.[90] A rash occurs in approximately 10 per cent of patients, mostly during the first 8 weeks of therapy, but less than 10 per cent of the cases evolve into a serious reaction. Data from a population-based registry of Stevens-Johnson syndrome and toxic epidermal necrolysis yielded an incidence estimate of only 3 in 10 000 for lamotrigine.[91] The incidence of rash is higher with higher initial doses and when lamotrigine is added to valproic acid.[84,92] It appears that a reduction in the recommended starting dose (see below) of lamotrigine was associated with a significant reduction in the incidence of serious rashes.[92] Patients who had developed a rash have been

successfully rechallenged.[93] The other side-effects of lamotrigine include somnolence, dizziness, headache, diplopia, nausea and vomiting. Other reported adverse effects include insomnia, tic disorders or tourettism,[94,95] as well as multiorgan dysfunction with disseminated intravascular coagulation.[96] Finally, it appears that lamotrigine can exacerbate myoclonic seizures. This has been observed in patients with juvenile myoclonic epilepsy,[97] severe myoclonic epilepsy of infancy,[98] and at high dose in one patient with Lennox-Gastaut syndrome.[99]

PHARMACOKINETICS, INTERACTIONS, DOSAGE

Valproic acid inhibits the metabolism of lamotrigine, and thus decreases the dosage requirements, whereas enzyme-inducing drugs increase the dosage requirements. As a consequence, the appropriate dosage of lamotrigine varies substantially as a function of co-medication. In addition, in order to reduce the risk of serious skin reactions, a low initial dose and slow titration schedule are necessary. The current initial dosage recommendations for lamotrigine in children as a function of pre-existing medication regimen are summarized in Table 22A.1. The initial recommended dose is 0.4 mg/kg per day in children taking lamotrigine in monotherapy or with drugs that do not influence lamotrigine kinetics, such a gabapentin, topiramate, benzodiazepines, tiagabine, levetiracetam or zonisamide.

Topiramate

EFFICACY

Topiramate has revealed itself to be a useful drug that is effective in various forms of pediatric epilepsy. Topiramate has been shown to be effective against focal-onset seizures in adults[100–102] as well as in children.[103] Additional double-blind studies have demonstrated the efficacy of topiramate against generalized tonic-clonic seizures without focal origin[104] and against the seizures associated with the Lennox-Gastaut syndrome.[105] In the study on generalized tonic-clonic seizures, a subgroup of patients had juvenile myoclonic epilepsy. In those patients, topiramate was far superior to placebo against the generalized tonic-clonic seizures. In a pilot study, a positive response to topiramate was also found in the treatment of infantile spasms.[106]

SIDE-EFFECTS

In terms of adverse effects caused by topiramate, children do not seem to differ substantially from adults. The effects on the central nervous system are dominated not by sedation, but by cognitive impairment. The effect on cognition is characterized mostly by psychomotor slowing, impaired concentration, confusion and language

Table 22A.1 *Recommended initial dosage schedule for lamotrigine in children*

	Weeks 1–2	Weeks 3–4	Maintenance
>12 years			
With valproic acid	25 mg QOD	25 mg QD	100–200 mg per day
Monotherapy	25 mg QD	25 mg BID	100–400 mg per day
With inducing AEDs	50 mg QD	50 mg BID	300–500 mg per day
2–12 years			
With valproic acid	0.15 mg/kg per day	0.3 mg/kg per day	1–5 mg/kg per day
Monotherapy	0.4 mg/kg per day	0.8 mg/kg per day	2–8 mg/kg per day
With inducing AEDs	0.6 mg/kg per day	1.2 mg/kg per day	5–15 mg/kg per day

BID, twice daily; QD, daily; QOD, every other day.

difficulties.[107,108] The cognitive effects are not necessarily related to dose or titration, seem to affect certain patients and not others, and may represent the most common reason to discontinue topiramate.[107] Other side-effects of topiramate may include anorexia, weight loss, paresthesias, nephrolithiasis and metabolic acidosis.[109–111] Hypohidrosis, or decreased ability to sweat, is a rare side-effect of topiramate which can lead to heat and exercise intolerance.[112] Recently, acute-angle glaucoma has been reported to physicians by the company that is marketing topiramate. One needs to look particularly for eye pain and redness of the eyes.

PHARMACOKINETICS, INTERACTIONS, DOSAGE

The pharmacokinetics of topiramate have been studied in children and, compared to adult values, topiramate clearance was found to be 50 per cent higher in children 7–17 years old[113] and 100 per cent higher in infants.[114] Although topiramate does not significantly affect the pharmacokinetics of other AEDs, enzyme-inducing drugs increase its clearance by a factor of about 2.[115] In children, the recommended initial titration for topiramate is 0.5 to 1.0 mg/kg per day, followed by weekly increases by 0.5 to 1.0 mg/kg per day up to a target dose of 4–6 mg/kg per day. Topiramate doses of 20 to 30 mg/kg per day have been effective and well tolerated in some young children.

Felbamate

EFFICACY

Felbamate was first released in North America in 1993, as the first new AED in 15 years. It has been shown to be effective against focal-onset seizures.[116] Felbamate was the first drug to be tested in a placebo-controlled trial in children with the Lennox-Gastaut syndrome.[117] It was significantly superior to placebo, particularly against the astatic seizures. Uncontrolled observations have suggested that felbamate may be effective against absence seizures,[118] infantile spasms[119–121] and acquired epileptic aphasia.[122]

SIDE-EFFECTS

Initially, the commonly recognized side-effects of felbamate were nausea, vomiting, anorexia, weight loss and insomnia. Unfortunately, during the first year of marketing, unacceptable numbers of patients treated with felbamate developed aplastic anemia[123] or hepatic failure.[124] This has markedly reduced the use of felbamate. Aplastic anemia seems to be less likely to occur in children. The youngest reported case was 13 years old, and the outcome was not fatal. Currently, the main indication for felbamate is in children with Lennox-Gastaut syndrome who have failed to respond to several other medications.

DOSAGE

The recommended initial dosage of felbamate in children is 15 mg/kg per day for 1 week. If tolerated, the dose can be increased to 30 mg/kg per day during the second week, and to 45 mg/kg per day during the third week. Frequent monitoring of the complete blood count and the liver enzymes is mandatory.

Gabapentin

EFFICACY

The clinical efficacy of gabapentin in the treatment of focal-onset seizures has been demonstrated in five placebo-controlled add-on trials[125] and one monotherapy trial[126] in adults, and one placebo-controlled add-on trial in children.[127] However, two double-blind, placebo-controlled studies in absence epilepsy demonstrated no efficacy of gabapentin.[128] In a double-blind, placebo-controlled study of benign epilepsy of childhood with centrotemporal spikes, 220 children were enrolled and received either gabapentin (30 mg/kg per day) or placebo.[129] The difference between gabapentin and placebo approached statistical significance in the intent-to-treat analysis ($p = 0.085$), and was statistically significant when the analysis was limited to evaluable patients ($n = 208$; $p = 0.0254$).

SIDE-EFFECTS

Somnolence, dizziness, ataxia and fatigue were the most common side-effects. Increased appetite and excessive weight gain may occur. Significant behavioral problems may occur in children.[130] Serious side-effects seem to be exceedingly rare.[131]

PHARMACOKINETICS, INTERACTIONS, DOSAGE

Gabapentin has pharmacokinetic properties that are clinically desirable: being entirely eliminated by the kidneys, and not bound to plasma proteins, it is neither the cause nor the object of pharmacokinetic interactions. Absolute bioavailability is saturable and is lower with higher single doses. The initial target dose of gabapentin in children is 30 mg/kg per day and it can be achieved within a few days. In order to achieve the maximal benefit from gabapentin, doses of 50–100 mg/kg per day may be necessary and well tolerated. There is no need to monitor serum levels of gabapentin; no therapeutic range has been recommended.

Vigabatrin

EFFICACY

Vigabatrin, or γ-vinylGABA, appears to be mainly effective against focal-onset seizures and infantile spasms. Controlled studies in adults have clearly demonstrated that vigabatrin reduces the frequency of complex partial seizures,[132,133] with little benefit against other seizure types.[132] Experience in children has been the subject of two reviews.[134,135] The best results were achieved against partial seizures.[136] The focus of interest for the use of vigabatrin in pediatric epilepsy has shifted toward infantile spasms. An add-on study was carried out in a total of 70 patients with infantile spasms.[137] A seizure reduction of at least 50 per cent was seen in 68 per cent of the patients, and 43 per cent became seizure free. Vigabatrin appeared to be particularly effective in patients with tuberous sclerosis. Vigabatrin was later shown to be significantly more effective than hydrocortisone in infantile spasms due to tuberous sclerosis.[138] Several other studies have documented the efficacy of vigabatrin as a first drug in the treatment of infantile spasms, particularly among those with structural brain anomalies and tuberous sclerosis.[139–143]

SIDE-EFFECTS

Initially, the main recognized side-effects of vigabatrin were sedation, agitation, insomnia, depression and weight gain. However, the use of vigabatrin has been later seriously limited by the relatively frequent occurrence of irreversible visual field constriction.[144] Most patients are subjectively asymptomatic. This effect has also been documented in children.[145,146] Vigabatrin may at times exacerbate seizures, predominantly among patients with nonprogressive myoclonic epilepsy and the Lennox-Gastaut syndrome.[147] Vigabatrin was also found to exacerbate absence seizures[148] and seizures in patients with Angelman syndrome.[149]

DOSAGE

The recommended dose of vigabatrin in children is usually 40–85 mg/kg per day, but higher doses have been used and well tolerated. Doses of 100–200 mg/kg per day may be necessary in infants treated for infantile spasms. Vigabatrin is not involved in any pharmacokinetic interaction.

Tiagabine

EFFICACY

So far, the published evidence suggests that the spectrum of efficacy of tiagabine is limited to seizures of focal onset. This efficacy has been demonstrated in several controlled trials in adults.[150,151] Significant efficacy, compared to placebo, was demonstrated mostly at doses of 32 mg/day and above. A single-blind add-on study was carried out in 52 children with various forms of epilepsy.[152] The median seizure reduction was 33 per cent at 4 months in patients with localization-related epilepsy, and 0 per cent in those with generalized epilepsy.

SIDE-EFFECTS

The side-effects of tiagabine are mostly dose-related central nervous system effects, such as dizziness, fatigue, somnolence, headache, tremor, difficulty in concentrating and depressed mood. There is no evidence of systemic or serious side-effects.[153] At least five cases of nonconvulsive status epilepticus have been attributed to tiagabine.[154,155] However, an epidemiological comparison led to the conclusion that tiagabine in recommended doses does not increase the risk of status epilepticus in patients with partial seizures.[156]

PHARMACOKINETICS, INTERACTIONS, DOSAGE

Tiagabine does not seem to affect the levels of other AEDs, but the enzymatic inducers carbamazepine, phenytoin and phenobarbital markedly shorten its elimination half-life. The half-life of tiagabine was found to be 3.2 h and 5.7 h in induced and uninduced children, respectively.[157] Despite its short half-life, tiagabine was found to be equally effective when given twice daily or three times daily, although it may be better tolerated when given three times daily.[158] A suggested titration schedule for tiagabine in children is to introduce the drug at an initial dose of 0.1 mg/kg per day for the first week. The dose can be increased by 0.1 mg/kg per day at intervals of 1–2 weeks up to a target dose of 0.5–1.0 mg/kg per day.

Zonisamide

EFFICACY

Several studies have established the efficacy of zonisamide against focal-onset seizures in adults[159–161] and in children.[162] In addition, there have also been reports suggesting successful treatment with zonisamide in patients with various generalized seizures, such as generalized tonic-clonic seizures, absences, and infantile spasms,[162–164] as well as in early infantile epileptic encephalopathy.[165] Zonisamide appears to have a specific indication in the treatment of progressive myoclonic epilepsy such as Unverricht-Lundborg disease[166,167] and Lafora disease.[168]

SIDE-EFFECTS

Among the side-effects of zonisamide, somnolence, ataxia and anorexia seem to be the most common.[159,160] Psychotic reactions have also been observed.[169] Allergic reactions can also occur. Zonisamide is a sulfonamide, and patients with a history of an allergic reaction to a sulfonamide should not be prescribed zonisamide. Nephrolithiasis can be associated with zonisamide treatment, and seems to occur more frequently in the USA and in Europe than in Japan.[170,171] Like topiramate, zonisamide can also cause oligohidrosis.[172,173]

PHARMACOKINETICS, INTERACTIONS, DOSAGE

The pharmacokinetics of zonisamide have been determined in adults.[174] Its relatively long half-life of 50–70 h is reduced by about 50 per cent by enzyme-inducing drugs.[175] Inversely, lamotrigine seems to inhibit the elimination of zonisamide.[176] The recommended initial titration of zonisamide in children is 1–2 mg/kg per day, to be increased by 1–2 mg/kg per day at intervals of 1–2 weeks, to a target dose of 4–8 mg/kg per day and a maximum of 12 mg/kg per day.

Levetiracetam

EFFICACY

At this time, published evidence regarding the efficacy of levetiracetam in double-blind studies is limited to focal-onset seizures in adults.[177–179] Levetiracetam appears to have good long-term efficacy, and to be well tolerated.[180] Efficacy of levetiracetam in children with focal-onset seizures and in patients with generalized epilepsy is being studied. In open-label trials, adult patients with chronic cortical myoclonus were successfully treated with levetiracetam.[181,182]

SIDE-EFFECTS

Overall, levetiracetam appears to be safe and well tolerated, without systemic or serious toxicity.[183] The most common side-effects are somnolence, asthenia and dizziness. Increasingly, behavioral problems are being recognized in association with levetiracetam, especially in children.[184,185] In four children with epilepsy, reversible psychosis with visual and auditory hallucinations, or persecutory delusions, developed after the introduction of levetiracetam.[186]

PHARMACOKINETICS, INTERACTIONS, DOSAGE

The pharmacokinetics of levetiracetam have been studied in 24 children, 6–12 years old.[187] The elimination half-life was 6.0 h, and the apparent body clearance was 30–40 per cent higher than in adults. An initial daily dose of 10 mg/kg can be prescribed in children. This dose can be increased by 10–20 mg/kg per day at intervals of 1–2 weeks, up to 40–60 mg/kg per day.

ADRENOCORTICOTROPIC HORMONE AND STEROIDS

Adrenocorticotropic hormone (ACTH) has established itself as a treatment of choice for infantile spasms with hypsarrhythmia. When effective, it not only controls the infantile spasms, but it also normalizes the EEG. Less commonly, ACTH is used in children with refractory epilepsies such as Lennox-Gastaut syndrome, and in the Landau-Kleffner syndrome. The indications for steroids in the treatment of epilepsy are the same as for ACTH. There are ongoing controversies as to whether ACTH is superior to steroids; whether ACTH should be used as soon as a diagnosis of West syndrome is made; and what represents the optimal dose and treatment duration with ACTH. In general, one half to two thirds of patients with infantile spasms will benefit significantly from either ACTH or steroid therapy. In a double-blind study, patients were randomized to prednisone or ACTH, with a corresponding oral or intramuscular placebo.[188] No difference in efficacy was found between ACTH and steroids. The success rate was not related to the duration of the epilepsy before the onset of treatment. In contrast, Lombroso[189] concluded that the long-term outcome was better with ACTH than with prednisone in patients with cryptogenic infantile spasms. In this, as well as in another report,[190] better results were obtained when ACTH therapy was initiated within the first month following the onset of spasms. Various initial doses and rates of tapering have been recommended. The initial daily dose usually lies between 110[189] and 150[191–192] U/m² body surface. Good results were recently reported with much lower doses of 4–26 U/m² per day.[193]

The initial dose of ACTH is given intramuscularly in two divided doses for 1–3 weeks. The dose is then reduced gradually and the total duration of treatment may vary from 3 weeks to 3 months. Therapy with ACTH is best started in the hospital. This will allow monitoring of blood glucose and blood pressure carefully, as well as teaching the parents to inject ACTH and to check for glycosuria. After discharge, blood pressure should be measured first daily, then every 2–3 days. Glycosuria and occult blood in stool should also be monitored. Steroids and ACTH are by no means harmless. A serious infection is the main concern, in addition to hypertension, hyperglycemia with glucosuria, and congestive heart failure.

Vitamin B6

The use of vitamin B_6, or pyridoxine, in the treatment of epilepsy has not been limited to cases of pyridoxine deficiency or dependency. The link between pyridoxine and epilepsy is most likely based on the fact that pyridoxine is an essential part of a coenzyme responsible for the synthesis of the inhibitory neurotransmitter GABA. Pyridoxine dependency, an autosomal recessive inborn error of metabolism, does not have characteristic clinical features and it should be considered in any child with cryptogenic refractory seizures up to the age of 2 years, including those with infantile spasms.[194] Most commonly, pyridoxine dependency presents with intractable seizures during the neonatal period. The diagnosis can be established by administering 50–100 mg of pyridoxine intravenously during a flurry of seizures, if possible while recording the EEG. If there is a good response within minutes to hours, this should be followed by an oral maintenance dose of 50–100 mg/day. The use of very high doses of pyridoxine (200–400 mg/kg per day) in patients with infantile spasms has been advocated.[195] Five responded within 2 weeks and were seizure free within 4 weeks. Besides gastrointestinal side-effects, which improved with dosage reduction, there were no serious adverse reactions. Considering the potentially serious side-effects of ACTH, steroids and valproic acid in this age group, pyridoxine is an attractive alternative. In a group of 18 patients, pyridoxine at lower doses (40–50 mg/kg per day) was combined with low doses of ACTH (0.4 U/kg per day). The success rate was similar to that achieved with high doses of ACTH.[196]

DRUG CHOICE AND TREATMENT PARADIGMS

The optimal choice of the first drug in a child with newly diagnosed epilepsy will be based on the seizure type or the syndrome diagnosis. In addition, adverse effects will be taken into consideration, in conjunction with the patient's age and gender. Drugs of first choice for different syndromes and seizure types are listed in Table 22A.2. The selected initial drug is almost invariably prescribed in monotherapy. According to the drug's specific titration schedule, the dose is increased progressively as long as the seizures still occur, and as long as the drug is tolerated. Unless an idiosyncratic reaction occurs at a relatively low dose, failure of the medication can be established with certainty only if the maximal tolerated (i.e. subtoxic) dose

has been achieved. The appropriate duration of treatment with a given drug at the usual therapeutic doses may vary as a function of the seizure frequency. In patients with frequent seizures, it may not take a long time to conclude that the drug is ineffective, whereas patients with occasional or irregular seizure occurrence may require a longer exposure to the drug before that conclusion is reached.

A certain proportion of patients will not become seizure free with the first medication. This may vary from as little as 20 per cent in benign idiopathic epilepsy syndromes, to almost 100 per cent in severe epilepsies. In those patients, the first monotherapy is usually replaced in an overlapping fashion by a second drug in monotherapy. There is now a much larger choice of drugs, and they are listed as drugs of second and third choices in Table 22A.2. These choices are not firmly established, and not supported by comparative trials of efficacy. Experience with the individual drugs and with their side-effects will often influence the choice. The proposed sequence may have to be reassessed periodically on the basis of new evidence. The third therapeutic step may be either a third drug in monotherapy or a combination of two drugs. Depending on the seizure type and the underlying cause of the epilepsy, alternative treatments such as epilepsy surgery or the vagus nerve stimulator may be considered long before all the drugs listed in Table 22A.2 are tried. In focal epilepsies, it is now common practice to consider the possibility of epilepsy surgery after two or three appropriate drugs have failed despite adequate trials.

MONITORING OF AED THERAPY

The therapeutic range of AED plasma levels is a useful guideline but, in many instances, clinical observation of efficacy and side-effects is more valuable. Applying the suggested therapeutic range of a drug rigidly may actually limit the potential benefit derived from the drug. Measurements of plasma levels are available for most AEDs, including many of the newer drugs. However, drug levels are ordered less frequently with the newer AEDs, not only because their therapeutic ranges have not been established, but also because the value of determining levels in general has been critically reassessed. There are valid indications for levels, especially if they can potentially answer a specific clinical question, such as whether the patient is compliant with medication intake; whether high therapeutic levels have been reached in a patient whose seizures are not controlled; whether pharmacokinetic interactions require dosage adjustments; whether possible side-effects can be attributed to one of the two or three drugs that a patient may be taking; and whether a patient's liver disease, kidney disease or pregnancy alter the drug's level. Also, once a

Table 22A.2 *Drug choice by epileptic seizures and syndromes in children*

Partial seizures with or without secondary generalization

First choice:	Carbamazepine/oxcarbazepine
Second choice:	Gabapentin, lamotrigine, topiramate, valproic acid
Third choice:	Levetiracetam, tiagabine, zonisamide, phenytoin, phenobarbital
Consider:	Benzodiazepine, primidone, acetazolamide, vigabatrin, felbamate

Generalized tonic-clonic seizures

First choice:	Valproic acid, carbamazepine, phenytoin
Second choice:	Topiramate, lamotrigine
Third choice:	Phenobarbital, primidone

Absence seizures

Before age 10 years:

First choice:	Ethosuximide (if no convulsions), valproic acid
Second choice:	Lamotrigine
Third choice:	Topiramate, methsuximide, acetazolamide, benzodiazepine

After 10 years:

First choice:	Valproic acid
Second choice:	Lamotrigine
Third choice:	Ethosuximide, topiramate, zonisamide, methsuximide, acetazolamide, benzodiazepine

Juvenile myoclonic epilepsy

First choice:	Valproic acid
Second choice:	Lamotrigine, topiramate, clonazepam
Third choice:	Phenobarbital, primidone, levetiracetam, zonisamide

Lennox–Gastaut and related syndromes

First choice:	Valproic acid
Second choice:	Topiramate, lamotrigine
Third choice:	Ketogenic diet, benzodiazepine, phenobarbital, felbamate
Consider:	Ethosuximide, methsuximide, levetiracetam, zonisamide, VNS, ACTH or steroids

Infantile spasms

First choice:	ACTH, vigabatrin
Second choice:	Valproic acid, topiramate
Third choice:	Lamotrigine, tiagabine, benzodiazepine
Consider:	Pyridoxine, zonisamide

Benign epilepsy with centrotemporal spikes

First choice:	Sulthiame, gabapentin, valproic acid
Second choice:	Carbamazepine
Third choice:	Lamotrigine, topiramate, phenobarbital

patient is well stabilized and seizure free after titration of the medication, it may be appropriate to measure a blood level as a baseline for future reference.

In addition to drug levels, monitoring of AED therapy may include additional monitoring of other laboratory parameters, in particular complete blood count (CBC) and liver enzymes. These tests may be helpful to identify certain alterations such as thrombocytopenia, leukopenia, or progressive elevation of liver enzyme values. However, routine periodic determination of liver enzymes and CBC is unlikely to identify early stages of serious reactions such as severe liver disease or bone marrow toxicity.[197] A high index of suspicion based on monitoring for early clinical evidence of severe reactions is probably more reliable. Precise instructions should be given to patients and parents regarding the symptoms to be monitored, and appropriate tests should be ordered in case of clinical suspicion. For instance, in patients taking valproic acid who experience vomiting and abdominal pain, amylase and lipase should be determined in addition to liver enzymes, because of the possibility of pancreatitis. Other examples are the determination of serum sodium levels in patients on oxcarbazepine who have mental status changes or increased seizures, or looking for microscopic hematuria in patients who take topiramate or zonisamide and experience flank pain suggestive of a kidney stone. Baseline CBC and determination of liver enzymes before introduction of a drug may serve as a baseline for future reference and as a screening for patients with preexisting abnormalities. Institutionalized patients with multiple caregivers should have routine blood monitoring on an annual basis. These patients, especially if they are on enzyme-inducing drugs, are at risk for a vitamin D-deficient state and should receive vitamin D supplements. Recommendations regarding folic acid supplementation in female patients of childbearing age taking valproic acid have been outlined in the section on valproic acid. Finally, routine monitoring of CBC and liver enzyme is important in patients taking felbamate.

KEY POINTS

Phenobarbital

- **Spectrum of efficacy:** generalized tonic-clonic seizures; simple and complex partial seizures without or with generalization; generalized convulsive and simple or complex partial status epilepticus; juvenile myoclonic epilepsy; neonatal seizures; prophylaxis of febrile seizures
- **Possible side-effects:** sedation and drowsiness, hyperactivity, aggressiveness, irritability, allergic rashes and hypersensitivity reactions, osteoporosis in immobilized children due to accelerated vitamin D metabolism, vitamin K-deficient hemorrhagic disease in neonates
- **Dosage:** Titration: not necessary. Maintenance dose: 2–8 mg/kg per day

Phenytoin

- **Spectrum of efficacy:** generalized tonic-clonic seizures, simple and complex partial seizures without or with generalization, generalized convulsive status epilepticus, simple or complex partial status epilepticus, and neonatal seizures
- **Possible side-effects:** nystagmus, ataxia, gingival hyperplasia, hypertrichosis or hirsutism, allergic reactions, hypersensitivity syndrome, pseudolymphoma, polyneuropathy
- **Dosage:** Titration: not necessary. Maintenance dose: 5–8 mg/kg per day, higher in infants

Carbamazepine and oxcarbazepine

- **Spectrum of efficacy:** simple and complex partial seizures, primarily or secondarily generalized tonic-clonic seizures
- **Possible side-effects:** allergic rash, leukopenia, hyponatremia, dizziness, diplopia, ataxia, and vomiting
- **Dosage:** Titration: 5–10 mg/kg per day, increased by 5–10 mg/kg per day at weekly intervals. Maintenance dose: 30 mg/kg per day not unusual in children, especially in combination therapy.

Valproic acid

- **Spectrum of efficacy:** simple and complex partial seizures, primarily or secondarily generalized tonic-clonic seizures, absences, myoclonic seizures, juvenile myoclonic epilepsy, Lennox-Gastaut syndrome, infantile spasms, progressive myoclonic epilepsy, febrile seizures, neonatal seizures
- **Possible side-effects:** tremor, drowsiness and lethargy, encephalopathy, nausea, vomiting, anorexia, increased appetite and excessive weight gain, potentially fatal hepatotoxicity, pancreatitis, thrombocytopenia, increased hair loss, facial or limb edema, noctural enuresis, menstrual irregularities, polycystic ovaries, neural tube defect in the newborn
- **Dosage:** Titration: 10–15 mg/kg per day, increased by 5–10 mg/kg per day at weekly intervals. Maintenance dose: 20–60 mg/kg per day

Ethosuximide

- **Spectrum of efficacy:** absence seizures
- **Possible side-effects:** upset stomach, hiccups
- **Dosage:** Titration: 10 mg/kg per day, increased by 10 mg/kg per day at weekly intervals. Maintenance dose: 30–40 mg/kg per day

Lamotrigine

- **Spectrum of efficacy:** simple and complex partial seizures, without or with secondary generalization, absences, generalized tonic-clonic seizures, myoclonic seizures, Lennox-Gastaut syndrome, possibly infantile spasms
- **Possible side-effects:** rash that may evolve into Stevens-Johnson syndrome, somnolence, dizziness, headache, diplopia, nausea and vomiting, insomnia, tics or tourettism
- **Dosage:** Slow titration is mandatory and rate depends on other AEDs administered (see Table 22A.1)

Topiramate

- **Spectrum of efficacy:** simple and complex partial seizures, with or without secondary generalization, generalized tonic-clonic seizures, Lennox-Gastaut syndrome, juvenile myoclonic epilepsy, infantile spasms
- **Possible side-effects:** cognitive impairment, anorexia, weight loss, paresthesias, nephrolithiasis, metabolic acidosis, hypohidrosis, acute-angle glaucoma
- **Dosage:** Titration: 0.5–1.0 mg/kg per day, followed by weekly increases by 0.5–1.0 mg/kg per day up to a target dose of 4–6 mg/kg per day. Maintenance dose: up to 30 mg/kg per day

Felbamate

- **Spectrum of efficacy:** simple and complex partial seizures, without or with secondary generalization, Lennox-Gastaut syndrome, absences, juvenile myoclonic epilepsy, infantile spasms
- **Possible side-effects:** nausea, vomiting, anorexia, weight loss, insomnia, aplastic anemia, hepatic failure
- **Dosage:** Titration: 15 mg/kg per day, increased to 30 mg/kg per day during the second week, and to 45 mg/kg per day. Maintenance dose: 45–60 mg/kg per day

Gabapentin

- **Spectrum of efficacy:** simple and complex partial seizures, without or with secondary generalization, rolandic epilepsy
- **Possible side-effects:** somnolence, dizziness, ataxia, and fatigue, increased appetite and excessive weight gain, behavioral problems

- **Dosage:** Titration: 10 mg/kg per day, increased by 10 mg/kg per day at intervals of 3 days to initial target dose of 30 mg/kg per day. Maintenance dose: 50–100 mg/kg per day

Vigabatrin

- **Spectrum of efficacy:** simple and complex partial seizures, without or with secondary generalization, generalized tonic-clonic seizures, infantile spasms
- **Possible side-effects:** sedation, agitation, insomnia, depression, weight gain, irreversible visual field constriction
- **Dosage:** 40–200 mg/kg per day

Tiagabine

- **Spectrum of efficacy:** simple and complex partial seizures, without or with secondary generalization, and possibly infantile spasms
- **Possible side-effects:** dizziness, fatigue, somnolence, headache, tremor, difficulty concentrating, depressed mood
- **Dosage:** Titration: 0.1 mg/kg per day for the first week, increased by 0.1 mg/kg per day at intervals of 1–2 weeks up to a target dose of 0.5–1.0 mg/kg per day

Zonisamide

- **Spectrum of efficacy:** partial seizures without or with secondary generalization, generalized tonic-clonic seizures, progressive myoclonic epilepsy, absence seizures, infantile spasms, Lennox-Gastaut syndrome
- **Possible side-effects:** somnolence, ataxia, anorexia, psychotic reactions, allergic rash, nephrolithiasis, oligohidrosis
- **Dosage:** Titration: 1–2 mg/kg per day, to be increased by 1–2 mg/kg per day at intervals of 1–2 weeks, to a target dose of 4–8 mg/kg per day and a maximum of 12 mg/kg per day

Levetiracetam

- **Spectrum of efficacy:** partial seizures, simple and complex, without or with secondary generalization
- **Possible side-effects:** somnolence, asthenia, dizziness, behavioral problems, psychosis
- **Dosage:** Titration: 10 mg/kg per day, increased by 10–20 mg/kg per day at intervals of 1–2 weeks, up to 40–60 mg/kg per day

REFERENCES

1. Mitchell W, Chavez J. Carbamazepine versus phenobarbital for partial onset seizures in children. *Epilepsia* 1987; **28**: 56–60.
2. Mattson R, Cramer JA, Collins JF, *et al.* Comparison of carbamazepine, phenobarbital, phenytoin and primidone in partial and secondarily generalized tonic-clonic seizures. *New England Journal of Medicine* 1985; **313**: 145–151.
3. Shaner MD, McCurdy S, Herring M, Gabor A. Treatment of status epilepticus: a prospective comparison of diazepam and phenytoin versus phenobarbital and optional phenytoin. *Neurology* 1988; **38**: 202–207.
4. Crawford TO, Mitchell WG, Fishman LS, Snodgrass SR. Very high-dose phenobarbital for refractory status epilepticus in children. *Neurology* 1988; **38**: 1035–1040.
5. Gal P, Toback J, Boer H, Erkan N, Wells T. Efficacy of phenobarbital monotherapy in treatment of neonatal seizures – relationship to blood levels. *Neurology* 1982; **32**: 1401–1404.
6. Painter MJ, Scher MS, Stein AD, *et al.* Phenobarbital compared with phenytoin for the treatment of neonatal seizures. *New England Journal of Medicine* 1999; **341**: 485–489.
7. Wolf S, Forsythe A. Behavior disturbance, phenobarbital and febrile seizures. *Pediatrics* 1978; **61**: 728–731.
8. Farwell JR, Lee YJ, Hirtz DG, *et al.* Phenobarbital for febrile seizures – effects on intelligence and on seizure recurrence. *New England Journal of Medicine* 1990; **322**: 364–369.
9. Pitlick W, Painter M, Pippenger C. Phenobarbital pharmacokinetics in neonates. *Clinical Pharmacology and Therapeutics* 1978; **23**: 346–350.
10. Gal P, Toback J, Erkan N, Boer H, Henry R. The influence of asphyxia on phenobarbital dosing requirements in neonates. *Developments in Pharmacological Therapy* 1984; **7**: 145–152.
11. Heimann G, Gladtke E. Pharmacokinetics of phenobarbital in childhood. *European Journal of Clinical Pharmacology* 1977; **12**: 305–310.
12. Bourgeois BFD, Dodson WE, Ferrendelli JA. Primidone, phenobarbital and PEMA: I. Seizure protection, neurotoxicity and therapeutic index of individual compounds in mice. *Neurology* 1983; **33**: 283–290.
13. Bourgeois BFD, Dodson WE, Ferrendelli JA. Primidone, phenobarbital and PEMA: II. Seizure protection, neurotoxicity and therapeutic index of varying combinations in mice. *Neurology* 1983; **33**: 291–295.
14. Oleson OV, Dam M. The metabolic conversion of primidone to phenobarbitone in patients under long-term treatment. *Acta Neurologica Scandinavica* 1967; **43**: 348–356.
15. Oxley J, Hebdige S, Laidlaw J, Wadsworth J, Richens A. A comparative study of phenobarbitone and primidone in the treatment of epilepsy. In: Johannessen SI, Morselli PL, Pipenger CE, *et al.* (eds) *Antiepileptic Therapy. Advances in Drug Monitoring.* New York: Raven Press; 1980: 237–245.
16. Powell C, Painter MJ, Pippinger CC. Primidone therapy in refractory neonatal seizures. *Journal of Pediatrics* 1984; **105**: 651–654.
17. Sapin J, Riviello J, Grover W. Efficacy of primidone for seizure control in neonates and young infants. *Pediatric Neurology* 1988; **4**: 292–295.
18. Herranz JL, Armijo JA, Artega R. Clinical side effects of phenobarbital, primidone, phenytoin, carbamazepine, and

valproate during monotherapy in children. *Epilepsia* 1988; **29**: 794–804.

19. Painter MJ, Pippinger C, Wasterlain C, *et al.* Phenobarbital and phenytoin in neonatal seizures: metabolism and tissue distribution. *Neurology* 1981; **31**: 1107–1112.

20. Dodson WE. Phenytoin elimination in childhood: effect of concentration dependent kinetics. *Neurology* 1980; **30**: 196–199.

21. Bourgeois BFD, Dodson WE. Phenytoin elimination in newborns. *Neurology* 1983; **33**: 173–178.

22. Dodson WE. The nonlinear kinetics of phenytoin in children. *Neurology* 1982; **32**: 42–48.

23. Mattson RH, Cramer JA, Collins JF, Dept. of VA Epilepsy Cooperative Study No. 264 Group. A comparison of valproate with carbamazepine for the treatment of complex partial seizures and secondarily generalized tonic-clonic seizures in adults. *New England Journal of Medicine* 1992; **327**: 765–771.

24. Verity CM, Hosking G, Easter DJ. A multicentre comparative trial of sodium valproate and carbamazepine in pediatric epilepsy. The Paediatric EPITEG Collaborative Group. *Developmental Medicine and Child Neurology* 1995; **37**: 97–108.

25. Snead OC, Hosey LC. Exacerbation of seizures in children by carbamazepine. *New England Journal of Medicine* 1985; **313**: 916–921.

26. Glauser TA, Nigro M, Sachdeo R, *et al.* Adjunctive therapy with oxcarbazepine in children with partial seizures. The Oxcarbazepine Pediatric Study Group. *Neurology* 2000; **54**: 2237–2244.

27. Isojärvi JIT, Huuskonen UEJ, Pakarinen AJ, Vuolteenaho O, Myllylä V V. The regulation of serum sodium after replacing carbamazepine with oxcarbazepine. *Epilepsia* 2001; **42**: 741–745.

28. Braathen G, Theorell K, Persson A, Rane A. Valproate in the treatment of absence epilepsy in children. *Epilepsia* 1988; **29**: 548–552.

29. Callaghan N, O'Hare J, O'Driscoll D, O'Neill B, Dally M. Comparative study of ethosuximide and sodium valproate in the treatment of typical absence seizures (petit mal). *Developmental Medicine and Child Neurology* 1982; **24**: 830–836.

30. Sato S, White BG, Penry JK, *et al.* Valproic acid versus ethosuximide in the treatment of absence seizures. *Neurology* 1982; **32**: 157–163.

31. Ramsay RE, Wilder BJ, Murphy JV, *et al.* Efficacy and safety of valproic acid versus phenytoin as sole therapy for newly diagnosed primary generalized tonic-clonic seizures. *Journal of Epilepsy* 1992; **5**: 55–60.

32. Iivanainen M, Himberg JJ. Valproate and clonazepam in the treatment of severe progressive myoclonus epilepsy. *Archives of Neurology* 1982; **39**: 236–238.

33. Siemes H, Spohr HL, Michael T, Nau H. Therapy of infantile spasms with valproate: results of a prospective study. *Epilepsia* 1988; **29**: 553–560.

34. deSilva M, MacArdle B, McGowan M, *et al.* Randomised comparative monotherapy trial of phenobarbitone, phenytoin, carbamazepine, or sodium valproate for newly diagnosed childhood epilepsy. *Lancet* 1996; **347**: 709–713.

35. Rantala H, Tarkka R, Uhari M. A meta-analytic review of the preventive treatment of recurrences of febrile seizures. *Journal of Pediatrics* 1997; **131**: 922–925.

36. Gal P, Oles KS, Gilman JT, Weaver R. Valproic acid efficacy, toxicity and pharmacokinetics in neonates with intractable seizures. *Neurology* 1988; **38**: 467–471.

37. Marescaux C, Warter JM, Micheletti G, *et al.* Stuporous episodes during treatment with sodium valproate: report of seven cases. *Epilepsia* 1982; **23**: 297–305.

38. Dinesen H, Gram L, Anderson T, Dam M. Weight gain during treatment with valproate. *Acta Neurologica Scandinavica* 1984; **70**: 65–69.

39. Bryant A, Dreifuss FE. Valproic acid hepatic fatalities. III. U.S. experience since 1986. *Neurology* 1996; **46**: 465–469.

40. Asconapé JJ, Penry JK, Dreifuss FE, Riela A, Mirza W. Valproate-associated pancreatitis. *Epilepsia* 1993; **34**: 177–183.

41. Delgado MR, Riela AR, Mills J, Browne R, Roach S. Thrombocytopenia secondary to high valproate levels in children with epilepsy. *Journal of Child Neurology* 1994; **9**: 311–324.

42. Haidukewych D, John G, Zielinski JJ, Rodin EA. Chronic valproic acid therapy in incidence of increases in venous plasma ammonia. *Therapeutic Drug Monitoring* 1985; **7**: 290–294.

43. Ettinger A, Moshe S, Shinnar S. Edema associated with long-term valproate therapy. *Epilepsia* 1990; **31**: 211–213.

44. Choonra IA. Sodium valproate and enuresis. *Lancet* 1985; **1**: 1276.

45. Margraf JW, Dreifuss FE. Amenorrhea following initiation of therapy with valproic acid. *Neurology* 1981; **31**: 159.

46. Isojarvi JI, Laatikainen TJ, Knip M, *et al.* Obesity and endocrine disorders in women taking valproate for epilepsy. *Annals of Neurology* 1996; **39**: 579–584.

47. Luef G, Abraham I, Trinka E, *et al.* Hyperandrogenism, postprandial hyperinsulinism and the risk of PCOS in a cross sectional study of women with epilepsy treated with valproate. *Epilepsy Research* 2002; **48**: 91–102.

48. Lindhout D, Meinardi H. Spina bifida and in utero exposure to valproate. *Lancet* 1984; **2**: 396.

49. Omtzigt JGC, Los FJ, Grobbee DE, *et al.* The risk of spina bifida aperta after first-trimester exposure to valproate in a prenatal cohort. *Neurology* 1992; **42**(Suppl. 5): 119–125.

50. Wegner C, Nau H. Alteration of embryonic folate metabolism by valproic acid during organogenesis. *Neurology* 1992; **42**(Suppl. 5): 17–24.

51. Gugler R, Schell A, Eichelbaum M, Froscher W, Schulz HU. Disposition of valproic acid in man. *European Journal of Clinical Pharmacology* 1977; **12**: 125–132.

52. Perucca E, Gatti G, Frigo GM, *et al.* Disposition of sodium valproate in epileptic patients. *British Journal of Clinical Pharmacology* 1978; **5**: 495–499.

53. Cloyd JC, Fischer JH, Kriel RL, Kraus DM. Valproic acid pharmacokinetics in children. IV. Effects of age and antiepileptic drugs on protein binding and intrinsic clearance. *Clinical Pharmacology and Therapeutics* 1993; **53**: 22–29.

54. Devinsky O, Leppik I, Willmore LJ, *et al.* Safety of intravenous valproate. *Annals of Neurology* 1995; **38**: 670–674.

55. Giroud M, Gras D, Escousse A, Dumas R, Venaud G. Use of injectable valproic acid in status epilepticus: a pilot study. *Drug Investigations* 1993; **5**: 154–159.

56. Wheless J, Venkataraman V. Safety of high intravenous valproate loading doses in epilepsy patients. *Journal of Epilepsy* 1998; **11**: 319–324.

57. Sato S, Dreifuss FE, Penry JK. Prognostic factors in absence seizures. *Neurology* 1976; **26**: 788–796.

58. Rowan AJ, Meijer JWA, de Beer-Pawlikowski N, van der Geest P, Meinardi H. Valproate-ethosuximide combination therapy for refractory absence seizures. *Archives of Neurology* 1983; **32**: 797–802.

59. Snead OC. The neuropharmacology of epileptic falling spells. *Clinical Neuropharmacology* 1987; **10**: 205–214.

60. Snead OC, Hosey LC. Treatment of epileptic falling spells with ethosuximide. *Brain and Development* 1987; **9**: 602–604.

61. Mireles R, Lcppik IE. Valproate and clonazepam comedication in patients with intractable epilepsy. *Epilepsia* 1985; **26**: 122–126.

62. Vassella F, Pavlincova E, Schneider HJ, Rudin HJ, Karbowski K. Treatment of infantile spasms and Lennox-Gastaut syndrome with clonazepam. *Epilepsia* 1973; **14**: 165–175.

63. Obeid T, Panayiotopoulos CP. Clonazepam in juvenile myoclonic epilepsy. *Epilepsia* 1989; **30**: 603–606.

64. Congdon PJ, Forsythe WI. Intravenous clonazepam in the treatment of status epilepticus in children. *Epilepsia* 1980; **21**: 97–102.

65. Bittencourt PRM, Richens A. Anticonvulsant-induced status epilepticus in Lennox-Gastaut syndrome. *Epilepsia* 1981; **22**: 129–134.

66. Andre M, Boutroy MJ, Dubruc C, *et al*. Clonazepam pharma-cokinetics and therapeutic efficacy in neonatal seizures. *European Journal of Clinical Pharmacology* 1986; **30**: 585–589.

67. Sher PK. Alternate-day clonazepam treatment of intractable seizures. *Archives of Neurology* 1985; **42**: 787–788.

68. Dreifuss F, Farwell J, Holmes G, *et al*. Infantile spasms. Comparative trial of nitrazepam and corticotropin. *Archives of Neurology* 1986; **43**: 1107–1110.

69. Wyllie E, Wyllie R, Cruse RP, Rothner AD, Erenberg G. The mechanism of nitrazepam-induced drooling and aspiration. *New England Journal of Medicine* 1986; **314**: 35–38.

70. Murphy JV, Sawaski F, Marquardt KM, Harris DJ. Deaths in young children receiving nitrazepam. *Journal of Pediatrics* 1987; **111**: 145–157.

71. Rintahaka PJ, Nakagawa JA, Shewmon DA, Kyyronen P, Shields WD. Incidence of death in patients with intractable epilepsy during nitrazepam treatment. *Epilepsia* 1999; **40**: 492–496.

72. Robertson MM. Current status of the 1,4- and 1,5-benzo-diazepines in the treatment of epilepsy: the place of clobazam. *Epilepsia* 1986; **27**: S27–41.

73. Allen JW, Oxley J, Robertson M, *et al*. Clobazam as adjunctive treatment in refractory epilepsy. *British Medical Journal* 1983; **286**: 1246–1247.

74. Allen JW, Jawad S, Oxley J, Trimble M. Development of tolerance to anticonvulsant effect of clobazam. *Journal of Neurology, Neurosurgery and Psychiatry* 1985; **48**: 284–285.

75. Dulac O, Figueroa D, Rey E, Arthuis M. Monotherapie par le clobazam dans les epilepsies de l'enfant. *La Presse medicale* 1983; **12**: 1067–1069.

76. Keene DL, Whiting S, Humphreys P. Clobazam as an add-on drug in the treatment of refractory epilepsy in childhood. *Canadian Journal of the Neurological Sciences* 1990; **17**: 317–319.

77. Feely M, Gibson J. Intermittent clobazam for catamenial epilepsy. *Journal of Neurology, Neurosurgery and Psychiatry* 1984; **47**: 1279–1282.

78. Sanders J, Patsalos P, Oxley J, *et al*. A randomized, double-blind, placebo-controlled, add-on trial of lamotrigine in patients with severe epilepsy. *Epilepsy Research* 1990; **6**: 221–226.

79. Messenheimer J, Ramsay R, Willmore L, *et al*. Lamotrigine therapy for partial seizures: a multicenter, placebo-controlled, double-blind, cross-over trial. *Epilepsia* 1994; **35**: 1131–20.

80. Gilliam F, Vazquez B, Sackellares J, *et al*. An active-control trial of lamotrigine monotherapy for partial seizures. *Neurology* 1998; **51**: 1018–1025.

81. Brodie M, Richens A, Yuen A. Double-blind comparison of lamotrigine and carbamazepine in newly diagnosed epilepsy. *Lancet* 1995; **345**: 476–479.

82. Steiner T, Dellaportas C, Findley L, *et al*. Lamotrigine monotherapy in newly diagnosed untreated epilepsy: a double-blind comparison with phenytoin. *Epilepsia* 1999; **40**: 601–607.

83. Wallace SJ. Add-on trial of lamotrigine in resistant childhood seizures. *Brain and Development* 1990; **12**: 734.

84. Besag FMC, Wallace SJ, Dulac O, *et al*. Lamotrigine for the treatment of epilepsy in childhood. *Journal of Pediatrics* 1995; **127**: 991–997.

85. Motte J, Trevathan E, Arvidsson JF, *et al*. Lamotrigine for generalized seizures associated with the Lennox-Gastaut syndrome. *New England Journal of Medicine* 1997; **337**: 1807–1812.

86. Beran R, Berkovic S, Dunagan F, *et al*. Double-blind, placebo-controlled, crossover study of lamotrigine in treatment-resistent generalised epilepsy. *Epilepsia* 1998; **39**: 1329–1333.

87. Frank L, Enlow T, Holmes G *et al*. Lamictal (lamotrigine) monotherapy for typical absence seizures in children. *Epilepsia* 1999; **40**: 973–979.

88. Veggiotti P, Cieuta C, Rey E, *et al*. Lamotrigine in infantile spasms. *Lancet* 1993; **344**: 1375–1376.

89. Timmings P, Richens A. Efficacy of lamotrigine as monotherapy for juvenile myoclonic epilepsy: pilot study results [abstract]. *Epilepsia* 1993; **34**(Suppl. 2): S160.

90. Schlienger R, Knowles S, Shear N. Lamotrigine-associated anticonvulsant hypersensitivity syndrome. *Neurology* 1998; **51**: 1172–1182.

91. Messenheimer J. Efficacy and safety of lamotrigine in pediatric patients. *Journal of Child Neurology* 2002; **17**: 2S34–42.

92. Wong IC, Mawer GE, Sander JW. Factors influencing the incidence of lamotrigine-related skin rash. *Annals of Pharmacotherapy* 1999; **33**: 1037–1042.

93. Tavernor S, Wong I, Newton R, Brown S. Rechallenge with lamotrigine after initial rash. *Seizure* 1995; **4**: 67–71.

94. Lombroso C. Lamotrigine-induced tourettism. *Neurology* 1999; **52**: 1191–1194.

95. Sotero de Menezes MA, Rho JM, Murphy P, Cheyette S. Lamotrigine-induced tic disorder: report of five pediatric cases. *Epilepsia* 2000; **41**: 862–867.

96. Chattergoon D, McGuigan M, Koren G, Hwang P, Ito S. Multiorgan dysfunction and disseminated intravascular coagulation in children receiving lamotrigine and valproic acid. *Neurology* 1997; **49**: 1442–1444.

97. Biraben A, Allain H, Scarabin JM, Schuck S, Edan G. Exacerbation of juvenile myoclonic epilepsy with lamotrigine. *Neurology* 2000; **55**: 1758.

98. Guerrini R, Dravet C, Genton P, *et al*. Lamotrigine and seizure aggravation in severe myoclonic epilepsy. *Epilepsia* 1998; **39**: 508–512.

99. Guerrini R, Belmonte A, Parmeggiani L, Perucca E. Myoclonic
    status epilepticus following high-dosage lamotrigine therapy.
    Brain and Development 1999; **21**: 420–424.
100. Tassinari CA, Michelucci R, Chauvel P, *et al.* Double-blind,
    placebo-controlled trial of topiramate (600 mg daily) for the
    treatment of refractory partial epilepsy. *Epilepsia* 1996; **37**:
    763–768.
101. Ben-Menachem E, Henriksen O, Dam M, *et al.* Double-blind,
    placebo-controlled trial of topiramate as add-on therapy
    in patients with refractory partial seizures. *Epilepsia* 1996;
    37: 539–543.
102. Faught E, Wilder B, Ramsay R, *et al.* Topiramate placebo-
    controlled dose-ranging trial of refractory partial epilepsy
    using 200-, 400- and 600-mg daily doses. *Neurology* 1996;
    46: 1684–1690.
103. Elterman R, Glauser T, Wyllie E, *et al.* A double-blind,
    randomized trial of topiramate as adjunctive therapy for partial-
    onset seizures in children. *Neurology* 1999; **52**: 1338–1344.
104. Biton V, Montouris G, Ritter F, *et al.* A randomized, placebo-
    controlled study of topiramate in primary generalized tonic-
    clonic seizures. *Neurology* 1999; **52**: 1330–1337.
105. Sachdeo R, Glauser T, Ritter F, *et al.* A double-blind,
    randomized trial of topiramate in Lennox-Gastaut syndrome.
    Neurology 1999; **52**: 1882–1887.
106. Glauser T, Clark P, Strawsburg R. A pilot study of topiramate
    in the treatment of infantile spasms. *Epilepsia* 1998; **39**:
    1324–1328.
107. Tatum WO, French JA, Faught E, *et al.* Postmarketing
    experience with topiramate and cognition. *Epilepsia* 2001;
    42: 1134–1140.
108. Martin R, Kuzniecky R, Ho S, *et al.* Cognitive effects of
    topiramate, gabapentin, and lamotrigine in healthy young
    adults. *Neurology* 1999; **52**: 321–327.
109. Shorvon S. Safety of topiramate: adverse events and
    relationships to dosing. *Epilepsia* 1996; **37**(Suppl. 2): S18–22.
110. Wilner A, Raymond K, Pollard R. Topiramate and metabolic
    acidosis. *Epilepsia* 1999; **40**: 792–795.
111. Takeoka M, Holmes GL, Thiele E, *et al.* Topiramate and
    metabolic acidosis in pediatric epilepsy. *Epilepsia* 2001; **42**:
    387–392.
112. Arcas J, Ferrer T, Roche M, Martinez-Bermejo A, Lopez-
    Martin V. Hypohidrosis related to the administration of
    topiramate to children. *Epilepsia* 2001; **42**: 1363–1365.
113. Rosenfeld W, Doose D, Walker S, Baldassarre J, Reife R. An
    open-label, single-center, pharmacokinetic and tolerability
    study of topiramate adjunctive therapy in pediatric patients
    with epilepsy. *Epilepsia* 1995; **36**(Suppl. 3): S158.
114. Glauser T, Miles M, Tang P, Clark P, McGee K, Doose D.
    Topiramate pharmacokinetics in infants. *Epilepsia* 1999;
    40: 788–791.
115. Bourgeois BFD. Drug interaction profile of topiramate.
    Epilepsia 1996; **37**(Suppl. 2): S14–17.
116. Bourgeois BFD, Leppik IE, Sackellares JC, *et al.* Felbamate:
    a double-blind controlled trial in patients undergoing
    presurgical evaluation of partial seizures. *Neurology* 1993;
    43: 693–696.
117. The Felbamate Study Group in Lennox-Gastaut Syndrome.
    Efficacy of felbamate in childhood epileptic encephalopathy
    (Lennox-Gastaut syndrome). *New England Journal of
    Medicine* 1993; **328**: 29–33.
118. Devinsky O, Kothari M, Rubin R, *et al.* Felbamate for absence
    seizures. *Epilepsia* 1992; **33**(Suppl. 3): 84.
119. Hurst D, Rolan T. The use of felbamate to treat infantile
    spasms. *Journal of Child Neurology* 1995; **10**: 134–136.
120. Stafstrom C. The use of felbamate to treat infantile spasms.
    Journal of Child Neurology 1996; **11**: 170–171.
121. Hosain S, Nagarajan L, Carson D, *et al.* Felbamate for
    refractory infantile spasms. *Journal of Child Neurology* 1997;
    12: 466–468.
122. Glauser T, Olberding L, Titanic M, Piccirillo D. Felbamate in
    the treatment of acquired epileptic aphasia. *Epilepsy
    Research* 1995; **20**: 85–89.
123. Kaufman D, Kelly J, Anderson T, Harmon D, Shapiro S.
    Evaluation of case reports of aplastic anemia among patients
    treated with felbamate. *Epilepsia* 1997; **38**: 1265–1269.
124. O'Neil M, Perdun C, Wilson M, McGown S, Patel S.
    Felbamate-associated fatal acute hepatic necrosis. *Neurology*
    1996; **46**: 1457–1459.
125. Leiderman D. Gabapentin as add-on therapy for refractory
    partial epilepsy: results of five placebo-controlled trials.
    Epilepsia 1994; **35**: S74–76.
126. Chadwick D, Anhut H, Greiner M, *et al.* A double-blind trial
    of gabapentin monotherapy for newly diagnosed partial
    seizures. *Neurology* 1998; **51**: 1282–1288.
127. Appleton R, Fichtner K, LaMoreaux L, *et al.* Gabapentin as
    add-on therapy in children with refractory partial seizures:
    a 12-week, multicentre, double-blind, placebo-controlled
    study. Gabapentin Paediatric Study Group. *Epilepsia* 1999;
    40: 1147–1154.
128. Trudeau V, Myers S, LaMoreaux L, *et al.* Gabapentin in naive
    childhood absence epilepsy: results from two double-blind,
    placebo-controlled, multicenter studies. *Journal of Child
    Neurology* 1996; **11**: 470–475.
129. Bourgeois B, Brown L, Pellock J, *et al.* Gabapentin
    (neurontin) monotherapy in children with benign childhood
    epilepsy with centrotemporal spikes (BECTS): a 36-week,
    double-blind, placebo-controlled study. *Epilepsia* 1998;
    39: 163.
130. Wolf S, Shinnar S, Kang H, Gil K, Moshé S. Gabapentin
    toxicity in children manifesting as behavioral changes.
    Epilepsia 1995; **36**: 1203–1205.
131. McLean M, Morrell M, Willmore L, *et al.* Safety and
    tolerability of gabapentin as adjunctive therapy in a large,
    multicenter study. *Epilepsia* 1998; **40**: 965–972.
132. Tassinari CA, Michelucci R, Ambrosetto G, Salvi F. Double-
    blind study of vigabatrin in the treatment of drug-resistant
    epilepsy. *Archives of Neurology* 1987; **44**: 907–910.
133. French JA, Mosier M, Walker S, Sommerville K, Sussman N.
    A double-blind, placebo-controlled study of vigabatrin three
    g/day in patients with uncontrolled complex partial seizures.
    Vigabatrin Protocol 024 Investigative Cohort. *Neurology*
    1996; **46**: 54–61.
134. Gram L, Sabers A, Dulac O. Treatment of pediatric epilepsies
    with γ-vinyl GABA (Vigabatrin). *Epilepsia* 1992; **33**(Suppl. 5):
    26–29.
135. Appleton RE. The role of vigabatrin in the management of
    infantile epileptic syndromes. *Neurology* 1993; **43**: S21–23.
136. Uldall P, Alving J, Gram L, Hogenhaven H. Vigabatrin in
    childhood epilepsy: a 5-year follow-up study. *Neuropediatrics*
    1995; **26**(5): 253–256.

137. Chiron C, Dulac O, Beaumont D, *et al*. Therapeutic trial of vigabatrin in infantile spasms. *Child Neurology* 1991; **6**(Suppl. 2): 2552-2559.

138. Chiron C, Dumas C, Jambaque I, Mumford JP, Dulac O. Randomized trial comparing vigabatrin and hydrocortisone in infantile spasms due to tuberous sclerosis. *Epilepsy Research* 1997; **26**: 389-395.

139. Aicardi J, Mumford J, Dumas C, Wood S. Vigabatrin as initial therapy for infantile spasms: a European retrospective survey. Sabril IS Investigator and Peer Review Groups. *Epilepsia* 1996; **37**: 638-642.

140. Vigevano F, Cilio M. Vigabatrin versus ACTH as first-line treatment for infantile spasms: a randomized, prospective study. *Epilepsia* 1997; **38**: 1270-1274.

141. Appleton RE, Peters AC, Mumford JP, Shaw DE. Randomised, placebo-controlled study of vigabatrin as first-line treatment of infantile spasms. *Epilepsia* 1999; **40**(11): 1627-1633.

142. Granström M, Gaily E, Liukkonen E. Treatment of infantile spasms: Results of a population-based study with vigabatrin as the first drug for spasms. *Epilepsia* 1999; **40**: 950-957.

143. Elterman RD, Shields WD, Mansfield KA, Nakagawa J. Randomized trial of vigabatrin in patients with infantile spasms. Neurology 2001; **57**: 1416-1421.

144. Miller NR, Johnson MA, Paul SR, *et al*. Visual dysfunction in patients receiving vigabatrin: clinical and electrophysiologic findings. *Neurology* 1999; **53**: 2082-2087.

145. Vanhatalo S, Paakkonen L. Visual field constriction in children treated with vigabatrin. *Neurology* 1999; **1**: 1713-1714.

146. Gross-Tsur V, Banin E, Shahar E, Shalev RS, Lahat E. Visual impairment in children with epilepsy treated with vigabatrin. *Annals of Neurology* 2000; **48**: 60-64.

147. Lortie A, Chiron C, Mumford J, Dulac O. The potential for increasing seizure frequency, relapse, and appearance of new seizure types with vigabatrin. *Neurology* 1993; **43**(Suppl. 5): S24-27.

148. Panayiotopoulos CP, Agathonikou A, Ahmed Sharoqi I, Parker APJ. Vigabatrin aggravates absences and absence status. *Neurology* 1997; **49**: 1467.

149. Kuenzle C, Steinlin J, Wohlrab G, Boltshauser E, Schmitt B. Adverse effects of vigabatrin in Angelman syndrome. *Epilepsia* 1998; **39**: 1213-1215.

150. Richens A, Chadwick D, Duncan J, *et al*. Adjunctive treatment of partial seizures with tiagabine: a placebo-controlled trial. *Epilepsy Research* 1995; **21**: 37-42.

151. Kalviainen R, Brodie MJ, Duncan J, *et al*. A double-blind, placebo-controlled trial of tiagabine given three-times daily as add-on therapy for refractory partial seizures. Northern European Tiagabine Study Group. *Epilepsy Research* 1998; **30**: 31-40.

152. Uldall P, Bulteau C, Pedersen SA, Dulac O, Lyby K. Tiagabine adjunctive therapy in children with refractory epilepsy: a single-blind dose escalating study. *Epilepsy Research* 2000; **42**: 159-168.

153. Leppik IE, Gram L, Deaton R, Sommerville KW. Safety of tiagabine: summary of 53 trials. *Epilepsy Research* 1999; **33**: 235-246.

154. Schapel G, Chadwick D. Tiagabine and non-convulsive status epilepticus. *Seizure* 1996; **5**: 153-156.

155. Ettinger AB, Bernal OG, Andriola MR, *et al*. Two cases of nonconvulsive status epilepticus in association with tiagabine therapy. *Epilepsia* 1999; **40**: 1159-1162.

156. Shinnar S, Berg AT, Treiman DM, *et al*. Status epilepticus and tiagabine therapy: review of safety data and epidemiologic comparisons. *Epilepsia* 2001; **42**: 372-379.

157. Gustavson L, Boellner S, Granneman G, *et al*. A single-dose study to define the tiagabine pharmacokinetics in pediatric patients with complex partial seizures. *Neurology* 1997; **48**: 1-6.

158. Biraben A, Beaussart M, Josien E, *et al*. Comparison of twice- and three times daily tiagabine for the adjunctive treatment of partial seizures in refractory patients with epilepsy: an open label, randomized, parallel-group study. *Epileptic Disorders* 2001; **3**: 91-100.

159. Schmidt D, Jacob R, Loiseau P, *et al*. Zonisamide for add-on treatment of refractory partial epilepsy: a European double-blind trial. *Epilepsy Research* 1993; **15**: 67-73.

160. Leppik IE, Willmore LJ, Homan RW, *et al*. Efficacy and safety of zonisamide: results of a multicenter study. *Epilepsy Research* 1993; **14**: 165-173.

161. Faught E, Ayala R, Montouris GG, Leppik IE. Randomized controlled trial of zonisamide for the treatment of refractory partial-onset seizures. *Neurology* 2001; **57**: 1774-1779.

162. Kumagai N, Seki T, Yamawaki H, *et al*. Monotherapy for childhood epilepsies with zonisamide. *Japanese Journal of Psychiatry and Neurology* 1991; **45**: 357-359.

163. Suzuki Y, Nagai T, Ono J, *et al*. Zonisamide monotherapy in newly diagnosed infantile spasms. *Epilepsia* 1997; **38**: 1035-1038.

164. Yanai S, Hanai T, Narazaki O. Treatment of infantile spasms with zonisamide. *Brain and Development* 1999; **21**: 157-161.

165. Ohno M, Shimotsuji Y, Abe J, Shimada M, Tamiya H. Zonisamide treatment of early infantile epileptic encephalopathy. *Pediatric Neurology* 2000; **23**: 341-344.

166. Henry TR, Leppik IE, Gumnit RJ, Jacobs M. Progressive myoclonus epilepsy treated with zonisamide. *Neurology* 1988; **38**: 928-931.

167. Kyllerman M, Ben-Menachem E. Long-term treatment of progressive myoclonic epilepsy syndromes with zonisamide and n-acetylcysteine. *Epilepsia* 1996; **37**(Suppl. 5): 172.

168. Yoshimura I, Kaneko S, Yoshimura N, Murakami T. Long-term observations of two siblings with Lafora disease treated with zonisamide. *Epilepsy Research* 2001; **46**: 283-287.

169. Miyamoto T, Kohsaka M, Koyama T. Psychotic episodes during zonisamide treatment. *Seizure* 2000; **9**: 65-70.

170. Leppik IE. Zonisamide. *Epilepsia* 1999; **40**(Suppl. 5): 23-29.

171. Kubota M, Nishi-Nagase M, Sakakihara Y, *et al*. Zonisamide-induced urinary lithiasis in patients with intractable epilepsy. *Brain and Development* 2000; **22**: 230-233.

172. Shimizu T, Yamashita Y, Satoi M, *et al*. Heat stroke-like episode in a child caused by zonisamide. *Brain and Development* 1997; **19**: 366-368.

173. Okumura A, Ishihara N, Kato T, *et al*. Predictive value of acetylcholine stimulation testing for oligohidrosis caused by zonisamide. *Pediatric Neurology* 2000; **23**: 59-61.

174. Buchanan RA, Bockbrader JN, Chang T, Sedman AJ. Single- and multiple-dose pharmacokinetics of zonisamide. *Epilepsia* 1996; **37**(Suppl. 5): 172.

175. Ojemann LM, Shastri RA, Wilensky AJ, *et al.* Comparative pharmacokinetics of zonisamide (CI-912) in epileptic patients on carbamazepine or phenytoin monotherapy. *Therapeutic Drug Monitoring* 1986; **8**: 293–296.

176. McJilton J, DeToledo J, DeCerce J, *et al.* Cotherapy of lamotrigine/zonisamide results in significant elevation of zonisamide levels. *Epilepsia* 1996; **37**(Suppl. 5): 173.

177. Cereghino JJ, Biton V, Abou-Khalil B, *et al.* Levetiracetam for partial seizures: results of a double-blind, randomized clinical trial. *Neurology* 2000; **55**: 236–242.

178. Ben-Menachem E, Falter, European Levetiracetam Study Group. Efficacy and tolerability of levetiracetam 3000 mg/d in patients with refractory partial seizures: A multicenter, double-blind, responder-selected study evaluating monotherapy. *Epilepsia* 2000; **41**: 1276–1283.

179. Grant R, Shorvon SD. Efficacy and tolerability of 1000–4000 mg per day of levetiracetam as add-on therapy in patients with refractory epilepsy. *Epilepsy Research* 2000; **42**: 89–95.

180. Krakow K, Walker M, Otoul C, Sander JW. Long-term continuation of levetiracetam in patients with refractory epilepsy. *Neurology* 2001; **56**: 1772–1774.

181. Frucht SJ, Louis ED, Chuang C, Fahn S. A pilot tolerability and efficacy study of levetiracetam in patients with chronic myoclonus. *Neurology* 2001; **57**: 1112–1114.

182. Krauss GL, Bergin A, Kramer RE, Cho YW, Reich SG. Suppression of post-hypoxic and post-encephalitic myoclonus with levetiracetam. *Neurology* 2001; **56**: 411–412.

183. French J, Edrich P, Cramer JA. A systematic review of the safety profile of levetiracetam: a new antiepileptic drug. *Epilepsy Research* 2001; **47**: 77–90.

184. Bourgeois BFD, Holder DL, Valencia I, *et al.* Open-label assessment of levetiracetam efficacy and adverse effects in a pediatric population. *Epilepsia* 2001; **42**(Suppl. 7): 53–54.

185. Gustafson MC, Ritter FJ, Frost MD, Karney VL, Hoskin C. Clinical experience with levetiracetam treating refractory, symptomatic seizures in children. *Epilepsia* 2001; **42**(Suppl. 7): 55.

186. Kossoff EH, Bergey GK, Freeman JM, Vining EPG. Levetiracetam psychosis in children with epilepsy. *Epilepsia* 2001; **42**: 1611–1613.

187. Pellock JM, Glauser TA, Bebin EM, *et al.* Pharmacokinetic study of levetiracetam in children. *Epilepsia* 2001; **42**: 1574–1579.

188. Hrachovy RA, Frost JD, Kellaway P, *et al.* Double-blind study of ACTH vs. prednisone in infantile spasms. *Journal of Pediatrics* 1983; **103**: 641–645.

189. Lombroso CT. A prospective study in infantile spasms: Clinical and therapeutic correlations. *Epilepsia* 1983; **24**: 135–158.

190. Singer WD, Rabe EF, Haller JS. The effect of ACTH therapy on infantile spasms. *Journal of Pediatrics* 1980; **96**: 485–489.

191. Snead OC, Benton JW, Hosey LC, *et al.* Treatment of infantile spasms with high-dose ACTH: Efficacy and plasma levels of ACTH and cortisol. *Neurology* 1989; **39**: 1027–1031.

192. Baram TZ, Mitchell WG, Tournay B, *et al.* High-dose corticotropin (ACTH) versus prednisone for infantile spasms: a prospective, randomized, blinded study. *Pediatrics* 1996; **97**: 375–379.

193. Ito M, Aiba H, Hashimoto K, *et al.* Low-dose ACTH therapy for West syndrome. Initial effects and long-term outcome. *Neurology* 2002; **58**: 110–114.

194. Mikati MA, Trevathan E, Krishnamoorthy KS, Lombroso CT. Pyridoxine-dependent epilepsy: EEG investigations and long-term follow-up. *Electroencephalography and Clinical Neurophysiology* 1991; **78**: 215–221.

195. Pietz J, Benninger C, Schäfer H, *et al.* Treatment of infantile spasms with high-dose vitamin B6. *Epilepsia* 1993; **34**: 757–763.

196. Takuma Y, Seki T, Hirai K. A study of a new treatment for intractable epilepsy with infantile spasms and related disorders using a combination of high-dose pyridoxal phosphate and low dose ACTH. *Brain and Development* 1990; **12**: 641.

197. Pellock J, Willmore L. A rational guide to routine blood monitoring in patients receiving antiepileptic drugs. *Neurology* 1991; **41**: 961–964.

22B

The ketogenic diet

EILEEN PG VINING AND ERIC H KOSSOFF

In recent years, the ketogenic diet has emerged as an important alternative therapy for intractable epilepsy in children. This is a stringently controlled diet that provides nutrition predominantly as fats so that ketosis is maintained on a long-term basis. Many studies have demonstrated its efficacy in a wide range of seizure disorders and we have a better understanding of side-effects, how to deal with them, and potential long-term problems, but the mechanism of action is still unclear.

BACKGROUND

Until the 20th century there were few effective treatments for epilepsy. Prayer and fasting had been advocated as therapy since at least biblical times. In the early 20th century attention turned to the fasting component and led to Wilder's original publication in 1921 that outlined a ketogenic diet.[1] On the basis of earlier studies of metabolism in diabetics, he recognized that fasting produced ketosis, which could be sustained by a diet that contained an excess of ketogenic foods (fats) rather than antiketogenic foods (proteins and carbohydrates). He and colleagues at the Mayo Clinic recommended an energy-restricted diet that provided approximately 1 g/kg per day of protein, a small amount of carbohydrates and more than 90 per cent of energy intake as fats.[2]

The diet was used extensively for about 20 years until the advent of specific anticonvulsants, particularly phenytoin, provided treatment that was easier to use. The diet then fell into disuse, except in a few centers that cared for children with very refractory epilepsy, where it remained a therapy of last resort. The diet underwent a major revival in the mid-1990s, following the publicity that resulted from a campaign launched by The Charlie Foundation.[3]

BASIC SCIENCE

The initial theories that acidosis, dehydration or hyperlipidemia were responsible for the efficacy of the diet have largely been abandoned and newer work has focused on the role of ketones as they affect both neurons and astrocytes.

Schwartzkroin[4] reviewed a variety of hypotheses that might explain the efficacy of the diet via alteration of the inhibitory-excitation balance. The diet might change the energy metabolism of the brain, cell properties, neurotransmitter function, neuromodulators or the extracellular environment of the brain. A number of investigators are beginning to develop models to approach these issues and hopefully provide an explanation for the mechanism of action of the diet. This could ultimately lead to more specific and effective treatments than the diet formulation currently in use.

CLINICAL EFFICACY

Numerous retrospective studies have described the efficacy of the diet. Its revival in the mid-1990s led to prospective studies that have provided more conclusive evidence of efficacy. In order to demonstrate that the diet could be adequately prescribed and maintained in a variety of clinical settings, a multicenter study was initiated involving seven sites that were trained to use the Hopkins form of the classic diet.[5] Fifty-one children with intractable epilepsy, aged 1–8 years, were enrolled and placed on a classic 4:1 ratio diet (4 g fat:1 g combined protein and carbohydrate). At 1 year, 40 per cent of the original group had a greater than 50 per cent decrease in seizures, with 47 per cent of the children staying on it for that length of time. It appeared that there were no major differences between centers' abilities to manage the diet.

The efficacy was very similar in a larger study of 150 children who also were followed through 1 year on the diet: 50 per cent had a greater than 50 per cent decrease and 27 per cent had more than 90 per cent improvement.[6] In these studies there was no relationship between seizure control and age, gender or seizure type. This cohort was subsequently evaluated 3–6 years later to examine the long-term impact of the diet.[7] Only 15 children remained on the diet. The group of 83 children who had remained on the diet at 1 year continued to do well. Forty-one (27 per cent) still had more than 90 per cent improvement from their original baseline seizure frequency. In addition, there had been a major reduction in anticonvulsant medication. These and other studies were reviewed by a Blue Cross and Blue Shield Technical Advisory Board, leading to their conclusion that, 'The diet's effectiveness in providing seizure control for children with difficult-to-control seizures has remained as good or better than any of the newer medications.'[8]

More recently, a retrospective study described the efficacy of the diet in the treatment of 23 children with infantile spasms, of whom 74 per cent had not responded to ACTH or steroids.[9] Thirteen (57 per cent) had more than 50 per cent improvement at 1 year and remained on the diet, and three were seizure free. Younger children and those who had been on fewer medications appeared to do better.

DIET PROTOCOL

The ketogenic diet is a medical therapy that must be individualized for each child. Many factors are considered in determining the ratio to be used, the amount of energy intake and the fluids to be administered. Children who are at periods when growth is maximal are often started at 3:1 ratio diets in order to be able to provide more protein. Adolescents are also routinely started at a 3:1 ratio in order to be able to liberalize their meals slightly. Calculation of the energy intake is generally based at 75 per cent of the daily recommended intake for age. This is modified by many factors and is influenced greatly by whether the child is at their ideal body weight. If the child is significantly overweight, the diet is calculated to produce weight loss. Children who are very hypotonic and immobile require less food energy, while children who are spastic and expending a great deal of energy even when immobile require higher energy intake. Fluids are generally calculated to meet 80 per cent of daily needs.

Once the diet ratio, energy intake and fluid content have been calculated, an individualized plan is created. If the child is an infant on formula or is tube fed, the feedings will be calculated using a combination of fats including Microlipid (Mead Johnson) and oils, protein (Ross Carbohydrate-free Concentrate), carbohydrate usually as polycose (Ross), and water. Older children will usually be given a number of menus that will provide for three meals and a snack. A typical breakfast might consist of egg cooked with butter and herbs, bacon and 'hot chocolate' (cream and chocolate flavoring). A computer program for calculating the various components of each meal was created a number of years ago by a group of our parents. This is routinely used by our dietician and by families who wish to be more flexible in creating a variety of meals for their children. We encourage older children to adapt their favorite foods to a ketogenic diet. Creativity has abounded and has resulted in ketogenic forms of pizza, tacos, spaghetti, bagels, muffins, ham sandwiches and cheesecake. The diet is routinely supplemented with calcium (Calcimix 500 mg) and multivitamins and minerals (Unicap-M). Occasionally additional supplementation with zinc or carnitine may be considered when hair changes occur or when children seem particularly listless, hypotonic or constipated.

Although there are published accounts of introduction of the ketogenic diet without fasting and as an outpatient, our center continues to prefer admitting the child during fasting and initiation of foods.[10] We know that some children will be controlled rapidly in that setting and feel that this results in greater confidence and hopefully compliance with the diet. We also believe that the complete switch-over to ketogenic foods is facilitated by this withdrawal. Children can become symptomatic during this period (hypoglycemia, vomiting), and monitoring and treatment are facilitated in an inpatient setting. The support structure of the hospital setting is also important to parents in this difficult period for their child. Finally, there is an intensive educational process that must be accomplished during these few days as families become competent in assessing the level of ketosis, preparing the diet and monitoring for side-effects. Over the years, a standardized approach to initiation of the diet has been developed and we have established a critical pathway protocol that makes the process easier for families, nurses, the dietician and physicians.[11] A summary of the plan is shown in Table 22B.1.

Optimizing the diet to achieve the best possible seizure control includes regular reassessment and formal clinic visits at 3, 6 and 12 months. Our dietician and nurse are available for ongoing management and routinely carefully monitor weight loss/gain, compliance with the

Table 22B.1 *Overview of admission for initiation of the ketogenic diet*

Day	Care	Nutrition
Minus 1	History/physical Introductory class	Begin fasting after dinner

Day 1	Admit to hospital
	Classes continue
	Dextrostix every 6 h ; if <40 mg/dL every 2 h;
	  Glucose <25 mg/dL give 30 mL
	  orange juice; follow
	Use carbohydrate-free medications
		Fast
		Fluids restricted to 60–75 mL/kg per day;encourage
		  drinking

Day 2	Continue monitoring Classes continue	Continue fluids Fast until dinner then 1/3 of the usualcalories given as 'eggnog'
Day 3	Continue monitoring until tolerating meals Classes continue	Continue fluids Breakfast and lunch: 1/3 of calculated meal as 'eggnog' Dinner: 2/3 of calculated meal as 'eggnog'
Day 4	Classes continue	Breakfast and lunch: 2/3 of calculated meal as 'eggnog' Dinner: Full ketogenic diet meal
Day 5	Discharge review: medications, vitamins, monitoring, follow-up	Breakfast: Full ketogenic diet meal Have 2 'eggnog' meals prepared for travel

diet and intercurrent illnesses. Follow-up laboratory work includes routine chemistries, lipid profile, urinalysis and urine calcium and creatinine measurements. If the child has gained weight, energy intake may need to be decreased. If the child is not maintaining good ketosis, the ratio may need to be adjusted and inadvertent consumption of carbohydrates (medicines, even skin lotions) must be evaluated. Frequently, we will advise fasting for 12–24 h to boost ketosis.

It is our practice to suggest discontinuation of therapy when a patient has been seizure free for 2 years (whether on the diet or on medication). Discontinuation of the diet should be gradual. The initial step can be to lower the ratio to 2 or 2.5:1. We then advocate increasing the portions of foods that are on the diet, and finally liberalizing carbohydrates. Substituting whole milk, then 2 per cent, and then 1 per cent milk and finally adding carbohydrates is an alternative approach. The decision to discontinue the diet is more difficult when patients have had major, but not complete, improvement and families do not wish to alter an apparent fragile balance. If the child is healthy and growing modestly we will generally continue the diet.

DIFFICULTIES WITH DIET: SHORT- AND LONG-TERM

In the period of diet initiation, hypoglycemia, vomiting and dehydration can occur but are usually manageable. When children refuse food, we try substituting foods that may be preferable. In some children, behavioral issues may be a factor that should be addressed.

The most common problems are gastrointestinal. Constipation can usually be managed with increased fluids, stool softeners, the use of some medium-chain triglycerides and laxatives when necessary. When intercurrent vomiting or diarrhea occurs, parents must carefully manage fluids to prevent dehydration and severe acidosis.

Families and primary care physicians are often very concerned about growth. The diet is calculated to provide minimally adequate nutrition, and that is reflected in our recent evaluation of growth. In a prospective study of 237 children that were followed for an average of 1 year on the diet, growth remained within normal parameters. When growth measurements were normalized for age and sex, the weight fell initially but then generally stabilized, except in children who were initially overweight, in whom it continued to decline. Linear growth was not adversely impacted initially but did continue to decline over a 2-year period. Very young children appeared to grow less well on the diet, and their nutrition must be very carefully managed.[12]

Renal stones have been reported in approximately 5 per cent of children on the ketogenic diet.[13] They appear to be more prevalent where there is a positive family history. Although carbonic anhydrase inhibitor anticonvulsants (topiramate, zonisamide and acetazolamide) have an associated risk of kidney stones, the combination does not seem to increase the risk above that of the diet alone.[14] However, children with a family history of kidney stones or prior renal abnormalities may be at higher risk and should have their urines routinely alkalized by PolycitraK (2 mEq/kg per day, divided dose twice daily). Fluids are routinely liberalized in these patients. In all our patients, regardless of other medications, we monitor the spot urine calcium:creatinine ratio. If it exceeds 0.2, we recommend alkalinizing the urine with PolycitraK. When stones develop they are managed in a standard fashion and frequently children are maintained on the diet.[15]

The lipid profile of children on the ketogenic diet is usually abnormal.[16] Long term use of the diet is associated with less marked changes. Most children are on the diet for a limited period of time and it is unclear what impact, if any, the diet will have on the overall health of the child.

A variety of other problems have been described in anecdotal reports. These include: hypoproteinemia, Fanconi's renal tubular acidosis, elevated liver enzymes, cardiomyopathy, prolonged QT interval, pancreatitis, bruising and vitamin deficiency.[17-21] Children on the diet must be carefully followed and any deterioration should be carefully investigated to determine if it could be related to some aspect of the ketogenic diet. Clearly, the diet can be abandoned if it appears to be implicated in a significant side-effect, and can also be reinstituted when the condition has resolved.

KEY POINTS

- The ketogenic diet is an **effective alternative therapy** for intractable epilepsy
- Most **side-effects** can be managed without requiring discontinuation of the diet
- The ketogenic diet **requires a skilled, committed team** to be effective
- **Clinical studies** are required to examine a number of issues:
  - how to minimize the impact of the diet on **growth**
  - would certain **nutritional elements** enhance seizure control?
  - is such stringent **control of energy intake** necessary?
  - the effectiveness of the diet in **specific seizure types** (e.g. infantile spasms) and epilepsy syndromes
- The **mechanism of action** of the diet is still unclear
- An understanding of the mechanism of action may allow the development of a **more specific and less restrictive** treatment
- The ketogenic diet must be made **more widely available**

REFERENCES

1. Wilder RM. The effect of ketonemia on the course of epilepsy. *Mayo Clinic Bulletin* 1921; **2**: 307.
2. Peterman MG. Ketogenic diet in epilepsy. *JAMA* 1925; **84**: 1979.
3. Abrahams J. *An Introduction to the Ketogenic Diet: A Treatment for Pediatric Epilepsy* (videotape). Santa Monica, CA: The Charlie Foundation, 1994.
4. Schwartzkroin PA. Mechanisms underlying the anti-epileptic efficacy of the ketogenic diet. *Epilepsy Research* 1999; **37**: 171–180.
5. Vining EPG, Freeman JM, Ballaban-Gil K, *et al.* A multi-center study of the efficacy of the ketogenic diet. *Archives of Neurology* 1998; **55**: 1433–1437.
6. Freeman JM, Vining EPG, Pillas DJ, *et al.* The efficacy of the ketogenic diet – 1998: a prospective evaluation of intervention in 150 children. *Pediatrics* 1998; **102**: 1358–1363.
7. Hemingway C, Freeman JM, Pillas DJ, Pyzik PL. The ketogenic diet: a 3 to 6 year follow-up of 150 children enrolled prospectively. *Pediatrics* 2001; **108**: 898–905.
8. Lefevre F, Aronson N. Ketogenic diet for the treatment of refractory epilepsy in children: a systematic review of efficacy. *Pediatrics* 2000; **105**: e46.
9. Kossoff EH, Pyzik PL, McGrogan JR, Vining EPG, Freeman JM. Efficacy of the ketogenic diet for infantile spasms. *Pediatrics* 2002; **109**: 780–783.
10. Wirrell EC, Darwish HZ, Williams-Dyjur C, Blackman M, Lange V. Is a fast necessary when initiating the ketogenic diet? *Journal of Child Neurology* 2002; **17**: 179–182.
11. Freeman JM, Kelly MT, Freeman JB. *The Ketogenic Diet: A Treatment for Epilepsy.* New York: Demos, 2000.
12. Vining EPG, Pyzik P, McGrogan J, *et al.* Growth of children on the ketogenic diet. *Developmental Medicine and Child Neurology* 2002; **44**: 796.
13. Herzberg GZ, Fivush BA, Kinsman SL, Gearhart JP. Urolithiasis associated with the ketogenic diet. *Journal of Pediatrics* 1990; **117**: 743–745.
14. Kossoff EH, Pyzik PL, Furth SL, *et al.* Kidney stones, carbonic anhydrase inhibitors, and the ketogenic diet. *Epilepsia* 2002; **43** (10): 1168–1171.
15. Furth SL, Casey JC, Pyzik PL, *et al.* Risk factors for urolithiasis in children on the ketogenic diet. *Pediatric Nephrology* 2000; **15**: 125–128.
16. Kwiterovich PO Jr, Vining EPG, Pyzik P, Skolasky R Jr, Freeman JM. Effect of a high-fat ketogenic diet on plasma levels of lipids, lipoproteins, and apolipoproteins in children. *JAMA* 2003; **290**: 912–920.
17. Hahn TJ, Halstead LR, DeVivo DC. Disordered mineral metabolism produced by ketogenic diet therapy. *Calcified Tissue International* 1979; **28**: 17–22.
18. Stewart WA, Gordon K, Camfield P. Acute pancreatitis causing death in a child on the ketogenic diet. *Journal of Child Neurology* 2001; **16**: 682.
19. Berry-Kravis E, Booth G, Taylor A, Valentino LA. Bruising and the ketogenic diet: evidence for diet-induced changes in platelet function. *Annals of Neurology* 2001; **49**: 98–103.
20. Best TH, Franz DN, Gilbert DL, Nelson DP, Epstein MR. Cardiac complications in pediatric patients on the ketogenic diet. *Neurology* 2000; **54**: 2328–2330.
21. Ballaban-Gil K, Callahan C, O'Dell C, *et al.* Complications of the ketogenic diet. *Epilepsia* 1998; **39**: 744–748.

Vagal nerve stimulation

JEROME V MURPHY AND SARA HUDSON

HISTORY OF VAGAL NERVE STIMULATION

Stimulation of the vagal nerve was shown in the 1960s to influence EEG activity in laboratory animals,[1,2] and in 1972 by Zabara to block induced vomiting in a dog.[3] Zabara subsequently demonstrated that stimulation of the left vagal nerve controlled seizures induced in dogs with intravenous phenylenetetrazol.[4] A similar effect was shown by others in different animal models of epilepsy.[5–8] The left vagal nerve was used because its fibers are predominantly afferent. Following an open pilot study of 16 refractory patients,[9] two double-blinded, active control studies in patients at least 12 years old with intractable partial seizures showed the efficacy of vagal nerve stimulation (VNS).[10,11] In the long-term studies and in postapproval reports, the number of patients with at least a 50 per cent reduction in seizures approaches 50 per cent.[12,13]

MECHANISM OF ACTION

The mechanism of action of VNS is poorly understood. Fos staining of rats undergoing VNS demonstrates synaptic activation of thalamus, hypothalamus and amygdala, areas that can inhibit epileptic discharges.[14] Efficacy of the VNS in rats is lost if the nucleus ceruleus is chemically ablated.[15] PET in humans has shown changes in blood flow to specific forebrain and brainstem nuclei.[16] There was a correlation between the alteration of blood flow in the thalamus and suppression of seizure activity. Cerebrospinal studies of patients receiving VNS have shown changes suggesting activation of the neurotransmitters GABA, serotonin and dopamine.[17,18] The basis for the increased benefit from VNS observed over the first 18 months of stimulation is not clear.

TECHNICAL ASPECTS

Vagal nerve stimulators have been implanted by neurosurgeons, otolaryngologists and vascular surgeons. The generator is programmed to a duty cycle of tolerated settings using a computer-attached wand. The stimulation parameters that can be varied include the routine and on-demand currents; the duration of stimulation and period between stimulations; the pulse width; and the pulse frequency. Commonly used duty cycles are 30 s on and 5 min off, as used in the preapproval studies; 30 s on and 3 min off, based on laboratory observations;[19] and rapid cycle, 7 s on and 12 s off.[20] We have generally used the 30 s/3 min duty cycle and changed to rapid cycle if the patient has shown no benefit after a year.

VNS has also been shown to shorten a seizure.[21] A strong magnet, which can be worn on the belt or on the wrist, is swiped over the generator during a seizure and releases a preset magnet current. In our first 100 implanted patients, 34 of the 70 families on whom magnet use information was available reported that the magnet had aborted or shortened a seizure.

The present generator, Model 101, has an 8–12 year life. The life of the generator will vary with the duty cycle and the use of the on demand, magnet-induced current.

Replacement requires only a chest incision to insert and connect a new generator.

PATIENT SELECTION

VNS has been approved in the USA as adjunctive therapy for medically refractory partial seizures in patients at least 12 years old, but approval in the European Community has no limitations on seizure types or patient age. In an open study of 60 children between 3 and 18 years of age,[22] the responder rate was very similar to those described in adults[10–13] with the median reduction in seizure frequency for the group as a whole increasing over time to 43 per cent at 18 months (see Figure 22C.1). Reported

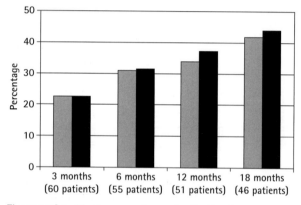

Figure 22C.1 *Median percentage reduction in seizure frequency in 60 children under 19 years of age. Gray bars, actual; black bars, intent to treat.*

Table 22C.1 *Adverse events in > 10 per cent of patients per epoch*

Epoch (months)	Event	% of Patients
0–3	Fever	26.7
	Cough	25.0
	Headache	23.3
	Voice alteration	21.7
	Congestion/cold	20.0
	Infection	18.3
	Vomiting	18.3
	Pharyngitis	13.3
	Nausea	11.7
3–6	Voice alteration	14.6
	Headache	12.7
	Congestion/cold	12.7
	Fever	10.9
6–12	Fever	15.7
	Headache	15.7
	Congestion/cold	13.7
	Voice alteration	13.7
12–18	Voice alteration	13.0

adverse events diminished over time. The only persistent adverse event was voice alteration during the generator discharge (see Table 22C.1).[22] VNS has also been reported to be as effective in children and adults with primary generalized epilepsies[23] as in partial seizures. Improved seizure control has also been reported in patients with Lennox-Gastaut syndrome,[24–27] hypothalamic hamartomas[28] and tuberous sclerosis complex.[29] However, VNS was reported to be ineffective in 10 children older than 3 years with infantile spasms.[30]

VNS is generally considered after a patient has failed three appropriately used antiepileptic drugs. Focal resection is generally preferred if the patient is a suitable candidate. There have been no comparative studies with the ketogenic diet, but VNS is associated with fewer side-effects and is tolerated better, particularly by children over 5 years of age. There is no contraindication to VNS. Although no comparative trials have been undertaken, VNS would appear to be preferable to corpus callosotomy in terms of cost, efficacy and potential adverse effects.[31] Cost-effectiveness studies have been very favorable.[32–34] In a group of 19 children with therapy resistant epilepsy, the cost was estimated to have been recovered within 2.3 years.[32]

ADVERSE EFFECTS

The infection rate in the preapproval studies was 1.1 per cent.[35] Three of the first 100 devices implanted at our institution became infected, requiring removal of the generator, antibiotic therapy and reimplantation. Adverse effects in children have included fever, cough, headache, voice alteration, congestion/cold, infection, vomiting, pharyngitis and nausea. These were present during the first 3 months of stimulation and only voice alteration during stimulation was reported at 12–18 months of therapy (Table 22C.1).[22] None of these adverse effects resulted in discontinuation of VNS.

Less common side-effects have included atropine-responsive bradycardia, which was reported intraoperatively in several adults but did not recur with continued VNS use.[36] Transient vocal cord paralysis occurred in our 128th patient. Concern has been raised about the possibility of aspiration during stimulation.[37] In 8 patients studied during normal stimulation and during the highest tolerated stimulation, aspiration of barium below the vocal cords was not induced.[38] Twenty-four hour Holter monitoring, gastrin levels and pulmonary functions demonstrated no changes in a double-blinded randomized study.[11]

The leads on the vagus are heated and may cause tissue injury if exposed to MRI. It is recommended that MRI head scans be performed using a closed head coil system. MRI scans of the body and diathermy are contraindicated because of the potential for thermal injury to the vagal nerve.

PATIENT AND PHYSICIAN RESOURCES

There is a registry containing data from more than 5000 implanted patients from 796 centers, with a follow-up more than 1 year in approximately 20 per cent of the patients (*cyberonics.com* or *efa.org*). The registry permits registered physicians to examine the data for results in patients with a similar epileptic profile before implanting a patient.

> ## KEY POINTS
>
> - VNS has been **approved** in the USA as adjunctive therapy for medically refractory partial seizures in patients at least 12 years old, but approval in the European Community has no limitations on seizure types or patient age
> - VNS has also been reported to be as **effective** in children and adults with primary generalized epilepsies as in partial seizures. Improved seizure control has also been reported in patients with Lennox-Gastaut syndrome, hypothalamic hamartomas and tuberous sclerosis complex
> - The **left vagal nerve** is stimulated because its fibers are predominantly afferent
> - The **stimulation parameters** that can be varied include the routine and on-demand currents; the duration of stimulation and period between stimulations; the pulse width; and the pulse frequency. Commonly used cycles are 30 s on/5 min off, 30 s on/3 min off, and 7 s on/12 s off (rapid cycle)
> - A strong **magnet**, which may be worn on the belt or on the wrist, can be swiped over the generator during a seizure and releases a preset magnet current, which has been shown to shorten a seizure
> - **Adverse effects** in children have included fever, cough, headache, voice alteration, congestion/cold, infection, vomiting, pharyngitis and nausea. Voice alteration during stimulation tends to be the only persistent adverse effect
> - It is recommended that **MRI head scans** be performed using a closed head coil system in patients with a VNS. MRI scans of the body and diathermy are contraindicated due to the potential for thermal injury to the vagal nerve

REFERENCES

1. Chase MH, Sterman MB, Clemente CD. Cortical and subcortical patterns of response to afferent vagal stimulation. *Experimental Neurology* 1966; **16**: 36–49.
2. Chase MH, Nakamura Y, Clemente CD, Sterman MB. Afferent vagal stimulation: neurographic correlates of induced EEG synchronization and desynchronization. *Brain Research* 1967; **5**: 236–249.
3. Zabara J, Chaffee RB Jr, Tansy MF. Neuroinhibition in the regulation of emesis. *Space Life Science* 1972; **3**: 282–292.
4. Zabara J. Inhibition of repetitive seizures in canines by repetitive vagal stimulation. *Epilepsia* 1992; **33**: 1005–1012.
5. Woodbury JW, Woodbury DM. Vagal stimulation reduces the severity of maximal electroshock seizures in intact rats: use of a cuff electrode for stimulating and recording. *Pacing and Clinical Electrophysiology* 1991; **14**: 94–107.
6. Woodbury DM, Woodbury JW. Effects of vagal stimulation on experimentally induced seizures in rats. *Epilepsia* 1990; **31**(Suppl. 2): S7–19.
7. Lockard JS, Congdon WC, DuCharme LL. Feasibility and safety of vagal stimulation in monkey model. *Epilepsia* 1990; **31**(Suppl. 2): S20–26.
8. McClachlan RS. Suppression of interictal spikes and seizures by stimulation of the vagus nerve. *Epilepsia* 1993; **34**: 918–923.
9. Penry JK, Dean JC. Prevention of intractable seizures by intermittent vagal stimulation in humans: Preliminary results. *Epilepsia* 1990; **31**(Suppl. 2): S40–43.
10. Ben-Medachem E, Manon-Espailat R, Ristanovic R, *et al.* Vagus nerve stimulation for treatment of partial seizures: 1. A controlled study of effect on seizures. *Epilepsia* 1994; **35**: 616–626.
11. Handforth A, DeGiorgio CM, Schacter SC, *et al.* Vagus nerve stimulation therapy for partial-onset seizures. A randomized active-control trial. *Neurology* 1998; **51**: 48–55.
12. Morris GL, Mueller WM. The Vagus Stimulation Study Group E01–E05. *Neurology* 1999; **53**: 1731–1735.
13. DeGiorgio CM, Schacter SC, Handforth E, *et al.* Prospective long-term study of vagus nerve stimulation for the treatment of refractory seizures. *Epilepsia* 2000; **41**: 1195–1200.
14. Naritoku DK, Terry WJ, Helfert RH. Regional induction of *fos* immunoreactivity in the brain by anticonvulsant stimulation of the vagus nerve. *Epilepsy Research* 1995; **22**: 53–62.
15. Krahl SE, Clark KB, Smith DC, Browning RA. Locus ceruleus lesions suppress the seizure-attenuating effects of vagus nerve stimulation. *Epilepsia* 1998; **39**: 709–714.
16. Henry TR, Votaw JR, Pennell PB, *et al.* Acute blood flow changes and efficacy of vagus nerve stimulation in partial epilepsy. *Neurology* 1999; **51**: 1166–1173.
17. Ben-Menachem E, Hamberger A, Hedner T, *et al.* Effects of vagus nerve stimulation on amino acids and other metabolites in the CSF of patients with partial seizures. *Epilepsy Research* 1995; **20**: 221–227.
18. Hammond EJ, Uthman BM, Wilder BJ, *et al.* Neurochemical effects of vagus nerve stimulation in humans. *Brain Research* 1992; **583**: 300–303.
19. Takaya M, Terry W, Naritoku DK. Vagus nerve stimulation induces a sustained anticonvulsant effect. *Epilepsia* 1996; **37**: 1111–1116.

20. DeGiorgio CM, Thompson J, Lewis P, *et al*. Vagal nerve stimulation: analysis of device parameters in 154 patients during the long-term XE5 study. *Epilepsia* 2001; **42**: 1017–1020.

21. Hammond EJ, Uthman BM, Reid SA, *et al*. Vagus nerve stimulation in humans – neurophysiological studies and electrophysiological monitoring. *Epilepsia* 1990; **31**(Suppl. 2): S51–59.

22. Murphy JV. The Pediatric VNS Study Group. Left vagal nerve stimulation in children with medically refractory epilepsy. *Journal of Pediatrics* 1999; **134**: 563–566.

23. Labar D, Murphy J, Tecoma E, EO4VNS Study Group. Vagus nerve stimulation for medication-resistant generalized epilepsy. *Neurology* 1999; **52**: 1510–1512.

24. Ben-Menachem E, Hellstrom K, Waldton C, Augustinsson LE. Evaluation of refractory epilepsy treated with vagus nerve stimulation for up to 5 years. *Neurology* 1999; **52**: 1265–1267.

25. Hosain S, Nikalov B, Harden C, *et al*. Vagus nerve stimulation treatment for Lennox-Gastaut syndrome. *Journal of Child Neurology* 2000; **15**: 509–512.

26. Frost M, Gates J, Helmers SL, *et al*. Vagal nerve stimulation in children with refractory seizures associated with Lennox-Gastaut syndrome. *Epilepsia* 2001; **42**: 1148–1152.

27. Aldenkamp AP, Van de Veerdonk SHA, Majoie HJM, *et al*. Effects of 6 months of treatment with vagus nerve stimulation on behavior in children with Lennox-Gastaut syndrome in an open clinical and nonrandomized study. *Epilepsy and Behavior* 2001; **2**: 343–350.

28. Murphy JV, Wheless JW, Schmoll CM. Left vagal nerve stimulation in six patients with hypothalamic hamartomas. *Pediatric Neurology* 2000; **23**: 167–168.

29. Parain D, Menniello MJ, Berquen P, *et al*. Vagal nerve stimulation in tuberous sclerosis complex patients. *Pediatric Neurology* 2001; **25**: 213–216.

30. Fohlen MJ, Jalin C, Pinard J-M, Delalande OR. Results of vagal nerve stimulation 10 children with refractory infantile spasms (abstract). *Epilepsia* 1998; **39**(Suppl. 6): 170.

31. Schmidt D, Bourgeois B. A risk-benefit assessment of therapies for Lennox-Gastaut syndrome. *Drug Safety* 2000; **22**: 467–477.

32. Majoie HJM, Berfelo MW, Aldenkamp AP, *et al*. Vagus nerve stimulation in children with therapy resistant epilepsy diagnosed as Lennox-Gastaut syndrome. *Journal of Clinical Neurophysiology* 2001; **18**(5): 419–428.

33. Boon P, Vonck K, D'Have M, *et al*. Cost-benefit analysis of vagus nerve stimulation for refractory epilepsy. *Acta Neurologica Belgica* 1999; **99**: 275–280.

34. Boon P, Vonck K, Vanderkerkchove T, *et al*. Vagus nerve stimulation for medically refractory epilepsy; efficacy and cost-benefit analysis. *Acta Neurochirurgica* 1999; **141**: 447–452.

35. Bruce DA, Alksne JF, Bernard E. Implantation of a vagal nerve stimulator for refractory partial seizures: surgical outcomes of 454 study patients. *Epilepsia* 1998; **39**(Suppl. 6): 92–93.

36. Asconape JJ, Moore DD, Zipes DP, *et al*. Bradycardia and asystole with the use of vagal nerve stimulation for the treatment of epilepsy: a rare complication of intraoperative device testing. *Epilepsia* 1999; **40**: 1452–1454.

37. Lundgren J, Ekberg O, Olsson R. Aspiration: a potential complication to vagus nerve stimulation. *Epilepsia* 1998; **39**: 998–1000.

38. Schallert G, Foster J, Lindquist N, Murphy JV. Chronic stimulation of the vagal nerve in children: effect on swallowing. *Epilepsia* 1998; **39**: 1113–1114.

22D

Surgery

CHARLES E POLKEY

Pediatric epilepsy surgery presents different pathological substrates and technical challenges from adult surgery. It requires a multidisciplinary approach that involves the cooperation and understanding of the parents and caregivers.[1]

PATHOLOGICAL SUBSTRATES OF INTRACTABLE EPILEPSY

Various pathologic substrates are suitable for resective surgery. However, the same pathologic abnormality may be localized, diffuse or multifocal and therefore not always amenable to resection (Table 22D.1).

Malformations of cortical development (MCD)

Embryonic development between 6 and 16 weeks determines the production of a normal organized cerebral cortex. Disturbance of migration, cell differentiation,

Table 22D.1 *Cortical dysplasia: distribution of abnormalities in 90 patients (per cent)*

Bilateral localized	20
Unilateral	36
Diffuse	44

Based on Guerrini et al.[2]

programmed cell death and synaptic elimination produces a wide variety of malformations (see Chapter 4C). The surgical targets are focal cortical dysplasia and hemimegalencephaly.

Focal cortical dysplasia and hemimegalencephaly often present at an early age. In 68 patients with focal cortical dysplasia who were operated before the age of 18 years, the mean age of seizure onset was 7 months. The lesions were predominantly extratemporal (88 per cent) and 21 per cent underwent surgery before the age of 2 years.[3] MCD are often associated with other neurologic abnormalities. In 109 patients under 19 years of age with MCD, 75 per cent had seizures, 68 per cent developmental delay or intellectual disability, and 48 per cent abnormal neurological findings.[4] Only 20 per cent of these patients had the potential surgical targets of focal cortical dysplasia or hemimegalencephaly.

Hamartomas are defined as normal tissue in an abnormal situation or as an abnormal arrangement of normal elements. The hypothalamic hamartoma has come to prominence because of recent advances in the recognition and treatment of the lesion.

Tuberous sclerosis and variants

Neville reviews the neurocutaneous syndromes that include epilepsy in their expression.[5] Apart from Sturge-Weber syndrome, the most important of these is tuberous sclerosis. Cortical tubers, subependymal nodules and giant cell astrocytomas close to the foramen of Monro are the main manifestations in the brain. Among 23 children aged 3 years or less, operated for drug-resistant epilepsy, one patient (4 per cent) had tuberous sclerosis. A resectable focus was located in 16 patients among 21 children with multiple tubers on MRI.[6]

Arteriovenous malformations

These usually present with hemorrhage in childhood. Among 160 children with arteriovenous malformations, 80 per cent presented with hemorrhage.

Cavernoma

These small vascular lesions, easily seen on MRI, are angiographically occult. They present with either epilepsy or hemorrhage. The incidence in children is low. In a community study that examined imaging findings in 488 of 613 children with epilepsy, only 1 of the 62 patients with a structural lesion had a cavernoma.[7] Epilepsy was the presenting feature in 6 of 7 children in one series[8] and in 12 of 22 in another.[9]

Sturge-Weber syndrome

Sturge-Weber syndrome is characterized by a flat, facial angioma affecting at least the first branch of the trigeminal nerve, with ipsilateral leptomeningeal vascular anomalies and ipsilateral vascular lesions of the choroid. Homolateral cerebral hemiatrophy develops together with corticosubcortical calcifications.

Developmental delay is associated with early seizure onset and intensity of seizures. In one study, 75 per cent of patients had seizure onset in the first year of life, and 83 per cent of these patients had developmental or academic problems.[10]

In surgical series, between 13 per cent and 22 per cent of patients have Sturge-Weber syndrome. In a multicenter study of 333 hemispherectomies there were 8 per cent with Sturge-Weber syndrome.[11]

Cerebrovascular infarction

There are many causes of stroke in childhood. A study of 73 children with stroke, after the neonatal period up to 17 years of age, showed that recurrent seizures were associated with delayed onset of initial seizures and cortical involvement as documented by neuroradiological studies. The surgical treatment of these patients usually involves a major resection or hemispherectomy.

Glial tumors

According to Aicardi, 0.2–0.3 per cent of children with epilepsy have brain tumors.[12] A study from Rochester found that tumors accounted for epilepsy in 1 per cent of children aged less than 15 years.[13] These tumors are commonly astrocytomas, which are usually low-grade; oligodendrogliomas rarely present in children with seizures.[14] In the Childhood Brain Tumor Consortium database, the incidence of epilepsy in the children with supratentorial tumors was age-dependent: 22 per cent in those <1 year of age and 68 per cent in those >15 years of age.[15]

Mixed tumors including dysembryoplastic neuroepithelial tumors (DNET)

These lesions contain both neuronal and glial elements. The commonest mixed tumors are the dysembryoplastic neuroepithelial tumor (DNET) and the ganglioglioma. The DNET is a heterogenous mixed glial tumor with three distinct cell types.[16] Gangliogliomas accounted for 1–4 per cent of pediatric brain tumors. The mean age at presentation in 99 children with gangliogliomas was 9.5 years and 49 per cent of children presented with partial epilepsy.[17]

Infections and their consequences

Infection of the CNS may result in permanent brain injury and epilepsy. In a study of 300 children with partial seizures, 20 patients had lesions attributable to an infectious process.[18] Similarly, 26 of 185 children who suffered acute bacterial meningitis had a persisting neurological deficit and half of these had late seizures.[19]

Rasmussen's encephalitis

This condition, usually involving one hemisphere, affects mainly children but has been described in adolescents and adults[20] (see Chapter 11E). The child usually presents between 4 and 8 years of age with seizures. These very often are unilateral focal motor seizures that become very difficult to control. This is accompanied by an increasing hemiparesis, in part ictal, and intellectual deterioration. There are corresponding neuroradiological changes with increasing hemispheric atrophy. The disease may burn out leaving a profound hemiplegia, hemianopia and epilepsy, or it may stop at any intermediate stage.[21]

Rasmussen's disease was the underlying diagnosis in 24 (4 per cent) of our 652 resections and in 10 of the 37 patients who underwent hemispherectomy before the age of 16 years. Similarly, Rasmussen's disease was the pathologic substrate in 25 per cent of 333 hemispherectomies in a multicenter study.[11]

Mesial temporal sclerosis (MTS)

In MTS there is neuronal loss in the mesial temporal structures, especially in the hippocampus with severe neuronal loss in the subfields CA1, 3 and 4, with preservation of the resistant sector CA2. Although the neuronal loss is predominantly unilateral, in 10–15 per cent it was bilateral and severe.[22] The pathogenesis of MTS is discussed in Chapter 5.

MTS in children is less common in the younger age groups but has been identified on MRI in a child aged 3 months and in a surgically resected specimen at the age of 2 years. MTS was demonstrated radiologically in 27 per cent of 30 children less than 14 years old with newly diagnosed temporal lobe epilepsy.[23] Indeed, MTS is a relatively uncommon pathologic finding in children operated on at less than 12 years of age. MTS in children is commonly associated with dual pathology. Thus, 79 per cent of 34 children and adolescents with MTS had a combination of mild MTS and mild to moderate cortical dysplasia.[24]

Trauma

Focal resection is not particularly effective in children with traumatic brain injury. Severe head injury tends to be diffuse and affect multiple sites. Assessment of 25 patients with posttraumatic epilepsy found that 16 (80 per cent) could not be adequately localized, and 5 of the remaining 9 patients had MTS.[25] Those with MTS had all been injured before 5 years of age.

SELECTION OF SURGICAL CANDIDATES

The primary aim in patient selection is to demonstrate that a localized resection is likely to result in a significant chance of improved seizure control and an acceptable level of morbidity and mortality. If a resection is not possible then a functional procedure, such as corpus callosotomy or subpial transection, can be considered. There are five surgically remediable syndromes:[26]

- mesial temporal epilepsy
- lesional partial epilepsy
- diffuse hemispheric syndromes
- secondary generalized epilepsy in infants and small children
- secondary generalized epilepsy in older patients.

The selection process consists of three steps:

- establish the epileptic nature and intractability of the patient's illness
- match the patient to one of the remediable syndromes

- consider a functional intervention if the patient is not suitable for resective surgery.

The International League Against Epilepsy's Subcommission on Surgery suggested that drug resistance should be defined by inadequate response to a minimum of two first-line drugs, either as monotherapy or in combination, as appropriate to the epileptic syndrome. Although they recommended at least 2 years of treatment in adults, they recognized that a period of 2 years may be too long in children and recommended that the long-term effects on development should be considered when timing surgical intervention.[27]

Selection for resective surgery depends upon the demonstration of concordant data from a variety of sources, including:

- clinical history, including both interictal history to characterize the background cerebral disorder and the ictal history to localize the origin of the seizures
- neuroradiological investigations, of which the structural gold standard is MRI; this can be supplemented by functional imaging including SPECT, PET and fMRI
- neurophysiological investigations, both interictal studies to investigate background changes, and ictal recordings including videotelemetry
- neuropsychological investigations to reveal deficits in cognitive function allowing localization of cerebral pathology, and to predict the effects of cerebral resection
- quality of life and psychiatric assessments; the latter is especially useful in older children.

Clinical history

Time devoted to this will be well repaid; the previous medical history, especially of neurological events, should be covered and a description of the seizures obtained from the patient and an independent observer. Careful history-taking can establish the nature and location of the cerebral pathology. In 100 children with temporal lobe epilepsy, Ounsted noted the age of their first seizure and age of onset of chronic epilepsy, the presence or absence of certain clinical events and their overall IQ once the chronic epilepsy had been established.[28] By these simple enquiries he divided the children into three groups (Table 22D.2). These mirror fairly accurately the division into perinatal damage, mesial temporal sclerosis and tumors and malformations, which are now recognized with MRI.[28]

Although a patient may experience simple partial seizures, complex partial seizures and secondary generalization, the seizure onset should be able to be localized. This data should be congruent with any postictal neurological deficit, such as a Todd palsy. Exceptionally, the seizure

Table 22D.2 *Details of patients with TLE studied by Ounsted[29]*

	Children with cerebral insult	Children with bouts of status	Children with neither	All children
n	35	32	33	100
Median age of seizure onset	36 months	16 months	58 months	28 months
Median age of onset of temporal lobe seizures	68 months	46 months	96 months	64 months
Verbal IQ	76	78	104	
Performance IQ	82	79	102	
Full-Scale IQ				87

activity may spread to the opposite hemisphere and result in an inappropriate deficit. Speech deficits when the seizure is in the dominant hemisphere, or ictal automatisms with nondominant involvement, have localizing value, as does the occurrence of contralateral dystonic posturing in some temporal lobe seizures.

Engel has described the syndrome of mesial temporal lobe epilepsy.[26] There is an increased incidence of febrile convulsions in these patients. The onset of chronic seizures usually occurs between 5 and 10 years of age, the seizures can remit, reappearing in adolescence or early adult life, and secondary generalization is uncommon. If the febrile convulsion was severe, there may have been a period of hemiparesis, which, if accurately recorded or recalled, is of considerable lateralizing value. Simple partial seizures (auras) occurring alone are common. The aura is usually autonomic or psychic, the commonest being a rising epigastric aura or an aura of fear. Even quite young children, if given the opportunity, can describe these events. The complex partial seizure usually begins with a behavioral arrest or stare, there are oroalimentary automatisms and there may be contralateral limb dystonic posturing. In children less than 6 years old with seizures of temporal lobe origin, atypical semiology may occur with asymmetric motor phenomena, posturing similar to that seen in frontal lobe seizures and head nodding.

The neurological examination often demonstrates minimal or no abnormality.

Neuroradiological studies

Structural MRI and various functional studies are most often used. These can pose technical challenges in infants and smaller children and considerable expertise is often required to achieve a meaningful result.

MRI

The epilepsy protocols used for MRI require several sequences and can be time-consuming, necessitating a general anesthetic in younger children (see Chapter 19A).

Two sequences are of particular interest in presurgical evaluation:

- the **T1–volume sequences** allow a detailed structural examination
- the **fluid attenuated inversion recovery sequence** (FLAIR) can reveal lesions in otherwise normal MRI examinations, particularly subtle cortical dysplasia and tubers.

MRI examination has been shown both in adults and in children to be useful for demonstrating the underlying pathology and also as a predictor of surgical outcome. The ability to demonstrate a lesion on MRI depends on the pathology. A diagnostic MRI was obtained in 17 of 18 children with either focal cortical dysplasia or hemimegalencephaly and corresponded to the histological diagnosis in 16.[30] The radiological features in cortical dysplasia include abnormal gyral formation, abnormal cortical thickening, loss of gray-white differentiation and abnormal signal on T2 weighted images. A discrete MRI abnormality is associated with a better outcome than a normal MRI in children undergoing extratemporal epilepsy surgery.

In most temporal lobe series, depending upon the age of the patients, there will be a significant incidence of MTS. The radiological features of MTS are atrophy of the hippocampus, a signal change on T2 sequences and on FLAIR sequences, where it can be especially dramatic, and sometimes a loss of gray-white differentiation in the anterior temporal cortex. Four series of pediatric temporal lobe surgery with differing proportions of pathological substrates are summarized in Table 22D.3. The incidence of MTS varies between 31 per cent and 57 per cent. In a study of MTS in children and adolescents two groups of 17 patients, older or younger than 12 to 13 years, were analyzed.[24] Approximately half of the patients had atrophy involving the whole hippocampus in both groups. In the remaining patients the atrophy was focal in the head or body. FLAIR showed subtle abnormalities of the ipsilateral temporal neocortex in all the children, but only 60 per cent of the adolescents. Evidence of dual pathology, in the form of mild to moderate cortical dysplasia was

Table 22D.3 *Comparison of pathology in four pediatric series of temporal lobe resections*

Reference	n	% MRI positive	% of patients with this substrate in the resected specimen			
			MTS	Other	Nonspecific	Dual pathology
14	28	84	39.3	42.8	?	?
15	22	59	43	52*	5	?
16	42	64	31	52.4	16.6	19
13	53	76	57	19	24	17

*This includes 28.5 per cent with gliosis.

seen in 79 per cent of both groups, but did not affect the surgical outcome.

Functional imaging – radioisotope studies

There are limitations to the use of radioactive compounds in children. With improvement in structural MRI, these methods are used mainly as confirmatory methods of localization or in cases where the evidence is discordant.

The use of PET is almost entirely interictal. The most useful ligands are a glucose analogue, 2-deoxy-2[^{18}F]fluoro-D-glucose (FDG-PET) and a benzodiazepine receptor binding compound, [^{11}C]flumazenil (FMZ-PET) (see Chapter 19B). There is good correlation, for lateralization, between the presence of hippocampal sclerosis and hypometabolism on both FDG-PET and FMZ-PET. The latter shows a smaller area, and both may show bilateral disease. FDG-PET can indicate the severity of damage, and correlated with seizure outcome and intellectual function, in unilateral Sturge-Weber syndrome.[31] α-[^{11}C]Methyl-L-tryptophan has been used to identify epileptogenic tubers in tuberous sclerosis. If the findings on structural MRI, FMZ-PET and FDG-PET are coregistered, the FMZ-PET abnormality covers a larger area than the structural lesion and tends to correspond to the area of spiking, whereas FDG-PET covers an even larger area.

Focal areas of hypometabolism with FDG-PET have been demonstrated children with infantile spasms. PET showed localized abnormalities in all 23 patients and was the only investigation to localize the abnormality in 14 of the 23 patients. Focal resections were performed in all patients and 15 became seizure free (65 per cent).[32] Abnormal PET findings are not necessarily stable and the disappearance of foci on re-examination at 1 year has been described.[33] Among 67 patients with infantile spasms, 66 per cent had some asymmetric features in their clinical assessments, neurophysiological investigations or radiological findings. Nine of these patients were operated and PET studies were important in localizing the surgical target in two cases without MRI abnormalities.[34]

In SPECT the injected tracer measures regional cerebral blood flow (rCBF). The tracer is fixed within the brain between 15 s and 40 s after intravenous injection and remains fixed for some hours, allowing later imaging. Premixed versions of the tracer are available for rapid injection. As a focal seizure progresses, local cerebral blood flow at first increases and then decreases. Rapidly propagating seizures, such as those from the frontal lobe, may generalize before the tracer reaches the brain region, making localization impossible. A study of 71 admissions of 59 children, aged 18 months to 17 years, showed that appropriate injections were achieved on 48 occasions.[35] There were 46 scans and 42 of these studies (93 per cent) were localizing. Cross *et al.* studied 35 children who underwent surgery: 13 children had hippocampal sclerosis, 11 showed interictal hypoperfusion and 8 ictal hyperperfusion. There were 8 children with cortical dysplasia, all of whom showed ictal hyperperfusion. Their conclusion that ictal SPECT probably adds little to the information from interictal SPECT is interesting.[36]

SPECT studies may be useful in patients without MRI abnormality, or to prevent intracranial recording.

fMRI

These investigations rely on changes in the MRI signal related to the proportion of deoxyhemoglobin in the blood. This BOLD (blood oxygenation level dependent) signal can then be coregistered with appropriate structural MRI sequences.[37] Motor mapping in both adults and children is accurate when compared with intraoperative findings. Although we have found this method reliable in intact patients with small lesions, the movement artifact has been a considerable problem in patients with hemiplegia or hemiparesis.

Clinical neurophysiology

Focus localization is possible with interictal scalp recording, especially if there are sleep recordings with appropriate electrode placements. A lateralized focus is present in 64 per cent of children, rising to 96 per cent where a structural lesion, such as MTS, was a selection criterion. Videotelemetry can confirm the nature of the patients' habitual seizures. It can also distinguish multiple seizure types and nonepileptic events. Thus, unless the interictal scalp findings are very clear, videotelemetry should be undertaken.

Subdural recordings are probably used more often in children than in adults. In the younger age groups, where cortical neuronal migration disorder is common, the extent of the pathology, the epileptogenic zone and the functional importance of abnormal cortex may need to be assessed. Subdural recordings are most useful in non-lesional epilepsies. They have not been used in our hemispherectomy candidates and only rarely in those with temporal lobe epilepsy.

Platinum electrodes are available commercially from four contact strips to large 8×8 arrays. Patients with indwelling electrodes should have antibiotic cover from insertion until at least 24 h after removal. Intracranial electrodes carry risks of infection, edema and hemorrhage. Subdural strip electrodes have a very low risk and no complications were reported in 300 cases.[38] More complications arise when larger subdural arrays are used. In our center significant complications were seen in 24 per cent of 93 patients implanted with 20-, 32- or 64-contact mats. Infection was seen in 13 per cent, there was transient neurological deterioration in 8 per cent, and significant subdural hematomas in 2 per cent. Subdural grids may be complicated by aseptic meningitis, which can be severe. Local cerebral swelling can be a problem, especially in patients who have been previously operated at that site, and in whom tedious dissection of adhesions has been necessary. Most of the infection occurs locally within the wound and in the extradural space, and meningitis or encephalitis has not been seen. The likelihood of infection increases with prolonged implantation, which should therefore be kept to a minimum. In one study, expected adverse events, such as fever, CSF leakage, nausea and headache, occurred in 41 per cent of patients and unexpected adverse events occurred in 5 per cent.[39] In contrast, Duchowny reported no adverse effects in 45 adolescents and children implanted with subdural electrodes and found the technique practical and relatively safe.[40] Depth electrodes have only been used very occasionally in children and there is one report of depth electrode exploration to locate a medial frontal focus in a 12-year-old child.

MAGNETOENCEPHALOGRAPHY

Magnetoencephalography (MEG) constructs equivalent dipoles from magnetic signals in the brain. These dipoles can then be coregistered with appropriate MRI sequences to provide magnetic source imaging (MSI). Because of the expense of setting up and maintaining this facility, especially when the number of recording channels is high, this is a scarce resource. Minassian et al. described this investigation in 11 children with extratemporal, nonlesional

epilepsy. In 10 patients the interictal epileptiform discharges were congruent with the ictal onset zone, as revealed by chronic subdural recording.[41]

Neuropsychological assessment

This is important both in localization and in the prediction of outcome of cerebral resections. Because of variations in age and developmental status, this assessment requires a skilled and experienced team. Oxbury describes in detail the appropriate tests to assess intellectual function and memory.[42] Holthausen analyses the nature and development of hemispheric defects.[43]

Speech and language testing is important in the surgical management of epilepsy. The gold standard for language dominance is the intracarotid sodium amytal test (ISA). This test needs cooperation from the child, limiting its use in younger children and in those with limited intellectual capacity. Two groups, using intravenous anesthesia for the insertion and manipulation of the angiographic catheter, have obtained meaningful results in children aged between 5 and 16 years.[44,45] Language dominance was established in 63 per cent of children and memory status in 64 per cent; those who failed were younger. It is difficult, even in experienced centers, to obtain a meaningful result from the ISA test in children less than 10 years old.

None of the noninvasive alternatives, including transcranial stimulation, PET studies and MEG studies, are used regularly. fMRI may be a noninvasive alternative for establishing speech laterality. The tests used, and the validity of testing, are discussed by Bookheimer.[37] The area of activation is more extensive in children and there is also more right hemisphere activation. A patient has been described whose language area remained inactivated for 2 weeks after a bout of partial status.[46]

Phased selection

The children proceed from one phase to the next until it is clear that a particular operation is appropriate or that no surgery is possible. At each investigation, especially where there is discomfort or risk, a full discussion is essential, not only of that procedure, but also of where it will lead. Table 22D.4 illustrates the procedure and the phased selection of 120 children.

SURGICAL PROCEDURES

Epilepsy surgery in children, especially in the younger age group, should be performed by a pediatric neurosurgeon in a center specializing in epilepsy surgery. An agreement

Table 22D.4 *Fate of 120 children admitted to a presurgical assessment programme*

Phase 1A
Clinical history and review of previous notes
Routine and sleep EEG with appropriate scalp lead placements
MRI – epilepsy protocol – GA if necessary
Neuropsychological and developmental assessment
Quality of life and neuropsychiatric assessment

Phase 1B
Videotelemetry with scalp leads
Videotelemetry with minor invasive leads
   sphenoidal leads
   subtemporal subdural strips
Advanced MRI protocols, e.g. T2 mapping, volumetrics
Functional brain imaging
   PET
   ictal SPECT
   fMRI
   MEG
Intracarotid sodium amytal (Wada) test

Phase 2
Videotelemetry with major invasive electrodes (subdural mats – depth electrodes)
Appropriate hypothesis
Observation of seizures and electrophysiological correlates
Stimulation to determine epileptic thresholds
Stimulation to obtain functional information such as motor and sensory function or speech and language

	Stop	Operate	Go to next phase
Phase 1A	17	40	63
Phase 1B	18	23	22
Phase 2	2	20	

regarding the benefits and risks of the procedure should be made between the epilepsy surgery team, the parents and the child where appropriate. Most parents will accept a reasonable risk and the inevitability of some cognitive or other changes in exchange for a reasonable prospect of seizure control. In adults the series of reported patients are large and contain a high proportion of temporal lobe resections. By contrast, in children there are age-related risks, the proportion of extratemporal resections is greater and the number of patients reported, especially in the younger age groups, is smaller. After 10 years of age, the morbidity and mortality probably approximates to that of adult or mixed series. In modern epilepsy surgery operative mortality is commendably low. There was only 1 death from hematoma in 654 procedures in Sweden between 1990 and 1995.[47] In the King's/Maudsley series from 1976 to 2001 there have been 818 procedures resulting in 7 perioperative deaths (0.86 per cent). Nonneurological morbidity in the form of infection or intracranial

hematoma is equally low and the incidence of infection is around 0.5 per cent.

There was no mortality in 32 children undergoing frontal lobe surgery, and transient neurological or surgical complications in only 4 patients.[48] There were complications in 7 per cent of 42 children undergoing temporal lobectomy.[49] One would expect more problems in the younger patients. In patients aged less than 3 years at surgery, Duchowny *et al.* reported a surgical mortality of 6 per cent in 31 children[40] whereas Sugimoto reported no mortality in 23 children.[50] Certain procedures might be expected to have greater morbidity and mortality. However, the technique of hemispherectomy, which involves major tissue resection, has been modified to become safer in the last 10–15 years. Resection of hypothalamic hamartoma, where access is difficult, had no mortality and low morbidity, especially the transcallosal approach.[51]

Outcome measures for epilepsy surgery are not easy. The scale proposed by Engel in 1987 (Table 22D.5), has been generally accepted.[52] Recently, an alternative scheme has been proposed in which the number of seizure-free days is measured. Seizure counting, by whatever means, is only one outcome measure and changes in cognitive function, neurologic development, and psychiatric abnormalities are also important to measure. Improvements in quality of life paralleled seizure relief on the Engel outcome scale in 64 patients undergoing epilepsy surgery before the age of 18 years.[53] The responsibilities of the epilepsy surgery team extend beyond the surgery and involve rehabilitation and careful, long-term follow-up.

Resective procedures

The principles of resective surgery are complex. Areas can be defined in relation to focal epilepsy such as the irritative zone, the lesional zone, etc. as outlined by Luders.[54] The most important of these is the epileptogenic zone, defined as **the cortical region that may generate seizures**. The total resection of this epileptogenic zone is necessary and sufficient to control seizures. However, the methodology is not yet available to define the epileptogenic zone adequately and the practical results of surgery support the notion that this is a limited working concept. In pediatric epilepsy surgery, in which a high proportion of patients have malformations of cortical development and where the whole lesion may not be demonstrated, even with very sophisticated brain imaging, some of the neurophysiological properties associated with the epileptogenic zone may be a means of recognizing the true extent of the pathology. Chassoux *et al.* describe the value of neurophysiological signatures in identifying areas of focal cortical dysplasia. In patients operated for frontal lobe epilepsy, including some children and adolescents,

Table 22D.5 *Engel outcome scale*[26]

Class I	Seizure free
A	Completely seizure free
B	Auras only since surgery
C	Some seizures after surgery, but seizure free for at least 2 years
D	Atypical generalized convulsion with antiepileptic drug withdrawal
Class II	*Rare seizures ('almost seizure free')*
A	Initially seizure free, but rare seizures now (2–3 per year)
B	Rare seizures since surgery
C	More than rare seizures since surgery, but rare seizures for at least 2 years
D	Nocturnal seizures only, which do not cause disability.
Class III	*Worthwhile improvement*
A	Worthwhile seizure improvement (70–90 per cent reduction in seizure frequency)
B	Prolonged seizure free intervals, amounting to half the follow-up period but not less than 2 years.
Class IV	*No worthwhile improvement*
A	Significant seizure reduction
B	No appreciable changes
C	Seizures worse

the best results were obtained when seizure patterns associated with focal cortical dysplasia had been eliminated from the postresection electrocorticogram.[55]

There have been varying reports on the usefulness of chronic subdural recording to identify the epileptogenic zone. Where there was a diffuse lesion or no discrete lesion, identification of the epileptogenic zone seems to improve outcome or make a good outcome possible. A study of 75 patients less than 12 years old, using both the anatomical lesion and interictal and ictal neurophysiological data, noted that complete resection of the epileptogenic zone was associated with a good outcome.[56] Fukuda *et al.* showed that the epileptogenic zone was within the lesion in focal cortical dysplasia, whereas it was perilesional in DNET, and that it was necessary to identify and remove the epileptogenic areas for a good outcome.[57] However, in 6 of 15 children with gangliogliomas studied with subdural grids, the extent of resection of areas of ictal onset did not correspond with outcome whereas completeness of resection of the tumor did.[58] Similarly, in 17 of 34 children with brain tumors who underwent chronic subdural recording, only 2 had a distinct ictal onset zone that could be identified and resected.[59] Finally, a discrete lesion on preoperative imaging was the best predictor of a good outcome In 31 patients less than 3 years of age, and in nonlesional cases, the extent of cortical removal did not correlate with the seizure outcome.[40]

In conclusion, resective surgery should be based on removal of the lesion in patients with a discrete lesion. Where there is no discrete lesion, both acute and chronic neurophysiologic recording may be helpful in determining the extent of the resection.

Temporal lobe resections

The selection criteria for temporal lobe surgery are similar in children and adults. The MRI, seizure semiology, neurophysiological findings and other data should be concordant. Dual pathology is more common in children and may be a significant factor in planning the resection. The seizure outcome, especially in younger children, is determined by the pathological substrate. It is important to remove the mesial temporal structures adequately. Spencer's approach through the temporal horn, exposed by a limited anterior temporal resection, is probably the most effective.[60] We have performed temporal lobectomy in 67 children aged 16 years or less, and selective amygdalo-hippocampectomy in 4, with no operative deaths. Three patients sustained limb weakness, transient in one and leaving a mild functional deficit in the other two patients. Two patients had significant visual field defects. The cognitive outcome depends upon the pathology. Patients with earlier onset epilepsy and those with lower preoperative IQ scores show less cognitive decline following surgery. Children of normal intelligence, with a discrete lesion in the dominant temporal lobe, are likely to suffer a decline in language function and verbal memory, which may not recover. If there is a preoperative deficit, it is likely to remain. There is little evidence that surgical technique affects this outcome, although selective amygdalo-hippocampectomy may have less effect on verbal function. Improvement in behavior following temporal lobe resections can occur and psychiatric problems are not common, particularly in young children. Five of the 70 children on whom we have performed temporal lobectomy have experienced psychiatric problems, and four of these five children were aged over 12 years. The problems included depression in two children, psychosis in two and another syndrome in one child. The results of surgery, after comparable and substantial periods of follow-up, appear better in children than in adults. The outcome with regard to seizures is influenced by the age of the patient and the pathological substrate. A beneficial result was seen in 26 of 29 patients (90 per cent) who underwent temporal lobectomy, most of whom had mesial temporal scleriosis.[61] Our own results from temporal lobectomy are presented in Table 22D.6.

In conclusion, temporal lobectomy in suitable pediatric candidates will produce seizure freedom in approximately 65 per cent of patients and significant relief in a further 20 per cent. The physical and cognitive morbidity is low and improvement in quality of life can be expected.

Table 22D.6 *Comparison of the results of temporal lobe resection in adults and children*

	Children	Adults
n	71	247
Engel 1A	42.2%	25.5%
Engel 1	64.8%	56.6%
Improved (Engel 3A or better)	84.5%	81.4%
Not improved (Engel 3B or worse)	15.5%	16.2%
Died	0%	2.4%
Follow-up	2–24 years (mean 7.24)	2–23 years (mean 6.55)

Extratemporal resection

Extratemporal resections involve mostly the frontal lobe and are commoner in children than in adults. MRI may demonstrate lesions that cross lobar boundaries, or are closely related to eloquent cortex, posing the dilemma of whether lesionectomy will produce a good outcome or whether it is necessary to remove surrounding, apparently epileptogenic cortex. This raises the two issues of whether resection of the surrounding cortex will risk a significant neurological or intellectual deficit, and whether lesionectomy based upon MRI findings will suffice. If a lesion is very discrete, even if it is located within primary motor or sensory cortex, then lesionectomy is unlikely to produce a permanent deficit although a transient one may occur. If the lesion is diffuse, as sometimes seen in neuronal migration disorders, or there is no structural abnormality on adequate MRI examination, then the epileptogenic zone may be located partly or entirely within eloquent cortex. Careful mapping using subdural electrodes may be necessary to predict the effects of a resection accurately, or to plan an alternative strategy such as multiple subpial transection.

Extratemporal surgery has a less good outcome than temporal lobe surgery in terms of seizure outcome and complications. In a series of patients operated under 18 years of age, 54 per cent were seizure free (Engel 1A), 69 per cent were in Engel's category 1 and there was a significant improvement in 84 per cent.[62] This group emphasized that identification of eloquent areas by mapping or other means and careful surgical technique minimized neurological complications. Important technical points included careful endopial dissection, using an ultrasonic aspirator, preservation of the remote vascular supply and minimal manipulation of the white matter. Their mortality and morbidity was low. One perioperative death occurred from unexplained swelling following a frontal lobectomy (2 per cent); five patients had an increased or new motor deficit (8 per cent), three patients a sensory deficit (5 per cent), and two patients a complete homonymous hemianopia (3 per cent). Nonneurological complications occurred in eight

patients (12 per cent). We have 42 patients aged 17 years or less who underwent extratemporal resections, 16 of whom had resections involving the frontal lobe (38 per cent). There were five patients with an increased or *de novo* hemiplegia (19 per cent) and one had a visual field defect (4 per cent). Motor deficits occurred only in patients with cortical dysplasia and did not complicate removal of indolent tumors. Overall 15 per cent were completely seizure free (1A), 27 per cent were Engel 1, 73 per cent were improved and 27 per cent unimproved.

Frontal lobe resections make up most of the extratemporal resections in both mixed and pediatric series and up to 60 per cent of patients become seizure free. The removal of a discrete lesion detectable by MRI is associated with the most satisfactory outcome. Resection of focal neoplasms carries the best prognosis. Resections in, or adjacent to, the supplementary motor area result in transient neurologic deficits in 89 per cent of patients, virtually all of which resolve leaving at most a subtle motor handicap.

There are few studies of resections from eloquent areas in children. Resections from these areas should be designed to minimize or eliminate potential neurological and intellectual deficits. In young children, where cooperation with noninvasive tests may be difficult, subdural mapping and intraoperative evoked motor and sensory potentials may be necessary. Pathological lesions may change the normal distribution of functional areas. With central lesions, a different disposition of central activation makes conventional assumptions about the location of functioning areas unreliable, particularly in patients with cortical dysplasia.[63]

In conclusion, extratemporal resection, even from eloquent areas of cortex, can be beneficial. There are varying degrees of success and the neurological morbidity is dependent upon the nature and location of the underlying pathological substrate, the identification of eloquent areas by mapping or other means, and on careful surgical technique.

Hypothalamic hamartoma

This lesion is associated with precocious puberty and epilepsy. Two epileptic syndromes are associated with hypothalamic hamartoma. One presents in early childhood with gelastic epilepsy, multiple seizure types, severe intractability, developmental delay and a severe behavior disorder. The other presents at a later age with gelastic and complex partial seizures that tend not to secondarily generalize. This second group usually has normal intellect and behavior.

SPECT studies and intralesional recordings show that these lesions are intrinsically epileptogenic. Surgical procedures that do not deal with the lesion directly, such as callosotomy, temporal lobectomy or vagus nerve stimulation, have been shown to be of no value. The results of surgery are much better in patients with precocious puberty, where the success rate is high and the complications low. This may relate to the fact that those with precocious puberty tend to be associated with pedunculated (parahypothalamic) lesions and those without precocious puberty with sessile (intrahypothalamic) lesions.[64]

The approaches to these lesions have included:

- destruction by minor invasive or noninvasive means
- surgical disconnection rather than volume resection
- total or subtotal resection by an open surgical approach.

Radiofrequency destruction of a hamartoma was associated with complete remission in one child.[65] Improvement in seizure control, but not seizure freedom, was described in two children treated by gamma knife radiosurgery.[66] Four of eight patients in a multicenter study were rendered seizure free and the other four had improved seizure control.[67] In addition, behavior was improved in two patients. Of 13 children aged between 14 months and 19 years who had a combined disconnection and resection,[68] 5 became seizure free (Engel class 1) and only 1 patient was not improved. One child sustained a hemiplegia. The relationship of the lesion to the interpeduncular cistern and the walls of the hypothalamus influences the outcome of total or subtotal resection of the lesion. A transcallosal, interforniceal, transventricular approach with stereotactic assistance was used in 17 children, in whom 9 had precocious puberty.[69] All of the lesions were sessile and 7 were predominantly intraventricular. Ten patients were seizure free after surgery and 6 of the remaining seven were improved (Engel 3A or better). There were no permanent major complications and the morbidity included mild residual hemiparesis in 1 patient, persistent appetite stimulation in 3, and persistent short-term memory problems in 6. There was marked improvement in behavior and quality of life in 15 of these 17 patients. Seizure freedom correlated with normal preoperative intellect and absence of secondarily generalized epilepsy but not with extent of resection.[69]

The choice of surgical approach to hypothalamic hamartomas depends upon the type of epilepsy and the location and size of the lesion.

Hemispherectomy

The indications for hemispherectomy are intractable epilepsy secondary to gross unilateral hemispheric disease. The hemisphere disease should be sufficient to give, or to anticipate, a severe hemispheric neurological deficit including a visual field defect. There are four pathological substrates: atrophic lesions, Rasmussen's disease, hemimegalencephaly and a residual miscellany of lesions such as Sturge-Weber disease. Neuroimaging is important in demonstrating the etiology of the hemispheric

disease and to confirm the structural integrity of the other hemisphere. Although the lesion is unilateral, there may be bilateral cognitive dysfunction. Indeed, Krynauw, who reported the first series of hemispherectomy for epilepsy, suggested that dementia was a primary indication for surgery.[70] The neurophysiological response of the affected hemisphere may be limited and there may be more neurophysiological abnormalities in the unaffected hemisphere. Videotelemetry may occasionally be necessary to confirm the origin of the seizures.

A major selection criterion is the extent to which hemisphere function, especially language, is preserved or transferred. This is influenced by the age of onset of the seizures and the speed of progression of the disease. Early studies of sensorimotor function suggested that function worsened in about 7 per cent of patients after hemispherectomy. Holthausen et al. noted that patients with acquired lesions could not actively extend their fingers and had very marked pyramidal signs after hemispherectomy. In contrast, patients with developmental lesions, such as hemimegalencephaly, were able to actively extend and flex their fingers after operation and had only mild pyramidal signs.[39]

The effects of hemispherectomy on speech and language are complex. The age at the time of hemispheric insult, the prior speech development and the length and severity of the seizure disorder prior to surgery all influence the ability of the brain to reorganize function. Up to around 5 years of age the hemispheres are equipotential in the development of speech and language. Forcing verbal and nonverbal functions into one hemisphere results in a 'crowding' effect whereby nonverbal function is less well developed to allow more verbal development. If the epileptiform activity affects the unaffected hemisphere following surgery, this also interferes markedly with reorganization and cognitive outcome. Speech and language outcome is less good in patients with hemimegalencephaly or late onset of Rasmussen's disease in the dominant hemisphere. The preoperative development quotients influenced outcome in patients with cortical dysgenesis who underwent hemispherectomy. Those with a preoperative developmental quotient >50 had a chance to attain normal development whereas those with a quotient <10 never did.[71] A high preoperative development quotient and a seizure-free outcome were the best predictors of a good cognitive outcome. A comparison of preoperative and postoperative nonverbal communication found that the patients were less good at nonverbal communication than controls but tended to improve to the control level after operation, independent of the side of operation.[72] In six children with Rasmussen's disease, who had developed normal language development before undergoing left hemispherectomy between ages 7 and 14 years, there was a considerable improvement in their receptive language function at 1 year but expressive language functions remained severely impaired.[73] Expressive language function appears to do better in those with a developmental rather than an acquired etiology. In cortical dysgenesis there can be a poor developmental and intellectual performance from the beginning, which will only improve if part of the poor intellectual performance is due to seizure activity.

The original technique of hemispherectomy, first described by Dandy and subsequently by Krynauw,[70] consisted of removal of the whole hemisphere except the basal ganglia. Hoffmann used the technique of hemidecortication, at the level of the main white matter tracts.[74] Until the introduction of functional hemispherectomy by Rasmussen, hemispherectomy fell into decline because of the scale of the surgery and the late delayed complication of cerebral hemosiderosis.[75] There are now three techniques which rely upon microsurgical ventricular access resulting in a less extensive and shorter operation. They all involve the same disconnection with complete division of the corpus callosum, isolation of the frontal and temporal lobes by division of the appropriate fiber tracts anteriorly and posteriorly, division through the internal capsule and in some cases resection of the insular cortex. All of these techniques are easy in patients with atrophic lesions but are more difficult in those with hemimegalencephaly, where the anatomy is usually distorted and the landmarks displaced. Modern neuronavigation systems have lessened this difficulty.

The mortality and morbidity of these operations is low. There were 3 deaths in 63 patients undergoing functional hemispherotomy: 1 unexplained, 1 secondary to venous infarction and 1 with diffuse swelling.[76] Three patients needed shunts and there was 1 infection. Hemispherotomy or peri-insular hemispherectomy is the preferred operation, especially in infants, because of shorter operating times and reduced blood loss. Kestle and colleagues compared hemidecortication in 5 patients and peri-insular hemispherotomy in 11. On all measures such as blood loss,

postoperative fever, ventriculoperitoneal shunt insertion and length of postoperative stay in hospital, patients subjected to peri-insular hemispherotomy did better.[77]

The first Palm Desert symposium in 1985 reported that 77 per cent became seizure free and only 5 per cent failed to benefit from hemispherectomy[52] (see Table 22D.7). A multicenter retrospective study of 328 hemispherectomies found that seizure relief rate varied with etiology and to a lesser extent with surgical technique[11] (see Table 22D.7). Outcome was related to the completeness of disconnection, although those with dysplasia did worse with all techniques. Decortication was the worst technique with all pathologies.[11] It is generally accepted that behavior and intellectual performance also improve when the seizures are controlled.

Stereotactic radiosurgery

This technique uses radiation directed at a target with a stereotactic frame, and in young children requires general anesthesia. It has been used in children for many years for the treatment of arteriovenous malformations and tumors. The treatment of epilepsy with radiosurgery was pioneered by Barcia-Salorio and it has been used by Regis and others in the treatment of mesial temporal sclerosis and hypothalamic hamartoma.[78,79] The effect of the radiosurgery may take some months and the procedure may cause brain swelling. The long-term risks from complications such as radiation necrosis and possible tumor induction are unknown but probably small. In one study, 31 patients, aged from 1 to 25 years, with nonprogressive lesions <2.0 cm in diameter were treated with the gamma knife.[80] At follow-up, 12 patients had an Engel class 1 outcome (39 per cent), 2 had an improvement (6 per cent) and in 9 there was no improvement (55 per cent). The Miami group, using this technique, rendered a child with an insular lesion seizure free, and in two children with hypothalamic hamartoma, one obtained complete seizure control and the other had a >90 per cent reduction in seizure frequency.[81]

FUNCTIONAL SURGERY

Functional procedures are designed to ameliorate the clinical manifestations of seizures by modification of the neuronal pathways, but they rarely abolish seizures. Currently there are two useful procedures: division of the corpus callosum, and interruption of intracortical connections by multiple subpial transections. Experimental treatments under study include local brain cooling, localized drug delivery through implanted pump systems, and local repair either with gene therapy or with neural transplantation.

Table 22D.7 *Aetiology and seizure relief from hemispherectomy. Results of Holthausen Multicentre Study[11]*

	n	Per cent seizure free
Technique		
Hemispherotomy	56	86
Adams modification	60	78
Functional hemispherectomy	109	66
Anatomical hemispherectomy	42	64
Decortication	61	61
Aetiology		
Sturge-Weber	28	82
Hemiatrophy	44	77
Rasmussen's	83	77
Vascular	46	76
Other	28	68
Cortical dysplasia	99	57

Division of the corpus callosum

Introduced in 1940, and modified to a staged procedure in the 1970s, corpus callosotomy is effective chiefly against drop attacks although other generalized seizures also respond. MRI studies have shown that a 70–80 per cent disconnection is effective. Sequential radiofrequency lesions and stereotactic radiosurgery have been used to make the lesion but are not established techniques.

Corpus callosotomy is associated with a significant morbidity. Transient complications were recorded in 30 per cent of 26 children, all of which resolved within 3 months.[82] Four instances of transient hemiparesis were reported in a study of 20 patients.[83] Transient mutism, which always recovered completely, was reported in 28 per cent of another series.[84] Among our 28 patients undergoing anterior callosotomy there was one perioperative death from pneumonia and two instances of acute anterior cerebral ischemia with no long-term effects. A few patients had transient limb weakness and one an extradural hematoma. In summary, the mortality is between 0 and 6 per cent, permanent neurological deficit is less than 5 per cent, and transient deficit up to 30 per cent.

The indications for corpus callosotomy are not well established. Drop attacks, intractable generalized seizures and episodes of status are the epileptic conditions most likely to be helped. Most patients who benefit have bilateral synchronous discharges in the resting scalp EEG. Only drop attacks show major benefit and these remit in 70–100 per cent of patients. There is a tendency for the results of callosotomy to decline after the first 2 years but the drop attacks do not usually return to their preoperative severity.

Multiple subpial transection (MST)

Morrell noted that the horizontal (tangential) fibers of the cortex propagated the epileptic discharge and the vertical (radial) fibers subserved function. He proposed that division of the horizontal fibers at regular intervals in a cortical epileptic focus would curtail the epileptic discharges but preserve function.[85] This procedure has been shown to be useful where an epileptic focus involves eloquent cortex such as in primary motor or sensory cortex or language cortex, in Landau-Kleffner syndrome, and in some children with multifocal epilepsy.

MST with and without resection was performed in 84 patients and 49 per cent of the combined group became seizure free as did 37 per cent of those treated with MST alone. Serious neurological deficit occurred in 7 per cent.[86] A multicenter meta-analysis of MST in 211 patients demonstrated that this technique was effective against both generalized and partial seizures.[87] EEG localization, age at epilepsy onset, duration of epilepsy, and location of MST were not significant predictors of outcome for any kinds of seizures after MST, with or without resection. New neurologic deficits were observed in 23 per cent of MST with resection and 19 per cent of those without resection.[87] A relapse rate of 19 per cent after several years has been reported.

MST has also been used to control refractory status epilepticus.[88] In addition, MST with resection was used in seven children with malignant rolandic-sylvian epilepsy.[89] Three children became seizure free and the remaining four had rare seizures. Shimizu described the use of MST with and without resection in 31 children in whom the focus was in unresectable speech or motor cortex. Of the 25 cases followed for >1 year, there was no morbidity or mortality, 10 patients had an Engel group 1 or 2 outcome, and 3 had no benefit.[90] Shimizu also demonstrated hyperexcitability in an area of cortical dysgenesis in the right central motor cortex using transcranial magnetic stimulation. Following MST, the seizures were controlled and the hyperexcitability was abolished.[91] MST has been used by ourselves and others to treat Rasmussen disease, but no patient has achieved complete seizure control.[92,93]

Landau-Kleffner syndrome (acquired epileptic aphasia) is characterized by the development between 4 and 7 years of age of a persistent aphasia and behavioral disorder in association with seizures (see Chapter 13). The untreated patient makes a slow and imperfect recovery and, if the patient has been mute for more than 1 year, a severe and permanent language disability will follow. Morrell believed that in some cases of Landau-Kleffner syndrome a single sylvian focus produced, through secondary epileptogenesis, a severe bilateral EEG disturbance in sleep. This EEG disturbance prevented the development of speech in the secondarily affected hemisphere. In 1995, he described improvements in language and behavior in 12 of 14 patients treated with MST.[94] Although many of these patients have severe diffuse bilateral epileptiform discharges, MST appears to be most appropriate in those patients with Landau-Kleffner syndrome in whom the epileptiform activity can be demonstrated to be arising unilaterally, usually from deep within the sylvian fissure. The pentothal suppression test, intracarotid sodium amytal (Wada) test and MEG have been used to identify the driving hemisphere. Morrell operated on nine patients on the left side and five on the right;[94] we have carried out seven left-sided operations and three right-sided operations. Children with a severe bilateral EEG disturbance in sleep for more than 36 months do not have normal language outcome. Thus, MST should be considered in any child with Landau-Kleffner syndrome who has had a severe bilateral EEG disturbance in sleep for more than 2 years and who is not responsive to steroids or other medication, particularly when behavior is severely disturbed and seizures are frequent.[95]

Improvement in language function and behavior and improvement in the EEG are the criteria for a good outcome in these patients. Only 4 of 18 treated in Chicago failed to improve and only 1 of our 10 patients came into that category. In retrospect, our failure probably related to poor selection.

Comparison of preoperative and postoperative language scores in the Rush patients showed significant improvement after surgery. The later the tests were given after surgery the better the result, and the shorter the period between language deterioration and surgery the greater the improvement.[96] Four of our patients had a transient deterioration some months after surgery with increased seizures, deterioration or halting of language improvement and deterioration in EEG. Three patients improved after a short time, one needed restoration of anticonvulsant medication, another underwent reoperation. Provided that the selection is rigorous we anticipate that 70 per cent of patients with Landau-Kleffner syndrome will benefit, especially if the surgery is carried out promptly.

Patil has used MST in more difficult cases. In 15 patients he excised dominant seizure foci remaining after MST and 9 became seizure free (60 per cent).[97] In patients with multifocal and bihemispheric foci, using MST with other techniques, he reported that 9 of 19 patients became seizure free, or had rare seizures.[98] In 50 children with autistic spectrum disorder, Lewine and Patil identified epileptiform activity using MEG in 41 children (82 per cent). There was an improvement in the autistic features and language in 12 of the 18 patients who had MST.[99] The selection of patients who might benefit is clearly difficult, and the use of MST in the management of autistic spectrum must be considered speculative at this time.

STIMULATION

Because of reliable hardware and longer battery life, this is now a practical method of treatment. Three methods are available: indirect stimulation of the brain through the vagus nerve, stimulation of localized deep brain targets using technology proven in the treatment of movement disorder, and the possibility of direct cortical stimulation for which the technology is available.

Vagus nerve stimulation

Vagus nerve stimulation is described in Chapter 22C and has also been reviewed by Polkey[100] and Wilder.[101]

Deep brain and cortical stimulation

Stimulation of both cerebellar hemispheres was described in 1973. Later targets have been the subthalamic nucleus, the centromedian nucleus and the anterior nucleus of the thalamus, and latterly the temporal cortex. Lesions such as hypothalamic hamartomas have also been stimulated. None of these methods has yet proved to be of value and they are not in general use. The topic was reviewed by Fisher[102] in 1997 and Velasco[103] in 2001.

REOPERATION

Reoperation is inevitable in an epilepsy surgery practice as concepts of epilepsy change and new technologies emerge. Patients should be assessed against the present indications for resective surgery with the same rigor that would be applied to a first operation. In the temporal lobe, this comes down to a lesion. In the frontal lobe, the neurophysiological findings, both in the investigation phase and at operation, may have greater importance. Two factors of significance were found in 21 patients who underwent a second resective operation.[104] No patient with a history of CNS infection that predated the epilepsy was rendered seizure free. If the ictal EEG was concordant with the previous ictal EEG and MRI findings then all reoperated patients either became seizure free or had at least a 95 per cent reduction in seizures. In adult or mixed series of patients the outcome from resective reoperation is around 44 per cent seizure-free and 25 per cent not affected, and when there is a structural lesion that has been missed or incompletely removed, then 80–90 per cent became seizure-free. Unexpected morbidity is variable between the series and may be higher than in first operations.

In a retrospective study of reoperation in 20 children from Miami, extension of the initial resection was carried out in eight patients and 66 per cent became seizure free. Five patients underwent a corticectomy or lobectomy remote from the first operation and four patients had a multilobar resection which may have 'included' the original resection site. Four of these nine patients (44 per cent) became seizure free. Finally, three patients underwent hemispherectomy and two became seizure free. However, there was unexpected morbidity in three of the four patients who underwent multilobar resection.[105] These findings are consistent with previous accounts of reoperation, which should be seriously considered as part of an epilepsy surgery program and offered to patients with appropriate indications.

KEY POINTS

- Surgical treatment of intractable childhood epilepsy is a **safe and practical** practice when carried out in experienced centers by a pediatric multidisciplinary team
- It is essential to achieve an **understanding between the team, patient and parents or caregivers** regarding the nature of the problem and a realistic account of the solution
- The patient should proceed through those parts of a **staged investigation program** necessary to decide about the possibility and nature of the surgical procedure
- **Resective procedures** are well established, carry the possibility of complete cure and have acceptable levels of mortality and morbidity
- **Functional procedures** can alleviate epilepsy and produce significant improvements in development and quality of life in appropriate cases
- Surgical options should be **reconsidered** when one procedure fails
- It is particularly important that there should be an adequate **follow-up and aftercare program** in children following epilepsy surgery

REFERENCES

1. Taylor DC, Cross JH, Harkness W, Neville BG. Defining new aims and providing new categories for measuring outcome of epilepsy surgery in children. In: Tuxhorn I, Holthausen H, Boenigk H (eds) *Paediatric Epilepsy Syndromes and their Surgical Treatment*. London: John Libbey, 1997; 17–25.
2. Guerrini R, Dravet C, Bureau M, Mancini J, Canapicchi R, Livet MO, Belmonte A. Diffuse and localised dysplasias of the cerebral cortex: Clinical presentation, outcome and proposal for a morphologic MRI classification based on a study of 90 patients. In: Guerrini R, Andermann F, Canapicchi R, Roger J, Zifkin BG, Pfanner P (eds) *Dysplasias of Cerebral Cortex and Epilepsy*. Philadelphia: Lippincott-Raven, 1996; 255–269.
3. Kloss S, Pieper T, Pannek H, Holthausen H, Tuxhorn I. Epilepsy surgery in children with focal cortical dysplasia (FCD): results of long-term seizure outcome. *Neuropediatrics* 2002; **33**(1): 21–26.
4. Leventer RJ, Phelan EM, Coleman LT, *et al*. Clinical and imaging features of cortical malformations in childhood. *Neurology* 1999; **53**(4): 715–722.
5. Neville BG. Neurocutaneous syndromes. In: Oxbury JM, Polkey CE, Duchowny M (eds) *Intractable Focal Epilepsy*. London: Saunders: 2000; 225–232.
6. Koh S, Jayakar P, Dunoyer C, *et al*. Epilepsy surgery in children with tuberous sclerosis complex: presurgical evaluation and outcome. *Epilepsia* 2000; **41**(9): 1206–1213.
7. Berg AT, Testa FM, Levy SR, Shinnar S. Neuroimaging in children with newly diagnosed epilepsy: A community-based study. *Pediatrics* 2000; **106**(3): 527–532.
8. Buckingham MJ, Crone KR, Ball WS, Berger TS. Management of cerebral cavernous angiomas in children presenting with seizures. *Child's Nervous System* 1989; **5**(6): 347–349.
9. Di Rocco C, Iannelli A, Tamburrini G. Cavernomas of the central nervous system in children. A report of 22 cases. *Acta Neurochirurgica (Wien)* 1996; **138**(11): 1267–1274.
10. Sujansky E, Conradi S. Sturge-Weber syndrome: age of onset of seizures and glaucoma and the prognosis for affected children. *Journal of Child Neurology* 1995; **10**(1): 49–58.
11. Holthausen H, May TW, Adams CBT, *et al*. Seizures post hemispherectomy. In: Tuxhorn I, Holthausen H, Boenigk H (eds) *Paediatric Epilepsy Syndromes and their Surgical Treatment*. London: John Libbey, 1997; 749–773.
12. Aicardi J. Epilepsies as a presenting manifestation of brain tumors and other selected brain disorders. In: *Epilepsy in Children*. New York: Raven Press, 1994; 334–353.
13. Hauser WA, Annegers JF, Kurland LT. Incidence of epilepsy and unprovoked seizures in Rochester, Minnesota: 1935–1984. *Epilepsia* 1993; **34**(3): 453–468.
14. Riviello JJ, Honavar M, Holmes GL. Tumors and partial seizures. In: Oxbury JM, Polkey CE, Duchowny M (eds) *Intractable Focal Epilepsy*. London: Saunders: 2000; 196–212.
15. Gilles FH, Sobel E, Leviton A, *et al*. Epidemiology of seizures in children with brain tumors. The Childhood Brain Tumor Consortium. *Journal of Neurooncology* 1992; **12**(1): 53–68.
16. Crone NE, Hao L, Hart J Jr, *et al*. Electrocorticographic gamma activity during word production in spoken and sign language. *Neurology* 2001; **57**(11): 2045–2053.
17. Johnson JH, Jr, Hariharan S, Berman J, Sutton LN, Rorke LB, Molloy P *et al*. Clinical outcome of pediatric gangliogliomas: ninety-nine cases over 20 years. *Pediatr Neurosurg* 1997; **27**(4): 203–207.
18. Wang PJ, Liu HM, Fan PC, *et al*. Magnetic resonance imaging in symptomatic/cryptogenic partial epilepsies of infants and children. *Chung-Hua Min Kuo Hsiao Erh Ko i Hsueh Hui Tsa Chih* 1997; **38**(2): 127–136.
19. Pomeroy SL, Holmes SJ, Dodge PR, Feigin RD. Seizures and other neurologic sequelae of bacterial meningitis in children. *New England Journal of Medicine* 1990; **323**(24): 1651–1657.
20. Hart YM, Andermann F, Fish DR, *et al*. Chronic encephalitis and epilepsy in adults and adolescents: a variant of Rasmussen's syndrome? *Neurology* 1997; **48**(2): 418–424.
21. Andermann F. *Chronic Encephalitis and Epilepsy*. Boston: Butterworth-Heinemann, 1991.
22. Margerison JH, Corsellis JAN. Epilepsy and the temporal lobes. clinical, electroencephalographic and neuropathological study of the brain in epilepsy, with particular reference to the temporal lobes. *Brain* 1966; **89**: 499–534.
23. Sztriha L, Gururaj AK, Bener A, Nork M. Temporal lobe epilepsy in children: etiology in a cohort with new-onset seizures. *Epilepsia* 2002; **43**(1): 75–80.
24. Mohamed A, Wyllie E, Ruggieri P, *et al*. Temporal lobe epilepsy due to hippocampal sclerosis in pediatric candidates for epilepsy surgery. *Neurology* 2001; **56**(12): 1643–1649.
25. Marks DA, Kim J, Spencer DD, Spencer SS. Seizure localization and pathology following head injury in patients with uncontrolled epilepsy. *Neurology* 1995; **45**(11): 2051–2057.

26. Engel J Jr, Cascino GD, Shields WD. Surgically remediable syndromes. In: Engel JJ, Pedley TA (eds) *Epilepsy: A Comprehensive Textbook.* Philadelphia: Lippincott-Raven, 1998; 1687–1696.

27. Binnie CD, Polkey CE. Commission on Neurosurgery of the International League Against Epilepsy (ILAE) 1993–1997: recommended standards. *Epilepsia* 2000; **41**(10): 1346–1349.

28. Ounsted C, Lindsay J, Norman J. *Biological Factors in Temporal Lobe Epilepsy.* London: Heinemann, 1966.

29. Ounsted C, Lindsay J, Norman J. *Biological Factors in Temporal Lobe Epilepsy.* London: Heinemann, 1996.

30. Woo CL, Chuang SH, Becker LE, *et al.* Radiologic–pathologic correlation in focal cortical dysplasia and hemimegalencephaly in 18 children. *Pediatric Neurology* 2001; **25**(4): 295–303.

31. Kiley MA, Oxbury JM, Coley SC. Intracranial hypertension in Sturge-Weber/Klippel-Trenaunay-Weber overlap syndrome due to impairment of cerebral venous outflow. *Journal of Clinical Neurosciences* 2002; **9**(3): 330–333.

32. Chugani HT, Shewmon DA, Shields WD, *et al.* Surgery for intractable infantile spasms: neuroimaging perspectives. *Epilepsia* 1993; **34**: 764–771.

33. Metsahonkala L, Gaily E, Rantala H, *et al.* Focal and global cortical hypometabolism in patients with newly diagnosed infantile spasms. *Neurology* 2002; **58**(11): 1646–1651.

34. Kramer U, Sue WC, Mikati MA. Focal features in West syndrome indicating candidacy for surgery. *Pediatric Neurology* 1997; **16**(3): 213–217.

35. O'Brien TJ, Zupanc ML, Mullan BP, *et al.* The practical utility of performing peri-ictal SPECT in the evaluation of children with partial epilepsy. *Pediatric Neurology* 1998; **19**(1): 15–22.

36. Cross JH, Hartley L, Harkness W, *et al.* Correlation of single photon emission computed tomography with pathology and seizure outcome in children undergoing epilepsy surgery. *Neuropathology and Applied Neurobiology* 2002; **28**(2): 159–160.

37. Bookheimer SY, Cohen MS. Functional MRI. In: Engel J, Pedley TA (eds) E*pilepsy: A Comprehensive Textbook.* Philadelphia: Lippincott-Raven, 1997; 1053–1065.

38. Wyler AR, Walker G, Somes G. The morbidity of long term seizure monitoring using subdural strip recording. *Journal of Neurosurgery* 1991; **74**: 734–737.

39. Swartz BE, Rich JR, Dwan PS, *et al.* The safety and efficacy of chronically implanted subdural electrodes: a prospective study. *Surgical Neurology* 1996; **46**(1): 87–93.

40. Duchowny M, Jayakar P, Resnick T, *et al.* Epilepsy surgery in the first three years of life. *Epilepsia* 1998; **39**(7): 737–743.

41. Minassian BA, Otsubo H, Weiss S, *et al.* Magnetoencephalographic localization in pediatric epilepsy surgery: comparison with invasive intracranial electro-encephalography. *Annals of Neurology* 1999; **46**(4): 627–633.

42. Oxbury S. Neuropsychological evaluation – children. In: Engel JJ, Pedley TA (eds) *Epilepsy: A Comprehensive Textbook.* Philadelphia: Lippincott-Raven, 1998; 989–999.

43. Holthausen H, Strobl K, Pieper T, Teixeira VA, Oppel F. Prediction of motor functions post hemispherectomy. In: Tuxhorn I, Holthausen H, Boenigk H (eds) *Paediatric Epilepsy Syndromes and their Surgical Treatment.* London: John Libbey, 1997; 785–798.

44. Masters LT, Perrine K, Devinsky O, Nelson PK. Wada testing in pediatric patients by use of propofol anesthesia. *American Journal of Neuroradiology* 2000; **21**(7): 1302–1305.

45. Hamer HM, Wyllie E, Stanford L, *et al.* Risk factors for unsuccessful testing during the intracarotid amobarbital procedure in preadolescent children. *Epilepsia* 2000; **41**(5): 554–563.

46. Jayakar P, Bernal B, Santiago ML, Altman N. False lateralization of language cortex on functional MRI after a cluster of focal seizures. *Neurology* 2002; **58**(3): 490–492.

47. Rydenhag B, Silander HC. Complications of epilepsy surgery after 654 procedures in Sweden, September 1990–1995: a multicenter study based on the Swedish National Epilepsy Surgery Register. *Neurosurgery* 2001; **49**(1): 51–56.

48. Kral T, Kuczaty S, Blumcke I, *et al.* Postsurgical outcome of children and adolescents with medically refractory frontal lobe epilepsies. *Child's Nervous System* 2001; **17**(10): 595–601.

49. Sinclair DB, Wheatley M, Aronyk K, *et al.* Pathology and neuroimaging in pediatric temporal lobectomy for intractable epilepsy. *Pediatric Neurosurgery* 2001; **35**(5): 239–246.

50. Sugimoto T, Otsubo H, Hwang PA, *et al.* Outcome of epilepsy surgery in the first three years of life. *Epilepsia* 1999; **40**(5): 560–565.

51. Rosenfeld JV, Harvey AS, Wrennall J, Zacharin M, Berkovic SF. Transcallosal resection of hypothalamic hamartomas, with control of seizures, in children with gelastic epilepsy. *Neurosurgery* 2001; **48**(1): 108–118.

52. Engel J. Outcome with respect to epileptic seizures. In: Engel J (ed.) *Surgical Treatment of the Epilepsies.* New York: Raven Press, 1987; 553–571.

53. Keene DL, Loy-English I, Ventureyra EC. Long-term socioeconomic outcome following surgical intervention in the treatment of refractory epilepsy in childhood and adolescence. *Child's Nervous System* 1998; **14**(8): 362–365.

54. Luders H, Awad IA. Conceptual considerations. In: Luders H (ed.) *Epilepsy Surgery.* New York: Raven Press, 1992; 51–62.

55. Chassoux F, Devaux B, Landre E, *et al.* Stereoelectro-encephalography in focal cortical dysplasia: a 3D approach to delineating the dysplastic cortex. *Brain* 2000; **123**(8): 1733–1751.

56. Paolicchi JM, Jayakar P, Dean P, *et al.* Predictors of outcome in pediatric epilepsy surgery. *Neurology* 2000; **54**(3): 642–647.

57. Fukuda M, Kameyama S, Tomikawa M, *et al.* [Epilepsy surgery for focal cortical dysplasia and dysembryoplastic neuroepithelial tumor]. *No Shinkei Geka* 2000; **28**(2): 135–144.

58. Khajavi K, Comair YG, Prayson RA, *et al.* Childhood ganglioglioma and medically intractable epilepsy. A clinicopathological study of 15 patients and a review of the literature. *Pediatric Neurosurgery* 1995; **22**(4): 181–188.

59. Khajavi K, Comair YG, Wyllie E, *et al.* Surgical management of pediatric tumor-associated epilepsy. *Journal of Child Neurology* 1999; **14**(1): 15–25.

60. Spencer DD, Spencer SS, Mattson RH, Williamson PD, Novelly RA. Access to the posterior medial temporal structures in the surgical treatment of temporal lobe epilepsy. *Neurosurgery* 1984; **15**: 667–671.

61. Grattan-Smith JD, Harvey AS, Desmond PM, Chow CW. Hippocampal sclerosis in children with intractable temporal lobe epilepsy: detection with MR imaging. *AJR* 1993; **161**(5): 1045–1048.

62. Cataltepe O, Comair YG. Complications of extratemporal epilepsy surgery in infants and children. In: Tuxhorn I,

Holthausen H, Boenigk H (eds) *Paediatric Epilepsy Syndromes and their Surgical Treatment*. London: John Libbey, 1997; 709–725.

63. Marusic P, Najm IM, Ying Z, *et al*. Focal cortical dysplasias in eloquent cortex: functional characteristics and correlation with MRI and histopathologic changes. *Epilepsia* 2002; **43**(1): 27–32.

64. Arita K, Ikawa F, Kurisu K, *et al*. The relationship between magnetic resonance imaging findings and clinical manifestations of hypothalamic hamartoma. *Journal of Neurosurgery* 1999; **91**(2): 212–220.

65. Fukuda M, Kameyama S, Wachi M, Tanaka R. Stereotaxy for hypothalamic hamartoma with intractable gelastic seizures: technical case report. *Neurosurgery* 1999; **44**(6): 1347–1350.

66. Koo B, Ham SD, Sood S, Tarver B. Human vagus nerve electrophysiology: a guide to vagus nerve stimulation parameters. *Journal of Clinical Neurophysiology* 2001; **18**(5): 429–433.

67. Regis J, Bartolomei F, de Toffol B, *et al*. Gamma knife surgery for epilepsy related to hypothalamic hamartomas. *Neurosurgery* 2000; **47**(6): 1343–1351.

68. Fohlen M, Jalin C, Delalande O. Surgical treatment of hypothalamic hamartoma in children with refractory epilepsy. *Epilepsia* 2000; **41**: S183.

69. Harvey AS, Fereman JL, Rosenfeld JV, Zacharin M, Wrennall JA, Bailey CA, Berkovic SF. Postoperative course and seizure outcome following transcallosal resection of hypothalamic hamartoma in seventeen children with intractable gelastic epilepsy. *Epilepsia* 2001; **42**(Suppl. 7): 216.

70. Krynauw RA. Infantile hemiplegia treated by removing one cerebral hemisphere. *Journal of Neurology, Neurosurgery and Psychiatry* 1950; **13**: 243–267.

71. Maehara T, Shimizu H, Kawai K, *et al*. Postoperative development of children after hemispherotomy. *Brain and Development* 2002; **24**(3): 155–160.

72. Caplan R, Guthrie D, Shields WD, *et al*. Early onset intractable seizures: nonverbal communication after hemispherectomy. *Journal of Developmental and Behavioral Pediatrics* 1992; **5**: 348–355.

73. Boatman D, Freeman J, Vining E, *et al*. Language recovery after left hemispherectomy in children with late-onset seizures. *Annals of Neurology* 1999; **46**(4): 579–586.

74. Hoffman HJ. Hemispherectomy. In: Tuxhorn I, Holthausen H, Boenigk H (eds) *Paediatric Epilepsy Syndromes and their Surgical Treatment*. London: John Libbey, 1997; 739–742.

75. Rasmussen T. Hemispherectomy for seizures revisited. *Canadian Journal of Neurological Science* 1983; **10**: 71–78.

76. Villemure JG, Vernet O, Delalande O. Hemispheric disconnection: callosotomy and hemispherotomy. *Advances and Technical Standards in Neurosurgery* 2000; **26**: 25–78.

77. Kestle J, Connolly M, Cochrane D. Pediatric peri-insular hemispherotomy. *Pediatric Neurosurgery* 2000; **32**(1): 44–47.

78. Barcia-Salorio JL, Barcia JA, Roldan P, Hernandez G, Lopez-Gomez L. Radiosurgery of epilepsy. *Acta Neurochirurgica – Supplementum* 1993; **58**: 195–197.

79. Regis J, Bartolomei F, Hayashi M, *et al*. The role of gamma knife surgery in the treatment of severe epilepsies. *Epileptic Disorders* 2000; **2**(2): 113–122.

80. Whang CJ, Kwon Y. Long-term follow-up of stereotactic gamma knife radiosurgery in epilepsy. *Stereotactic and Functional Neurosurgery* 1996; **66**(Suppl. 1): 349–356.

81. Dunoyer C, Ragheb J, Resnick T, *et al*. The use of stereotactic radiosurgery to treat intractable childhood partial epilepsy. *Epilepsia* 2002; **43**(3): 292–300.

82. Pinard JM, Delande, Jambaque I, *et al*. Anterior and total callosotomy in epileptic children: Prospective one-year follow-up study. *Epilepsia* 1991; **32**(Suppl. 1): 54.

83. Phillips J, Sakas DE. Anterior callosotomy for intractable epilepsy: outcome in a series of twenty patients. *British Journal of Neurosurgery* 1996; **10**(4): 351–356.

84. Quattrini A, Del Pesce M, Provinciali L, *et al*. Mutism in 36 patients who underwent callosotomy for drug-resistant epilepsy. *Journal of Neurosurgical Sciences* 1997; **41**(1): 93–96.

85. Morrell F, Whisler WW, Bleck TP. Multiple subpial transection. A new approach to the surgical treatment of focal epilepsy. *Journal of Neurosurgery* 1989; **70**: 231–239.

86. Smith MC. Multiple subpial transection in patients with extratemporal epilepsy. *Epilepsia* 1998; **39**(Suppl. 4): S81–89.

87. Spencer SS, Schramm J, Wyler A, *et al*. Multiple subpial transection for intractable partial epilepsy: an international meta-analysis. *Epilepsia* 2002; **43**(2): 141–145.

88. D'Giano CH, Del CG, Pomata H, Rabinowicz AL. Treatment of refractory partial status epilepticus with multiple subpial transection: case report. *Seizure* 2001; **10**(5): 382–385.

89. Otsubo H, Chitoku S, Ochi A, *et al*. Malignant rolandic-sylvian epilepsy in children: diagnosis, treatment, and outcomes. *Neurology* 2001; **57**(4): 590–596.

90. Shimizu H, Maehara T. Neuronal disconnection for the surgical treatment of pediatric epilepsy. *Epilepsia* 2000; **41**(Suppl. 9): 28–30.

91. Shimizu T, Maehara T, Hino T, *et al*. Effect of multiple subpial transection on motor cortical excitability in cortical dysgenesis. *Brain* 2001; **124**(7): 1336–1349.

92. Morrell F, Whisler WW, Smith MC. Multiple subpial transection in Rasmussen's encephalitis. In: Andermann F (ed.) *Chronic Encephalitis and Epilepsy: Rasmussen's Syndrome*. Boston: Butterworth-Heinemann, 1991; 219–233.

93. Schramm J, Aliashkevich AF, Grunwald T. Multiple subpial transections: outcome and complications in 20 patients who did not undergo resection. *Journal of Neurosurgery* 2002; **97**(1): 39–47.

94. Morrell F, Whisler WW, Smith MC, *et al*. Landau-Kleffner syndrome. Treatment with subpial intracortical transection. *Brain* 1995; **118**(6): 1529–1546.

95. Robinson RO, Baird G, Robinson G, Simonoff E. Landau-Kleffner syndrome: course and correlates with outcome. *Developmental Medicine and Child Neurology* 2001; **43**(4): 243–247.

96. Grote CL, Van Slyke P, Hoeppner JA. Language outcome following multiple subpial transection for Landau-Kleffner syndrome. *Brain* 1999; **122**(3): 561–566.

97. Patil AA, Andrews R, Torkelson R. Isolation of dominant seizure foci by multiple subpial transections. *Stereotactic and Functional Neurosurgery* 1997; **69**: 210–215.

98. Patil AA, Andrews RV, Torkelson R. Surgical treatment of intractable seizures with multilobar or bihemispheric seizure foci (MLBHSF). *Surgical Neurology* 1997; **47**(1): 72–77; discussion 77–78.

99. Lewine JD, Andrews R, Chez M, *et al*. Magnetoencephalographic patterns of epileptiform activity in children with

regressive autism spectrum disorders. *Pediatrics* 1999; **104**: 405–418.

100. Polkey CE. Brain stimulation for epilepsy. In: Oxbury JM, Polkey CE, Duchowny M (eds) *Intractable Focal Epilepsy*. London: Saunders, 2000; 751–760.

101. Wilder BJ. Vagal nerve stimulation. In: Engel JJ, Pedley TA (eds) *Epilepsy: A Comprehensive Textbook*. Lippincott-Raven, 1998; 1353–1358.

102. Fisher RS, Mirski M, Krauss GL. Brain stimulation. In: Engel JJ, Pedley TA (eds) *Epilepsy: A Comprehensive Textbook*. Philadelphia: Lippincott-Raven, 1997; 1867–1875.

103. Velasco M, Velasco F, Velasco AL. Centromedian-thalamic and hippocampal electrical stimulation for the control of intractable epileptic seizures. *Journal of Clinical Neurophysiology* 2001; **18**(6): 495–513.

104. Holmes MD, Wilensky AJ, Ojemann LM, Ojemann GA. Predicting outcome following reoperation for medically intractable epilepsy. *Seizure* 1999; **8**(2): 103–106.

105. Shaver EG, Harvey AS, Morrison G, *et al.* Results and complications after reoperation for failed epilepsy surgery in children. *Pediatric Neurosurgery* 1997; **27**(4): 194–202.

Behavioral therapy

JOANNE DAHL

PSYCHOLOGICAL TREATMENT OF EPILEPSY

The approach to the child with an epileptic seizure disorder requires consideration of two very important dimensions. The first is the one on which most medical and surgical professionals focus: the predisposition of a low seizure threshold, or the underlying pathology. The second is the pattern of internal or external factors which influence the occurrence of seizures. Recent psychological studies have contributed knowledge on the presentation of seizures at particular times and in particular places, and on how this information can be used to benefit quality of life. An overview of these contributions is presented, with the aim that children with epilepsy may receive more adequate understanding of their situations and treatment.

BEHAVIORAL ANALYSIS

The framework of the cognitive behavior therapy model is based on functional contextualism. This is built on a health, rather than illness, model, with the implication that the child can only be understood and treated if the surrounding context, at both macro and micro levels, is understood. At the macro level, it is important to investigate and understand the life directions valued by the child. The importance of life dimensions, e.g. relationships with family, friends, opposite sex, school and leisure-time activities, physical health and spirituality is determined. These may be conceptualized as a 'life compass' towards which all activities should progress. The goal of therapy is to help the child to build skills necessary to 'influence' life in activities in these valued directions. If occurrence of, or fear of, seizures is reported as a barrier to acting towards valued life directions, exposure to seizures or fear of seizures will probably be a part of treatment. The belief that, firstly, seizures must be controlled; and, secondly, valued life directions can be pursued, is likely to lead to an unnecessarily low quality of life. Challenging the 'occupation' of epilepsy in the child's life is central in therapy.

At the micro level, the context of the seizure behavior chain needs to be understood. The behavioral diagnosis serves to map out the interaction of the seizure behavior in relation to its context, involving both psychological and physical reactions as well as the environment. Behavior analysis operationalizes seizures in terms of: discriminative stimuli or antecedents; seizure response; and consequences of the seizure behavior. In terms of the learning paradigm, the critical issue is the **function** of the seizure in the life of the child.

ANTECEDENTS

Antecedents may be external or internal stimuli which precede and are correlated to seizure occurrence. In this model, antecedents are assumed to be conditioned to seizure start: after a number of associations between this particular stimulus and the seizure response, a predictable constellation, a **behavior chain**, emerges. According to the learning model, these antecedent stimuli may be coincidental and irrelevant, but, through conditioning, obtain seizure-eliciting qualities. Investigating the unique pattern of seizure-eliciting stimuli serves two purposes: prediction and influence. Reliability of prediction enables the child and family freedom of choice in their responses, rather than feelings of victimization and passive acceptance of seizure occurrence. Behavioral treatment strategies focus on helping the individual to build alternative ways of responding to seizure-eliciting stimuli. For those who display specific, identifiable and reproducible signals, fairly simple and effective treatment methods have been developed and evaluated. Early studies showed how children with reflex epilepsy could become desensitized by means of systematic and gradual exposure to these stimuli.[1] More recently, using similar methods of exposure to specific seizure-triggering stimuli as nonpharmacological alternative treatment, it was found that, for people with idiopathic generalized epilepsy and those with photosensitive seizures, this exposure-based treatment was as effective as drug therapy; and gave positive experiences of self-control.[2] For many, seizure antecedents are less specific, with emotions of fear, anxiety, anticipatory stress or drowsiness. A general common denominator exists in situations or states where there are shifts in cortical activity.[3] Getting up from or going to bed, coming home from school, relaxing from a strenuous task, or anticipating a challenging task are examples. Here, behavioral treatment methods focus on teaching the person to arouse or focus cortical activity contingent upon these 'risk' signals. Treatment methods include the use of meditation and yoga;[4] relaxation,[5,6] with the aim of focusing cortical activity; inhaling aromas,[7] for a general arousal of cortical activity; and breathing control.[8] Fear and anxiety are commonly associated with seizure occurrence,[3,9] so several studies have focused on exposure-based treatment.[10,11] The most important issues are:

- identification of functional categories of seizure eliciting and inhibiting stimuli
- systematic exposure to specific stimuli below seizure eliciting levels
- establishment of a repertoire for correcting shifts of cortical activity
- training in application of countermeasures, e.g. changes in arousal levels contingent upon any pre-seizure signal.

SEIZURE RESPONSE

The seizure itself informs critically on the parts of the brain influenced and on the order of such influence. It is valuable to study carefully seizure behavior from the very first visible or sensory sign, the **preictal phase**, through the peak of the seizure, the **ictal phase**, to the end, into the **postictal period**. It is important to know how the first signs are perceived; reactions to these signs; how consciousness and emotions are influenced throughout the seizure; and the times involved in each phase. This information will provide clues to possible methods of interruption of the chain of seizure behavior. Ways in which the child and/or the parents have already tried to interrupt an ongoing seizure must also be investigated. Seizure control refers to an individual's ability to influence the character or duration of the seizure response. Examples are the ability to postpone, elicit, abort, shorten, lengthen and adapt seizure expression to the situation. Most individuals attempt to develop seizure control techniques and experience some degree of control. The commonest spontaneous methods are for partial seizures: restraint of motor phenomena (74 per cent), stimulation of areas of sensation (77 per cent), use of visual (22 per cent), auditory (85 per cent), or, olfactory (32 per cent) stimuli, applied relaxation (78 per cent) and/or talking to oneself (89 per cent).[3] Many children report being able to trigger seizures: commonly through imitation of seizure movements, and/or exposing themselves to identified seizure eliciting stimuli.[3,9] These could be more generally described as means of generating general arousal or reduction of cortical activity. On the whole, children and/or parents have considerable experience in methods of triggering, prevention, interruption, change or postponement of seizures. This information should be carefully documented, and, if possible, replicated in an EEG laboratory. The nature of this seizure response provides the clinician with direct guidelines on how to interrupt the chain of seizure behavior. Much work has been done in the EEG and slow cortical potential feedback areas on teaching generation of antiepileptic brain activity contingent upon early seizure signals.[12] Important issues to investigate in individual ability to control seizures are:

- belief of the child or family in their influence (prediction, triggering, postponement, alteration, interruption) on seizure occurrence
- appearance, possible replication, and effectiveness of this influence
- reasons for initiating or not initiating seizure control.

CONSEQUENCES OF SEIZURES

If the reactions of the child and those around can be categorized as avoidance of demands, special attention or benefits, escape from an adverse situation, or stimulating, then seizures may be considered 'functional.' This implies that the child has learned to use seizures as a means of influencing the environment. Attempting to influence one's environment towards valued goals is a healthy sign. However, if such attempts have long-term negative effects they are considered dysfunctional, since the results are not in the intended long-term direction. Detection of the pattern of seizure consequences, positive and negative, short- and long-term, in the form of a functional analysis is essential. Whether a consequence is positive or negative, short-term or long-term, can only be determined in relation to the child's valued directions. If the child has learned that 'allowing' a seizure to occur in a school examination results in alleviation of that demand, this is a short-term positive consequence, giving temporary relief from an adverse situation. However, 'allowing' seizures to occur in a test situation makes the long-term valued direction of doing well in school more difficult to attain, and thus must be considered dysfunctional with respect to the life compass. The function of the seizure is included in the treatment program by reinforcing the child's long-term valued directions and helping the child to take small steps towards them, rather than towards short-term symptom alleviation. The most important points to consider relating to the consequences of seizures are the immediate and long-term effects of seizure occurrence on the child's valued directions; the types of patterns of functions that seizure occurrence present; the skills necessary for building of more functional means of obtaining long-term goals.

KEY POINTS

- Psychological diagnosis and treatment of children with epileptic seizure disorders entails the exploration of **patterns of internal or external factors** which influence seizure occurrence and utilizes this information to best aid the child and family towards empowerment
- This is done by investigating:
  - patterns of **precursors to seizure occurrence**
  - the nature of **seizure behavior**
  - any means of **influencing the chain** of seizure behavior: triggering, preventing, postponing, shortening or interrupting
  - the **consequences, effects or function** of seizure occurrence
- Treatment of the child with seizure disorders aims at helping the child build the skills necessary to progress in **valued life directions**. Exposure to seizures or fear of seizures is commonly included in treatment as this is believed to be a barrier to valued activities

REFERENCES

1. Forster F. *Reflex Epilepsy. Behavior Therapy and Conditioned Reflexes*. Springfield, IL: Charles C. Thomas, 1977.
2. Wolf P, Okujava N. Possibilities of non-pharmacological conservative treatment of epilepsy. *Seizure* 1999; **8**: 45–52.
3. Dahl J. *Epilepsy: A Behavior Medicine Approach to Assessment and Treatment in Children*. Göttingen: Hofgrefe & Huber, 1992.
4. Ranaratban S, Sridharan K. Yoga for epilepsy. *Cochrane Library*, Issue 1. Oxford: Update Software, 1999.
5. Puskarich C, Whitman S, Dell J, *et al*. Controlled examination of effects of progressive relaxation training on seizure reduction. *Epilepsia* 1992; **33**: 675–680.
6. Dahl J, Melin L, Lund L. Effects of a contingent relaxation program on adults with refractory epileptic seizures. *Epilepsia* 1987; **28**: 125–132.
7. Betts T. An olfactory counter measures treatment for epileptic seizures using a conditioned arousal response to specific aromatherapy oils. *Epilepsia* 1995; **36**(Suppl. 3): 130–131.
8. Fried R. Breathing training for the self-regulation of alveolar CO_2 in the behavioral control of idiopathic epileptic seizures. In: Mostofsky DI, Loyning Y (eds). *The Neurobehavioral Treatment of Epilepsy*. New Jersey: Lawrence Erlbaum, 1993.
9. Spector S, Goldstein L, Cull C, Fenwick P. *Precipitating and Inhibiting Epileptic Seizures: A Survey of Adults with Poorly Controlled Epilepsy*. London: International League Against Epilepsy, 1994.
10. Devinsky O, Cox C, Witt E, Ronsaville D. Ictal fear in temporal lobe epilepsy, association with interictal behavioral changes. *Journal of Epilepsy* 1991; **4**: 231–238.
11. Spector S. Foots A, Goldstein L. Reduction in seizure frequency as a result of group intervention for adults with epilepsy. *Epilepsia* 1995; **36**(Suppl. 3): S130.
12. Martinovic Z. Adjunctive behavioral treatment in adolescents and young adults with juvenile myoclonic epilepsy. *Seizure* 2001; **10**: 42–47.

23

Cognitive aspects

DOROTHÉE GA KASTELEIJN-NOLST TRENITÉ AND ANNE DE SAINT-MARTIN

The onset of epilepsy occurs before the age of 20 years in 60 per cent of patients, and one third have their first seizure when in junior school. The appearance of epilepsy in childhood often interferes with normal cognitive development and with academic achievement.[1] Several studies have shown that children with epilepsy perform less well at school than their healthy peers. This occurs even during periods without clinical seizures and in children with idiopathic epilepsy including the so-called 'benign' partial epilepsies.[2–5] In studies on twins[6] differences were found between pairs with and without epilepsy and, within twins, if only one had epilepsy. In a recent long-term follow-up study in newly diagnosed epilepsy patients, it was not only shown that schooling achievement was lower in epilepsy patients compared to the general population, but also that age at onset during the high school period had the most negative impact regardless of the duration of active epilepsy.[7] Furthermore, neuropsychological impairment, such as memory disturbance, visuospatial and verbal deficits has been demonstrated in children even with very well-controlled epilepsy, such as absence epilepsy and benign partial epilepsies without any obvious problem in academic achievement.[8,9] Estimates of prevalence rate of learning problems range from 5 to 50 per cent.[10] The interindividual differences are striking in most studies; intraindividual variance in performance is also more often found in children with epilepsy.[11,12]

Parents, teachers and doctors are often asked how cognitive dysfunction can be assessed, prevented or treated in children with epilepsy. There is often uncertainty about the relationship between the learning disorder and epilepsy. Clinicians and researchers have identified several variables that influence learning and cognitive function, such as age at onset of seizures, duration of epilepsy, type and frequency of seizures, and subclinical epileptiform EEG discharges. Differences in etiology, such as a progressive brain disease, localized or generalized brain damage after a trauma, or a meningoencephalitis, may also influence learning problems. The underlying brain disease or damage generally has a much greater negative effect on learning problems than the associated epileptic seizures. However, in at least 50 per cent of children with epilepsy no etiologic factor can be determined[1] and a genetically determined susceptibility is likely.[13] In addition to the influence of the epileptic disorder itself, antiepileptic treatment (AEDs) can also affect cognition. Another negative influence is the impact of epilepsy on social functioning, which in turn decreases school performance.[14] Finally, all of the above-mentioned factors – epileptic (sub)clinical seizures, underlying brain dysfunction with cognitive deficits, AEDs, social stigma and low self-esteem – can lead to behavioral changes in the child, thus worsening cognitive performance and learning. It is therefore not surprising that many questions concerning this topic still have to be answered.[15]

Although the various determinants are interrelated, it is nevertheless possible to give an impression of the impact of the various factors involved. Since the beginning of the 20th century, and especially in the last 25 years, many studies have been performed.

TESTS

Intelligence tests

Sullivan and Gahagan[16] investigated 103 children with epilepsy using the Binet–Simon intelligence test and observed that the average IQ of the children with epilepsy was 92.4 whilst that of a normal control group was 105. The IQ was relatively higher in children whose epilepsy appeared after the age of 6 years and in children with only 'minor seizures'. It was also recognized in the 1940s that different intelligence tests, such as the Pintner-Cunningham and Binet-Simon tests, could give different results in the same children with epilepsy;[17] use of the Pintner-Cunningham test gave overall better results. This difference appeared to be mainly due to the time factor in the Binet-Simon test, which led to the conclusion that children with epilepsy suffer from psychomotor slowing more than normal children.

Since the 1970s, the WISC (Wechsler Intelligence Scale for Children) and more recently the WISC-R (Wechsler Intelligence Test for Children-Revised) have been used most often. Various studies have demonstrated that IQ levels of children with epilepsy tend to be below the population mean.[18,19] Rutter et al. found a distribution of intelligence in children with epilepsy closely resembling the normal distribution values.[20] However, it should be noted that the children investigated all attended normal schools and showed a mild form of epilepsy. The IQ score of the epileptic child is influenced by the type, frequency and severity of epileptic seizures as well as by the etiology.

Analysis of sub-test scores reveals below-average scores especially in vocabulary (fluency, verbal language skill), coding or digit-symbol (attention, sensory-motor coordination) and information (verbal language skill). Furthermore, a relatively high test-retest variability can be found in repeated IQ testing. During a mean follow-up period of 10 years, positive or negative fluctuations as high as 10 points in verbal or performance sub-tests were observed in children with epilepsy at any IQ level.[19,21] In both studies a steady rise in IQ was observed in the children in remission in contrast to those with continued epileptic seizures. However, no significant relationships were found between age, sex, etiology, EEG abnormalities, seizure type, frequency or duration of epilepsy and the verbal IQ, performance IQ or Full-Scale IQ. A higher initial verbal IQ and early onset of epilepsy correlated with lower performance-IQ at follow-up.

Ellenberg et al. studied IQ before and after the onset of seizures in 62 children between the age of 4 and 7 years.[22] No differences in IQ were found at 7 years of age between the children with seizures and the controls, when matched for initial IQ at 4 years of age, sex, race and socio-economic status. The neurological and developmental status before onset of the seizures appeared to be the major determinant of outcome and the seizures themselves did not appear to result in intellectual deterioration.

Wallace et al. investigated the outcome at 8 or 9 years of age in children whose first seizure had occurred with fever between 2 months and 7 years.[23] The IQs of the total group showed normal means and distribution. However, some sub-groups performed less well: lower social class and persisting neurological abnormality correlated with lower level of neuropsychological functioning. Girls appeared to be much more affected than boys when they had a history of recurrent seizures. Furthermore, girls, especially those with right-sided seizures, carried a poor prognosis if the attacks had started early in life (between 13 and 18 months).

Apart from factors such as age at onset and duration of epilepsy, differences can be found in performance depending on seizure type. Generalized tonic-clonic seizures have a greater impact than short-lasting partial seizures. Neuropsychological investigations should therefore not be performed within a few days of a generalized tonic-clonic convulsion. Fedio and Mirsky found specific disorders of attention and constructional apraxia in children with generalized tonic-clonic convulsions, compared to those with partial seizures.[24] Similar findings were reported by Giordani et al.:[25] patients with a partial epilepsy showed better results on the sub-tests of the WISC-R (picture arrangement, coding, block design and object assembly) than did those with a generalized epilepsy. These performance sub-tests require visual spatial problem solving and sequencing in addition to attention and concentration.

One would expect children with an epileptic focus in the left or right temporal lobe to show hemisphere-specific dysfunction. The left side of the brain is generally specialized in verbal information processing and the right in visuospatial information processing. Indeed, some studies have demonstrated hemisphere-specific dysfunctions in patients with epileptic-foci in the left versus right temporal lobe.[24,26] However, laterality is difficult to investigate. Firstly, one has to select children who have exclusively seizures that originate and stay confined to the region of the epileptic brain focus. Most children with partial epilepsy also have secondarily generalized seizures. In addition, ictal EEG recordings often demonstrate that both the right and left temporal region or other regions (loci) can act as the seizure origin or become involved as soon as epileptic brain activity spreads. In order to select children with 'pure' localization-related seizures, detailed seizure histories and ictal video-EEG are necessary. Secondly, and especially in children, functional reorganization or plasticity may occur if selected areas of the brain are dysfunctional.[27] This is more likely to occur in children who become epileptic at an early age. Some intellectually handicapped children, for example, who have severe neuronal loss in one hemisphere, show epileptic seizures arising in their relatively good functioning side of the brain while the other side functions less well and is nonepileptogenic. Thus, even children who show a consistent epileptic focus are not necessarily a homogenous population. Furthermore, the most often used psychological test, the WISC, does not provide a consistent and reliable index of lateralization (see above). Factors such as a lower intelligence, seizures and drug intoxication have a negative influence particularly on nonverbal sub-tests of the WISC. Bailet and Turk found that children with epilepsy scored significantly lower on the coding subtest when compared with healthy controls and children with migraine.[5] These confounding factors must thus be taken into consideration in intelligence testing.

Unnoticed seizures or subclinical EEG discharges during testing may also have an impact on outcome of particular sub-tests. We investigated 21 schoolchildren with or without a history of seizures or social-emotional or educational problems.[28] They were selected because they showed focal or generalized, subclinical epileptiform EEG discharges in the waking state. The children were all investigated using the Revised Amsterdam Child Intelligence Test (RAKIT) with continuous EEG-video monitoring. The mean IQ of the 21 children was 87.4, which is significantly lower than the standard normal value for this test battery (mean 100, standard deviation 15). The test profile was significantly abnormal, mainly as a result of poor performance on a paired-associates task, requiring short-term verbal learning. In this test the child is asked to reproduce the proper names of animal pictures after 1 min and 5 min. Item performances of all sub-tests were impaired during epileptiform discharges, with the exception of the sub-test that involved recall of material learned previously (long-term memory). These data help to explain some of the test-retest variability observed in children with epilepsy.

Neuropsychological tests

Attention and concentration deficits are often recognized as a particular problem in children with epilepsy.[2] In one study, the teachers described 36 of the 85 children with epilepsy as lethargic, dull and apathetic.[29] Reaction time and psychomotor speed, as measured by simple and choice reaction time tests, are markedly increased in children with epilepsy.[30] Oostrom et al. did not find slowing in 51 newly diagnosed children, who were investigated before the start of drug treatment and 3 and 12 months later.[12] However, they made more errors on the computerized tasks and showed more variance in performance when compared to healthy controls. In addition, there was a striking difference between epilepsy patients. Behavioral abnormalities, subclinical epileptiform discharges and the underlying etiology may have contributed to these differences. Remarkably, twice as many children with epilepsy as

healthy controls needed educational assistance at school. Finally, using a computerized visual-search task (CVST), Alpherts and Aldenkamp demonstrated that speed of information processing was often lower in children with epilepsy than in controls.[31]

Although clinical observations more than 100 years ago suggested a relationship between memory disturbances and epilepsy,[32] there are limited data on the effect of epilepsy on memory. In the studies performed, it has been shown that memory impairment is particularly found in patients with partial complex seizures of temporal lobe origin: verbal memory impairment in patients with left-sided temporal foci; and nonverbal memory impairment in patients with right-sided foci.[24,33] Memory impairment has also been found during the occurrence of epileptiform-EEG discharges using short-term memory tasks.[34] Anti-epileptic drugs such as phenytoin have also been shown to influence memory negatively.[35]

ACADEMIC ACHIEVEMENT

General

In 122 epileptic children with an IQ of at least 70 (WISC-R), Seidenberg et al. demonstrated less academic achievement than expected based on IQ.[3] Arithmetic and spelling were the most affected, followed by reading comprehension and word recognition. Older children were further behind in their achievement levels in all areas than younger children. Earlier age at seizure onset, longer duration of epilepsy and the presence of generalized seizures were associated with poor arithmetic achievement scores. Other factors, such as number of AEDs, did not influence the results.

Primary school children with idiopathic partial and generalized types of epilepsy and an IQ of at least 80 (WISC-R) were followed for about 3 years with repeated testing and were compared with healthy controls and children with migraine by Bailet and Turk.[5] The epilepsy group performed consistently worse over the years in reading, spelling and arithmetic. No difference was seen between those with new-onset epilepsy and those with pre-existing disease.

Austin et al. compared scholastic achievement (reading, arithmetic, language and vocabulary) and behavior (Achenbach scale) in 117 epileptic children and 108 children with asthma.[11] Both groups of children were treated for at least 1 year with medication and none had presumed intellectual deficits or significant developmental delay. Boys with a high seizure frequency performed particularly poorly. At follow up after 4 years, twice as many children with epilepsy (44 per cent) as with asthma (23 per cent) were found to have repeated one or more grades. The children with epilepsy continued to perform significantly worse in all achievement areas, particularly those with a high seizure frequency.[36] Surprisingly, no improvement in achievement was seen in those children who had a clear improvement in seizure control. This may imply that either the underlying neurological dysfunction causes an irreversible learning deficit regardless of the seizure frequency (secondary effect of the brain dysfunction), or that the seizures themselves, if appearing at a crucial time in development, lead to irreparable underachievement. The last hypothesis is supported by epidemiological studies in Finland[1] and in the Netherlands.[7] Medical and psychosocial outcomes of 243 patients (diagnosed between 1953 and 1967) were evaluated with a questionnaire. School achievement appeared to be significantly different from the general Dutch population for both men and woman; only 35 per cent of the epilepsy group has completed high school (low and high levels included) versus 65 per cent of the Dutch population as a whole. Surprisingly, the number of epilepsy patients having a university degree did not show such a big difference (10 vs. 16 per cent). Furthermore, to ascertain the impact of having epilepsy at school age (preschool being under 6 years, school being 6–18 years and post-school being over 18 years) we compared the different epilepsy characteristics in a sample of 243 patients. There were no significant differences between the groups with respect to duration of seizures (on average 20 years) and duration of medication (on average 25 years). Children who were diagnosed with epilepsy at less than 6 years of age achieved lower education levels than would be expected ($p = 0.014$). The majority of these children achieved no better than 'lower professional education'. In children who were diagnosed with epilepsy at school age (6–18 years), this tendency was more marked ($p = 0.0003$). There was no correlation between schooling achievement and the occurrence of epilepsy after the age of 18 years ($p = 0.22$). Thus, having seizures and using AEDs during the school period seems a major determinant of the level of schooling achievement that is finally attained.

Specific

READING AND ARITHMETIC

Rutter et al. found that 18 per cent of the children with epilepsy were 2 years or more below grade level in reading comprehension, although their IQ scores were average or better.[20] Boys showed more reading impairment than girls. This sex difference in reading ability was not found in arithmetic skills by Seidenberg.[3] However, Austin et al. observed clear deficits in boys in all academic areas and especially in the boys with a high seizure frequency.[11]

Children with epileptiform EEG abnormalities scored lower on reading and spelling tests than those of the same intelligence without epileptiform EEG abnormalities.[5]

Left-sided epileptiform discharges especially may influence reading performance.[34,37] However, neither Seidenberg nor Camfield found a consistent relationship between a left-sided EEG focus and reading disabilities. Seidenberg's patients with right focal epileptiform discharges performed less well in reading comprehension but had a preserved reading rate. A possible explanation could be that memorizing the spatial component of reading is impaired. Camfield et al. found lower scores on mental arithmetic in children with left-temporal foci.[26] However, we did not observe a difference between left- and right-sided discharges with regard to arithmetic.[34]

With the exception of the last mentioned study, none of the above-mentioned studies simultaneously correlated epileptiform discharges in the EEG with test performance. Furthermore, the findings of Stores and Hart[37] and of Kasteleijn-Nolst Trenité[38] are consistent with the concept that advanced reading is generally supported by the left hemisphere, whereas arithmetic is a function supported by both hemispheres.[39] Arithmetic underachievement is also a common finding in learning disabled and intellectually disabled children without epilepsy.[40]

Not only children but also adolescents with epilepsy showed poorer comprehension of reading than their controls matched for age, sex and general ability.[41] The lowest overall reading scores were found in patients with myoclonic seizures, partial seizures with secondary generalization or generalized tonic–clonic seizures. This is more or less in agreement with Seidenberg et al.,[3] who found that children with both generalized tonic-clonic and absence seizures did less well than others.

SPELLING

Jennekens-Schinkel et al. compared the writing-to-dictation results between mildly epileptic children of at least average intelligence attending an ordinary elementary schools with normal controls.[42] Epileptic boys, followed by epileptic girls and then control boys, made the highest number of errors. Children with epilepsy made significantly more letter-perseveration errors, made more corrections and left more errors uncorrected (performance errors). Other variables, such as type of epilepsy, were not found to influence the error-rates. Epileptic boys were also more impaired in spelling in the study by Bailet and Turk.[5]

SUBCLINICAL EPILEPTIFORM EEG DISCHARGES AND COGNITION

Assessment

Although epileptiform discharges lasting 10 s or less are often not observed to have a clinical correlate, they can nevertheless disturb cognition, as first demonstrated by

Schwab in 1939.[43] He demonstrated that during generalized discharges some patients had a slowed reaction to a visual stimulus while others did not respond at all. Many authors have subsequently demonstrated transitory cognitive impairment (TCI) during epileptiform EEG discharges. The tasks used have included simple motor reaction tasks, such as tapping or writing, and more complex tasks, such as forward or backward subtraction, simple or choice-reaction time-tests, and short-term memory tests. Most tests were performed during epileptiform discharges evoked by hyperventilation or photic stimulation (reviewed by Aarts et al.[44]).

The likelihood of demonstrating cognitive impairment during a generalized spike-wave discharge depends on the complexity of the task: choice reaction time-tests and short-term memory tests are more sensitive than simple motor tasks such as finger tapping. Although cognitive impairment can be demonstrated during discharges lasting only 0.5 s, the likelihood increases greatly if the discharges last more than 3 s. Examination of the effect of discharges on cognition is complicated because performance of the task influences the epileptiform discharges. Schwab observed that an illuminated visual stimulus shortened the duration of the discharges, unless the discharges were longer than 10 s.[43] In general, cognitive activity reduces the frequency and duration of spontaneous epileptiform EEG discharges.[45] Hutt et al. observed an interaction between level of performance and frequency of EEG discharges.[46] Of particular interest is the observation that mental activities, particularly writing and written calculation but also mental calculation and reading, can provoke epileptiform discharges in some children, often accompanied by myoclonic and absence seizures.[47] This phenomenon was seen almost exclusively in children and adolescents with an IGE. The study of cognitive impairment during subclinical EEG discharges is of practical as well as scientific importance. Such discharges may contribute to educational problems and could even contribute to accidents and be hazardous in traffic situations.

Transitory cognitive impairment (TCI) has been demonstrated using a self-pacing, microcomputer-generated short-term memory task with continuous EEG recording.[44] This test is similar to Corsi's blocks test[48] and has a nonverbal version (a maximum of seven colored rectangles) and a verbal version (a maximum of seven names of common animals). The stimuli are presented randomly on the screen with changing colors and the presentations and responses are all automatically annotated on the EEG. After visual identification of type and location of epileptiform discharges the number of correct or incorrect answers per patient and per session can be compared with occurrence or absence of the epileptiform discharges in that particular child. This design, in which the patient serves as his or her own control, eliminates possible confounding influences e.g. types of epilepsy,

etiology or medication. We investigated a total of 70 children (34 boys, 36 girls) between 6 and 15 years of age with this modified Corsi blocks test. These children were selected because a routine EEG had shown at least one subclinical EEG discharge every 5 min and at most every 5 s. TCI in either or both tasks was found in a total of 47 per cent of the children. Right-sided discharges impaired performance in 50 per cent of the test sessions and had more profound influence on the visual spatial task. Left-sided discharges appeared to exert greater influence on the verbal task. This study demonstrated that short lasting and even isolated generalized and focal epileptiform EEG discharges that looked as if they were subclinical appeared to influence cognitive functioning.[34]

We have studied the consequences of TCI on academic achievement in 20 children with subclinical epileptiform EEG discharges, who were asked to perform 10 min of reading, arithmetic and writing, with a period of rest as baseline, all under continuous video-EEG monitoring[49] (see Figure 23.1). Reading errors comprised repetitions, corrections, hesitations, omissions, additions and words read wrongly. Reading and arithmetic quotients were calculated on the basis of the child's academic achievement (a positive quotient meant better achievement than expected according to age and education). The mean reading and arithmetic quotients were 0.7 and 0.73 respectively, compared to 1.0 in normal control populations. High discharge rates tended to be associated with low scholastic performance, particularly in arithmetic. Surprisingly, the discharge rate was found to be lower at rest than during the three task domains. The reading and arithmetic tests were presented at three levels of difficulty. The highest discharge rate occurred when reading and arithmetic were performed at the student's level. Reading efficiency was significantly reduced during discharges, and more reading errors were made when the discharge length was longer than 3 s. The children with predominantly left-sided discharges performed significantly less well on reading tasks than children with right-sided discharges, i.e. the left-sided discharge group performed at a level of about 2 years below expected school level, and children with right-sided discharges at a level of 1 year below expected school level. These group differences were not found in arithmetic quotients: all three groups performed on levels about 1 year below the school level. The results were thus in accordance with those obtained with the short-term memory test (Corsi) and also in agreement with those of Stores and Hart,[37] but not with those of Camfield et al.[26] Neither of these studies, however, correlated simultaneous EEG discharges with test performance.

The incidence of subclinical epileptiform discharges while awake in normal or epileptic children is unknown. Petersén and Eeg-Olofsson reported that approximately 10 per cent of children with a history of seizures have epileptiform activity in their EEG.[50] However, routine EEG

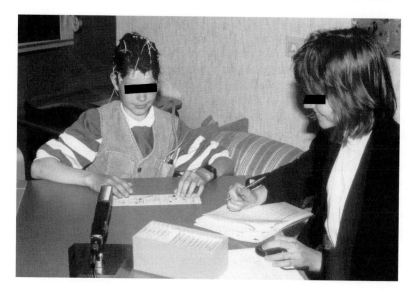

Figure 23.1 *The psychologist tests this patient with subclinical epileptiform discharges under continous EEG and video recording. Applied tests are not only neuropsychological tests, but also simple reading and arithmetic tasks. Afterwards a correlation can be made between exact time of occurrence of focal or generalized epileptiform discharges in the EEG and errors in performance.*

recordings are obtained normally from patients lying on a bed with closed eyes. No data are available concerning the influence of rest, learning and exercise on the frequency of epileptiform discharges. Similarly, the impact of EEG discharges during sleep has not been explored, although learning difficulties are a well-recognized feature in children who have continuous spikes and slow waves during sleep.

Rolandic epilepsy as a model

Rolandic epilepsy is a good model in which to study the consequences of underlying epileptic activity on cognition. This epilepsy occurs in childhood, has no underlying brain lesion, resolves spontaneously at adolescence, and does not necessarily require treatment. This 'benign' syndrome is characterized by few seizures but paradoxically by abundant focal interictal EEG abnormalities, activated by sleep.[51] Although it has an excellent long-term prognosis, many authors have demonstrated the existence of subtle cognitive impairments, sometimes more evident with oromotor or speech-transient acquired deficits, during the active phase.[9] The relevance of these subtle dysfunctions, as well as their correlation with seizures or interictal EEG abnormalities, remains unclear.

We have conducted a prospective study involving children with idiopathic focal epilepsy with rolandic spikes in which the patients were followed longitudinally with repeated sleep EEG and neuropsychological evaluations, until recovery.[52] Based on early EEG characteristics, we divided the patients into an active group and a control group. Frequent seizures, a drop in school performance, acquired behavioral disorders or cognitive deficit, and a major EEG abnormality characterized the active group. A small number of seizures, a good academic achievement and few EEG abnormalities characterized the control

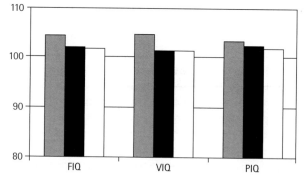

Figure 23.2 *Longitudinal evolution of FIQ, VIQ and PIQ in the control group characterized by few seizures, few EEG abnormalities (20/27). Gray bars, onset; black bars, active phase; white bars, recovery.*

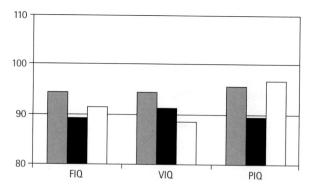

Figure 23.3 *Longitudinal evolution of FIQ, VIQ, and PIQ in the active group, characterized by abundant interictal abnormalities and slow focus (7/27). Gray bars, onset; black bars, active phase; white bars, recovery.*

group. The active group had a significant acquired cognitive decline, which resolved when the child had outgrown the epilepsy (Figures 23.2–23.7). This decline was mainly observed on performance IQ and those IQ subtests that

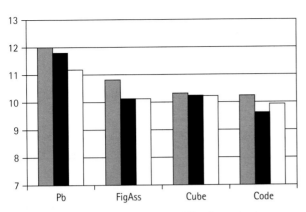

Figure 23.4 *Longitudinal evolution of IQ subtests in the control group (2/27). Gray bars, onset; black bars, active phase; white bars, recovery.*

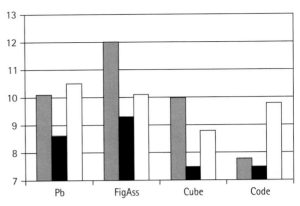

Figure 23.7 *Longitudinal evolution of IQ subtests in the active group (7/27). Gray bars, onset; black bars, active phase; white bars, recovery.*

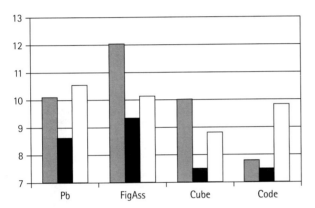

Figure 23.5 *Longitudinal evolution of IQ subtests in the active group (7/27). Gray bars, onset; black bars, active phase; white bars, recovery.*

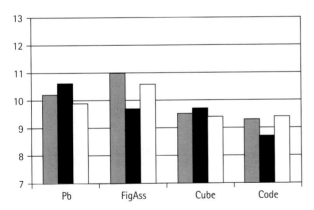

Figure 23.6 *Longitudinal evolution of IQ subtests in treated patients of the control group (VPA). Gray bars, onset; black bars, active phase; white bars, recovery.*

involve working memory and executive functioning. We also observed a deficit of sustained attention during the active phase of the epilepsy. Executive functions, controlled by the frontal lobe, seem more vulnerable to epileptic dysfunction during their maturation and their impairment

may interfere with learning (processing).[53] In a similar study, Deonna *et al.*[9] followed 19 children with rolandic epilepsy and three with benign occipital epilepsy for 1–3 years using repeated EEGs and neuropsychological testing. Although no persistent cognitive stagnation or regression was observed, nine of the 22 children had school difficulties needing adjustment. Eight of the nine showed isolated weaknesses in particular areas of cognition. Interestingly, transient cognitive impairments were found in the active phase in seven out of these eight patients and these correlated in time with worsening of the EEG. We also compared the longitudinal cognitive evolution between the control group and the active group treated by the same treatment (valproate). No decline was observed in the control group, while a transient decline was observed in the active group (Figures 23.5 and 23.7). Drugs can provoke attention deficits and a slower reaction time, especially when given as polytherapy.[30] However, our study showed a direct effect of the epilepsy, independent of the treatment consequences, as both groups received the same treatment during the active phase of the epilepsy.

Cognitive disorders may occur in patients with idiopathic partial epilepsies who do not exhibit overt seizures but show only abundant interictal epileptiform EEG discharges. In our study, certain EEG patterns were associated with a poor cognitive evolution.[52] We found a significant correlation between the persistence of abundant spike-waves during sleep and cognitive disturbances. Disturbances of higher cortical functions were also strongly correlated with morphological organization and location of interictal abnormalities. A permanent slow wave focus is usually associated with a structural brain lesion and is uncommon in idiopathic epilepsy. However, such a focus was present in seven children. An intermittent focal slow activity may appear in the same regions as spike-waves during periods of abundant spike-waves. Slow EEG activity reflects hypersynchronous GABAergic inhibitory and postsynaptic potentials and suggests that cortical inhibition is increased. During the active phase of rolandic epilepsy, cortical inhibition, powerful enough to control initiation of ictal activity, may also produce a disorganization within the epileptic cortex, rendering it temporarily unavailable for physiologic processing.

Treatment

The ultimate evidence that TCI is caused by subclinical EEG discharges in certain children is the finding that performance improves after suppression of the EEG discharges. Aarts *et al.* demonstrated this in a 13-year old boy who complained of difficulty with his schoolwork.[44] In his EEG repeated runs of generalized sharp waves or irregular spike-wave activity were seen and TCI was demonstrated using the Corsi test. Because of repeated errors he never advanced beyond a series length of two blocks or two words. Following intravenous injection of diazepam, epileptiform activity was completely suppressed. After 15 minutes, performance-testing was repeated and he was able to give correct answers to series of three blocks. One hour later, while his epileptiform activity was still absent and he felt less drowsy, he managed to respond correctly to series of four blocks. In a double-blind controlled trial of valproic acid in 6 children with subclinical EEG discharges and well-controlled or no seizures, cognitive performance increased significantly in 2 of the 4 patients who showed a good suppression of EEG discharges. The other 2 had either no change or a lowering in school performance that was considered to be due to a behavioral disturbance induced by the valproic acid. Thus, some, but not all, of the children who were treated with valproic acid and had subsequent suppression of clinical EEG discharges showed an increase in cognitive performance. In a similar study of 12 children treated with valproic acid or clobazam, 2 children dropped out because of side-effects but 8 of the other 10 children showed an improvement in performance on the Neale reading test, digit-span and Bender time.[54] However, no improvement in neuropsychologic functioning was observed in a randomized, double-blind, placebo controlled, single-crossover trial of valproic acid in 8 children between 6 and 12 years of age with significant learning and behavioral problems and abundant subclinical EEG discharges.[55] There may have been a methodological problem in this study, which used a simple crossover design, in that valproic acid shows a pharmacodynamic effect even 6 weeks after withdrawal.[56] In addition, only half of the children had a relative decrease in EEG discharges and the dosage of valproic acid may have been too low for these patients.

In conclusion, seizures and subclinical epileptiform discharges can definitely cause cognitive deficits in children with idiopathic (including benign) and cryptogenic epilepsy, and this effect is independent of the AED treatment. Interestingly, an effect of the subclinical discharges on cognition can be demonstrated in only 40–50 per cent of children. It is difficult to predict which children might benefit from medication, but a slow wave focus has been shown to correlate with transient cognitive dysfunction.

ANTIEPILEPTIC DRUGS

General

AEDs can prevent epileptic seizures but do not cure the epilepsy. No consensus exists on whether treatment should be started immediately after the first seizure, or after a second or further seizure, or whether no treatment at all should be used. The timing of AED withdrawal in treated children is also debated.[57] If AEDs had only very minor side-effects, these dilemmas would not arise. However, AEDs are psychoactive, and parents report behavioral side-effects in about 6 per cent of normal intelligent children and adolescents receiving AEDs.[58] Children are especially sensitive to cognitive side-effects such as slowness but paradoxical effects such as hyperactivity and psychosis have also been reported with phenobarbital, valproic acid, lamotrigine and levetiracetam.[59,60] Rapid initiation of the dose and preexisting neuropsychological deficits are risk factors for such effects.[60,61] Paradoxical side-effects are usually obvious and result in a change in medication but, in intellectually disabled children, can be difficult to differentiate from the behavioral regression that sometimes accompanies suppression of seizures.

The main cognitive side-effects of AEDs demonstrated in the laboratory involve attention, psychomotor speed and memory.[62] These are usually dose-dependent, occur more often in patients on polytherapy and occur more often with certain drugs.[59] Well-controlled studies on cognitive side-effects of AEDs are, however, lacking in children. It is likely that the effect on cognitive functioning will become a more important issue in the development of new AEDs. Patients and parents consider side-effects as an important reason for withdrawal of medication, more so than the treating physician.[63] Nonetheless, it is clear that the negative cognitive effects of AEDs are often relatively minor compared to the disruptive effect of seizures and subclinical epileptiform EEG discharges, except for those who experience a paradoxical change in behaviour.

Specific

The introduction of AEDs such as valproic acid and carbamazepine changed the treatment of epilepsy significantly. A major advantage of valproic acid and carbamazepine appeared to be that the children became more active.[64]

In order to assess systematically the cognitive side-effects of phenytoin, carbamazepine, valproic acid and clobazam, without confounding epilepsy variables, Trimble and Thompson performed double-blind placebo-controlled studies in healthy adult volunteers, who took the drugs for a period of 2 weeks and had tests of short-term memory, speed and decision-making.[64,65] All drugs showed a negative influence on performance, even within the therapeutic ranges. However, phenytoin had a negative effect on all tests, whereas the other drugs did not impair memory function. Similarly, volunteers receiving gabapentin performed worse on 15 per cent of test items whereas those receiving clobazam performed worse on 40 per cent of test items than when on no medication.[66] An even greater difference was seen with lamotrigine: lamotrigine users performed worse than on placebo on only about 3 per cent of the test items.[67] In a parallel comparison trial of single-dose and 4-week administration of gabapentin, topiramate and lamotrigine the greatest negative effects were observed in those receiving topiramate. The topiramate group's verbal fluency rate dropped an average of 50 per cent per subject, compared with a negligible change for the other two AED groups, whereas a threefold error rate increase occurred on the visual attention task (these persons also reported speech and language dysfunction as well as attentional difficulties with numbness of face and lips). During the steady-state phase topiramate users performed relatively worse on tests of verbal memory and psychomotor speed, compared with the baseline condition.[68] Only short-term effects of the drugs (<4 weeks) can be investigated in healthy and adult volunteers, and from drug development studies it is known that epileptic patients can react differently in terms of side-effects in relation to attained blood levels.[69]

In a matched control study in 622 newly diagnosed epileptic patients of 18 years and older, a comparison of the influence of four AEDs (**carbamazepine, phenytoin, phenobarbital or primidone**) with regard to behavioral and cognitive effects was carried out. Smith found interrelations between age, education and IQ.[70] When the data were controlled for these factors, no dramatic differences were found in performance between the four drug groups. The carbamazepine group showed significantly fewer cognitive effects than the others. If age, education and IQ seem to be important confounding factors in adult studies, this certainly must be of great importance in studies in children. Therefore, the effect of drugs should be investigated in children who serve as their own controls.

Vining et al. investigated 21 children of normal intelligence and with relatively mild seizure-disorders in a double-blind crossover study, to measure the effects of phenobarbital and valproic acid on cognitive functioning.[71] The children had different types of seizures (tonic–clonic seizures or partial complex seizures); the EEGs

before the study entry were normal in 5 patients, slightly abnormal in 9 and markedly abnormal in 7 of the cases. Ten boys and 11 girls underwent a complete neuropsychological battery, including the WISC before entry of the trial: the mean Full-Scale IQ was 94.0 (standard deviation 14.4). Most of the children were already receiving medication before the study, including phenobarbital, phenytoin, primidone or carbamazepine. Both continuous performance reaction tests, as measure of vigilance and concentration, as well as complete neuropsychological testing, were repeatedly carried out. The design (two 6-month double-blind crossover periods) was such that the children served as their own controls. There was no statistical difference in seizure control between the valproic acid and phenobarbital period. However, children receiving phenobarbital performed less well ($p < 0.01$) on four tests of neuropsychological functioning, i.e. block-design (timed constructional praxis), performance IQ, Full-Scale IQ and Berkeley paired-association learning tasks (attention and short-term learning). Thus, valproic acid gave significantly less cognitive impairment in children than phenobarbital. This study demonstrated that different AEDs could have a different effect on higher cortical functioning, even at lower or average dosages. Another more recent study by Williams et al.[72] revealed no difference in cognition in 37 children (age 6–17) with newly diagnosed epilepsy (22 partial epilepsy), after a 6-month successful treatment with monotherapy with carbamazepine (17),valproic acid (11), ethosuximide (4), lamotrigine (2), gabapentin (2) or phenytoin (1), as compared to children with diabetes mellitus. One of the reasons might be that the interindividual differences resulted in statistical regression to the mean. Comparison within patients might be more informative in this respect. This study nevertheless shows that, in general, at least the short-term effects of most AEDs are negligible.

A number of studies have been performed using the design of discontinuation of AEDs in children. Riva and Devoti[73] selected 16 children with different types of epilepsy who had been seizure free for at least 2 years, had been receiving phenobarbital monotherapy for 4–9 years, and all had blood level ranges between 15 and 40 mg/L. The phenobarbital dosage was reduced by half and EEGs were repeated every 3 months. Those in whom the EEG continued to have no epileptiform discharges and had a well-organized background ($n = 9$) were assessed neuropsychologically a second time, 6 months to 4 years later. Improvement was found in the Performance Intelligence subtests of the WISC and attention test with letters, numbers and figures (Barrage Test). Interestingly, in general the tests with clear time limitations improved, while the level of performance stayed unchanged (age adapted) when the children in the phenobarbital period were given no time limit. It thus seems that a particular effect of phenobarbital in children is reversible slowness. Similarly, in a study of 70 seizure-free children in whom the WISC-R was administered before and 1 and 7 months after withdrawal of monotherapy with carbamazepine ($n = 25$), phenobarbital ($n = 22$) and valproic acid ($n = 23$), children receiving phenobarbital had lower initial IQ scores, which increased slightly after discontinuation of the drug, particularly the digit span and block design subtests.[74]

Although the benzodiazepines, diazepam, clonazepam and more recently clobazam have been used frequently as AEDs in children, little research has been done on their cognitive effects. The benzodiazepines have been investigated thoroughly in animal models, healthy volunteers (e.g. in driving tests)[75] and psychiatric patients, but not in epileptic patients. Benzodiazepines can cause sedation, with a resulting impairment of various cognitive effects, particularly just after introduction of the drug, after which time some tolerance to the side-effects occurs.

Side-effects are more common at higher drug dosages. In patients receiving phenytoin or carbamazepine monotherapy,[77] psychomotor deterioration was observed at higher concentrations of both phenytoin and carbamazepine. In a similar study on 46 children with well-controlled seizures receiving sodium valproate monotherapy, those children with generalized epilepsy and those receiving less than 20 mg/kg per day performed best.[76]

We have limited data as to which of the older drugs are preferable in children, although clobazam seems to be the drug of first choice in this respect.[30] A number of new AEDs, such as lamotrigine, gabapentin, tiagabine, topiramate, zonisamide and levetiracetam are now available in many countries. In general, well-performed trials on cognitive effects in children are lacking, especially for the newer drugs. There is a clear need to develop specific neuropsychological instruments and standardized designs to be included in the randomized controlled trials on new antiepileptic drugs.[78] Ratings by parents and teachers on changes in behavior and academic achievements are also very important measures and can also be used in daily clinical practice.

SUMMARY

It is well recognized that children with epilepsy have a higher risk of deficits in cognitive functioning. In several studies over the past 25 years, it has been shown that children with epilepsy, boys more than girls, perform worse at school than their healthy peers and also perform worse than children with other chronic diseases, such as asthma or migraine. Their academic progress is affected particularly when the seizures persist. Furthermore, their academic achievement seems to be dependent on age at onset of the epilepsy in the schooling period.

Many different factors contribute to cognitive impairment, and most of these are interrelated. Seizures are a sign or symptom, and epilepsy cannot be considered a disease entity. Consequently, it is very difficult to compare the various studies performed in children with epilepsy with respect to more detailed variables. At one end of the scale are children with severe brain damage; at the other end are otherwise normal intelligent children without detectible brain dysfunctions except the occurrence of epileptiform EEG discharges. Recent studies in children with idiopathic partial epilepsies, e.g. rolandic and occipital epilepsies have elegantly shown that

- seizures and epileptiform discharges cause cognitive deficits, independent from medication
- great variability in performance and outcome on follow-up can be found even in these supposedly homogeneous groups.

Underlying brain 'damage' has a continuous negative influence on cognitive functioning. In contrast, epileptic seizures and subclinical EEG discharges influence cognitive functioning intermittently, which may contribute to the commonly observed test-retest variability and the clear interindividual variance. Generalized seizures have more impact than partial ones, unless the duration of the partial seizure is long. After a seizure, a child can catch up with his or her previous level of functioning. However, if the number or severity of the seizures is high, the influence can be very substantial. AED treatment generally decreases the number of seizures and subclinical EEG discharges and thus has a positive influence on cognitive functioning. Several studies have indeed shown a beneficial effect of suppression of epileptiform EEG discharges on learning and cognition in the laboratory and in daily life, in about 50 per cent of children with idiopathic and cryptogenic epilepsy. Unfortunately, we cannot predict yet which children might benefit from AEDs. Standardized psychological measurements during EEG recordings, in combination with parents' and teachers' questionnaires before and after drug treatment, will objectify the impact of drug treatment in the individual child.

The type of drug, rate of titration, and daily dosage influence the negative effects of AEDs on cognition. Very few well-controlled studies have been performed and the effects on cognitive functioning of interactions between the various AEDs are even less well known. In clinical practice individual differences are striking. In general, drug-related cognitive side-effects are less than the cognitive effects of seizures and discharges, except in the child with a preexistent mental impairment or a behavioral disturbance. Psychosocial factors may also have an impact on cognitive functioning. The above-mentioned factors help to explain why the literature on the cognitive aspects in children with epilepsy is often contradictory and confusing. Ideally, studies should be performed in homogenous groups of children with epilepsy. Alternatively, if children are used as their own control, differences in etiology, seizure type and medication are no longer important variables.

In the clinical assessment of children with epilepsy, it is of the utmost importance to carry out psychological investigations when the children are medically stable. This means postponing assessment when the child has had a clear change in seizure frequency or seizure type, or is withdrawing or changing medication. The neuropsychologist should also be aware of the type of epilepsy, frequency and severity of seizures, including the last occurring seizure, as well as type of medication. The tests should at least include assessment of motor speed, attention and concentration, learning, memory and higher executive functioning. Academic achievement tests (reading, spelling and arithmetic) must be part of the tests employed. Observation from parents and teachers is very important and could be standardized. Eventually, combination of all the above-mentioned information will give a complete picture of the intellectual ability and functioning of the child. However, one must always bear in mind that many children with epilepsy have no impairment in cognitive functioning and that not all problems arising at school can be ascribed to epilepsy or medication.

KEY POINTS

Neuropsychologic testing:
- Epileptic children have on average a **lower IQ** than their healthy peers and patients with 'chronic' diseases such as asthma and migraine
- Contradictory results in the same cognitive outcome measures in some studies could be due to the **differences in patient characteristics** such as etiology, age at onset, type of epilepsy, severity of epilepsy and behavioral problems
- Children with **uncontrolled seizures**, particularly those with generalized tonic-clonic seizures, have a lower IQ than seizure-free children
- Performance on **nonverbal subtests** is more impaired than on verbal tests, mainly due to the disproportionate effect of psychomotor slowing on nonverbal tasks
- The high test-retest variability observed in many studies may be due to the effect of **unnoticed seizures or subclinical epileptiform EEG discharges** occurring during the testing or instruction phase
- Generalized tonic-clonic seizures have a great impact on cognitive function, and neuropsychological investigations should not be performed within a few days of a generalized tonic-clonic convulsion

Academic achievement:
- Children with epilepsy **do less well at school** than their healthy peers and children with a chronic disease such as asthma or migraine.
- Epileptic children make **less academic progress**, especially when the seizures are not controlled
- **Boys** with epilepsy are more vulnerable than girls
- Occurrence of consistent **left**-sided epileptiform EEG discharges impairs reading
- Final academic levels are lower when the **onset of the epilepsy** occurs during school age

Subclinical epileptiform EEG discharges:
- Subclinical epileptiform discharges can cause **transient cognitive dysfunction** in children with idiopathic (including benign) and cryptogenic epilepsy
- An effect of the subclinical discharges on cognition can be demonstrated in **only 40–50 per cent** of children
- A **slow wave focus** appears to be a predictive factor for transient cognitive dysfunction
- In order to know whether suppression of the EEG discharges is beneficial to the child, **standardized EEG and cognitive performance measures** before and after use of medication are necessary

Antiepileptic drugs:
- The main cognitive side-effects of AEDs demonstrated in the laboratory involve **attention, psychomotor speed and memory**
- **Withdrawal of phenobarbital** has been shown to reverse slowness and result in a slightly higher IQ
- Using the **lowest possible dosage and monotherapy** minimizes cognitive side-effects
- Rapid escalation of the dosage and preexisting neuropsychological deficits are **risk factors** for cognitive side-effects
- **Paradoxical side-effects** of AEDs are usually obvious; more subtle cognitive changes are more difficult to recognize
- In **intellectually disabled children**, paradoxical side-effects can be difficult to differentiate from the behavioral regression that may be associated with suppression of seizures.
- Many **newly developed AEDs** appear to have fewer cognitive side-effects and some seem to be more psychostimulant than suppressant
- Because of the **confounding variables**, the cognitive effect of drugs should be investigated in children who serve as their own controls
- **Neuropsychological measures** should be reported in the results of randomized controlled trials of AEDs

> • **Ratings by parents and teachers** on changes in behavior and academic achievement are important measures that should be used in controlled trials of AEDs and can also be incorporated into daily clinical practice

ACKNOWLEDGMENTS

The research on subclinical EEG discharges was supported by a grant from the CLEO (Commissie Landelijk Epilepsie Onderzoek). We would like to thank Professor D.J. Bakker and Dr. B.M. Siebelink for their critical comments.

REFERENCES

1. Sillanpää M, Jalava M, Kaleva O, Shinnar S. Long-term prognosis of seizures with onset in childhood. *New England Journal of Medicine* 1998; **11**(338); 1715–1722.

2. Stores G. School children with epilepsy at risk of learning and behaviour problems. *Developmental Medicine and Child Neurology* 1978; **20**: 502–508.

3. Seidenberg M, Beck N, Geisser M, *et al*. Academic achievement of children with epilepsy. *Epilepsia* 1986; **27**: 753–759.

4. Staden U, Isaacs E, Boyd SG, Brandl U, Neville BGR. Language dysfunction in children with Rolandic epilepsy. *Neuropediatrics* 1998; **29**: 242–248.

5. Bailet LL, Turk WR. The impact of childhood epilepsy on neurocognitive and behavioural performance: a prospective longitudinal study. *Epilepsia* 2000; **41**(4): 426–431.

6. Lennox WG, Collins AL. Intelligence of normal and epileptic twins. *American Journal of Psychiatry* 1945; **99**: 174–180.

7. Shackleton DP, Kasteleijn-Nolst Trenité DGA, de Craen AJM, Vandenbroucke JP, Westendorp RGJ. Living with epilepsy: Long term prognosis and psychosocial outcomes. *Neurology* 2003; **61**; 64–70.

8. Pavone P, Bianchini R, Trifiletti RR, *et al*. Neuropsychological assessment in children with absence epilepsy. *Neurology* 2001; **56**: 1047–1051.

9. Deonna T, Zesiger P, Davidoff V, *et al*. Benign partial epilepsy of childhood: a longitudinal neuropsychological and EEG study of cognitive function. *Developmental Medicine and Child Neurology* 2000; **42**: 595–603.

10. Thompson PJ. Educational attainment in children and young people with epilepsy. In: Oxley J, Stores G (eds) *Epilepsy and Education*. London: Medical Tribune Group, 1987; 15–24.

11. Austin KJ, Huberty TJ, Huster GA, Dunn DW. Academic achievement in children with epilepsy or asthma. *Developmental Medicine and Child Neurology* 1998; **40**: 248–255.

12. Oostrom KJ, Schouten A, Kruitwagen CL, Peters AC, Jennekens-Schinkel A. Attention deficits are not characteristic of school children with newly diagnosed idiopathic or cryptogenic epilepsy. *Epilepsia* 2002; **43**(3): 301–310.

13. Doose H, Neubauer BA, Petersen B. The concept of hereditary impairment of brain maturation. *Epileptic Disorders* 2000; **2**(Suppl. 1): S45–9.

14. Oostrom KJ, Schouten A, Olthof T, Peters AC, Jennekens-Schinkel A. Negative emotions in children with newly diagnosed epilepsy. *Epilepsia* 2000; **41**(3): 326–331.

15. Cornaggia CM and Gobbi G. Learning disability in epilepsy: definitions and classification. *Epilepsia* 2001; **42**(Suppl. 1): 2–5.

16. Sullivan EB, Gahagan L. On intelligence of epileptic children. *Genetic Psychology Monographs* 1935; **17**: 309–375.

17. Ledeboer BCh. Over epilepsieën by kinderen; een klinische studie van het epilepsie-vraagstuk. Thesis, 1941 [in Dutch].

18. Farwell JR, Dodrill CB, Batzel LW. Neuropsychological abilities of children with epilepsy. *Epilepsia* 1985; **26**: 395–400.

19. Bourgeois BFD, Prensky AL, Palkes HS, Talent BK, Busch SG. Intelligence in epilepsy: a prospective study in children. *Annals of Neurology* 1983; **14**: 438–444.

20. Rutter M, Graham P, Yule W. *A Neuropsychiatric Study in Childhood*. Philadelphia: Lippincott, 1970.

21. Rodin EA, Schmaltz S, Twitty G. Intellectual functions of patients with childhood epilepsy. *Developmental Medicine and Child Neurology* 1986; **28**: 25–33.

22. Ellenberg JH, Hirtz DG, Nelson KB. Do seizures in children cause intellectual deterioration? *New England Journal of Medicine* 1986; **314**(17): 1085–1088.

23. Wallace SJ, Cull AM. Long-term psychological outlook for children whose first seizure occurs with fever. *Developmental Medicine and Child Neurology* 1979; **21**: 28–40.

24. Fedio P, Mirsky AF. Selective intellectual deficits in children with temporal lobe or centrencephalic epilepsy. *Neuropsychologia* 1969; **7**: 287–300.

25. Giordani B, Berent S, Sackellares JC, *et al*. Intelligence test performance of patients with partial and generalized seizures. *Epilepsia* 1985; **26**(1): 37–42.

26. Camfield PR, Gates R, Ronen G, *et al*. Comparison of cognitive ability, personality profile and school success in children with epilepsy with pure right versus left temporal lobe EEG foci. *Annals of Neurology* 1984; **15**: 122–126.

27. Schwartzkroin PA. Plasticity and repair in the immature central nervous system. Chapter 9 in: Schwartzkroin PA, Moshé SL, Noebels JL, Swann JW (eds) *Brain Development and Epilepsy*. New York: Oxford University Press, 1995.

28. Siebelink BM, Bakker DJ, Binnie CD, Kasteleijn-Nolst Trenité DGA. Psychological effects of subclinical epileptiform EEG discharges in children. II. General intelligence tests. *Epilepsy Research* 1988; **2**: 117–121.

29. Holdsworth L, Whitmore K. A study of children with epilepsy attending ordinary schools. I: Their seizure patterns, progress and behaviour in school. *Developmental Medicine and Child Neurology* 1974; **16**: 746–758.

30. Mitchell WG, Zhou Y, Chavez JM, Guzman BL. Effects of antiepileptic drugs on reaction time, attention, and impulsivity in children. *Pediatrics* 1993; **91**(1): 101–105.

31. Alpherts WCJ, Aldenkamp AP. Computerized neuropsychological assessment in children with epilepsy. In: Aldenkamp AP, Dodson WE (eds) *Epilepsy and Education; Cognitive Factors in Learning Behavior*. New York: Raven Press, 1990; S35–40.

32. Gowers WR. *Epilepsy and Other Chronic Convulsive Diseases: Their Causes, Symptoms and Treatment*. New York: William Wood, 1885. American Academy of Neurology reprint series, vol. I.

33. Lavadas E, Umilta C, Provinciali L. Hemisphere-dependent cognitive performances in epileptic patients. *Epilepsia* 1979; **20**: 493–502.

34. Kasteleijn-Nolst Trenité DGA, Smit AM, Velis DN, Willems J, Van Emde Boas W. On-line detection of transient neuropsychological disturbances during EEG discharges in children with epilepsy. *Developmental Medicine and Child Neurology* 1990; **32**: 46–50.

35. Thompson PJ, Huppert FA, Trimble MR. Phenytoin and cognitive functions: effects on normal volunteers and implications for epilepsy. *British Journal of Clinical Psychology* 1981; **20**: 155–162.

36. Austin KJ, Huberty TJ, Huster GA, Dunn DW. Academic achievement in children with epilepsy or asthma. *Developmental Medicine and Child Neurology* 1999; **41**: 473–497.

37. Stores G, Hart J. Reading skills of children with generalized or focal epilepsy attending ordinary school. *Developmental Medicine and Child Neurology* 1976; **18**: 705–715.

38. Bakker DJ, Vinke J. Effects of hemispheric-specific stimulation on brain activity and reading in dyslectics. *Clinical and Experimental Neuropsychology* 1985; **7**(5): 505–525.

39. Levin HS, Spiers PA. Acalculia. In: Heilman KM, Valenstein E (eds) *Clinical Neuropsychology*. New York: Oxford University Press, 1985; 97–115.

40. Strang J, Rourke BP. Adaptive behavior of children who exhibit specific arithmetic disabilities and associated neuropsychological abilities and deficits. In: Rourke BP (ed.) *Neuropsychology of Learning Disabilities. Essentials of Subtype Analysis*. New York: Guildford, 1985; 302–331.

41. Clement MJ, Wallace SJ. A survey of adolescents with epilepsy. *Developmental Medicine and Child Neurology* 1990; **32**: 849–857.

42. Jennekens-Schinkel A, Linschooten-Duikersloot EMEM, Bouma PAD, Peters ACB, Stijnen, T. Spelling errors made by children with mild epilepsy: writing-to-dictation. *Epilepsia* 1987; **28**(5): 555–563.

43. Schwab RS. A method of measuring consciousness in petit mal epilepsy. *Journal of Nervous and Mental Diseases* 1939; **89**: 690–691.

44. Aarts JHP, Binnie CD, Smit AM, Wilkins AJ. Selective cognitive impairment during focal and generalized epileptiform EEG activity. *Brain* 1984; **107**: 293–308.

45. Vidart L, Geier S. (1967) Enregistrements télé-encephalographiques chez des sujets épileptiques pendant le travail. *Revue Neurologique* 1967; **117**: 475–480.

46. Hutt SJ, Newton S, Fairweather H. Choice reaction time and EEG activity in children with epilepsy. *Neuropsychologia* 1977; **15**: 257–267.

47. Matsuoka H, Takahashi T, Sasaki M, *et al.* Neuropsychological EEG activation in patients with epilepsy. *Brain* 2000; **123**(2): 318–330.

48. Milner B. Interhemispheric differences in the localization of psychological processes in man. *British Medical Bulletin* 1971; **27**: 272–277.

49. Kasteleijn-Nolst Trenité DGA, Bakker DJ, Binnie CD, Buerman A, van Raaij M. Psychological effects of subclinical epileptiform EEG discharges. I. Scholastic skills. *Epilepsy Research* 1988; **2**: 111–116.

50. Petersén I, Eeg-Olofsson O. The development of the electroencephalogram in normal children from the age of 1 through 15 years. Non-paroxysmal activity. *Neuropädiatrie* 1971; **2**: 247–304.

51. Beaussart M. Benign epilepsy of children with Rolandic (centro-temporal) paroxysmal foci: a clinical entity. Study of 221 cases. *Epilepsia* 1972; **13**: 795–811.

52. Massa R, Saint-Martin A de, Carcangiu R, *et al.* EEG criteria predictive of cognitive complications in idiopathic focal epilepsy with rolandic spikes. *Neurology* 2001; **57**: 1071–1079.

53. Metz-Lutz M, Kleitz C, de Saint-Martin A, *et al.* Cognitive development in benign focal epilepsies of childhood. *Developmental Neuroscience* 1999; **21**: 182–190.

54. Marston D, Besag F, Binnie CD, Fowler M. Effects of transitory cognitive impairment on psychosocial functioning of children with epilepsy: a therapeutic trial. *Developmental Medicine and Child Neurology* 1993; **35**: 574–581.

55. Ronen GM, Richards JE, Cunningham C, Secord M, Rosenbloom D. Can sodium valproate improve learning in children with epileptiform bursts but without clinical seizures? *Developmental Medicine and Child Neurology* 2000; **42**(11): 751–755.

56. Rowan AJ, Binnie CD, Warfield CA, *et al.* The delayed effect of sodium valproate on the photoconvulsive response in man. *Epilepsia* 1979; **20**: 61–68.

57. Bouma PA, Peters AC, Brouwer OF. Long term course of childhood epilepsy following relapse after antiepileptic drug withdrawal. *Journal of Neurology, Neurosurgery and Psychiatry* 2002; **72**(4): 507–510.

58. Harbord MG. Significant anticonvulsant side-effects in children and adolescents. *Journal of Clinical Neuroscience* 2000; **7**(3): 213–216.

59. Trimble MR, Cull C. Children of school age: the influence of antiepileptic drugs on behaviour and intellect. *Epilepsia* 1988; **29**(Suppl. 3): S15–19.

60. Kossoff EH, Bergey GK, Freeman JM, Vining EP. Levetiracetam psychosis in children with epilepsy. *Epilepsia* 2001; **42**(12): 1611–1613.

61. Helmstaedter C, Wagner G, Elger CE. Differential effects of first antiepileptic drug application on cognition in lesional and non-lesional patients with epilepsy. *Seizure* 1993; **2**: 125–130.

62. Bourgeois BFD. AEDs, learning, and behavior. *Epilepsia* 1988; **39**(9): 913–921.

63. Kasteleijn-Nolst Trenité DGA, Rentmeester TW, Scholtes FBJ, *et al.* Perimarketing surveillance of lamotrigine in the Netherlands: doctors' and patients' viewpoints. *Pharmacy World and Science* 2001; **23**(1): 1–5.

64. Trimble MR, Thompson PJ. Anticonvulsant drugs, cognitive function, and behavior. *Epilepsia* 1983; **24**(Suppl. 1): S555–563.

65. Thompson PJ, Trimble MR. Anticonvulsant serum levels: relationship to impairments of cognitive functions. *Journal of Neurology, Neurosurgery and Psychiatry* 1983; **46**: 227–233.

66. Meador KJ, Loring DW, Ray PG, *et al.* Differential cognitive effects of carbamazepine and gabapentin. *Epilepsia* 1999; **40**(9): 1279–1285.

67. Meador KJ, Loring DW, Ray PG, *et al.* Differential cognitive and behavioural effects of carbamazepine and lamotrigine. *Neurology* 2001; **56**: 1177–1182.

68. Martin R, Kuzniecky R, Ho S, *et al.* Cognitive effects of topiramate, gabapentin, and lamotrigine in healthy young adults. *Neurology* 1999; **52**: 321–327.

69. Kasteleijn-Nolst Trenité DGA, Emde Boas W Van, Groenhout CM, Meinardi H. Preliminary assessment of the efficacy of Org 6370 in photosensitive epileptic patients: paradoxical enhancement of photosensitivity and provocation of myoclonic seizures. *Epilepsia* 1992; **33**(1): 135–141.

70. Smith DB. Anticonvulsants, seizures and performance: The Veteran's Administration experience. In: Trimble MR and Reynolds EH *Epilepsy, Behaviour and Cognitive Function.* Chichester: John Wiley & Sons Ltd, 1987; 67–78.

71. Vining EPG, Mellits ED, Dorsen MM, *et al.* Psychologic and behavioural effects of antiepileptic drugs in children: a double-blind comparison between phenobarbital and valproic acid. *Pediatrics* 1987; **80**(2): 165–174.

72. Williams J, Bates S, Griebel ML, *et al.* Does short-term antiepileptic drug treatment in children result in cognitive or behavioural changes? *Epilepsia* 1998; **39**: 1064–1069.

73. Riva D, Devoti M. Discontinuation of phenobarbital in children: effects on neurocognitive behaviour. *Pediatric Neurology* 1996; **14**(1): 36–40.

74. Chen Y, Chow JC, Lee I. Comparison of the cognitive effect of antiepileptic drugs in seizure-free children with epilepsy before and after drug withdrawal. *Epilepsy Research* 2001; **44**: 65–70.

75. Mortimer RG, Howat PA. Effects of alcohol and diazepam, singly and in combination, on some aspects of driving performance. In: O'Hanlon JF, de Gier JJ (eds) *Drugs and Driving.* London: Taylor & Francis, 1986; 163–178.

76. Aman MG, Werry JS, Paxton JW, Turbot T. Effect of sodium valproate on psychomotor performance in children as a function of dose, fluctuations in concentration and diagnosis. *Epilepsia* 1987; **28**(2): 115–124.

77. Aman MG, Paxon JW, Werry JS. Fluctuations in steady-state phenytoin concentrations as measured in saliva in children. *Pediatric Pharmacology* 1983; **3**: 87–94.

78. Cochrane HC, Marson AG, Baker GA, Chadwick DW. Neuropsychological outcomes in randomised controlled trials of antiepileptic drugs: a systematic review of methodology and reporting standards. *Epilepsia* 1998; **39**(10): 1088–1097.

24

Psychiatric aspects

SHARON DAVIES AND ISOBEL HEYMAN

THE PSYCHIATRY OF EPILEPSY IS IMPORTANT

Children with epilepsy are at increased risk for mental health problems when compared to both the general population, and to those with chronic illnesses not involving the central nervous system (CNS). Children with both epilepsy and structural CNS abnormality are more likely than not to have psychopathology.[1] The impact and burden of this psychiatric morbidity contributes significantly to the overall disability.

This chapter addresses the detection and assessment of mental health problems; outlines the common diagnoses and their specific treatments, and reviews types of emotional and behavioral disorder which seem particularly common in children with epilepsy. If progress through the social, emotional and educational challenges of childhood and adolescence is attended by mental health difficulties, early detection and assertive treatment are essential. A multidisciplinary approach is normally required.

RISK FACTORS

Structural brain abnormality is the strongest risk factor. Other predictors can be broadly divided into seizure factors, cognitive factors, effects of antiepileptic drugs (AEDs), social, and family factors. Seizure frequency or degree of cognitive impairment may be acting as markers for the severity or pervasiveness of underlying CNS disorder. Direct causality for any specific factor is difficult to establish as interaction is invariable (see Figure 24.1). Some specific risk factors where there is reasonable evidence for association and some suggestions for mechanism are discussed.

Chronic illness

Children suffering from chronic illnesses of any sort could be more prone to mental illness, secondary to distress, stigma, pain, effects on peer relationships or education. However, the presence of a brain disorder and/or intellectual impairment is a major contributory factor[2] to psychopathology when compared with, for example, cystic fibrosis,[3] diabetes,[4] cardiac disorders,[5] rheumatoid arthritis[6] and asthma.[7] Severity of physical disability has little effect, but psychopathology varies directly with the level of intellectual disability. Even children with seizures of recent onset have increased rates of behavioral problems, as do children in the 6-month period before the onset of seizures.[8,9]

All these studies support a strong and direct 'brain-behavior' link in epilepsy, and indicate that children with epilepsy should be screened for emotional and behavioral problems. The more such problems are seen as an integral component of the disability of epilepsy, the more likely they are to be detected and treated as part of routine care.

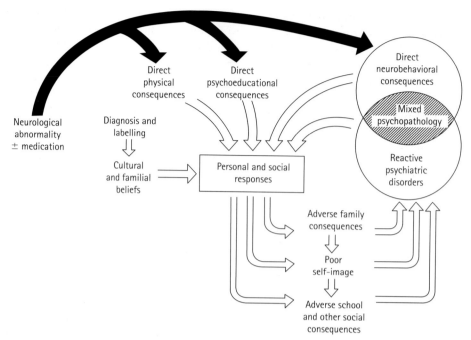

Figure 24.1 *A simplified representation of organic (black arrows) and psychosocial pathways (white arrows) from brain to behavioral abnormalities. Reproduced from R Goodman, Brain disorders in M Rutter, E Taylor and L Hersov (eds),* Child and Adolescent Psychiatry *2002 with the permission of Blackwell Publishing Ltd.*

Stigma

Very young children and their peers may take an unconcerned view of epilepsy and its associated symptoms, but the realization that they 'differ' from classmates or friends develops. Likewise, other children begin to notice and comment on obvious seizures, the need to take medication or absence from school. Teasing, unkind mimicry, bullying or, more subtly, incorrect and unhelpful assumptions about the child, can result. Much work has been done to consider whether the child with epilepsy is truly stigmatized, and whether this represents a risk to mental health.

Stigma occurs when a particular aspect of an individual's behavior or character is perceived negatively and used to define that person in a negative way. Much has been written about how stigma relates to issues of identity, and how a framework 'stigma theory' might be helpful in understanding causes and consequences of stigmatization.[10] Stigma theory has been invoked to help explain why the psychosocial burden of a diagnosis of epilepsy seems greater than for other chronic diseases.[11] When a 'social visibility' scale measured how often children with epilepsy were identified by teachers because of emotional and behavioral concerns, no evidence was found of stigma, unless the epilepsy was complicated by learning disability or other neurological abnormality.[12] Peer rejection may be consequential on psychiatric disorders, rather than representing risks for their development.[1] However, the subsequent social isolation will add to the disability.

Stigma is socially constructed, and stigmatized identities change over time, but epilepsy and certain psychiatric disorders remain 'stigmatized' to a large extent. However, stigma associated with epilepsy seems to be decreasing in many cultures. Nevertheless, the child with behavioral problems or learning disabilities in combination with epilepsy may well be identified as a 'problem' child by both peers and adults.

Learning disability

Both global and specific learning disabilities are associated with higher rates of childhood psychiatric disorder. These contribute to the increased risks of psychiatric problems in children with epilepsy.[13] Low average Full-Scale IQ and specific reading retardation (dyslexia) are commoner than in control children.[1,14] Even when IQ is discounted, those with epilepsy experience more academic problems and underachievement[15,16] (Chapters 13, 23). The group with epilepsy, learning disability and behavioral problems is the most challenging to support, medically, socially and educationally, and exemplifies the cumulative burden of risk in children with epilepsy.

SEIZURE FACTORS

Seizures themselves may have a direct effect on emotions and behavior. Mental state changes before, during and after a seizure can include behavioral change in the prodromal/preictal phase, acute change during the epileptic seizure itself, and also postictally. Emotional, cognitive and behavioral abnormalities can be associated with ictal activity that is apparent on EEG recording, but is not identifiable as an overt seizure. In some instances, parents are able to predict ensuing seizures through recognizable behavioral changes in the child. Increased irritability, changes in motor activity, reduced concentration, and increased aggression and other behavioral changes are sometimes noted as much as a day in advance. Other children become anxious before a seizure. With some seizure types the aura may include intense feelings of fear or unease.

Whether extreme behavioral changes can occur during the seizure itself is controversial. Some seizure types can be associated with complex and apparently volitional behaviors, but, in general, EEG recordings taken during behavioral outbursts in children with and without epilepsy fail to reveal acute seizures. Postictal behavioral changes can be quite prolonged; children can be drowsy, uncooperative, irritable and even aggressive.

The severity of seizures and the age at which epilepsy began may be important predictors of mental health problems. Inadequate seizure control has been linked to behavioral disturbances by some authors.[4,17–19] Greater seizure frequency is associated with more behavioral problems, whereas, with good seizure control, the psychosocial impact of epilepsy is minimized.[20] The lag of academic performance behind expectations based on IQ and age is greater with earlier onset of seizures, higher total number of seizures and multiple seizure types.[21] However, seizure variables may largely reflect the severity of underlying CNS pathology.

Are some seizure types and syndromes particularly associated with psychopathology?

It is difficult to establish whether particular seizure types are associated with increased risk of behavioral disturbance. Overall, complex partial epilepsy has been more strongly associated with psychiatric disorder than generalized epilepsy. In particular, temporal lobe epilepsy (TLE) is usually thought of as being highly associated with psychiatric disturbance, though there is great variability in the psychiatric manifestations of TLE in adults.[22]

Temporal lobe epilepsy (TLE)

In a study specifically of children with TLE, only 15 per cent were free from psychological problems.[23] Nearly 50 per cent suffered from catastrophic rage attacks, hyperkinesis or these combined. The rate of hyperkinesis was several times greater if TLE was associated with structural brain abnormality. However, in studies comparing children with TLE with those with other seizure types, it is less clear that TLE is more strongly associated with behavioral or emotional problems. When normal controls are compared with children with complex partial seizures (CPS) and primary generalized epilepsy (PGE), no differences in rates of psychiatric disorder are found between the two epilepsy groups. Nor are differences detected in the type of psychopathology, casting doubt on earlier views that children with CPS have externalizing disorders and those with PGE internalizing disorders. The epilepsy groups had significantly higher rates of psychiatric problems compared to a nonepileptic group.[24]

Factors such as gender, IQ and lateralization of the seizure focus may have greater influence on the risk of psychiatric disorder. In epilepsy surgery patients, those with right-sided lesions have higher rates of autistic spectrum disorder.[25] Boys (but not girls) with TLE have been found to be more at risk of behavioral disorder if the EEG showed left temporal spikes.[26] Other studies have not found gender to be significant.[27] In summary, issues of gender, age, IQ, EEG variables, societal reactions to epilepsy, and treatment variables may be just as important risk factors for psychopathology as seizure types and related variables.[17,28]

AURAS

Auras associated with TLE can cause subjective feelings of anxiety and panic. In general, patients with frequent or multiple auras have higher rates of psychiatric problems.[29] *Déjà vu*, forced thinking and disturbances of higher function are rarely reported in children, but, if asked directly, children can give compelling accounts of these unusual and often distressing experiences.

Frontal lobe epilepsy

Frontal lobe seizures can be bizarre and are particularly prone to misdiagnosis as pseudo-seizures, sleep disorders or behavioral problems.[30] Odd movements such as rocking, thrashing, cycling motion of the legs, turning or arching backwards and noises (laughing, screaming, swearing, squealing, etc.) may occur. They may be exclusively nocturnal and of brief duration with no period of postictal drowsiness. Clinical experience suggests that children with frontal lobe abnormalities such as cortical dysplasia, and associated epilepsy, may have particular problems with hyperactive, disinhibited and disruptive behavior.

ANTIEPILEPTIC DRUGS

All medications that act on the central nervous system have the potential to alter behavior, emotions and cognition.

Young people may be more at risk of these. All antiepileptic drugs (AEDs) have anecdotal reports of unwanted behavioral side-effects, but it can be difficult to implicate particular medications. High degrees of variability in cognitive function for individuals at different time points may confound attempts to assess the effects of AEDs on cognition.[31] However, an unexpected change should always lead to consideration of drug effects.

Changes in behavior attributed to drugs may emerge in relation to the epilepsy, or an underlying neurological disorder. Neuropsychological deficits occur even when structural brain abnormality is excluded or controlled for, and even if patients are not taking AEDs, suggesting that fundamental disorders of attention and impaired alertness may be characteristic in epilepsy, irrespective of treatment.[32] Some AEDs are more associated with mental state changes than others. Individuals taking more than one drug have increased chances of cognitive or behavioral side-effects.[33] Of the older AEDs, phenobarbital was most often associated with adverse behavioral side-effects, particularly aggression, hyperactivity and depression.[34,35] However, behavioral change is not always negative: it is suggested that carbamazepine may have an independent beneficial effect on cognition, behavior or mood.[36] The psychopharmacological effects of AEDs are exploited in their use as mood stabilizers and in treatment of aggressive behavior, particularly in children with learning disability.

Limited evidence on newer AEDs[37,38] suggests psychosis, depression, agitation, aggressivity, irritability or hyperactivity may be precipitated in 9–30 per cent of children who receive vigabatrin.[39–41] These changes appear to be reversible with dose reduction and seem to be more likely if the patient is intellectually disabled or has a past history of behavioral problems. Gabapentin has been implicated in the development of hyperactivity and aggression in children with learning disability: discontinuation has resulted in resolution of behavior difficulties.[42] Topiramate has been reported to change behavior, but there is more evidence for cognitive side-effects.[43] Medication side-effects should always be considered if there is a behavioral change, and it is important to take parents' or teachers' impressions seriously. However, often after careful clinical analysis, it is difficult to implicate the AED in the behavior change, more than, for example, fluctuations in seizure control, or an upset at school. This uncertainty is in line with attempts made to study objectively the evidence for a clinically significant effect of AEDs on behavior, where an unequivocal causal relationship is methodologically difficult to establish.[44] However, taking a collaborative and experimental approach with the family on exploring the relationship between drugs and behavior is essential in maintaining their confidence through any future drug changes which may be necessary.

FAMILY AND SOCIAL FACTORS

Children with epilepsy are vulnerable to the same adverse social and family factors as other children. A child with a chronic disorder can impact on a family's emotional and financial well-being, which may in turn exacerbate any developmental or behavioral problems experienced by the child. Multiple variables contribute to the psychosocial problems: physical (disability, restriction of activities, side effects of medications, fatigue), psychological (feeling different from peers, depression or anxiety about illness, worries about the future, lack of independence) social (multiple hospital visits/stays, stressors on parents and siblings, restricted social life).

Those children who have an additional diagnosis of conduct disorder are likely to have the same adverse family factors as are associated with conduct disorder in the general population.[45] These include increased family stress, less family mastery, less extended family social support and poorer family functioning (less intrafamily esteem and communication). Divorce or separation in parents increases rates of childhood depression and behavioral problems.[18,27,46] An Impact of Paediatric Epilepsy Scale[20] revealed that the parents of children with epilepsy are more stressed, and have lower self-esteem and more emotional problems than expected, but these findings are not always replicated.[47] It has been suggested that the psychosocial impact on families depends on the severity of the epilepsy, the complexity of clinical management, the meaning of the illness to child and family; restrictions in the child's and family's activities, the child and family's coping abilities and the levels of social support and resources.[47]

In all studies on family factors, it is difficult to define mechanisms or to attribute directions of effects. For example, if depression in a parent is associated with increased behavioral disturbance in a child, is this because the parental depression contributes to the child's disorder, or because this particular child has such severe epilepsy with co-morbid behavioral disorder that it is overwhelming and distressing to the parent? There is some evidence that psychiatric morbidity in the mothers of children with chronic, but not newly diagnosed, epilepsy is relevant.[47] In clinical practice, it is likely that both mechanisms operate, and that treatment or support for parents may facilitate their coping skills. It is usual in child psychiatry to emphasize the importance of family factors in the emergence of emotional and behavioral problems, but the brain-behavior links are likely to be more important in epilepsy. For example, although absence epilepsy has generally been thought to have a low impact on family or child functioning, it can be associated with poor psychosocial outcome, behavior problems, high rates of unplanned pregnancy, academic difficulties and occupational underachievement.[6] Similarly, although poor psychosocial outcome in the general population is strongly associated with social and family adversity, and clearly children with epilepsy are not immune to these influences, they may also be subject to other unusual risks. Neurotoxicity from AEDs has been highlighted as a predictor of poor quality of life, although this clearly interacts strongly with disease severity and chronicity.[48]

ADOLESCENCE

Adolescence is always a challenging stage. For those with chronic illness, there may be particular difficulties with managing specifically medical aspects, e.g. taking medication. Psychosocial implications relate to the predicament of negotiating independence and identity in the context of a chronic physical illness, where the possibilities of stigma, reduced independence, interference with social functions and peer relations, lowered self-esteem and mood, and impaired cognition exist.[48] Compared with control subjects, adolescents with epilepsy have a larger discrepancy between actual and ideal self-images: they estimate their chances of success in school as poorer and have poorer body and self-image concepts.[49] They tend to limit themselves in choice of profession and education in a way not proportionate to their disease and possibilities.[50] With intractable epilepsy or additional neurological impairments, successful separation from the parents is more difficult or impossible. Understandably, parents can also find it difficult to allow appropriate increases in independent activity, thereby provoking arguments and oppositional behavior as well as preventing developmentally appropriate social interactions.

Typical adolescent activities such as staying up late and experimenting with drugs and alcohol, may worsen seizure control or provoke family battles. Side-effects of AEDs can become more of an issue, especially for girls. For example, with valproic acid there are possibilities of hair loss, excess weight gain, menstrual irregularities and polycystic ovary syndrome; and with enzyme-inducing AEDs, reduced efficacy of oral contraception. There is a high rate of unplanned pregnancy in young women with epilepsy.[6] Battles around compliance can occur as adolescents attempt to exert more control over their healthcare. Adolescents may not be well catered for in pediatric or child psychiatry services, and a strong case can be made for dedicating specialized multidisciplinary services for this age group.[51]

DETECTION, ASSESSMENT AND TREATMENT OF THE COMMON CHILD PSYCHIATRIC DISORDERS

Children with epilepsy are subject to the same psychiatric disorders as those in the general childhood population.

Unusual emotional or behavioral disorders are not generally seen. Trying to establish which mechanisms are most significant is less important than making clear diagnoses and implementing effective treatment. A brief summary of the most important mental health problems of children follows.[52,53] In a population study, among children with uncomplicated epilepsy, 13 per cent had emotional disorder, 7.5 per cent conduct disorder, 5 per cent mixed disorder and 2 per cent hyperkinetic disorder. There was no association between epilepsy and a specific syndrome so, as in the general population, children with epilepsy suffered most commonly from emotional and conduct problems.[1,4] In an epidemiological study in the UK in 1999, this finding was confirmed, but children with 'complicated' epilepsy (defined as having additional neurological problems) had especially high rates of attention deficit hyperactivity disorder and autistic spectrum disorder.[54]

Classification

The adequacy of current diagnostic categories in psychiatry for fully describing the behavioral consequences of epilepsy in children has been questioned.[55] Aggressive behavior, temper tantrums, disinhibition and hyperactivity do not easily fit into diagnostic categories. However, making a *Diagnostic and Statistical Manual*/International Classification of Disease (DSM/ICD) diagnosis is a rigorous way to frame thinking, allows a clear mechanism for review and informs prognosis and treatment. In a study of the appropriateness of ICD 10 diagnostic categories in adults and children with epilepsy,[56] it was concluded that, in a patient with 'a clear sensorium' ICD 10 psychiatric diagnoses could be applied, alongside the diagnosis of epilepsy, but concerns about the limitations of the current systems were expressed and further research was urged.

Assessment

Psychiatric assessments are distinct components of evaluation, and require input from specialist mental health professionals. Diagnosis must take account of the child's developmental stage, since thorough psychiatric assessment necessitates understanding of the child's cognitive strengths and weaknesses. Furthermore, a formulation of the emotional and behavioral issues requires an integration of the child's epilepsy history and current epilepsy symptoms. Assessment ideally involves meeting the child, individually and with the parents/carers, as well as gathering information from teachers and other professionals involved with the child to establish whether behavioral or emotional problems occur only at school, where perhaps the child's learning problems have not been recognized.

Table 24.1 *Identifying emotional and behavioral problems*

Epilepsy review

Has there been a change in seizure type, severity, frequency?
Are there significant EEG changes without related seizures?
Is the behavior change peri-ictal?
Has there been a medication change, and might the drug
   be having behavioral side-effects?

Psychiatric review

Does the child have an additional psychiatric diagnosis?
Is it possible to determine any factors which might be
   contributing to this?

Behavioral analysis

Is the behavior situational? (Need accounts from parents,
   carers, school, etc.)
Are there identifiable antecedents and consequences to
   particular behaviors?
What has worked in modifying the behavior?

Family review

Does the family have adequate support/respite, etc.?
Does the family have realistic expectations?
Are parents overprotective/overindulgent, etc.?

Educational review

Is the child's cognitive level known? If not, psychometry is
   usually helpful
Does the child have specific learning disabilities?
What are the particular challenges in the classroom setting?
How much special/statutory help does the child receive?

Table 24.2 *Suggested structure for child psychiatric assessment*

Current problems/parental concerns
Direct question screen for symptoms
Disruptive/hyperactive
Emotional
Relationships (family and peer)
Developmental history
Emergence of emotional and behavioral problems
Relationship to epilepsy/medication etc.
Developmental milestones (especially social/emotional)
Family history (especially psychiatric disorder)
Past psychiatric history
Medical/epilepsy history and relationship to psychiatric
   symptoms
Overall impairment experienced as a result of psychiatric
   problems
Use of standardized questionnaires and rating scales
Formulation (suggest use of Axis system such DSM-IV)
   Axis I: Clinical disorders
   Axis II: Personality disorders and learning disability
   Axis III: General medical conditions
   Axis IV: Psychosocial and environmental problems
   Axis V: Global assessment of functioning

Patchy cognitive strengths and weaknesses can be difficult to appreciate and lead to frustration both at home and in school. Understanding the developmental context of the child is essential. A scheme for this general assessment is given in Table 24.1.

A thorough screening for emotional and behavioral symptoms can be facilitated by use of standardized psychiatric/psychological instruments such as the Strengths and Difficulties Questionnaire.[57] It can be helpful to think about a child's symptoms in a series of domains (see Table 24.1). Disorder-specific instruments can give additional help with the assessment process, and may be useful for monitoring treatment response.[58,59]

A full family history is important for establishing the living arrangements for the child, relationships with other family members and siblings, and to screen for familial risks for mental illness.

A suggested structure for child psychiatric assessment is given in Table 24.2.

SPECIFIC PSYCHIATRIC DISORDERS AND EPILEPSY

The diagnostic features and main treatments of common childhood disorders are summarized here. More unusual conditions seen in young people with epilepsy are discussed in more detail.

Conduct disorder and oppositional defiant disorder

Disruptive behavior disorders are the most common reason for parents to seek help. Diagnostic criteria range from repetitive and persistent hostile and defiant patterns of behavior (oppositional defiant disorders), progressing to violation of the basic rights of others or breaking major age-appropriate norms or rules (conduct disorders). True conduct disorder is probably less problematic in general, as many young people with epilepsy are quite highly monitored by parents and less likely to engage in particularly socialized forms of disorder. However, early disruptive behavior disorders are risk factors for later delinquency, and for adult violence and criminality. Genetic and environmental variables contribute to this association, and it may be that epilepsy has a further influence in some individuals. One study of delinquent adolescents suggested that the combination of psychomotor epilepsy with psychiatric symptoms is particularly associated with violence.[60] A constellation of problem behaviors, including irritability, aggression and temper tantrums, which do not easily fit into diagnostic categories, is common. Parents may not feel confident in setting appropriate boundaries for behavior, unwittingly exacerbating disruptive behaviors. Parent training is effective in children with oppositional defiant disorder, and similar approaches could be equally effective in children with epilepsy.[61] Behavior modification in the home and at school remains the most effective treatment for behavior disorders, and seeking expert advice for undertaking behavioral analysis, and design of behavioral programs is often worthwhile. Medication for disruptive behavior does not usually provide long-term benefit, although medical treatment of coexistent ADHD can be helpful.

Attention deficit/hyperactivity disorder (ADHD)

ADHD is the name given to a triad of symptoms of inattention, hyperactivity and impulsivity persisting to a degree that is maladaptive and developmentally inappropriate. Pervasiveness of symptoms or impairment is required to make a diagnosis. Symptoms of ADHD are common in children with epilepsy, especially those with structural brain abnormalities. Responses to stimulant medication are variable, the hyperactivity often showing improvement following improved seizure control. It is possible that, in some children, persistent interictal abnormal epileptiform activity on EEG is associated with symptoms of hyperactivity that respond to an increase in AED dosage. Methylphenidate is considered the first-line medication for ADHD. Although there is a theoretical risk of lowering the seizure threshold, there is little systematic evidence for this. One small study of children with ADHD and epilepsy found them to be as responsive to methylphenidate as those without epilepsy, with no increase in seizures.[62] Treatment should be started with a low dose, which is increased slowly with careful monitoring of therapeutic response and side-effects, especially where seizures are continuing.[63]

Depression

In pediatric epilepsy populations, about 25 per cent show increased ratings on depression inventories.[64,65] Direct questioning of the child is very important. Psychological treatments (Chapter 22E) have proven efficacy in young people.[66] Pharmacologic treatment should also be considered. Tricyclic antidepressants should probably be avoided because they risk lowering of the seizure threshold. There are now several trials showing good responses to selective serotonin reuptake inhibitors (SSRI) in childhood depression.[67] Citalopram has the least propensity for drug interactions, which may be important with co-medication with AEDs. Although citalopram may have the least risk of this, the SSRIs also have the potential to lower the seizure threshold, and should be used cautiously. Attempted suicide is 15 times commoner in adolescents with epilepsy than in the general population.[68] The attempts are more medically serious, with more

premeditation and more serious suicidal intent. Treatment with phenobarbital may be particularly associated with depression and suicidality. In children, seizure type and lateralization seem to be weak indicators of psychopathology in general, and of depression in particular. Significant predictors of depression seem to be the young person's attitudes to epilepsy, satisfaction with family relationships and having a poor sense of control of their own lives.[65]

Anxiety disorders

The common anxiety disorders include generalized anxiety disorder, specific phobias, obsessive compulsive disorder and social phobias. All anxiety disorders are commoner than expected in young people with epilepsy, but there is little detailed information on specific or unusual forms. Clinical observation suggests a frequent tendency to cling to one or both parents, particularly at bedtime. These types of difficulties can usually be approached with behavioral and family interventions, bearing in mind the (often justifiable) fears of seizures occurring during the night.

Generalized anxiety disorder is characterized by pervasive feelings of worry that are difficult to control and are accompanied by physical symptoms such as restlessness, muscle tension, impaired concentration, sleep disturbance or fatigue. Sometimes fear, anxiety or even panic-like symptoms can be part of an aura, or the seizure itself. However, anxiety is common: 16 per cent of children with epilepsy have significant anxiety symptomatology.[64] The first line of treatment is cognitive behavioral therapy (Chapter 22E). In severe or resistant cases, SSRIs can be effective.[69]

Specific fears and phobias are usually highly responsive to a behavioral approach, with graded exposure to the feared stimulus and subsequent desensitization being the treatment of choice. Panic disorder, defined as recurrent panic attacks with subsequent worry about the onset of further attacks or their consequences, is very rare in prepubertal children.[70] It is not known whether panic is commoner than expected in young populations with epilepsy.

Obsessive compulsive disorder is characterized by persistent intrusive, repetitive, distressing thoughts, and associated ritualized behavior which often seem to reduce anxiety. There may be some differences from other anxiety disorders since there seems to be a stronger relationship with brain disorder, particularly basal ganglia abnormalities. The population prevalence is about 1 per cent in people under 18 years old. The obsessions and compulsions can significantly impair a child's functioning, through diversion from more important activities and causing marked distress. The first-line treatment should be cognitive behavioral therapy, but this disorder is also highly responsive to SSRIs.[71] Though many children with epilepsy have 'obsessive' type problems, these are often not truly obsessive compulsive disorder, and may be personality traits or autistic spectrum symptoms.

Autistic spectrum and language disorders

Autism and autistic spectrum disorders are characterized by qualitative impairments in reciprocal social interaction and patterns of communication, and by restricted, stereotyped, repetitive ranges of interests and activities. Affected children have an increased rate of epilepsy.[72] There is little systematic study of autistic features in children with epilepsy, but clinical observation suggests that one or more components of the autistic triad are relatively common in children with severe epilepsy and learning difficulties. In particular, abnormalities of social understanding and empathy are over-represented, even if diagnostic criteria for autism or Asperger's syndrome are not fully met. In patients undergoing temporal lobectomy, young people with right-sided temporal lobe pathologies are many times more likely to have conditions in the autistic spectrum than those with left-sided lesions.[25] The Landau-Kleffner syndrome (Chapter 13) presents with loss of receptive and expressive language skills, associated with EEG changes, and, in the majority of cases, seizures. Behavioral changes are common with the onset of language loss but it is unclear if these children show impairments in reciprocal social communication of the qualitative nature associated with autism.[73] Infantile spasms are associated with increased rates of autism.[74] Coexistence of tuberous sclerosis could be instrumental in some cases, since individuals with both tuberous sclerosis and epilepsy are at very high risk for an autistic spectrum disorder.[75]

Psychosis

In the general population, psychosis is rare in prepubertal children, becoming commoner in later adolescence. Psychosis is always a serious mental illness, and requires specialist psychiatric assessment and treatment. Core symptoms of an acute psychotic episode are delusions, hallucinations (usually auditory) and thought disorder. Antipsychotic drugs are often needed, and all have the potential to reduce the seizure threshold, but treating the psychosis remains paramount, and can usually be achieved without significant increase in seizures. However, clozapine is associated with a significant risk of precipitating seizures and should be used with caution.[76]

PSYCHIATRIC DISORDERS PARTICULARLY ASSOCIATED WITH EPILEPSY

Epileptic psychosis

Epilepsy and schizophrenia are both relatively common disorders in adult populations. Some researchers have argued that any association is spurious.[77] However, overall, it appears that in later adolescence, epilepsy confers vulnerability to psychotic disorders. These include a chronic interictal psychosis closely resembling schizophrenia, **schizophrenia-like psychoses of epilepsy** (SLPE), and episodic psychotic states. SLPE resembles schizophrenia in phenomenology, has a similar course, is as responsive to antipsychotic medication and appears to be largely uninfluenced by concurrent seizure activity.[78] However, unlike probands with schizophrenia, the prevalence of schizophrenia in family histories of those with SLPE is similar to the general population. Liability to SLPE appears to be unrelated to epilepsy severity and often occurs when seizure frequency is declining. Whether or not it is a distinct nosological entity remains somewhat controversial but more recent studies lend strong support to the notion that SLPE is a unique disorder.[79]

Episodic psychoses

Postictal psychosis is the commonest of the episodic psychoses. Characteristically it arises after seizure exacerbations, especially in clusters accompanied by secondary generalization. There is usually a lucid interval of 12–72 h with subsequent deterioration of the mental state with affective, schizophrenic or confusional elements. Spontaneous resolution generally occurs and may be associated with increased epileptic activity or slowed dominant rhythm.[80] Compared with SLPE there is a later age of onset of epilepsy and psychosis and patients report more seizure clustering and ictal fear. Bilateral EEG discharges are seen more often in those with postictal psychoses than in nonpsychotic controls or SLPE.[81]

Other episodic psychoses, occurring less commonly, include those induced by AEDs and those arising during periods of improved seizure control. The latter are associated with the phenomenon of forced normalization (FN) where normalization of EEG leads to emergence of psychosis. It may be particularly prone to occur when new AEDs are added.[82] The issue of forced normalization in children needs further study, in particular to establish whether it might manifest with behavioral change rather than typical psychotic episodes.

Pathogenesis

Temporal lobe epilepsy (TLE) appears to be a greater risk factor for psychosis than idiopathic generalized epilepsy (IGE). Cerebral localization and lateralization has been the topic of much discussion, with an association of psychosis with left temporal foci reported,[83] but it may be that cerebral dominance is the more important predictor.[84] Functional neuroimaging may further elucidate any possible association between localization of seizure focus and risk of psychosis.[85] The neuropathology of the underlying lesion is also relevant. In adults, gangliogliomas were more strongly associated with psychosis than other underlying pathologies.[86,87] The stage of cerebral maturation at which a lesion develops seems more relevant than the neuropathological characteristics: lesions arising pre-or perinatally seem to present greater risks for psychosis.[88]

Epilepsy surgery and psychosis

In well-selected adult patients, psychosis is not a contraindication to surgery. Preoperatively a diagnosis of SLPE has been associated with a left temporal focus but 85 per cent of *de novo* psychoses arising postoperatively follow right temporal surgery. Although this has not received much attention in pediatric epilepsy surgery, the risk of postoperative psychosis may become increasingly relevant for the older adolescent.

Psychosis and pediatric populations

In pediatric populations, the rare occurrence of psychosis may be an unusual AED-related event. Acute psychotic episodes, which have been reported after initiation of levetiracetam therapy, resolve with cessation or dose reduction.[89] Nevertheless, overall, it has been suggested that 10 per cent of children with TLE develop psychosis by adulthood, with rage attacks and hyperkinesis increasing the risk.[90] The psychosis may resolve spontaneously and may be associated with increased epileptic activity or slowed dominant rhythm. Formal thought disorder (illogical thinking) occurs significantly more often in children with CPS than in those with IGE or absences, or in nonepileptic children. Severity of illogical thinking relates to global cognitive dysfunction.[91] One report on children with seizures and interictal schizophrenia-like symptoms found the presentation was similar to that in adults, but the children had frequent seizures while psychotic. All had epilepsy for 5–9 years before onset of psychotic symptoms.[92]

PSEUDO-SEIZURES

Definition

Nonepileptic seizures are 'attacks' that are mistaken for epilepsy. They may be physiological or psychological in origin, but are not associated with abnormal cortical electrical discharges. Chapter 2 describes the organic causes of nonepileptic attacks. In addition, there are some psychiatric episodes to be considered. These include panic attacks, hyperventilation in the context of anxiety, depersonalization and derealization phenomena, mannerisms and stereotypies. Some unusual psychotic phenomena could be mistaken for pseudo-seizures. Rarely, children may present in dissociative states following severe trauma, such as sexual abuse. Münchausen syndrome by proxy occasionally needs to be considered.[93]

A pseudo-seizure is a nonepileptic attack of psychological origin. Other names such as **psychogenic seizures**, **hysteroepilepsy**, **hysterical seizures** and **nonepileptic attack disorder** have been applied. All can be seen as equally stigmatizing, and pseudo-seizure is the term most often used in the literature. Pseudo-seizure is not a psychiatric diagnosis in itself; a diagnosis of conversion disorder (DSM IV or ICD 10) is usual. Varying degrees of conscious motivation may be implicated, but, importantly, these attacks are not considered to be deliberate or due to malingering.

Diagnostic issues

Differentiating pseudo-seizures from physical and psychiatric causes of episodic abnormal behavior as well as distinguishing between pseudo-seizures and true epilepsy can be very challenging. There are no absolutely pathognomonic clinical signs that enable reliable differentiation. Pseudo-seizures are strongly suggested by a high frequency of seizures, especially of prolonged duration and with poor responses to AEDs, in otherwise normal young people. At the same time, it is important to recognize that nonconvulsive status epilepticus can manifest in odd and inappropriate behavior, which may not readily be recognized as epilepsy-related.[94] Frequent seizures and poor responses to medication also occur in true epilepsy, and may be related to the underlying neurological abnormality, suboptimal treatment or progressive cerebral pathology. The bizarre nature of the attack is also thought to be suggestive, but seizures of frontal or temporal lobe origin can involve changed behavior, including altered mood states, speech and language changes, unusual perceptual experiences, laughing or

Table 24.3 *Pseudo-seizures*

In favor of pseudo-seizures	Somewhat against pseudo-seizures	Diagnostic measures
Disjointed nonphysiological progression of pattern of attack Absence of EEG change during convulsive episode Prompt clinical and EEG recovery from a generalized convulsive episode No rise in plasma prolactin following convulsive episode Disorientation in person after an attack Nonorganic amnesia Occurrence confined to company of 'significant' other people Never any independent witnesses Attacks readily induced by suggestion Change in nature of attacks following observation of attacks in other people Habitual somatic reactions to stress	No obvious reasons for pseudo-seizures Psychologically well adjusted other than concern about occurrence of attacks Developmental or family predisposition to epilepsy or other physical disorder Other episodes or physical signs suggestive of organic pathology	Detailed description of attacks from first subjective or objective change whole sequence until full recovery Detailed account or times, dates and circumstances in which episodes occur Careful historical review Current physical condition Psychiatric assessment EEG monitoring (including frontal regions) during a number of attacks (repeated if necessary) Possibly plasma prolactin estimation Evaluation of all the above in light of the forms that pseudo-seizures can take and the many conditions with which pseudo-seizures can be confused

Reproduced from G. Stores, Practitioner review: Recognition of pseudoseizures in children and adolescents. *Journal of Child Psychology and Psychiatry* 40; **6**: 851–857 with the permission of Blackwell Publishing Ltd.

running, without any 'convulsive' features. In CPS, some awareness can be preserved, even during such dramatic episodes, but preserved awareness would be suspicious in the context of a generalized seizure. Abrupt onset of the attack without warning, and abrupt termination without postattack confusion, sleepiness or EEG abnormality, often considered typical of pseudo-seizures, are seen consistently in mesial frontal seizures. Postictal 'resistive violence' can occur in postictal confusional states.[95] Incontinence, tongue biting or other injuries are not reliable distinguishing features. Physical signs such as absent corneal reflexes and upgoing plantar responses are difficult to elicit reliably during a convulsive episode. Pseudo-seizures during feigned sleep have been reported.[96] Emotional triggers or precipitants may be more often thought to be more associated with pseudo-seizures, but there is evidence that life-events, stress or emotion can also trigger true seizures.[97] Likewise, the emotional response of a young person to their seizures is very variable, and neither high levels of distress or apparent indifference help distinguish between epileptic and nonepileptic seizures.

Features in favor of or against a diagnosis of pseudo-seizures, with measures required for a diagnosis, have been suggested (see Table 24.3).

Investigations

Many investigations have been suggested, but these must be used in conjunction with clinical and EEG evidence. Plasma prolactin levels rise approximately 5–10 times in the initial 20–60 min after generalized tonic-clonic seizures. With other seizure types, this test is prone to false positives and false negatives and can be normal after repeated seizures or convulsive status.[98]

EEG evidence

Brief EEG recordings, taken between episodes, are of no value and can be misleading. Some simple partial epilepsies or mesial frontal seizures may not be accompanied by ictal abnormalities when recordings are taken from scalp electrodes. Nonspecific abnormalities may be difficult to interpret, or unrelated to the nature of the patient's attacks. A diagnosis of pseudo-seizures is firmest if the event is captured on video-EEG and is not associated with any EEG abnormality. Inpatient video-EEG monitoring is useful, but, particularly for children, prolonged ambulatory EEG monitoring is preferable. This could be combined with video recording or systematic observer description of attacks. It is important to record a number of attacks, since, if there are multiple types, some may be true epilepsy. Many people with pseudo-seizures also have epileptic seizures:[99] in one pediatric series, epilepsy was found in most of those with pseudo-seizures.[100] Such co-morbidity is higher when learning disability is also present.[101]

Clinical presentation

Pseudo-seizures can mimic the whole range of epileptic seizures. In adolescents, the clinical picture is more likely to resemble that in adults, whereas in younger children prolonged staring and unresponsiveness may be the usual presentation.[102] In children and young people with both epilepsy and pseudo-seizures, the two types of event are often very different, and patient and family education can be facilitated by review of videotaped events, if available.

Pediatricians and child psychiatrists are often asked whether altered behavior in a child might be epilepsy. In general, careful clinical history taking is the most useful way of distinguishing epileptic from nonepileptic events.[103]

Importance

Pseudo-seizures are an important problem, resulting in significant impairment for the child and leading to treatment which is inappropriate, ineffective, costly and possibly toxic. Misdiagnosis as status epilepticus can occur and high-dose intravenous treatment and its attendant risks can be problematic, or even result in unnecessary intubation and ventilation.[104] Nonepileptic seizures account for about 20 per cent of intractable seizure disorders, and are often more frequent and disabling than true epilepsy. Similarly, there are obvious medical consequences as well as adverse psychological and social implications of confusing true epilepsy with pseudo-seizures. Correct diagnosis is the essential first step in management. The use of EEG-video telemetry as the 'gold standard' in diagnosis of pseudo-seizures (with some exceptions) has resulted in increased study of their characteristics. However, there has been little systematic work in children and adolescents. Extrapolation from the adult literature may provide some guidance.[105]

Epidemiology

Pseudo-seizures were found in 7 per cent of paediatric patients having video EEG monitoring at the Cleveland Clinic Foundation over a 6-year period.[106] Some were seen in children as young as 5 years of age, but most presented in late adolescence. The only population-based study estimates the incidence nonepileptic attacks of psychological origin to be 1.4 per 100 000 population and 3.4 per 100 000 in the 15–24 age group.[107] In hospital-based studies 5–20 per cent of patients with intractable epilepsy in outpatients and 10–40 per cent patients admitted for epilepsy monitoring are thought to have pseudo-seizures. In adults, pseudo-seizures are overwhelmingly a disorder of women: whether there is a similar sex-bias in children is not known.

Psychological characteristics and background of children and adolescents prone to pseudo-seizures

Some studies suggest a higher rate of sexual abuse in children with pseudo-seizures, while other series do not find that this or other adverse experiences discriminate consistently between patients with pseudo-seizures and those with true epilepsy.[108] A prospective study of children with specific, identified, psychological stressors found these did not immediately precede the onset of pseudo-seizures.[106] Rather, the onset tended to occur months or years after sexual or physical abuse, on a background of severe chronic family dysfunction. Recognition of distant psychosocial stressors may be useful in some individuals. However, the value of this approach is limited by the speculative nature of the connections made between past experiences and the nature of the attacks. Caution is required when making causal links between psychological stressors and the onset of pseudo-seizures and giving them diagnostic significance.

Anxiety, depressive, dissociative and somatoform disorders can be expected in some young patients.[109] In clinical practice, children with pseudo-seizures often have a current stressor. Particularly in those who also have epilepsy, aspects of daily life can be quite troublesome and cause significant distress. History-taking can sometimes establish particular situations when pseudo-seizures occur and lead to identification of a stressor such as bullying, or an unmet educational need. Children with unidentified social difficulties can tend to have pseudo-seizures when overchallenged socially. Addressing the cause through environmental manipulations, can be very powerful in reducing or eliminating attacks.

Treatment and outcome

Outcome is considered better in children than in adults.[110,111] In young people, pseudo-seizures may be related to transient stress and coping problems, rather than with more intractable personality issues.[111] Children and adolescents also have shorter durations of pseudo-seizures (5.5 months compared with 5.5 years) with no difference in outcome related to co-morbid psychiatric diagnosis.[110] Correct early diagnosis is associated with better outcome.[105]

There is a dearth of controlled studies on treatment in children. Close liaison between neurology and psychiatry, with clear communication of diagnosis and management plans to all professionals involved, especially family doctors and hospital emergency departments, is important.[113] The diagnosis of pseudo-seizures should be presented in a positive light,[114] with general management following lines as for abnormal illness behavior. These include helping the patient and family to think psychologically about some aspects of their difficulties, but avoiding polarizing the discussion into physical versus psychological. The approach must be nonjudgemental and often needs to focus on diffusing anxieties related to the diagnosis. A behavioral approach involving graded rehabilitation, which should include 'face-saving' explanations for the child and family, is suggested. Co-morbid psychiatric diagnoses such as depression should be treated. Subsequent investigations are limited, and the focus is on rehabilitation back to usual activities. Patient and family education and support are important, especially if true epilepsy is also present. Often the 'pseudo-' and 'true' events are very different. Families can be helped to distinguish the attacks by review of videotaped events, and learn to cope with pseudo-seizures in a different, ideally nonreinforcing, manner.

EPILEPSY SURGERY AND PSYCHIATRIC DISORDER

A selected group of children with intractable seizures, usually of focal origin and with a resectable brain lesion, may undergo surgery in attempts to control their epilepsy (see Chapter 22D). This group often has multiple risk factors for psychiatric disorder, and, indeed, has very high rates of emotional and behavioral problems. There is often considerable discussion as to whether surgery will have an impact on these symptoms. Psychiatrists may be involved both pre-and postoperatively, to assess individual children for mental health problems, and to discuss with the parents a realistic set of expectations in terms of seizure and behavioral outcome. There have been no systematic or controlled studies on the effects of epilepsy surgery on psychiatric symptoms in children and adolescents. The sparse available information on behavioral or quality of life always shows that positive benefits are highly correlated with reduction in severity of seizures. Improved attention span and social skills, and reduced hyperactivity, are reported.[115] Parents' reports of satisfaction with quality of life correlate significantly with good seizure outcome. Nonresective surgery (multiple subpial transection) was also reported to improve language and social skills temporarily, in a group of children with epilepsy-related autistic features.[116] Positive behavioral outcomes have also been reported following resective surgery.[117,118] Children who underwent hemispherectomy for severe epilepsy, were reported to have excellent relief from behavioral disorder. However, by contemporary standards, these studies are impaired by lack of systematic behavioral measures. Temporal lobectomy is the commonest surgical procedure for intractable seizures, but behavioral outcomes following this procedure have been little studied in children. In one early series,[119] positive seizure and behavioral outcome related to the presence of mesial temporal sclerosis as the underlying pathology. More recently, no changes in neuropsychological measures were found following temporal lobectomy, but improvement in internalizing symptoms and social interaction were suggested.[120]

EDUCATIONAL PROVISION FOR CHILDREN WITH EPILEPSY AND MENTAL HEALTH PROBLEMS

Rates of behavior problems are lowest, estimated at 12–23 per cent in normal population samples, such as children with epilepsy in normal schools or seen by family doctors. The figures rises to about 50 per cent in those attending outpatient epilepsy clinics and to 95 per cent in children with epilepsy requiring specialist inpatient treatment. Even children with idiopathic epilepsy have increased long-term risks for learning and behavioral problems, and these are amplified in children with structural brain lesions.[121] One of the most frequent dilemmas is finding the appropriate educational setting (see Chapter 23). Most manage in mainstream school, but many require specialist support or teaching at some stage. The presence of behavioral problems increases the likelihood that special schooling will be needed, and when behavioral and learning problems are combined, this is almost inevitable. Behavioral problems often impair the ability of mainstream schools to cope with the epilepsy itself.

KEY POINTS

- **Psychiatric disorder is common** in children with epilepsy
- Children with epilepsy should have access to **effective psychiatric diagnostic services** and treatments
- **Multidisciplinary working** can help prevent additional disability in children with epilepsy

---

REFERENCES

1. Rutter M, Graham P, Yule W. *A Neuropsychiatric Study in Childhood.* Clinics in Developmental Medicine No. 35/36. London: Heinemann, 1970.
2. Goodman R. Brain disorders. In: Rutter M, Taylor E (eds) *Child and Adolescent Psychiatry.* Oxford: Blackwell Science, 2002.
3. Breslau N. Psychiatric disorder in children with physical disabilities. *Journal of the American Academy of Child Psychiatry* 1985; **24**(1): 87–94.
4. Hoare P. The development of psychiatric disorder among schoolchildren with epilepsy. *Developmental Medicine and Child Neurology* 1984; **26**(1): 3–13.
5. McDermott S, Mani S, Krishnaswami S. A population-based analysis of specific behavior problems associated with childhood seizures. *Journal of Epilepsy* 1995; **8**: 110–118.

6. Wirrell EC, Camfield CS, Camfield PR et al. Long-term psychosocial outcome in typical absence epilepsy. Sometimes a wolf in sheeps' clothing. Archives of Pediatrics and Adolescent Medicine 1997; **151**(2): 152–158.

7. Austin JK, Smith MS, Risinger MW, McNelis AM. Childhood epilepsy and asthma: comparison of quality of life. Epilepsia 1994; **35**(3): 608–615.

8. Dunn DW, Austin JK, Huster GA. Behaviour problems in children with new-onset epilepsy. Seizure 1997; **6**(4): 283–287.

9. Austin JK, Harezlak J, Dunn DW, et al. Behaviour problems in children before first recognized seizures. Pediatrics 2001; **107**: 115–122.

10. Goffman E. Stigma. Notes on the Management of Spoiled Identity. New York: Prentice Hall, 1963.

11. Taylor DC. Epilepsy and prejudice. Archives of Disease in Childhood 1987; **62**(2): 209–211.

12. Britten N, Wadsworth MEJ, Fenwick PBC. Stigma in patients with early epilepsy: A national longitudinal study. Journal of Epidemiology and Community Health, 1984; **38**: 291–295.

13. Besag FM. Childhood epilepsy in relation to mental handicap and behavioural disorders. Journal of Child Psychology and Psychiatry 2002; **43**(1): 103–131.

14. Farwell JR, Dodrill CB, Batzel LW. Neuropsychological abilities of children with epilepsy. Epilepsia 1985; **26**(5): 395–400.

15. Holdsworth L, Whitmore K. A study of children with epilepsy attending ordinary schools. I: their seizure patterns, progress and behaviour in school. Developmental Medicine and Child Neurology 1974; **16**(6): 746–758.

16. Mitchell WG, Chavez JM, Lee H, Guzman BL. Academic underachievement in children with epilepsy. Journal of Child Neurology 1991; **6**(1): 65–72.

17. Hermann BP, Whitman S, Hughes JR, Melyn MM, Dell J. Multietiological determinants of psychopathology and social competence in children with epilepsy. Epilepsy Research 1988; **2**(1): 51–60.

18. Austin JK, Risinger MW, Beckett LA. Correlates of behavior problems in children with epilepsy. Epilepsia 1992; **33**(6): 1115–1122.

19. Schoenfeld J, Seidenberg M, Woodard A, et al. Neuropsychological and behavioral status of children with complex partial seizures. Developmental Medicine and Child Neurology 1999; **41**(11): 724–731.

20. Camfield C, Breau L, Camfield P. Impact of pediatric epilepsy on the family: a new scale for clinical and research use. Epilepsia 2001; **42**(1): 104–112.

21. Seidenberg M, Beck N, Geisser M, et al. Academic achievement of children with epilepsy. Epilepsia 1986; **27**(6): 753–759.

22. Paradiso S, Hermann BP, Robinson RG. The heterogeneity of temporal lobe epilepsy. Neurology, neuropsychology, and psychiatry. Journal of Nervous and Mental Diseases 1995; **183**(8): 538–547.

23. Ounsted C. Aggression and epilepsy rage in children with temporal lobe epilepsy. Journal of Psychosomatic Research 1969; **13**(3): 237–242.

24. Ott D, Caplan R, Guthrie D, et al. Measures of psychopathology in children with complex partial seizures and primary generalized epilepsy with absence. Journal of the American Academy of Child and Adolescent Psychiatry 2001; **40**(8): 907–914.

25. Taylor DC, Neville BG, Cross JH. Autistic spectrum disorders in childhood epilepsy surgery candidates. European Journal of Child and Adolescent Psychiatry 1999; **8**(3): 189–92.

26. Stores G. School-children with epilepsy at risk for learning and behaviour problems. Developmental Medicine and Child Neurology 1978; **20**(4): 502–508.

27. Hoare P, Kerley S. Psychosocial adjustment of children with chronic epilepsy and their families. Developmental Medicine and Child Neurology 1991; **33**(3): 201–215.

28. Whitman S, Hermann BP, Black RB, Chhabria S. Psychopathology and seizure type in children with epilepsy. Psychological Medicine 1982; **12**(4): 843–853.

29. Manchanda R, Freeland A, Schaefer B, McLachlan RS, Blume WT. Auras, seizure focus, and psychiatric disorders. Neuropsychiatry, Neuropsychology, and Behavioral Neurology 2000; **13**(1): 13–19.

30. Stores G, Zaiwalla Z, Bergel N. Frontal lobe complex partial seizures in children: a form of epilepsy at particular risk of misdiagnosis. Developmental Medicine and Child Neurology 1991; **33**(11): 998–1009.

31. Bourgeois BF, Prensky AL, Palkes HS, Talent BK, Busch SG. Intelligence in epilepsy: a prospective study in children. Annals of Neurology 1983; **14**(4): 438–444.

32. Bennett-Levy J, Stores G. The nature of cognitive dysfunction in school-children with epilepsy. Acta Neurologica Scandinavica 1984; **99**(Suppl.): 79–82.

33. Trimble MR. Anticonvulsant drugs and cognitive function: a review of the literature. Epilepsia 1987; **28**(Suppl. 3): S37–45.

34. Ounsted C. The hyperkinetic syndrome in epileptic children. Lancet 1955; **ii**: 303–311.

35. Brent DA, Crumrine PK, Varma R, Brown RV, Allan MJ. Phenobarbital treatment and major depressive disorder in children with epilepsy: a naturalistic follow-up. Pediatrics 1990; **85**(6): 1086–1091.

36. Thompson PJ, Trimble MR. Anticonvulsant drugs and cognitive functions. Epilepsia 1982; **23**(5): 531–544.

37. Trimble MR, Rusch N, Betts T, Crawford PM. Psychiatric symptoms after therapy with new antiepileptic drugs: psychopathological and seizure related variables. Seizure 2000; **9**(4): 249–254.

38. Besag FM. Behavioural effects of the new anticonvulsants. Drug Safety 2001; **24**(7): 513–536.

39. Wong IC. Retrospective study of vigabatrin and psychiatric behavioural disturbances. Epilepsy Research 1995; **21**(3): 227–230.

40. Ferrie CD, Robinson RO, Panayiotopoulos CP. Psychotic and severe behavioural reactions with vigabatrin: a review. Acta Neurologica Scandinavica 1996; **93**(1): 1–8.

41. Thomas L, Trimble M, Schmitz B, Ring H. Vigabatrin and behaviour disorders: a retrospective survey. Epilepsy Research 1996; **25**(1): 21–27.

42. Lee DO, Steingard RJ, Cesena M, et al. Behavioral side effects of gabapentin in children. Epilepsia 1996; **37**(1): 87–90.

43. Martin R, Kuzniecky R, Ho S, et al. Cognitive effects of topiramate, gabapentin, and lamotrigine in healthy young adults. Neurology 1999; **52**(2): 321–327.

44. Bourgeois BF. Antiepileptic drugs, learning, and behavior in childhood epilepsy. Epilepsia 1998; **39**(9): 913–921.

45. Grunberg F, Pond DA. Conduct disorders in epileptic children. *Journal of Neurology, Neurosurgery and Psychiatry* 1957; **20**: 65–68.

46. Austin JK. Childhood epilepsy: child adaptation and family resources. *Child and Adolescent Mental Health Nursing* 1988; **1**: 18–24.

47. Hoare P. Psychiatric disturbance in the families of epileptic children. *Developmental Medicine and Child Neurology* 1984; **26**(1): 14–19.

48. Devinsky O, Westbrook L, Cramer J, *et al*. Risk factors for poor health-related quality of life in adolescents with epilepsy. *Epilepsia* 1999; **40**(12): 1715–1720.

49. Viberg M, Blennow G, Polski B. Epilepsy in adolescence: implications for the development of personality. *Epilepsia* 1987; **28**(5): 542–546.

50. Rossi G, Bonfiglio S, Veggiotti P, Lanzi G. Epilepsy: a study of adolescence and groups. *Seizure* 1997; **6**(4): 289–295.

51. Appleton RE, Neville BG. Teenagers with epilepsy. *Archives of Disease in Childhood* 1999; **81**(1): 76–79.

52. Goodman R, Scott S. *Child Psychiatry*. Oxford: Blackwell Science, 1997.

53. Rutter M, Taylor E (eds). *Child and Adolescent Psychiatry*. Oxford: Blackwell Science, 2002.

54. Davies S, Heyman I, Goodman R. A population survey of mental health problems in children with epilepsy. *Dev Med Child Neurol* 2003; **45**: 292–295.

55. Taylor DC, Lochery M. Behavioral consequences of epilepsy in children. Developing a psychosocial vocabulary. *Advances in Neurology* 1991; **55**: 153–162.

56. Onuma T. Classification of psychiatric symptoms in patients with epilepsy. *Epilepsia* 2000; **41**(Suppl. 9): 43–48.

57. Goodman R. Psychometric properties of the Strengths and Difficulties Questionnaire (SDQ). *Journal of the American Academy of Child and Adolescent Psychiatry* 2001; **40**: 1337–1345.

58. Myers K, Winters NC. Ten-year review of rating scales. I: overview of scale functioning, psychometric properties, and selection. *Journal of the American Academy of Child and Adolescent Psychiatry* 2002; **41**: 114–122.

59. Myers K, Winters NC. Ten-year review of rating scales. II: Scales for internalizing disorders. *Journal of the American Academy of Child and Adolescent Psychiatry* 2002; **41**: 634–659.

60. Lewis DO, Pincus JH, Shanok SS, Glaser GH. Psychomotor epilepsy and violence in a group of incarcerated adolescent boys. *American Journal of Psychiatry* 1982; **139**(7): 882–887.

61. Scott S, Spender Q, Doolan M, Jacobs B, Aspland H. Multicentre controlled trial of parenting groups for childhood antisocial behaviour in clinical practice. *BMJ* 2001; **323**(7306): 194–198.

62. Feldman H, Crumrine P, Handen BL, Alvin R, Teodori J. Methylphenidate in children with seizures and attention-deficit disorder. *American Journal of Disease of Children* 1989; **143**(9): 1081–1086.

63. Gross-Tsur V, Manor O, van der Meere J, Joseph A, Shalev RS. Epilepsy and attention deficit hyperactivity disorder: is methylphenidate safe and effective? *Journal of Pediatrics* 1997; **130**(1): 40–44.

64. Ettnger AB, Weisbrot DM, Nolan EE, *et al*. Symptoms of depression and anxiety in paedatric epilepsy patients. *Epilepsia*, 1998; **39**(6): 595–599.

65. Dunn DW, Austin JK, Huster GA. Symptoms of depression in adolescents with epilepsy. *Journal of the American Academy of Child and Adolescent Psychiatry* 1999; **38**(9): 1132–1138.

66. Curry JF. Specific psychotherapies for childhood and adolescent depression. *Biological Psychiatry* 2001; **49**(12): 1091–1100.

67. Sampson SM, Mrazek DA. Depression in adolescence. *Current Opinion in Pediatrics* 2001; **13**(6): 586–590.

68. Brent DA. Overrepresentation of epileptics in a consecutive series of suicide attempters seen at a children's hospital, 1978–1983. *Journal of the American Academy of Child Psychiatry* 1986; **25**(2): 242–246.

69. Velosa JF, Riddle MA. Pharmacologic treatment of anxiety disorders in children and adolescents. *Adolescent Psychiatry Clinics of North America* 2000; **9**(1): 119–133.

70. Moreau D, Weissman MM. Panic disorder in children and adolescents: a review. *American Journal of Psychiatry* 1992; **149**(10): 1306–1314.

71. Rapoport JL, Inoff-Germain G. Treatment of obsessive-compulsive disorder in children and adolescents. *Journal of Child Psychology and Psychiatry* 2000; **41**(4): 419–431.

72. Berney TP. Autism – an evolving concept. *British Journal of Psychiatry* 2000; **176**: 20–25.

73. Robinson RO, Baird G, Robinson G, Simonoff E. Landau-Kleffner syndrome: course and correlates with outcome. *Developmental Medicine and Child Neurology* 2001; **43**(4): 243–247.

74. Riikonen R, Amnell G. Psychiatric disorders in children with earlier infantile spasms. *Developmental Medicine and Child Neurology* 1981; **23**(6): 747–760.

75. Bolton PF, Park RJ, Higgins JN, Griffiths PD, Pickles A. Neuro-epileptic determinants of autism spectrum disorders in tuberous sclerosis complex. *Brain* 2002; **125**: 1247–1255.

76. Miller DD. Review and management of clozapine side effects. *Journal of Clinical Psychiatry* 2000; **61**(Suppl. 8): 14–17.

77. Sachdev P. Schizophrenia-like psychosis and epilepsy: the status of the association. *American Journal of Psychiatry* 1998; 155(3): 325–336.

78. Toone BK, Garralda ME, Ron MA. The psychoses of epilepsy and the functional psychoses: a clinical and phenomenological comparison. *British Journal of Psychiatry* 1982; **141**: 256–261.

79. Bredkjaer SR, Mortensen PB, Parnas J. Epilepsy and non-organic non-affective psychosis. National epidemiologic study. *British Journal of Psychiatry* 1998; **172**: 235–238.

80. Logsdail SJ, Toone BK. Post-ictal psychoses. A clinical and phenomenological description. *British Journal of Psychiatry* 1988; **152**: 246–252.

81. Umbricht D, Degreef G, Barr WB, *et al*. Postictal and chronic psychoses in patients with temporal lobe epilepsy. *American Journal of Psychiatry* 1995; **152**(2): 224–231.

82. Yamomoto T, Pipo JR, Akaboshi S, Narai S. Forced normalization induced by ethosuximide therapy in a patient with intractable myoclonic epilepsy. *Brain and Development* 2001; **23**(1): 62–64.

83. Flor-Henry P. Psychosis and temporal lobe epilepsy. A controlled investigation. *Epilepsia* 1969; **10**(3): 363–395.

84. Barr WB, Ashtari M, Bilder RM, Degreef G, Lieberman JA. Brain morphometric comparison of first-episode schizophrenia and temporal lobe epilepsy. *British Journal of Psychiatry* 1997; **170**: 515–519.

85. Maier M, Mellers J, Toone B, Trimble M, Ron MA. Schizophrenia, temporal lobe epilepsy and psychosis: an in vivo magnetic resonance spectroscopy and imaging study of the hippocampus/amygdala complex. *Psychological Medicine* 2000; **30**(3): 571–581.

86. Taylor DC. Mental state and temporal lobe epilepsy. A correlative account of 100 patients treated surgically. *Epilepsia* 1972; **13**(6): 727–765.

87. Andermann LF, Savard G, Meencke HJ, *et al.* Psychosis after resection of ganglioma or DNET: evidence for an association. *Epilepsia* 1999; **40**: 83–87.

88. Roberts GW, Done DJ, Bruton C, Crow TJ. A 'mock up' of schizophrenia: temporal lobe epilepsy and schizophrenia-like psychosis. *Biological Psychiatry* 1990; **28**(2): 127–143.

89. Kossoff EH, Bergey GK, Freeman JM, Vining EP. Levetiracetam psychosis in children with epilepsy. *Epilepsia* 2001; **42**(12): 1611–1613.

90. Lindsay J, Ounsted C, Richards P. Long-term outcome in children with temporal lobe seizures. III: Psychiatric aspects in childhood and adult life. *Developmental Medicine and Child Neurology* 1979; **21**(5): 630–636.

91. Caplan R, Arbelle S, Guthrie D, *et al.* Formal thought disorder and psychopathology in pediatric primary generalized and complex partial epilepsy. *Journal of the American Academy of Child and Adolescent Psychiatry* 1997; **36**(9): 1286–1294.

92. Caplan R, Shields WD, Mori L, Yudovin S. Middle childhood onset of interictal psychosis. *Journal of the American Academy of Child and Adolescent Psychiatry* 1991; **30**(6): 893–896.

93. Meadow R. Neurological and developmental variants of Munchausen syndrome by proxy. *Developmental Medicine and Child Neurology* 1991; **33**(3): 270–272.

94. Stores G, Zaiwalla Z, Styles E, Hoshika A. Non-convulsive status epilepticus. *Archives of Disease in Childhood* 1995; **73**(2): 106–111.

95. Stores G. Practitioner review: Recognition of pseudoseizures in children and adolescents. *Journal of Child Psychology and Psychiatry* 1999; **40**(6): 851–857.

96. Thacker K, Devinsky O, Perrine K, Alper K, Luciano D. Nonepileptic seizures during apparent sleep. *Annals of Neurology* 1993; **33**(4): 414–418.

97. Verduyn CM, Stores G, Missen A. A survey of mothers' impressions of seizure precipitants in children with epilepsy. *Epilepsia* 1988; **29**(3): 251–255.

98. Yerby MS, van Belle G, Friel PN, Wilensky AJ. Serum prolactin in the diagnosis of epilepsy: sensitivity, specificity, and predictive value. *Neurology* 1987; **37**(7): 1224–1226.

99. LaFrance WC. How many patients with psychogenic nonepileptic seizures also have epilepsy? *Neurology* 2002; **58**(6): 990–991.

100. Holmes GL, Sackellares JC, McKiernan J, Ragland M, Dreifuss FE. Evaluation of childhood pseudoseizures using EEG telemetry and video tape monitoring. *Journal of Pediatrics* 1980; **97**(4): 554–558.

101. Kanner AM, Parra J, Frey M, *et al.* Psychiatric and neurologic predictors of psychogenic pseudoseizure outcome. *Neurology* 1999; **53**(5): 933–938.

102. Kramer U, Carmant L, Riviello JJ, *et al.* Psychogenic seizures: video telemetry observations in 27 patients. *Pediatric Neurology* 1995; **12**(1): 39–41.

103. Carmant L, Kramer U, Holmes GL, *et al.* Differential diagnosis of staring spells in children: a video-EEG study. *Pediatric Neurology* 1996; **14**(3): 199–202.

104. Pakalnis A, Paolicchi J, Gilles E. Psychogenic status epilepticus in children: psychiatric and other risk factors. *Neurology* 2000; **54**(4): 969–970.

105. Krumholz A. Nonepileptic seizures: diagnosis and management. *Neurology* 1999; **53**(5; Suppl. 2): S76–83.

106. Wyllie E, Glazer JP, Benbadis S, Kotagal P, Wolgamuth B. Psychiatric features of children and adolescents with pseudoseizures. *Archives of Pediatrics and Adolescent Medicine* 1999; **153**(3): 244–248.

107. Sigurdardottir KR, Olafsson E. Incidence of psychogenic seizures in adults: a population-based study in Iceland. *Epilepsia* 1998; **39**(7): 749–752.

108. Berkhoff M, Briellmann RS, Radanov BP, Donati F, Hess CW. Developmental background and outcome in patients with nonepileptic versus epileptic seizures: a controlled study. *Epilepsia* 1998; **39**(5): 463–469.

109. Goodyer IM. Epileptic and pseudoepileptic seizures in childhood and adolescence. *Journal of the American Academy of Child Psychiatry* 1985; **24**(1): 3–9.

110. Wyllie E, Friedman D, Luders H *et al.* Outcome of psychogenic seizures in children and adolescents compared with adults. *Neurology* 1991; **41**(5): 742–744.

111. Gudmundsson O, Prendergast M, Foreman D, Cowley S. Outcome of pseudoseizures in children and adolescents: a 6-year symptom survival analysis. *Developmental Medicine and Child Neurology* 2001; **43**(8): 547–551.

112. Andriola MR, Ettinger AB. Pseudoseizures and other nonepileptic paroxysmal disorders in children and adolescents. *Neurology* 1999; **53**(5; Suppl. 2): S89–95.

113. Bowman ES. Nonepileptic seizures: psychiatric framework, treatment and outcome. *Neurology* 1999; **53**(Suppl. 2): S84–88.

114. Shen W, Bowman ES, Markand ON. Presenting the diagnosis of pseudoseizure. *Neurology* 1990; **40**(5): 756–759.

115. Yang TF, Wong TT, Kwan SY, *et al.* Quality of life and life satisfaction in families after a child has undergone corpus callostomy. *Epilepsia* 1996; **37**: 76–80.

116. Nass R, Gross A, Wisoff J, Devinsky O. Outcome of multiple subpial transections for autistic epileptiform regression. *Pediatric Neurology* 1999; **21**: 464–470.

117. Lindsay J, Ounsted C, Richards P. Hemispherectomy for childhood epilepsy: a 36-year study. *Developmental Medicine and Child Neurology* 1987; **29**: 592–600.

118. Goodman R. Hemispherectomy and its alternatives in the treatment of intractable epilepsy in patients with infantile hemiplegia. *Developmental Medicine and Child Neurology* 1986; **28**: 251–258.

119. Davidson S, Falconer MA. Outcome of surgery in 40 children with temporal-lobe epilepsy. *Lancet* 1975; **i**: 1260–1263.

120. Williams J, Griebel ML, Sharp GB, Boop FA. Cognition and behavior after temporal lobectomy in pediatric patients with intractable epilepsy. *Pediatric Neurology* 1998; **19**: 189–194.

121. Bailet LL, Turk WR. The impact of childhood epilepsy on neurocognitive and behavioral performance: a prospective longitudinal study. *Epilepsia* 2000; **41**: 426–431.

25

Social aspects

DAVID W DUNN AND JOAN K AUSTIN

Children with epilepsy have more than a paroxysmal disorder that manifests as seizures requiring long-term antiepileptic therapy. They also have more behavioral problems and academic difficulties than other children and, upon reaching adulthood, may have less social and vocational success.[1,2] Aicardi[3] suggests that we consider epilepsy to be a pervasive, nonparoxysmal disorder that, even between episodes of seizures, adversely affects the central nervous system. Using Taylor's terminology, epilepsy is both an illness and a predicament for the child.[4] As an illness, epilepsy consists of seizures and the child's experience with seizures, laboratory studies, and medication. Epilepsy as an illness contributes to the child's definition of their role in society. As a predicament, epilepsy is a complex set of psychosocial problems that are unique to the individual child.

In this chapter we review the effects of epilepsy on the child, concentrating on the recent literature on quality of life (QOL), and the effects of this chronic illness on families. We consider the response of schools and society, emphasizing recent work on stigma as it affects the child with seizures. We assess the restrictions on sports and driving placed upon the child and review attempts to provide comprehensive, integrated treatment for the child with epilepsy.

QUALITY OF LIFE

Assessment with comprehensive instruments

Substantial recent effort has gone into defining and developing tools to measure QOL in children with epilepsy.

QOL includes physical, psychological, social, and academic functioning, all areas that may be adversely affected by childhood epilepsy. Though there are both generic and epilepsy-specific comprehensive assessment tools, most studies have focused on a single dimension of QOL. Psychological functioning has been studied substantially more than social and academic functioning. Limitations include predominant use of clinical samples, exclusion of children with learning disabilities (termed mental retardation in many studies), and a lack of studies on preschool children. Most of the new QOL scales have not been used beyond the initial validation studies.

The Child Health Questionnaire[5] is a new generic QOL scale that has strong psychometric properties as well as norms for age and gender. Several forms of this instrument exist and allow the assessment of both physical and psychosocial well being of the child by both the child and the parent. Gilliam et al.[6] used this instrument in a study of the outcome of epilepsy surgery in children. In comparison to normative samples, the children with recent surgery for seizure control had significantly worse QOL in physical functioning, general behavior, general health, self-esteem, and both emotional impact and time impact on parents.

Hoare and Russell[7] developed the Impact of Childhood Illness Scale, a 30-item scale that is completed by parents. Although it was designed to study the effect of epilepsy on QOL, the scale is generic enough to be used with any chronic illness. The four sections cover impact of illness, effect on child development and adjustment, impact on parents and impact on family. Hoare and Russell found that children with intractable seizures had a poorer QOL than children with well-controlled seizures, supporting construct validity for the scale. In a subsequent comparison of QOL in children with epilepsy versus children with diabetes mellitus, Hoare et al.[8] found that epilepsy had a significant adverse impact on QOL whereas diabetes was not associated with negative impact on QOL. Early onset of seizures, more frequent seizures and additional disabilities predicted more negative QOL for children with epilepsy.

Apajaslo et al.[9] have also designed a comprehensive QOL self-report measure that they tested on a small group of adolescents with epilepsy. The questionnaire had adequate content and construct validity and adequate test-retest reliability.

Several comprehensive QOL scales have been developed specifically for children and adolescents with epilepsy. The Quality of Life in Epilepsy Inventory for Adolescents (QOLIE-AD-48) is a 48-item scale that is completed by the adolescent.[10] It has a total summary score and 8 subscales: impact of epilepsy, memory and concentration, attitude toward epilepsy, physical functioning, stigma, social support, school behavior, and health perceptions. The scale was validated on a sample of adolescents 11–17 years of age. Initial studies have shown adequate internal consistency reliability, test-retest reliability, construct validity, and external validity. Devinsky et al.[11] evaluated 197 adolescents 11–17 years of age with the QOLIE-AD-48. Older age, lower socioeconomic status, more severe seizures, and side-effects from antiepileptic drugs (AEDs) were risk factors for lower QOL. Girls had lower scores on the Attitude toward Illness and Health Perceptions subscales than boys. Using a modification of the QOLIE-89 scale, Wildrick et al.[12] found that children and adolescents with well-controlled seizures had social worries, including fear of having a seizure in front of friends, and academic worries such as getting along with teachers, remembering assignments and grades.

Another comprehensive epilepsy-specific scale is the Quality of Life in Childhood Epilepsy questionnaire.[13] This 73-item parent-completed scale was validated on a sample of parents of children with epilepsy aged 4–18 years. The domains covered are physical function, cognitive function, emotional well-being, social function and behavior. It had good internal consistency reliability and construct validity. Sabaz et al.[14] used the QOLCE in a study of refractory epilepsy comparing children with and without intellectual disability. The children with epilepsy and intellectual disability had poorer QOL scores on the overall scale, attention, language, control/helplessness, physical restrictions, social interactions and social activities, and behavior scales. These results were independent of seizure frequency and number of AEDs.

A final example is the Impact of Pediatric Epilepsy Scale (IPES) developed by Camfield et al.[15] This brief 11-item parent-completed questionnaire was validated on a sample of parents of children 2–16 years of age. The scale has adequate internal consistency reliability and test-retest validity. Construct validity was supported when children with more severe illness were found to have poorer QOL as measured by the IPES than those with less severe illness.

Assessment with a battery of instruments

An alternative to developing a specific QOL scale for assessing children with epilepsy has been to utilize multiple measures for a comprehensive evaluation. Austin et al.[16] used this approach in comparing children with seizures to children with asthma on quality of life. The physical domain was assessed using a questionnaire covering frequency of seizures or asthmatic attacks, side-effects of medications and school absences. Measures of behavior included the Child Behavior Checklist (CBCL),[17] the Piers-Harris Self-concept Scales[18] and the Child Attitude toward Illness Scale.[19] Social domain included peer relations and social activity from the CBCL and satisfaction with family measured by the revised Family APGAR.[20] Academic performance was assessed with the Teacher Report Form and the school progress section both from the CBCL.[21] In a first study of 136 children with epilepsy and 134 children with asthma aged 8–12 years, they found that children with epilepsy had more impairment in psychological, social, and academic QOL domains whereas children with asthma were more compromised in the physical domain. The study was repeated 4 years later comparing QOL in children with active or inactive epilepsy to QOL in children with asthma.[22] The epilepsy group continued to have relatively more problems. Children with active epilepsy were doing more poorly than those with inactive epilepsy or the children with asthma. Children with inactive epilepsy were faring worse than both active and inactive asthma groups in school achievement, and were worse than children with inactive asthma in school progress and intellectual self-concept. In this sample, girls with more severe seizures were doing worse in measures of QOL.

Several groups have completed comprehensive assessments utilizing a variety of cognitive and neuropsychological assessments and the CBCL for evaluation of behavior. Weglage et al.[23] studied 40 children with centrotemporal spikes. Measures included neuropsychological and cognitive assessments, CBCL and EEGs. They found an association between lower IQ and frequency of spikes on EEG, and slightly more problems on CBCL total behavior, social problems, compulsive behavior and delinquency scores in the children with spikes than controls. Mandelbaum and Burack[24] used a neuropsychological battery of tests and the CBCL to compare children with differing seizure types. They found higher cognitive scores in children with partial seizures as compared to generalized seizures, and in children with convulsive seizures as compared to nonconvulsive seizures. Children with generalized nonconvulsive seizures had more impairment on the CBCL Internalizing scale than those with generalized convulsive and partial seizures. Schoenfeld et al.[25] evaluated 57 children aged 7–16 years with complex partial seizures and compared performance to siblings. They found significantly lower performance by the children with seizures on verbal and nonverbal memory, language, academic achievement, problem solving, mental efficiency and motor skills. Compared to siblings, the children with seizures had impairment on the CBCL with most differences in social problems, thought problems and attention problems. Seizure frequency in the past year was the strongest predictor of behavioral problems, and earlier age of onset was the best predicator of cognitive problems.

Three studies have assessed QOL in adults with seizure onset during childhood. In a prospective population-based study, Sillanpää et al.[26] followed 245 children with seizure onset prior to age 16 years for an average of 35 years. Individuals with uncomplicated epilepsy had fewer years of education, were more frequently unemployed, were less likely to be married and were less likely to have children than community controls. Even those whose seizures were in remission were less likely to be married or in a committed relationship or to have children when compared to controls. As expected, persons with complicated epilepsy were experiencing more problems than those with uncomplicated epilepsy. Similarly, Wirrell et al.[27] found that young adults who had developed absence seizures during childhood had significantly worse QOL than a comparison group who had juvenile rheumatoid arthritis. Compared to controls, the children with absence seizures were more likely to have failed a grade, required special education services, or failed to graduate from high school or attend college. By the young adult years, the patients with seizures had more mental health problems, unplanned pregnancies and social impairments than the adults with arthritis. In contrast, Kokkonen et al.[28] found no increase in psychiatric problems in a sample of young adults who had childhood-onset epilepsy had no more psychiatric problems than normal controls and fewer problems than a comparison group of adults with cerebral palsy or spina bifida.

Single-domain studies

There are numerous studies that examine a single domain of QOL in children with epilepsy. In a recent review, we were able to find 13 studies of psychosocial functioning and 7 studies of cognitive/academic functioning in children with epilepsy published between January 1994 and February 1999.[29] Strengths of these studies included large sample sizes and the use of standard measurements. In the psychosocial studies, the CBCL was the most commonly used instrument. Standard assessments of cognitive function and a variety of neuropsychological measures were used in both psychosocial and cognitive/academic studies. Most studies were cross-sectional in design and used a clinical sample. Two studies[30,31] employed an epidemiological approach. Mitchell et al.[32] used a longitudinal design in one psychosocial study and Austin et al.[33] did a 4-year follow-up assessment in an evaluation of academic achievement. Most studies excluded children who were mentally handicapped and children in the youngest age groups.

A consistent finding was an increased prevalence of emotional and behavioral problems (see Chapter 24). Children with epilepsy had more problems whether compared to children in the general population or to children with other chronic illnesses. In an epidemiological study conducted on the Isle of Wight, Rutter et al.[34] found that the children with uncomplicated epilepsy had four times the rate of behavioral problems seen in children in the general population. Hoare,[35] comparing behavioral problems in children with epilepsy to children with diabetes mellitus, found behavioral disturbance in 48 per cent of the children with seizures and 17 per cent of the children with diabetes. McDermott et al.[36] noted behavioral disorders in 31 per cent of children with epilepsy, 21 per cent of children with heart disease, and 8.5 per cent of the children in the control group. Austin et al.[16] used asthma as a comparison group and found the children with asthma had more physical problems, but the children with epilepsy had more psychosocial and academic problems. Studies of specific disorders have reported more attention-deficit/hyperactivity disorder, depression, and sleep disorders in children with seizures than in healthy controls.[37–39]

This increased risk of behavioral problems is present even in children with recent onset seizures. Hoare[35] found behavioral problems in 45 per cent of children with new-onset seizures currently treated with AEDs versus 10 per cent of a control group. Dunn et al.[40] reported behavioral problems as measured by CBCL in 24 per cent of children with new-onset seizures. In a sample of 224 children, Austin et al.[41] found that 32.1 per cent of the children with new-onset seizures were in the clinical or at-risk range on the total behavior problem score of the CBCL.

Academic performance and cognitive functioning is a second domain of QOL that has received considerable attention (see Chapter 23). Consistent findings are lower scores on intellectual assessments and academic underachievement in children with epilepsy. Cognitive abilities vary widely depending on etiology of seizures, presence of additional CNS damage, and epilepsy syndrome, and thus an overall average lower score in a large, heterogeneous sample of children with epilepsy is not unexpected. What is somewhat more surprising however, is the consistent finding of academic underachievement after controlling for intellectual functioning. The underachievement of the children with epilepsy is apparent in comparison to normal population or chronic illness controls. Seidenberg et al.[42] found significant underachievement in arithmetic in 32 per cent and in reading, spelling and word recognition tests in 10–16 per cent of the children with epilepsy. In a sample of children with epilepsy 5–13 years of age, Mitchell et al.[43] reported underachievement after adjusting for cognitive abilities in 31 per cent in math, 38 per cent in reading comprehension, and 32 per cent in spelling. Austin et al.[44] compared academic achievement in children with either epilepsy or asthma. At baseline, the children with epilepsy had significantly lower scores on tests of academic performance than the children with asthma. When the group was reassessed 4 years later, the children with both active and inactive epilepsy continued to perform more poorly than children with asthma.[33]

Risk factors for poor quality of life

Risk factors for a diminished QOL include demographic factors, seizure variables, neurological variables, side-effects of AEDs, and psychosocial response to epilepsy. Demographic factors most often implicated are age, age of onset of seizures and gender, though research on demographic factors has been inconsistent or has shown only modest effect.[30,45] Neurological damage has been a more definite risk factor. Children with uncomplicated epilepsy have more cognitive and behavioral problems than children with other chronic illnesses not involving the brain, and children with epilepsy and additional CNS damage have more problems than children with uncomplicated epilepsy.[34,46] Neuropsychological dysfunction, including problems with attention and memory, has been associated with behavioral problems in children with epilepsy.[47–50]

Seizure variables are possible risk factors for problems with QOL. The seizure syndromes associated with mental handicap and intractability are associated with more impaired QOL.[31,51] Data linking QOL to different seizure types in the child without mental handicap have been less consistent. Hoare found an association between focal EEG abnormalities and behavioral problems, but several others report little association between seizure type and behavior disturbance.[35,45,52,53] Seizure frequency and seizure severity are risk factors for impaired QOL, with poorer seizure control, increased seizure number, or more severe seizures associated with behavior problems in most studies[25,32,45,54] with only occasional exceptions.[51] AEDs have been minimally involved in decreasing QOL for children with epilepsy. Williams et al.[55] found no significant effect of short-term AED treatment on cognition or behavior in children with new-onset epilepsy. Aldenkamp et al.[56,57] noted more alertness in both child and parent's report, and improved psychomotor speed on neuropsychological testing after discontinuation of AEDs. No other changes were found on any cognitive or behavioral factors.

Psychosocial factors also have been associated with QOL outcomes. Family problems are associated with both behavior problems and academic underachievement in children with epilepsy.[32,45,58] The child's response to illness was a determinant of risk for impaired QOL. Austin and Huberty[19] found that positive attitudes toward having epilepsy were associated with fewer behavior problems, less depression and more positive self-concepts. Perceptions of an external or unknown locus of control in children with epilepsy were more frequent than in children with diabetes mellitus,[59] and have been associated with symptoms of depression in adolescents with seizures.[60]

THE IMPACT OF CHILDHOOD EPILEPSY ON THE FAMILY

Childhood epilepsy is a problem both for the child and the family. Research has demonstrated an impact of epilepsy on parents and siblings and associations between family factors and behavioral problems in children with epilepsy. Though the findings are generally consistent, Ellis et al.[61] have pointed out several shortcomings in the studies of families of children with epilepsy. Most of the studies used only the perceptions of the parent and not the child, selected families attending specialty clinics, and used single time assessments that may have obscured problems associated with continuing development in children and adolescents.

The family experiences the impact of epilepsy at the moment of the first seizure. Even a benign febrile seizure may be intensely frightening. Baumer et al.[62] found that more than half the parents witnessing a first febrile seizure thought their child was dying or likely to die. Ziegler et al.[63] listed sadness and grief, anxiety and fear and anger as possible first responses to the diagnosis of epilepsy in a child. They also note that denial and anger may prevent the formation of a therapeutic alliance and anxiety may compromise the understanding necessary for successful therapy. In a sample of 69 children with new-onset epilepsy, Oostrom et al.[64] found that 48 per cent of parents felt they were unable to continue their usual style of parenting. Shore et al.[65] assessed concerns and fears of parents of children with new-onset seizures. Worries about brain tumors, loss of intelligence, brain damage, death, or addiction to AEDs were present in over one third of mothers at both 3 and 6 months, and in one third of fathers at 3 months and one fifth at 6 months.

Parents of children with chronic seizures continue to be concerned about the effects of epilepsy on their child. Surveys have found that parents are worried about recurrent seizures, the cause of their child's seizures, side-effects of medication and need for restrictions of activities.[66–68] Arunkumar et al.[69] found that more than 30 per cent of parents of children with epilepsy listed medication side-effects, cognitive effects, potential injuries, independence and the future as concerns.

Epilepsy in childhood has been associated with disruption of family process. Austin[66] found that, when compared to families of children with asthma, the families of children with chronic epilepsy had lower levels of esteem and communication and less extended family social support. Kitamoto et al.,[70] in a study from Japan, noted that parents of children with uncomplicated epilepsy were more rejecting of their children compared to normal standards. Mothers of children with complicated epilepsy were anxious and overprotective and fathers were rejecting. In a study of families in India, Thomas and Bindu[71] noted frustration, guilt, anger, and depression in family members of children with epilepsy. Hodes et al.[72] described more emotional overinvolvement and a trend to more hostility toward children with epilepsy than to siblings. Brown and Jadresic[73] found that higher levels of expressed emotion in parents of children with epilepsy were directly related to seizure number. In contrast, Hoare and Kerley[58] did not find an increase in psychiatric difficulties or disturbed marital relationships in parents of children with epilepsy.

The presence of seizures in a child also may have an adverse effect on siblings. Hoare[74] found more behavioral problems in siblings of children with chronic seizures than in children in the general population and siblings of children with new-onset seizures. Mims[75] noted a trend for increased externalizing behavior in siblings of children with frequent seizures compared to siblings of children with infrequent seizures or control children. Mims also found that most siblings of children with both frequent and infrequent seizures had worries or concerns about seizures. This suggests that more severe seizures may be a stress for both parents and siblings.

The family environment has been associated with the behavioral outcome in children with epilepsy. Both Hoare and Kerley[58] and Austin et al.[45] described an association between family stress and impaired behavior in children with seizures. Austin et al.[45] showed associations between family mastery and social support respectively, and child behavior. Austin also has reported an association between lower scores in family adaptation and resources and poor psychosocial adaptation of the child.[66] Carlton-Ford et al.[30] found that the combination of family factors and additional childhood disabilities had a major effect on childhood behavior. Mitchell et al.[32] noted a substantial association between family acculturation and behavior. They found that factors involved in acculturation were associated with parental fears and negative attitudes.

The family factors associated with childhood behavior may have arisen in response to seizures, may have preceded the seizures or, if present prior to seizures, may have been exacerbated by the stress of a new illness. In a sample of families of children with new-onset epilepsy, Oostrom et al.[64] found that longstanding behavior problems in the child and family troubles such as marital discord, divorce or psychiatric illness in another family member were associated with poor adaptation of the child to seizures.

Several studies have shown the importance of the interaction between parent and child in predicting behavioral problems in children with seizures. Parental suppression of aggression and sexuality has been related to slow social development of the child[76] and autocratic style in the mother to withdrawal of the child.[77] Lothman and Pianta[78] found that mother's support and affective availability were predictors of childhood adjustment and competence, whereas parental overcontrol[79] and maternal criticism and hostility[72] have been associated with childhood behavioral problems. These are most likely styles present before the onset of seizures that may have become more pronounced with the stress of a chronic illness.

CHILDHOOD EPILEPSY AND THE COMMUNITY

Stigma

The impact of epilepsy extends beyond the child and the family to the surrounding community. Members of the community may have limited understanding of epilepsy and therefore the child and family are forced to deal with stigmatization. People with epilepsy report that dealing with stigma and the resultant prejudicial responses from others is one of their biggest challenges. Even children with new-onset seizures and their parents were found to be concerned about stigma. In a study of new-onset seizures by Austin et al., the children reported feeling different from their peers and feared teasing or rejection if they should have a seizure in front of their peers.[80] Their parents worried about whether they should disclose the fact that their child had seizures for fear that responses of others would be negative.[81]

Although there are few studies that focus on the effects of stigma in children and adolescents with epilepsy, stigma has been found to have detrimental effects. Westbrook et al.[82] studied 64 adolescents with epilepsy and found poorer self-esteem in those who had higher perceptions of stigma. A surprising finding in this study was that most of the adolescents did not feel particularly stigmatized by their epilepsy nor did they believe it affected their ability to date or have friends. On the other hand, over half of them reported that they kept their epilepsy a secret from others and a majority reported that they either never or rarely talked about their epilepsy with others. These findings suggest that these adolescents felt uncomfortable revealing to others that they had epilepsy, which also could reflect perceived stigma.

Findings from a large survey of general population adolescents in the USA conducted by the Epilepsy Foundation suggest that adolescents with epilepsy do face a social environment characterized by stigma.[83] Almost three quarters of the 19 441 respondents thought that youth with epilepsy would be more likely to get picked on or bullied by others. A large majority of the respondents believed that having epilepsy would or could lead to unpopularity. Only one third of the respondents stated that they would date someone with epilepsy. The fact that fewer than half of the respondents reported that they would disclose epilepsy to others if they had the condition suggests that these adolescents perceive that epilepsy leads to negative social consequences. These findings help explain the reluctance on the part of adolescents and parents of children with epilepsy to disclose to others.

Public beliefs and knowledge about epilepsy are thought to influence the amount of stigma associated with epilepsy. Often public perceptions are based on incomplete or inaccurate information. The survey of general population teenagers in the USA showed a lack of familiarity with and knowledge about epilepsy. Of seven common health conditions, these adolescents were least familiar with epilepsy. In addition, most held misconceptions about epilepsy and the people who have the condition. Only 51 per cent of the respondents were sure that epilepsy was not contagious, only 47 per cent thought that young people with epilepsy could attend regular schools and only 42 per cent believed that people with epilepsy were able to work.[83]

This lack of knowledge about epilepsy could result in an unsafe environment for adolescents if they should have a seizure in front of their peers. A majority of the respondents in the survey reported that they would not know what to do if someone had a seizure. Even though one third of the respondents indicated that they would know what to do if someone had a seizure, because of the nature of the survey, the accuracy of their perception could not be verified.

Comprehensive care for the child with epilepsy

The child and family begin their interaction with the larger community in the emergency room, hospital or physician's office. At least in more developed countries, patients have access to modern technology and medical care. Comprehensive care centers are available, though managed care insurance systems and geographic location may limit access. In contrast, services for epilepsy are much more variable in developing countries.[84] As an example, with the exception of South Africa, there is limited availability of neurologists, EEG and neuroimaging in most of sub-Saharan Africa. Medication costs are also a major concern in developing countries.

In developed countries, most audits of epilepsy care have found that families of children with epilepsy are satisfied with the medical care given their children. The deficits identified by parents are in communication, information

and psychosocial care.[68,85,86] Suurmeijer[87] found that one third of parents or partners of people with epilepsy were dissatisfied with access to clinic personnel and communication. Shore et al.[65] in a survey of parents of children with new-onset epilepsy, reported dissatisfaction with information received and noted that there was only minimal decrease in dissatisfaction between 3 months and 6 months after onset of seizures. Approximately half the parents continued to report strong needs for information. In an audit of a tertiary children's epilepsy unit, Robinson et al.[68] found that, even though 45 of 50 parents were fairly or very satisfied with services, 42 of 50 wanted more information or resources, including responses to their concerns about etiology of seizures, side-effects of medication and restrictions of activities. There may be a disparity between physicians' perception of patients needs and parents' concerns, with physicians overestimating parents' concerns about seizures and medications and underestimating their concerns about psychosocial care.[88]

Studies of children with epilepsy have also identified a need for improved communication. In a large survey of children with epilepsy, Brown[89] found that half the children did not feel they understood what their doctor had said while explaining their seizures and one third said their doctor never explained epilepsy to them. McNelis et al.[90] in a study of children with new-onset seizures, found that approximately one third of the children were less than satisfied with the care received and half reported need for additional information. More than half said they needed help in deciding how to talk to others about seizures and how to handle seizures at school. Comparing children with epilepsy to children with asthma or diabetes, Houston et al.[91] noted less knowledge of illness and more reluctance to talk to friends about their illness in the children with epilepsy. In contrast to most other studies, Norrby et al.[92] found no difference in well-being in a comparison of 31 children with epilepsy 9–13 years of age and 342 age-matched healthy controls. They thought that clinic's attention to information needs might have resulted in a better outcome for children with epilepsy.

A response to the additional nonmedical needs of parents could take several forms. Ziegler et al.[63] described the use of a psychosocial consultant in a comprehensive epilepsy clinic to help with assessment, promote adaptation to epilepsy at each stage of development and aid the neurologist in diagnosis of co-morbid behavioral conditions. Robinson et al.[68] described establishing parent and adolescent groups to deal with the psychosocial concerns discovered in their audit of a comprehensive epilepsy clinic for children. Lewis et al.[93,94] developed a large-group educational program that resulted in improved knowledge of epilepsy in children and mothers and a reduction in maternal anxiety about seizures. Austin et al.[95] have used a small-group approach to provide educational and emotional support. Other studies have shown that individual and group psychotherapy for adolescents with intractable seizures may be used to assess emotionally based seizure precipitants and teach relaxation or self-control techniques with a resultant decrease in seizure frequency and improved self-concept[96] (see Chapter 22E).

Restrictions for children and adolescents with epilepsy

Parents and children generally receive their initial information on appropriate restrictions in activities from the medical community. Most restrictions placed on the child with seizures are intended to minimize the risk of injury or death. In the home, the general recommendations are to not allow a young child to be in the bath alone, to leave bathroom doors unlocked and to shield fireplaces and stoves (cookers).[97,98] Overnight stays and travel are permitted as long as there is a responsible person aware of the child's seizures and medical care accessible.

The recommendations on sports have varied. The International League Against Epilepsy (ILAE) suggests allowing the child to participate in all sports and extracurricular school activities with the exception of scuba diving and skydiving.[98] The American Academy of Pediatrics recommends avoidance of contact sports such as football and soccer for children with poorly controlled seizures, but recommends no limitations for children with well-controlled seizures.[99] Most agree that swimming should be allowed but only under careful supervision. Data addressing the question of seizure recurrence with exercise are limited. Nakken et al. found that epileptiform discharges on EEG decreased in 20 of 26 children monitored during exercise and increased or did not change in 5 children.[100] These 5 children had experienced seizures during or soon after exercise in the past, suggesting that restrictions need to be individualized and the child monitored for individual response to exercise.

One concern about restrictions is the manner in which they are implemented. Some children with seizures may be limited excessively. Kirsch and Wirrell[101] found no increase in risk of injury for cognitively normal children with epilepsy. Carpay et al.[102] found restrictions placed on 83 per cent of children with seizures during the past year, but found no association between restrictions and seizure type or frequency.

Driving is a concern for the adolescent with seizures. Unfortunately, younger patients with seizures have a relatively higher risk for traffic accidents and this increased risk is greater than that seen in older individuals with seizures.[103] Risk factors for accidents include noncompliance with AEDs, shorter seizure-free intervals, absence of an aura and prior accidents not related to seizures.[104] The laws vary from country to country and, in the USA, from state to state. State laws set an average of 6 months free of seizures before obtaining a driver's license.[105] The impact

on adolescents is significant. Clement and Wallace[106] found that only two thirds of adolescents with epilepsy expected to ever drive, versus almost all the adolescents in a control group.

Epilepsy and schools

Accommodations within the school system may be necessary for children with epilepsy. Beyond extra help for memory or attention problems or special class placement for learning disability, children may need additional services because of seizures. Lanfear and Rashid[107] described an effort by two nurses with special expertise in epilepsy to teach epilepsy awareness and medication management to school nurses. They were able to develop protocols for children with intractable seizures, including training in the use of rectal diazepam. The program was successful, allowing the children to remain in school. Freeman et al.[108] developed a more extensive program that involved initial needs assessment, counseling, evaluation of classroom placement and vocational training. They were able to reduce the dropout and grade failure rates to half what they were in the regular school system. They also found that the children who participated in the program were less likely to be either out of school or unemployed after graduation. The cost of the program was approximately 10 per cent greater than that spent on the average student in the system.

One problem for children with epilepsy in the regular school system may be the teacher's lack of knowledge of epilepsy. Hanai[67] found that teachers in Japan were more likely to favor restrictions for involvement in physical education and school activities for children with epilepsy than were parents. Only 20 per cent of teachers knew that children needed to take medication exactly as prescribed by physicians and 65 per cent indicated a need for more information about seizures. Parents of 52 per cent of the children with seizures in regular classes and 9 per cent of the children in special classes had not informed the school of their child's epilepsy. A study from Thailand found that 38 per cent of teachers said they had no knowledge of epilepsy and 15 per cent believed that all children with epilepsy should be in special classes. Only 11.4 per cent knew appropriate seizure first-aid.[109]

Support groups

Support groups can address many of the needs of children with seizures and their parents. Lee[110] suggests that these groups developed in response to insufficient care for patients. These support groups have given patients information about their condition, assistance in obtaining services and social contacts to reduce isolation and stigma. With continuing growth, the support groups have also empowered patients. They provide education to the public and advocacy for patients. The public visibility of these organizations has helped obtain equal rights for patients with epilepsy and public funding for research in the causes and treatment of seizures. Epilepsy associations are now available throughout the world. In addition to the ILEA, as of 2000 there were 50 national epilepsy associations.[1] The support groups are limited by their need to be constantly raising funds for programming and occasionally by the poor fit between an individual child and family and the majority of members of the local support group. Overall, the epilepsy support groups have contributed to significant improvement in quality of life for patients with seizures.

KEY POINTS

- Comprehensive instruments for the **assessment of quality of life** in children with epilepsy include generic tools and epilepsy-specific instruments
- Quality of life in children and adolescents with epilepsy can be measured using a **battery of instruments** assessing attitudes, cognitive function, academic achievement, and psychological functioning
- Children with epilepsy have more **cognitive and behavioral problems** than children with chronic illnesses not affecting the brain. Risk factors are neurological impairment beyond seizures, frequent or severe seizures, and psychosocial factors affecting the child or the family
- Seizures in children may result in **parental anxiety.** Family disruption is associated with behavioral problems in children with epilepsy
- **Stigma** is a significant problem in adolescents with epilepsy. Most adolescents in a general population survey felt that adolescents with epilepsy would be unpopular and most kept their seizures a secret. Teachers may have only a limited knowledge of epilepsy
- Children and adolescents with epilepsy are restricted from swimming alone, driving, and, when seizures are poorly controlled, from contact sports. **Excessive restrictions should be avoided** in children and adolescents with well-controlled seizures

REFERENCES

1. Baker GA, Jacoby A. Quality of life. In: *Epilepsy: Beyond Seizure Counts in Assessment and Treatments*. Amsterdam: Harwood Academic Publishers, 2000.
2. Ettinger AB, Kanner AM. *Psychiatric Issues in Epilepsy*. Philadelphia: Lippincott Williams & Wilkins, 2001.
3. Aicardi J. Epilepsy as a non-paroxysmal disorder. *Acta Neuropediatrica* 1996; **2**: 249–257.
4. Taylor DC. The components of sickness: diseases, illnesses and predicaments. In: Apley J, Ounsted C (eds) *One Child*. London: Heinemann Medical, 1982: 1–13.
5. Landgraf JM, Abetz L, Ware JE. *The CHQ User's Manual*. Boston: The Health Institute, New England Medical Center, 1996.
6. Gilliam F, Wyllie E, Kashden J, *et al.* Epilepsy surgery outcome: comprehensive assessment in children. *Neurology* 1997; **48**: 1368–1374.
7. Hoare P, Russell M. The quality of life of children with chronic epilepsy and their families: preliminary findings with a new assessment measure. *Developmental Medicine and Child Neurology* 1995; **37**: 689–696.
8. Hoare P, Mann H, Dunn S. Parental perception of the quality of life among children with epilepsy or diabetes with a new assessment questionnaire. *Quality of Life Research* 2000; **9**: 637–644.
9. Apajaslo M, Sintonen H, Holmberg C, *et al.* Quality of life in early adolescence: a sixteen-dimensional health-related measure. *Quality of Life Research* 1996; **5**: 205–211.
10. Cramer JA, Westbrook LE, Devinsky O *et al.* Development of the Quality of Life in Epilepsy Inventory for Adolescents: the QOLIE-AD-48. *Epilepsia* 1999; **40**: 1114–1121.
11. Devinsky O, Westbrook L, Cramer J, *et al.* Risk factors for poor health-related quality of life in adolescents with epilepsy. *Epilepsia* 1999; **40**: 1715–1720.
12. Wildrick D, Parker-Fisher S, Morales A. Quality of life in children with well-controlled epilepsy. *Journal of Neuroscience Nursing* 1996; **28**: 192–198.
13. Sabaz M, Cairns DR, Lawson JA, *et al.* Validation of a new quality of life measure for children with epilepsy. *Epilepsia* 2000; **41**: 765–774.
14. Sabaz M, Cairns DR, Lawson JA, Bleasel AF, Bye AM. The health-related quality of life of children with refractory epilepsy: a comparison of those with and without intellectual disability. *Epilepsia* 2001; **42**: 621–628.
15. Camfield C, Breau L, Camfield P. Impact of pediatric epilepsy on the family: a new scale for clinical and research use. *Epilepsia* 2001; **42**: 104–112.
16. Austin JK, Smith MS, Risinger MW, McNelis AM. Childhood epilepsy and asthma: comparison of quality of life. *Epilepsia* 1994; **35**: 608–615.
17. Achenbach TM. *Manual for the Child Behavior Checklist/4–18*. Burlington, VT: University of Vermont Department of Psychiatry, 1991.
18. Piers EV. *Piers-Harris Children's Self-Concept Scale, Revised Manual*. Los Angeles: Western Psychological Services, 1984.
19. Austin JK, Huberty TJ. Development of the Child Attitude Toward Illness Scale. *Journal of Pediatric Psychology* 1993; **18**: 467–480.
20. Austin JK, Huberty TJ. Revision of the Family APGAR for use by 8-year-olds. *Family Systems Medicine* 1989; **7**: 323–327.
21. Achenbach TM. *Manual for the Teacher Report Form and 1991 Profile*. Burlington VT: University of Vermont Department of Psychiatry, 1991.
22. Austin JK, Huster GA, Dunn DW, Risinger MW. Adolescents with active or inactive epilepsy or asthma: a comparison of quality of life. *Epilepsia* 1996; **37**: 1228–1238.

23. Weglage J, Demsky A, Pietsch M, Kurlemann G. Neuropsychological, intellectual, and behavioral findings in patients with centrotemporal spikes with and without seizures. *Developmental Medicine and Child Neurology* 1997; **39**: 646–651.

24. Mandelbaum DE, Burack GD. The effect of seizure type and medication on cognitive and behavioral functioning in children with idiopathic epilepsy. *Developmental Medicine and Child Neurology* 1997; **39**: 731–735.

25. Schoenfeld J, Seidenberg M, Woodard A, *et al.* Neuropsychological and behavioral status of children with complex partial seizures. *Developmental Medicine and Child Neurology* 1999; 41(11): 724–731.

26. Sillanpää M, Jalava M, Kaleva O, Shinnar S. Long-term prognosis of seizures with onset in childhood. *New England Journal of Medicine* 1998; **338**: 1715–1722.

27. Wirrell EC, Camfield CS, Camfield PR, Dooley JM, Gordon KE, Smith B. Long-term psychosocial outcome in typical absence epilepsy. *Archives of Pediatric and Adolescent Medicine* 1997; **151**: 152–158.

28. Kokkonen E, Kokkonen J, Saukkonen A. Do neurological disorders in childhood pose a risk for mental health in young adulthood? *Developmental Medicine and Child Neurology* 1998; **40**: 364–368.

29. Austin JK, Dunn DW. Children with epilepsy: quality of life and psychosocial needs. *Annual Review of Nursing Research*, 2000; **18**: 26–47.

30. Carlton-Ford S, Miller R, Brown M, Nealeigh N, Jennings P. Epilepsy and children's social and psychological adjustment. *Journal of Health and Social Behavior* 1995; **36**: 285–301.

31. Steffenburg S, Gillberg C, Steffenburg U. Psychiatric disorders in children and adolescents with mental retardation and active epilepsy. *Archives of Neurology* 1996; **53**: 904–912.

32. Mitchell WG, Scheier LM, Baker SA. Psychosocial, behavioral and medical outcomes in children with epilepsy: a developmental risk factor model using longitudinal data. *Pediatrics* 1994; **94**: 471–477.

33. Austin JK, Huberty TJ, Huster GA, Dunn DW. Does academic achievement in children with epilepsy change over time? *Developmental Medicine and Child Neurology* 1999; **41**: 473–479.

34. Rutter M, Graham P, Yule W. *A Neuropsychiatric Study in Childhood*. Philadelphia: Lippincott, 1970.

35. Hoare P. The development of psychiatric disorder among school children with epilepsy. *Developmental Medicine and Child Neurology* 1984; **26**: 3–13.

36. McDermott S, Mani S, Krishnaswami S. A population-based analysis of specific behavior problems associated with childhood seizures. *Journal of Epilepsy* 1995; **8**: 110–118.

37. Dunn DW, Austin JK. Behavioral issues in pediatric epilepsy. *Neurology* 1999; **53** (Suppl. 2): S96–100.

38. Stores G, Wiggs L, Campling G. Sleep disorders and their relationship to psychological disturbance in children with epilepsy. *Child: Care, Health and Development* 1998; **24**: 5–19.

39. Cortesi F, Giannotti F, Ottaviano S. Sleep problems and daytime behavior in childhood idiopathic epilepsy. *Epilepsia* 1999; **40**: 1557–1565.

40. Dunn DW, Austin JK, Huster GA. Behavior problems in children with new-onset epilepsy. *Seizure* 1997; **6**: 283–287.

41. Austin JK, Harezlak J, Dunn DW *et al.* Behavior problems in children before first recognized seizures. *Pediatrics* 2001; **107**: 115–122.

42. Seidenberg M, Beck N, Geisser M *et al.* Academic achievement of children with epilepsy. *Epilepsia* 1986; **27**: 753–759.

43. Mitchell WG, Chavez JM, Lee H, Guzman BL. Academic underachievement in children with epilepsy. *Journal of Child Neurology* 1991; **6**: 65–72.

44. Austin JK, Huberty TJ, Huster GA, Dunn DW. Academic achievement in children with epilepsy or asthma. *Developmental Medicine and Child Neurology* 1998; **40**: 248–255.

45. Austin JK, Risinger M, Beckett LA. Correlates of behavior problems in children with epilepsy. *Epilepsia* 1992; **33**: 1115–1122.

46. Breslau N. Psychiatric disorder in children with physical disabilities. *Journal of the American Academy of Child and Adolescent Psychiatry* 1985; **24**: 87–94.

47. Hermann BP. Neuropsychological functioning and psychopathology in children with epilepsy. *Epilepsia* 1982; **23**: 545–554.

48. Williams J, Griebel ML, Dykman RA. Neuropsychological patterns in pediatric epilepsy. *Seizure* 1998; **7**: 223–228.

49. Semrud-Clikeman M, Wical B. Components of attention in children with complex partial epilepsy with and without ADHD. *Epilepsia* 1999; **40**: 211–215.

50. McCarthy AM, Richman LC, Yarbrough D. Memory, attention and school problems in children with seizure disorders. *Developmental Neuropsychology* 1995; **11**: 71–86.

51. Hoare P, Mann H. Self-esteem and behavioral adjustment in children with epilepsy and children with diabetes *Journal of Psychosomatic Research* 1994; **38**: 859–869.

52. Whitman S, Hermann BP, Black RB, Chhabria S. Psychopathology and seizure type in children with epilepsy. *Psychological Medicine* 1982; **12**: 843–853.

53. Caplan R, Arbelle S, Magharious W *et al.* Psychopathology in pediatric complex partial and primary generalized epilepsy. *Developmental Medicine and Child Neurology* 1998; **40**: 805–811.

54. Hermann BP, Whitman S, Dell J. Correlates of behavior problems and social competence in children with epilepsy, aged 6–11. In: Hermann B, Seidenberg M (eds) *Childhood Epilepsies: Neuropsychological, Psychosocial and Intervention Aspects.* New York, John Wiley & Sons, 1989: 143–157.

55. Williams J, Bates S, Griebel ML, *et al.* Does short-term antiepileptic drug treatment in children result in cognitive or behavioral changes? *Epilepsia* 1998; **39**: 1064–1069.

56. Aldenkamp AP, Alpherts WCJ, Blennow G *et al.* Withdrawal of antiepileptic medication in children – effects on cognitive function. *Neurology* 1993; **43**: 41–50.

57. Aldenkamp AP, Alpherts WCJ, Sandstedt P *et al.* Antiepileptic drug-related cognitive complaints in seizure-free children with epilepsy before and after drug discontinuation. *Epilepsia* 1998; **39**: 1070–1074.

58. Hoare P, Kerley S. Psychosocial adjustment of children with chronic epilepsy and their families. *Developmental Medicine and Child Neurology* 1991; **33**: 201–215.

59. Mathews WS, Barabas G. Perceptions of control among children with epilepsy. In: Whitman S, Hermann BP (eds) *Psychopathology in Epilepsy: Social Dimensions.* New York, Oxford University Press, 1986: 162–182.

60. Dunn DW, Austin JK, Huster GA. Symptoms of depression in adolescents with epilepsy. *Journal of the American Academy of Child and Adolescent Psychiatry* 1999; **38**: 1132–1138.

61. Ellis N, Upton D, Thompson P. Epilepsy and the family: a review of the current literature. *Seizure* 2000; **9**: 22–30.

62. Baumer JH, David TJ, Valentine SJ, Roberts JE, Hughes BR. Many parents think their child is dying when having a first febrile seizure. *Developmental Medicine and Child Neurology* 1981; **23**: 462–464.

63. Ziegler RG, Erba G, Holden L, Dennison H. The coordinated psychosocial and neurologic care of children with seizures and their families. *Epilepsia* 2000; **41**: 732–743.

64. Oostrom KJ, Schouten A, Kruitwagen CLJJ, Peters ACB, Jennekens-Schinkel A. Parents' perceptions of adversity introduced by upheaval and uncertainty at the onset of childhood epilepsy. *Epilepsia* 2001; **42**: 1452–1460.

65. Shore C, Austin J, Musick B, Dunn D, McBride A, Creasy K. Psychosocial care needs of parents of children with new-onset seizures. *Journal of Neuroscience Nursing* 1998; **30**: 169–174.

66. Austin JK. Childhood epilepsy: child adaptation and family resources. *Journal of Child and Adolescent Psychiatric and Mental Health Nursing* 1988; **1**: 18–24.

67. Hanai T. Quality of life in children with epilepsy. *Epilepsia* 1996; **37**: 28–32.

68. Robinson RO, Edwards M, Madigan C, Ledgar S, Boutros A. Audit of a children's epilepsy clinic. *Developmental Medicine and Child Neurology* 2000; **42**: 387–391.

69. Arunkumar G, Wyllie E, Kotagal P, Ong HT, Gilliam F. Parent- and patient-validated content for pediatric quality-of-life assessment. *Epilepsia* 2000; **41**: 1474–1484.

70. Kitamoto I, Kurokawa T, Tomita S, Maeda Y, Sakamoto K, Ueda K. Child-parent relationships in the care of epileptic children. *Brain and Development* 1988; **10**: 36–40.

71. Thomas SV, Bindu VB. Psychosocial and economic problems of parents of children with epilepsy. *Seizure* 1999; **8**: 66–69.

72. Hodes M, Garralda ME, Rose G, Schwartz R. Maternal expressed emotion and adjustment in children with epilepsy. *Journal of Child Psychology and Psychiatry* 1999; **40**: 1083–1093.

73. Brown SW, Jadresic E. Expressed emotion in the families of young people with epilepsy. *Seizure* 2000; **9**: 255–258.

74. Hoare P. Psychiatric disturbance in the families of epileptic children. *Developmental Medicine and Child Neurology* 1984; **26**: 14–19.

75. Mims J. Self-esteem, behavior, and concerns surrounding epilepsy in siblings of children with epilepsy. *Journal of Child Neurology* 1997; **12**: 187–192.

76. Hartlage LC, Green JB. The relation of parental attitudes to academic and social achievement in epileptic children. *Epilepsia* 1972; **13**: 21–26.

77. Ritchie K. Research note: interaction in the families of epileptic children. *Journal of Child Psychology and Psychiatry* 1981; **22**: 65–71.

78. Lothman DJ, Pianta RC. Role of child-mother interaction in predicting competence of children with epilepsy. *Epilepsia* 1993; **34**: 658–669.

79. Carlton-Ford S, Miller R, Nealeigh N, Sanchez N. The effects of perceived stigma and psychological over-control on the behavioral problems of children with epilepsy. *Seizure* 1997; **6**: 383–391.

80. Austin JK. Concerns and fears of children with seizures. *Clinical Nursing Practice in Epilepsy* 1993; **1**: 4–6.

81. Austin JK, Oruche UM, Dunn DW, Levstek DA. New-onset childhood seizures: parents' concerns and needs. *Clinical Nursing Practice in Epilepsy* 1995; **2**: 8–10.

82. Westbrook LE, Bauman LJ, Shinnar S. Applying stigma theory to epilepsy: A test of a conceptual model. *Journal of Pediatric Psychology* 1992; **17**: 633–649.

83. Austin JK, Shafer PO, Deering JB. Epilepsy familiarity, knowledge, and perceptions of stigma: report from a survey of adolescents in the general population. *Epilepsy and Behavior* 2002; **3**: 368–375.

84. Jallon P. Epilepsy in developing countries. *Epilepsia* 1997; **38**: 1143–1151.

85. Williams J, Sharp GB, Griebel ML, *et al.* Outcome findings from a multidisciplinary clinic for children with epilepsy. *Children's Health Care* 1995; **24**: 235–244.

86. Webb DW, Coleman H, Fielder A, Kennedy CR. An audit of pediatric epilepsy care. *Archives of Diseases of Childhood* 1998; **79**: 145–148.

87. Suurmeijer TPBM. Quality of care and quality of life from the perspective of patients and parents. *International Journal of Adolescent Medicine and Health* 1994; **7**: 289–302.

88. Coulter DL, Koester BS. Information needs of parents of children with epilepsy. *Developmental and Behavioral Pediatrics* 1985; **6**: 334–338.

89. Brown SW. Quality of life: a view from the playground. *Seizure* 1994; **3**: 11–15.

90. McNelis A, Musick B, Austin J, Dunn D, Creasy K. Psychosocial care needs of children with new-onset seizures. *Journal of Neuroscience Nursing* 1998; **30**: 161–165.

91. Houston EC, Cunningham CC, Metcalfe E, Newton R. The information needs and understanding of 5–10-year old children with epilepsy, asthma or diabetes. *Seizure* 2000; **9**: 340–343.

92. Norrby U, Carlsson J, Beckung E, Nordholm L. Self-assessment of well-being in a group of children with epilepsy. *Seizure* 1999; **8**: 228–234.

93. Lewis MA, Salas I, de la Sota A, Chiofalo N, Leake B. Randomized trial of a program to enhance the competencies of children with epilepsy. *Epilepsia* 1990; **31**: 101–109.

94. Lewis MA, Hatton CL, Salas I, Leake B, Chiofalo N. Impact of the children's epilepsy program on parents. *Epilepsia* 1991; **32**: 365–374.

95. Austin JK, McNelis AM, Shore CP, Dunn DW, Musick B. A feasibility study of a family seizure management program: 'Be Seizure Smart'. *Journal of Neuroscience Nursing* 2002; **34**: 30–37.

96. Dahl J, Brorson L, Melin L. Effects of a broad-spectrum behavioral medicine treatment program on children with refractory epileptic seizures: an 8-year follow-up. *Epilepsia* 1992; **33**: 98–102.

97. Austin JK, deBoer HM. Disruptions in social functioning and services facilitating adjustment for the child and adult. In: Engel J, Pedley TA (eds) *Epilepsy: A Comprehensive Textbook*. Philadelphia, Lippincott-Raven, 1997: 2191–2201.

98. Commission of Pediatrics of the ILAE. Restrictions for children with epilepsy. *Epilepsia* 1997; **38**: 1054–1056.

99. Committee on Sports Medicine. Recommendations for participation in competitive sports. *Pediatrics* 1988; **81**: 737–739.

100. Nakken KO, Løyning A, Løyning T, Gløersen G, Larsson PG. Does physical exercise influence the occurrence of epileptiform EEG discharges in children? *Epilepsia* 1997; **38**: 279–284.

101. Kirsch R, Wirrell E. Do cognitively normal children with epilepsy have a higher rate of injury than their nonepileptic peers? *Journal of Child Neurology* 2001; **16**: 100–104.

102. Carpay HA, Vermeulen J, Stroink H, *et al.* Disability due to restrictions in childhood epilepsy. *Developmental Medicine and Child Neurology* 1997; **39**: 521–526.

103. Hansotia P, Broste S. Epilepsy and traffic safety. *Epilepsia* 1993; **34**: 852–858.

104. Krauss GL, Krumholz A, Carter RC, Li G, Kaplan P. Risk factors for seizure-related motor vehicle crashes in patients with epilepsy. *Neurology* 1999; **52**: 1324–1329.

105. Krauss GL, Ampaw L, Krumholz A. Individual state driving restrictions for people with epilepsy in the US. *Neurology* 2001; **57**: 1780–1785.

106. Clement MJ, Wallace SJ. A survey of adolescents with epilepsy. *Developmental Neurology and Child Neurology* 1990; **32**: 849–857.

107. Lanfear JH, Rashid C. Who cares for students with epilepsy in mainstream education? *Seizure* 1998; **7**: 189–192.

108. Freeman JM, Jacobs H, Vining E, Rabin CE. Epilepsy and inner city schools: a school-based program that makes a difference. *Epilepsia* 1984; **25**: 438–442.

109. Kankirawatana P. Epilepsy awareness among school teachers in Thailand. *Epilepsia* 1999; **40**: 497–501.

110. Lee P. Support groups for people with epilepsy. In: Baker GA, Jacoby A. (eds) *Quality of Life in Epilepsy: Beyond seizure counts in assessment and treatment.* Amsterdam: Harwood Academic Publishers, 2000: 273–281.

26

Special centers for childhood epilepsy

FRANK MC BESAG

Segregation of people on the basis of a disease or disorder is no longer either accepted or acceptable. The current emphasis is on ensuring that children with epilepsy lead lives that are as normal as possible. There should be no hint of institutionalization in management. Most children have well-controlled seizures, attend mainstream schools and do not require much attention from the specialist services. To meet their needs adequately, a significant minority need additional help and a few require a short or longer-term placement in a special center.

HISTORY OF THE SPECIAL CENTERS

The belief that epilepsy might be a bad influence on others, or might even be infectious, continued well into the twentieth century.[1] One of the earliest recorded establishments with a more caring attitude was founded at the end of the fifteenth century, when a 'hospice for epileptics' was provided in Alsace. In 1867, a particularly influential center was established in a farmhouse near the town of Bielefeld, Germany. This was the beginning of the famous Bethel Center. Subsequently the colonies at Meer en Bosch, Heemsteede, Netherlands and Filadelfia, Dianalund, Denmark were founded. Based on the Bethel experience, several centers opened in the UK. Some of these continue to form a nucleus for intensive work, including research and assessment. They have a particular role to play for people with difficult epilepsy. A number of other European centers have similar wide-ranging remits.

Attitudes have changed in important ways. The epilepsy center is no longer viewed as a place where people can be segregated from society. Instead, it enables people with problematic epilepsy to fulfill a greater role within society by offering specialist assessment, treatment, education and rehabilitation. In the UK, this philosophy has successively grown out of a number of reports including the 1944 Education Act, the Warnock Report,[2] which greatly influenced the subsequent 1981 Education Act, and the 2001 Special Educational Needs and Disability Act. These emphasize the importance of educating children in mainstream schooling, wherever this is feasible, whilst acknowledging the important role of special schools for those with difficulties.

EPILEPSY AND EDUCATIONAL DIFFICULTIES

In children, the management of epilepsy almost inevitably impinges on education (see also Chapters 13, 16, 23). Early publications[3–7] revealed educational difficulties in a high proportion. The Isle of Wight Study[8] found an excess of reading retardation around 10 years of age. Subsequent reports have expanded knowledge in this field.[9–14] In the UK, the best epidemiological investigation has been the National Child Development Study, which was based on a cohort of 17 733 children born in 1 week in 1958.[15–17] When epilepsy was present, 37 per cent of affected children were receiving additional special educational help by age 16 years. In Finland, early reviews concluded that 27.5 per cent children with epilepsy did not complete their basic education, or required schooling in establishments for learning disability[18,19] and later studies suggest that many other children could benefit from individualized specialist reassessment of the effects of epilepsy on their learning.[20] It seems that about half of those with epilepsy will experience some educational difficulty and a smaller proportion, perhaps about one third, will not remain in mainstream schooling. However, a much smaller group, less than 1 per cent, attend the epilepsy special centers or schools.

REASONS FOR REFERRAL

The reasons for referral to an epilepsy specialist school or center are given in Table 26.1, and those relating to 'difficult epilepsy' in Table 26.2.[21,22] Distinctions must be made between residential centers for children with epilepsy, offering the possibility of intensive, medium-term or long-term multidisciplinary intervention, and outpatient services, which are sometimes also referred to as centers. Most of the following comments refer to the four residential centers in the UK, which are listed in Table 26.3. Residential schools for those with epilepsy are distinguished from other facilities by the emphasis on allowing full participation in educational and social activities with a suitable peer group. Relationships with the community, both locally and further afield, are also strongly encouraged. In principle, this is no different from the ideal situation in any other school. However, in the special center, the training and experience of the staff, together with specialist medical back-up, enable a broader curriculum and a much wider range of activities to be offered.

A further important distinction relates to reviews of antiepileptic drugs (AEDs). Admitting a child to an acute hospital for 2–3 weeks to 'sort out their AEDs' is often counter-productive. It may falsely raise the expectations of the family, and disrupt the child's routine by admission to circumstances where it is difficult to provide a 'normal' environment offering a full range of facilities, including education, recreation, leisure, a peer group and opportunities for interaction with the outside world. In contrast, the staff in the residential center have the opportunity of observing the child in a number of different situations over a period of some weeks, before instituting any changes. In general, assessment of changes in AEDs cannot be hurried. Sometimes a child may continue with severe epilepsy for several weeks and then suddenly make a response, even becoming seizure-free. In such circumstances, a hasty judgment about the efficacy of the drug could lead to erroneous conclusions and the child might be denied the opportunity of improving. In recent years, the introduction of many new drugs has increased the chances of achieving a good response, but has also led to greater complexity in the potential for adverse effects, including effects on learning and behaviour.[23,24] All epilepsy centers, whether residential or not, should offer a multidisciplinary approach, capable of assessing the whole child. Failure to acknowledge aspects other than epilepsy results in a poor service to the child and family.[25]

The center can also fulfill a role in pre- and post-surgical rehabilitation of children undergoing surgical treatment for epilepsy. Abolition of seizures may imply a major change in life-role. Some children and teenagers find it very difficult to come to terms with this, and require much support. There is a worthwhile trend to use the centers much more for short-term assessment and intervention. In the past, agencies have tended only to consider referring a child if the epilepsy has been severe for many years and if there has been a major failure to progress, either in terms of response to treatment or in educational and social development. There is a place for a different model, in which the child is recommended

Table 26.1 *Problems leading to referral*

'Difficult' epilepsy
Other medical conditions
Poor cognitive abilities
Behavioral difficulties
Poor integration with peer group
Family and social dysfunction
Psychiatric difficulties
Multiple problems

Table 26.2 *Components of 'difficult' epilepsy*

Frequent seizures
Injury in seizures
Risk of status epilepticus
Variable seizure frequency
Postictal problems
Antiepileptic drug problems
Inadequate control
Epilepsy that is difficult to recognize

Table 26.3 *Special centers for childhood epilepsy in the UK*

Park Hospital, Oxford	Outpatient services, short and medium-term intensive inpatient assessment
David Lewis Centre, Cheshire	Medium-term intensive assessments in a designated assessment center and long-term placements
St Elizabeth's School, Much Hadham, Hertfordshire	Long-term placements
National Centre for Young People with Epilepsy (NCYPE), Lingfield, Surrey	Medium-term and long-term placements; short and medium-term assessments; rehabilitation following neurosurgery

early, as soon as the epilepsy begins to interfere in a major way with quality of life, and as soon as it is clear that the problem is unlikely to be solved rapidly using local services. Such a child might stay in a center for approximately 6–12 months, during which a major AED review could be undertaken. Even if the review were not complete at the end of that period, there would be reasonable expectations that it would be so advanced that plans could be continued in the community. Towards the end of the assessment period, an around-the-table case review is recommended. This provides the opportunity for documentation of the child's special needs, taking into account the effect(s) of any interventions which have taken place at the center, and for future planning. In difficult cases, with highly resistant epilepsy or, when there are other major problems, longer-term placement might be appropriate. This model of medium-term assessment is already available in some of the centers in the UK (see Table 26.3).

The centers also have a major role to play in research and teaching. Investigation of new AEDs can be conducted much more safely when children are being continually observed in an establishment which has an on-site doctor and full EEG and nursing facilities. Important research into drug treatment, cognitive changes and behavioral disturbance in children with epilepsy has already been conducted. The centers may often combine with epilepsy associations in holding courses for teachers, doctors, other staff and patients. It is important that the specialist knowledge gained is shared.

OUTCOME

The major changes in the patterns of referral to the centers make it difficult to draw firm conclusions about outcome. Previously a much larger proportion of children were referred and employment rates in the general population were higher. Consequently, against the general background of relatively poor outcomes for people with epilepsy, the results were relatively good.[26,27] Recently, the tendency has been to refer only those with particularly difficult epilepsy. These young people often have other special needs which prevent them from entering open employment. The current suggestion is that the epilepsy center should be used more often for short-term assessments and rehabilitation, including those related to surgery. If this becomes accepted, with the result that children are referred earlier and stay for relatively shorter periods, the outcome should be particularly good. There is relatively little chance of a satisfactory outcome if a child is referred after years of neurological, educational and social damage following recurrent bouts of inadequately treated, prolonged status epilepticus.

KEY POINTS

- Most children with epilepsy should attend a **mainstream school** and do not need the services of an epilepsy special center
- It is important to recognize that a large proportion of children with epilepsy, approximately half of the total number, have some **educational difficulty**: professionals must offer the additional support that such children require
- A relatively small proportion needs the **specialist services** of an epilepsy center
- **Waiting** until the child and family have suffered many years of severe epilepsy, fragmented education and grossly restricted quality of life should be discouraged
- **Early recognition** of problematic epilepsy, early referral, intensive assessment and appropriate specialist management allow a much better chance of returning to the local community and re-establishing a satisfactory quality of life

REFERENCES

1. Grant RH. Special centres. In: Reynolds EH, Trimble MR (eds) *Epilepsy and Psychiatry*. Edinburgh: Churchill Livingstone, 1981; 347–361.
2. Warnock M. *Report of the Committee of Enquiry into the Education of Handicapped Children and Young People*. London: HMSO, 1978.
3. Pond DA, Bidwell BH. A survey of epilepsy in fourteen general practices II: social and psychological aspects. *Epilepsia* 1960; **1**: 285–299.
4. Ounsted C, Lindsay J, Norman R. *Biological Factors in Temporal Lobe Epilepsy*. London: Spastics Society/Heinemann Medical, 1966.
5. Green JB, Hartlage LC. Comparative performance of epileptic and nonepileptic children and adolescents. (On tests of academic, communicative and social skills). *Diseases of the Nervous System* 1971; **32**: 418–421.
6. Holdsworth L, Whitmore K. A study of children with epilepsy attending ordinary schools. I: their seizure patterns, progress and behaviour in school. *Developmental Medicine and Child Neurology* 1974; **16**: 746–758.
7. Pazzaglia P, Frank-Pazzaglia L. Record in grade school of pupils with epilepsy: an epidemiological study. *Epilepsia* 1976; **17**: 361–366.
8. Rutter M, Graham P, Yule W. *A Neuropsychiatric Study in Childhood*. London: Heinemann Medical, 1970.
9. Stores G. Cognitive function in children with epilepsy. *Developmental Medicine and Child Neurology* 1971; **13**: 390–393.
10. Stores G. Behaviour disturbance and type of epilepsy in children attending ordinary school. In: Penry JK (ed.)

Proceedings of Eighth International Symposium. New York: Raven Press, 1977; 245–249.

11. Stores G. School-children with epilepsy at risk for learning and behaviour problems. *Developmental Medicine and Child Neurology* 1978; **20**: 502–508.

12. Stores G. Problems of learning and behaviour in children with epilepsy. In: Reynolds EH, Trimble MR (eds) *Epilepsy and Psychiatry.* London: Churchill Livingstone, 1981; 33–48.

13. Stores G, Hart J, Piran N. Inattentiveness in schoolchildren with epilepsy. *Epilepsia* 1978; **19**: 169–175.

14. Stores G, Hart JA. Proceedings: Reading skills of children with generalized and focal epilepsy attending ordinary school. *Electroencephalography and Clinical Neurophysiology* 1975; **39**: 429–430.

15. Ross EM, Peckham CS, West PB, *et al.* Epilepsy in childhood: findings from the National Child Development Study. *BMJ* 1980; **280**: 207–210.

16. Verity, CM, Ross EM. Longitudinal studies of children's epilepsy. In: Ross EM, Reynolds EH (eds) *Paediatric Perspectives in Epilepsy.* Chichester: John Wiley, 1985; 133–140.

17. Kurtz Z, Tookey P, Ross E. The epidemiology of epilepsy in childhood. In: Ross E, Chadwick D, Crawford R (eds) *Epilepsy in Young People.* Chichester: John Wiley, 1987; 13–21.

18. Sillanpaa M. Social functioning and seizure status of young adults with onset of epilepsy in childhood. An epidemiological 20-year follow-up study. *Acta Neurologica Scandinavica* 1983; (Suppl. 96): 1–81.

19. Sillanpaa M. Prognosis of children with epilepsy. In: Sillanpaa M, Johannessen SI, Blennow G, *et al.* (eds) *Paediatric Epilepsy.* Petersfield: Wrightson, 1990; 341–368.

20. Airaksinen EM, Matilainen R, Mononen T, *et al.* A population-based study on epilepsy in mentally retarded children. *Epilepsia* 2000; **41**: 1214–1220.

21. Besag FMC. The role of special centres for children with epilepsy. In: Oxley J, Stores G (eds) *Epilepsy and Education. A Medical Symposium on Changing Attitudes to Epilepsy in Education.* London: Medical Tribune Group, 1986; 65–71.

22. Besag FMC. Schooling the child with epilepsy. In: *The Royal College of General Practitioners Members' Reference Book,* 1988; 370–372.

23. Besag FMC. Behavioural effects of the new anticonvulsant drugs. *Drug Safety* 2001; **24**: 513–536.

24. Besag FMC. Childhood epilepsy in relation to mental handicap and behavioural disorders. *Journal of Child Psychology and Psychiatry and Allied Disciplines* 2002; **43**: 103–131.

25. Taylor DC. The components of sickness: diseases, illnesses, and predicaments. *Lancet* 1979; **2**: 1008–1010.

26. Harrison RM, Taylor DC. Childhood seizures: a 25-year follow up. Social and medical prognosis. *Lancet* 1976; **1**: 948–951.

27. Sillanpää M, Jalava M, Kaleva O, Shinnar S. Long-term prognosis of seizures with onset in childhood [see comments]. *New England Journal of Medicine* 1998; **338**: 1715–1722.

27

The adolescent with epilepsy

KEVIN FARRELL

The teenage years span the period between the dependence of childhood and the autonomy of adult life. This transition poses major challenges for all adolescents but is particularly challenging for those with epilepsy. The uncertainty of when a seizure may occur, the side-effects of medications, the associated educational difficulties that are common in children with epilepsy, the parental tendency toward overprotection and the social stigma of epilepsy all contribute to the challenges faced by the teenager with epilepsy.

SOCIAL ISSUES

Adults with epilepsy often cite social difficulties and employment difficulties as greater problems than the seizures themselves. Some of these problems are clearly related to cognitive abnormalities. However, many of the difficulties stem from adverse experiences during childhood and teenage years. Adolescents often feel uncomfortable disclosing to their peers that they have epilepsy.[1] Some children with epilepsy have difficulty forming and maintaining friendships, develop poor self-esteem and become socially isolated. Activities that promote the development of friendships can be useful, for example involving the child in extracurricular youth activities.

Many parents have difficulty allowing the teenager with epilepsy to have the amount of freedom and responsibility that is necessary for the development of self-sufficiency. The physician may contribute to this problem by failing to respect the increasing autonomy that exists in the second decade of life. As patients enter their teenage years,

decision-making needs to move away from the parents to the child. The precise age at which this occurs will depend on the cognitive and emotional maturity of the individual. However, failure of the physician to recognize the increasing independence of teenagers can contribute to the social difficulties and lack of control experienced subsequently by many adults with epilepsy. At medical appointments, younger teenagers with epilepsy should be seen both alone and in the presence of a parent. The eventual aim is for the older teenager to be able to visit the physician alone, an arrangement that should be encouraged whenever possible.

RESTRICTIONS AND FREEDOMS

The development of independence requires teenagers with epilepsy to recognize that the diagnosis imposes certain restrictions. It is more likely that they will adhere to limitations if they are involved in their formulation.

Sports and other restrictions

The risk of having a seizure while in the water has usually been stressed throughout childhood, and most teenagers can appreciate the importance of always having a 'buddy' when swimming, and notifying a lifeguard at the pool. Certain other sports, such as scuba diving or hang-gliding, are clearly not activities that are safe for a person with epilepsy. However, most sporting activities impose only a slightly increased risk, if any, and this is generally considered to be acceptable given the self-esteem that is created by involvement in sporting activities. Whether or not to take a particular risk must be weighed against the benefits of the activity, and is a philosophical rather than a medical issue. The physician can provide valuable input, but those who receive the benefit and take the risk should normally make the decision. As an example, in the author's practice most parents of younger children and most teenagers with epilepsy will choose to continue certain sports, such as snowboarding and skiing, provided that the epilepsy is reasonably well controlled.

Driving

Obtaining a license to drive is considered by many teenagers to be a 'rite of passage'. It is important that teenagers be advised of the local regulations about driving and epilepsy well before the age at which they might want to drive. The situation where an older teenager arrives at the clinic with car keys and inadequately controlled seizures is a challenge best avoided. Some jurisdictions require that the physician be satisfied not only that the seizures are controlled but also that the teenager is compliant with medication. Discussion of these issues in the early teenage years allows the individual to come to terms with the situation and can be a powerful incentive for medication compliance.

Alcohol

Alcohol per se has an anticonvulsant effect. However, its use may be associated with a withdrawal effect, altered drug metabolism, a tendency to forget to take medication and sleep disturbance. The combination of alcohol use and sleep deprivation is particularly likely to provoke seizures, especially in patients with idiopathic generalized epilepsies.[2] The use of alcohol by teenagers is widespread, and a balanced discussion of the risks of its use is likely to be more effective than outright proscription.[3]

Recreational drugs

There are limited data on the risks of recreational drugs in patients with epilepsy. Marijuana appears to offer a protective effect,[4] but its use may be associated with poor compliance with antiepileptic medication and problems with motivation. Cocaine, amphetamine, heroin, phencyclidine, ecstasy and γ-hydroxybutyrate are proconvulsant.[4,5]

FUTURE EMPLOYMENT

Children with epilepsy are at particular risk of failing to reach their educational and vocational goals.[6] Educational difficulties are often due to cognitive dysfunction occurring as a result of the underlying brain abnormality that is responsible for the epilepsy. The side-effects of medications may also contribute to learning difficulties. There is evidence that early assessment of the educational needs of the child, together with modification of classroom placement and vocational assessment, can have a significant impact on educational achievement and employment. Although many schools have programs designed to promote the integration of teenagers with disabilities into the workforce, very few are sensitive to the needs of children with epilepsy. It is our practice to ensure that children with school difficulties have an educational assessment in the elementary school years.

Post-secondary school planning should begin by at least 15 years of age. Ideally, some form of vocational assessment should be obtained in order that planning of further training can take place. Employer discrimination is another factor that may prevent individuals reaching their employment potential. Local Epilepsy Societies can play an important role in the education of employers and the establishment of job opportunities for young adults with epilepsy.

MEDICAL ISSUES

Natural history of epilepsies

Knowledge of the natural history of the adolescent's epilepsy type can be very helpful in the establishment of realistic expectations.

TYPICAL ABSENCE SEIZURES

These remit during childhood or adolescence in 94 per cent of patients.[7] However, generalized tonic-clonic seizures (GTCS) develop in 16–44 per cent of those with typical absence seizures (see Chapter 11A). In one series of patients with childhood or juvenile absence epilepsy, who were followed until 20–52 years of age, GTCS occurred in 74 per cent of those with juvenile absence epilepsy but only 25 per cent of those childhood absence epilepsy and only 16 per cent of those with onset before 9 years of age.[8] The presence of photosensitivity or polyspike-wave discharges on the EEG increases the risk of GTCS.[9] In patients with childhood absence epilepsy, posterior rhythmic delta activity is associated with a lower risk of GTCS.[7,10] When GTCS occur, they usually start between 5 and 10 years after the onset of the absence seizures[11] and are often easily controlled with medication.[8]

JUVENILE MYOCLONIC EPILEPSY (JME)

JME is associated with good seizure control in 80–90 per cent of patients receiving an appropriate antiepileptic drug (AED).[11] However, withdrawal of medication nearly always results in a recurrence of seizures, even in patients who have had several years of seizure control.[10]

MESIAL TEMPORAL SCLEROSIS

Patients with temporal lobe seizures associated with mesial temporal sclerosis present often in later childhood or adolescence with complex partial seizures. The prognosis for seizure control with medication is generally poor, whereas temporal lobectomy in appropriate patients is associated with control of complex partial seizures in 80–90 per cent of patients.[12] The increasing availability of high-resolution MRI has led to the recognition of these patients at a relatively early age. It is important that the poor prognosis of medical treatment in such patients be recognized early and that appropriate referral is made to a surgical center.

Improving control

Many paroxysmal events in teenagers are non-epileptic, and it is not uncommon for children to be mistakenly diagnosed as having epilepsy and treated with AEDs. Recognition of the true nature of these events is based largely on the history and it is important to reconsider the diagnosis in all teenagers with poorly controlled seizures (see Chapter 2).

Problems with compliance can be anticipated in many teenagers with epilepsy, and are due to a variety of factors. Comparison of drug levels obtained at the same time of day may help to detect this problem. Denial of the epilepsy and a strong desire to fit in with peers are normal features of adolescent development. Teenagers are usually reluctant to be seen taking medications during the day, and a twice-daily dose schedule should be used wherever possible. Rebellion against parental involvement is not an uncommon factor, and education of the parents can be as important as education of the teenager. In this context, the physician can act as a useful role model by seeing a teenager alone. Complacency regarding good seizure control can also be an important factor and can result in poor compliance and a recurrence of the seizures. Finally, concern over side-effects may be a potent factor. Practices that promote self-sufficiency are likely to lessen problems with compliance. For example, explanation that the licensing authority will approve a driving license only when the teenager has demonstrated an ability to take the medicine consistently can be a powerful inducement for compliance.

The teenage years are an appropriate time to review the AED regimen and consider possible side-effects. This is particularly appropriate for teenage girls, who should be informed of the potential teratogenic effects and the effects of AEDs on contraception (see below).

Epilepsy surgery can dramatically improve seizure control in many patients whose seizures are intractable to AEDs. It has been estimated that only a small fraction of those who might benefit from this approach are referred for surgical assessment.[13] The advances in neuroimaging have improved the detection of focal brain abnormalities. Thus, mesial temporal sclerosis may now be identified radiologically in early childhood, particularly in children with a history of a neurologic insult or febrile seizure.[14] Children with the electroclinical and radiologic features of mesial temporal lobe sclerosis who have seizures that are not controlled despite a trial of three appropriate AEDs should be referred to a center specializing in pediatric epilepsy surgery. The most common pathological lesion in patients selected for focal extratemporal resection is focal cerebral dysgenesis. It is important that such children be referred to a center that specializes in pediatric epilepsy surgery and has experience in invasive monitoring. Delaying the surgery until adult life denies the possibility of the adolescent growing up in a seizure-free environment, which in turn compromises both emotional development and employment potential.

WOMEN'S ISSUES

Contraception, pregnancy planning, teratogenicity and the influence of the menstrual cycle on seizure control are areas that are ideally introduced in early teenage years. It is important to provide teenagers with written information on these topics.[15] Providing a list of reliable websites allows teenagers to obtain information that they feel uncomfortable discussing with the physician (see Table 27.1).

Contraception

Hormonal contraception is less effective when taken with AEDs that induce hepatic microsomal metabolism (see Table 27.2). Women receiving enzyme-inducing AEDs should use contraceptives containing at least 50 μg of the estrogenic component, or change to an antiepileptic medication that does not influence steroid metabolism or to a nonhormonal method of contraception (Table 27.2).

Pregnancy

Approximately 30 per cent of adolescent pregnancies are unplanned. Consequently, teenagers should be counseled as early as possible on the effects of pregnancy on epilepsy and on the effects of epilepsy and AEDs on the developing fetus. Pregnancy alters the pharmacokinetics of many AEDs and therefore can influence seizure control. Women

Table 27.1 *Helpful websites for teenagers*

General

www.epilepsy.org.uk/upbeat/index.html	Epilepsy Action (British Epilepsy Association)	This site specializes in general information on epilepsy and has a special section on problems faced by teenagers
www.epilepsyfoundation.org/	Epilepsy Foundation of America	This site has been developed by the major organization in the US dedicated to the welfare of people with epilepsy. It provides general information on epilepsy and has sections in English and Spanish

Antiepileptic medications

www.aesnet.org/aed/index.cfm	American Epilepsy Society	This site provides reliable information on the antiepileptic drugs available in the United States

Women's issues

www.epilepsy.org.uk/info/women.html	Epilepsy Action (British Epilepsy Association)	This site specializes in general information on epilepsy and has a special section on women's issues
www.aafp.org/afp/20021015/1489.html	American Academy of Family Physicians	This site is designed for family physicians and uses technical language but provides an excellent review of women's issues in epilepsy

Table 27.2 *Effect of antiepileptic medications on oral contraceptive efficacy*

Medications that lessen oral contraceptive efficacy
- Carbamazepine
- Ethosuximide (possibly)
- Felbamate
- Phenytoin
- Phenobarbital
- Primidone
- Oxcarbazepine
- Topiramate

Medications that do not lessen oral contraceptive efficacy
- Clobazam, clonazepam, nitrazepam
- Gabapentin
- Levetiracetam
- Lamotrigine
- Tiagabine
- Valproate
- Zonisamide

with epilepsy who do not take AEDs have a slightly higher risk of having a child with a life-threatening congenital abnormality or one that requires medical or surgical treatment to lead a normal life. The baseline risk of a major malformation is ~2 per cent in the normal population but is increased to 5–6 per cent in mothers receiving a single AED and to 10 per cent in women taking two AEDs.[16] Neural tube defects occur in 1–2 per cent of children exposed *in utero* to valproic acid and in 0.5–1 per cent of children exposed to carbamazepine polytherapy.[17] There is a twofold increase in minor congenital anomalies, which occur in 7–15 per cent of infants exposed to AEDs.[18]

The pathophysiologic basis of AED teratogenesis is poorly understood but may involve reduction in folic acid concentration, disturbances in folic acid-mediated biochemical processes, or both.[17] Thus, it is recommended that folic acid supplementation be provided to all women of childbearing potential. The recommended dosage range is 0.4–4 mg per day, with many neurologists using 1 mg per day.[17]

WHO SHOULD LOOK AFTER THE TEENAGER WITH EPILEPSY?

The patterns of epilepsy care vary widely, even across the so-called 'developed' world. In some countries psychiatrists play a major role in management of patients with epilepsy, whereas elsewhere neurologists or pediatricians are the specialists most involved. As the evidence base of epilepsy accumulates, it is becoming increasingly apparent that many neurologists, pediatricians and psychiatrists are inadequately informed and experienced to provide optimal care to patients with epilepsy. Consequently, the optimal arrangement for the care of the teenager will depend in large part on the expertise that exists in that region.

Physicians with a particular interest in epilepsy in the adolescent and young adult should ideally see the teenager with epilepsy. In countries where specialist involvement is strictly defined by age, the formation of a 'transition clinic' staffed by both pediatric and adult specialists may permit the special needs of the teenager to be addressed and a smooth transition made to adult care. This approach may be less important in places where the specialist treats both children and adults with epilepsy.

It is important that the care of adolescents with epilepsy be based primarily on their specific needs. Although there are many important medical issues that relate to teenagers, the burden of epilepsy involves particularly social issues. As such, expertise in emotional and social issues and in preparation for employment are skills needed by those who care for teenagers with epilepsy. Education of the patient and family is very important. Most physicians have limited expertise in these areas and have time constraints that compromise their ability to address these issues adequately. Involvement of other professionals with an interest in epilepsy, such as nurses, educators or social workers, working in concert with the physician, is probably the most cost-effective way to deliver the care that is needed. Networking with the local epilepsy association and other support organizations in the region may also facilitate the development of a comprehensive plan for a teenager with epilepsy.

- Only a small fraction of children and teenagers who might benefit from **epilepsy surgery** are referred for surgical assessment
- **Delaying epilepsy surgery** until adult life denies the possibility of growing up in a seizure-free environment, which compromises both emotional development and employment potential
- Hormonal **contraception** is less effective when taken with AEDs that induce hepatic microsomal metabolism
- The baseline risk of a major **malformation** is ~2 per cent in the normal population but is increased to 5–6 per cent in mothers receiving a single AED and to 10 per cent in women taking two AEDs
- **Folic acid supplementation** should be provided to all women of childbearing potential

KEY POINTS

- Parents should be encouraged to allow a teenager with epilepsy to have the amount of freedom and responsibility that is necessary for the development of **self-sufficiency**
- As patients enter their teenage years, **decision-making** needs to move away from the parents to the child
- Most **sporting activities** impose only a slightly increased risk to the teenager with epilepsy, and the benefits of involvement in sporting activities generally outweigh the risks
- It is important that teenagers are advised of the local regulations pertaining to **driving** and epilepsy well before the age at which they might want to drive
- The combination of **alcohol use and sleep deprivation** is particularly likely to provoke seizures, especially in patients with idiopathic generalized epilepsies
- **Post-secondary school planning** should begin by at least 15 years of age and some form of vocational assessment should be obtained for vulnerable individuals
- Local **epilepsy societies** can play an important role in the education of employers and the establishment of job opportunities for young adults with epilepsy
- **Non-epileptic episodes** are sometimes misdiagnosed as epilepsy in teenagers and it is important to consider this possibility in all teenagers with poorly controlled 'seizures'

REFERENCES

1. Westbrook LE, Bauman LJ, Shinnar S. Applying stigma theory to epilepsy: A test of a conceptual model. *Journal of Pediatric Psychology* 1992; **17**: 633–649.
2. Wolf P, Okujava N. Possibilities of non-pharmacologic treatment of epilepsy. Seizure 1999; **8**: 45–52.
3. Smith PE, Wallace SJ. Taking over epilepsy from the Paediatric neurologist. *J Neurology Psychiatry* 2003; **74** (Suppl. 1.i): 37–41.
4. Ng SK, Brust JC, Hauser WA, Susser M. Illicit drug use and the risk of new-onset seizures. *American Journal of Epidemiology* 1990; **132**: 47–57.
5. O'Dell LE, Li R, George FR, Ritz MC. Molecular serotonergic mechanisms appear to mediate genetic sensitivity to cocaine-induced convulsions. *Brain Research* 2000; **863**: 213–224.
6. Sillanpää M, Jalava M, Kaleva O, Shinnar S. Long-term prognosis of seizures with onset in childhood [see comments]. *New England Journal of Medicine* 1998; **338**: 1715–1722.
7. Oller-Daurella L, Sanchez ME. Evolucion de las auscensias tipicas. *Revue Neurologique* (Barcelona) 1981; **9**: 81–102.
8. Loiseau P, Duché B, Pédespan J-M. Absence epilepsies. *Epilepsia* 1995; **36**: 1182–86.
9. Loiseau P, Panayiotopoulos CP, Hirsch E. Childhood absence epilepsy and related syndromes. In: Roger J, Bureau M, Dravet C, *et al.* (eds) *Epileptic Syndromes in Infancy, Childhood and Adolescence*, 3rd edn. London: John Libbey, 2002; 285–303.
10. Loiseau P, Pestre M, Dartigues J-F, *et al.* Long term prognosis in two forms of childhood epilepsy: typical absence seizures and epilepsy with Rolandic (centrotemporal) EEG foci. *Annals of Neurology* 1983; **13**: 642–648.
11. Thomas P, Genton P, Gelisse P, Wolf P. Juvenile myoclonic epilepsy. In: Roger J, Bureau M, Dravet C, *et al.* (eds) *Epileptic Syndromes in Infancy, Childhood and Adolescence*, 3rd edn. London: John Libbey, 2002; 335–355.
12. Engel J Jr, Williamson PD, Wieser H-G. Mesial temporal lobe epilepsy. In: Engel J Jr, Pedley TA (eds) *Epilepsy:*

A Comprehensive Textbook. Pliadelphia: Lippincott-Raven, 1997; 2417–2426.

13. Blume WT. Temporal lobe epilepsy surgery in childhood: rationale for greater use. *Canadian Journal of the Neurological Sciences* 1997; **24**(2): 95–98.

14. Harvey AS, Grattan-Smith JD, Desmond PM, Chow CW, Berkovic SF. Febrile seizures and hippocampal sclerosis: frequent and related findings in intractable temporal lobe epilepsy of childhood. *Pediatric Neurology* 1995; **12**(3): 201–206.

15. Nordli Jr, DR. Special needs of the adolescent with epilepsy. *Epilepsia* 2001; **42**(Suppl. 8): 10–17.

16. American Academy of Neurology. Practice parameter: management issues for women with epilepsy (summary statement). Report of the Quality Standards Subcommittee of the American Academy of Neurology. *Neurology* 1998; **51**: 944–948.

17. Morrell, MJ. Guidelines for the care of women with epilepsy. *Neurology* 1998; **51**(Suppl. 4): S21–27.

18. Gaily E, Granstrom ML. Minor anomalies in children of mothers with epilepsy. *Neurology* 1992; **42**(4; Suppl. 5): 128–131.

Index